S0-BXW-678

# Handbook of ABUSABLE DRUGS

Handbook of

# ABUSABLE DRUGS

KENNETH BLUM, Ph.D.
Professor
Department of Pharmacology
University of Texas
Health Science Center

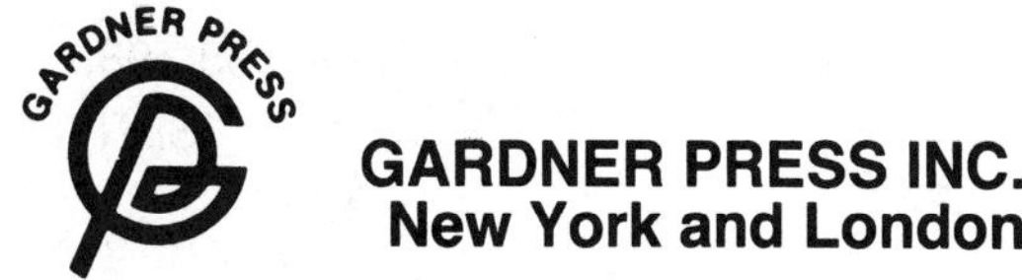


GARDNER PRESS INC.
New York and London

Gardner Press, Inc.
19 Union Square West
New York 10003

All foreign orders except Canada and South America to:
Afterhurst Limited
Chancery House
319 City Road
London N1, United Kingdom

**Library of Congress Cataloging in Publication data**

Blum, Kenneth.
Handbook of abusable drugs.

Includes bibliographies and index.
1. Substance abuse—Handbooks, manuals, etc.
2. Psychotropic drugs—Handbooks, manuals, etc.
I. Title. [DNLM: 1. Substance abuse. 2. Psychotropic drugs. 3. Psychopharmacology. 4. Drugs. QV 77 B658h]
RC564.B58 1983 615′.78 83-5667
ISBN 0-89876-036-4

Book Design by Raymond Solomon

Printed in The United States of America

THE AUTHOR dedicates this work to some very special people as well as to a few specific causes:

To my devoted family: Arlene, my wife; Jeffrey and Seth, my sons, who I hope will learn from these writings and not allow certain temptations of life, especially psychoactive chemicals, to take control of their destinies.

To those unfortunate young people who allow drugs and alcohol to contribute in part to their self-inflicted demise.

To the National Foundation on Addictive Disease for continued success in their pursuit of research and education in the biogenetics of human compulsion.

To the children of drug and alcohol abusers, potential victims of a devastating disease who require special societal consideration and loving care.

## "A FRIENDLY ADDICTION"

Life to most may just
    be a fling.
To some with special
    care it has
    real meaning—

At times the world
    outside may seem
So strange, so
    far and so
    uncaring—

Fantasies can come true
    if special friends
    around you believe
    in it, too—

So don't fret or
    ever regret what
    you have done,
    as long as there is
Benefit for even one—

Search your soul
    for something new, but
    tread carefully day by day, 'cause
    "Addiction" may be a step away—

Plan your life,
    but don't stop dreaming.
One day you may find
    it full of meaning—

Special friends
Need love and care,
    and like a drug
    may be an "Addiction."
But might serve
    as a useful prescription—

KB

# PUBLISHER'S ACKNOWLEDGMENTS

The publication of this major work is the result of the effort, skill, and support of many individuals and firms. Special recognition is given to those who gave their professional best to this book:

Dr. Giancarlo Guideri, who reviewed all the proofs for pharmacological accuracy. To Drs. Bernard Segal, Maurice Hirst, J. M. Khanna, John C. Crabbe, James F. Maddux, Seymour Ehrenpreis, Maharaj K. Ticku, Charles Walton, David Smith, Thomas F. Burks, Larry Ereshefsky, Sidney Cohen, Thomas Gentry, Charles Bowden, Allan Collins, A. H. Briggs, Susan Dalterio, and R. Ramanjaneyulu who read all or parts of the book for comments.

Raymond and Sidney Solomon, of Publishers Creative Services Inc., who designed the format and coordinated the production.

Evelyn Tucker, professional copyeditor, whose expertise and humanistic intelligence have very few equals.

Aldo Pellini, for his superb artwork in the diagrams and formulas.

Charles and Marian Klamkin, for their competence in proofing the final stages and for preparing the indexes.

Pauline and George Monette, of the Twin Company and their staff for their extraordinary skill, effort, and patience in typesetting this work.

Brian Payne, John Paeglow and staff of the Hamilton Printing Company for their fine job of printing and binding.

Lewis Falce and Staff of Algen Press for their excellent job of jacket printing.

Marsha Ross, Lance Rembar and Aaron Spungin of Gardner Press for their fine administrative and supportive efforts beyond the call of duty.

And, finally, we thank all fellow publishers and others for use of selections of their material. We apologize for any possible omission of proper credit, permissions or other oversights. A work of this enormity involves months of effort to perfect.

# Author's Acknowledgments

Obviously, without the enthusiastic support of many dedicated individuals this book could not have been written and produced.

The author gratefully acknowledges the following individuals: Dr. Arthur H. Briggs, Chairman, Department Pharmocology, University of Texas Health Science Center, San Antonio, Texas, for continued encouragement and academic support; Dr. David A. Kronick, Ellen Hanks, Pat Brown and other University of Texas Health Science librarians for assisting in compiling and proofreading the references list; Ms. Deluvina Hernandez, Marilyn Wilson, Sheri Wilke, Georgetta Neal, Naomi Rodriguez, Reesa Bowen, and Thelma Pacheco for expert typing of the manuscript; Jeffrey Blum, Seth Blum, and Georgetta Neal for compiling the extensive drug list; Arlene Blum and Georgetta Neal for proofreading the manuscript; Dr. R. Ramanjaneyulu and Gloria Martinez for their expert rewriting of certain portions of the manuscript; Dr. Giancarlo Guideiri of New York Medical College for acting as the chief pharmocologic advisor to the project; Leonard Delallo for assistance in reviewing chemical formulas of the various drugs cited in the text; Robert Ochoa for assisting in proofreading and editing of the manuscript; James E. Tilton for the development of concepts regarding the writing of the preface; Dr. Tom Payte, a San Antonio addiction expert, for permission to utilize his schematic of the "Anatomy of a Fix"; Dr. William Stanvinohoa and Dr. Jack Wallace of the University of Texas Health Science Center for his consultation and permission to utilize certain unpublished writings concerned with the overview of the current status of toxicology in the United States; Dr. Arthur H. Briggs and Sanford Futterman for their permission to utilize certain unpublished writings regarding solvent abuse in America and psychedelics, respectively. Dr. Ralph Ryback, a well-known authority in the clinical aspects of alcoholism for permission to utilize certain unpublished writings on the history of alcohol abuse in society. Dr. Jane Newitt and others for their views on drugs in the future. Dr. Silva Sankar, PJD Publishing, New York, for the utilization of numerous tables on LSD from his well known authoritative work *LSD: A Total Study*; Dr. Maurice Hirst, of the University of Western Ontario, London, Canada, for special permission to utilize certain unpublished writings concerned with the history of pharmacology as a discipline as well as historical data relevant to worldwide drug abuse; Dr. John Morgan, of the City College of New York, for his initial critique of the first draft of the manuscript developed for the National Institute on Drug Abuse.

The author of this work would like to acknowledge my fellow career teachers in Addiction for their dedication and fine work in the field of drug abuse teaching to the medical profession.

Certainly, the author is grateful to all his relatives and special friends, especially to his sister Barbara Damesak; Paul Newman; Ramon Valadez; Henry Martel; Gerald Warshofsky; Andrew Steinhauer, among others, who provided the motivation to work diligently into the early morning hours and successfully complete this sometimes almost impossible task.

A very special thanks to Marc Katz, of Katz's Delicatessen, Austin, Texas, a place where many hours of writing of the manuscript occurred and whose enthusiasm for the endeavor and good food stimulated the creativity of the author.

Last but not least, a very special acknowledgement to Gardner Spungin, the publisher of this work, a man with great vision and wisdom, whose inspiration, enthusiasm, patience, guidance, and constant hands-on advice provided not only the impetus to continue but a special kind of love which will always be cherished and remembered.

# Contents

**Chapter 13**
**TRANQUILIZING AGENTS**

# Preface

It is well established that drug and alcohol abuse and alcoholism constitute a major health, economic, and social problem throughout the world. In the United States alone, more than ten million people are affected by the dilemma and phenomenology of alcohol abuse and approximately 200,000 of them will die prematurely each year from a variety of ethanol-related pathologies and factors—including cirrhosis, cancer, heart disease, suicide, and homicide, as well as highway fatalities and other accidents. If those are the facts concerning a legally sanctioned substance, what might we expect for the other drugs of abuse? Certainly the economics alone provide enough impetus for an investment by all concerned to understand the biologic and sociologic aspects of abusable drugs. Without question, there should be a commitment by the United States and other governments to wage war against drug misuse and abuse.

It is not easy to work toward the eradication of illegal psychoactive drug use. However, to be effective in this mammoth task, neither magic nor luck is necessary. Instead, extraordinary knowledge of the fundamental aspects of how drugs work on the body; how social elements affect their use; and how their use affects society is a minimum requirement. A fundamental understanding of the entity of substance abuse requires knowledge acquired through painstaking research by dedicated scientists, as well as by behavioral scientists working to unravel the mysterious motivation to explore psychoactive chemicals.

As Albert Einstein pointed out in the mid-1930s: "It has often been said, and certainly not without justification, that the man of science is a poor philosopher."

There was a time, not too long ago, when the scientist who ventured philosophic opinions about the nature of human beings and the implications of their actions for society was considered to be overreaching the bounds of his or her own expertise. "Stick to facts" was often the retort to scientists who strayed from statistical charts and graphs into the realm of speculative conjecture about human behavior.

With the passage of years, however, and with the dawning recognition of the total impact of science on human lives and human institutions, it has become apparent that science, in and of itself, is not enough to cope with the quest for knowledge. J. Robert Oppenheimer expressed his feelings about this matter when he declared:

> But the image that comes to my mind is . . . of an essentially infinite world, knowable in many different ways; and all these paths of knowledge are interconnectable, and some are interconnected, like a great network—a great network between people, between ideas, between systems of knowledge—a reticulated kind of structure which is human culture and human society.

The purpose of this book is to point out linkages between scientific phenomena and social behavior. More specifically, this book illustrates what is referred to as social pharmacology—the exploration of the interrelationships among chemical agents (drugs), consciousness (a person), and social systems (society).

The various abusable drugs detailed in this work are so complex in terms of their biologic interactions that, for any one individual to provide a meaningful analysis of the field, certain information had to obtained from various sources to serve as the basis of this most complete reference book. This treatise provides the reader with a detailed, critical review of the biochemical, pharmacologic, and sociologic aspects of drugs of abuse. Each chapter presents an authoritative and integrated discussion of a particular substance abuse problem, but with a unique and charismatic approach. The book was an outgrowth of a request by NIDA to compile all available data on the pharmacology and toxicology of commonly abused drugs. First written in 1977 and revised in 1982, it also was refereed by two experts in the field, and then further revised accordingly.

This volume is divided into 21 chapters, arranged in logical sequence from the introduction to "social pharmacology," to simple definitions of euphoria, compulsive drug use, tolerance, dependence, and withdrawal. Then the book delineates and further analyzes the contemporary drug scene and motives for substance use, and details the pharmacodynamic properties of drugs and their routes of administration. Basic pharmacologic considerations and principles of drug action are also discussed. A pharmacologic classification of abusable drugs is presented, and each prototype drug—such as narcotics, narcotic-antagonists, methadone, internal opiates, alcohol, sedative-hypnotic stimulants, tobacco, cannabis, hallucinogens, anti-anxiety agents, psychotropic agents, and over-the-counter drugs—is treated separately in great detail. The book concludes with a complete analysis of potential drug and alchohol interactions, and drug abuse, in the year 2001.

Such unique features as a "Drug Index," a glossary of both "street" and scientific terms, fingertip drug charts for the student, and federally mandated drug schedules are also included. The book is fully referenced, with over 3500 selected references. Unlike most volumes of this size, this work truly represents the current state of the art, including referenced material for the current year, 1983. Another interesting aspect is that the approaches to the various drug mechanisms are not typically "stale" and conservative, but somewhat speculative in part and stimulating for the interested research scientist or research-oriented social scientists. Additionally, the treatment and prevention sections for each prototype drug represent the current state of the art, so that those involved with treatment programs or alcohol and chemical dependency can utilize the information to best advantage. The clinical sociologist may not require all the material contained in this volume (structural formulas, drug mechanisms), but for the most part will find the reading fascinating and informative, as well as of practical value to his or her clinical practice.

Drug use, abuse, and misuse are unquestionably a major problem in our society, and the growth of this problem has created a most complex task for the educator. The focus of national attention on the drug dilemma in recent years is due in part to a magnified public awareness and to the increased availability of pharmaceutical and other intoxicating agents, which can be readily obtained over the counter at pharmacies and from illegitimate street sources. Growing experimentation "in the streets" is commonplace, especially with alcohol as the drug. The "drug culture," as the newspapers and magazines call it, does not belong just to the kids. Everyone is in it together.

The ultimate goal of this work is an attempt to come closer to the definition of Oppenheimer's "great network," which must exist between systems of knowledge—between the pharmacologic analysis and the sociologic phenomena that mark our journey through space and time.

What major area of activity is unaffected by drugs today? The great bureaucracies of health, education, and law enforcement gear themselves up in massive array to deal with the sociologic aspects of drug-affected behavior. National policy is fashioned to deal with the problem in terms of international trade and law enforcement.

The subject matter of this book is of both theoretic and practical importance, and should serve as an excellent reference source for behavioral scientists, clinicians, pharmacologists, biochemists, and other scientists, as well as for lay people interested in and charged with understanding the phenomenology of the substance abuse problem. I feel that this account will make a substantial contribution toward the reduction, and eventual eradication, of drug and alcohol abuse, because it provides a framework of knowledge, a necessary requisite.

However, unless a holistic approach is offered by those who are striving to develop the answers to resolve the drug dilemma, then we will continue to present a fragmented, disjointed portrait of drug and alcohol abuse—notable in its academic and scientific perceptions, but seriously lacking in sociologic insight that can be applied to everyday life. Once again, to quote Dr. Einstein:

> The whole of science is nothing more than a refinement of everyday thinking. It is for this reason that the critical thinking of the physicist cannot possibly be restricted to the examination of the concepts of his own specific field. He cannot proceed without considering critically a much more difficult problem, the problem of analyzing the nature of everyday thinking.

I hope that this work will stimulate my scientific colleagues to continue their important research on all drugs, and, at the same time, encourage them to begin to consider their findings in broader terms that can be applied to the society in which they practice their science. This is a book not only about drugs and molecules, but about human needs and strivings.

Certainly, I have diligently labored to provide the most complete compendium on abusable drugs possible, realizing that scientific inquiry will result in new information that eventually will make this work historical in nature and incomplete; however, for the most part, it will serve as a reference source for many years to come. In this regard, it is noteworthy that, as Saint Paul remarked, "We know in part and we prophesy in part." May the words on these pages serve as a point of departure and not as finite solution to the intriguing problem of abusable drugs.

K.B.

# Handbook of ABUSABLE DRUGS

# Chapter 1

# The Background for Abuse

## A. INTRODUCTION

In the beginning, probably long before humans planted crops, they already had knowledge of the local plants that could alter their consciousness. Certainly there are reports that not only were pain-relieving and sleep-producing herbs known, but also, in some regions, dissociating or hallucinogenic drugs were identified and held in high esteem. There are accounts of peyote pilgrimages from Canada down to Texas or northern Mexico, and of pituri trails running for hundreds of miles. The search for botanicals has become a universal drive.

Since human beings have been aware of themselves and of the need to master their environment, they have also been aware of illness and pain, as well as death. To aid in coping with distress, they have developed helping systems, and individuals have been chosen to carry out the rituals that the culture prescribes as helping. These systems developed first within the family, and have survived as wisdom passed down through generations.

A given plant, at different times, can be viewed as an ornament, as food, as a spice, or as a sacred ritual substance with special powers. A plant not only can play a role in personal, family, or community religious life, but can become a medication given by grandmothers or dispensed or prescribed by physicians. Dr. George Meyer[1] has stated:

> The same plant can be a healing medication, an economic or political tool (as in the Spice Wars or Opium Wars), or even an illegal drug whose use, now called abuse, can be reason for severe punishment. Over the years, commonly used plants such as coffee, tea or tobacco, although controversial, have survived these issues of use and abuse.

Health professionals, charged with finding new drugs for the eradication of mental disease, utilize highly sophisticated stereochemists' computerized scanning of potentially consciousness-altering molecular configurations. This kind of technology overshadows the down-to-nature search for mind-altering roots, leaves, and cacti, which still continues. However, through high technology, it is possible to produce, from electric charges and atomic arrangements of the compound, a drug that will allay distress, achieve self-transcendence, induce pleasure, or simply intoxicate. Such advanced knowledge can work for human good, or ill. There are psychedelic chemists so knowledgeable that they keep a molecule ahead of the law by bringing forth compounds not yet covered by legislation.

Today life brings turmoil and uncertainty. We have seen rapid social change and an erosion of established values and beliefs. According to a President's Commission on Mental Health, a fourth of the citizens of the United States suffer from some form of severe emotional stress. Another study shows that 80 percent of all Americans feel the need to reduce stress in their daily lives. There is obviously a compelling desire for people to understand better the forces of stress that affect them. There is also, certainly, a need to understand the physiologic and chemical "coping mechanisms" that are available. People want to know how they can reduce the harmful impact of stress on their physical and mental well-being. Many of us are living with unease, frustration, anxiety, and depression. Traditional sources of information on how to cope with daily stress are no longer available, or effective, in the same way they were for previous generations. The family unit is largely fragmented and diluted as a source of authoritative advice and counsel. The role of organized religion has also been diminished considerably by the struggle to live in these corrupt times. Even the family doctor has given way to the family psychologist, the marriage counselor, and the financial consultant.

Many of us have come to expect instant relief from notions and feelings, and, if necessary, to look for instant pleasure that is chemically induced. Cohen[2] points out that:

> The cultural taboos against drugs for enjoyment and fun have been breached by more citizens than ever before. Add to this the enhanced precision of synthetic compounds that will do it better, and we have a situation that is not about to go away.

In the past 20 years, since the psychedelic '60s, the drug scene has been changing—but not improving.

At the more general level of social change, we find a drawn-out period of adolescence, in which young people simply need more time and many more diversified experiences to achieve a healthy, integrated personality. As our society becomes more interrelated by communication, transportation, and mobility, they require more time for trial-and-error experimentation and exploration to avoid the conformity and drabness they fear. The social, educational, and intellectual pressures on young people are greater than ever before. They, as well as we, must perform, produce, and achieve in the context of larger institutions. Over the years, an economy of abundance has developed, but the ethic of hard work continues to dominate our ideals, if not our motivations.

If we add to all of these conditions the discontent with the direction our country is taking—the adoption of policies that have not been able to keep pace with the rising expectations of minority groups, the periodic thrusts of the civil rights movements, and the outstanding achievements in technology, with the comparative neglect of needed social reforms—the result is disenchantment with and alienation from our sociopolitical system.

The point to be made here is that drugs—and a greater inclination to try them, once or twice or perhaps sporadically—conveniently fit into these social changes by allowing us to manipulate moods; by representing a feeling toward society, whether a protest or a challenge to find something better; and, most important, by simply providing fun for the user.

Why are certain drugs abused? Why should one drug be preferred over another, although both belong to the same pharmacologic class? What kinds of emotional experiences are sought by abusers of drugs? These are just a sampling of the questions raised by the phenomenon of drug use and misuse, and it is the behavioral scientist, pharmacologist, psychologist, physician, and social worker, among other professionals, who are challenged to provide the answers.

All substances of abuse either raise or lower consciousness and enhance or depress mood. The varieties of changes in awareness range from a complete obliteration of consciousness, such as large doses of central nervous system (CNS) depressants can bring, to a vast intensification of awareness, such as experienced in the LSD state.

Will a drug be abused even if it has unpleasant properties? Some individuals may be deterred by a vile-tasting or -smelling concoction, or by one that produces a gastrointestinal upheaval, but others will indulge. *Datura stramonium*, also known as jimson weed, is unpleasant but it still has its devotees. Nutmeg and mace (*Myristica fragrians*) are difficult to swallow in intoxicating doses, but some manage to do so. The first cigar or the first injection of opiate is quite unpleasant, but people persist and acquire tolerance of the side effects. Peyote cactus (*Lophophora williamsii*) is far from enjoyable, in terms of going down and coming back up; nevertheless it is sought after. Drugs, like people, are not always predictable. Neither is the view of society.

According to J.P. Smith,[3] by both social custom and law, society defines what we mean by "drugs" and differentiates these from "chemicals," which are called toxins, poisons, and even beverages. In times with slow rates of social change, we find rather general agreement throughout a society on what is to be called a drug, the nature of the drug abuse problem, and what society should do about it. But the times in which we now live are seeing very rapid social change, so that many elements of society are out of touch with each other, if not in sharp conflict. The phrase "bring us together" is popular, and for good reason. We need more consensus—reasoned, deliberate consensus—than we now have in the drug area. And, if this is not possible, at least a small amount of tolerance for human foibles will go a long way toward getting us started in the right direction.

At this point, you may feel that you are being served a dish of platitudes when you expected to dine on something more substantial. Be assured that these are not platitudes, but recommendations for careful analysis of the problem before we decide what the problem really is. This is the attitude with which we should consider the question of drugs and society.

The individuals who fit into our picture are certainly not the hard-line addicts on heroin, morphine, paregoric, or barbiturates. Our discussion is centered on broad trends rather than on a small percentage of pathologic individuals. The broad trends are more adequately described in terms of drug use and abuse than of drug dependence or addiction. Far fewer persons are actually dependent on drugs than abuse them, especially if a legal definition of abuse, with all of its limitations, is adopted.

Agreement appears to exist as to the presence of the three major elements in the drug abuse problem: the drugs, the people who use them, and the social forces shaping, and in turn being influenced by, both of these.

A recently coined term that fits the study of all three of these elements is *social pharmacology*; it now awaits a new depth in its definition, delineation, and role in the psychotropic drug abuse field.

Probably the first question that arises is: How widespread is the use of stimulants, depressants, hallucinogens, and narcotics? Our difficulty here is that we have an enormous number of studies, all providing proximate answers to the question, but for different groups of people, in different regions of the country, using different methods of study and survey, and done at different times.

Several tentative conclusions may be drawn from these drug use studies. Marihuana appears to attract the greatest experimentation and narcotics the least, with other drugs falling in between. Males tend to experiment more than females; persons who are better educated and of a higher class socioeconomically tend to "try out" drugs more frequently than persons who are less educated and from lower socioeconomic classes. (The question of extent is further detailed in Chapter 2.) Furthermore the comparison of drugs of abuse with recreational drugs reveals the lack of consistency in society's approach to both. A person may be a confirmed alcoholic and be regarded as "sick" in our society. But one who habitually uses marihuana (i.e., is dependent on it psychologically) will be viewed as a criminal, not a sick person, even if the social liability of both persons is much the same. The attitude of many people is that society does not need either one, but that we already have ten million alcoholics, so why create a comparable class of potheads? And so the arguments go on. It is well to remember that what is called a recreational drug here not only has a legal but also an informal social base—the behavior of millions of individuals who happen to prefer a particular drug. At some point, the law will begin to reflect the behavior and attitudes of such people.

While such a scheme as this necessarily oversimplifies a great deal by focusing on drugs, it does characterize the general attitude of many, if not most, persons in Western society: that the drugs a doctor prescribes for you are "good," even if serious side effects occur; and that drugs self-administered in private are "bad," per se, even if some of the consequences are beneficial. Finally, recreational drugs are not called drugs because we do not like to admit that directly changing our moods or feelings has some social benefits, as well as liabilities.

Terminology in any field can pose potential problems. In this book, *drug abuse* refers to the use, usually by self-administration, of any drug in a manner that deviates from the approved medical or social patterns within a given culture. The term conveys the notion of social disapproval and it is not necessarily descriptive of any particular pattern of drug use or its potential adverse consequences.

Nonmedical drug use is a less pejorative term, but is so general that it encompasses behaviors ranging from the occasional use of alcohol to the compulsive use of opioids, and includes behaviors that may or may not be associated with any adverse effects. Nonmedical drug use may be the experimental use of a drug on one or a few occasions because of curiosity about its effects or to conform to the expectations of peer groups. It may involve the casual or "recreational" use of modest amounts of a drug for its pleasurable effects, or the use may be circumstantial—that is, certain drug effects are sought because they are helpful in particular circumstances, as when students or truck drivers take amphetamines to alleviate fatigue. These various forms of nonmedical use may then lead to more intensive use, in terms of frequency or amount, and in some cases to patterns of compulsive drug use.

## B. ADDICTION AND DEPENDENCE

In any discussion of drug abuse, the terms *addiction* and *physiologic* and/or *psychologic dependence* need to be well delineated. It is suggested that the interested reader refer to other work for greater detail, as well as to Chapter 2 of this book.

### 1. Euphoria[2]

Since the dawn of time, many human beings have, consciously or unconsciously, attempted to relieve the painful state of mind known as *aphoria* through either traditional or non-traditional medical approaches. The ultimate goal has been not only to reduce psychic pain, but to replace it with the unique feeling of being "high," which has become generally known in the medical field as *euphoria*. Historical records point towards the fact that in almost every distinct culture, society has accepted and sanctioned the use of herbs, plant extracts, elixirs, mixtures, powders and even synthesized chemicals as euphoriants. In further support of this concept there is a United States patent pending on the use of a mushroom product identified as a recreational euphoriant. In this regard one is reminded of Huxley's suggestion to actively search for a substance which relieved one's aphoria was non-addictive and non-toxic, produced no hangover, and was relatively short in duration. He called this substance *soma*.

Pharmacologically, it is extremely difficult to describe the exact neurochemical events which must occur in the brain consistently whenever one transcends from the aphoric to the euphoric state. According to most pharmacologists, the state of euphoria is not simply the reduction of physiologic or psychic pain; indeed, it is the positive experience of feeling right with oneself and the surrounding universe. In terms of pharmacologic mechanisms, certain euphoria-inducing drugs produce similar states through dissimilar neuro-pathways. For example, cocaine or amphetamines act via stimulations of the reward centers in the septal area of the brain. Interestingly, microinjections of Norepinephrine, a chemical in the brain released by cocaine or amphetamines, and electrical stimulations of the septal area of the brain both induce elation similar to intense euphoric states. Another form of euphoria is via reduction of tension and anxiety. For example, antianxiety drugs like the benzodiazepines (Librium- or Valium-types), acting through the so-called GABA-Benzodiazepine receptor complex, produce euphoria states. Other forms of euphoria include the reduction of sometimes unwanted and disturbing sexual drives, hunger, and psychic emptiness.

Opium and its known derivatives, working over endorphinergic (internal opiate) mechanisms, elicit such responses.

Depressants, such as alcohol and solvent inhalants, also produce euphoric states by depressing the inhibitory controls over behavior and mood. To some people the impairment of such mental functions as rational thought, memory, or judgment might even be experienced as enjoyable or euphoric.

## 2. Addictive Behavior and Addiction

The best definition of addiction, an arbitrary term, is that by Dr. Jaffe[4]:

> A behavioral pattern of compulsive drug use, characterized by overwhelming involvement with the use of a drug, the securing of its supply and a high tendency to relapse after withdrawal.

Any person who has a tendency to devote considerable amounts of time to the use of a drug, and whose behavioral activities center upon acquiring it, can be safely labeled as addicted to and obsessed with that drug. Addiction, however, does not refer to a physical drug dependency as defined by the World Health Organization. It is concerned with a quantitative rather than a qualitative sense of drug use. It is possible to be physically dependent on a drug without being addicted, and vice versa. It is not possible, however, to make a distinction and state precisely where compulsive drug use becomes an addiction. Addiction as defined here is in reference to a behavioral tendency to seek, secure, and use a drug with the possibility of relapse after withdrawal.

## 3. Compulsive Drug Use or Abuse

The various reasons for drug use and its subsequent social, personal, physical, and psychologic implications are complex factors yet to be determined. Among these factors, one of the most difficult problems that predisposes a compulsive drug use is the individual's need to use a drug to achieve a state of well-being or to feel "normal." Ranging from a mild desire to an intense need to use a drug, this indulgence in its most severe form may result in a chronic relapsing disease. Consequently there is a behavioral obsession to procure and use the drug. This type of behavioral dependency precedes *compulsive drug use* and *compulsive drug abuse*. The two terms can be used interchangably with the understanding that *drug abuse* is without reference to whether the drug is licit or illicit. Under certain circumstances *drug use* implies any drugs, whereas drug abuse specifies illicit drug use.

In certain circles, drug abuse refers to the use of any drug that is not legally prescribed by the medical profession, such as the occasional use of marihuana, LSD, or peyote. However, the more informed circles would ascribe to the idea that drug abuse should refer to the abuse of any drug, whether it is licit or illicit. Thus drug use would not be limited to the occasional ingestion of LSD, even though this is an illicit substance.

## 4. Psychological Dependence

The chronic abuse of psychoactive drugs usually leads to what has been termed psychological or psychic dependence. This condition, which is common to all types of long-term drug and alcohol abuse, reflects the user's attitude and the intensity of the habit—that is, the need to seek a particular substance over and over again. In fact, the degree of psychologic dependence dictates the associated use or abuse of a substance necessary to maintain an "optimal state" of well-being.[4] The overall magnitude or degree of the resulting psychologic dependence varies significantly from person to person, i.e., with the individuality of the user.

An example of a mild form of psychologic dependence is one in which the drug maintenance level is not very intense and requires only the infrequent imbibing of the substance, such as practiced by the occasional drinker of alcohol or the once-a-month smoker of marijuana. On the other end of the scale, the more severe type of psychologic dependence becomes, in many chronic abusers, an obsession, whereby the drug—rather than the individual's emotional makeup, mind, or ethics—dictate overall lifestyle. This obsession with the drug can lead to an amoral existence and many times results in criminal activity. Although for the most part the psychologically dependent person does not want to inflict harm on others, he or she will do so if it becomes a necessity to acquire money for the drug. In America today the compulsion for such substances is a prime reason why both women and men turn towards prostitution or permit their children to be sexually exploited for money.[5]

From a clinical point of view, one could assign an estimated rather than a precise value to the degree and intensity of the individual's psychologic dependence—namely, mild, moderate, or marked. The determinants of the degree of addiction include the liability of abuse of the drug; the strength of the reinforcing qualities of the drug; first impressions of the drug-experience; drug-related excitement, especially its sexual-arousal action; and its cost. The illusion of how wonderful the individual will feel on the drug and even the excitement of the procurement of it reduce the chance of the eradication of the drug from the user's life.[6]

When an individual loses the interest in, and drive and motivation for, normal drug-free living, the practitioner is faced with a serious and frustrating task.

In the view of some workers, psychologic dependence develops as a result of the "rewards" the user obtains from the drug experience. Being psychologically dependent on a drug implies that the user will assign priorities to actions involving the procurement of the drug. It suggests that the individual has come to prefer the illusions of excitement and enrichment that surround the experience and will not easily sever the relationship with the newly found ally.[6]

The person who gets satisfaction from the first use of a drug tends to use it again and again. This continued repetition may make it necessary to utilize the drug as an instrument in adjusting to life, relying upon it for fulfillment that others achieve without the help of drugs. When this occurs, the user is psychologically dependent upon the drug. This type of dependence is the least amenable to cure because that individual, in the deep involvement with drugs, may have lost the interest, the drives, and the motivations that lie at the root of normal living.

## 5. Physiologic Factors in Drug Dependence[7]

Any distinction between the psychologic and physiologic aspects of drug dependence is, to a certain extent, artificial. The so-called physiologic aspects of drug dependence, tolerance and physical dependence, are widely recognized; yet the biochemical nature of these conditions and their relation to the psychologic aspects of drug dependence are far from clear. A vast amount of research is needed on the nature of drug dependence.

### *a. Tolerance*

Tolerance is a condition in which the body cells protect themselves against toxic substances by developing resistance to them. Tolerance is manifested when repeated doses of the same amount of a drug become diminishingly effective and progressively larger doses are required to secure the desired effect.

### *b. Physical Dependence*

Physical dependence is a condition in which the body has adjusted to the presence of a drug and, when forced to function without the drug, reacts with a characteristic illness, called *abstinence syndrome* or *withdrawal illness*. Although the nature of the physical revulsion has been recognized for years, its cause has never been scientifically established. One theory that is widely held is the theory of *homeostasis*,[8] which relates both tolerance and withdrawal illness to the action of forces that try to keep the body's processes in balance. When a person takes a drug that has a depressant effect, the autonomic nerve centers, according to the theory, try to compensate for the drug's effect through changes in the activity of the central nervous system. To experience the depressant effect of the drug, that person then must take more of it to overcome these compensatory forces. When the drug is discontinued, these factors are suddenly released, and the body undergoes the period of readjustment called withdrawal illness.

The physiologic aspects of drug dependence

may be overcome by appropriate medical treatment. Thus the drug user's claim of physical dependence on a drug, although representing a need that may be bona fide at the onset of withdrawal symptoms, appears from a long-range point of view to be a rationalization, rather than a reason, for the continued use of the drug. The long-term psychologic factors are more compelling than the immediate physiologic factors in the maintenance of drug dependence.

## 6. Drugs as Behavior Reinforcers[9]

At this time societal pressures dictate and facilitate our coping mechanisms by directing the pervasive use of drugs. Just as an aspirin will cure our headaches, a similar rationale can be applied to "cure" our everyday stress and strain through the use of drugs. The problems associated with using drugs for nonmedicinal purposes and to help us "make it through the night," to lift our spirits, to feel "good," indeed require abstract reasoning for their solution and a great deal of intellectual stimulation. They encompass a whole world of complexities surrounding the individual and society as a whole. After this absolute prerequisite of thought concerning drug use we have begun to realize that drugs are readily available and seem to offer simplistic solutions to the myriad of problems that face humankind. To some it seems that the rather sudden concern on the part of government and the general population is based more on the fear of having a stereo or color TV stolen than on any real concern for the life of any single addict.

With regard to some aspects of addiction, drug dependence is the common factor whether it is on opiates or alcohol. The main concern is the drug's use regardless of its type. At this point, society tends to view the heroin addict far more negatively than the alcoholic or the marihuana user, for example. The opinion seems to be that we have enough dope addicts so to compound the problem is nonsense. The opiate user differs far less from the general population than is generally assumed. Drug dependence should be approached with the understanding that there are multiple causative and contributing factors. The more one understands this, the more one appreciates the awesome complexities of the disorder—if one accepts it as a disorder. One should realize that the contemporary hard-core criminal addicts are far more products of societal actions than of their basic personalities or of the pharmacology of heroin. Certainly treatment programs, whether methadone drugfree (nonnarcotic), therapeutic community, or spiritual alternatives, should direct their efforts to improving the quality of life, providing meaningful options while facilitating change, and giving individuals a choice in determing what they will do with the rest of their lives.

Whether people are searching for that something "other" or yearning to go beyond themselves, or attempting to escape, there is a tendency to use nonmedicinal drugs such as opioids, barbiturates, alcohol, volatile solvents, CNS stimulants, nicotine, and caffeine. An inclination to take drugs is characteristic of humans, and of other mammals as well. Laboratory animals, like humans, quickly learn to self-administer most nonmedicinal drugs.

Factors involved in drug-induced reward or "self-administration" (via a lever) of a particular substance by an animal include a) overall abuse liability or euphorgenic properties of the substance; b) load factors, or the amount of work required to obtain the dose; c) schedule of reinforcement; d) previous exposure to the drug, e.g., in the prenatal state; e) route of administration and size of dose. This observation omits physical dependence and preexisting psychopathology as prerequisites for initiating drug use. The result is that drugs become a reinforcer and predispose the compulsive tendency of drug use.

## 7. General Tolerance and Physical Dependence

Tolerance of, and physical dependence on drugs are not necessarily dependently "linked" but possibly occur via different and independent phenomena. Scrutiny of the pharmacological literature reveals controversy on this important subject. Some investigators have proposed a derivative description of research models supporting a "linked" mechanism for tolerance and physical dependence. However, not all drugs that produce tolerance equally cause physical dependence in the user. A good example of this is those drugs chronically administered such as anticholinergics, chlorpromazine, cyclazocine (a synthetic narcotic antagonist), and imipramine. In contrast, both tolerance and physical dependence develop in the chronic abusers of narcotics, alcohol, and hypnotics.

Sociologically, a major problem experienced by the (nonmedicinal) abusers of psychoactive chemicals, related to the phenomena of tolerance and physical dependence, results in a "Catch 22" situation, in which he or she must balance the body's increased requirement for, or tolerance of, the drug with the spiralling increase in dosage and, therefore, increased cost.

What tolerance does in our bodies is not clearly defined. How it develops and the risks involved can be speculated on more precisely. The elusiveness in defining tolerance is compounded when we realize that a narcotic drug will produce tolerance of that drug by some parts of our bodies and not by others. The net effect of tolerance is therefore not evenly distributed.

The danger of adaptation to drugs such as opioids brings forth both physical and social problems. Opioid tolerance is attributed mainly to some form of adaptation of cells in the nervous system to the drug action ("pharmacodynamic," "tissue," or "cellular" tolerance). Other characteristics in opioid-tolerant animals are decreased duration and intensity of the analgesic, euphorigenic, sedative, and other CNS depressant effects; marked elevation in the average lethal dose; increased metabolic rate of opioids; and less depression of brain concentrations of morphine and methadone that produce severe depression in nontolerant animals.

Building tolerance to opioids may compel the user to increase the search for the drug, and repeatedly to use the drug to achieve the same euphoric state initially experienced. The drug may be illicit and add to the problems the user already faces. If the drug is expensive, an economic burden is inevitable. A more serious consequence may be the toxic level acquired in the process of achieving the desired drug effect.

Tolerance develops only after a drug is used again before the total effect of a previous dosage has disappeared and the drug is completely eliminated. A person may increase the level of intake of the drug to get another "rush" immediately following the first dose. The dangerous end result is a tolerance to massive doses of the drug to achieve the sought-after euphoric level.

Similar rapid tolerance development is seen with amphetamine and other classes of drugs. Unlike opiates, no physical withdrawal symptoms are observed. It is theoretically possible for an individual to use morphine once every 48 to 72 hours for an entire lifetime, always experiencing the same effect and never having to increase the dosage or experience any form of withdrawal sickness.

To discontinue use of the drug requires knowledge concerning the individual tolerance threshold, physiology, environment, and the actual dose of the drug administered. The tolerance threshold of the addicted individual refers to the amount of the narcotic required to maintain a state of physiologic normality. It can be increased or decreased, either by continued administration of doses in excess of the tolerance threshold, or by giving doses of less than the established tolerance level. Detoxification aims to reduce the individual's physical and emotional discomfort. It is simply a process of using progressively smaller doses to allow the tolerance threshold to be reduced eventually to zero.

Whether a person goes "cold turkey" or experiences a gradual detoxification, the severity of the withdrawal symptoms will depend largely on the individual physiology, the threshold tolerance, and the actual dose of the drug administered.

### *a. Adaptation to Hypnotics and Narcotics* [2,11]

The mechanisms involved with drug-induced tolerance are not clearly understood. However, numerous reports in the scientific literature suggest that certain endogenous chemicals may be responsible for and/or mediate in the cell's ability to adapt to the drug. Certain neurotransmitters, neuropeptides, neucleotides and trace metals have been cited for their actions related specifically to the tolerance phenomenon.

It is well established that genetics may play a significant role as a determinant in both animal and human responsiveness or sensitivity to psychoactive drugs. Specifically, both rats and mice have been selectively bred for differences in their inherent tolerance or inborn resistance to alcohol, barbiturates, glutethamide, meprobamate, and opiates. In a sense, this may help explain why some individuals appear to be more sensitive than others with regard to overall drug effects.

Another important pharmacodynamic parameter of tolerance to hypnotic and opiate-like substances is drug-disposition and concomitant blood levels. Examples of this can be obtained from studies which evaluate the concentrations of alcohol and barbiturates in tolerance and non-tolerant animals. Animals tolerant of barbiturates or alcohol show much less sedation and motor impairment than do non-tolerant animals at equivalent blood concentrations.

Cellular adaptation of psychoactive drugs varies with respect to the specific target organ. For example, although there is tolerance to the chronic abuse of opiates on the gastrointestinal actions, there is no tolerance to the pupillary effects of narcotics. Additionally, there is tolerance to opiates with respect to carbon dioxide mediated respiratory responses, whereby there is less tolerance in those animals otherwise tolerant to alcohol or barbiturates, as evidenced by the fact that no dramatic elevation of the lethal blood concentration is observed.

The duration and intensity of a particular drug is determined by a) metabolism or degradation of the substance, and b) pharmocodynamic tolerance. In tolerant animals a swifter enzymatic degradation can be observed with the use of short-acting barbiturates (e.g., pentobarbital, hexobarbital), alcohol and certain nonbarbiturate hypnotics.

### *b. Abstinence Syndrome*

Simplifying the characteristics of any form of drug abstinence is far from an easy task. There are too many factors intertwined to unveil a simple solution. Individuals have different psychologic and physiologic makeups and the drug is therefore left to that variable. For the sake of helping to contribute valid data on drug withdrawal, and ultimately to assist those suffering from drug addiction and subsequent withdrawal symptoms, some generalized information can be noted.

Sometimes a drug will alleviate or modify symptoms, but after chronic administration is halted, the initial symptoms experienced will again surface. However, these symptoms (termed withdrawal symptoms) are now harder to deal with because the pleasurable experience due to the symptom modification is no longer available.

Some researchers have reported a pattern in which abstinence reactions of some drugs were observed to be like a rebound effect. The drugs reported include opioids, general depressants of the CNS (alcohol, barbiturates, and related hypnotics), amphetamines, nicotine, and opioid antagonists. Chlorpromazine, imipramzine, and cyclazocine may also have rebound effects, however, these drugs have distinct withdrawal symptoms of their own.

Morphine depresses the polysynaptic reflexes, and the flexor and crossed extensor spinal reflexes, but after withdrawal the opposite is experienced. General depressants increase the seizure threshold but during withdrawal spontaneous seizures are observed. Blum and associates[12] have suggested that the hyperexcitability, alteration of body temperature, seizure activity, and other symptoms associated with alcohol withdrawal may be the result of the formation of tetrahydroisoquinoline alkaloid (condensation product of acetaldehyde and dopamine) and the subsequent release of this substance following withdrawal of alcohol exposure (see Table 1-1). Amphetamines prescribed for fatigue, to curb appetite, and to counteract depression are frequently associated with the opposite effects after withdrawal. The most severe consequence is a lack of energy and depression. Heavy smoking of nicotine, often used to calm general nervousness and to suppress anger, manifests itself in increased irritability after its withdrawal. These observations of reactions following drug abstinence should help us to understand drug-withdrawal reactions and the extent of the various drugs' usefulness, and perhaps to find better alternatives to their use.

### *c. Cross-Dependence*

Under certain circumstances, it is true that it may benefit the drug addict to substitute one drug for another (potent to less potent) to suppress ''harsh'' symptoms associated with abstinence reactions of narcotic drugs. For example, if a long-acting drug such as methadone is substituted over several days for morphine, abrupt discontinuation produces a withdrawal syndrome characteristic of the long-acting drug rather than of morphine. The idea is to utilize the concept termed *cross-dependence*. Cross-dependence refers to the potential of one drug to take the place of another, and to suppress the symptoms of physical dependence of the substituted drug. Both will have the same general pharmacologic effects, however, the degree of cross-dependence varies from partial to complete.

Almost any potent opioid will show cross-dependence with other opioids. Alcohol may partially suppress the symptoms of barbiturate withdrawal.[12] Studies using animal models show high cross-dependence among general CNS depressants and a moderate degree of cross-dependence among most sedative hypnotics (e.g., paraldehyde, chloral hydrate, meprobamate, chlordiazepoxide) and with alcohol and barbiturates. Evidence shows some cross-dependence between barbiturate and volatile anesthetics. Most observations in clinical reports are in agreement; however, well-controlled studies are necessary.

Because long-acting drugs have longer half-lives, the withdrawal symptoms are generally less severe but more protracted.[13–16] This is an important clinical aspect of cross-dependence and of methadone, phenobarbital, and chlorodiazepoxide. The concept of cross-dependence is utilized when the heroin addict uses alcohol or methadone to achieve his/her euphoria when heroin is unavailable.

### *d. Meaning of Cross-Dependence*

The term *cross-dependence* refers to the extension of physical dependence to the other drugs of a particular class. When the specific drug to which the subject develops physical dependence is not available, the subject tends to

**TABLE 1-1**
**Withdrawal Syndromes**

| | Types of Withdrawal[2] | | |
|---|---|---|---|
| | *Narcotic** | *Depressant**†* | *Stimulant***‡* |
| Piloerection | X | | |
| Lacrimation | X | | |
| Rhinorrhea | X | | |
| Diarrhea | X | | |
| Muscle spasm | X | | |
| Muscle pain | X | | X |
| Nausea, vomiting | X | X | |
| Delirium, hallucinations | X | X | |
| Convulsions | X | X | |
| Insomnia | X | X | |
| Sweating | X | X | |
| Tremors | | X | |
| Psychic depression | | | X |
| Hyperphagia | | | X |
| Hypersomnia | | | X |

*Opium derivatives and synthetic narcotics.
†**Hypnotics, sedatives, anxiolytics, alcohol.
‡*** Amphetamines, anoretics, cocaine.

(From Cohen, S. *The Substance Abuse Problems*. Haworth Press, New York, 1981, p. 6.) With permission use other drugs of the same class or a related class to alleviate the withdrawal symptoms. For instance, a barbiturate addict who is unable to obtain the drug tends to look for another depressant, such as alcohol. The effect of the new drug, however, will be unsuccessful in reducing the withdrawal symptoms caused by the discontinuation of the original drug. Instances of heroin addicts unsuccessfully depending upon barbiturates in the absence of heroin are numerous unless doses of the barbiturate cause unconsciousness. The phenomenon of cross-dependence is of practical importance to physicians in treating cases of drug addiction, for purposes of gradual withdrawal of a drug. Heroin addicts are commonly given methadone, which is a narcotic drug with a relatively long duration of action. The daily dose of methadone is gradually reduced so that, in about ten days, narcotic intake can be stopped completely and all physical dependence on narcotics will have been lost. Alcoholics are usually put on treatment with a depressant such as diazepam (Valium), which has a longer duration of action than alcohol. It is increasingly common for a person to be addicted to more than one drug. (For example, heroin addicts simultaneously use barbiturates.) Gradual withdrawal in such cases can be accomplished by attempting either a simultaneous withdrawal of both the drugs, or by a sequential withdrawal (i.e., withdrawal of one drug first while keeping the dose of the other drug high until the first drug is completely withdrawn).

### *e. Cross-Tolerance*

Tolerance to a particular drug is said to occur when the effects produced by a given dose of the drug are less than those normally expected. Cross-tolerance is the extension of this phenomenon to all the drugs belonging to the class. For instance, if a person develops tolerance to diazepam (Valium), cross-tolerance to all the other drugs of the benzodiazepine class might develop, resulting in the gradual increase of the daily dosage. This is a sad situation for both the physician and the patient. However, the development in recent years of drugs belonging to different classes but having the same pharmacologic properties has solved the problem of cross-tolerance in a variety of drugs, such as the analgesics, antidepressants, and barbiturates.

Statistical data show that when narcotic addicts develop cross-tolerance, they tend to subject themselves to abrupt abstinence from the drug or go to the physician for a supervised withdrawal. The reason for this tendency is that the tolerance and physical dependence are temporarily lost due to withdrawal of the narcotic drug, and after a short gap the addict jumps back to the regular dose to enjoy the normal effects of the drug. Other reasons to enter into supervised withdrawal include: (1) not enough money to sustain drug habit; (2) lack of ability to continue self injection—pathologic changes of largest veins; (3) concern that level of dependence has become unmanageable, having transferred from a minor habit (e.g., weekend use of opiates) to a more major phase of daily use; (4) lack of availability of drugs of good quality.

The biochemical changes that occur as tolerance develops are not as yet completely understood. It is suggested that during cross-tolerance the drug is metabolized and inactivated in a fast process before the structure-related pharmacologic properties are visualized. It has been demonstrated that in the case of prolonged administration of barbiturates, the production of the constituent enzymes of the liver that are responsible for the metabolic inactivation of the barbiturates was considerably enhanced. With regard to this older view, the "state-of-the-art" concept of cross-tolerance would not support it. In fact, this enhancement is not specific; these enzymes deactivate many substances, both drugs and normal body constituents. This would produce a "cross-tolerance" between drugs of different classes, which is far too general.

Another concept is that the drug molecules are subjected to intracellular binding processes that diminish the tissue responses. This phenomenon of pharmacodynamic tolerance and the concept of immobilization of the drug molecules by intracellular binding sound promising although not much direct evidence to demonstrate the effects is available to date.

The term *metabolic tolerance* refers to an enhanced ability of the body to inactivate a drug as a consequence of repeated exposure to it. The terms *pharmacologic, tissue*, and *pharmaco-*

*dynamic tolerance* refer to the concept that through repeated exposure to a drug, the responding cells of a tissue somehow accommodate to the drug's continued presence in such a way that the drug elicits a weaker cellular response.[5]

Ross and associates[17] demonstrated a biochemical cross-tolerance between ethanol and morphine. Both morphine and ethanol deplete regional brain calcium. Animals that were pretreated with either morphine or ethanol, when challenged with one or the other, showed marked tolerance to the brain-calcium-depleting effects of these agents. Although other work has also supported the cross-tolerance between alcohol and opiates,[18] some does not.[19]

There is evidence that tolerance and its development require the production of protein. This may be associated with more specific enzymes than those of the liver. Other mechanisms may involve down-regulations of receptors, changes in ion fluxes in neurons, and development of nonfunctional binding sites. This is an important aspect that requires more thoughtful research.

### 8. Relapse and protracted Abstinence

Following an extensive reevaluation of recovery problems associated with opiate withdrawal, various investigators[20,21] discovered long-term physiologic and psychologic abnormalities that, in some cases, persist weeks after abstinence. This syndrome has been termed "protracted abstinence" and is immediately relieved by small amounts of narcotics. According to Martin[22] during the protracted abstinence phase most individuals are more vulnerable and may be more prone to turn to opioids for their reinforcing effects.

## C. SUMMARY

After carefully searching the literature to obtain a reasoned consensus about drug dependence, the freshest and most up-to-date view on the subject is derived from the writings of Segal.[23] He states that:

> Drug dependence should be viewed as a continuum starting from a low degree of dependence seen in experimental or social usage, and ranging to physical dependency or addiction. The compulsive extreme of drug dependence may lead to disorders or defects of behavior with serious implications for the public safety, health and welfare. Many forms of drug dependence, however, do not carry adverse social consequences, as is illustrated by the widespread chronic use of substances such as tobacco and coffee. Heavy and prolonged chronic use of tobacco and coffee may damage organ systems and result in injury to individual health, but they do not induce a physical dependence or result in anti-social behavior, even upon prolonged or excessive use. This factor distinguishes these two drugs from other dependence-producing drugs.
>
> Drug dependence or addiction can thus be considered from two points of view: one relates to the interaction between the drug and the individual; the other to the interaction between drug abuse and society. The first viewpoint is concerned with drug dependence and the interplay between the pharmacological actions of the drug and the psychological status of the individual. The second—the interaction between drug abuse and society—is concerned with the interplay of a wide range of conditions: environmental, sociological and economic. Investigation of drug abuse is currently proceeding along these two lines, as well as studying the interrelationship of these two dimensions. The achievement of a greater understanding of the nature of drug-taking behavior and drug dependence should help in the development of more effective intervention, treatment and prevention strategies to help in dealing with the adverse consequences of drug dependency.

## REFERENCES


1. Meyer, G.F. The art of healing: Folk medicine, religion and science. In G. Meyer, K. Blum, and J.C. Cull, eds., *Folk Medicine and Herbal Healing*. Springfield, Ill.: Thomas, 1981, p. 5.
2. Cohen, S. *The Substance Abuse Problems*. New York: Haworth, 1981.
3. Smith, J.P. Drug abuse; data and debate. In P.H. Blachly, ed., *Society and Drugs: A Short Sketch*. Springfield, Ill.: Thomas, 1970, p. 169.
4. Jaffe, J.M. Drug addiction and drug abuse. In L.S. Goodman and A. Gilman, eds., *The Pharmacological Basis of Therapeutics*, 5th ed. New York: Macmillan, 1975, p. 284.
5. Hofmann, F.G. *A Handbook on Drug and Alcohol Abuse: The Biomedical Aspects*. New York: Oxford, 1975.
6. Jaffe, J.H. Drug addiction and drug abuse. In L.S. Goodman and A. Gilman, eds., *The Pharmacological Basis of Therapeutics*, 4th ed. New York: Macmillan, 1970, p. 276.

7. Seevers, M.H. Psychopharmacological elements of drug dependence. *JAMA* 206:1263, 1968.
8. Hug, C.C. Characteristics and theories related to acute and chronic tolerance development. In S.J. Mulé and H. Brill, eds., *Chemical and Biological Aspects of Drug Dependence*. Cleveland, Ohio: CRC, 1972, p. 307.
9. Narcotic Drug Addiction. (Public Health Service Pub. No. 1021; Mental Health Monograph No. 2). Washington, D.C.: Department of Health, Education and Welfare, 1963, p. 4.
10. Schuster, C.R., and Thompson, T. Self administration of and behavior dependence on drugs. *Ann. Rev. Pharmacol* 9:483, 1969.
11. Kalant, H., LeBlanc, A. E., and Gibbins, R.J. Tolerance to, and dependence on, some non-opiate psychotropic drugs. *Pharmacol. Rev.* 23:135, 1971.
12. Blum, K., et al. Possible role of tetrahydroisoquinoline alkaloids in post-alcohol intoxication states. *Ann. N.Y. Acad. Sci.* 273:234, 1976.
13. Fraser, H.F. Criteria for evaluating physical dependence and overall abuse potential of drugs in man. In S.J. Mulé and H. Brill, eds., *Chemical and Biological Aspects of Drug Dependence*. Cleveland, Ohio: CRC, 1972, p. 85.
14. Isbell, H., et al. Liability of addiction to 6-dimethylamino 4-4-diphenyl-3-Heptanone (methadone) in man, experimental addition to methadon. *Arch. Intern. Med.* 82:362, 1948.
15. Wulff, M.H. The barbiturate withdrawal syndrome: A clinical and electroencephalographic study. *Electroenceph. Clin. Neurophysiol.* Suppl. 14:1, 1959.
16. Hollister, L.E., Montzenbecker, F.P., and Degan, R.O. Withdrawal reactions from chlordiazepoxide (Librium). *Psychopharmacologia*, 2:63, 1961.
17. Ross, D.H. Selective action of alcohols on cerebral calcium levels. *Ann. N.Y. Acad. Sci.*, 273:280, 1976.
18. Khanna, J.M., et al. Cross-tolerance between ethanol and morphine with respect to their hypothermic effects. *Eur. J. Pharmacol.* 59:145, 1979.
19. Miceli, D., Marfaing-Jallat, P., and LeMagnen, J. Failure of naloxone to affect initial and acquired tolerance to ethanol in rats. *Eur. J. Pharmacol.* 63:327, 1980.
20. Dole, V.P. Narcotic addiction, physical dependence and relapse. *N. Engl. J. Med.* 286:988, 1972.
21. Cushman, P., and Dole, V.P. Detoxification of rehabilitated and methadone-maintained patients. *JAMA* 226:747, 1973.
22. Martin, W.R., et al. Methadone—A reevaluation. *Arch. Gen. Psychiatry* 28:286, 1973.
23. Segal, B. Drug use and addiction: A review of the problem. Personal communication, 1982.

## SUGGESTED READINGS

### Monographs and Reviews

Brecher, E.M. *Licit and Illicit Drugs*. The Consumers Union report on narcotics, stimulants, depressants, inhalants, hallucinogens, and marijuana, including caffeine, nicotine, and alcohol. Boston: Little, Brown, 1972.

Cohen, S. Psychotomimetic agents. *Ann. Rev. Pharmacol.* 7:30, 1967.

Connell, P.H. *Amphetamine Psychosis* (*Maudsley Monographs no. 5*) Institute of Psychiatry. London: Chapman & Hall, 1958.

Dole, V.P. Biochemistry of addiction. *Ann. Rev. Biochem.* 39:821, 1970.

Domino, E.F. Neuropsychopharmacology of nicotine and tobacco smoking. In W.L. Dunn, Jr., ed., *Smoking Behavior: Motives and Incentives*. Washington, D.C.: Winston, 1973, p. 5.

Efron, D.H., Holmstedt, B., and Kline, N.S., eds., *Ethnopharmacologic Search for Psychoactive Drugs*. Proceedings of a symposium held in San Francisco, Calif., Jan. 28-30, 1967. (Public Health Service Pub. No. 1645) Bethesda, Md., Dept. of Health, Education and Welfare, 1967.

Essig, C.F. Addiction to non-barbiturate sedatives and tranquilizing drugs. *Clin. Pharmacol. Ther.* 5:334, 1964.

Essig, C.F. XIV. Addiction to barbiturate and nonbarbiturate sedative drugs. *Res. Publ. Assoc. Res. Nerv. Ment. Dis.* 46:188, 1968.

Farnsworth, N.R. Hallucinogenic plants. Various chemical substances are known to be the hallucinogenic principles in many plants. *Science* 162:1086, 1968.

Freed, E.X. Drug abuse by alcoholics: A review. *Int. J. Addict.* 8:451, 1973.

Freedman, D.X. The psychopharmacology of hallucinogenic agents. *Ann. Rev. Med.* 20:409, 1969.

Glasscote, R.M., et al. *The Treatment of Drug Abuse: Programs, Problems, Prospects*. Washington, D.C.: Joint Information Service of the American Psychiatric Assn. and the National Assn. for Mental Health, 1972.

Goldstein, A. Heroin addiction and the role of methadone in its treatment. *Arch. Gen. Psychiatry* 26:291, 1972.

Harris, L.S. General and behavioral pharmacology. *Pharmacol. Rev.* 23:285, 1971.

Hawkins, R.D., and Kalant, H. The metabolism of ethanol and its metabolic effects. *Pharmacol. Rev.* 24:67, 1972.

Hollister, L.E. Marihuana in man: Three years later. *Sci. Wash.* 172:21–29, 1971.

Hug, C.C. Characteristics and theories related to acute and chronic tolerance development. In S.J. Mulé and H. Brill, eds. *Chemical and Biological Aspects of Drug Dependence.* Cleveland, Ohio: CRC, 1972, p. 307.

Kalant, H., LeBlanc, A.E., and Gibbins, R.J. Tolerance to, and dependence on, some non-opiate psychotropic drugs. *Pharmacol. Rev.* 23:135, 1971.

Kalant, O.J. *The Amphetamines: Toxicity and Addiction.* Springfield, Ill.: Thomas, 1966.

Kupperstein, L.R., and Sussman, R.M. A bibliography on the inhalation of glue fumes and other toxic vapors—A substance abuse practice among adolescents. *Int. J. Addict.* 3:177–19, 1968.

Lewin, L. *Phantastica; Narcotic and Stimulating Drugs: Their Use and Abuse.* London: Paul, Trench, Trubner, 1931. (Tr. of 2d German ed., 1924.)

Lifer, C.S. Chemical characteristics of drugs inducing physical and/or psychic dependence to alcohol. In S.J. Mulé and H. Brill, eds. *Chemical and Biological Aspects of Drug Dependence.* Cleveland, Ohio: CRC, 1972, p. 135.

Lundwall, L., and Baekeland, F. Disulfiram treatment of alcoholism. *J. Nerv. Ment. Dis.* 153:381, 1971.

Malick, J.B., and Bell, R.M. *Endorphins: Chemistry, Physiology, Pharmacology, and Clinical Relevance.* New York: Dekker, 1982.

*Marihuana and Health: Second Annual Report to Congress.* Washington, D.C.: U.S. Department of Health, Education, and Welfare, 1972.

McWilliams, S.A., and Tuttle, R.J. Long-term psychological effects of LSD. *Psycholol. Bull.* 79:341, 1973.

Meyer, R.D. *Guide to Drug Rehabilitation: A Public Health Approach.* Boston: Beacon, 1972.

Musto, D.F. *The American Disease.* New Haven, Conn.: Yale Univ. Press, 1973.

Nagle, D.R. Anesthetic addiction and drunkenness: A contemporary and historical survey. *Int. J. Addict.* 3:25–40, 1968.

Nahas, G.G. *Marihuana: Deceptive Weed.* New York: Raven, 1973.

National Commission on Marihuana and Drug Abuse. *Marihuana: A Signal of Misunderstanding: First Report.* Washington, D.C.: U.S. Government Printing Office, 1972.

National Commission on Marihuana and Drug Abuse. *Drug Use in America: Problem in Perspective: Second Report.* Washington, D.C.: U.S. Government Printing Office, 1973.

*Non-medical Use of Drugs with Particular Reference to Youth.* Report of the special Committee on Drug Abuse, Council on Community Health Care, Canadian Medical Association. *Canad. Med. Assoc. J.* 101:804, 1969.

President's Commission on Law Enforcement and Administration of Justice. Task Force on Narcotics and Drug Abuse. *Narcotics and Drug Abuse; Annotations and Consultants' papers. Task Force Report.* Washington, D.C.: U.S. Government Printing Office, 1967.

Sapira, J.D. The narcotic addict as a medical patient. *Am. J. Med.* 45:555, 1968.

Shuster, L. Tolerance and Physical Dependence. In D.H. Clanvet, ed., *Narcotic Drugs: Biochemical Pharmacology.* New York: Plenum, 1971, pp. 408.

Stimson, G.V. *Heroin and Behaviour: Diversity Among Addicts Attending London Clinics.* New York: Wiley, 1973.

Thornton, W.E., and Thornton, B.P. Narcotic poisoning: a review of the literature. *Am. J. Psychiatry* 131:867, 1974.

Way, E.L. Some biochemical aspects of morphine tolerance and physical dependence. In S. Fisher and A.M. Freedman, eds., *Opiate Addiction: Origins and Treatment.* Washington, D.C.: Winston, 1973, p. 99.

WHO Expert Committee on Drug Dependence: Twentieth Report. (World Health Organization Technical Report Series no. 551) Geneva, World Health Organization, 1974.

Wikler, A. *Opiates and Opiate Antagonists. A Review of Their Mechanisms of Action in Relation to Clinical Problems* (Public Health Monograph no. 52) Washington, D.C.: U.S. Government Printing Office, 1958.

Wikler, A. Theories related to physical dependence. In S.J. Mulé and H. Brill, eds., *Chemical and Biological Aspects of Drug Dependence.* Cleveland, Ohio: CRC, 1972, p. 359.

Wilmarth, S.A., and Goldstein, A. *Therapeutic Effectiveness of Methadone Maintenance Programs in the U.S.A.* Geneva: World Health Organization, 1974.

Wood, W.G., and Elias, M.F. *Alcoholism and Aging Advances in Research.* Boca Raton, Fla.: CRC Press. 1982.

## Articles

Council on Mental Health and Committee on Alcoholism and Drug Dependence. Dependence on cannabis (marhihuana). *JAMA* 201:368, 1967.

Council on Mental Health and Committee on Alcoholism and Drug Dependence. Dependence on LSD and other hallucinogenic drugs. *JAMA* 202:47, 1967.

Dimijian, G.G., and Radelat, F.A. Evaluation and treatment of the suspected drug user in the emergency room. *Arch. Intern. Med.* 125:162, 1970.

Dishotsky, N.I., et al. LSD and genetic damage. *Science* 172:431, 1971.

Dole, V.P. Methadone maintenance treatment for 25,000 heroin addicts. *JAMA* 215:1131, 1971.

Ferraro, D.P., and Grilly, D.M. Lack of tolerance to 9-tetrahydrocannabinol in chimpanzees. *Science* 179:490, 1973.

Flowers, N.C., and Horan, L.G. Nonanoxic aerosol arrhythmias. *JAMA* 219:33, 1972.

Gessa, G.L., Tagliamonte, A., and Tagliamonte, P. Aphrodisiac effect of p-chlorophenylalanine. *Science* 171:706, 1971.

Goodman, S.J., and Becker, D.P. Intracranial hemorrhage associated with amphetamine abuse. *JAMA* 212:480, 1970.

Gowdy, J.M. Stramonium intoxication: Review of symptomatology in 212 cases. *JAMA* 221:585, 1972.

Griffith, J.D., et al. Dextroamphetamine: Evaluation of psychomimetic properties in man. *Arch. Gen. Psychiatry* 26:97, 1972.

Gold, M.S., Pottash, A.L.L., Sweeney, D.R., Davies, R.K., and Kleber, H.D. Clonidine decreases opiate withdrawal—related anxiety: Possible opiate noradrenergic interaction in anxiety and panic. *Subs. Alc. Act./mis.* 1(2):239, 1980.

Hamilton, M.G., and Hirst, M. Alcohol-related tetrahydroisoquinolines: pharmacology and identification. *Subs. Alc. Act./mis.* 1(2):121, 1980.

Holzman, R.S., and Bishko, F. Osteomyelitis in heroin addicts. *Arch. Intern. Med.* 75:693, 1971.

Hopkins, G.B. Pulmonary angiothrombotic granulomatosis in drug offenders. *JAMA* 221:909, 1972.

Jacobson, C.B., and Berlin, C.M. Possible reproductive detriment in LSD users. *JAMA* 222:1367, 1972.

Jaffe, J.H., and Senay, E.C. Methadone and l-methadyl acetate: Use in management of narcotics addicts. *JAMA* 216:1303, 1971.

Jaffe, J.H., et al. Methadyl acetate vs. methadone: A double-blind study in heroin users. *JAMA* 222:437, 1972.

Kreuz, D.S., and Axelford, J. Delta-9-tetrahydrocannabinol: localization in body fat. *Science* 179:391, 1973.

Le Dain, G. *Final Report of the Commission of Inquiry Into the Non-Medical Use of Drugs*. Ottawa, Canada, 1973.

Lemberger, L., Crabtree, R.E., and Rowe, H.M. II-hydroxy-delta-9-tetrahydrocannabinol: Pharmacology, disposition, and metabolism of a major metabolite in man. *Science* 177:62, 1972.

Lemberger, L., Silberstein, S.D., Axelrod, J., and Kopin, I.J. Marihuana: Studies on the disposition and metabolism of delta-9-tetrahydrocannabinol in man. *Science* 170:1320, 1970.

Lemberger, L., et al. Delta-9-tetrahydrocannabinol: Temporal correlation of the psychologic effects and blood levels after various routes of administration. *N. Engl. J. Med.* 286:685, 1972.

Lerner, P. The precise determination of tetrahydrocannabinol in marihuana and hashish. *Bull. Narc.* 21:39, 1969.

Lewis, R., Gorbach, S., and Altner, P. Spinal pseudo-monas chondro-osteomyelitis in heroin users. *N. Engl. J. Med.* 286:1303, 1972.

Lieber, C.S. Liver adaptation and injury in alcoholism. *N. Engl. J. Med.* 288:356, 1973.

Lindell, T.D., Porter, J.M., and Langston, C. Intraarterial injections of oral medications. A complication of drug addiction. *N. Engl. J. Med.* 287:1132, 1972.

Louria, D.B. Medical complications of pleasure-giving drugs. *Arch. Intern. Med.* 123:82, 1969.

Maugh, T.H. 2d. Narcotic antagonists: The search accelerates. *Science* 177:249, 1972.

McGlothlin, W.H., Sparkes, R.S., and Arnold, D.O. Effect of LSD on human pregnancy. *JAMA* 212:1483, 1970.

Mechoulam, R. Marihuana chemistry. *Science* 168:1159, 1970.

Mechoulam, R., et al. Chemical basis of hashish activity. *Science* 169:611, 1970.

Melges, F.T., et al. Marihuana and temporal disintegration. *Science* 168:1118, 1970.

Melges, F.T., et al. Marihuana and the temporal span of awareness. *Arch. Gen. Psychiatry* 24:564, 1971.

Mikes, F., and Waser, P.G. Marihuana components: Effects of smoking on delta-9-tetrahydrocannabinol and cannabidiol. *Science* 172:1158, 1971.

Miller, R.R., Feingold, A., and Paxinos, J. Propoxyphene hydrocholoride: A critical review. *JAMA* 312:996, 1970.

Neal, J.M., Sato, P.T., and Howald, W.N. Peyote alkaloids: Identification in the Mexican cactus pelecyphora aselliformis ehrenberg. *Science* 176:1131, 1972.

Newman, L.M., et al. Delta-9-tetrahydrocannabinol and ethyl alcohol: evidence for cross-tolerance in the rat. *Science* 175:1022, 1972.

Olsen, R.W., and Snowman, A.M. Chloride-dependent enhancement by barbiturates of γ-aminobutynic acid receptor binding. *J. Neuroscience* 2(12):1812, 1982.

Owen, N.L. Abuse of propoxyphene. *JAMA* 216:2016, 1971.

Pillard, R.C. Marihuana. *N. Engl. J. Med.* 283:294, 1970.

Preston, A.J., and Muecke, E.G. A dose of Spanish fly. *JAMA* 214:591, 1970.

Reich, P., and Hepps, R.B. Homicide during a psychosis induced by LSD. *JAMA* 219:869, 1972.

Richter, R.W., et al. Acute myoglobinuria associated with heroin addiction. *JAMA* 216:1172, 1971.

Rubin, E., and Lieber, C.S. Alcoholism, alcohol and drugs. *Science* 172:1097, 1971.

Teresa, M., *et al.* Lack of cross-tolerance in rats among (−)delta-9-transtetrahydrocannabinol (delta 9-THC), Cannabis extract, mescaline and lysergic acid diethylamide (LSD-25). *Psychopharmacologia* 13:332, 1968.

Steinberg, A.D., and Karliner, J.S. The clinical spectrum of heroin pulmonary edema. *Arch. Intern. Med.* 122:122, 1968.

Tashkin, D.P., Shapiro, B.J., and Frank, I.M. Acute pulmonary physiologic effects of smoked marihuana and oral delta-9-tetrahydrocannabinol in healthy young men. *N. Engl. J. Med.* 289:336, 1973.

Taylor, G.J., 4th and Harris, W.S. Cardiac toxicity of aerosol propellants. *JAMA* 214:81, 1970.

Taylor, G.J., 4th and Harris, W.S. Glue sniffing causes heart block in mice. *Science* 170:866, 1970.

Taylor, R.L., Maurer, J.I., and Tinklenberg, J.R. Management of "bad trips" in an evolving drug scene. *JAMA* 213:422, 1970.

Tennant, F.S., Jr., and Groesbeck, C.J. Psychiatric effects of hashish. *Arch. Gen. Psychiatry* 27:133, 1972.

Tennant, F.S., Jr., and Prendergast, T.J. Medical manifestations associated with hashish. *JAMA* 216:1965, 1971.

Young, D.J. Propoxyphene suicides. Report of nine cases. *Arch. Intern. Med.* 129:62, 1972.

Zaks, A., et al. Naloxone treatment of opiate dependence. A progress report. *JAMA* 215:2108, 1971.

Chapter 2

# Some General Social Pharmacologic Aspects of Substance Abuse

## A. DRUG ABUSE IN A MODERN SOCIETY

The topic of contemporary drug abuse encompasses the modes of administration, effects, and side effects of a wide variety of drugs available today. The complexity of the drug scene is confusing not only to the person who uses the drugs, but also to the professionals working to treat the drug abuser. Much remains to be understood in the field of drug abuse. One of the objectives of this comprehensive treatise, therefore, is to provide the basics required to understand the patterns of drug abuse and to suggest a plausible solution to eliminate the problem.

The use of a drug that is not legally or socially sanctioned, without proper regard for its pharmacologic actions, is called *drug abuse*. Such an abuse would undoubtedly result in effects that are harmful to the individual and to the society. It is sometimes intriguing to ponder whether the application of a drug is positively destructive or is constructive for society. The Inca Indians chew coca leaves to increase their endurance.[1] A student uses dextroamphetamine to study all night for an exam. Are these instances to be listed as drug abuse? Does social drinking come under abuse of ethyl alcohol? The answers to these questions depend upon the individual. Some observers[2] assert that the connotation of drug abuse represents only a cultural aspect of judgment or a biased accusation. However, the use of some drugs such as the amphetamines in high doses is considered abuse in any cultural frame of reference. (The prolonged use of amphetamines in high doses invariably produces a progressive organic brain syndrome.) The concept of abuse also depends on cultural values.

Generally, an over-indulgence in drugs that do not alter consciousness or are not psychoactive is termed ''misuse'' rather than ''abuse.'' Furthermore, the terms ''drug abuse'' and ''drug dependence'' are not necessarily related or interdependent. The diabetic who requires insulin may be "drug dependent" but certainly is not considered to be "drug abusive." Additionally, clinicians may over-prescribe antibiotic medications such as penicillin, and treat eating disorders with diuretics or heart abnormalities with digitalis.[3] These constitute instances of drug misuses.

The ancient distinction[4] between the mind and the body brings up two distinctly rigid concepts of drug dependence—psychologic dependence and physical dependence.

Physical dependence on a drug results in a physiologically disruptive withdrawal illness after abrupt discontinuation of the drug following prolonged use. Such drugs that cause physical addiction include the opiates (pain killers), barbiturates (sleeping pills), tranquilizers [diazepam (Valium), chlordiazepoxide (Librium)], ethanol, and some nonbarbiturate sedatives. On the other hand, psychologic drug dependence will result in a mental craving for the drug when the drug is discontinued, as a result of habit formation. The habit assumes so enormous an importance to the individual that the addict may go back to the drug even after years of successful abstinence. Some point out that psychologic dependence precedes physical dependence. Studies on the action of central neurotransmitters have led to the theory of "noradrenergic reward" in which the pleasurable drug effects appear to occur in association with the potentiation of the catecholamine action at the central synapses, although the mechanism of potentiation might vary with different drugs. If this theory is right, it implies that the psychologic dependence on a drug occurs in association with a physicochemical change at the central synapse.[4] The gap is not fully bridged by this theory, however, as psychologic dependence also embodies the concept of dependence on established habit patterns; thus one may become dependent on a drug or on any often-repeated behavior such as eating a hearty breakfast each morning, or sex, or collecting items, or gambling. Society does not have a compelling interest in repetitive behavior until it becomes self-destructive. In other words, we do not worry about the addiction of collecting until we begin to collect people, as beautifully depicted in the movie *The Collector*.

## B. DRUG ABUSE PATTERNS

The medically unsupervised use of drugs and certain other substances for such purposes as changing one's mood, producing novel sensations or experiences, or changing the user's perception of self and the world, is termed "drug abuse".

The intensely subjective nature of the abuse phenomenon restricts the observer's understanding and analysis of the patterns of experience. Thus one has to rely on the reports from the addicts themselves or on the conclusions drawn from the behavior of the addicts to acquire basic knowledge of the concept. Numerous patterns of drug abuse exist, depending upon a number of factors, such as the emotional needs of the individual, the nature of the effects of the drug, and accessibility to the drug. To determine a person's pattern of drug abuse, one should know first what drug or drugs are being used. Some use just one drug such as marihuana or alcohol. Others use one drug primarily, but try to supplement it with another for improved effects. A heroin addict, for instance, might prefer to take a barbiturate or an amphetamine together with heroin to experience strange or enhanced effects. Some addicts use two or more drugs in a sequential pattern. One might switch to a depressant drug after a prolonged use of a stimulant drug. Scarcity of a drug might force the user to change to a substitute drug. A heroin addict might attempt to alleviate the symptoms of withdrawal by using a barbiturate when heroin is not available. Some addicts exhibit preferences for a variety, and thus develop a dependence on those drugs gradually.[5]

The pattern of abuse changes with age. At the age of 10, a person might start with "glue sniffing" and smoking marihuana. At 15, that person might switch to intravenous injections of heroin. Such a sequence of events, though frequent, is far from inevitable. The explanation as to why some drug users exhibit such a pattern of drug abuse changing only with age, while others do not, might depend more upon motivation factors than anything else. Some drugs that are, in fact, mixtures of two or more drugs, are sold as single drugs under different (often misleading) names, and the buyer does not inquire about the composition of the drug before buying and using it. Moreover, the seller actually may not know, and buyers are often overly trusting in terms of their drug purchases. A major danger is the problems associated with the so-called "look-alike drugs."

### *Trends in Substance Abuse*

In the substance abuse arena, all sorts of shifts have been noted for each abused chemical agent. A federal report,[6] as discussed by Dr. Sidney Cohen,[7] provides us with some estimates of the current substance abuse situation.

ALCOHOL

As might be expected, beverages containing alcohol are the most widely used and abused of the psychoactive substances. More than nine million people are believed to have definite problems in connection with their drinking. Alcoholic women are becoming more visible in American society, and the preponderance of male alcoholics over females seems to be diminishing.

Younger people are drinking more, with 6 percent of high school seniors consuming alcohol-containing beverages daily. Drinking patterns established during adolescence are believed to carry over to adulthood with some regularity. More than 200,000 deaths are reported yearly as alcohol-related. This constitutes 8 percent of all the deaths in this country. The past 15 years have shown a 30 percent increase in alcohol consumption.

TOBACCO

Tobacco is second to alcohol in its widespread use. Fifty-five million Americans smoke cigarettes daily. It is estimated that more than 300,000 citizens die prematurely each year from illnesses related to smoking. Currently about 22 percent of youths and 40 percent of adults are regular smokers, and these figures are essentially unchanged since 1974. What has changed drastically has been smoking by high school females. Their rate now approximates that of high school males. By age 12, one out of five youngsters smokes. The hope of a few years ago that the younger generation would not indulge as much in establishment drugs has not come to pass.

MARIHUANA

Cannabis is the most commonly used illegal drug. The rates are highest among 18 to 25-year-olds, but its use is spreading to those younger and older. About 16 million Americans have used marihuana during March [1978]. Of these, four million are between 12 and 17 and 8.5 million are in the 18- to 25-year-old age group. Ten percent of high school seniors are daily users. Very few deaths due to marihuana use are recorded.

HEROIN

The number of those addicted to heroin has stabilized during the past few years at about a half-million people. It should be recalled that there was a ten-fold increase in heroinism between 1960 and 1969—from about 60,000 to more than 600,000. This was followed by a slow decline and then a leveling off during the mid-1970s.

Heroin potency in street material is now down to 5 percent, and the cost per pure milligram of heroin has risen to about $2. The increased price and decreased potency are believed to reflect a diminished availability. These factors make heroin less attractive to novices and tend to move addicts into treatment. Heroin-related deaths and the number of emergency room visits involving this drug are down, another sign that the numbers involved are either stabilized or decreasing.

METHADONE

Methadone as a drug of abuse derives from its use as a maintenance treatment for about 80,000 clients. Since it is effective for about 24 to 35 hours during maintenance therapy, take-home supplies are given to those patients who are given the privilege of visiting the clinic only two or three times weekly.

Some of these supplies may be sold off; less frequently clinic robberies or sales by staff are sources of street methadone. More than 200 methadone-related deaths were reported in 1977, half of which were in New York City. This represents a decrease over previous years due to a tightening-up of take-home regulations. When LAAM, the longer acting methadone analogue, becomes available, this problem should be further reduced or eliminated entirely.

BARBITURATES

The source of black market barbiturates and other hypnotics is usually from prescribed materials, but they are supplemented with illegitimately manufactured products. Barbiturate deaths have been decreasing gradually since 1970 when physicians started prescribing the safer benzodiazepines more often for sleep. For example, in 1970 there were 1,873 barbiturate deaths due to suicide. In 1975 the numbers decreased to 1,036, despite a slight rise for all suicides from 23,488 in 1970 to 27,063 in 1975. Additional federal efforts are underway to curb the abuse of the barbituric acid derivatives and related drugs.

MINOR TRANQUILIZERS

Ninety million prescriptions for minor tranquilizers were filled in 1977, a slight decrease from the previous year. Although the majority of these drugs were used for proper indications, a number of patients and nonpatients misused and abused the anxiolytics by taking large quantities to achieve a state of intoxication or unconsciousness. A quarter of all drug-related emergency room visits is connected with tranquilizer use. The number of deaths due to anxiolytics alone is relatively small, but when used in combination with alcohol or other sedatives anxiolytics' depressant effects are enhanced.

AMPHETAMINES

Amphetamines and other appetite suppressant prescription drugs accounted for almost 17 million prescriptions in 1977. Most of these were properly used for narcolepsy, minimal brain dysfunction and, in short courses, for weight control. Four million of these prescriptions were for amphetamines of which 85 percent were for long-term weight control, a practice that has been demonstrated not to be effective. In addition, an unknown amount of illicit amphetamines is available. Their level of abuse is holding steady, and the intravenous injection of large amounts, the speedfreak phenomenon noted during the late 1960s, almost has disappeared. Nevertheless, the amphetamines remain a potential item of increased abuse.

COCAINE

Cocaine use continues to increase, with most of those who indulge doing so sporadically. This pattern may be due to high cost and relative unavailability. The average purity has dropped to 30 percent cocaine, whereas a few years ago 90 to 100 percent cocaine was the product most often available on the illicit market. The number of occasional recreational cocaine users and also of "coke-heads" will predictably increase during the next few years.

LSD AND OTHER HALLUCINOGENS

LSD, DMT, and other hallucinogenic drugs have declined in use since the mid-1960s, although they have, by no means, disappeared from the drug scene. Emergency room visits in connection with hallucinogens also have become much less frequent. However, there is one exception. Phencyclidine (PCP, Angel Dust) not only is increasing in usage, but the results of its ingestion are a matter of considerable concern to health care and law enforcement officials. The person under the influence of phencyclidine is more apt to engage in unpredictable, violent behaviors than have been encountered with other hallucinogens. The individual may present a variety of neurologic and psychiatric toxic reactions that are neither easily diagnosed nor treated.

INHALANTS

The sniffing of commercial products containing volatile solvents or the contents of aerosol sprays is a juvenile practice that does not always terminate when one becomes an adult. The practice is not decreasing: indeed, among high school seniors, it has been gradually increasing during the last few years. Acute lethality (sudden sniffing death) and chronic organ damage have been documented. At present, the following products are popular in various regions of the country: gold and bronze spray paints, Texas shoeshine aerosols, lacquer thinner, the volatile nitrates, gasoline, clear plastic spray, Transgo transmission fluid, and PAM, an aerosol spray.

SPECIAL POPULATIONS AT RISK

Certain groups vulnerable to overinvolvement with drugs have been identified. The ratio of female to male drug abusers is rising, particularly with regard to alcohol, sedatives, tranquilizers and certain other psychochemicals. Youths have shown dramatic increases in the abuse of all drugs during the past decade. In recent years, the increase continues for cocaine, marihuana, and phencyclidine. The elderly are a group at risk in the misuse of sedative prescription drugs singly and in combination. Geriatric patients in some long-term care facilities may be exposed to poor or improper prescribing practices to their detriment.

Ethnic minorities usually are over-represented in drug abuse survey data, and special prevention and treatment measures must be devised to deal with this serious issue. All of these populations at risk will require careful, thoughtful planning to reduce the prevalence of their dysfunctional drug use.

On the question of substance abuse trends, Cohen states[7]:

As we reflect on the implications of the current trends in the abuse of various psychochemicals, no clear pattern can be discerned. If we use the analogy of a few years ago, the "war on drugs" has resulted in neither victory nor defeat. We seem to be engaged in a sort of trench warfare where hard-earned gains on one salient are cancelled out by losses in another sector. Barring some unforeseen breakthrough, the tough, obstinate battling will continue, with the final issue remaining in doubt for years to come.

It may be, as some believe, that a significant degree of the drug problem will remain with us—and that it will never recede to the lower levels of the good old days. They claim that the quality of life, especially for the young, will have to change markedly before the abuse of drugs will revert to more acceptable levels.

The changes will have to be in the direction of enhanced aspirations, goals that are not compatible with the overuse of drugs, and hopes for the future that include emotional and physical growth, not impairment. Such a shift in the value system of youth is not impossible. It has happened before, and it is happening now to an all-too-small number of young people.

But what about the great majority?

Will it take a modern Children's Crusade—a spiritual renaissance dominated by some charismatic leader? Or can we work our way to a more sober, less stoned society through research and development? The final solution is evidently in prevention, but the large-scale prevention of substance abuse is a remote prospect at this time.

## C. THE DRUG EXPERIENCE

Various substances that are used or abused have quite different psychological and physiological effects. For the abusable psychotropics the prime actions usually induce states of euphoria complete with disturbances of so-called normal mental function. These impairments might require clinical attention. The exact nature of the particular drug experience depends on a number of factors such as (psychological) set and (sociological) setting; previous experience with a certain class of drug; psychological frame of the individual; and the drug dose and route-of-administration. Various types of psychological experiences have included marihuana-induced pleasure states, profound sadness, loss of memory, loss of time and distance perception, and loss of reality. Other substances, such as psychedelic mushrooms or LSD, distort reactions to sensory stimuli. Stimulant drugs such as amphetamines enhance the libido while depressants such as narcotics might reduce the sex drive in some users. Another depressant, alcohol, may induce violence in certain prone individuals.

## D. REASON FOR PSYCHOTROPIC DRUG ABUSE[5]

Humans seem to be consumed with the search for pleasure states. To many, reality provides a stable but sometimes boring and frustrating experience, with increases in cost of living, unemployment, and other societal pressures. There is also an enhancement of mental disturbance and a general feeling in some of ill-being. The now-accepted view that there is ''better living through chemistry'' provides an impetus—and rationalization—for so-called ''pleasure seekers.'' It is well known that there are certain drugs which can distort the perception of self and the environment. The major reasons for psychotropic drug abuse are to (a) distort the reality that is disagreeable to the subject, and b) create a better ''reality,'' substituting ''bad'' for ''good'' feelings. High doses of barbiturates depress the psyche so much that they precipitate a psychosis, in which the abuser loses contact with reality. Interestingly, drug users often seem to consciously or unconsciously seek death through the abuse of drugs.

With abusable drugs there are not only profound psychological effects observed but physiological ones as well. Sometimes small changes in the systemic blood pressure and temperature go unnoticed by the user whereby other actions such as photosensitivity, tremors, headache, nausea and vomiting cannot be ignored.

At this point, it would be appropriate to document some recent concepts about the use and misuse of psychoactive agents.

Kandel et al.[8] studied and reported on the antecedents of adolescent initiation into stages of drug use. These authors point out that many theories of drug dependence make some conception of individual pathology (biogenetic predisposition) a primary explanation, whereas others stress social factors. In the pathologic conception,[9,10] recent pharmacogenetic theories of substance-seeking behavior are receiving support derived from both animal[11] and human[12] experimentation. However, it should be noted that either conceptualization may apply to different stages of the process of the involvement in drug behavior; social factors play a more important role in the early states, except where genetics is involved (see references 9 and 10), and psychophysical factors may become important in the later ones.

Findings from the work of Kandel et al.[8] suggest that situational and interpersonal factors are most important for initiation into a behavior. They also found that intrapsychic factors are most important for increased involvement or participation in that behavior. Other studies suggest that adolescents use a variety of substances in response to interpersonal influences, both by peers and by parents.

Peer influences have been reported as a cause of drinking,[13] smoking,[14] and using marihuana[15] as well as other illicit drugs. Parental influences have been claimed for liquor,[16] cigarettes,[14] and illicit drugs.[17] Low academic levels,[18] school absences, and involvement in delinquent activities have been found to be associated with the use of marihuana or other illicit drugs[19] or of alcohol.[20] Depression[21] and alienation[22] have been stressed as important factors in the use of marihuana and other illicit drugs. Rebelliousness, which has been reported to be a good predictor of illicit drug use,[23] has been particularly emphasized as a factor in drinking.[16] Radical political ideology and lack of religiosity has been associated with use of illicit drugs[24] and of alcohol[25]

## E. RELATIONSHIP BETWEEN POTENCY, TOLERANCE, DOSAGE, AND ROUTE OF ADMINISTRATION[6]

The intensity of a drug's effects is determined, to an important degree, by the dose used. Drugs subject to abuse that also have legitimate therapeutic uses are commonly employed by drug-dependent individuals in quantities considerably larger than the conventional doses prescribed by physicians. An addict's daily intake of pentobarbital (Nembutal), for example, might well be 20 to 30 times greater than the dose of this drug ordinarily prescribed as an aid to sleep. For those drugs to whose effects appreciable refractoriness (tolerance) develops, the user eventually must increase the dose to obtain the original intensity of effect. The narcotics abuser, in particular, continually faces this problem: The development of tolerance requires a larger dose; the larger dose produces, in time, more tolerance, which means the dose must be increased again, and so on. Even in patterns of drug abuse that are free of the problem of tolerance, drug users often deliberately increase their intake to intensify the drug experience.

The intensity of a drug's effects also depends, in part, on the route of administration. The effects of a drug are likely to be more intense, but of briefer duration, when it is injected than when it is taken by mouth, and, in most cases, the effects will appear more rapidly. Users of heroin have learned that the most pleasurable experience with heroin is obtained by intravenous injection, and many users of amphetamine have come to the same conclusion.

If we assume that the effects produced by a drug are approximately the same on each occasion of use, we must then attempt to account for the great variability known to exist in the nature of the drug experience.

Why are some alcoholics effusive and convivial, whereas others are abusive and belligerent? Why do only some users of amphetamine become sexually aroused while under the influence of the drug? Why are some LSD "trips" good and others bad? No truly satisfactory answer can be given to this type of question. We believe that the nature of a drug experience is influenced by the user's response to the drug's effects. The response, we believe, is determined, in turn, by the user's general personality structure and particular emotional state at the time the drug is taken. This is a complex matter, and one that is poorly understood, as there is much that is unknown about the development and structure of personality and the determinants of various emotional states.

## F. DRUG ADMINISTRATION ROUTES[5]

The history of drug abuse dates back many centuries before Christ.[26] The early drug addicts used only the most readily available orifices of the body—the mouth and the nose—as routes of drug administration. The whole scene of drug abuse was revolutionized with the advent of the hypodermic syringe in the mid-19th century. The most widely employed modes of administration of drugs into the body now include oral (by mouth), nasal (by inhalation through nose), intravenous, subcutaneous, and sublingual.

Oral administration of a drug results in delayed effects, and to a less than maximal degree. However, a large oral dose can produce a greater effect than a small intravenous one. In contrast, the effects develop rapidly by injection and are maximum when the intravenous route is used. The drugs subject to abuse cannot exert their effects completely until the effective doses reach the site of action (which is usually the CNS) through the bloodstream. The rate at which they reach the principal sites of action governs the onset as well as the intensity of their effects. Consequently the route of administration plays a very important role in any application of drugs. Another factor that affects the efficacy of a drug is its fate after entering the bloodstream. The drug molecules may be carried to the liver, where they are metabolized and inactivated. They may be carried to the kidney and be excreted. They may be carried to certain indifferent tissues, such as the skeletal muscle or depot fat, where they exert no observable effect. Sometimes the molecules are bound to the plasma proteins and are temporarily immobilized. How rapidly a drug can exert its effects thus depends upon all the factors described and is directly proportional to how easily the drug is accessible to its receptor sites within or on the surface of the cells.

When a drug is injected subcutaneously (directly beneath the skin), the relatively sparse distribution of blood vessels in that area restricts the rate of its entry into the bloodstream. However, when a drug is injected into the muscle (intramuscularly), the process of its entry into the bloodstream is faster than through the subcutaneous injection but slower than via an intravenous injection.

In the case of certain drugs that exist in the gaseous state or are easily volatilized into the gaseous state, inhalation may be the only mode of administration. The onset of effects is more rapid than with a subcutaneous or intramuscular injection, but not as rapid as an intravenous injection. Finally, another method of administration is to place the drug tablet under the tongue and allow it to dissolve completely in saliva. The richly vascularized mucous membrane of the oral cavity absorbs the solution of the drug quickly. This is more efficient than oral ingestion of the drug, and is the method used by PCP addicts. Additionally, there is also the unusual use of windowpane LSD via the sublinqual route, which should be mentioned.

## G. FACTORS AFFECTING DRUG EFFECTS[5]

### 1. The Placebo Response

A substance that contains inert material having no biological action is considered a placebo when administered to patients who are told that it is an active drug. Usually, the typical, so-called "placebo effect" produces positive results in approximately 30% of subjects tested. The reason for the "placebo effect" is supposedly a strong belief or anticipation. In support of this statement, it has been reported that in post-surgical patients with severe pain, at least one third were reported to feel relief after a placebo was injected instead of an analgesic.

Novice individuals who are told that they are smoking good-grade marihuana act "stoned" even if they are smoking very poor or weak marihuana. Experienced users reject marihuana of poor quality, after testing its effects and are willing to pay as much as $150 per ounce for stronger material. There are other examples of how experienced and novice differ in their ability to adequately assess the pharmacological nature of a substance. The smoking of dried banana skins further exemplifies this notion. While novice users praise the effects of the smoke from dried banana skins, experienced drug aficionados reject the practice.

### 2. Drug Dosage

Most pharmacologists are taught very early in their careers to become aware of the dangers involved in drug responses, especially if only the effects of a single dose are known, rather than a full range of doses. To that end, drug-induced responses are tested in both animals and humans, utilizing a wide variety of doses and subsequently plotting a "dose-response curve" (see chapter 3).

Usually, the greater the dose the more intense its effects. However, this may not always be the case. Certain drugs do not have a dose-dependent effect. For example, marihuana has biphasic effects; i.e., lower doses have been known to induce excitation, whereas (in mice) higher doses produce sedation. Unexpectedly, small doses of LSD may produce panic states in novice users and have little or no effect on experienced individuals. Furthermore, there are numerous factors that significantly alter dose-dependent responses.

### 3. Elements of the Drug Experience[5]

The actual effects produced by any psychoactive substance are more or less dependent on four elements: 1) the pharmacological nature of the drug 2) the genetic make-up of the user 3) the environment in which the drug is consumed, and 4) the psychological state of the user.

These elements constitute a holistic view of the overall outcome of the drug experience. The pharmacology dictates the profound behavioral as well as physiological effects, the genetic element dictates the magnitude or intensity of the above effects, the environment or set and setting mediates the quality of the experience, and the psychological state prior to the use of the drug may control the actual ''type'' of the experience either euphoric or aphoric in nature.

Dr. Timothy Leary, the infamous former Harvard University professor, after ''turning on'' hundreds of college students to the world of psychedelics, especially LSD, realized the importance of proper guidance and social setting. In this regard, Leary insisted that novice users of LSD have a ''guide'' with them while under the influence of it. Throughout the United States, experienced LSD users volunteered to turn on other individuals to the drug and act as their guide. These guides were trained in the art of ''talking-down'' (a term which will be described in more detail in Chapter 18) and in the use of tranquilizers like chlorpromazine and even valium as treatment methods employed during so-called ''bad'' trips.

### 4. The Setting[5]

The importance of the *social setting* has been previously mentioned. The setting, if it is not right or comfortable, could significantly turn a pleasurable drug experience or a so-called ''good trip'' into a frightening and even sometimes horrifying experience, or ''bad trip.'' However, not all abusable drugs are so dependent on the setting for the final quality of the experience.

#### *a. Marihuana*

The smoking of marihuana is a good example of the importance of the setting. This fact is even more significant for the novice smoker compared to the experienced marihuana aficionado because the naive user does not know what to expect and the experience may differ from what is anticipated. The setting of it, if proper, will usually eliminate fears, reduce stress, and provide comradeship. This theory, of course, directly contradicts its illegal status; the laws against smoking marihuana are cited by marihuana users as the promoting of a double standard by a predominant culture of alcohol-users.[30] The enhancing of a pleasurable marijuana experience usually occurs when the drug is used among friends in a relaxed atmosphere. But if the user, sitting around with friends and smoking and listening to music, is suddenly confronted with a loud knock at the door and the admonition, ''It's the police!'', certainly he/she will quickly descend from a *euphoric* to an *aphoric* state.

#### *b. LSD*

The social setting as well as the psychological set of the LSD user are very important in determining the quality and type of the LSD-induced experience.

#### *c. Narcotics*

Unlike marijuana and LSD, opiate-like drugs attenuate the user's responsiveness to external stimuli. Most heavy narcotic users are indifferent to the world around them and thus setting has much less or little influence on the quality of the drug experience.

### *d. CNS Depressants of the Sedative-Hypnotic Type*

The drug experience derived from CNS depressants, such as sleeping remedies of the barbiturate type, when used in a quiet setting, usually induces somnolence. However, if it is taken in a noisy environment, the individual may experience intoxication and stupor without associated drowsiness. This is another example of how a setting could alter an expected outcome.

## 5. Predilection to Drug Abuse[5]

In this context, the term *predilection* infers a favorable inclination or susceptibility towards psychotropic abuse. Although the exact nature of this predilection has been adequately defined, research continues to unravel this most perplexing problem. The two questions which must be answered systematically are: a) what brain chemicals are possibly in excess or deficit in potentially prone candidates? b) what biological markers exist that can assist in predicting high at-risk groups or individuals? Consensus in the literature reveals that certain mental states such as depression and schizophrenia are caused in part by a deficit of Norepinephrine and an excess of dopamine, respectively. Additionally, there are theories describing deficits of brain-internal opiates called endophines occuring in compulsive disease such as alcohol and drug-seeking behavior.

It is believed by psychologists and pharmacologists that the so-called "compulsive personality" consists of two important elements, psychological and genetic. Hoffmann[5] points out that scientists as of yet have not been successful in providing the clinician with a reasonable and definitive explanation of drug abuse etiology. Currently, there exists some novel treatment approaches which are based upon existing neurochemical and pharmacological research on both animals and humans. These include, among others, acupuncture, hypnosis and biofeedback.

Scientists who have investigated the possibility that there is a distinct "psychological compulsive personality" which leads to drug abuse have not been able to distinguish this type of personality between users and nonusers of psychoactive drugs. However, it is generally agreed that since certain mental states are due to neurotransmitter dysfunctions, many individuals would take street drugs to delay or prevent the precipitation of active psychosis as well as relieving their psychic pain. (The author does not condone such a harmful and unsupervised practice.)

Although some progress has been made,[31] for the most part we are ignorant about underlying psychotic factors relevant to predisposition of drug abuse; however, a comparable degree of ignorance also impedes our full understanding of criminal behavior, compulsive overeating, and homosexuality.

Segal[32] suggests that "successful prevention and alleviation of drug-taking behaviors is most likely to occur when specific patterns of drug use and motives are considered in the context of the total coping and personality style of the individual." Segal further points out that it is extremely important to provide more desirable alternative involvements for youth that are more rewarding than drug experiences and incompatible with dependence on chemicals.

Efforts to delineate the factors that contribute to vulnerability have included studies of the personalities and family structures of different types of drug users, and the roles of peer groups, social factors, and economic conditions in generating tension and frustration. In some cases, constitutional and genetic factors have been identified that might be responsible either for abnormal states of tension or for unusually positive or negative responses to drug use or drug withdrawal.[33] But it would appear that for any given pattern of continued drug use, the outcome is the result of an interaction among social, biologic, and environmental factors.[34]

## REFERENCES

1. Goth, A. *Medical Pharmacology; Principles and Concepts*, 7th ed. St. Louis: Mosby, 1974, p. 299.
2. Snyder, S.H., Faillace, L., and Hollister, L. 2,5-dimethoxy-4-methyl-amphetamine (STP): A new hallucinogenic drug. *Science* 158:669, 1967.

3. Jelliffe, R.W., et al. Death from weight-control pills. A case report with objective postmortem confirmation. *JAMA* 208:1843–7, 1969.
4. Collier, H.O.J. The experimental analysis of drug dependence. *Endeavour* 31:123, 1972.
5. Hofmann, F.G. *A Handbook on Drug and Alcohol Abuse: The Biomedical Aspects.* New York: Oxford, 1975, p. 3.
6. *Drug Use, Patterns, Consequences and the Federal Response: A Policy Review.* Office of Drug Abuse Policy, Executive Office of the President, March 1978.
7. Cohen, S. *The Substance Abuse Problems.* New York: Haworth Press, 1981, p. 170.
8. Kandel, D.B., Kessler, R.C., and Margulies, R.Z. Antecedents of adolescent initiation into stages of drug use: A developmental analysis. In D.B. Kandel, ed., *Longitudinal Research on Drug Use: Empirical Findings and Methodological Issues.* Washington, D.C.: Hemisphere, 1978.
9. Goodwin, D. *Is Alcoholism Hereditary?* New York: Oxford, 1976.
10. Blum, K., et al. Psychogenetics of drug seeking behavior. *Subst. Alcohol Action Misuse* 1:255, 1980.
11. Blum, K., et al. Reduced leucine-enkephalin-like immunoreactive substance in hamster basal ganglia after long term exposure. *Science* 216:1425, 1982.
12. Genazzani, A.R., Nappi, G., and Facchinetti, F. Central deficiency of beta-endorphin in alcohol addicts. *J. Clin. Endocrinol. Metab.* 55:583, 1982.
13. Cahalan, D., and Room, R.L. Problem drinking among American men. New Brunswick, N.J.: Publications Division, Rutgers Center of Alcohol Studies, 1974.
14. Williams, T. *Summary and Implications of Review of Literature Related to Adolescent Smoking.* Bethesda, Md.: U.S. Department of Health, Education and Welfare, National Clearinghouse for Smoking and Health, 1971.
15. Brook, J., Lukoff, I., and Whiteman, M. Correlates of adolescent marihuana use as related to sex, age and ethnicity. *Yale J. Biol. Med.* 50:383, 1977.
16. Bacon, M., and Jones, M. *Teen-Age Drinking.* New York: Cromwell, 1968.
17. Smart, R.G., and Fejer, D. Drug use among adolescents and their parents: Closing the generation gap in mood modification. *J. Abnorm. Psychol.* 79:153–160, 1971.
18. Smith, G.M., and Fogg, C.P. Teenage drug use: A search for causes and consequences. In R.G. Simmons, ed., *Research in Community and Mental Health.* Vol. I. Greenwich, Conn.: JAI Press, 1979.
19. Jessor, R., and Jessor, S.L. *Problem Behavior and Psychosocial Development: A Longitudinal Study on Youth.* New York: Academic Press, 1977.
20. Wechsler, H., and Thum, D. Teen-age drinking, drug use and social correlates. *Q. J. Studies Alc.* 34:1220–1227, 1973.
21. National Commission on Marihuana and Drug Abuse. *Drug Use in America: Problem in Perspective.* Washington, D.C.: U.S. Government Printing Office, 1973.
22. Mellinger, G.D., Somers, R.H., and Manheimer, D.I. Drug use research items pertaining to personality and interpersonal relations: A working paper for research investigators. In D.J. Lettieri, ed., *Predicting Adolescent Drug Abuse: A Review of Issues, Methods and Correlates.* National Institute on Drug Abuse. Washington, D.C.: U.S. Government Printing Office, 1975, p. 299.
23. Smith, C.M., and Fogg, C.P. Teenage drug use: A search for causes and consequences. In D.J. Lettieri, ed., *Predicting Adolescent Drug Abuse: Review of Issues, Methods and Correlates.* National Institute on Drug Abuse. Washington, D.C.: U.S. Government Printing Office, 1975, p. 277.
24. Johnson, B.D. *Marihuana Users and Drug Subcultures.* New York: Wiley, 1973.
25. Maddox, G.L., and Bevode, C. *Drinking Among Teen-Agers; a Sociological Interpretation of Alcohol Use by High School Students.* New Brunswick, N.J.: Rutgers Center for Alcohol Studies, 1964.
26. Hofmann, F.G. *A Handbook on Drug and Alcohol Abuse: The Biomedical Aspects.* New York: Oxford, 1975, pp. 29–67.
27. Schultes, R.E. Hallucinogens of plant origin. *Science* 163:245, 1969.
28. Smith, D.E. The use of LSD in the Haight-Ashbury. Observations at a neighborhood clinic. *Calif. Med.* 110:472, 1969.
29. Smith, D.E., and Rose, A.J. The use and abuse of LSD in Haight-Ashbury. *Clin. Pediatr.* 7:317, 1968.
30. Kales, A., et al. Drug dependency. Investigations of stimulants and depressants. *Ann. Intern. Med.* 70:591, 1969.
31. Segal, B., Hobfoll, F., and Croner, F. Patterns of reason for drug use among detained and adjudicated juveniles. *Int. J. Addictions* (in press).
32. Segal, B. Drugs and youth: A review of the problem. Lecture presented at Dohto University, Japan, Nov. 1980.

33. Goodwin, D.W., et al. Alcohol Problems in adoptees raised apart from alcoholic biological parents. *Arch. Gen. Psychiatry* 28:238, 1973.
34. Blum, K., et al. A social pharmacological approach to drug-seeking behavior. *J. Psychedelic Drugs* 13:369, 1981.

## SUGGESTED READINGS

### Monographs, Reviews, and Books

Non-medical use of drugs, with particular reference to youth. *Can. Med. Assoc.* 101:72, 1969.

Louria, D.B. *The Drug Scene*. New York: McGraw-Hill, 1968.

Jaffe, J.H. Drug addiction and drug abuse. In L. Goodman and A. Gilman, eds., *The Pharmacological Basis of Therapeutics*, 4th ed. New York: Macmillan, 1970, p. 276.

Cohen, M., et al. Effect of actinomycin D on morphine tolerance. *Proc. Soc. Exp. Biol. Med.* 119:381, 1965.

Collier, H.O.J. Tolerance, physical dependence and receptors. A theory of the genesis of tolerance and physical dependence through drug-induced changes in the number of receptors. *Adv. Drug Res.* 3:171, 1966.

The addictive states. A. Wikler, ed., Baltimore: Williams & Wilkins, 1968 (*Res. Pub. Assoc. Res. Nerv. Ment. Dis.* 46).

Mulé, S.J., and Brill, H., eds. *Chemical and Biological Aspects of Drug Dependence*. Cleveland, Ohio: CRC, 1974.

Schucket, M.A. *Drug and Alcohol Abuse (A Clinical Guide to Diagnosis and Treatment)*. New York: Plenum, 1979.

Weil, A., and Rosen, W. *Chocolate to Morphine: Understanding Mind Addicting Drugs*. Boston: Houghton Mifflin, 1983.

Solomon, J. *Alcohol and Clinical Psychiatry*. New York: Plenum, 1982.

Chapter 3

# Basic Pharmacologic Considerations and Principles

## A. DEFINING PHARMACOLOGY AND TOXICOLOGY[1]

Never before have chemical agents exerted such a dynamic impact on human life through both our internal and external environment. If we do not ingest them to cure or prevent illness, then we are exposed and subjected daily to their influence in countless other ways—through the pollutants we breath, through the treated foods we eat, through the pesticides sprayed on the nation's crops, and through the soaps and detergents we use to keep ourselves and our possessions clean but that all too often are released into the country's streams and waterways. No wonder that the subject of pharmacology, the study of the effects of chemicals on biologic systems, is of increasing interest to both the scientist and the lay person.

Chemical agents not only provide the structural basis and energy supply for living organisms, but also regulate their functional activities. The interactions between potent chemicals and living systems contribute to the understanding of life processes and, in addition, afford effective methods for the treatment, prevention, and diagnosis of many diseases. Chemical compounds used for these purposes are *drugs*, and their actions on living systems are referred to as *drug effects*.

Pharmacology is the term applied to that broad science encompassing all aspects of information relating to the actions of chemical substances on living systems. It is a discipline of biology and is closely related to other disciplines, particularly to physiology and biochemistry.

One of the areas of this broad science, and possibly of greatest interest to humans and their survival, is *toxicology*, the study of the harmful effects of chemicals of all types. The increasing exposure of a large number of people, not only to potent new therapeutic agents, but also to potent licit and illicit chemical agents in our environment, has created a wider and more personal interest in pharmacology and toxicology than has ever existed before. All of us are involved because there is no way to escape exposure to many chemicals. For example, all human beings have a DDT burden. This is not necessarily a result of personal use of DDT, but of a world environment that now contains sufficient quantities effectively to contaminate all animal life.

## B. TRANSLATING ANIMAL DRUG EXPERIMENTATION TO THE HUMAN ORGANISM[1]

The data pertinent to pharmacology and toxicology are collected from many areas, with levels of complexity ranging from simple chemical reactions to the intricate relationships involved in the functioning of the human brain. Since most of the intense interest in pharmacology is centered on the human being, the action of chemicals in the human being is of primary importance. However, there are major problems involved with the study of chemical actions in humans. They include the possibility of causing toxic reactions, permanent injury, or even death, balanced against the need to obtain well-controlled scientific results. Because of the moral and scientific difficulties inherent in experimentation with humans, most information on the biologic effects of chemicals is obtained from animals. Modern pharmacology and toxicology rely on the view that information obtained from experimentation with animals is applicable to the human being. The screening and development of new therapeutic agents are based mostly on this premise. In most instances, extrapolation from experiments on animals is adequate. But in a few cases, the human being shows responses that could not be predicted from animal experiments, or could be predicted only with difficulty or from hindsight. Generally it is these areas in which the controversy rises to a high pitch. For example, thalidomide is a teratogen, that is, a drug that will cause abnormalities in the fetus. In human beings, a dose of 1 mg/kg of thalidomide each day will produce changes, whereas the rabbit requires 30 mg/kg/day and the rat is unaffected by doses up to 4000 mg/kg each day.[2]

Extrapolation from animal data to data for human beings also encounters difficulty in the use of numbers. A total of perhaps several thousand animals are exposed to a drug to study its possible toxic effects, but when that drug is introduced into widespread human use via federal regulations that control phased development of a new drug, the number exposed quite often is measured in millions. Therefore it is quite possible to see effects in human beings that were not found in the animals. And the toxic events that do occur in a small percentage of the animals studied could be very important when extrapolated to usage of the drug by millions of people. Regulations in the United States and Canada are sufficiently restrictive to have suppressed new drug development to the degree that North America is a second-class continent in the area of new and innovative drugs, but that is another issue. Other difficulties arise, especially when dealing with the pharmacologic and behavioral effects of psychotropic agents. In the case of these potent pharmacologic agents, the profound psychologic effects are determined by social setting and social set. In the investigation with laboratory animals, it is very difficult to control for this important parameter, and thus many sound scientific experiments may be translated wrongly to the human condition. Furthermore, in experiments concerned with the problem of substance abuse, it becomes increasingly important to keep in mind the difference between the dosage of a drug that is used in the street and that employed by the pharmacologist to obtain physiologic, pharmacologic, or behavioral effects.

It is perhaps true to say that those experiments in animals that have taken social setting (and social set?) into account have identified that the environment has a profound impact on the intensity of drug effects. The problem in most studies is not that they are unable to control the social environment, but that they tend to ignore it completely. Needless to say, social behavior in animals does not readily extrapolate to that in humans, but then behavior is not the same as ''setting'' either.

## C. BASIC MECHANISMS OF DRUG ACTION[1]

The study of the effects of chemicals is done first on small animals. The pharmacologist must establish a chemical's major effects. Drugs are usually characterized by such major biochemical or physiologic effects in the body. Categories such as analgesics, which decrease the feeling of pain, and antibiotics, which kill bacteria, are but descriptions of primary major effects. Pharmacologists have searched for years for chemicals that have a beneficial effect only; virtually all those that are used as drugs have a wide range of unwanted effects as well. We tend to minimize these therapeutically unwanted effects by calling them side effects, but, with improper use of a drug, they can become its major impact. For the evaluation and comparison of drugs, the scientist must attempt to quantitate their effects; that is, to assign numbers and values. Effects usually are related to dosage and are characterized in terms of maximum usefulness, variability, and selectivity.

Most drugs differ from inert chemicals or food in their potency, selectivity, and structural specificity. Digitoxin, reserpine, atropine, LSD, PCP, and penicillin are a few examples of potent, selective, and structurally specific compounds. A few milligrams of these drugs can alter normal or pathologic physiology or, as in the case of penicillin, can rid the body of invading microorganisms.

Potency immediately suggests an interaction with a biologic control system; selectivity points to a favored localization or affinity for some site of action. Finally, structural specificity brings to mind an interaction of the drug with some cellular constituent that is "complementary" to it in three-dimensional space.

Much of experimental pharmacology suggests that these suppositions are correct. Although the point is seemingly academic, an understanding of current views on the basic mechanisms of drug action should promote a way of thinking about drugs that will favor their correct use in therapeutics and, just as important, an understanding of the pharmacology of abusable drugs.

## D. THE DRUG RECEPTOR: A LOCK-AND-KEY CONCEPT

A drug receptor is a constituent of the cell that can specifically and reversibly bind to a drug molecule and is responsible for producing changes in the body's functions. The drug receptor interaction involves a reversible bond formation between the drug molecule and the site of binding in the receptor. This results in a chain of events that lead to a detectable response in the subject. The interaction is something like a key (drug) fitting into a lock (receptor) and the chain of events that follow is like the door being opened (the observable response).[3]

High specificity to a particular drug molecule is one of the important characteristic features of the drug receptor. Even a minute change in the molecular structure of the drug molecule greatly alters the response of the receptor cell. For instance, amphetamine and methamphetamine are two potent CNS stimulants that differ slightly in their chemical structures, but methamphetamine produces much greater behavioral stimulation than amphetamine. An explanation suggested for this is that the methamphetamine fits best into the receptor in the central nervous system and is less rapidly degraded by monoamine oxidase.

The idea that any drug could act as a "magic bullet" and magically and instantaneously relieve a physical malady is probably erroneous. In this regard, there is no such thing as a magic bullet that somehow affects a specific target organ. Instead selectivity of drug action is more a function of the location of the drug receptors, the strength of the drug's attachment to the receptor, and the consequences of the interaction between drug and receptor than it is a property of drugs being selectively distributed to a very small area of the body.

In 1878 Langley initially proposed the receptor concept. Subsequently, Paul Erlich widely used the concept in his chemotherapy studies. Langley's investigations included the impact on saliva secretion by the antagonists atropine and pilocarpine. His early hypotheses focused on an unknown substance in nerve endings or glands which could combine with those drugs. Erlich perceived the combination as either reversible or irreversible, with receptors identified as "groups of protoplasmic macro-molecules."[4]

Thus, for arsenicals, the mercapto group would be a receptor, although covalent bond formation is not a common drug–receptor interaction. Ehrlich recognized that many potent drugs can be removed easily from tissues, and therefore must form reversible combinations with receptors.

According to current concepts,[5] drug–receptor interactions may be of the following types:

1. Drugs may inhibit enzymes.

2. Some steroid hormones may act by derepressing a length of inactive DNA, leading to the synthesis of new proteins.

3. Drugs may act as coenzymes. The epinephrine receptor complex acts on adenyl cyclase.

4. Drugs may alter the permeability characteristics of cell membranes by interaction with permeases or carrier mechanisms.

Some drug effects are often attributed to a primary interaction with enzymes on the basis of insufficient evidence. Inhibition of an enzyme by a drug in the test tube can be misleading. Its effect in the body may depend upon an entirely different action. Nevertheless, in a few cases, effects undoubtedly are a result of enzymatic action. The anticholinesterases, such as physostigmine, the organophosphorus compounds and carbonic anhydrase inhibitors, such as acetazolamide (Diamox), and the monoamine oxidase inhibitors, such as iproniazid, exert many pharmacologic effects as a consequence of enzyme inhibition. Also, disulfiram (Antabuse) causes severe effects in a person who drinks alcohol because it blocks the enzyme that catalyzes the oxidation of acetaldehyde, a toxic product of alcohol degradation. The antimetabolites, of great interest in the chemotherapy of infections and cancer, compete with normal metabolites for an enzyme.

## E. POTENCY, SLOPE, MAXIMUM EFFECT, AND VARIABILITY

A drug is said to be potent when it has great biologic activity per unit weight. The situation of the dose–response curve along the dose axis is an expression of the potency of the drug. A typical dose–response curve (Figure 3-1) demonstrates three pertinent characteristics of the drug: its potency (from the position of the curve on the horizontal axis or the abscissa), its slope (the degree of intensification of response with a given increase in dose), and the dose required to produce the maximum effect.

### *a. Potency*

In television commercials and advertisements in popular magazines and newspapers, we have all seen the statement that one drug is more potent than another. How important is this, and what does it mean? Certainly potency would be influenced by many factors to be discussed in this chapter—absorption, distribution, metabolism, and excretion. For example, if two drugs are investigated for their sedative actions, but only one passes the blood–brain barrier (a physiologic barrier governing the entry of a drug into the brain), that drug will be the more potent.

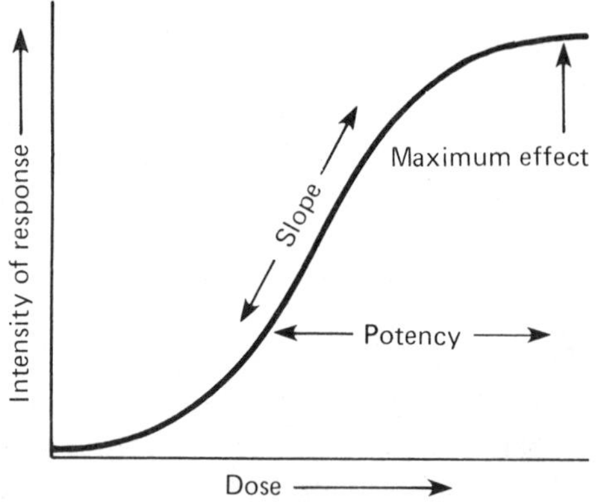


**Figure 3–1. Three principal components of the dose–response curve: potency, slope, and maximum effect. (After Fingl, E., and Woodbury, D.M. General principles. In L.S. Goodman and A. Gilman, eds., *The Pharmacological Basis of Therapeutics,* 5th ed. New York: Macmillan, 1975, Fig. 1–6, p. 25. With permission.)**

Furthermore, if two other drugs were capable of producing sedation, but one was capable of exerting this effect at half the dose level of the other, the first drug would be considered the more potent. The concept of potency is not an extremely important characteristic of a drug, since it makes little difference whether the effective dose is 0.1 gram or 10 grams, as long as the drug is administered in an appropriate dose and undue toxicity is not observed at that dose (a factor termed safety). This argument would negate the concept that the more potent the drug, the better it is. High potency, in fact, may be a disadvantage more than an advantage, since an extremely potent drug may also be much more toxic and dangerous.

### *b. Slope*

Slope is the central linear portion of the dose–response curve and is one of the variables that must be considered in determining the relative safety of a drug. A steep dose–response curve (for a CNS depressant) implies that there is a smaller difference between the dose that produces death and the dose that causes mild sedation than would be observed with a depressant that had a lower slope. The steeper the slope, the smaller the increase in dose is needed to go from a minimal response to a maximal effect. Additionally, the issue here is not the desired dose–effect curve, but its proximity to dose–effect curves of adverse and life-threatening reactions. Steepness on its own is not of significance if there is a high therapeutic index, a ratio between toxic dose and beneficent dose.

### *c. Maximum Effect*

The maximum effect produced by a drug, even at very large dosage, is termed its *ceiling effect* and is referred to as its maximum efficacy or, simply, *efficacy*. The peak of the dose–response curve indicates the maximum effect produced by a drug. Not all pain relievers (analgesics), for example, are capable of exerting the same level of analgesia. Morphine has sufficient efficacy to provide relief from intense pain that aspirin, even at massive doses, is incapable of relieving. It is important to note that potency and maximum effect of the drug are two separate considerations, and, although one compound may be less potent than another, it may still be capable of exerting a greater maximal effect.

### *d. Variability*

Since it is known that drug effects are never identical in all patients, or even in a given patient on different occasions, the final important factor to be considered in a dose–response curve is *variability*. The dose of a drug that will produce a given response in a number of animals will vary considerably. Figure 3-2 illustrates a Gaussian (bell-shaped) distribution of drug variability in a population of subjects. Note that, for a given response, some individuals will require only a small amount of the drug, whereas others will require much more than what is considered normal. Because of the phenomenon of variability of drug effects, it is extremely important that the dose of any drug be individualized, and thus generalization about "average doses" is very risky and meaningless.

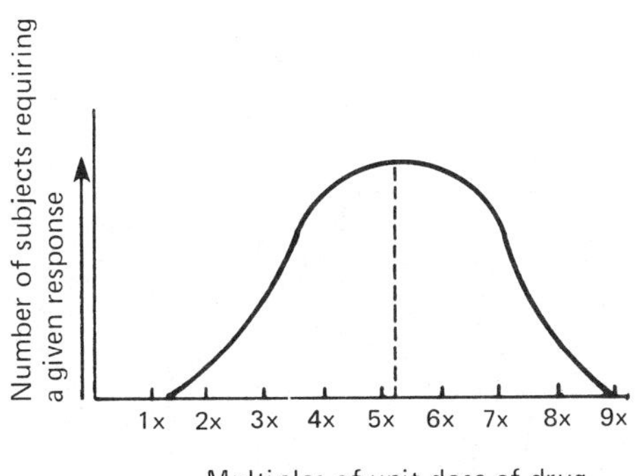


**Figure 3–2. Biologic variation in susceptibility to drugs. This curve is a Gaussian distribution, with the dose of drug plotted against the number of subjects requiring a given dose for a given response to occur. Note that, for a given response, some individuals will require only a small amount of the drug, whereas others will require much more than what is considered normal. (After Julien, R.M., *A Primer of Drug Action*, 2nd ed. San Francisco: Freeman, 1978, p. 264. With permission.)**

## F. MEASUREMENT OF POTENCY AND EFFICACY[3,5]

Madison Avenue's dramatizations of various brand comparisons on television often bombard the layman with claims of stronger potency—evidencing that Brand A is a "better" drug than Brand B. The confusion of the concepts of potency and efficacy illustrates a classic dilemma in therapeutics, wherein the issue of potency is overemphasized at the expense of a valid consideration of drug efficacy. As Goth[3] has pointed out, the relative potencies of drugs is of minor importance to the physician, while the concept of greater efficacy holds the key to the real worth of one drug compared to another.

The log dose-response curve that plots drug dosage against a measured effect can indicate drug potency at any point on the traditional sigmoid curve. However, the effective $dose_{50}$ ($ED_{50}$) is the relevant factor for comparative purposes. Thus, while Figure 3-3 portrays parallel dose-response curves for drugs A and B, the $ED_{50}$ of Drug B may far exceed that of drug A, resulting in a claim of greater potency for drug A. Madison Avenue to the contrary, the reality is that potencies are compared based on doses producing the same effect, rather than based on effects produced by the same dosage—a distinction clearly drawn by both Goth and Juиen.[3,5]

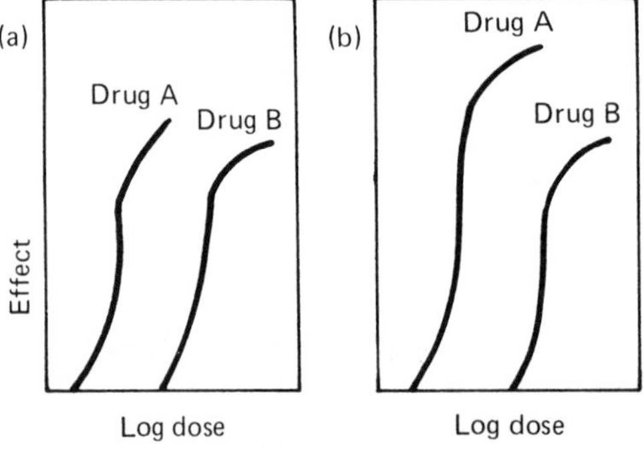


**Figure 3–3. Log dose–response curves illustrating the difference between potency and efficacy. A—Drug A is much more potent than drug B, but both have the same maximal effect. B—Drug A is not only more potent, but has a greater efficacy. It produces a higher peak effect than drug E.**

## G. SPECIFICITY[3]

One of the primary aims of therapeutics is the discovery of drugs with low side-effects and high specificity of action. A common misconception that is not consistent with experience maintains that a drug's relative effect on the organ site is dependent primarily on the density of the drug's distribution and concentration at the site.

For the most part, it is evident that it is the number and density of the receptors at the organ site, rather than of the drug's density and concentration, that dictate the magnitude of the resultant action.

The same holds true in terms of antidote development. That is, the greater the specificity of the drug, the better the chances that it can be blocked effectively by a receptor antagonist.

One pertinent example applies to Myodystrophy (Steinert's Disease), resulting in a deficiency of acetycholine at the receptor sites—a condition which has been corrected by the application of a drug at the organ site which mimics the action of the acetycholine substance at the receptors.

This type of selective binding to specific sites was accomplished with the opiates, and specific opiate receptor binding in vertebrate central and peripheral neural tissue has been identified.[6,7] This finding has clinical importance in that it provides the pharmacologist with a tool for studying the mechanism of action of the opiates and characterizing the differences that could be obtained with other drugs that cause CNS depression, such as barbiturates. The latter drugs do not selectively bind to opiate receptors. Although similarities exist between narcotic drugs and sedative-hypnotics, there are also distinct differences, which may be explained by their specific binding characteristics. Additional description of multiple opioid receptors is found elsewhere in this book.

## H. STRUCTURAL RELATIONSHIPS

Goldstein,[7] through vigorous experimentation, has concluded that the three-dimensional structure of the drug molecule is a determining factor in a drug's ability to bind to receptor sites. Stereoisomers have greatly different potencies. For example, d-amphetamine (dexedrine) is significantly more potent as a behavioral excitant relative to either the racemic amphetamine sulfate or the l-isomer of amphetamine. Goldstein[7] further points out that isomeric drugs interact with the receptor at a definite configurational site similar to an active site on an enzyme.

## I. PARTIAL AGONIST, AGONIST, AND ANTAGONIST

A drug is said to be an agonist when it exhibits affinity to a receptor site and efficacy in producing the required drug effects. An antagonist is one that competes with the drug (agonist) for the receptor site but fails to produce the drug effects as efficiently as the agonist, that is, the agonist has both affinity and efficacy, and the antagonist has affinity but not efficacy. The phenomenon is called competitive antagonism. Thus when a log dose–response curve is plotted for the agonist in the presence of an antagonist, the antagonist shifts the dose–response curve of the agonist to the right in a parallel way without a shift in the maximum (Figure 3-4). Naloxone, as an antagonist to morphine (the agonist), is a good example of this.

The partial agonists are the drugs that lie somewhere between the pure agonists and the pure antagonists. They exhibit affinity for the same receptor but have only partial efficacy. Diethanolamine,[8] a structural analog of ethanol, is a good example as a partial agonist to ethanol.

Diethanolamine was found[8,9] to produce a parallel shift to the right of the dose–response curves for ethanol, without depressing the max-

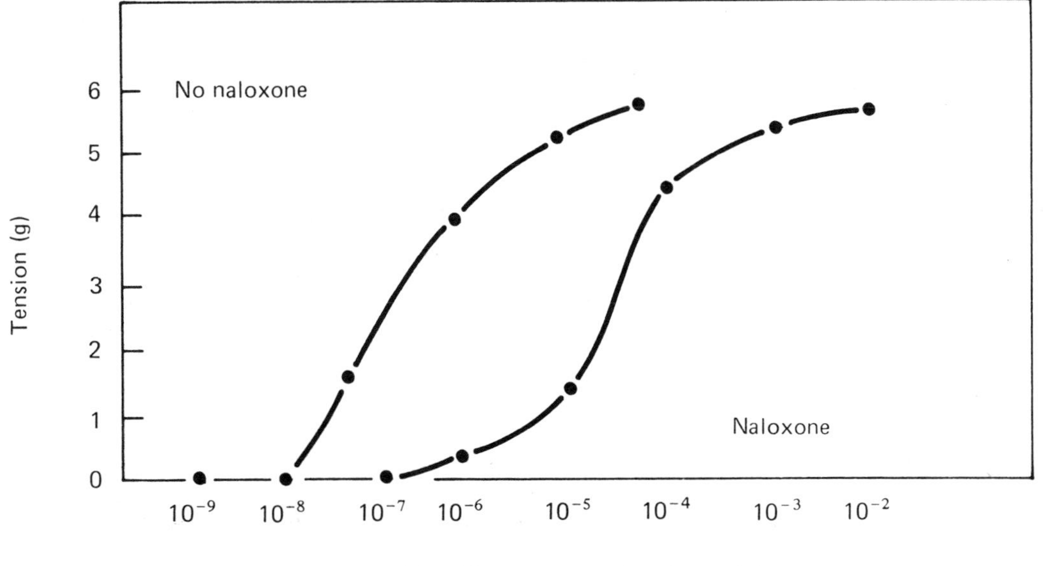


**Figure 3–4. Effect of morphine on tension development of guinea pig ileum. Naloxone, a competitive antagonist, caused a parallel shift of the log dose–response curve. (Adapted from Goth, A. *Medical Pharmacology*, 7th ed. St. Louis: Mosby, 1976, p. 8. With permission.)**

$$HN\begin{cases} CH_2{-}CH_2{-}OH \\ CH_2{-}CH_2{-}OH \end{cases}$$

**(a) Diethanolamine**

$$CH_3CH_2OH$$

**(b) Ethanol**

imum response. This finding suggests that the inhibitory action of diethanolamine to ethanol appears to be competitive in nature. However, in the same study, it was found that diethanolamine produces narcosis by itself (see Figure 3–5). A partial agonist should depress the maximum response if mixed with a full agonist, as well as produce a submaximal effect on its own. Thus diethanolamine is a pseudo-"partial" agonist or a "weak agonist–antagonist" to ethanol.

## J. ANTAGONISM OF THE NONCOMPETITIVE TYPE

When a combination of two drugs produces a parallel shift in the log dose–response curve without a shift in the maximum, as in the case of naloxone and morphine, it is evidence for common receptor interaction on a competitive basis. However, if increasing the concentration

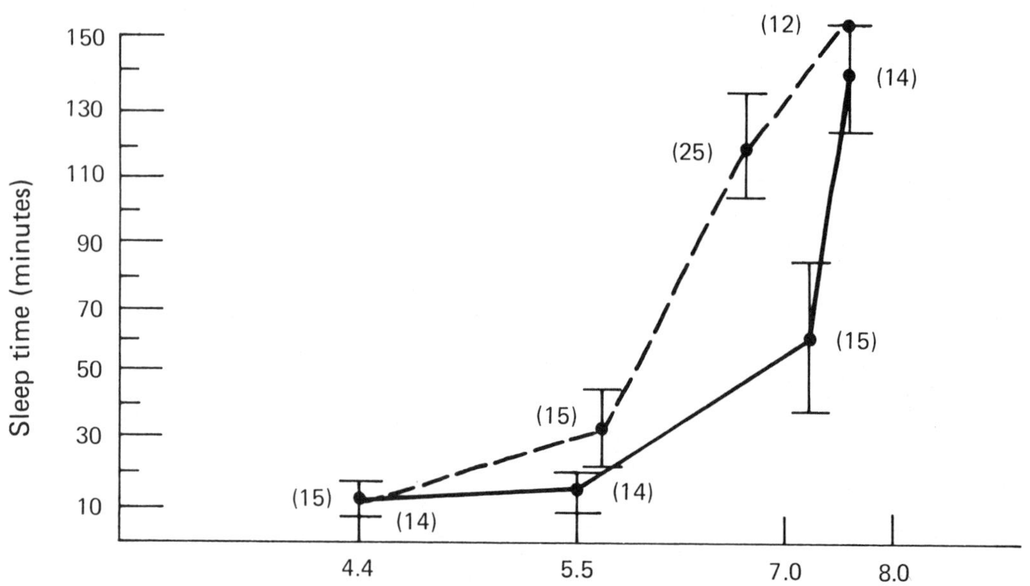


**Figure 3–5. Log dose–response curves for ethanol-induced sleep time in mice.**
**- - -Saline (equivalent volume to diethanolamine-rutin) injected I.P. two hours prior to ethanol.**
**——Diethanolamine-rutin, 5.2 mM/kg, injected I.P. two hours prior to ethanol.**
**Shown are mean values (± SEM as vertical bars). The number of mice used is indicated in parentheses at each plot point.**

of an agonist does not fully overcome the inhibition induced by an antagonist, the antagonism is considered noncompetitive. In the latter case, the net effect will be a decrease in the maximum height of the log dose–response curve, which is probably attributable to a reduced number of drug-receptor complexes.

## K. TRENDS IN FUNDAMENTAL PHARMACOLOGY

The new and fast growing branch of pharmacology that involves the study of the mechanisms of drug action is affording many interesting findings. Great strides in the study of drug receptors are taking place, including many successful attempts to isolate the specific receptors to some of the drugs. The opiate and benzodiazepine receptors are being studied in detail through the use of radiolabeled drug molecules.[10] Attempts also are being made to unfold the structure of the receptor macromolecule itself and thus correlate the structure–activity relationships and the drug–receptor interactions.

## L. SUMMARY OF THE CORRELATION OF THE AMOUNT OF CHEMICAL GIVEN AND BIOLOGIC EFFECTS[1]

As stated, there is no single characteristic relationship between the amount of chemicals given and the effect. The dose–effect relationship is established by giving a series of increasing doses and measuring the intensity of response. This is then plotted on the abscissa as dose and on the ordinate as intensity of effect. The median effective dose ($ED_{50}$) is the dose that will produce the desired effect in half of the subject people or animals. Because of the interaction of so many biochemical, physiologic, and psychologic systems, the dose–effect relationship in human beings can become quite complex. The graphic representation of the relationship may be linear, curved either way, or in the shape of an "S." Simple dose–effect curves can be characterized in four ways.

1. Potency is the amount of chemical required to produce the effect. Potency is not a very important characteristic of a drug. It becomes important only when the required dose is too large to be given conveniently.
2. Slope of the dose–effect relationship defines how sensitive the resultant effect is to the size of the dose. If the slope is quite steep, very little change in the dose will cause a large change in the effect, and the choice of a dose for the proper effect will be more difficult.
3. Maximum efficacy is the maximum effect produced by the drug, even at very large dosages. In some drugs, this can be seen as a plateau or flattening of the dose–effect line, and with some, other factors may intervene and the side effects may become so severe as to limit the effective dose.
4. Variability is always with us, and drug effects are never the same in all animals or patients, or even in the same patient at different times.

Depending on the status of the various systems, the response to a drug can vary tremendously. The best way to monitor dosage is through the use of chemical measurement of the amount of a drug in the patient's blood and clinical observation of the drug's effects.

The toxicity of the chemical or drug must be studied. A chemical's toxicity is reported as median lethal dose ($LD_{50}$); this is the amount of chemical in weight of drug per weight of animal required to kill one half of the animals. The $LD_{50}/ED_{50}$ ratio is called the therapeutic index. This relationship is interesting to pharmacologists because it gives some initial indication of the safety of a drug.

High toxicity does not necessarily mean that the chemical will cause a large number of deaths; for example, aspirin and salicylates, low in relative toxicity (oral $LD_{50}$ is 1500 mg/kg in rats), are the leading cause of death in children, due to accidental poisoning. For the years 1964–1967, U.S. Poison Control Centers indicated that ingestion of aspirin by children under 5 years of age was reported 16,887 times, while the ingestion of insecticides was reported only 2120 times. The widespread distribution of aspirin contributes to the incidence, as does the ability of children to mimic our drug-taking activity. Most certainly, a factor in its control is the respect and fear we show for the known poisonous substance.

In conclusion, the concept of intrinsic activity of drugs is helpful in understanding adverse drug effects (see Ariens, 1964). Although it is true in some cases that a drug of low potency will produce the same effect in very high doses as lower doses of another, more potent drug of the same type, this is not always the case. Some drugs have a higher intrinsic activity than others, and produce effects of a magnitude that cannot be achieved by the weaker drug at any dose. It is doubtful, for example, that mescaline or psilocybin, at any dose, could produce the exact intense psychotomimetic effect of a substantial dose of LSD.

## M. PHARMACOKINETICS

To be effective, a drug needs not only the specific chemical conformation for activity, but also several secondary characteristics: it must reach the site where it can act, it must not be unacceptably toxic, and it must be excreted adequately. The physiochemical factors in the transfer of drugs across membranes are depicted in Figure 3–6.

## N. PHARMACOKINETICS AND METABOLISM

### 1. Absorption[1]

The time required for an effect to occur after chemical administration, the latency, is primarily determined by the route of administration and the rate of absorption and distribution of the chemical. Intravenous administration is the most rapid and inhalation the next most rapid route; oral administration and absorption through the skin are the slowest routes of administration.

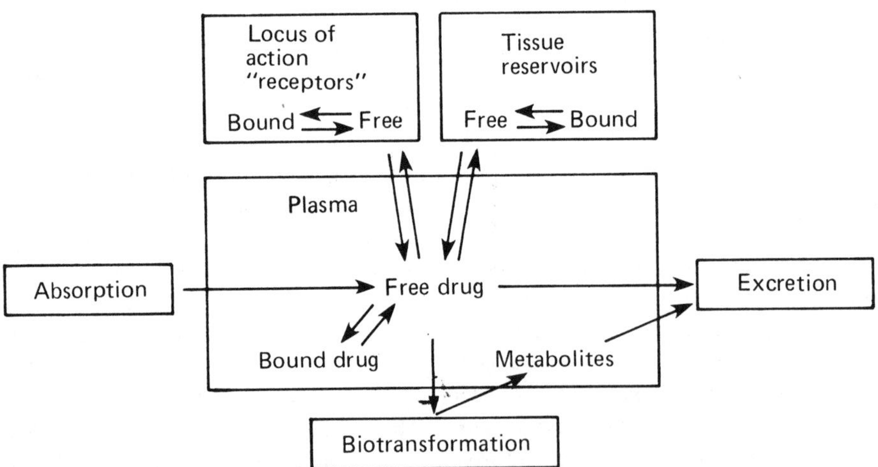


**Figure 3–6. Schematic representation of the interrelationship of the absorption, distribution, binding, biotransformation, and excretion of a drug and its concentration at its locus of action. Possible distribution and binding of metabolites are not depicted. (From L.S. Goodman and A. Gilman, eds. *The Pharmacological Basis of Therapeutics*, 6th ed. New York: Macmillan, 1980, p. 3. With permission.)**

Absorption from all sites is dependent upon the solubility of the chemical. Chemicals in solution are more rapidly absorbed than those given in solid form.

## 2. Distribution[1]

After the drug is absorbed and reaches the plasma of the blood, it must pass through the capillary wall, through processes of diffusion and filtration. Fat-soluble substances diffuse through the wall, whereas fat-insoluble compounds must be able to pass through holes or pores in the capillary wall. Drugs are not uniformly distributed in the body, and binding to protein in the plasma, concentration in body fat, and the hurdle of the blood–brain barrier contribute to the unequal distribution.

## 3. Metabolism[1]

The four chemical reactions generally involved in the transformation of chemicals or drugs are oxidation, reduction, hydrolysis, and conjugation of reaction.

These rates have an important bearing on the biologic activity of the chemical. The rate of metabolism is a major variable that influences intensity of effect and duration. A number of drugs—phenobarbital, for example—can increase the activity of the drug-metabolizing enzymes in the liver. This stimulation of drug metabolism can decrease the intensity and duration of response to the stimulation of the drug itself, and also to certain related drugs.[11] For example, a daily dose of 300 mg of diphenylhydantoin to ten patients resulted in an average blood plasma level of 12.3 mg/liter. When combined with 120 mg of phenobarbital for prolonged periods, the plasma level of diphenylhydantoin was only 3.5 mg/liter because of the increased metabolism.[11]

## 4. Excretion

Excretion of drugs is primarily through the kidney, but some excretion occurs through the feces. Large molecules are proportionally excreted into feces, for example, tetracyclines, steroids, and bile salt analogs. Small amounts of some drugs can be excreted through the lungs and by the sweat glands with saliva, tears, and so forth.

## 5. Factors that Modify the Therapeutic Dose of a Drug

a. Body weight. For precise adjustment of dosage, the dose per unit weight is used and is usually expressed as milligrans of a drug per kilogram of body weight. For some drugs, body surface area is a more precise index than is body weight.

b. Age. Children are quite often more sensitive to drug effects and the elderly adult may respond uniquely to drugs.

c. Sex. The metabolism of drugs may sometimes differ between the sexes.

d. Metabolism and excretion rate. These can vary and change the intensity and duration of drug effect.

e. Physiologic or pathologic status of the individual. This will have great influence on the drug effect.

f. Drug interaction. The effect of drugs may be modified by the administration of another drug or chemical.

## 6. Interaction of Drugs in the Body

### *a. Overdose*

This is a relatively common toxic reaction. It can occur for many reasons.

1. There is a desire to commit suicide.
2. The potency of the drug is greater than expected.
3. The rates of metabolism vary among individuals. The daily dose of a drug may give the proper response, cause severe toxicity, or have no effect at all. For example, the antidepressant drug desmethylimipramine (DMI) was given to three subjects in doses of 75 mg/day. Only one subject showed signs of increasing euphoria, and after five days, it was found that

this individual had plasma levels of DMI four times higher than the other two, less-reacting subjects.[12]

4. Synergy—a combination of drugs can have more than an additive effect.

5. Plasma-protein: displacement of one bound drug by another.

### *b. Drug Idiosyncrasy*

This is a genetically determined abnormal reaction to a drug. Understanding of the idiosyncratic reactions requires knowledge of three things:

1. The mechanism of how the usual drug effect is altered in the genetically abnormal person.
2. The biochemical abnormalities that constitute an expression of a genetic defect.
3. The pattern of inheritance of the genetic abnormality.

Most drug idiosyncrasies are discovered by chance when a drug is given to a person who carries a genetic trait determining the idiosyncratic response. Because of the complexity of brain function and the drugs that modify it, it is reasonable to speculate that there are intrinsic differences in responses to these agents. We would expect to find corresponding differences in the habitual use of these drugs. For example, study of the coffee drinking, ethanol use or abuse, and smoking habits of twins suggests that the use of these drugs is subject to genetic influence.[13,14]

### *c. Drug Allergy*

This is defined as an altered degree of susceptibility caused by a primary exposure to a foreign substance and manifested in a reaction to a subsequent exposure to the same thing. For a chemical to produce an allergic response, a prior sensitizing contact is required, either with the same compound or one that is closely related to it. Also, a period of time is required, usually about a week or so, for the synthesis of drug-specific antibodies. Examples: penicillin[15] and tobacco.[16]

### *d. Chemical Mutagenesis*

It is possible for a chemical to produce a permanent, characteristic change in a human reproductive cell. This alters the hereditary constitution of the individual. Continual genetic change is thus introduced into the species, unless the alteration is incompatible with survival. Example: caffeine.[17]

### *e. Chemical Carcinogenesis*

Cancer is a malignant, unrestrained growth of cells that can occur spontaneously or can be induced by radiation, viruses, and chemicals. Example: tobacco smoking and lung cancer.[18]

### *f. Chemical Teratogenesis*

It should be noted that, in most cases, drugs taken by the pregnant woman cross the placenta and therefore are potentially capable of producing an adverse drug reaction in the fetus.[19] Adverse reactions are difficult to predict in adults, and even more difficult to predict in the fetus or the neonate.[20] Some chemicals affect the cells of a developing embryo in such a way that defects are produced. If the embryonic sperm or egg cells escape damage, only the embryo itself will be affected. Substances that cause abnormal fetal development are called teratogens. Examples: thalidomide[21] and alcohol.[22]

### *g. Accumulation*[23]

If the elimination of a drug is slow and its administration frequent enough that the intake exceeds elimination, the amount of drug in the body increases until a new equilibrium is reached between intake and output. In other words, the drug accumulates in the body.

Drugs that are slowly metabolized or strongly bound to plasma proteins are likely cumulated because of slow elimination. (DDT is a good example.)

In this regard, marihuana is a good example of a drug that has the property of being slowly metabolized,[24] and, in fact, it takes about eight days completely to remove the active constituent, tetrahydrocannabinol (THC), from the body, and thus this substance will accumulate in the body.

### *h. Tachyphylaxis*[23]

Tachyphylaxis usually is a very rapidly developing tolerance. It manifests itself when a drug, upon rapid consecutive administration, each time produces smaller quantitative effects. However, tachyphylaxis does not have to be rapid (e.g., tachyphylaxis to organomercural diuretics can take several weeks).

Amphetamine is an example of a drug that produces tachyphylaxis, especially for its blood pressure effects. This drug depletes the stores of endogenous active substances, such as norepinephrine (NE). If such a drug is repeatedly administered before the stores are replenished, there will be less or no action.

In therapeutic practice, frequently more than one drug is administered at the same time. Two drugs, given at the same time, may either (1) act entirely independently on two sites: (2) produce similar actions on the same organ, synergism (Greek: *syn* = together; *ergo* = work); or (3) oppose each other's action, antagonism (Greek: *anti* = against; *ago* = act).

1. Synergism.[23] There are various ways for two drugs to act in concert:

a. Summation. The two drugs have similar actions that are simply additive, for example, histamine and acetylcholine in small amounts each causes a fall of the arterial blood pressure in the dog upon intravenous administration (although they do not act upon the same receptor). If the two drugs are injected together, the blood pressure change is simply an addition of the action of the two individual drugs.

Another example of synergism is the very common combination of alcohol and sleeping pills (barbiturates) or antianxiety drugs such as chlordiazepoxide (Librium) or diazepam (Valium).

b. Potentiation. The presence of drug A enhances the action of drug B. If drug A, the potentiator, has its own action similar to that of B, the combined action of A plus B will be greater than the simple algebraic sum of the action of the two; for example, it has been found that certain amino acids,[25] biogenic amines,[26,27] metabolites,[28,29] and Antabuse[26] could potentiate ethanol-induced narcosis. It has been reported that cocaine potentiates amphetamine-induced intensification of "conflict" behavior in rats.[30]

## 7. Termination of Drug Action[23]

Most drugs are useful if their action is temporary. An anesthetic drug is of great value in rendering a patient unconscious for the performance of complex surgical operations, but it is expected that its action will terminate and the patient will awaken after the operation. Aspirin is useful to relieve a headache, but it would be highly undesirable to carry 300 mg of aspirin in one's system forever (many people consume, during their lifetime, kilogram quantities of some drugs). It is appropriate, therefore, to summarize the various ways by which a drug action can be terminated in the body.

### *a. Elimination of the Drug from the Body*[23]

1. The drug can be eliminated unchanged through the lungs or kidneys, or by the sweat glands, saliva, bile, and so on.

2. The drug can be converted into another form, which is then rapidly eliminated. As most active drugs are fat-soluble, the body, through a special enzyme system, can convert them into water-soluble compounds, which the kidneys excrete rapidly.

3. Many drugs are metabolized in the body into inactive forms.

### *b. Termination of Drug Action Without Elimination from the Body*[23]

1. Highly fat-soluble drugs can be redistributed within the body. A typical example is thiopental, a so-called ultrashort-acting barbiturate that is suitable for intravenous anesthesia in humans. If it is injected intravenously, the drug rapidly enters the brain and produces anesthesia. But soon it is taken up in the fat tissues of the body, causing the blood level to fall. Concom-

itantly, the concentration of the drug decreases in other tissues, including the brain. This is the way in which the anesthetic action is quickly terminated.

2. The body can acquire resistance to the drug by developing tachyphylaxis or tolerance, such as with heroin, alcohol, barbiturates, LSD, amphetamine, or tobacco. A distinction could be made as to which psychoactive agents produce a form of tolerance or tachyphylaxis. Some investigators[30] believe that the CNS stimulants and hallucinogenic compounds produce tachyphylaxis rather than tolerance, whereas the CNS depressants, such as sedative-hypnotics, opiates, and alcohol, produce tolerance, not tachyphylaxis.

3. A drug action can be terminated by the administration of an antagonist, either chemical or functional. For example, naloxone is a narcotic antagonist that could terminate the action of opiates. High-dose methadone also could antagonize the effects of heroin by receptor blockade rather than a "pure" antagonistic action.

## O. SUMMARY

An understanding of the basic principles governing the effects of drugs on the physiology of animals and humans is extremely important. Without this basic information, we will be unable to deal with the phenomenology of drug use or abuse.

In the following chapters, the pharmacologic and medical aspects of certain types of drugs of abuse are presented in a nonjudgmental manner.

The terminology one uses is of minor importance, so long as the reader understands the context in which it is used. A drug will be described as addicting only if it is known that physical dependence upon its effects can develop. A drug will be described as habituating only if no physical dependence upon its effects has been demonstrated satisfactorily, regardless of the schedule of use. Drug abuse and drug dependence will refer only to the abuse of or dependence on the drugs specifically considered.

## REFERENCES


1. Stavinoha, W.B. How foreign chemicals act in biological systems. In K. Blum and A.H. Briggs, eds., *Drugs: Use or Abuse (A Manual)*. San Antonio: University of Texas Health Science Center, 1973.
2. de C. Baker, S.B., and Davey, D.G. The predictive value for man of toxicological test of drugs in laboratory animals. *Br. Med. Bull.* 26:208, 1970.
3. Goth, A. *Medical Pharmacology; Principles and Concepts*, 7th ed. St. Louis: Mosby, 1974.
4. Langley, J.N. On the physiology of the salivary secretion. Part II. On the mutual antagonism of Atropin and Pilocarpin, having especial reference to their relations in the sub-maxillary gland of the cat. *J. Physiol.* 1:339, 1878.
5. Julien, R.M. *A Primer of Drug Actions*, 2nd ed. San Francisco: Freeman, 1978.
6. Pert, C.B., and Snyder, S.H. Opiate receptor: Demonstration in nervous tissue. *Science* 179:1011, 1973.
7. Goldstein, A. The search for the opiate receptor. In G.H. Acheson, ed., *Pharmacology and the Future of Man; Proceedings of the Fifth International Congress on Pharmacology*. Basel: Karger, 1973, p. 140.
8. Blum, K., et al. Diethanolamine: A possible weak agonist-antagonist to ethanol. *Eur. J. Pharmacol.* 19:218, 1972.
9. Geller, I., et al. Protection against acute alcoholic intoxication with diethanolamine-rutin. *Res. Commun. Chem. Pathol. Pharmacol.* 1:383, 1970.
10. Braestrup, C., and Squires, R.F. Pharmacological characterization of benzodiazepine receptors in the brain. *Eur. J. Pharmacol.* 48:263, 1978.
11. Burns, J.J., et al. Application of drug metabolism to drug toxicity studies. *Ann. N.Y. Acad. Sci.* 123:273, 1965.
12. Broeid, B.B., Cosmides, G.J., and Rall, D.P. Toxicology and biomedical sciences. *Science* 148:1547, 1965.
13. Conterio, F., and Chiarelli, B. Study of inheritance of some daily life habits. *Heredity* 17:347, 1962.
14. Goldstein, A., Aronow, L., and Kalman, S. *Principles of Drug Action: The Basis of Pharmacology*. New York: Hoeber, 1968.
15. Bierman, C.S., Pierson, W.E., Zeitz, S.J., et al. Reactions association with ampicillin therapy. *JAMA* 220:1098, 1972.
16. Hosen, H. Tobacco sensitivity. *Ann. Allergy* 29:608, 1971.

17. Ostertag, W., Duisberg, E., and Sturmann, M. The mutagenic activity of caffeine in man. *Mutat. Res.* 2:293, 1965.
18. *The Health Consequences of Smoking*; supplement to the 1967 Public Health Service Review. (PHS Pub. No. 1696-2). Washington, D.C.: U.S. Department of Health, Education and Welfare, 1969.
19. Moya, F., and Thorndike, V. Passage of drugs across the placenta. *Am. J. Obstet. Gynecol.* 84:1778, 1962.
20. Brent, R.L. Protecting the public from teratogenic and mutagenic hazards. *J. Clin. Pharmacol.* 12:61, 1972.
21. Melling, G.W., and Katzenstein, M. The saga of thalidomide. *N. Engl. J. Med.* 267:1184, 1962.
22. Smith, D.W., Jones, K.L., and Hanson, J.W. Perspectives on the cause and frequency of the fetal alcohol syndrome. *Ann. N.Y. Acad. Sci.* 273:138, 1976.
23. Cutting, W.C. *Handbook of Pharmacology: The Actions and Uses of Drugs*. New York: Appleton-Century-Crofts, 1962, chaps. 1–6.
24. Hofmann, F.G. *A Handbook on Drug and Alcohol Abuse: The Biomedical Aspects*. New York: Oxford, 1975, p. 179.
25. Blum, K., Wallace, J.E., and Geller, I. Synergy of ethanol and putative neurotransmitters: Glycine and serine. *Science* 176:292, 1972.
26. Blum, K., et al. L-Dopa: Effect of ethanol narcosis and brain biogenic amines in mice. *Nature* 242:407, 1973.
27. Rosenfeld, G. Potentiation of the narcotic action and acute toxicity of alcohol by primary aromatic monoamines. *Q. J. Stud. Alcohol* 21:584, 1960.
28. Blum, K., et al. Synergy of ethanol and alcohol-like-metabolites: Tryptophol and 3,4-dihydroxyphenylethanol. *Pharmacology* 9:294, 1973.
29. Blum, K., et al. Ethanol narcosis in mice: Serotonergic involvement. *Experientia* 30:1053, 1974.
30. Geller, I., Hartmann, R.J., and Blum, K. The effects of low-dose combinations of D-amphetamine and cocaine on experimentally induced conflict in the rat. *Curr. Therap. Res.* 14:220, 1972.

## Articles

Butler, T.C. Introduction: Termination of drug action by elimination of unchanged drug. *Fed. Proc.* 17:1158, 1958.

Deneau, G.A., and Seevers, M.H. Pharmacological aspects of drug dependence. *Adv. Pharmacol. Chemother.* 3:267, 1964.

Isbell, H., and Fraser, H.F. Addiction to analgesics and barbiturates. *Pharmacol. Exp. Ther.* 99:355, 1950.

Möhler, H., and Okada, T. Properties of 3H-diazepam binding to benzodiazepine receptors in rat cerebral cortex. *Life Sci.* 20:2101, 1977.

Rosenberg, D.E., et al. Observations on direct and cross tolerance with LSD and d-amphetamine in man. *Psychopharmacologia* 5:1, 1963.

Seevers, M.H., and Deneau, G.A. Physiological aspects of tolerance and physical dependence. In: W.S. Root and F.G. Hoffman, eds., *Physiological Pharmacology*. New York: Academic, 1963, p. 565.

Veldstra, H. Synergism and potentiation with special reference to combination of structural analogues. *Pharmacol. Rev.* 8:339, 1956.

## Reviews

Albert, A. *Selective Toxicity*, 3rd ed. New York: Wiley, 1965.

Ariens, E.J. *Molecular Pharmacology: The Mode of Action of Biologically Active Compounds*, vol. 1. New York: Academic, 1964.

Burgen, A.S.V. Receptor mechanisms. *Ann. Rev. Pharmacol.* 10:7, 1970.

Burger, A., and Parulkar, A.P. Relationships between chemical structure and biological activity. *Ann. Rev. Pharmacol.* 6:19, 1966.

Feigerbaum, J.F., Fishman, R.H.B., and Yanai, J. Mechanisms of dopamine antagonism by morphine in rodents. *Subs. Alc. Act./Mis.* 3(6):307, 1982.

Furchgott, R.F. Receptor mechanisms. *Ann. Rev. Pharmacol.* 4:21, 1964.

Gourley, D.R.H. Basic mechanisms of drug action. *Fortschr Arzneimittelforsch.* 7:11, 1964.

Mautner, H.G. The molecular basis of drug action. *Pharmacol Rev.* 19:107, 1967.

## General References

Clark, A.J. *General Pharmacology* (*Handbuch der Experimentellen Pharmakologie*, vol. 4.) Berlin: Springer-Verlag, 1937.

Croxatto, R., and Huidobro, F. Fundamental basis of the specificity of pressor and depressor amines in their vascular effects. V. Theoretical fundaments; drug receptor linkage. *Arch. Int. Pharmacodyn. Ther.* 106:207, 1956.

Ferguson, J. Use of chemical potentials as indices of toxicity. *Proc. Roy. Soc. (Biol.)* 127:389, 1939.

Goldstein, A., Aronow, L., and Kalman, S. *Principles of Drug Action*, 2nd ed. New York: Wiley, 1974.

Hurwitz, L., and Suria, A. The link between agonist action and response in smooth muscle. *Ann. Rev. Pharmacol.* 11:303, 1971.

Katz, B. Microphysiology of the neuro-muscular junction. The chemo-receptor function of the motor end-plate. *Bull. Johns Hopkins Hosp.* 102:296, 1958.

Loh, H.H., and Ross, D.H., eds. *Neurochemical Mechanisms of Opiates and Endorphins* (*Advances in Biochemical Pharmacology*, vol. 20). New York: Raven, 1979.

Paton, W.D.M. A theory of drug action based on the rate of drug-receptor combination. *Proc. Roy. Soc. (Biol.)* B 154:21, 1961.

Paton, W.D.M. Receptors as defined by their pharmacological properties. In R. Porter and M. O'Connor, eds., *Molecular Properties of Drug Receptors; a CIBA Foundation Symposium*. London: Churchill, 1970.

Paterson, S.J., Robson, L.E., and Kosterlitz, H.W. Classification of opioid receptors. *Brit. Med. Bull.* 39(1):31, 1983.

Pauling, L. A molecular theory of general anesthesia. *Science* 134:15, 1961.

Pert, C.B., and Snyder, S.H. Opiate receptor: demonstration in nervous tissue. *Science* 179:1011, 1973.

Porter, R., and O'Connor, M., eds. *Molecular Properties of Drug Receptors*; a Ciba Foundation Symposium. London: Churchill, 1970.

Schild, H.O. Introduction. In H. deJonge, ed., *Quantitative Methods in Pharmacology*. Amsterdam: North-Holland, 1961.

Stephenson, R.P. A modification of receptor theory. *Br. J. Pharmacol.* 11:379, 1956.

Triggle, D.J. *Chemical Aspects of the Autonomic Nervous System*. London: Academic Press, 1965.

Waud, D.R. Pharmacological receptors. *Pharmacol. Rev.* 20:49, 1968.

Chapter 4

# Classification of Psychoactive Drugs

In this chapter, we briefly review the different classifications of centrally acting drugs. For additional material on this subject, the interested reader should refer to the *Handbook on Drugs and Alcohol Abuse: Biomedical Aspects*,[1] and an article by Jean Paul Smith.[2]

## A. DRUG PROBLEMS

Drug problems may be classified into three types.

### 1. Type I

The first type of drug problem arises from the unintended side effects of "medically prescribed drugs" and "over-the-counter preparations." Most of the "magic" aura comes from their use by the medical and paramedic professions to alleviate human ills. There are, however, adverse reactions to medically or self-prescribed compounds that are harmful and costly to the individual and society. These attract less attention than the other types of problems, probably because there is more social acceptance of the original need—the treatment of ills and maladies—that led to the administration or consumption of the preparation. As a corollary, vulnerability to the more powerful analgesics and sleep inducers exposes several professional groups, such as physicians and nurses, to increased risks of abuse.

### 2. Type II

The second category of problem is the broad and vague area called abuse, dependence, or addiction. It is loosely defined by the means by which a person acquires the drug, the individual's intended use, and the physical effects. Illicit purchase from a dealer of supplies to maintain a habit is the prototype of the abuse pattern, however limited it is as an example. By definition, drugs used in this manner are not socially sanctioned but are taken by choice rather than on the basis of a recommendation by a professional. And more important, the effect sought is to alter the individual's perception of reality. Research has not delineated the origins of personality dynamics for abuse, and there is a serious question as to whether genetic predispositions or early personality signs of drug abuse proneness exist at all.[3] Street drugs that are not diverted from legitimate channels of pharmaceutic production and distribution very often contain additives, contaminants, or toxic materials of immediate concern. "If a sizable amount of DMT powder does not get you, a little strychnine thrown in may do the job." The sad part of this is that some users may interpret a harrowing experience, which is psychologically disruptive, as simply a "wild trip." If one is looking for reasons why people should stay away from these drugs, the lack of information about the content and effects of possible contaminants are two very good ones.

### 3. Type III

The third category of drug effects that are of interest may be termed the recreational use of drugs, or drugs for which there is no prohibition or social sanction against their use. They are, from the standpoint of the law, neutral, even though restrictions on their distribution may somewhat decrease their abuse. Alcohol, tobacco, caffeine, and cola are examples of recreational drugs, and some contend that marihuana is more a recreational drug than a drug of abuse, although the evidence for this is scanty. Recreational drugs are those which the individual decides may be used for relaxation to get away from the stresses and strains of life.

## B. DRUG CLASSIFICATION

Drugs are classified into various groups on the basis of some of their primary properties (such as their therapeutic use, the anatomic site of action, their chemical structure). The main objective of such classifications is to give the user a brief idea of a drug's nature and applicability. Among many classifications, the following modes are important: (1) classification based on the anatomic site of action, for example, drugs acting on the central nervous system; (2) classification based on pharmacologic action, for example, analgesics, tranquilizers; (3) classification based on biochemical mechanism of action, for example, monoamine oxidase inhibitors; and (4) classification based on chemical structure, for example, barbiturates, benzodiazepines.

The salient pharmacologic aspects of use and abuse are in general the same for all the drugs belonging to a particular class or group. This helps the user to predict the effective applicability of any drug on the subject (patient). For instance, if an individual develops physical dependence to a particular drug, the possibility of physical dependence to other drugs of the same class can be predicted, and the physician can switch to a drug with the same pharmacologic properties but one that belongs to another class. This phenomenon is particularly useful in the treatment of tolerance to or physical dependence on drugs.

Certain classifications based on the pharmacologic properties of some of the drugs are too broad to facilitate any prediction of their effects. For instance, too little is known about the mechanism of action of drugs such as LSD, marihuana, and mescaline, which are classified as "hallucinogens." Even though they are basically similar in their effects, knowledge of the pharmacologic properties of any one of these drugs cannot be unequivocally extended to the other members of the same group (see Table 4-1).

### 1. Opioids

Drugs belonging to this group are used mainly as pain relievers (analgesics). They are also used occasionally to prevent diarrhea and reduce coughing. Prolonged use of narcotics results in tolerance and physical dependence.

Narcotics are divided into three subgroups based on their origin. These are (1) naturally occurring narcotics—the opium alkaloids morphine and codeine; (2) semisynthetic narcotics—the derivatives of morphine and codeine such as heroin, oxymorphone, metopon, hydrocodone, and oxycodone; (3) wholly synthetic narcotics—meperidine, methadone, levorphanol, and their analogs. The most recently introduced synthetic narcotics are the benzomorphan compounds such as phenazocine.

**TABLE 4–1**

**Comparison of Selected Effects of Commonly Abused Drugs***

| *Drug Category* | *Physical Dependence* | *Characteristics of Intoxication* | *Characteristics of Withdrawal* | *"Flashback" Symptoms* | *Masking of Symptoms of Illness or Injury During Intoxication* |
|---|---|---|---|---|---|
| Opiates | Marked | Analgesia with or without depressed sensorium; pinpoint pupils (tolerance does not develop to this action); patient may be alert and appear normal; respiratory depression with overdose | Rhinorrhea, lacrimation, and dilated, reactive pupils, followed by gastrointestinal disturbances, low back pain, and waves of gooseflesh; convulsions not a feature unless heroin samples were adulterated with barbiturates | Not reported | An important feature of opiate intoxication, due to analgesic action with or without depressed sensorium |
| Barbiturates | Marked | Patient may appear normal with usual dose, but narrow margin between dose needed to prevent withdrawal symptoms and toxic dose is often exceeded and patient appears "drunk," with drowsiness, ataxia, slurred speech, and nystagmus on lateral gaze; pupil size and reaction normal; respiratory depression with overdose | Agitation, tremulousness, insomnia, gastrointestinal disturbances, hyperpyrexia, blepharoclonus (clonic blink reflex), acute brain syndrome, major convulsive seizures | Not reported | Only in presence of depressed sensorium or after onset of acute brain syndrome |
| Nonbarbiturate sedatives glutethimide (Doriden) | Marked | Pupils dilated and reactive to light; coma and respiratory depression prolonged; sudden apnea and laryngeal spasm common | Similar to barbiturate withdrawal syndrome, with agitation, gastrointestinal disturbances, hyperpyrexia, and major convulsive seizures | Not reported | Same as in barbiturate intoxication |

*Modified from Dimijian, G.G., *Drug Ther.* 1:7, 1971. (With permission.)
(From Goth, A. *Medical Pharmacology*, 7th ed. C.V. Mosby, St. Louis, 1975.)

**TABLE 4–1**

**Comparison of Selected Effects of Commonly Abused Drugs (continued)**

| *Drug Category* | *Physical Dependence* | *Characteristics of Intoxication* | *Characteristics of Withdrawal* | *"Flashback" Symptoms* | *Masking of Symptoms of Illness or Injury During Intoxication* |
|---|---|---|---|---|---|
| Antianxiety ("minor tranquilizers") | Marked | Progressive depression of sensorium as with barbiturates; pupil size and reaction normal respiratory depression with overdose | Similar to barbiturate withdrawal syndrome, with danger of major convulsive seizures | Not reported | Same as in barbiturate intoxication |
| Ethanol | Marked | Depressed sensorium, acute or chronic brain syndrome, odor on breath, pupil size and reaction normal | Similar to barbiturate withdrawal syndrome, but with less likelihood of convulsive seizures | Not reported | Same as in barbiturate intoxication |
| Amphetamines | Mild to absent | Agitation, with paranoid thought disturbance in high doses; acute organic brain syndrome after prolonged use; pupils dilated and reactive; tachycardia, elevated blood pressure with possibility of hypertensive crisis and CVA; possibility of convulsive seizures | Lethargy, somnolence, dysphoria, and possibility of suicidal depression; brain syndrome may persist for many weeks | Infrequently reported | Drug-induced euphoria or acute brain syndrome may interfere with awareness of symptoms of illness or may remove incentive to report symptoms of illness |
| Cocaine | Absent | Paranoid thought disturbance in high doses, with dangerous delusions of persecution and omnipotence; tachycardia; respiratory depression with overdose | Similar to amphetamine withdrawal | Not reported | Same as in amphetamine intoxication |

†Meprobamate (Equanil), chlordiazepoxide (Librium), diazepam (Valium), ethchlorvynol (Placidyl)l and ethinamate (Valmid).

**TABLE 4–1**

**Comparison of Selected Effects of Commonly Abused Drugs (continued)**

| *Drug Category* | *Physical Dependence* | *Characteristics of Intoxication* | *Characteristics of Withdrawal* | *"Flashback" Symptoms* | *Masking of Symptoms of Illness or Injury During Intoxication* |
|---|---|---|---|---|---|
| Marihuana | Absent | Milder preparations: drowsy, euphoric state with frequent inappropriate laughter and disturbance in perception of time or space (occasional acute psychotic reaction reported). Stronger preparations such as hashish: frequent hallucinations or psychotic reaction; pupils normal, conjunctivae injected (marihuana preparations frequently adulterated with LSD, tryptamines, or heroin) | No specific withdrawal symptoms | Infrequently reported | Uncommon with milder preparations; stronger preparations may interfere in same manner as psychotomimetic agents |
| Psychotomimetics (LSD, STP, tryptamines, mescaline, morning glory seeds) | Absent | Unpredictable disturbance in ego function, manifest by extreme lability of affect and chaotic disruption of thought, with danger of uncontrolled behavioral disturbance; pupils dilated and reactive to light | No specific withdrawal symptoms; symptomatology may persist for indefinite period after discontinuation of drug | Commonly reported as late as one year after last dose | Affective response or psychotic thought disturbance may remove awareness of, or incentive to report, symptoms of illness |
| Anticholinergic | Absent | Nonpsychotropic effects such as tachycardia, decreased salivary secretion, urinary retention, and dilated, nonreactive pupils plus depressed sensorium, confusion, disorientation, hallucinations, and delusional thinking | No specific withdrawal symptoms; mydriasis may persist for several days | Not reported | Pain may not be reported as a result of depression of sensorium, acute brain syndrome, or acute psychotic reaction |

## TABLE 4–1

### Comparison of Selected Effects of Commonly Abused Drugs (continued)

| *Drug Category* | *Physical Dependence* | *Characteristics of Intoxication* | *Characteristics of Withdrawal* | *"Flashback" Symptoms* | *Masking of Symptoms of Illness or Injury During Intoxication* |
|---|---|---|---|---|---|
| Inhalants‡ | Unknown | Depressed sensorium, hallucinations, acute brain syndrome; odor on breath; patient often with glassy-eyed appearance | No specific withdrawal symptoms | Infrequently reported | Same as in anticholinergic intoxication |

‡The term "inhalant" is used to designate a variety of gases and highly volatile organic liquids, including the aromatic glues, paint thinners, gasoline, some anesthetic agents, and amyl nitrite. The term excludes liquids sprayed into the nasopharynx (droplet transport required) and substances that must be ignited prior to inhalation (such as marihuana).

The effects of the narcotics can be reversed by the use of certain drugs known as the narcotic antagonists such as nalorphine (Nalline) and naloxone (Narcan). These antagonists can cause a fully developed withdrawal syndrome within 30 minutes in addicts. In 1975[3] opioids, termed endorphins, were found in both animal and human tissue. These internal opioids are discussed fully in Chapter 8.

## 2. Central Nervous System (CNS) Depressants

The CNS depressants are drugs that can depress the activity in all parts of the central nervous system. Repeated use of these drugs leads to a relatively low degree of tolerance but chronic use with a daily intake beyond the "threshold dose" causes death as a result of respiratory depression. The threshold dose is, however, specific to each drug. The withdrawal syndrome associated with addiction to these drugs commonly starts with a hyperactivity of the CNS, resulting in convulsions and psychotic agitation lasting for about a week. Not all the drugs belonging to the class of CNS depressants appear to have the same pharmacologic action, even though they produce the same therapeutic effect. However, the pharmacologic aspects of their abuse remain the same. The benzodiazepines belong to this category.

## 3. Sedative Agents[1]

Drugs used to produce sleep and calm down patients are classified under this group. Of these, the barbiturates are the most widely used. Phenobarbital, secobarbital (Seconal), and pentobarbital are representative examples. Some of the old and new nonbarbiturate hypnotics also included in this group are chloral hydrate, glutethimide (Doriden), and ethchlovynol (Placidyl).

## 4. Ethyl Alcohol[1]

Ethanol (often simply called "alcohol") resembles the general depressants in its pharmacologic effects. However, it has limited recognized therapeutic use. The most widely abused substance known, it poses serious problems to both addicts and physicians.

## 5. General Anesthetics[1]

Anesthetics can produce unconsciousness and muscular relaxation, and are used to facilitate certain surgical procedures. They are, in general, gaseous or highly volatile liquids and inhalation of their vapors results in a state of intoxication. These drugs are rarely abused.

It is interesting to note that the drugs that are widely abused are those that can predominantly depress the central nervous system (e.g., the narcotics). Strangely enough, the major tranquilizers such as chlorpromazine (Thorazine) are not commonly abused. The anesthetics do not result in any physical dependence.

However, nitrous oxide, which has been demonstrated to interact with the endogenous opiate receptors, has been known to induce psychologic dependence. This finding might result in a predictor for other general anesthetic abuse.

## 6. Central Nervous System Stimulants[1]

Drugs used to stimulate the CNS and act as physiologic rather than receptor antagonists to the CNS depressants belong to this class (see also analeptic drugs). They are generally used for the treatment of emotional depression, suppression of appetite, etc. Powerful convulsants such as pentylenetetrazole (Metrazole) and strychnine, as well as psychotic antidepressants such as imipramine (Tofranil) and tranylcypromine (Parnate), belong in this category. Some of the mood-elevating agents such as imipramine and CNS stimulants such as caffeine are subject to drug abuse. However, statistics indicate no alarming proportions of addiction to these stimulants. One reason they may be unpopular among drug users might be that they are slow in producing the desired effects.

The amphetamines are one group of stimulants that are commonly used by the addicts.

Their ready availability (e.g., methamphetamine) permits their wide use in large doses even though they are relatively less potent than the other CNS stimulants. These drugs do not cause physical dependence but result in toxic reactions when administered by intravenous injection. When taken orally, they are less dangerous. Certain alterations of the electroencephalogram have been observed in some chronic amphetamine abusers.

## 7. Cocaine

A natural component of the leaves of the coca plant, cocaine is the oldest known local anesthetic drug. The capability of cocaine to excite the CNS is the main untoward effect that discourages physicians from using it, but the same property lures many to abuse it. The effects of cocaine and amphetamine when abused are similar in many respects. Cocaine is discussed in more detail in Chapter 12 on stimulant drugs. Some of the synthetic local anesthetics such as procaine (Novacaine) and lidocaine (Xylocaine) have completely replaced cocaine because of their low CNS excitatory action.

It has been observed that procaine is present in fairly high quantities in brown heroin.[4] Dr. Whitehead and associates (formerly of the Haight Ashbury Medical Free Clinic) postulated that the action of procaine as a monamine oxidase inhibitor is the cause of its antidepressant characteristics.[5] Hence it may be used as a diluent in brown heroin for its antidepressant characteristics.

## 8. Psychedelic Drugs[1]

The terms psychotogenic or psychotomimetic are used somewhat carelessly in describing their apparent production of an artificial state of psychosis (schizophrenia). States of mind produced by these drugs range from ''schizoid'' to ''psychedelic,'' but a more accurate term could be ''semipsychotomimetic,'' as suggested by Hofmann.[1] Scientific evidence does not clearly support the claims of insightful self-revelation and mind-expansion made by proponents of these hallucinogens.

The disciplines of scientific scrutiny appear to have been unevenly and shabbily applied to these substances, resulting in loose classification procedures and a tendency to lump all hallucinogens together in a ''stew pot'' of supposition and hypothesis. A myriad of tentative and uncertain conclusions are blended with an altogether unsatisfactory methodology that is yet to achieve good, solid pharmacological data about the nature of the hallucinogenic experience.

Although no physical dependence has been demonstrated, there is no lack of examples of significant tolerance among frequent users.[6]

## REFERENCES


1. Hofmann, F.G. *A Handbook on Drug and Alcohol Abuse: The Biomedical Aspects*, 2nd ed. New York: Oxford, 1983, p. 16.
2. Smith, J.P. *What Are Drugs? A Search for Personal Concensus Resource Book for Drug Abuse Education*, 2nd ed. National Clearinghouse for Drug Abuse Information. Washington, D.C.: U.S. Government Printing Office.
3. Goldstein, A. Opioid peptides (endomorphins) in pituitary and brain. *Science* 113:1081, 1976.
4. Blum, K. Depressive states induced by drugs of abuse: Clinical evidence, theoretical mechanism(s) and proposed treatment. Part II. *Psychedel. Drugs* 8(3):235, 1976.
5. Bucci, L. Procaine, a monoamine oxidase inhibitor in schizophrenia. *Dis. Nerv. Sys.* 34:389, 1973.
6. Inaba, D., et al. *Pharmacological and Toxicological Perspectives of Commonly Abused Drugs*, R.F. Dendy, ed. (NIDA, Medical Monograph 5). Washington, D.C.: U.S. Government Printing Office, 1979.

Chapter 5

# Narcotics

In this chapter, we explore the pharmacologic actions of narcotic drugs and the sociologic implications of opiate abuse.

## A. DEFINITION OF NARCOTIC DRUGS

The narcotic drugs include some of our most valuable medicines, as well as some of the most abused. The term *narcotic* originally referred to opium and the drugs made from opium, such as heroin, codeine, and morphine. Opium is obtained from the opium poppy; morphine and codeine are extracted from opium, and heroin is made chemically from morphine. Medical science subsequently synthesized drugs that have properties similar to heroin, codeine, or morphine. These drugs are also classified as narcotic drugs. To clarify terminology further, "opiate" refers to opium and its derivatives, whereas "opioid" refers to any substance of natural or synthetic origin that has morphine-like effects.

Federal law classifies the coca leaf and a chemical derived from it, cocaine, as narcotics, but these drugs are stimulants and medical science does not consider them narcotics. Cocaine is treated in Chapter 12.

### 1. Medicinal Uses

Natural and synthetic morphine-like drugs are effective pain relievers. They are among the most valuable drugs available to physicians and are widely used for short-term acute pain resulting from surgery, fractures, burns, and the like, as well as to reduce suffering in the later stages of terminal illnesses, such as cancer.

While Sir William Osler's reference to morphine as "God's own medicine" is a favorite quote of medical authors, there is little argument with the astonishing growth of the multi-billion-dollar pharmaceutical industry. Massive scientific and economic investments have been poured into the vigorous quest for a non-addicting, non-toxic pain-killer that can be bottled and marketed to the masses.

Controversy continues to swirl around the ethical issues debated among proponents of ample dosage to relieve deathbed sufferers of acute diseases and others of more conservative ilk who are suspect of analgesic relief that results in a severe aftermath of hard-core addiction. This is a dilemma that continues to challenge physicians in their weighing of humanistic and Hippocratic imperatives.

1. *Analgesia.* Intense pain can be relieved significantly by parenteral doses of morphine

which avoid the muddling of brain functions or respiratory problems.

2. *Sedative Action*. Few argue against the valid uses of narcotics for pre-operative sedation aimed at pain relief. However, there is growing reluctance to encourage routine use of narcotics in patients who are free of pain but need assistance to achieve sleep or a tranquil state. Drugs other than narcotics are available for such purposes.

3. *Antitussive Actions*. Supermarket shelves hold many examples of non-narcotic, non-addictive agents for cough suppression, despite the obvious efficiency of opiates for this task.

4. *Dyspnea*. It has been noted by Goodman and Gilman in their landmark work on pharmacological therapeutics that morphine provides dramatic relief for certain forms of dyspnea and pulmonary edema.

5. *Gastrointestinal*. Regarding diarrheal disorders, synthetic opiods, including diphenoxylate, are proving effective agents for decrease of bowel motility. The opiates remain in the forefront of treatment for these intestinal disorders.

Generally these drugs depress the central nervous system (CNS) to produce a marked reduction in sensitivity to pain, create drowsiness, and reduce physical activity. Other effects can include nausea and vomiting, constipation, itching, flushing, constriction of pupils, and respiratory depression.

Manufacture and distribution of medicinal opiates are stringently controlled by the federal government through laws designed to keep these products available only for legitimate medical use. Those who distribute the drugs are registered with federal authorities and must comply with specific record-keeping and drug-security requirements.

## 2. Substances of Abuse

The abuse of narcotic drugs dates from ancient times. The appeal of opioid-like drugs lies in their ability to reduce sensitivity to both psychologic and physical stimuli and to produce a sense of euphoria. They dull fear, tension, and anxiety. Under the influence of opioids the user is usually lethargic and indifferent to the environment and personal situation.

Chronic use leads to both physical and psychologic dependence. Tolerance develops and ever-increasing doses are required to achieve the desired effect. As the need for the drug increases, the user's activities become increasingly drug-centered.

When the drug supplies are cut off, withdrawal symptoms may develop. Characteristically they include nervousness; anxiety; sleeplessness; yawning; running eyes and nose; sweating; enlargement of the pupils; "gooseflesh"; muscle twitching; severe aches in back and leg muscles; hot and cold flashes; vomiting; diarrhea; increased breathing rate, blood pressure, and temperature; and a feeling of desperation and an obsessional desire to secure a "fix." The intensity of withdrawal symptoms varies with the degree of physical dependence and the amount of drug customarily used. Typically the symptoms begin about four to eight hours after the last dose. They increase in intensity and reach a peak in 36 to 72 hours, then gradually diminish over the next five to ten days, although insomnia, nervousness, and muscle aches and pains may last for several weeks.[1]

However, in contrast, experience with Vietnam soldiers using heroin has shown that, in many cases, its prolonged use and then abrupt cessation when they returned to the United States did not result in typical withdrawal symptoms or in reuse.[2]

Drug users live with the perpetual threat of an overdose. This can happen in various ways. A drug-dependent person may miscalculate the strength of the dose, or the drug may be stronger than it was represented to be at the time the user bought it. Death from narcotic overdosage is caused by respiratory failure.

Although the possibility of death from an overdose of narcotics is an ever-constant danger for the drug taker, usually the harmful effects are indirect. Because these dependent persons do not feel hungry, they often suffer from malnutrition. Because they are preoccupied with the drug taking, they usually neglect themselves.

They are more apt to contract infections because of their poor nutritional status. Also, the fact that they may inject contaminated drugs intravenously and are likely to be using poor or unsterile injection techniques may result in serious or fatal septicemia (blood poisoning), hepatitis, and abscesses at the site of injection, as well as in internal organs.

Brief descriptions of heroin as a drug of abuse and other opioids are given in the following.

### *a. Heroin*

Heroin is a white or brown powder known to the addict as H, horse, caballo, white stuff, white lady, Harry, joy powder, doojee, surag, scag, or smack. It produces an intense euphoria, making it the most popularly abused narcotic. Similar to all narcotic drugs, a tolerance develops rapidly and the abuser must ingest increasingly larger quantities to get any "kicks."

Heroin is administered in a variety of ways, including sniffing ("snorting"), smoking, and injection under the skin ("joy popping") or into a vein ("mainlining"). For the latter two methods, the powder is liquified before it is administered. The first emotional reaction is an easing of fears and relief from worry. This is often followed by a state of inactivity bordering on stupor ("on the nod").

Heroin is synthesized from morphine and, weight for weight, is up to ten times more potent in its pharmacologic effects. Pure heroin is "cut" or diluted by the trafficker with such substances as milk sugar or quinine, or both.

The drug sold to the addict as heroin usually contains one part of heroin plus nine parts or more of other substances.

In New York, among the estimated 100,000 heroin addicts, more than 900 fatalities attributable to drugs occurred in 1969. In that city, for the age group 15 to 35, drug abuse is now the leading cause of death. According to Michael M. Baden, Deputy Chief Examiner, the majority of fatalities result from an acute reaction to the intravenous injection of a mixture containing heroin.[3] The magnitude of the problem is illustrated further by Du Pont's estimate that in 1969 16,800 persons, or 2.2 percent of the population of Washington, D.C., were addicted to heroin.[4]

In 1975, further studies by Haberman and Baden[5] on 1954 sample death cases in New York revealed that of those reported as deaths from unnatural causes, 500 were homicide victims, 300 were suicides, about 400 were fatally injured in motor vehicles or other accidents, and more than 500 died directly of narcotism or alcoholism. Among the 1954 sample cases, almost 600 were identified as alcoholics, over 300 as narcotic abusers, and some 200 as having both conditions.

### *b. Morphine*

For many years, morphine was the drug of choice for the relief of pain. It is called white stuff, M, hard stuff, morpho, junk, and Miss Emma by street drug users, and is used by them when heroin is difficult to obtain. Euphoria can be produced with small doses. Tolerance and physical dependence build up rapidly.

### *c. Codeine*

More commonly abused in the form of cough preparations, codeine is less addictive than morphine or heroin and less potent, in terms of inducing euphoria. When withdrawal symptoms occur, they are less severe than with the more potent drugs.

### *d. Hydromorphone (Dihydromorphinone)*

This drug is made from morphine. Although it is almost as potent as heroin, its use does not seem to produce the same thrill as mainlining heroin does.

### *e. Oxycodone (Dihydrohydroxycodeinone)*

This drug is made from codeine. It is classified as a drug with high addiction potential. Although effective orally, most users dissolve tablets in water, filter out the insoluble binders, and mainline the active drug.

### *f. Meperidine*

A product of chemical laboratories rather than poppy fields, this drug was claimed to be without addicting potential when first produced. Experience, however, has proved otherwise (as it did with morphine and heroin). Dependence on this drug is slower to develop and less intense than with morphine.

### *g. Methadone*

Methadone was invented by German chemists in 1941, when the supply of morphine to Germany ran low. It has many properties similar to those of morphine, among which are the ability to relieve pain and to produce physical and psychologic dependence. A major difference between it and morphine and heroin is that when it is taken orally, under medical supervision, it prevents withdrawal symptoms for approximately 24 hours, but is quite addictive when taken by itself over the years.

## B. HISTORY OF OPIATE USE[6]

The poppy plant, *Papaver somniferum*, is indigenous to Asia Minor. Its medical use stretches beyond recorded history. As early as the fourth century B.C., a Sumerian tablet referred to the "joy plant," which most likely was the opium poppy. In the third century B.C., Theophastus mentioned the use of poppy juice.

The classical literature of Virgil and Ovid refers to the sleep-producing poppy. Both the Greek god of sleep, Hypnos, and the Roman god of sleep, Somnos, usually wore or carried poppies, and sometimes an opium container. Greek mythology suggests that Ceres created the poppy so that she could sleep and forget that her daughter had been given to Pluto.

The entire plant was initially ground by the Greeks and named meconium. Later the extraction of opium was differentiated from meconium, and the Greek word for the extract of the juice *opius* (meaning "little juices") came into written records.[7] Galen, the great Greek physician, thought opium quite useful because it "resists poison and venomous bites, cures chronic headache, vertigo, deafness, epilepsy, apoplexy, dimness of sight, loss of voice, asthma, coughs of all kinds, spitting of blood, tightness of breath, colic, the lilac poison, jaundice, hardness of the spleen stone, urinary complaints, fever, dropsies, leprosies, the trouble to which women are subject, melancholy and all pestilences."[8]

Knowledge of the Greek use of opium died with the decline of the Roman empire, but the Arab world used opium extensively as a social drug, as the Koran forbids the use of alcohol. The Arab physician Avicenna employed opium in his medical practice, and his writings, along with those of Galen, were the basis of medical education in Europe as the Renaissance began. In the 16th century, Paracelsus and his followers spoke the praises of opium and, later, Dr. Thomas Sydenham, the father of clinical medicine, said that "without opium, the healing arts would cease to exist."

Arabic traders introduced opium to the Chinese, who employed it mainly in the control of dysentery. When tobacco was introduced into China, smoking became almost universal. However, because tobacco was considered an evil, the emperor issued an edict prohibiting the use of American tobacco. The spread of opium abuse throughout China did not take place until the latter part of the 18th century when Portuguese, English, and American traders established a profitable business in the drug. For Chinese silver, the British traded Indian opium, which was more potent than the Chinese opium. As early as 1729, Yung Cheng issued an edict forbidding the sale of opium,[9] but it was ineffective. Russell and Company of Boston and New York ran a fleet of Chinese clippers, or opium clippers, and did extensive trading in China. Beginning in 1838, the Chinese again vigorously tried to suppress opium use, and even destroyed all the opium found on British and American ships. In retaliation, the British Parliament sent a squadron of ships to subdue the Chinese in what has been called the first opium war. The British won, and through the 1842 Treaty of Nanking established the port of Hong Kong and secured an indemnity of $21 million for the destroyed opium. This increased facilities for the subsequent phenomenal growth of opium importation, which by 1850 had reached 4000 tons a year.[10] In Europe, in 1806, Frederich Sertürner, a pharmacist assistant, published his report of the isolation of the primary active ingredients in opium, which he named morphium—after Morpheus, the god of dreams. The availability of the pure substance for therapy led to greater medical use, and the development of the hypodermic syringe in 1853 made it possible to deliver the undiluted morphine quickly into the body for rapid relief from pain. In the United States, the Civil War stimulated the wide use of the opiates and, after 1850, the importation of Chinese laborers introduced opium smoking to this country. These occurrences combined, at the turn of the century, with the normal medical use—both as physician-prescribed medicine and as patent medicine—to produce an addiction rate in the United States of around 1 percent of the population. At this time, the high rate of "morphinism" was not considered a social problem. As Lindersmith[12] points out: "Little emphasis was placed on the effect of evil association, and dope peddlers were not mentioned because they were rare or non-existent. The public had an altogether different conception of drug addiction. The habit was not approved, but neither was it regarded as criminal. It was usually looked upon as a vice or personal misfortune, much as alcohol is looked upon today by the uninformed public. Narcotic users were pitied rather than loathed as criminals or degenerates; an attitude which still prevails in Europe." In China, the rampant drug use resulting from the lucrative opium business forced Great Britain and China, in 1908, to agree to stop the shipment of opium into China. In 1909, in the United States, President Theodore Roosevelt called the first opium conference in an effort to establish greater international regulation of the opium trade. Later, mainly to support international commitments, the Harrison Narcotic Act was passed in 1914.[12] This was a regulatory and revenue measure, but the court decisions and the government regulations that evolved around the law, together with the attitude of law enforcement officials, brought about a change in the attitude of society toward the dependent opium user.

It might be interpreted by some that the strong enforcement of the Harrison Act by the Treasury Department drove the use of heroin underground and may have been responsible for the illicit trafficking that is still with us. Thus the addict became a criminal.

## C. CHEMISTRY, COMPOSITION, AND SOURCE

### 1. Chemistry and Classification of Opiate Analgesics[13]

Narcotic analgesics can be divided into five categories:

a. *Natural opium alkaloids*
   Morphine
   Codeine
b. *Synthetic derivatives of opiates*
   Dihydromorphinone (Dilaudid)
   Heroin
   Methyldihydromorphinone (metopon)
   Hydrocodone (Hycodan)
c. *Synthetic opiate-like drugs*
   Phenazocine (Prinadol)
   Meperidine (Demerol)
   Alphaprodine (Nisentil)
   Anileridine (Leritine)
   Piminodine (Alvodine)
   Diphenoxylate (with atropine, as Lomotil)
   Methadone (Dolophine)
   Levorphanol (Levo-Dromoran)
d. *Synthetic opiate-like drugs of low-addiction liability and potency*
   Propoxyphene (Darvon)
   Ethoheptazine (Zactane)
   Pentazocine (Talwin)
e. *Narcotic antagonists*
   Nalorphine (Nalline)
   Levallorphan (Lorfan)
   Naloxone hydrochloride (Narcan)
   Pentazocine (Talwin)
   Cyclazocine
   Cyclorphan
   Naltrexone

While the preceding litany of opiate analgesics appears varied and diverse, there is a root similarity among them which the addict knows

From: Goth, A. *Medical Pharmacology*, 11th ed. St. Louis: The C. V. Mosby Co., 1984 well. All these substances are powerful pain suppressants, antagonized by nalorphine and levallorphan.[14] All can and are substituted for each other by the addict who is capable of interchanging one for the other quite readily. As would be expected from scrutiny of their chemical formulas, the substances share a common ring structure, γ-phenyl-N-methyl-piperidine, as indicated in the accompanying chart from Goth's "Medical Pharmacology."[13]

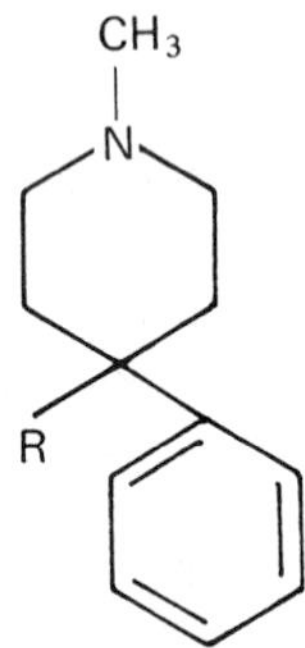


**γ-phenyl-N-methylpiperidine**

The analgesics are generally categorized according to their sources.

### *Natural Opium Alkaloids*

The poppy plant, long a symbol of worldwide religious, mythical and botanical significance, is the natural source of opium. The unripened seed capsule of *Papaver somniferum*, slashed with shallow cuts by harvesters, exudes a milky substance that turns reddish-brown and gummy overnight. This substance, when scraped from the pod, is collected and shaped into balls which comprise the raw opium that is a mainstay of the Third World's commodities market and the backbone of the industrialized world's underground economy.

The juice from the fruit is dried and powdered, becoming the form of the drug most people think of when they hear the term "opium." Powdered opium contains about 10 percent morphine and 0.5 percent codeine. The alkaloids make up about 25 percent of opium by weight (phenanthrenes and benzylisoquinolines). Table 5–1 shows the major constituents.

## 2. Morphine Chemistry

Sertürner is considered the father of morphine chemistry because he isolated morphine from opium in 1803. However, it was not totally synthesized until 1952,[15] which confirmed the structure proposed by the scientists Gulland and Robinson in 1925.

Other natural opiate derivatives are derived by modification of the two hydroxyl groups, one phenolic and the other alcoholic, of the morphine structure. Codeine is simply obtained by the substitution of phenolic hydroxy to make methylmorphine. Diacetylmorphine is heroin, and in dihydromorphine, the alcoholic hydroxyl is replaced by a ketone oxygen and the double bond adjacent to it is eliminated. Most potent

**TABLE 5–1**
**Constituents of Opium**

| Class | Alkaloid | Percentage |
|---|---|---|
| 1. Benzylisoquinoline | Narceine | 0.3 |
| | Narcotine | 6.0 |
| | Papaverine | 1.0 |
| 2. Phenanthrene | Thebaine | 0.2 |
| | Codeine | 0.5 |
| | Morphine | 10.0 |

Adapted from Goodman, L. S., and Gillman, A. *The Pharmacological Basis of Therapeutics* (2nd ed.). New York: Macmillan, 1955, p. 217.

semisynthetic alkaloids are synthesized by substitutions in the hydroxyl groups. However, the narcotic antagonist naltrexone is obtained by substituting the $CH_3$ group on the nitrogen by this radical:

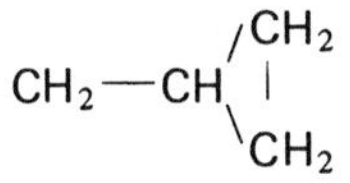

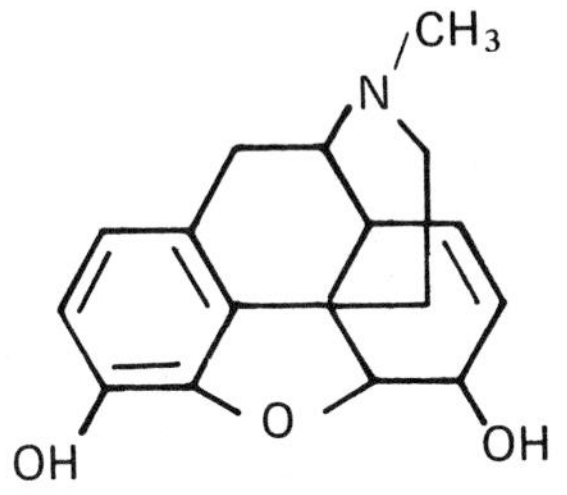

$$CH_2{-}CH\langle^{CH_2}_{CH_2}|$$

$CH_3$ N O OH OH

**Morphine**

The subcutaneous dosage range of morphine sulfate is 8 to 15 mg. This salt is available in 1-ml ampules or in varying tablet sizes.

## D. OPIOID PHARMACOLOGY

The classification of analgesics as narcotic and nonnarcotic is based on legal considerations. From a medical standpoint, it would be more useful to classify them as "strong" and "mild," as what the physician is interested in is the capability of a drug to relieve "severe" or "moderate" pain. Most of the narcotic analgesics are strong and most of the nonnarcotics are mild, however, the traditional classification is followed in this discussion.

As previously mentioned, opium has been used throughout recorded history. The chemist has succeeded in modifying the structures of the opium alkaloids and in creating related drugs. Although morphine is still a very important narcotic analgesic, some of the synthetic drugs are welcome additions to therapeutics. The great incentive for the development of new analgesics has been the possible dissociation of the analgesic from the euphoriant effects of these drugs and the elimination of addiction liability. Some success has been achieved in these efforts and in the synthesis of opiate antagonists and related peptidyl opiates and potential use of natural amino acids, that inhibit the breakdown of the "internal opioids."

### 1. Pharmacokinetics and Metabolism

The opiates are absorbed from the gastrointestinal tract, but not in a predictable manner. They are effective by injection. Upon injection, opiates leave the bloodstream and are concentrated primarily in the kidney, lung, liver, and spleen. The skeletal muscle does not receive as high a concentration as the organs, but because of the great mass of muscle relative to the size of the organs, most of the opiates in the body is in the muscle and there are very low concentrations in the CNS. Excretion is a relatively unimportant method for limiting the effects of morphine and its response and duration of effect. The predominant metabolic changes include dealkylation, conjugation, hydroxylation, and hydrolysis.[16]

### 2. Pharmacologic Properties

Morphine and its surrogates produce their major effects on the CNS and the bowel. The older literature on the opium alkaloids has been reviewed by Reynolds and Randall,[17] with additional reviews by Winter,[18] Lim,[19] Martin,[20] Domino,[21] and Lewis and associates.[22] Opioid actions and uses have also been the subject of a number of symposia,[23,27] monographs,[28,29] edited volumes,[30-32] and books.[33]

#### *a. Opiate Receptors*

The pharmacologic actions of morphine and related opiates are extremely complex. Although great advances have been made, the exact mechanisms by which opioids exert their effects remain uncertain. The definitive research showing that all vertebrates have built-in anti-pain compounds in the CNS is one of the most exciting discoveries in the field of drug abuse, and, in fact, in all of neurochemistry. Furthermore these compounds act on specific receptor sites at nerve cell synapses, the same binding sites occupied by the drugs we call narcotics.

Research of the past 50 years has demonstrated the high degree of specificity of opiate action. It has become evident that these must be highly specific binding sites or receptors on nerve cells in particular locations in the nervous system.

These receptors would be fashioned like locks, to accept only key-shaped internal or injected compounds with pain-relieving or euphoriant effects, such as opiate-like molecules. Slight modifications of the structure of opiates, or of their electric charges, will not permit a ''fit'' with the receptor molecule, and all narcotic activity will be lost.

Stereospecific saturable receptors for opioids and opioid antagonists have been studied in vertebrate neural tissues by several investigators.[34-37] The distribution of these receptors in the nervous system does not correlate precisely with the distribution of any one putative neurotransmitter or any recognized neural subsystem, although the limbic system and periaqueductal gray matter, areas that may play a role in opioid analgesia, are particularly enriched.[38,39] It is likely that the receptors thus far studied will prove to be heterogeneous or multiple in nature.[40,41] In addition, opiate receptors have been found in all vertebrates, but not in invertebrates, indicating that they are an adaptive advance by nature at a fairly high stage of evolution.[29]

In a general way, the distribution of opiate receptors in the brain resembles the distribution of a neurotransmitter. For example, dopamine is packaged in granules of certain nerve endings; its overall distribution in the brain is patchy, with small regions of high concentrations and other areas with no detectable amounts at all. Dopamine receptors are distributed to correspond with the dopamine in nerve endings, as a neurotransmitter, when it is released, has to combine with its specific receptor in order to cause its typical biologic effect; for the endogenous opioid, it might be euphoria or relief of pain.

It is known that minor manipulations of the spacial configuration of a narcotic can change it from a strong narcotic agonist to a narcotic antagonist that will prevent any narcotic from producing its effects. This occurs because a narcotic antagonist such as naltrexone can displace or prevent an agonist such as morphine from occupying the available narcotic receptor sites.

The unusually high structural specificity of the opiates and of the opiate receptors, as well as the actual presence of the receptors and their distribution, which suggested they might be neurotransmitter receptors, raised the evolutionary question as to why they should exist. Other neurotransmitter receptors are activated by endogenous neurotransmitters, and so logically it would seem that there are natural opioid substances that activate the opiate receptors. Thus the search for an ''endogenous ligand'' of the opiate receptor began (*ligand* means a molecule that binds to a receptor).

### *b. Internal Opioid Compounds*

In 1975, two substances were discovered in pig brain that have the pharmacologic actions of morphine, heroin, and related opiates. The substances were small peptides, consisting of a chain of five amino acids. One of the substances had the sequence tryosine-glycine-glycine-phenylalanine-methionine, whereas the other peptide differed only in that the amino acid leucine was present in the fifth position instead of methionine. The former was called methionine-enkephalin and the latter leucine-enkephalin. Today it is documented that, under certain conditions, leucine-enkephalin possesses higher opioid activity than methionine-enkephalin.[42] Other research uncovered much longer peptides in the pituitary gland. One was identified as a 31-amino-acid peptide and was called beta-endorphin. The first five amino acids of this peptide are identical to methionine-enkephalin.

It is noteworthy that these are not the only opioid peptides, but the chemical structures of some of the others have not yet been identified. For example, there is another peptide in the pituitary gland and also a small nonpeptide in the brain that are much like morphine in their chemical properties.

In terms of defining the internal opioid compounds, *endorphin* is used in a generic sense to mean any morphine-like peptide. The specific term beta-endorphin refers to the long pituitary peptide noted above. The term *enkephalin* refers to the small brain peptides, both methionine-enkephalin and leucine-enkephalin.

More detailed information concerning this subject is presented in Chapter 8, and the interested reader should refer to a selected bibliography on the topic.[43-47]

## E. EFFECTS ON ORGAN SYSTEMS

Morphine and the morphine-like analgesic agents produce major effects on the CNS and the gastrointestinal system.

The outstanding effect of morphine in humans is the relief of pain. This action is very selective; other senses are altered very little or not at all. Although morphine is effective for all types of pain, it is more so against continuous dull pain than against sharp intermittent pain. In the study of analgesic action in humans, pain is separated into two components: (1) as a specific sensation, which you feel; and (2) as suffering, or how you react to the specific sensation. Morphine and other morphine-like compounds decrease the perception of pain, and also alter the individual's reaction to it.

The latter effect is undoubtedly part of the euphoria. The patient is aware of the pain but is not bothered by it. The administration of morphine to certain individuals, particularly to those not experiencing pain, may result in an unpleasant experience consisting of mild anxiety, or even fear, and frequently nausea, sometimes with vomiting. This state is called dysphoria. Sleep is produced with larger doses of morphine, but the central depressant actions of morphine do not decrease anticonvulsant activity or cause slurred speech or significant motor incoordination, as do the barbiturates. A person's respiratory center is quite sensitive to the actions of morphine, and death from morphine overdose is attributable to respiratory failure. Morphine can contract bronchial smooth muscle, thereby decreasing the patient's ability to obtain oxygen. It also will constrict the pupil of the human eye, and pinpoint pupils are of diagnostic value. In opiate dependence, tolerance does not develop to this effect of morphine. Morphine can cause excitation in some individuals. It is particularly excitatory in horses, and has been used extensively in horse racing.

### 1. Specific Central Actions

#### *a. Respiration*

In 1961, Papadopoulos and Keats showed that although therapeutic doses of morphine reduce the response to carbon dioxide inhalation as well as lessening respiratory minute volume, the respiratory rate is only slightly changed.[48] In contrast, higher doses induce severe carbon dioxide retention as a result of respiratory depression. The method of administration of morphine is a determinant in the overall effect on the respiratory system. For example, following intravenous injection, maximal depression of respiration occurs within five minutes, whereas following the intramuscular route the response could be delayed for 60 minutes or more.[49] Although acute morphine poisoning produces stoppage of respiration and subsequent death, tolerance is known to occur in the chronic abuser not only to analgesic and euphoric actions of the drug, but in the respiratory center as well.

#### *b. Pupils*

It is well known that the CNS is the site of action for morphine-induced pupillary constriction. In those animals excited by morphine, such as cats, pupillary dilation is observed. Unlike with its analgesic, euphoric, and respiratory actions, addicts do not develop tolerance to the pupillary effects of morphine, and during withdrawal their pupils become dilated.

#### *c. Vomiting Action (Emesis)*

In 1954 it was reported[51] that the emetic action of morphine was mediated in dogs through the chemoreceptor trigger zone in the medulla. Morphine is a known dopamine receptor agonist[30] and thus it is not surprising that the dopamine agonist, apomorphine, obtained by the chemical modification of morphine, is a potent activator of the chemoreceptor trigger zone and is used clinically to induce vomiting.

### d. *CNS Stimulation*

In women and in certain animals, morphine induces CNS excitation. In some men, morphine injections may cause vomiting and delerium. In cats, it has been determined that lesions in the hypothalamus are required to block this unusual violent action of morphine, whereas decortication does not prevent it.

## 2. Other Actions

Miscellaneous effects of morphine include bronchial, cardiovascular, antidiuretic, biliary, gastrointestinal, and metabolic actions.

### a. *Bronchial Actions*

Although the exact cause of death of asthmatic patients as a result of morphine injections is unknown, it has been speculated that it is due to the bronchial smooth muscle contraction actions of morphine rather than its depressing effect on the respiratory center.

### b. *Actions on the Heart*

Over a decade ago, Fennessy and Rattray[52] reported on the cardiovascular effects of morphine in rodents. They suggested that in large doses, the narcotic lowered blood pressure reflexively by initiating afferent activity in the vagus nerve. The fall in blood pressure as a result of high doses of morphine—or central vasomotor depression—may also involve hypoxia. In support of the parasympathetic mechanism, the depressor response to intravenous morphine can be pharmacologically eliminated (or abolished) by the ganglionic blocking agent hexamethonium and reduced (but not abolished) by the muscurinic receptor blocker atropine. Additionally, it has been speculated that morphine-induced hypotension may be due to either a direct action to the heart or histamine release.

Clinically it is important to be aware of the fact that in therapeutic doses morphine has either no or minimal actions on the heart. This becomes important when the drug is given to relieve pulmonary edema and pain of mycardial infarction in cardiac patients.

### c. *Antidiuretic Action*

Morphine causes the release of the antidiuretic hormone and therefore inhibits micturition. In addition, morphine also decreases the perception of the stimulus for micturition. Another contributing factor is that morphine is known to contract the urethra and the detrusor muscle of the bladder, thereby enhancing vesicle sphincter tone.

Because of morphine's analgesic action it is useful in the relief of ureteral colic, and therapeutic doses of the drug do not significantly alter uterine contractions during labor.

### d. *Biliary Tract Actions*

The increase in intrabiliary pressure due to morphine is probably not mediated via a muscarinic receptor since atropine (a muscarinic receptor antagonist) does not affect resulting severe spasms of the biliary tract.

### e. *Gastrointestinal Actions*

It is well known that in street circles the addict complains about morphine-induced constipation. Tolerance to this effect of morphine occurs in the addict slowly, if at all. The exact effects of the centrally mediated actions of morphine on the gastrointestinal tract include stopping propulsive contractions in the bowels, increasing anal sphincter tone, increasing reabsorption of water, and drying the feces. For these reasons, morphine is useful in the treatment of diarrhea.

### f. *Effects on Metabolism*

Many years ago Bodo and co-workers[53] discovered that total sympathectomy prevents the rise in blood sugar induced by morphine injection. Another metabolic action of morphine is to decrease total oxygen consumption. The disposition and metabolism of morphine have been reviewed in other standard texts.[1]

## F. TOXICITY

### 1. Acute Toxicity

In acute morphine poisoning, the individual is comatose and cyanotic, with slow respiration and pinpoint-size pupils.

The management of such a patient is quite different from that of the barbiturate-poisoned patient. First, central stimulant drugs such as picrotoxin or pentylenetetrazole (Metrazol) should not be used, since there is experimental evidence of their lack of antidotal value. Morphine, in contrast to the barbiturates, has many excitatory actions and may be synergistic with the convulsants.

The major development in the treatment of acute morphine poisoning has been the discovery of the antidotal action of nalorphine or naltrexone.

Respiration and circulation can be improved in patients suffering from morphine overdose by intravenous injection of 5 to 10 mg of the narcotic antagonist nalorphine. The dosage may be repeated but should not exceed a total of 40 mg.

Naloxone hydrochloride (Narcan) and naltrexone are narcotic antagonists of great importance, and are discussed further in Chapter 6.

Most opiate-dependent individuals take heroin. However, heroin, by the time it reaches the user, is grossly contaminated with such things as starch, quinine, baking soda, and mannitol. Its strength is seldom known and thus it is not surprising that heroin overdose accounts for about 1 percent of the deaths of heroin users. Nonsterile drugs and equipment, and faulty techniques, cause much damage. Hepatitis was the most frequent complication observed by Louria and his associates, and was seen in 42 of the 100 cases of complications of heroin dependence studied by this group. Bacterial infection of the heart occurs quite often, and is more often fatal than hepatitis. Acute pulmonary congestion and edema are also frequent findings.[54]

In a study of 200 patients admitted to the Bernstein Institute Medical Unit, which cares solely for narcotic-dependent persons, reasons for admission were acute hepatitis, 30.5 percent; infections, 27.5 percent; detoxification, 11.5 percent; pulmonary disease, 6 percent; overdose, 5 percent; and venereal disease, 3.5 percent.[55] In 1970–1971, the Dallas County Medical Examiner's Office investigated 41 cases in which toxicologic analysis revealed the presence of propoxyphene. Ten had died from propoxyphene alone, and 12 were victims of a propoxyphene–alcohol combination. The number of victims of propoxyphene–alcohol was the same as that from combined barbiturates and alcohol during the same period—an important warning of the dangers of combining alcohol with propoxyphene.[56]

### 2. Chronic Toxicity

Prolonged misuse of opiates usually results in physical dependence, withdrawal, and tolerance to the actions of the narcotic being abused.

#### *a. Physical Dependence*

Physical dependence is an adaptive state produced by the chronic use of a drug, where that continued use is necessary for the maintenance of normal nervous system functions. If the administration of the drug is stopped, or its action is affected by a specific antagonist, intense physical disturbance occurs. This is referred to as withdrawal symptoms or the abstinence syndrome.[57] Morphine produces a strong physical dependence. The withdrawal symptoms appear a few hours after the last dose and reach peak intensity in 36 to 72 hours. The time of onset, peak intensity, and duration of the withdrawal phenomenon vary with the degree of dependence, the characteristics of the drug, and the individual using it. Methadone has effects that last much longer than those of morphine, and has a much slower and less traumatic withdrawal syndrome. Administration of a specific antagonist, such as nalorphine, promptly precipitates a rapid and intense withdrawal syndrome. One reason for the great emphasis upon withdrawal is probably the ease with which it can be observed and described. Paton[58] believes that the withdrawal phenomenon, although important medically, has no central importance in dependence.

The classic 1950s' stereotype of "cold turkey" withdrawal is epitomized by popular entertainment formats such as Sinatra's portrayal of his character's agonizing withdrawal process from heroin in the film "The Man with the Golden Arm." That portrayal is not indicative of the contemporary heroin experience.

Today's chronic heroin user develops only a mild degree of physical dependence on heroin, reflecting the common practice of extreme dilution so evident on the streets.

As pointed out by Louria, "the addict admitted to a medical ward for withdrawal or a medical complication can usually be treated with mild sedation without resorting to substitute narcotics such as methadone hydrochloride . . ."[59]

To achieve a significant level of physical dependence, it is generally agreed that today's user would probably spend up to $200 per day and more for heroin purchased in quest of an effective high.

Cross-addiction is a common phenomenon with today's heroin user, whether "speedballing" with the entertainment world's deadly intravenous combination of heroin and cocaine, or indulging simultaneously with barbiturates and alcohol.

This compounding of substances may reflect not only the general dissatisfaction with diluted heroin effects today, but also indicates a willingness to experiment with various combinations in order to produce "novel experiences."

Barbiturate usage, in combination with heroin, demands careful monitoring during withdrawal periods. Whether the barbiturates are manufactured by legitimate pharmaceutical companies or bought on the streets as unknown products of "basement labs," the result may be a user with a so-called heroin dependence whose real physical dependence is on barbiturates.

The classic cycle of the chronic heroin user is the three-fold transition among states described as "high, straight and sick."[60] In today's diluted heroin environment, it takes ever-increasing amounts of the drug to achieve a satisfactory "high," especially for a user with moderate tolerance. The cycle demands more dollars from the user to chase an even more intense escape from his "sick" state into his "high" state.

In general, today's user has been "conned" by repeated dilution into an imagined state of physical dependence on heroin, forced to steal to support greater purchases of diluted heroin. In reality, the problems of dependence are more likely to reside in cross-addictive experiences with alcohol, barbiturates or other substances.

### *b. Abstinence Syndrome*

There is considerable information available concerning the characteristics of withdrawal to narcotics.[61,62] The person dependent on these drugs seeks them for their euphorogenic effects as well as to ward off the unpleasant withdrawal syndrome that occurs about four to eight hours after the last dose, and which reaches a peak at 36 to 72 hours. Depending on the severity of the withdrawal syndrome, disturbances will subside in five to ten days.

At first, the seeking of euphorogenic effects is the reason for repeated use of the drug. Warding off withdrawal does not come into play until the individual has received a number of doses of the narcotic. Once the dependence is established, the fear of withdrawal becomes a predominant reason for the continued use. In many instances, the opiate-dependent individual will maintain the "addiction" to avoid withdrawal.

For decades, physicians could not decide whether the withdrawal syndrome was primarily organic or psychic in nature. It is now generally accepted that the syndrome has both voluntary and involuntary components.

The withdrawal syndrome can be precipitated by the injection of a narcotic antagonist, such as naloxone, or by the abrupt cessation of the drug (opiate). The withdrawal syndrome will appear almost immediately following an antagonist injection but takes hours after the final dose of an opiate is administered.

The opiate withdrawal is characterized by abdominal pain, irritability, cold sweats, yawning, gooseflesh, diarrhea, nausea, perspiration, and vomiting. These effects will be noticed within the first 24 hours of abstinence. They are uncomfortable but not life threatening, in healthy individuals. The user may also fall asleep for several hours. ''Rebound'' excitability of the CNS, manifested by pupillary dilation, increases in heart rate, a rise in blood pressure, involuntary twitching and kicking, and spontaneous sexual orgasms, may occur. Tremors and pain in the back of extremities are common complaints. Leukocytosis often develops. A user can lose ten pounds in 24 hours and also suffer from disturbances in acid-base balance and dehydration.

A number of medical disorders can complicate matters and increase the severity of withdrawal. These disorders include arthritis, damage to the liver (cirrhosis), peptic ulcer, ulcerative colitis, epilepsy, and diabetes. A number of cardiovascular diseases such as congestive heart failure, severe hypertension, and anginal syndrome, as well as respiratory disease or asthma and pneumonia, also can potentiate the danger of withdrawal.

### *c. Protracted Abstinence*

In some individuals mild physiologic disturbances can persist for over six months. Martin and associates[63] have termed this period the ''protracted'' phase. According to their studies, the protracted phase begins between the sixth and ninth week and is characterized by alterations in pupil diameter, body temperature, and blood pressure. The same group[64] measured urine catecholomines during the protracted period and reported that urinary epinephrine output was highest during the first week of withdrawal, then continued at a lower level, but was still significantly elevated for 16 weeks. In addition, daily urine output was depressed for the first several weeks of narcotic withdrawal.

### *d. Tolerance*

Tolerance is an adaptive state of diminished response to a drug so that a larger dose is required to produce the initial response. Tolerance need not develop to all the effects of the drug. Both dependence and drug abuse may occur without tolerance. With the morphine-type analgesics, tolerance evolves primarily to the respiratory depressant, analgesic, sedative, and euphoregenic effects. The rate of tolerance development depends on the pattern of use. Intermittent use lessens the possibility of development of tolerance while continuous use increases it. However, the dose is still limited, and even in the tolerant opiate-dependent individual, death from an overdose will result from respiratory depression. Significant tolerance does not develop to the constipating effect on the bowel. Meperidine-dependent individuals do not develop significant tolerance to its excitatory activity. Individuals who are tolerant to one of the opiate analgesics will be tolerant to the others; this is called cross-tolerance, as previously defined. Tolerance is rapidly lost upon withdrawal of the opiates, so that reinstitution of the drug at the prewithdrawal dose may result in overdose (OD). In this regard, chronic users have been known to take as much as 4 grams of a drug in 24 hours—far greater than the lethal dose for a nontolerant person. The duration of tolerance is one to two weeks, and following this period of abstinence, the individual again responds to a small dose of the drug. Dependent users may die as a consequence of taking their usual large dose of morphine after a period of abstinence during which they have lost their tolerance.

### *e. Tests To Establish the Ability of a Drug To Cause Dependence*

There is evidence to suggest that the overall abuse liability of some of the analgesics related to the opioid antagonists is lower than that of morphine. The implications of the differences in abuse potential for the choice of agents in therapy are discussed in the following.

To establish the ability of a drug to cause dependence, such animals as mice, cats, dogs, or monkeys can be used.[65,66] In mice, a rapid and simple procedure is to implant a pellet containing 75 mg of morphine under the skin. After a few days, abstinence signs are observable upon removal of the pellet, but much more dramatic effects can be obtained by using naloxone to precipitate withdrawal. The abstinence syndrome in the mouse includes defecation, urination, sniffing, increased motor activity, tremors, and, most characteristically, stereotyped jumping. The jumping response can be used in studying the degree of dependence. Median effective doses of naloxone can be determined easily—the greater the degree of dependence, the lower the median effective dose of naloxone. Alternatively, dependence intensity can be qualified by a graded response; that is, the total jump attempts after a fixed dose of naloxone during a set time period.

To gain a finer assessment of the ability of a drug to cause dependence, tests can be carried out in monkeys. A number of objective behavioral measures can be used, including operant behavior. Physiologic measurements, such as the study of marked changes in temperature produced by narcotic withdrawal in the monkeys, as well as the ability of narcotics to reverse the effects of morphine withdrawal, have been used. Studies have also been carried out in baboons. The baboons first were prepared for self-administration of the narcotic by means of an intravenous catheter. They then were subjected to a continuous experimental program to study the adaptation, the establishment of initial drug dependence, drug substitution, and experiments to determine the amount of drug required to establish stable-state dependence.

For trials in humans, former opiate-dependent persons from addiction research centers were used as subjects. These former users, who were in good physical condition, volunteered for the experiment while serving their terms. The studies were carried out to determine: (1) the effects of the drugs and the reactions of the subject to them in comparison with morphine or another drug in the user's experience; (2) the ability of the drug to substitute for morphine in a morphine-dependent person; and (3) the ability of the drug to produce tolerance and dependence on prolonged administration.[64]

## G. ABUSE OF OPIATES[67]

"The sufferer is tremulous and loses his self-command: he is subject to fits of agitation and depression. He has a haggard appearance . . . as with other agents, a renewed dose of the poison gives temporary relief, but at the cost of future misery." This is not an account of the action of heroin or morphine on someone addicted to it, but of the effects of coffee as described by a distinguished pharmacologist at the turn of the century. Tea was thought to be equally harmful, and to cause "hallucinations which may be alarming in their intensity." The now popular habit of drinking tea at breakfast was considered by many doctors to be hazardous in the extreme. "An hour or two after breakfast at which tea has been taken . . . a grievous sinking feeling . . . may seize the sufferers, so that speech is an effort. The speech may become weak and vague and by miseries such as these the best years in life may be spoilt." Knowledge of the action of the drugs contained in tea and coffee has come a long way since these early years, but ignorance, prejudice, and fear still haunt our understanding of many other drugs. Scientists are not immune to these fears and prejudices, and even may have to adopt some of them as working hypotheses before they can progress.

This does not mean that we have no hard facts concerning drug dependence. On the contrary, they are available from a wide range of disciplines—from pharmacology to sociology.

Curiosity, rather than a search for oblivion, is the reason most heroin users first experimented with the drug, according to a survey of 106 addicts in the United Kingdom and the United States conducted by J.H. Willis of Guy's Hospital, London. These users had all been admitted to the hospital for treatment, and had been administering heroin to themselves daily for at least six months. Other reasons given for first trying heroin were a search for relief of a depressed mood or the desire to elevate one's mood above normal. About a third of the subjects recalled that their first experience with heroin had been unpleasant.

Nobody knows how many people try heroin once and find this first taste so disagreeable that they do not persist, but those in the Willis sample reported that they began to inject themselves daily within one to six months of their first experience with heroin.

## 1. Number of Current Users and Comradeship[67]

Every opiate-dependent person is a potential focus of the spread of that dependence. Communities have been evaluated into which one or a small number of narcotic-dependent individuals moved and produced a spread of opiate use that resembled the pattern of a typhoid outbreak from an infected food handler. The moral question raised by this analogy is: If all the "junkies" could be removed from a community, would the infection naturally disappear? That question is being asked by government enforcement officials. It is not the goal here to pass judgment on this issue, but rather to describe, as lucidly as possible, the real street picture with special emphasis on the role of "comradeship."

In this regard, "turning on" and "scoring" are two of the terms used by drug takers to describe the different stages of a trip. The world of drugs is characterized by a language all its own. The person who knows these words, and wears the right clothes, belongs to the subculture and is accepted with little question. To consider drug dependence without reference to this aspect of the drug experience would be very misleading. Too often in the past, interest in users has been limited to the physical aspects of their dependence on drugs, and they have been treated as objects to be cured simply by getting them to stop being physically dependent on the drug. Many users who have been withdrawn from physical dependence go back to drugs—not simply because they lack will power, as sometimes suggested, but because all their friends are junkies and they identify strongly with them, or because of some underlying genetic disease.[68]

Records show that many such persons have had disturbing experiences of rejection or domination by parents. The drug scene provides a genuine escape into a group that accepts them with little question and provides a comradeship that they failed to find elsewhere. This comradeship is expressed not only by their common clothes and language, but also by the sharing of many things, often including the syringe used for injection. And it is this sharing of syringes that brings with it a danger of infection by the virus that causes jaundice—so much so that tracing jaundice sufferers has been found a good way to discover dependent drug users.

The comradeship of the drug user sharing drug and syringe is similar to that of the smoker who passes around a pack of cigarettes. Curiously, many tobacco smokers are unable to enjoy a cigarette if they are asked to smoke while blindfolded. Apparently, for many people, an important part of the smoking ritual is to be able to observe themselves performing. In the same way, the rituals of drug taking are important and afford some satisfaction in themselves—a conclusion that may seem scientifically dubious but is, in fact, supported by experiments on animals. This ritual aspect of drug taking may be particularly important among persons in the United States who obtain such small supplies of heroin that they seldom develop the severe physical withdrawal symptoms of the user of high doses.

As well as providing a ritual, drug use furnishes a ready identity for the users. According to Isidor Chein of the Research Center for Human Relations, New York University, the person's feelings can be summarized in this way: "You are a teacher. You are a cop. You are a parent, a man, a woman, a citizen, a voter, a landlord, a housewife. Me, I'm a junkie. A junkie is a person, not a thing." In this way, the user acquires an identity and a set of relationships that have some personal meaning.

Cure of dependence of the most severe type is possible, but it cannot be guaranteed. It is necessary not only to rid the body of the physical craving for the drug, but to provide rewarding alternatives in the hope that the drug itself will become progressively less rewarding.

## 2. Availability of the Drug

According to Cohen,[69] "Sufficient quantities of heroin exist within the national boundaries to provide all current 'addict' needs for the next two-to-three years. Estimates that no more than 10–15% of all contraband heroin is confiscated are possibly correct. . . . Local shortages may occur from time to time, but these will have an insignificant effect upon addict numbers." Substitutes for low supplies of heroin include codeine cough syrups, barbiturates and other sedatives, and methadone. Many chronic heroin users enter methadone detoxification programs in an effort to reduce the size of their daily requirement, which is a very popular way in which an opiate abuser deals with a drug "panic." We can assume from estimates by informed experimenters that 15 percent of all heroin addicts (about 75,000) are under treatment in methadone maintenance programs. This fact may have some relation to the leakage of methadone onto the street, which results in a direct expansion of total illicit opiate supplies. Cohen[69] further states that, "In some cities, like New York, methadone from illicit sources has constituted a black market commodity which satisfies the primary needs of a fair number of addicts and tides others over until their heroin connection is re-established." Certainly methadone diversion in New York, and possibly in other major U.S. cities, is a serious factor in the epidemiology of opiate abuse. And establishment of heroin maintenance clinics will similarly result in a catastrophic expansion of illicit heroin supplies. Furthermore, single-syndicate eradication will not produce more than a minor impact on the illicit market because multiple supply channels exist. The "British system," since it was changed in 1968, pumps more methadone to British addicts than heroin, so that approach is not helpful in terms of reducing opiate availability. The destruction of opium plantings is not the simple solution; a relatively small planting area will meet the needs of the nation's chronic opiate users, and this can be placed in remote, well-camouflaged terrain. Less than 100 tons of opium are required to yield the six to nine tons of heroin needed annually for the black marketplace in the United States.

## 3. Facts and Figures[70]

As has been previously stated, chronic illicit use of narcotics generally begins with sporadic experimentation involving free heroin furnished by friends. In a minority of users, initial experimentation leads to psychologic dependence, daily use, and, finally, a state of physical dependence. Tolerance gradually develops, and the amount of heroin injected daily slowly rises.

Commonly the initial illegal drugs used are alcohol and tobacco (the users being minors), then marihuana, then the hallucinogens and/or amphetamines, and finally heroin. Use of marihuana in no way induces progression to higher or harder drugs.[69,71,72]

The chronic user of narcotics exists in an addict subculture in which the entire day generally revolves around obtaining drugs or relaxing under their effect. Upon arising, there is the wake-up dose. Following this, the user will seek money to purchase additional drugs, often obtaining it through some sort of crime, and then will contact a trusted dealer to score (buy) enough heroin to last at least until the next morning.

Persons dependent on narcotics are usually unable to hold steady jobs that will pay enough to support a habit. For this reason, the addict must finance the drug intake by donations from relatives (spouse or parents) or friends, or by illegal means. The three most common criminal methods are burglary, prostitution, and the dealing of drugs.

This last method is of particular significance, as one way to support a habit is to develop a clientele of other drug users. Small-time users, who deal drugs to support their expensive habits, should be differentiated from the nondependent syndicate pushers who control the drug traffic and make the profits.[71,73]

It should be noted that all of the crimes cited are nonviolent. Users rarely engage in violence, not only because the drugs induce passivity, but also because police pursuit is less intense for nonviolent crimes. Thus the stereotype of the "dangerous dope fiend" is quite without foundation in fact. This is not to imply, however, that dependence-related crime is not important.

Narcotics-related burglary is extremely expensive for the public, as "fences" commonly give only one fifth of the value of stolen goods. This means that a $50-a-day habit requires $250 worth of goods a day to maintain. It has been estimated that in 1968, when over half the U.S. users were in New York, dependence-related crime cost that city $10 million per day.

Rather than being an effect of the narcotics themselves, burglary appears to be a direct result of the present U.S. narcotics laws, which stimulate the formation and continuance of the black market. This problem is not found with the system that has noncriminalized the use of narcotics.[73,75]

In recent years, a change in the patterns of narcotics use has appeared to be developing. There has apparently been a nationwide increase in both the number of dependent persons and the number of urban centers where illicit heroin is available.

The classic user once was a young, ghetto male, wearing long sleeves to cover the needle marks. He was unemployed, malnourished, had a short attention span, and, of course, noticeable miosis. The major exceptions were members of the medical profession who became dependent on Demerol (or morphine) rather than heroin, and generally attempted to keep working to maintain their proximity to hospital supplies.

Now increasing numbers of young people on all social levels are becoming involved with narcotics. Some are students; others work, deal drugs, or steal. However, despite this increase in the number of narcotic users, there are still relatively few users of illicit narcotics, compared with the tremendous number of people using other drugs.[76]

Problems associated with chronic use of narcotics can be summarized as follows:

1. Physical problems[60,61,72,77-81]

a. Direct

(1) No direct degenerative changes.

(2) Overdose (OD)—especially due to incorrect dosage supplied by dealer (pusher); a common cause of death; also encountered by inexperienced users.

(3) Withdrawal—a syndrome secondary to physical dependence.

b. Indirect—many disease states indirectly result from chronic heroin use.

(1) Hepatitis—a sometimes fatal liver disease transmitted by unsterile techniques and sharing of syringes.

(2) Tetanus (lockjaw)—very rare disease contracted by unsterile injection techniques.

(3) Abscess and thrombophlebitis (blood vessel inflammation)—due to unsterile techniques.

(4) SEB—subacute bacterial endocarditis (heart valve infection) due to unsterile techniques.

(5) Pulmonary emboli—involve minute areas of lung tissue; death results from clogging of blood vessels by materials used to cut heroin.

(6) Pulmonary edema—fluid congestion of lungs, cause unknown.

(7) Upper respiratory infection (especially pneumonia)—due to decreased resistance to infection.

(8) Malnutrition—due to lack of interest in food intake and lack of money to purchase food.

(9) Degenerative nerve changes—rare, possibly allergic in origin.

2. Psychological problems[70,79,82,83]

a. Release and/or increase of preexisting emotional problems.

b. Amotivation—loss of all drives (food, sex, advancement); only the drug is important, as it satisfies all drives by itself.

c. Paranoia—fear of anyone but other addicts; indirect result of criminalization.

d. Emotional dependence on drugs makes cessation of drug use extremely difficult.

3. Social problems[71,72,76]

a. Arrest—use of narcotics is illegal except with physician's prescription.

b. Alienation—user becomes immersed in an "addict" subculture and feels uncomfortable with previous friends or family.

c. Difficulty in finding and keeping a job—most employers refuse to consider known or ex-users for decent jobs.

## H. TREATMENT: PROBLEMS IN PERSPECTIVE

"The origin of all sciences is in the desire to know causes; and the origin of all false sciences and imposture is in the desire to accept false causes rather than none; or, which is the same thing, in the willingness to acknowledge our own ignorance."—William Hazlitt, 1829.

Beginning with the fact that very little is known about the factors that lead an individual to initiate use of dependence-producing drugs, it follows that many different kinds of treatment are espoused. These include penal methods, drug substitution, psychotherapy, and indifference. Most of the methods of treatment have a limited success with a limited number of people. As for a cure, no one has a solution that will always lead to a total cessation of misuse of drugs.[83] Future research, it is hoped, will provide the key; defects in the biochemical constitution of the brain are believed by some scientists to be the answer to why some people are more prone to dependence than others.[32,68,84]

The major approaches to treatment of the opiate-dependent individual are (1) maintenance clinics, (2) self-help programs, (3) use of opiate antagonists, (4) legal prohibition, and (5) benign neglect.

## 1. Maintenance Clinics

The patients are maintained on a synthetic opiate, usually methadone.[84] Methadone duplicates many of the effects of morphine, but it is longer acting and is effective when taken orally. It produces little or no euphoria. The patient receives a small dose each day, becomes tolerant to the drug's effect, and is stabilized at that dose. The patient is now tolerant to other opiates and the usual dose of heroin produces little or no effect. Since the patient is supplied with an opiate, there is no need for criminal activity to obtain narcotics. At present, we do not know whether the patient can ever be withdrawn from methadone. About 20 percent of all those in the programs in England generally learn to do without it. About 20 percent who remain in the programs, in general, function better and feel better. If the addict cannot do without the opiate, one can view maintenance as one would view insulin for the diabetic.[85] Methadone maintenance is an effective program for many, but not all, patients. M.J. Kreek,[86] in studies of patients having maintenance treatments with methadone in high doses of 80 to 100 mg daily, found minimal side effects and no toxic effects in her group, and Blinick et al.[87] found that in pregnancies observed in 105 narcotic-addicted women, while on methadone therapy, there were no maternal fatality complications and pregnancy was unremarkable. One third of the infants were premature by weight, but no serious effects were attributable to methadone. Follow-up revealed normal growth and development.[87] A disturbing report by Dobbs[88] indicates that in a random sample of 100 clinic patients receiving methadone maintenance treatment, a majority were still using heroin, and the patients who had been on treatment the longest showed evidence of a higher rate of heroin usage than recently admitted patients. Alcoholism often becomes a problem.[88]

The maintenance system in England deserves special note because of many misconceptions. The original program allowed physicians to prescribe heroin to certified British heroin-dependent persons. Although early reports were very promising, during 1969, 2782 addicts were reported, and in 1970 the number was 2661. In the analysis of the 1430 addicts at the end of 1970, 992 were employed.[89] England long ago considered and rejected the U.S. law enforcement approach. In 1920, when the Dangerous Act was first introduced to England, Walter Elliott, in Parliamentary debate, stated that to follow the American model of narcotics prohibition would be to court disaster.[90] However, even before all the statistics were compiled, authorities felt that the system had failed, and in 1968 it was replaced by a network of narcotic treatment clinics. Physicians were no longer allowed to prescribe heroin to British addicts. In contrast to the past, only approximately 16 percent of the new opiate abusers attending these certified clinics actually get heroin; the rest receive either nothing or methadone alone.

Dr. Reginald Smart[91] reports a number of negative aspects concerning the British system.

1. Illicit drug use and criminality have not disappeared from the British addict population. Because of the low doses of drugs prescribed by the clinics, addicts merely supplement their clinic supplies with street supplies.
2. There is no proof that heroin use has decreased in England. All that is known is that fewer prescriptions for heroin are being written.
3. The clinics have difficulty attracting and holding their clients. Half of the clients have used heroin for at least two years before first appearing at a clinic. Overall dropout rates are about 50 percent a year.
4. Illicit sales of heroin were found to have

increased after the clinics were established.

5. A substantial increase in the number of convictions for possession or trafficking of heroin has occurred since 1968.

6. The number of registered narcotic addicts in England over the past five years has remained constant at about 3000. According to Gould, the actual number of opiate addicts may be ten times as many.

7. In addition to these points, it should be noted that the addict mortality rate in England is 27 per 1000 per year, even higher than the U.S. rate. This occurs despite the sterile syringes and sterile heroin that are distributed there. A good number of the deaths are caused by unsterile techniques, which addicts persist in using in spite of the instructions and demonstrations given them in the clinics.

## 2. Self-Help Programs

The self-help programs are based on the assumption that a character defect causes drug abuse. The opiate abuser must show the genuineness of the desire to become drugfree. There is a parallel between the therapeutic community (TC) and Alcoholics Anonymous. In a TC, the ultimate punishment is exclusion from the group. Emphasis is placed on concentration, on the here and now of behavior. Total abstinence is demanded. Dependent patients are forced to accept responsibility for their behavior. Pressure is used to modify behavior and ex-users are utilized in the program.[92]

Unfortunately this is effective in only a small number of patients. In most TCs, between 50 and 90 percent of the applicants are rejected or quit at the initial stage. Among the programs are Daytop Village, Odyssey House, and Phoenix House.

## 3. Use of Opiate Antagonists

Specific opiate antagonists, such as the short-duration nalorphine, levallorphan, and naloxone, and the longer duration cyclazocine and naltrexone, are also used in therapy of dependence of the morphine type. A number of such compounds have been discovered that have minimal or no opioid effects, but do have the ability to block the effect of morphine. They either prevent the narcotics from producing an effect or, if given after the narcotic, terminate the effect. Thus the antagonists can precipitate abrupt withdrawal symptoms. The use of these compounds is based on the hypothesis that an antagonist that prevents opiate euphoria will eliminate drug-seeking and diminish the risk of dependence.[73,94] But because they do not overcome "drug hunger," the patient is constantly tempted to miss the dose and take heroin. Where long-term therapy is required, there is probably no reason to choose an opiate antagonist over methadone. The number of cases treated by this method remains small and further testing is needed. A double-blind study by Grosz involving the treatment of patients with propranolol confirmed the fact that propranolol reduces the residual drug hunger and blocks the euphoric effects of heroin. Propranolol and/or its metabolites act as narcotic antagonists; they have an extended duration, 40 to 80 hours, of narcotic antagonist action, and can be administered by mouth.[95] Grosz's studies were done with outpatients in an uncontrolled situation. A later inpatient study (double-blind) failed to confirm Grosz's findings.[96] Clonidine, another adrenergic acting compound, appears to be useful in the treatment of opiate withdrawal.

## 4. Legal Sanctions

Endorsement of laws against unsanctioned importation, growing, possession, and illicit use of opiates has been the primary means by which the United States has attempted to control opiate use. Laws against import have not been effective, with border seizure of heroin amounting to less than 5 percent of the estimated imports in 1970. And the price of heroin has been falling, indicating that there is a large supply. In England, the cost to the pharmacy is $0.00067 per milligram, whereas in the United States the street cost is $0.50 to $1.50 per milligram. The profit earned in domestic distribution is so great that it is unlikely that the risks can be increased enough to discourage it. In the United States, illicit use accounts for only about 50,000 pounds of opium each year, or about 1.5 percent of the total world production. The entire U.S. demand could probably be met by the production of opium poppies on just five to ten square miles of the earth's 16 million square miles of arable land.[96] A program based on suppression of production seems impossible to implement.

It appears that law enforcement will remain, for some time, a significant mechanism for gathering opiate users. The likelihood of the jailed drug user being given therapy is slight. One survey showed that 90 to 95 percent of those who leave prison without treatment relapse almost immediately into drug use. John Ingersoll, former director of the Bureau of Narcotics and Dangerous Drugs, has said that law enforcement is not curative, but is the first-aid agency of society. If we want a cure, then we have to go to the basic causes.[92]

### 5. Benign Neglect

Nationally well over 90 percent of all heroin users are not in any program at all.

#### *Approach to the Problem in Canada*

In Canada, the LeDain Report (see "Monographs") recommends that the impact of criminal law on those possessing drugs for personal use be minimized. The recommended treatment for opiate dependence is (1) hospitalization for treatment of acute effects, with gradual withdrawal using methadone; (2) individual or group psychotherapy, vocational guidance, job placement, and rehabilitation or maintenance on a narcotic antagonist; or if this therapy fails, (3) a choice for the user of methadone or other opiate maintenance or residence in a therapeutic community.

The pharmacology of certain specific agents used in the treatment of heroin use is presented in the narcotic antagonist section and in Chapter 7.

### 6. Treatment Modalities

Many treatment physicians raise the issue of the role of media advertising in encouraging the use of drugs. The heroin epidemic is only a symptom of a much greater malaise affecting society. Instead of solving our real problems by diligent effort, people have relied on the false belief in instant gratification with drugs like heroin. Certainly this fact becomes evident in the more than 225 million prescriptions for tranquilizers, sedatives, and energizers written by doctors in 1970. In today's chaotic world a seemingly easy solution is either the abuse of illicit narcotics or the overprescription of tranquilizers by careless physicians.

The WHO Expert Committee on Drug Dependence[96,97] stated in its "Eighteenth Report":

> The rehabilitation of former drug users, regardless of age, is, in most cases, a long and difficult process. Relapse must be expected and planned for. Success necessitates the adoption by the local community of mature and realistic attitudes and the avoidance of panic, moral condemnation and discrimination. Facilities for vocational training and sometimes the provision of sheltered work opportunities and hostels are useful in rehabilitation and help prevent relapse. Generally speaking, facilities for the registration, diagnosis, treatment, after-care, etc. of drug dependent individuals and groups shall be regarded as indispensible integrated parts of the health and social service structures of any community in which abuse exists.

## I. OTHER DERIVATIVES

### 1. Opium Alkaloids Other than Morphine

#### *a. Codeine*

Methylmorphine, or codeine, is medically used as an analgesic and a cough suppressant. The drug is usually given orally and is less potent as a pain reliever and sedative than morphine. However, it is difficult to demonstrate that it is any stronger than aspirin clinically.[80] If a dose of 120 mg of codeine is injected, it closely approximates 10 mg of morphine as an analgesic. In one study performed on postoperative patients, 60 mg of codeine given by mouth produced relief in 40 percent of the patients, whereas a placebo was effective in 33 percent.[1,80]

The pharmacologic effects of codeine, although much less intense, are similar to those of morphine. Codeine is not a good substitute to the experienced opiate addict because codeine produces only mild euphoria. There are two prime circumstances in which codeine is abused today. One concerns adolescent drug experimenters who purchase codeine-containing cough medicines and the other involves the heroin user who is temporarily unable to obtain that drug. As a related opiate the dependent individual may rely on cough medicines to postpone withdrawal. Other codeine congeners include hydrocodone (dihydrocodeinone, Hycodan, etc.), dihydrocodeine (Paracodin), and oxycodone (dihydrohydroxy-codeinone).

Tolerance to codeine develops more slowly than to morphine and it is also less addictive.

Codeine phosphate is widely used in oral doses of 15 to 64 mg for moderately severe pain, when the nonnarcotic analgesics prove ineffective. It is given by subcutaneous injection for severe pain.

Codeine is partly demethylated to morphine in the body and is partly changed to norcodeine. The conjugated forms of these compounds are excreted in the urine.

### *b. Synthetic Natural Opiates*

1. *Hydrocodone (Hycodan).* This drug is more effective as a cough suppressant than codeine but has a higher abuse liability. The usual dose is 5 to 15 mg given three to four times a day for adults.

2. *Dihydromorphinone (Dilaudid).* Because of its high potency, dihydromorphinone (Dilaudid) is not as frequently found on hospital formulary lists. It is up to ten times as potent an analgesic as morphine. Although less nauseating and constipating than morphine, it produces greater respiratory depression. Thus doses for hypodermic injection are 1/10 that of morphine, or 1 to 2 mg.

3. *Methyldihydromorphinone (Metopon).* This opiate drug is effective by oral administration but is more potent than morphine and potentially more dangerous.

4. *Pantopium (Pantopon).* This product is nothing more than a synthetic representation of the naturally existing alkaloids of opium. Those who ingest this drug are receiving a high dose of morphine since it contains 50 percent morphine per dose. It has no advantages over morphine taken by itself.

5. *Heroin or diacetylmorphine.* Heroin is often abused by the injection route. The drug has been approved in England but it is not legal in America. It is a powerful euphoriant and analgesic.

### *c. Synthetic Narcotic-like Drugs*

1. *Alphaprodine (Nisentil).* Structurally this drug is a piperidine derivative. The main advantage of this substance is its rapid onset of analgesic action. However, because of a short duration of action, it is not considered a superior agent.

2. *Anileridine (Levitine).* This drug is chemically related to meperidine but is slightly more potent. For severe pain, the adult oral dose is 25 to 50 mg and the intramuscular dose is 40 mg.

3. *Meperidine (Penthidine, Isonipercaine, Demerol, Dolantin).* Eisleb and associates first introduced meperidine as an atropine-type antispasmatic.

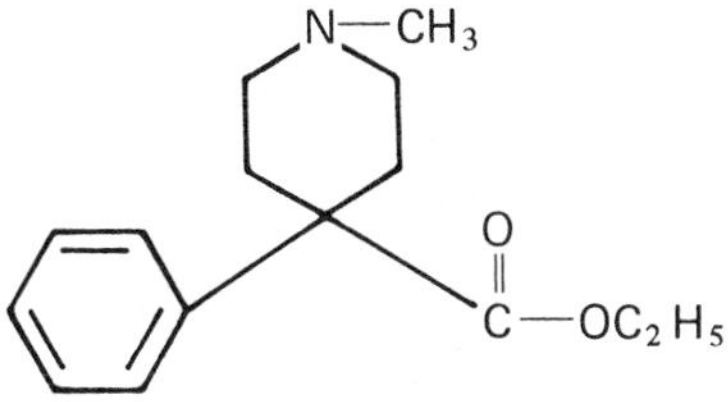

$N—CH_3$

O

$C—OC_2H_5$

**Meperidine**

In the 1950s, the drug was touted as a new nonaddicting analgesic agent with some advantages over morphine—little or no respiratory depression, and a spasmolytic rather than a spasmogenic action.

However, as it turns out, when the morphine and meperidine are compared in equianalgesic doses, the latter drug is just as depressant to respiration and as addictive. The analgesic is approximately ten times less potent than morphine. There are two properties that should reduce the abuse of the drug: (1) tissue irritation, and (2) very short duration of action.

Although nurses, physicians, and pharmacists in the past believed that the drug was "less addicting" than morphine, dependence does occur, and a withdrawal syndrome will develop rapidly, but will be brief. Abstinence is qualitatively similar to heroin and the first signs of withdrawal appear four to five hours after the last dose and maximum intensity is reached in 7 to 12 hours. With meperidine, the gastrointestinal disturbances are less intense than with other narcotics. However, CNS problems are more pronounced.

In fact, mydriasis, tremors, involuntary muscular activity, mental confusion, and even grand mal seizures may occur with high doses of meperidine. Intravenous injection of meperidine may be followed by severe hypotension, in part caused by histamine release.[1]

Addicts have been known to inject doses of 3000 to 4000 mg/day because of the development of tolerance. In nontolerant people, these doses produce respiratory depression followed by coma and death.

The liver plays a role in the metabolism of meperidine. In fact, the stimulatory effects of meperidine are probably due in part to the demethylated metabolite, normeperidine. In some cases, because the stimulatory actions are so prominent, barbiturates may be introduced to reduce the excitation.

It is well established that abuse of this drug is highest among health professionals. It is important to note that many regard meperidine as being a greater impairment to work (especially in hospitals) than other narcotics.

4. *Methadone (Amidon, Dolophine)*. Discovered in Germany during World War II, this drug has a similar pharmacologic profile to morphine although it is not related to it structurally (see Chapter 7).[84] We have devoted an entire chapter to methadone.

**Methadone**

5. *Piminodine (Alvodine) and Diphenoxylate (Lomotil)*. These two drugs are related to meperidine. Piminodine is recommended as an analgesic (oral or by injection), and diphenoxylate has been used for the control of diarrhea.

6. *Levorphanol (Levo-Dromoran)* The chemical structure of the levo and dextro form of Levorphanol is very similar to morphine. The

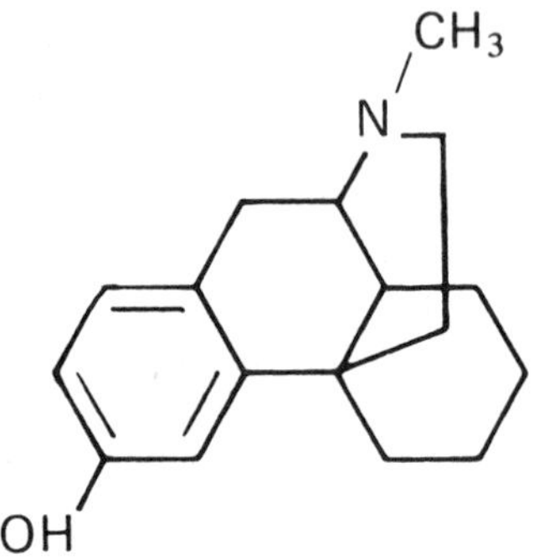


**Levorphanol**

Levo form is approximately 5 times as potent as a pain reliever as morphine. Although both dependence liability and central nervous system depression of the respiratory system are quite significant, its pharmacologic effects on the gastrointestinal tract (induction of constipation and emesis) are only moderate.

The dextro isomer, dextrorphan, has little analgesic action but possesses some antitussive properties.

7. *Dextromethorphan (Romilar)*. The methyl ether of dextrorphan, it has about the same antitussive potency as codeine, with no analgesic, euphoric, or respiratory-depressant properties. It is widely used as a cough suppressant. It is a harmless drug[100] relative to other narcotics.

## 2. Synthetic Opiate-like Drugs (Low Addiction Liability)

Propoxyphene and ethoheptazine are related to methadone and meperidine, respectively, but have much lower potency and dependence liability. Pentazocine is one of the narcotic antagonists with some analgesic potency and low dependence liability.

1. *Propoxyphene (Darvon).* Darvon compound, a combination of caffeine, aspirin, and phenacetin, is widely used as an analgesic. Pure propoxyphene is weaker than codeine.

Although propoxyphene can induce dependence, if we consider the number of individuals who have become addicted to the drug, it represents a small percentage relative to its use. A dose of 32 to 64 mg should reduce pain.

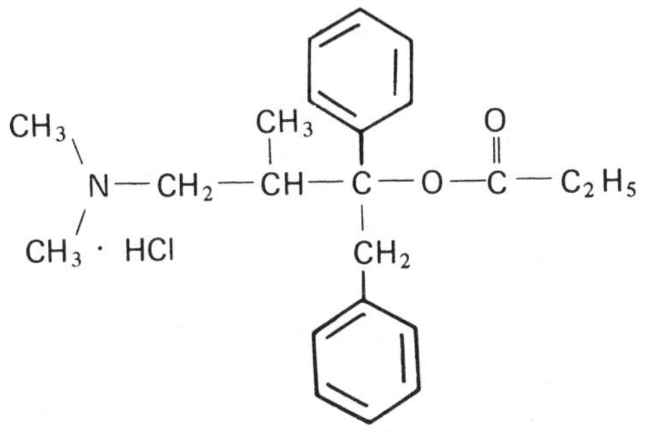

**Propoxyphene hydrocholoride**

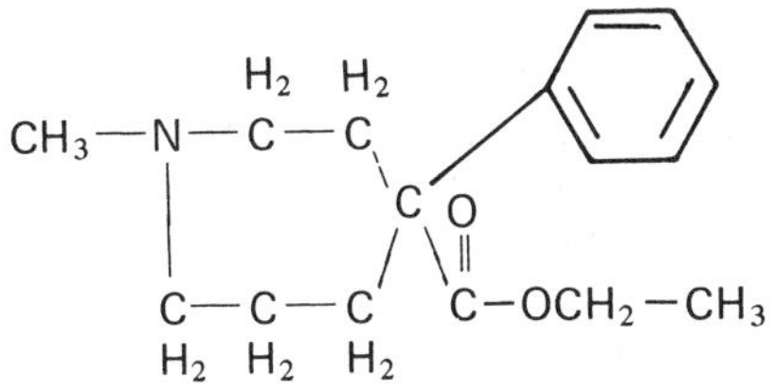

**Ethoheptazine**

Acute propoxyphene intoxication resembles morphine poisoning. The respiratory depression responds to the administration of a narcotic antagonist such as nalorphine.

The use of a derivative propoxyphene napsylate (Darvon-N) for the treatment of heroin and methadone dependence has been proposed.[101] As Dr. Inaba and associates[101] put it, "I got a yen for that Darvon-N."

An article by Tennant et al.[102] demonstrates that high-dose maintenance treatment with Darvon-N for 90 days is relatively complication-free. The drug appears to be particularly useful for the detoxification of heroin- and methadone-dependent individuals, and also as a short-term maintenance agent for heroin dependence.

2. *Ethoheptazine (Zactane).* This is related to meperidine and, like propoxyphene, is of low potency and dependence potential. It is not nearly as popular as the latter.

## 3. Pentazocine (Talwin)

An outcome of narcotic antagonist research, this drug is a synthetic analgesic chemically related to phenazocine which is at best a weak antagonist. For analgesic effects pentazocine is either subcutaneously or intramuscularly injected in 20–40 mg. doses.[102,103] Using morphine as a standard pain killer, pentazocine may be as effective as 10 mg. of the latter drug. Unlike most narcotic analgesics, larger doses are not more powerful, suggesting a flattened dose-response curve. One positive aspect of its use clinically is a rather low dependence liability but it is not very effective via the oral route.

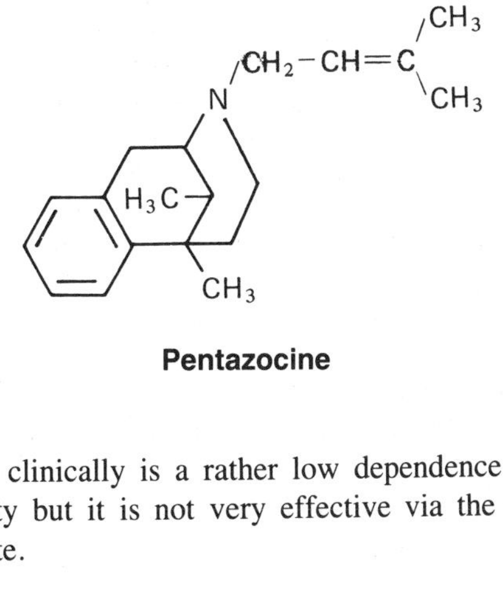

**Pentazocine**

## 3. Opioid Antagonists

An intensive search is under way for the "ideal" narcotic antagonist, namely, a pharmacologic agent that blocks the effects of opiates, has few or no side effects of its own, requires relatively infrequent administration, and is not prohibitively expensive to produce. No drug has yet met these criteria, but some have come close.[104] A number of agents are being tested.[105] Naltrexone is longer acting.[14]

As previously mentioned, the earliest known narcotic antagonists were nalorphine (Nalline) and levallorphan (Lorfan). Administration of a narcotic antagonist precipitates an abstinence syndrome if physical dependence on an opiate has become established. The use of antagonists is not without hazard, however. A severe abstinence syndrome may be precipitated that cannot be suppressed during the period of action of the antagonist, and the antagonist itself, except for naloxone, may further embarrass respiration that has been compromised by alcohol, barbiturates, or other nonnarcotic depressants. (See Chapter 6 for greater detail.)

An important issue that has been succinctly stated by Hofmann[61] is:

> To designate as narcotics only those drugs whose effects are similar to those of opium and its derivatives serves a valuable communicative purpose, for it enables succinct reference to be made to a specific and pharmacologically unique type of drug. But to categorize the misuse of heroin and of marihuana, for example, as forms of "narcotic addiction" is not only, in most respects, pharmacologically and medically absurd, but serves also to obscure or remove important qualitative and quantitative differences among various drugs subject to abuse that have been established after years of study. The more important consideration in this situation is not that the use of both heroin and marihuana is illegal and may harm the user and society, but that the salient pharmacological and medical aspects of the abuse of heroin differ markedly from those of the abuse of marihuana. The appropriate use of the term, narcotic, is one means of indicating these differences.

Physicians working in the drug abuse field should promote the above position and attempt to relate it clearly to less-informed individuals or representatives of institutions concerned with the "drug dilemma."

## REFERENCES


1. Jaffe, J.H., and Martin, W.R. Narcotic analgesics and antagonists. In A.G. Goodman and L.S. Gilman, eds., *The Pharmacological Basis of Therapeutics*. 5th ed. New York: Macmillan, 1975, p. 245.
2. Borne, P. *The Psychology and Physiology of Stress: With Reference to Special Studies of the Viet Nam War*. New York: Academic, 1969.
3. Abelson, P.H. Death from heroin. *Science* 168:1289, 1970.
4. Dupont, R.L. Profile of a heroin-addiction epidemic. *N. Engl. J. Med.* 285:320, 1971.
5. Haberman, P.W., and Baden, M.M. *Alcohol, Other Drugs and Violent Death*. New York: Oxford, 1978.
6. Stavinoha, W.B. Narcotics: Opiate and opiate-like analgesic agents. In K. Blum and A.H. Briggs, eds., *Drugs: Use or Abuse (A Manual)*. San Antonio: University of Texas Health Science Center, 1973, p. 26.
7. Macht, D.I. The history of opium and some of its preparations and alkaloids. *JAMA* 64:477, 1915.
8. Scott, J.M. *The White Poppy: A History of Opium*. New York: Funk & Wagnalls, 1969, p. 111.
9. Taylor, N. *Narcotics: Nature's Dangerous Gifts*. New York: Dell, 1969.
10. Fields, A., and Tararin, P.A. Opium in China. *Br. J. Addict.* 64:371, 1970.
11. Seevers, M.H. Drug addiction problems. *Sigma Xi Q.* 27:91, 1939.
12. Lindesmith, A.R. *Addiction and Opiates*. Chicago: Aldine, 1968.
13. Goth, A. *Medical Pharmacology: Principles and Concepts*, 8th ed. St. Louis: Mosby, 1974.
14. Archer, S. Historical perspective on the chemistry and development of naltrexone. In *Narcotic Antagonists: Naltrexone Pharmacochemistry and Sustained Release Preparations*. (NIDA Research Monograph 28) Washington, D.C.: NIDA, 1981, p. 3.
15. Small, L.F. *Chemistry of the Opium Alkaloids*. Supplement No. 103, Pub. Health Report. Washington, D.C.: U.S. Government Printing Office, 1932.
16. Way, E.L., and Adler, T.K. The pharmacologic implications of the fate of morphine and its surrogates. *Pharmacol. Rev.* 12:383, 1960.
17. Reynolds, A.K. *Morphine and Allied Drugs*. Toronto: University of Toronto Press, 1957.
18. Winter, C.A. The physiology and pharmacology of pain and its relief. In G. DeStevens, ed., *Medicinal Chemistry* (Analgetics, vol. 5). New York: Academic, 1965, p. 9.
19. Lim, R.K.S. A revised concept of the mechanism of analgesia and pain. In R.S. Knighton and P.R. Dumke, eds., *Pain*. Boston: Little, Brown, 1966, p. 117.
20. Martin, W.R. Analgesic and antipyretic drugs: Strong analgesics. In W.S. Root and F.G. Hofmann, eds., *Physiological Pharmacology: Volume 1, The Nervous System—Part A: Central Nervous System Drugs*. New York: Academic, 1963, p. 275. Also:
    Martin, W.R. Opioid antagonists. *Pharmacol. Rev.* 19:463, 1967.

21. Domino, E.F. IX. Effects of narcotic analgesics on sensory input, activating system and motor output. *Res. Publ. Assoc. Res. Nerv. Ment. Dis.* 46:117, 1968.
22. Lewis, J.W., Bentley, K.W., and Cowan, A. Narcotic analgesics and antagonists. *Ann. Rev. Pharmacol.* 11:241, 1971.
23. Pain: Proceedings of the International Symposium on Pain organized by the Laboratory of Psychophysiology, Faculty of Sciences, Paris, April 11–13, 1967. Soularic, A., Cahn, J. and Charpentier, J., eds. New York: Academic, 1968.
24. Wikler, A., ed., *The Addictive States.* Baltimore: Williams & Wilkins, 1968. (*Res. Pub. Assoc. Res. Nerv. Ment. Dis.* 46)
25. Clouet, D.H., ed., *Narcotic Drugs: Biochemical Pharmacology.* New York: Plenum, 1971.
26. Kosterlitz, H.W., Collier, H.O.J., and Villarreal, J.E., eds. *Agonist and Antagonist Actions of Narcotic Analgesic Drugs.* Baltimore: University Park Press, 1971.
27. Braude, M.C., et al., eds., *Narcotic Antagonists.* New York: Raven, 1974. (Advances in Biochemical Psychopharmacology, v8).
28. Rittenhouse, J.D., ed., *The Epidemiology of Heroin and Other Narcotics.* (NIDA Research Monograph 16). Rockville, Md.: National Institute on Drug Abuse, 1977.
29. Dupont, R.I., Goldstein, A., and O'Connell, J., eds. *Handbook on Drug Abuse.* Washington, D.C.: National Institute on Drug Abuse, 1979.
30. Loh, H.H., and Ross, D.H., eds., *Neurochemical Mechanisms of Opiates and Endorphins.* New York: Raven, 1979.
31. Herz, A., ed., *Developments in Opiate Research.* New York: Dekker, 1978.
32. Blum, K., ed., *Alcohol and Opiates: Neurochemical and Behavioral Mechanisms.* New York: Academic, 1977.
33. Cohen, S. *The Substance Abuse Problems.* New York: Haworth, 1981.
34. Goldstein, A., Lowney, L.I., and Pal, B.K. Stereospecific and nonspecific interactions of the morphine congener levorphanol in subcellular fractions of mouse brain. *Proc. Natl. Acad. Sci. U.S.A.* 68:1742, 1971.
35. Pert, C.B., and Snyder, S.H. Opiate receptors: Demonstration in nervous tissue. *Science* 179:1011, 1973. Also:
Pert, C.B., and Snyder, S.H. Opiate receptor binding of agonists and antagonists affected differently by sodium. *Molec. Pharm.* 10:868, 1974.
36. Simon, E.J., Hiller, J.M., and Edelman, I. Stereospecific binding of the potent narcotic analgesic [$^3$H]letorphine to rate-brain hemogenate. *Proc. Natl. Acad. Sci. U.S.A.* 70:1947, 1973.
37. Lowney, L.I., et al. Partial purification of an opiate receptor from mouse brain. *Science* 183:749, 1974.
38. Hiller, J.M., Pearson, J., and Simon, E.J. Distribution of stereospecific binding of the potent narcotic analgesic etorphine in the human brain: Predominance in the limbic system. *Res. Commun. Chem. Pathol. Pharmacol.* 6:1052, 1973.
39. Kuhar, M.J., Pert, C.B., and Snyder, S.H. Regional distribution of opiate receptor binding in monkey and human brain. *Nature* 245:447, 1973.
40. Martin, W.R., et al. The effects of morphine and nalorphine-like drugs in the nondependent and morphine-dependent chronic spinal dog. *J. Pharmacol. Exp. Ther.* 197:517, 1976.
41. Egan, T.M., and North, R.A. Both mu and delta opiate receptors exist on the same neuron. *Science* 214:923, 1981.
42. Vaught, J.L., Kotano, T., and Takemori, A.E. Interactions of leucine-enkephalin and narcotics with opioid receptors. *Mol. Pharmacol.* 19:236, 1981.
43. Frederickson, R.C. Enkephalin: Pentapeptides—A review of current evidence for a physiological role in vertebrate neurotransmission. *Life Sci.* 21:23, 1977.
44. Goldstein, A. Endorphins: physiology and clinical implications. *Ann. N.Y. Acad. Sci.* 311:49, 1978.
45. Hughes, J., and Kosterlitz, H.W. Opioid peptides. *Br. Med. Bull.* 33:157, 1977.
46. Snyder, S.H. Opiate receptors and internal opiates. *Sci. Am.* 236:44, 1977.
47. Terenius, L. Endogenous peptides and analgesia. *Ann. Rev. Pharmacol. Toxicol.* 18:189, 1978.
48. Papadopoulos, C.N., and Keats, A.S. Studies of analgesic drugs—VI: Comparative respiratory depressant activity on phenazocine and morphine. *Clin. Pharmacol. Ther.* 2:8, 1961.
49. Dripps, R.D., and Comroe, J.H., Jr. Clinical studies on morphine—I: the immediate effect of morphine administered intravenously and intramuscularly upon the respiration of normal man. *Anesthesiology* 6:462, 1945.
50. Wikler, A. Studies on the action of morphine on the central nervous system of the cat. *J. Pharmacol. Exp. Ther.* 80:176, 1944.
51. Wang, S.C., and Glaviano, V.V. Locus of

emetic action of morphine and hydergine in dogs. *J. Pharmacol. Exp. Ther.* 111:329, 1954.

52. Fennessy, M.R., and Rattray, J.F. Cardiovascular effects of intravenous morphine in the anesthetized rat. *Eur. J. Pharmacol.* 14:1, 1971.
53. Bodo, R.C., Tui, C., and Benaglia, A.E. Studies on the mechanism of morphine hyperglycemia: Role of the sympathetic nervous system with special reference to the sympathetic supply to the liver. *J. Pharmacol. Exp. Ther.* 62:88, 1938.
54. Louria, D.B., Hensle, T., and Rose, T. The major medical complications of heroin addiction. *Ann. Intern. Med.* 67:1, 1967.
55. White, A.G. Medical disorders in drug addicts. 200 consecutive admissions. *JAMA* 223:1469, 1973.
56. Sturner, W.Q., and Garriott, J.C. Deaths involving propoxyphene. A study of 41 cases over a two-year period. *JAMA* 223:1125, 1973.
57. Eddy, N.B., et al. Drug dependence: Its significance and characteristics. *Bull. WHO* 32:721, 1965.
58. Paton, W.D. Drug dependence: Pharmacological and physiological aspects. *J. R. Coll. Phys. Lond.* 4:247, 1970.
59. Louria, D.B. Medical complications of pleasure-giving drugs. *Arch. Intern. Med.* 123:82, 1969.
60. Dole, V.P., Nyswander, M.E., and Kreek, M.J. Narcotic blockade. *Arch. Intern. Med.* 118:304, 1966.
61. Hofmann, F.G. *A Handbook on Drug and Alcohol Abuse: The Biomedical Aspects.* New York: Oxford, 1975, p. 68.
62. Jaffe, J.H. Drug addiction and drug abuse. In L. Goodman and A. Gilman, eds., *The Pharmacological Basis of Therapeutics*, 4th ed. New York: Macmillan, 1970, pp. 276.
63. Martin, W.R., and Jasinski, P.R. Physiological parameters of morphine dependence in non-tolerance, early abstinence, protracted abstinence. *J. Psychiat. Res.* 7:9, 1969.
64. Eisenman, A.J., Sloan, J.W., Martin, W.R., Jasinski, P.R., and Brooks, J.W. Catecholomine and 17-hydroxycorticoid excretion during a cycle of morphine dependence in man. *J. Psychiat. Res.* 7:19, 1969.
65. Halbach, H., and Eddy, N.B. Tests for addiction (chronic intoxication) of morphine type. *Bull. WHO* 28:139, 1963.
66. Maickel, R.P., and Zabik, J.E. A simple animal test system to predict the likelihood of a drug causing human physical dependence. *Subst. Alcohol Actions Misuse* 1:259, 1980.
67. Jaffe, J.H. The swinging pendulum: The treatment of drug users in America. In R.I. Dupont, A. Goldstein, and J. O'Donnell, eds., *Handbook on Drug Abuse.* Washington, D.C.: National Institute on Drug Abuse, 1979, p. 3.
68. Schuckit, M.A. A theory of alcohol and drug abuse: A genetic approach. In D.J. Lettier, M. Sayers, and H.W. Pearson, eds., *Theories on Drug Abuse: Selected Contemporary Perspectives* (NIDA Research Monograph 30) Washington, D.C.: National Institute on Drug Abuse, p. 297, 1980.
69. Cohen, S. *The Substance Abuse Problems.* New York: Haworth, 1981, p. 175.
70. *Project Speed Syllabus.* Iowa Regional Medical Program, University of Iowa, 1971.
71. Jones R.T., Cannabis. In S.J. Mulé and H. Brill, eds., *Chemical and Biological Aspects of Drug Dependence.* Cleveland, Ohio: CRC Press, 1974, p. 65.
72. Jaffe, J.H. Narcotic analgesics. In L. Goodman and A. Gilman, eds., *The Pharmacological Basis of Therapeutics*, 4th ed. New York: Macmillan, 1970, p. 237.
73. Robbins, E.S., et al. College student drug abuse. *Am. J. Psychiatry* 126:1743, 1970.
74. Hekimian, J.J., and Gershon, S. Characteristics of drug abusers admitted to a psychiatric hospital. *JAMA* 205:125, 1968.
75. Louria, D.B. *The Drug Scene.* New York: McGraw-Hill, 1968.
76. Shure, E. *Crimes Without Victims; Deviant Behavior and Public Policy: Abortion, Homosexuality, Drug Addiction.* Englewood Cliffs, N.J.: Prentice-Hall, 1965.
77. Dimijian, C.G. Contemporary drug abuse. In A. Goth, ed., *Medical Pharmacology: Principles and Concepts*, 5th ed. St. Louis: Mosby, 1970, p. 277.
78. Dismukes, W., et al. Viral hepatitis associated with illicit parenteral use of drugs. *JAMA* 206:1048, 1968.
79. Dewey, W.L. Narcotic analgesics and antagonists. In S.J. Mulé and H. Brill, eds., *Chemical and Biological Aspects of Drug Dependence.* Cleveland, Ohio: CRC Press, 1974, p. 2501.
80. Morrison, W., et al. The acute pulmonary edema of heroin intoxication. *Radiology* 97:347, 1970.
81. Richter, R.W., and Rosenberg, R.N. Transverse myelitis associated with heroin addiction. *JAMA* 206:1255, 1968.
82. Solomon, P. Medical management of drug de-

pendence. *JAMA* 206:1521, 1968.
83. Bewley, T.H. Finding the way. *World Health* 1971, pp. 26–31.
84. Dole, V.P., and Nyswander, M. A medical treatment for diacetylmorphine (heroin) addiction. A clinical trial with methadone hydrochloride. *JAMA* 193:646, 1965.
85. Patch, V.D. Methadone. *N. Engl. J. Med.* 286:43, 1972.
86. Kreek, M.J. Medical safety and side effects of methadone in tolerant individuals. *JAMA* 223:665, 1973.
87. Blinick, G., Wallach, R.C., and Jerez, E. Pregnancy and narcotics addicts treated by medical withdrawal: The methadone detoxification program. *Am. J. Obstet. Gynecol.* 105:997, 1969.
88. Dobbs, W.H. Methadone treatment of heroin addicts. Early results provide more questions than answers. *JAMA* 218:1536, 1971.
89. Beedle, P. The patterns of drug abuse in the United Kingdom. *Adv. Exp. Med. Biol.* 20:114, 1972.
90. Transatlantic debate on addiction. *Br. Med. J.* 3:321, 1971.
91. Cohen, S. *Substance Abuse Problems.* New York: Haworth, 1981, p. 272.
92. *Dealing with Drug Abuse*; a report to the Ford Foundation. P.M. Wald and P.B. Hutt, Co-chairmen. New York: Praeger, 1972.
93. Fink, M., et al. Naloxone in heroin dependence. *Clin. Pharmacol. Ther.* 9:568, 1968.
94. Jaffe, J.H. Cyclazocine in the treatment of narcotic addiction. *Curr. Psychiatry Ther.* 7:147, 1967.
95. Grosz, J.H. Effect of propranolol on active users of heroin. *Lancet* 2:612, 1973.
96. Resnick, R.B., et al. Evaluation of propanolol in opiate dependence. *Arch. Gen. Psychiatry* 33:993, 1976.
97. *The Use of Cannabis. Report of a WHO Scientific Group.* (World Health Organization Technical Report Series No. 478) Geneva: World Health Organization, 1971.
98. Beecher, H.K. Appraisal of drugs intended to alter subjective responses, symptoms. *JAMA* 158:399, 1955.
99. Eisleb, O., and Schaumann, O. Dolantin, ein neuartiges Spasmolytikum und Analgetikum (Chemisches und Pharmakologisches). *Deutsch Med. Wschr.* 65:967, 1939.
100. Cass, L.J., Frederik, W.S., and Andosca, J.B. Quantitative comparison of dextromethorphan hydrobromide and codeine. *Am. J. Med. Sci.* 227:291, 1954.
101. Inaba, D.S., Newmeyer, J.A., and Gay, G.R. I got a yen for that Darvon-N: A pilot study on the use of propoxphene napsylate in the treatment of heroin addiction. *Am. J. Drug/Alcohol Abuse* 1:67, 1974.
102. Tennant, F.S., Tischler, M., Russell, R., et al. *Treatment of Heroin Addicts with Propoxyphene Napsylate.* Committee on Drug Dependence of the New York Academy of Science. Chapel Hill, N.C., March 23, 1973.
103. Beaver, W.T., et al. A comparison of the analgesic effects of pentazocine and morphine in patients with cancer. *Clin. Pharmacol. Ther.* 7:740, 1966.
104. Maugh, T.H. 2d Narcotic antagonists: The search accelerates. *Science* 177:249, 1972.
105. Zaks, A., et al. Naloxone treatment of opiate dependence. A progress report. *JAMA* 215:2108, 1971.
106. Ray, O., *Drugs, Society and Human Behavior.* St. Louis: The C.V. Mosby Co., 1983

## SUGGESTED READINGS

### Monographs and Reviews

Archer, S., Albertson, N.F., and Pierson, A.K. Structure-activity relationships in the opioid antagonists. In H.W. Kosterlitz, H.O.J. Collier, and J.E. Villarreal, eds., *Agonist and Antagonist Actions of Narcotic Analgesic Drugs.* Baltimore: University Park Pr., 1971, p. 25.

Beaver, W.T. Mild analgesics: A review of their clinical pharmacology, I. *Am. J. Med. Sci.* 251:576, 1966.

Beecher, H.K. *Measurement of Subjective Responses: Quantitative Effects of Drugs.* New York: Oxford, 1959.

Braenden, O.J., Eddy, N.B., and Halbach, H. Synthetic substances with morphine-like effect. Relationship between chemical structure and analgesic action. *Bull. WHO* 13:937, 1955.

Brogden, R.N., Speight, T.M., and Avery, G.S. Pentazocine: A review of its pharmacological properties, therapeutic efficacy and dependence liability. *Drugs* 5:6, 1973.

Bucher, K. Pathophysiology and pharmacology of cough. *Pharmacol. Rev.* 10:43, 1958.

Dole, V.P. Biochemistry of addiction. *Ann. Rev. Biochem.* 39:821, 1970.

Eckenhoff, J.E., and Oech, S.R. The effects of narcotics and antagonists upon respiration and circulation in man. A review. *Clin. Pharmacol. Ther.* 1:483, 1960.

Eddy, N.B., Halbach, H., and Braenden, O.J. Synthetic substances with morphine-like effect: Clinical experience; potency, side-effects, addiction liability. *Bull. WHO* 17:569, 1957.

Lasagna, L. The clinical evaluation of morphine and its substitutes as analgesics. *Pharmacol. Rev.* 16:47, 1964.

Le Dain, G. *Final Report of the Commission of Inquiry Into the Non-medical Use of Drugs.* Ottawa, Canada, 1973.

Lees, G.M., Kosterlitz, H.W., and Waterfield, A.A. Characteristics of morphine-sensitive release of neurotransmitter substances. In H.W. Kosterlitz, H.O.J. Collier, and J.E. Villarreal, eds., *Agonist and Antagonist Actions of Narcotic Analgesic Drugs.* Baltimore: University Park Pr., 1971, p. 142.

Lewin, L. *Phantastica; Narcotic and Stimulating Drugs: Their Use and Abuse.* London: Paul, Trench, Trubner, 1931. (Translation of the 2nd German ed., 1924)

Maddux, J.F., and Desmond, D.P. *Careers of Opioid Users.* New York: Praeger.

May, E.L., and Sargent, L.J. Morphine and its modifications. In G. DeStevens, ed., *Medicinal Chemistry* (Analgesics, Vol. 5.) New York: Academic, 1965, p. 123.

Merck Sharp and Dohme Research Laboratories. Medical Literature Dept. *Codeine and Certain Other Analgesic and Antitussive Agents: A Review.* Rahway, N.J.: Merck, 1970.

Miller, R.R., Feingold, A., and Paxinos, J. Propoxyphene hydrochloride: A critical review. *JAMA* 213:996, 1970.

Morley, J.S. Chemistry of opioid peptides. *Br. Med. Bull.* 39(1):5, 1983.

Mulé, S.J. Physiological disposition of narcotic agonists and antagonists. In D.H. Clouet, ed., *Narcotic Drugs: Biochemical Pharmacology.* New York: Plenum, 1971, p. 99.

Murphree, H.B. Clinical pharmacology of potent analgesics. *Clin. Pharmacol. Ther.* 3:473, 1962.

Musto, D.F. *The American Disease: Origins of Narcotic Control.* New Haven, Conn.: Yale University Press, 1973.

Salem, H., and Aviado, D.M., eds. *Antitussive Agents (International Encyclopedia of Pharmacology and Therapeutics,* Section 27.) Oxford: Pergamon, 1970.

Sapira, J.D. The narcotic addict as a medical patient. *Am. J. Med.* 45:555, 1968.

Scrafani, J.T., and Clouet, D.H. Biotransformations. In D.H. Clouet, ed., *Narcotic Drugs: Biochemical Pharmacology.* New York: Plenum, 1971, p. 137.

Sloan, J.W. Corticosteroid hormones. In D.H. Clouet, ed., *Narcotic Drugs: Biochemical Pharmacology.* New York: Plenum, 1971, p. 262.

Terry, C.E., and Pellens, M. *The Opium Problem.* New York: Bureau of Social Hygiene, 1928.

Way, E.L. II. Distribution and metabolism of morphine and its surrogates. *Res. Publ. Assoc. Res. Nerv. Ment. Dis.* 46:13, 1968.

Way, E.L., ed., *Endogenous and Exogenous Opiate Agonists and Antagonists.* New York: Pergamon, 1980.

Way, E.L., and Alder, T.K. *The Biological Disposition of Morphine and Its Surrogates.* Geneva: World Health Organization, 1962.

Way, E.L., and Shen, F.H. Catecholamines and 5-hydroxytryptamine. In D.H. Clouet, ed., *Narcotic Drugs: Biochemical Pharmacology.* New York: Plenum, 1971, p. 229.

Wikler, A. *Opiates and Opiate Antagonists: A Review of their Mechanisms of Action in Relation to Clinical Problems.* (Public Health Monograph Number 52.) Washington, D.C.: Public Health Service, 1958.

Winstock, M.V: In Peripheral tissues. In D.H. Clouet, ed., *Narcotic Drugs: Biochemical Pharmacology.* New York: Plenum, 1971, p. 394.

Chapter 6

# Pharmacology and Clinical Applications of Narcotic Antagonists

## A. INTRODUCTION

Morphine and related narcotics are such effective analgesics or pain killers that they are extensively used despite many side effects, which range from the merely unpleasant to the distinctly dangerous. Safe use of these drugs requires careful adjustment of dosage to provide desirable analgesia and euphoria without severe central nervous system (CNS), especially respiratory, depression. Thus it is almost unbelievable that a specific narcotic antagonist had been known for almost 40 years before the introduction of the antagonists into clinical medicine.[1]

As previously mentioned, narcotic antagonists are usually defined as chemical compounds that block the effects of opiate drugs. They block the analgesia, the euphoria, and all the physiologic changes, such as pupillary constriction, produced by agonist opiates. By blocking the effects, narcotic antagonists also prevent the development of physical dependence on and tolerance to opiate drugs.[2]

Opiate drugs range from morphine, heroin, and other agonists to antagonists such as naloxone and naltrexone. Between the pure agonists and the pure antagonists are drugs such as pentazocine, cyclazocine, and nalorphine, which have mixed agonist and antagonist effects.

The theory underlying narcotic antagonist treatment of heroin dependence is based on the concept of extinction. This assumes that the euphoriant effects of opiate drugs reinforce the self-administration of these drugs. If an ex-dependent person is given a narcotic antagonist and administers an agonist drug, that person will experience no effect—that is, no euphoria. This lack of reinforcement will gradually result in the extinction of heroin self-administration.[3,4] Interestingly, this very unique effect of extinction by an opiate antagonist has been reported for ethanol self-administration in monkeys and rodents.[5] With regard to alcohol treatments, the blockade produced by narcotic antagonists is different from that produced by disulfiram. The agent disulfiram (Antabuse) is a commonly used chemical for the treatment of alcoholism. It exerts its action not by blocking the effects of alcohol on receptor sites,[6] but by interrupting the metabolism of alcohol at the acetaldehyde stage. The build-up of acetaldehyde produces severe symptoms of nausea, vomiting, and hypotension. For some alcoholics, the knowledge that drinking will produce such symptoms may act as a deterrent to further consumption of alcohol. In contrast, narcotic antagonists exert their activity by blocking the access of agonists to the opiate receptor sites at the molecular level. Furthermore, antagonists do not produce symptoms when an agonist is administered. Rather, when opiate receptor sites are occupied by an antagonist, opiate agonists simply have no pharmacologic action.

## B. HISTORY

In 1915, Pohl[7] reported that N-allylnorcodeine antagonized the respiratory depressant effects of morphine. His findings were confirmed by Meissner in 1923[8] and Hart in 1941.[9] Synthesis[10–11] and pharmacology[12–13] of N-allylnormorphine or nalorphine (Nalline) were described in four papers appearing between 1941 and 1944. But, perhaps because the work was done in a search for a nonaddicting analgesic, its significance was not fully realized until Eckenhoff et al.[14] demonstrated in 1951 that nalorphine was an antidote for morphine poisoning in humans. Various workers later showed that it was effective against heroin, other morphine derivatives, and synthetic drugs such as methadone and meperidine. The other basic clinical pharmacologic properties of nalorphine were delineated in the report by Wikler et al. in 1953,[15] that nalorphine could precipitate the abstinence syndrome in morphine-dependent subjects, and in the report of Lasagna and Beecher, 1954,[16] who showed that nalorphine was as potent an analgesic as morphine in humans.

When the potential value of nalorphine was finally realized, many derivatives of morphine and other analgesics were investigated for antagonist activity. Numerous compounds with varying degrees of such activity have been synthesized, but only two others have been marketed. The pharmacology of levallorphan (Lorfan), the N-allyl derivative of levorphan, was described in 1952,[17] and naloxone (Narcan), the N-allyl derivative of oxymorphone, in 1961.[18] The latter is of special interest because it is a pure antagonist with no morphine-like (agonist) actions of its own. All other antagonists studied have varying degrees of agonist action. These agonist–antagonist compounds may be useful as analgesics. One, the benzomorphan pentazocine (Talwin), is marketed for this purpose.

## C. CHEMISTRY OF NARCOTIC ANTAGONISTS[19]

As far back as the early 1900s, scientists began to actively search for specific antidotes for various narcotic-induced responses. The early work was remarkable since at that time there was absolutely no knowledge of the mechanism of narcotic action. In fact, molecular pharmacology or receptology was not understood or researched. Chemists developed substances with narcotic antagonist qualities. N-method substitution with an allyl group in various opioids (codeine, morphine, levorphanol, oxymorphone iphenazone) produces compounds with antagonistic effects in most instances but not always. Complications arise when substances derived from these chemical manipulations result, for example, in products that are not simply pure antagonists but possess agonistic actions as well.

### 1. Structure–Activity

Useful antagonists are N-allyl or chemically equivalent derivatives or morphine congeners, levorphan congeners, or benzomorphan congeners. All are derived from the basic morphine structure, and to understand how a morphine derivative can antagonize such dissimilar chemical types as meperidine and methadone, we must consider the spatial configurations or shape of the molecules. According to Beckett and Casy,[20] the spatial configurations of the morphine-like analgesic molecules are very similar; all seem to fit a receptor provided with a negatively charged anionic site to attract the positively charged nitrogen atom on the analgesic molecule. The molecule is oriented on the receptor by a portion that projects into a cavity near the anionic site and is held to the receptor by physical forces applied to one or more of the rings that lie on the flat surface of the receptor adjacent to the cavity. The receptor will accept only molecules with levo configurations, thus accounting for the fact that the levo forms of analgesics, such as methadone and levorphan, possess analgesic activity and the dextro forms do not. (Levo and dextro forms are mirror images of each other.) The antagonists have the same stereochemical features as the analgesics and presumably compete with the analgesics for the receptor site. The reasons why the N-allyl group or its equivalent confers antagonist properties on the parent compounds, and, especially, the reasons why naloxone is a pure antagonist with virtually no agonist actions, are not known at present.

The chemistry and structure–activity relationship of opioid antagonists have been reviewed by Lewis and associates,[21] Archer and co-workers,[22] and Harris.[20] Structural formulas of nalorphine and levallorphan are shown in Figure 6–1. For greater detail, see Braude et al.[24]

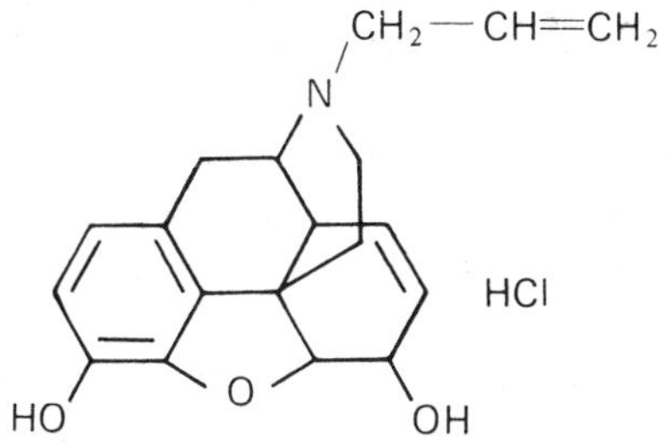

nalorphine hydrochloride

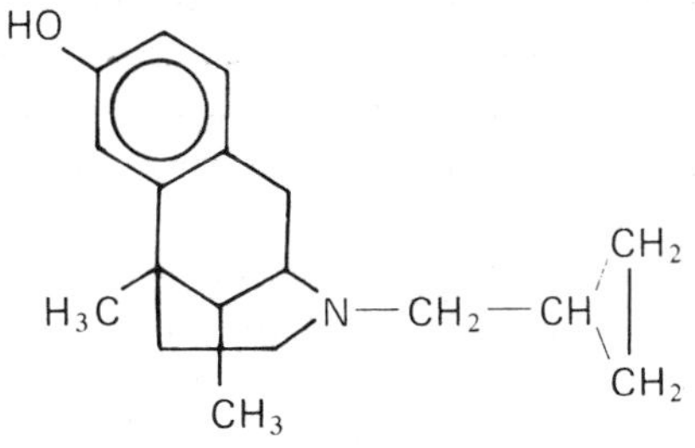

cyclazocine

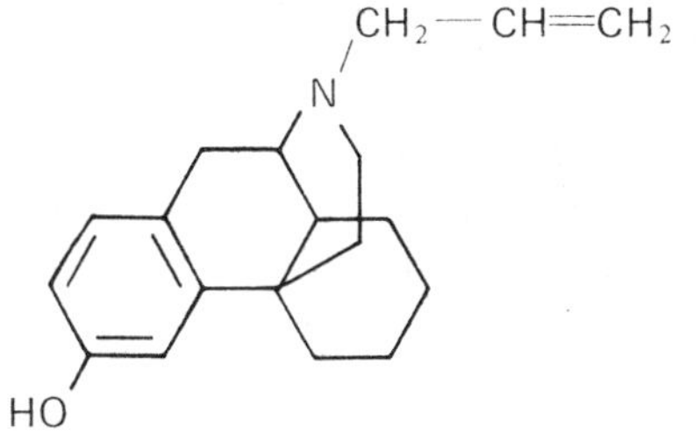

levallorphan

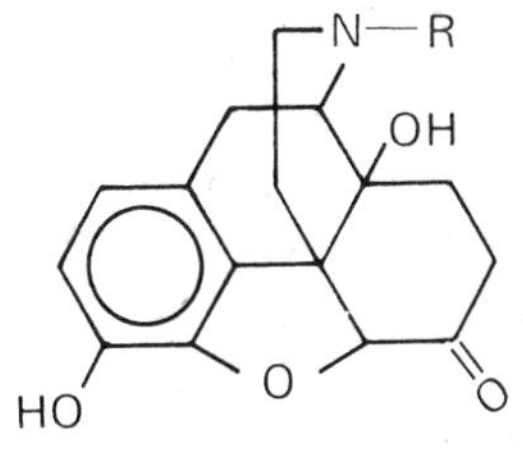

$R = -CH_2CH{=}CH_2$

naloxone

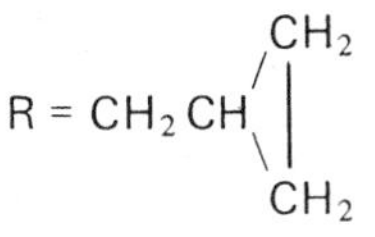

$R = CH_2CH<(CH_2)_2$ (cyclopropylmethyl)

naltrexone

**Figure 6–1**

## D. INTRODUCTION TO PHARMACOLOGY OF OPIOID ANTAGONISTS

In the exciting field of pharmacology there are certain drugs which are considered "agonists" and others are termed "antagonists." As previously mentioned, these two types of drug classes are not always independent, for some drugs constitute a mixed profile of the "agonist-antagonist" or the "partial-agonist" type. For example, Nalorphine, a well-known clinically useful opiate-antidote, is now considered to be a partial agonist. However, the term "opioid antagonist" to describe such drugs as Naloxone and Naltrexone which are pure antagonists present no difficulty. In contrast, such drugs as nalorphine, levallorphon, and cyclazocine, besides powerful antagonistic actions, also induce agonistic responses similar to those of morphine.

The pharmacologic actions of the antagonists differ markedly when they are given alone, as compared with when they are administered after or in combination with narcotics. In general, when agonist–antagonist compounds are administered to normal animals or humans, the effects are qualitatively similar to those of morphine, in that simultaneous stimulation and depression of different parts of the CNS occur. Naloxone differs from other antagonists in that normal or supranormal doses have no subjective or objective effects. On the other hand, all antagonists have a toxic effect in common—the ability to stimulate the CNS to the point of convulsions. Morphine-like compounds and all antagonists, including naloxone, kill rodents such as mice by CNS stimulation and convulsions. Both naloxone and naltrexone have become the most important narcotic antagonists because they have no apparent effects in doses far in excess of those needed to antagonize overdoses of narcotics.[25] In contrast,[15] small doses of agonist–antagonist compounds (5 to 15 mg of nalorphine) have been reported to produce pleasant relaxation and drowsiness, euphoria, dysphoria, daydreams, pinpoint pupils (miosis), nausea, giddiness, sweating, ataxia, droopy eyelids (pseudoptosis), and vomiting. Additional effects of large doses (30 to 75 mg of nalorphine) produce sweating, anxiety, and pressure of thoughts. Many of the symptoms are extremely unpleasant, but can be relieved by 100 to 250 mg of sodium pentobarbital. Respiratory depression, hypotension, and analgesia also may be produced by agonist–antagonist compounds, but with many of these compounds, incidence of dysphoria in patients with postoperative pain is rather high, as compared with morphine. Repeated daily administration of small doses of agonist–antagonist compounds is enjoyed by post-addicts until tolerance develops, but not daily administration of larger doses. Both tolerance and physical dependence have been demonstrated for these compounds, but the abstinence syndrome is qualitatively different from the morphine abstinence syndrome.[26] It appears that the agonist effects predominate at low doses, and it is possible that high doses are less pleasant because of antagonism of the depressant properties by the stimulant actions inherent in the molecules.

When antagonists are administered after an overdose of narcotics, an entirely different effect is obtained. Dogs severely depressed by morphine become alert within 60 seconds of an intravenous injection of an effective dose of an antagonist, exhibiting an apparently complete reversal of the morphine actions. On the other hand, antagonism of the lethal stimulant effects of narcotics in rodents has not been shown, although there is some evidence that naloxone affords some protection against convulsions in mice. In humans, the agonist actions of nalorphine or levallorphan may increase the depression in subjects minimally depressed by narcotics, but the drugs will antagonize the depressant effects of narcotics in patients who are comatose or semicomatose, an effect also observed with alcohol overdose.[27]

In the treatment of narcotic overdose, the superiority of naloxone as an antagonist is derived from its lack of agonist actions. It will reverse even minimal depression resulting from narcotics and, if the depression is attributable to some other drug, it will not be deepened by naloxone. If severe narcotic depression exists, an effective dose of naloxone will promptly reverse the depression. Respiration quickens and conscious patients may notice the loss of euphoria. If the patient is comatose, ventilation and hypotension will improve and the patient may awaken sufficiently to respond to usual auditory, tactile, or visual stimuli. The dose of antagonist may have to be repeated one or more times, at 90- to 120-minute intervals, since the action of most narcotics is longer than the action of naloxone.

In general anesthesia, utilizing the narcotic technique, respiratory depression can be combated with small doses of naloxone without appreciably lightening the anesthesia. In this situation, too much antagonist will reverse analgesia and require additional doses of narcotics or the substitution of another anesthetic agent.

Although narcotic antagonists effectively will reverse the depression produced by overdoses of narcotics, the effects of these compounds, when given to animals or humans who are tolerant or addicted to narcotics, are the sudden production of severe signs and symptoms of abstinence.[28] Abstinence phenomena can be precipitated by narcotic antagonists after administration of 15 mg of morphine four times daily for only two to three days. Peak effects occur in less than an hour, and subside over a period of several hours. The greater the tolerance, the greater is the severity of the abstinence phenomena produced by a given dose of antagonist. A severe reaction initially might include dilated pupils, sweating, rapid breathing, restlessness, nausea, and muscular aching, followed by yawning, tearing, running nose, and gooseflesh. Very small doses produce little more than dilated pupils and vague symptoms of discomfort, but large doses in highly dependent or tolerant-dependent subjects can result in a severe abstinence syndrome, which, unlike the abstinence syndrome following the withdrawal of a narcotic, occasionally may be fatal.

## E. PHARMACOKINETICS AND METABOLISM

High-purity antagonists such as naloxone and naltrexone have advantages over drugs that have both agonist and antagonist properties. Thus their main function is to block the agonist effect. Naloxone and naltrexone are almost pure antagonists; therefore, they seem to counteract CNS depression very effectively. They are most efficient when administered by different routes. Their duration of action or lasting effect differs when they are administered orally.

Naloxone is absorbed orally, but is only 1/50th as potent as when given parenterally. This is so because of its rapid metabolism in the liver.[29] Even an oral dose in excess of 1 gram is metabolized within 24 hours. Naltrexone, on the other hand, like cyclazocine, has cyclopropylmethyl substitution on the nitrogen and is more effective when administered orally. Its effect can last as long as 24 hours.[30] Apparently, when naloxone is metabolized in the liver, it rapidly conjugates with glucuronic acid as other small amounts of metabolites are simultaneously produced.[29] This same reasoning seems also appropriate for the effects of nalorphine. Like levallorphan, nalorphine is most effective during parenteral administration. Within a time span of three to four hours, nalorphine is found in the brain in amounts three to four times higher than the same dose of morphine. However, a rapid decrease is evident after four hours.

## F. BASIC PHARMACOLOGIC PROPERTIES

Great clinical benefits would be obtained if a new drug could be discovered which is safe, non-addicting, has few side effects, has strong potency with a high degree of selectivity, is of long duration, and is orally effective as a pure opiate antagonist. In terms of potential commercialization for the treatment of chemical dependency of the opiod type, the substance must be inexpensive or at least not prohibitively expensive to produce.

Naloxone, although it possesses some of the qualities, frequent administration prevents overall patient acceptability and clinical usefulness. Research is ongoing for long-acting pure narcotic antagonists. Naloxone is a prototype for the development of the ideal drug.

Pharmacologically it eliminates euphoria, nausea, respiratory depression, and the gastrointestinal disturbances induced by opiates. Furthermore, in the absence of opioids, naloxone is almost lacking in agonistic actions. Zaks and associates[32] reported that oral 1-gram amounts of naloxone failed to induce any significant subjective or physiological responses. Additionally, subcutaneous doses of up to 12 mg. result in little or no observable effects and even higher doses of up to 24 mg. produces only slight sedation. Martin and co-workers[30] reported that naltrexone has the important quality of being a pure antagonist with a longer duration than naloxone. Other longer acting antagonists will be discussed herein.

Nalorphine unlike "pure antagonists" produce an array of pharmacological actions in doses of 5 to 15 mg. which include morphine-like autonomic effects; lowering of body temperature; heart rate changes; $CO_2$-reduced sensitivity; anti-diuretic hormone (ADH) inhibition of release; constriction of the pupil; and analgesia at 10 to 15 mg. doses. In some patients nalorphine produces such unpleasant reactions as "crazy feelings," anxiety, marked hallucinations (visual), and the feeling of being drunk. Although the pain-relieving qualities of Nalorphine do not parallel increases in dose, the psychotiminetic affects are usually enhanced. Low doses in drug-free addicts produce a general dysphoric feeling closer to the alcohol and barbiturate experience than to the experience of morphine.

The agonistic effects of nalorphine are the result of kappa rather than mu receptor interaction.

## 1. Mechanisms of Action[18]

### *a. Pharmacologic View*

Studies by several researchers provide evidence that agonist and antagonist drugs function at the molecular level by binding, or not binding, stereospecifically to opioid receptor sites.

In the first study, by Goldstein and associates,[37] a large membrane-bound mouse brain proteolipid was extracted and partially purified to provide data on the stereospecific binding of the opiate receptors. They found that this proteolipid, approximately 60,000 daltons in mass, was like a major opiate receptor. It would bind selectively to agonist levorphanol, but would not easily bind to naloxone. Furthermore, the pharmacologic effects are the result of the agonist receptor binding and a consequent conformational change. Besides the opiate receptor there are second messengers that also respond to the display of pharmacologic effects due to the agonist or partial agonist properties.[36,38–40] In light of the stereospecific binding of agonist or antagonist to the opiate receptor, it is important to recognize and understand what the receptor itself is like. A study by Pert and Snyder[39] reveals that brain homogenate receptors seem dependent on the presence of sodium ions to determine either agonist or antagonist actions. Similar rationale is suggested by Ross and Cardenas,[41] but with calcium and/or calmodulin as key regulators of opiate receptor configuration. In the former study using sodium ions, the observation is that the nature of the receptor is largely dependent on the conformational change due to the sodium ion, which will, in turn, determine the presence of agonist or antagonist properties. In vitro, drugs having a mixture of agonist or antagonist properties could, hypothetically, exert their action in either direction. Their preference would depend on the special effect of sodium ions, which determine the form of the receptor, or its action at the allosteric site. Similar methods of experimentation may be useful in studying new compounds and testing for relative agonist and antagonist properties of drugs.

### *b. Clinical View*

Theories regarding the mechanisms of action of the narcotic antagonists[42] have been clouded by the fact that most are based on studies that have utilized agonist–antagonist-type compounds. It is likely that molecules of antagonist and narcotic vie competitively for cell receptor sites. Most of the phenomena described can be accounted for if it is assumed that the antagonist has a greater affinity for the receptor than the narcotic does. If naloxone is given to a subject who is mildly depressed by the narcotic, the effects of the narcotic will disappear. If the depression is severe, small doses of naloxone will antagonize the respiratory depressant effect of the narcotic, and larger doses will antagonize the analgesic and euphorigenic effects as well. This dose–action relationship clearly suggests that naloxone is competitively taking receptor sites away from the narcotic. Precipitation of abstinence effects in tolerant individuals also can be explained by displacement of the narcotic from the receptor sites by the antagonist, which, in effect, amounts to withdrawal of the narcotic medication.

An alternate hypothesis postulates that the antagonist acts through mechanisms responsible for physical dependence. This theory assumes that the relationship between physical dependence and the narcotic doses tolerated is paralleled by the relationship between the effectiveness of the narcotic antagonist and the depression produced by the narcotic. The theory assumes that the antagonist can produce some effects that are definitely more than substitutions for the effects of the narcotic. Production of withdrawal symptoms is an example of this, as is the fact that abstinence syndromes are usually opposite to the ordinary effects of narcotics.

Patients with narcotic depression treated successfully with antagonists may exhibit restlessness, dilated pupils, increased blood pressure, and rapid breathing, which are also components of the abstinence syndrome. In fact, this hypothesis is based on phenomena related to narcotic withdrawal. It may be related to the dualistic theory of narcotic action, which postulates simultaneous stimulation and depression of different centers in the CNS and assumes that withdrawal symptoms are due to persistence of the stimulant actions of the narcotic after the depressant effects have passed. Since the antagonists do not antagonize the stimulant actions of the narcotics, they might act by counteracting the depressant effects and thus unmasking the stimulant effects.[43] Obviously, as with narcotics, the mechanism of action of the narcotic antagonists is not completely understood.

## 2. Antagonist Effects

The advantages of naloxone as an antagonist easily surpass the effects of mixed agonist and antagonist properties displayed by nalorphine and other drugs of this type. For example, in situations where the causes for CNS and respiratory depression are not known and the patient may be at a risk, the advantage of pure antagonist drugs, including naloxone and especially naltrexone, cannot be overemphasized. Immediate effects are seen after the injection of naloxone in counteracting opioid drug actions. Its duration of action usually lasts for one to four hours, but varies depending on the dose that is used. Some of the rapidly exerted effects of naloxone include respiratory elevation, sedation, and the return of normal blood pressure. It is important to note that naloxone is known to elevate respiratory rates higher than before the opiate-induced respiratory depression. This is known as the ''overshoot'' phenomenon and is explained by the possible unwinding effect due to acute physical dependence. Small doses of 0.4 to 0.8 mg of naloxone exhibit respiratory elevation within one to two minutes. One milligram of naloxone completely blocks 25 mg of heroin.[32] Much higher doses (10–15 mg) are needed to reverse the psychotomimetic and dysphoria effects of nalorphine and cyclazocine.

The antagonist quality of naloxone is unquestionable. However, not all respiratory depressants are aided by its superior antagonist property. All other nonopioid CNS depressants, including alcohol and barbiturates, are apparently less affected by opioid antagonists. On the contrary, nalorphine-type antagonists are less efficient as antagonists, and may even contribute to the respiratory depression already there, caused by the CNS depressant. This is not to say that nalorphine is ineffective in opposing opioid effects. Like naloxone, when injected in doses of 5–10 mg, nalorphine exerts rapid antagonist properties, within one to two minutes in severe respiratory cases. Its effect can last from one to four hours. Similar to naloxone, nalorphine also antagonizes gastrointestinal effects and the morphine-induced antidiuretic, hypothermic, and antitussive effects may go unnoticed, since nalorphine also displays agonist properties.

Although it is known that nalorphine produces its own respiratory depressant effects which could add to already existing CNS depression induced by alcohol, barbiturates or other non-opioid drugs, other ''pure antagonists'' do not affect respiratory depression induced by those CNS depressants.

## 3. Clinical Pharmacologic Properties

The drug of choice for the treatment of opioid overdose, because of its pure antagonist properties, is naloxone. However, as soon as phase III clinical trials are completed, naltrexone will be the drug of choice. It is for this reason that the section on clinical pharmacology of opioid antagonists focuses on naltrexone instead of naloxone.

Naltrexone (N-cyclopropylmethyl-noroxymorphine), synthesized by Blumberg et al. in 1965,[45] has a longer duration of action and greater potency than its N-allyl congener, naloxone.[46] Naltrexone is also orally efficacious at significantly lower doses than naloxone.

### *a. Opiate Receptor Blockade*

In a paper by Vereby,[47] the time–action of opiate antagonist activity of naltrexone was evaluated in detoxified ex-opiate-dependent persons, using 25 mg of intravenous heroin challenges. A 100-mg naltrexone dose provided 95 percent blockade at 24 hours, 86.5 percent blockade at 48 hours, and 46.6 percent blockade at 72 hours. Following oral administration, naltrexone was rapidly and completely absorbed. Peak levels of naltrexone and its major metabolite, 6 beta-naltrexol, were reached one hour after the dose. According to Vereby, the high 6-beta-naltrexol plasma concentrations only one hour after drug administration indicate a rapid biotransformation process, converting a large fraction of the dose to less active metabolites. Over 70 percent of the dose was excreted in the 24-hour urine collection and less than 0.5 percent in the feces. Vereby and associates[47] also report that no change was observed in the rate of naltrexone disposition during chronic dosing versus acute dosing, indicating no metabolic induction. These authors conclude, on the basis of their studies, that the rapid achievement of steady-state naltrexone plasma levels eliminates the need for stepwise induction at the beginning of naltrexone treatment.

Opiate blockade by naltrexone can be observed by inspection of Figure 6–2, taken from a study by Vereby et al.[48]

### *b. Metabolism*

The major metabolite of naltrexone in humans is 6-beta-naltrexol, isolated by Cone in 1973,[49] and the structure was confirmed by Chatterjie et al. in 1974.[50] A minor metabolite, 2-hydroxy-3-methoxy-6-α-naltrexol (HMN), was isolated by Vereby et al.[51] and its structure was confirmed by Cone et al.[52]

Quantitatively 6-α-naltrexol is the most abundant metabolite formed and is excreted both free and conjugated. Naltrexone is mostly glucuronidated before excretion and HMN is found only in the free form.

The opiate antagonistic activity of 6-β-naltrexol varies from 1/50th to 1/12th of that of naltrexone,[53,54] depending on the species and methods used. Use of the opiate receptor binding assay from rat brain synaptosome preparations indicated that although HMN was antagonistic, the affinity to the opiate receptor was 1000 times less than that of the parent compound, naltrexone.

Typical urinary patterns of excretion of naltrexone and metabolites are depicted in Tables 6–1, 6–2, and 6–3.

Naloxone is also biotransformed extensively after oral administration, but into inactive glucuronides. Vereby[47] suggests that this fact may be the reason for naloxone's short time–action. The longer duration of action of naltrexone may be due to the formation of active metabolites 6-β-naltrexol and HMN. This occurs in much the same way as the formation of active metabolites prolongs the time–action of l-acetylmethadol, in contrast to methadone, which is converted into inactive metabolites.

## 4. Tolerance, Addiction and Abuse Potential

Basically, there is little or no abuse liability

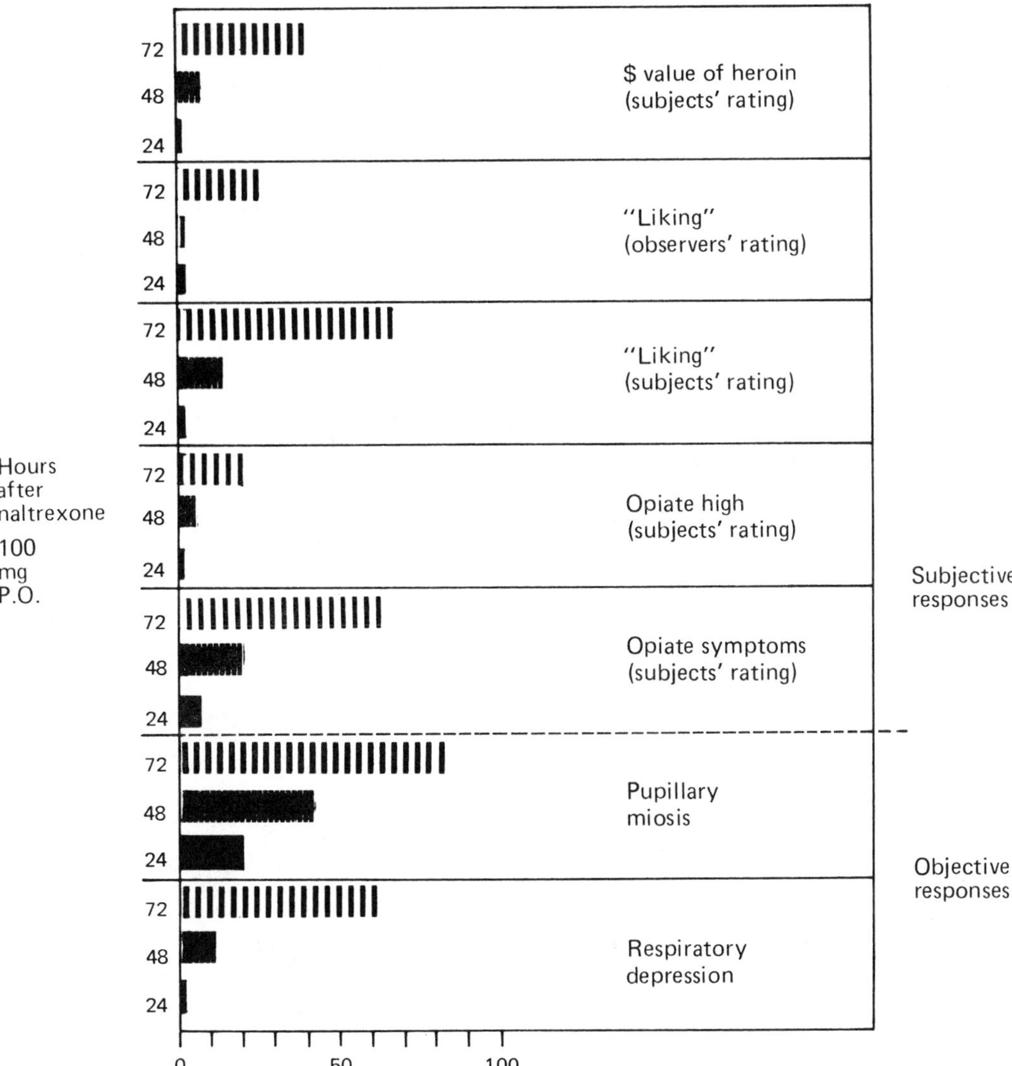


**Figure 6–2. The percent objective and subject responses are shown after 25 mg I.V. heroin, 24, 48, and 72 hours after 100 mg oral naltrexone. The 100 percent heroin responses were determined in the absence of naltrexone.**
**(From Vereby, K., et al.** *Clin. Pharmacol. Ther.* 20:315, 1976. With permission.)

with pure antagonists, but tolerance and potential addiction do develop to the agonistic effects of nalorphine and cyclazocine, representatives of the partial agonist type. Tolerance has been observed in patients under the influence of both nalorphine and cyclazocine, with regard to the dysphoric and other mental effects. In these tolerant individuals, 4 mg. of cyclazocine abolished the major pharmacologic actions of heroin and morphine.

Martin,[42] in a review of the literature revealed that cross-tolerance exists between various partial agonists such as cyclazocine and nalorphine. There is ample evidence that high-dose nalorphine and cyclazocine result in both tolerance and physical withdrawal symptoms.

However, there is not enough evidence to indicate that abrupt withdrawal of high-dose naloxone or naltrexone results in observable abstinence signs.

In the case of the nalorphine abstinence syndrome, there is a brief sensation which has been described as "electric shocks to the head" or, as Jaffe and Martin point out, "light-headedness" or "fainting spells."[19] Other noticeable signs include lacrimation, yawning, nose-running, chills, fever, diahhrea, and loss of appetite followed by a significant degree of weight reduction. All these symptoms, however, are less prominent than those observed with morphine. Certainly, there is no real craving or drug-seeking behavior for nalorphine as there is with morphine during the so-called "sick" phase of withdrawal.

**TABLE 6–1[47]**

**Concentration Ratio 6 α-Naltrexol/Naltrexone in 24 Hours**

| *Subjects* | *Acute* | *Chronic* |
|---|---|---|
| 1 | 3.4 | 2.5 |
| 2 | 3.6 | 4.0 |
| 3 | 3.6 | 3.3 |
| 4 | 2.7 | 3.4 |
| Mean | 3.3 | 3.3 |
| ± SD | 0.4 | 0.6 |

**TABLE 6–2**

**Urinary Excretion of Naltrexone and Metabolites, 24-Hour Collection[47] (Percent of Dose Excreted)**

| | **Naltrexone** | | **6 β-naltrexol** | | **2-hydroxy-3-methoxy 6 β-naltrexol** | |
|---|---|---|---|---|---|---|
| | *Free* | *Bound* | *Free* | *Bound* | *Free* | *Total* |
| Acute | 1.0 | 7.2 | 19.1 | 7.1 | 3.5 | 37.9 |
| Chronic | 1.1 | 15.0 | 29.0 | 17.5 | 7.6 | 70.2 |

**TABLE 6–3**

**Fecal Excretion of Naltrexone and Metabolites, 24-Hour Collection (Percent of Dose Excreted)**

| | *Naltrexone* | *6 β-naltrexol* | *2-hydroxy-3-methoxy 6 β-naltrexol* | *Total* |
|---|---|---|---|---|
| Acute | 0.13 | 1.9 | 0.08 | 2.1 |
| Chronic | 0.29 | 2.9 | 0.44 | 3.6 |

Following withdrawal from Pentazocine, profadol, or propiram, drug-seeking behavioral predispositions can be expected. The same withdrawal characteristics associated with nalorphine and morphine are present after withdrawal from Pentazocine. In the case of profadol or propiram abstinence, reactions similar to morphine are seen.

Quite simply, the range of effects produced by a drug determines the potential for abuse of that drug. This may include mainly physical dependence, unpleasant effects, desire for euphoric experience, and the absence of a drug-seeking or "craving." Morphine-type physical dependence is not supported by naloxone, nalorphine, naltrexone and cyclazocine, which are seen by post-addicts as either neutral or unpleasant in relation to subjective effects, failing to produce the range of physical dependence most often associated with drug-seeking behavior. Thus, their threshold for abuse potential is virtually non-existent. Profidal and propiram are exceptional in their capacity to precipitate abstinence at high levels of morphine physical dependence, while otherwise exhibiting morphine characteristics. Nonetheless, they are thought to possess an abuse potential nearing the level of morphine and related opioids.[29,33,42,55,56]

## G. CLINICAL APPLICATIONS

### 1. Treatment of Narcotic Poisoning[1]

The clinical applications of the narcotic antagonists are obvious. Naloxone or naltrexone ideally constitutes the therapy of choice in narcotic poisoning when severe respiratory, and possibly cardiovascular, depression exists. Methadone overdosage has been successfully treated with 0.4 mg of naloxone/30 minutes by I.V. drip overnight.[21] This method is preferable to repeated naloxone injections because it provides continuous reversal of the toxic effects of methadone, which may last for 24 hours. For overdose of shorter acting narcotics, an initial dose of 0.4 mg of naloxone may be given, preferably by the intravenous route. If necessary, the dosage may be repeated twice, at five-minute intervals, and again if depression recurs. Naloxone is such a specific narcotic antagonist that if there is no increase in ventilation or lightening of coma, some other cause for the depression should be considered. It is not very useful against depression resulting from barbiturates or similar drugs. Early reports to the contrary concerning nalorphine were founded on the stimulant action of high doses of the morphine-like drugs, including the antagonists, which had been noted in animal studies. If narcotic addiction is suspected, naloxone should be used cautiously, lest an abstinence syndrome be precipitated. A comatose, tolerant addict may respond to as little as 0.1 mg of naloxone.

In balanced anesthesia, the narcotic technique is increasing in popularity due to the suspicion that many of the newer halogenated inhalation agents are toxic to operating room personnel. Naloxone may be used for the treatment of narcotic depression during or following anesthesia. A dose as small as 0.1 mg may make the diagnosis, and only enough should be given to provide adequate ventilation; larger doses will reverse analgesia and more anesthesia will be required. One- or two-tenths milligram of naloxone is usually sufficient for narcotic depression in anesthesia. If two repetitions of this dose do not improve the situation, some other component of the anesthetic should be suspected. If naloxone is given postoperatively to reverse narcotic-induced respiratory depression, the patient should be watched carefully to make sure that the antagonist does not wear off, causing depression. Again, minimal doses of naloxone should be used to prevent reversal of the analgesic effect of the narcotic.

In obstetrics, naloxone may be used to prevent or treat depression in infants whose mothers have received doses of narcotic antepartum. If respiratory depression is present in the mother, 0.4 mg of naloxone should be administered at least ten minutes prior to delivery, if the infant is to benefit. To treat narcotic depression in the newborn whose mother has not received an antagonist, naloxone, 5 micrograms per kilogram (μg/kg), may be given in the umbilical vein.

The dose may be repeated twice at two-minute intervals if the infant has not responded.

## 2. Diagnosis of Opiate Dependence

In the past, the narcotic antagonist nalorphine in full antagonist doses was used to diagnose opiate-dependent and -tolerant abusers by its precipitation of severe withdrawal reactions. But this technique was dangerous and it was later discovered that small doses of the narcotic antagonist nalorphine (Nalline) would produce dilated pupils in narcotic-addicted individuals. This led to the development of the Nalline, or pupil, test for narcotic abuse. However, more recently urinalysis has for the most part replaced the "Nalline test." In 1973, Blachy[57] reported that naloxone could be utilized effectively to diagnose the degree of opiate dependence and used as a predictor to implement methadone maintenance treatment. It has also been observed that when naloxone is given with nalorphine, a more sensitive pupil test results.[58] Great advances will be made when newer antagonists are found that block both delta receptors and $\mu_1$ and $\mu_2$ or other opioid receptors as well. In the non-opioid user, naloxone or naltrexone alone will not cause any pupil effect.

## 3. Treatment of Narcotic Addiction by Continuous Blockade

Narcotic antagonists also have been used for the ambulatory treatment of abstinent dependent persons, since no tolerance develops to their antagonist actions and they block the euphoria sought by drug users who self-inject narcotics. As previously mentioned, their simple blocking action differs from that of disulfiram (Antabuse) in alcoholism in that alcohol produces very uncomfortable effects when taken by a patient on disulfiram. Naloxone and naltrexone are ideal drugs for narcotic blockade because of their lack of effects when given alone. Unfortunately 2.5 to 3 grams of naloxone are required to produce a 24-hour blockade against 50 mg of heroin when the naloxone is given orally.[59] Some hope has been expressed for partial blockade by naloxone in doses up to 800 mg per day,[60] but better results can be expected when a slow-release preparation is found that, after a single injection, can produce blockade for a period of days, weeks, or months. Indeed parenteral sustained-release naltrexone systems have been developed and await further clinical testing on humans.[61] The immediate future of naltrexone will see the completion of clinical testing and its marketing for general use. The real question is whether naltrexone, because of its pure antagonist effects, will be accepted by most patients willing to forfeit euphoria from heroin, or will be useful only as a crisis drug.

Cyclazocine, a long-acting antagonist with some agonist properties, has also been used to block the effects of injected narcotics.[62] The early studies were hampered by a high incidence of secondary effects, but doses have been raised to an effective level of 4 mg per day with the aid of the blockade of some side effects by oral naloxone. Four milligrams of cyclazocine a day will block 25 mg of heroin for about 20 hours. Recently it has been possible to raise the dose of cyclazocine to 20 mg per day, which will block 25 mg of heroin for up to 48 hours.

If drug dependence is an example of classical conditioning and therapy is an extinction of conditioned responses, treatment with narcotic blocking agents, such as methadone or narcotic antagonists, will be successful if patients who receive the blockading compound do not experience the euphoria, symptom relief, or physiologic effects of the narcotic when they attempt to self-administer it. Repeated disappointments following self-injection should lead to extinction of psychologic and physical aspects of dependence. With more than a decade of experience with this type of treatment of narcotic addiction, reports are beginning to appear that a fairly good percentage, perhaps as high as 50 percent, of patients may be withdrawn from treatment and remain free from narcotics for at least a year. It seems likely, however, that there always will be some patients who will require drug therapy for narcotic addiction until a better treatment is discovered. Certainly drug therapy for narcotic addiction leaves much to be desired and is highly controversial, but at least it has provided a new approach to treatment, with the consequent rethinking of the problem, which may eventually lead to a more permanent solution.

### 4. Antagonists as Analgesics

Finally, narcotic antagonists in which the agonist–antagonist ratio is high have some promise as strong analgesics. As noted earlier, nalorphine was shown to be, milligram for milligram, as potent as morphine, but it produces a high incidence of unpleasant mental effects. As a direct result of the finding that narcotic antagonists have analgesic properties, pentazocine (Talwin) was developed and is marketed as a strong analgesic for relief of moderate to severe pain.[63] It is an N-allyl derivative of phenazocine and has weak narcotic antagonist activity. It is about one third as potent as morphine and has side effects similar to those of morphine and related compounds. The incidence of subjective psychotomimetic effects produced by the usual therapeutic doses is lower than seen with nalorphine. The drug has a low but definite abuse potential. Pentazocine may seem a small step toward separating the analgesic from the dependence-producing properties of the narcotic analgesics, but it seems unlikely that a pure analgesic will be developed by manipulation of known molecules with morphine-like analgesic properties. Further advances in this field most likely will arise from the study of entirely different chemical types with analgesic action.

By way of summary, and because of the recent interest in narcotic antagonists from both a research and a treatment viewpoint, the history of the use of these agents for the treatment of heroin dependence is reviewed in the following section. Today these agents are also being used following detoxification with methadone.

## H. ANALYSIS OF THE USE OF NARCOTIC ANTAGONISTS IN TREATMENT OF DRUG DEPENDENCIES

As early as 1965, Martin, Wikler, and their colleagues decided to use narcotic antagonists in conjunction with good treatment programs in helping to treat opiate-dependent persons.[64,65] They focused primarily on the physical aspects of the problem: helping the addict to remain drugfree.

Drs. Martin and Wikler and colleagues have shown that animals and humans are abnormal for at least six months after cessation of daily use of opiates.[66] This may be part of the basis for the fact that there is a precipitated abstinence syndrome in some patients years after they get out of prison, when they go back to their old "copping" areas. The body has been made abnormal in some way. The essence of this theory is that if one protects the body from feeling any effects when a person takes opiates—and assuming the person is undergoing emotional and intellectual rehabilitation, is working or in job training, and has a reasonable education, a stable family life, and psychologic, psychiatric, medical, and dental care—the narcotic antagonists used for several months to several years may be of help during that early period without opiates. Neither Dr. Martin nor Dr. Wikler postulated that lifelong maintenance on narcotic antagonists would be needed. They see narcotic antagonists merely as chemotherapeutic adjuncts to a treatment program.

Over the years, since these important contributions by Martin and coinvestigators, the narcotic antagonists nalorphine, cyclazocine, naloxone, and naltrexone have been clinically employed and studied. A brief summary of their use and problems, as discussed by Dr. Arnold Schecter,[67] is presented here.

a. Nalorphine (Nalline)

Nalorphine was the first narcotic antagonist so used. It was not found to be useful in humans for conditioning from the use of opiates because, while it had some narcotic antagonist properties, it also had some morphine-like or agonist properties.[66] Therefore, people could become dependent to nalorphine and could feel some desired morphine-like symptoms.

b. Cyclazocine

The next drug used was cyclazocine.[68] It proved to be an almost but not quite pure narcotic antagonist. It was found that 4 mg blocked the effects of 15 mg heroin for up to 24 hours.[69] It became popular in the 1960's in about six treatment programs, including that of Dr. Jerome Jaffe and his colleagues in New York and Chicago[70] and Drs. Fink, Freedman, Resnick and others in New York City.[71]

Cyclazocine, taken orally, was obviously a very powerful narcotic antagonist, was relatively long-acting, but had certain disadvantages. A small percentage of patients would hallucinate and have racing thoughts, the latter like an amphetamine high, on cyclazocine when first placed on it. (This is referred to as a psychotomimetic or psychosis imitating effect of the drug.) This usually occurred on the first few days on the drug, during the induction phase. These unpleasant side effects made cyclazocine extremely unpopular among many patients and made inpatient induction a necessity. Very few patients want to be in a hospital for two-to-three weeks, first to become drug- (opiate) free and then to be gradually built up on cyclazocine. In addition, unlike methadone, which was becoming popular at exactly the same time, it was impossible to get high on the drug, which didn't really satisfy the drug craving in quite the same way that methadone did, although it was partly agonistic or morphine-like.

A finding by Fink, Freedman, Resnick and colleagues[71] at the New York Medical College in the '60's was that if naloxone, a completely pure narcotic antagonist, was given, it would alleviate the hallucinations and racing thoughts caused by cyclazocine, side effects which, presumably, were due to the agonistic action of the drug. They did not extend their findings far enough to use naloxone prophylactically, i.e. before the patient started taking cyclazocine, in order that there would never be any psychotomimetic effects. Presumably, the reasons for this were that the majority of the patients did not experience such effects and within five days, a gradual buildup of from 0 to 5 mg would be possible on cyclazocine. The next step, of course, would be to use naltrexone, a long-acting form of naloxone, prophylactically during cyclazocine induction routinely, to avoid dysphoric effects and yet continue using this very powerful (milligram for milligram) drug.

In addition, cyclazocine was not terribly popular because occasional patients would give their cyclazocine to methadone-maintenance patients or heroin addicts. The antagonists precipitate abstinence in a very fast, almost irreversible fashion, if given to someone who has not been gradually withdrawn from opiates and drug-free for a few days in advance. Thus, cyclazocine developed something of a bad street reputation. Also, programs centered around cyclazocine were competing with methadone programs and with drug-free therapeutic community programs, for the most part, in whatever cities they were found.

Cyclazocine programs and, later, naloxone programs, were also getting a bad reputation, because they were being used on prisoners in programs like Dr. Brahan's in Nassau County, New York, where prisoners with opiate problems were allowed to go to work after taking their narcotic antagonist and come back to the prison at the end of the day.

c. Naloxone (Narcan®)

Naloxone was tried next as a pure narcotic antagonist that had to be taken in doses of 3000 mg at one time, if the effect were to last to block 25 mg or more of intravenous heroin for 24 hours or more.[59] Such enormous doses were prohibitively expensive; thebain, from which the drug came, was in short supply and such large doses caused severe gastrointestinal distress, including nausea, vomiting and diarrhea. However, in conjunction with day-care programs, with the patient taking 800 mg of naloxone at the end of the day, to last until the next day, this treatment worked with limited success. Dr. Kleber and colleagues, at Yale in New Haven, Connecticut, seemed to have reasonable success in a young population with this method of therapy. Naloxone is normally used under Endo Laboratories' trade name of Narcan®, as the treatment of choice for narcotic overdose in emergency rooms. The drug is an extremely pure narcotic antagonist and seems to be very safe. Naloxone has, in fact, been tried in animals in long-acting depot preparations which have been prepared by Dr. Semour Yolles of the University of Delaware Chemistry Department and has been tested in dogs by Drs. William Martin, Virginia Sandquist and others at Lexington.[72,73] The drug, in a depot form, will block the effects of opiates for up to 21 days in animals. However, the polylactate and other forms in which the drug is now available have not yet been proven safe for human use. P.H. Marks et al.[74] used a biodegradable drug delivery system based on aliphatic polyester application to narcotic antagonists. They concluded, based on exploratory experiments with narcotic antagonists, that the polyacetate approach is feasible and that it is only necessary to optimize the various components to achieve a practical device.

d. Naltrexone

The next logical suggestion was presented by Dr. William Martin, when he spoke to Dr. Blumberg at Endo Laboratories and suggested that they try adding the chemical group (a cyclopropylmethyl group) that he thought was making cyclazocine long-acting to the naloxone molecule to see if naloxone, a pure antagonist, couldn't be made long-acting. Fortunately, it turned out that hallucinations were not caused by the cyclopropylmethyl group but, in fact, that group simply made naloxone very long-acting, and a new drug called at first Endo-1639A and now known as naltrexone was synthesized in 1963, at Endo Laboratories, by Dr. Matossian, at Dr. Harold Blumberg's suggestion.[36,45,75]

After extensive trials in dogs and then in limited trials in humans, conducted under the aegis of Drs. Martin, Jasinski, Mansky and other co-workers at the Lexington Addiction Research Center,[31] limited human trials were begun by Drs. Richard Resnick[77] and Arnold Schecter,[78] working independently, in January of 1973. Both groups of investigators found that naltrexone appears to be very safe medically, at least in the limited number of patients studied to date, that the patients received the drug very well, but that high intervention therapy appears necessary to retain patients in therapy and to obtain good habilitation or rehabilitation of the clients.

Interestingly enough, the patients who are in the narcotic antagonist program at the Downstate Medical Center/Kings County Hospital in Brooklyn are usually black or Puerto Rican males (these drugs have not yet been proven safe in women who may have children), who are articulate, upwardly-mobile and do not want to be on opiate maintenance for the rest of their lives. The drug's popularity is becoming markedly higher as outpatient induction becomes the method of choice. Three-day-a-week high-dose naltrexone is the primary method employed. At the Downstate Medical Center/Kings County Hospital, naltrexone induction usually takes place over a five-day period, with the patient stabilized at 125 mg of naltrexone which she/he then receives on Monday, Wednesday and Friday only. For four days a week, the patient is not required to come to the drug abuse program. This has met with reasonable popularity, but there is also something of a fear, particularly in the black population, that this program may be experimenting on them. By taking naltrexone daily for two months, Schecter was able to alleviate some of the fears by being a subject in a medical experiment. The emotionally more secure members of the population seem very desirous of receiving naltrexone as the last step before being opiate-free. This is particularly true of methadone maintenance patients, who have a great fear of not being able to make it in those first difficult months when the rate of relapse to illegal opiates is so high. While there has been a very vocal anti-methadone sentiment among Third World people, based on frequently justified fear and reaching almost hysterical limits at times, much of this fear must be considered legitimate, considering how disadvantaged minorities traditionally are treated.

## I. NARCOTIC IMMUNIZATION

In 1972 and 1973, Dr. Jerome Jaffe, the first director of the Special Action Office for Drug Abuse Prevention, an arm of the Executive Branch of the U.S. government, had suggested that narcotic antagonists could be used to "immunize" the population in a high-risk area such as Harlem, and that this could be done by giving shots of the long-acting drug to youngsters, or possibly even putting it in the drinking water in areas of high addiction. This proposal met with a marked outcry of protest among black and Puerto Rican New Yorkers, as an attempt to experiment on humans. In fact, the Tuskegee syphilis studies, conducted by the United States government, in which syphilitic black male patients were left untreated for the duration of their lives even though a cure for syphilis was known, provided real and frightening evidence to persons who did not relish further experiments on their bodies without their control or consent. As previously mentioned, scientists are actively engaged in studies concerned with the formation of antibodies directed toward opiate-like derivatives.[79]

## J. SIDE EFFECTS OF NARCOTIC ANTAGONISTS

There are certain problems associated with the clinical application of narcotic antagonists. For instance, the duration of action with earlier discovered agents such as nalorphine (Nalline) prompted the synthesis of longer acting substances such as naltrexone. Another problem is that naloxone (Narcan), for example, is only inertly active when given by the oral route. Side effects of therapeutic doses include dysphoria and, in some patients, hallucinations. In non-drug users,[61] cyclazocine induced side effects similar to those of the antidepressant drug imipramine (Tofranil). Narcotic antagonists with prominent "narcotomimetic" (agonistic) characteristics produce tolerance and physical dependence on regular usage, and a (relatively mild) withdrawal syndrome develops if intake is stopped or abruptly or markedly decreased. Certainly some of these problems can be circumvented when the sustained-release naltrexone product is made clinically available to the general public.

## K. SUMMARY

A meaningful assessment of the probable value of rehabilitation programs in which narcotic antagonists are used will require considerably more data than are available now. Clearly we need information about larger groups of patients and longer periods of time (i.e., years, not weeks or months, or treatment). And even these numbers will probably be of limited value only. As Martin et al. point out in reference to cyclazocine[64]: "Since this method of treatment controls only the pharmacological factors responsible for drug-seeking behavior, its effectiveness will be directly related to the importance of the pharmacological factors in the disease." Because it is believed that psychic and genetic factors are probably of much greater importance in the majority of patients than are pharmacologic ones, the success of narcotic antagonist programs will be determined largely by the nature of the "ancillary" services offered the patients, and by how competently these services are rendered. The underlying mechanisms for opiate-seeking behavior may involve both genetics and environment, and unless we delineate exactly how these elements mediate this compulsive behavior, eradication or indiscriminate drug misuse will be influenced only superficially.

## REFERENCES


1. Goth, A. *Medical Pharmacology*, 9th ed. St. Louis: Mosby, 1978, p. 297.
2. Archer, S. Historical perspective on the chemistry and development of naltrexone. In R.E. Willette and G. Barnett, eds., *Narcotic Antagonists: Naltrexone Pharmaco-Chemistry and Sustained Release Preparations*. (NIDA Research Monograph 28) Washington, D.C.: NIDA, 1981.
3. Martin, W.R., Gorodetzky, C.W., and McLane, T.K. An experimental study in the treatment of narcotic addicts with cyclazocine. *Clin. Pharmacol. Ther.* 7:455, 1966.
4. Dewey, W.L. Narcotic analgesics and antagonist. In S.S. Mulé and H. Brill, eds., *Chemical and Biological Aspects of Drug Dependence*. Cleveland, Ohio: CRC Press, 1974, p. 25.
5. Altshuler, H., Appelbaum, E., and Shippenberg, T.S. The effects of opiate antagonists on the discriminative stimulus properties of ethanol. *Pharmacol. Biochem. Behav.* 14:97, 1981.
6. Hiller, J.M., Angel, L.M., and Simon, E.J. Multiple opiate receptors: Alcohol selectively inhibits binding to delta receptors. *Science* 214(4519):468, 1981.
7. Pohl, J. Ueber das N-Allylcodein, einen Antagonisten des Morphins. *Z. Exp. Path. Ther.* 18:370, 1915.
8. Meissner, R. Ueber Atmungeserringende Heilmittel. *Z. Dtsch, Exp. Med.* 31:159, 1923.
9. Hart, E.R. N-allyl-norcodeine and N-allyl-normorphine: Two antagonists to morphine. *J. Pharmacol. Exp. Ther.* 72:19, 1941.
10. McCawley, E.L., Hart, E.F., and Marsh, D.F. The preparation of N-allylnormorphine. *J. Am. Chem. Soc.* 63:314, 1941.
11. Weijlard, J., and Ericksen, A.E. N-allylnormorphine. *J. Am. Chem. Soc.* 64:869, 1942.
12. Hart, E.R., and McCawley, E.L. The pharmacology of N-allylnormorphine as compared with morphine. *J. Pharmacol. Exp. Ther.* 82:339, 1944.
13. Unna, K. Antagonistic effect of N-allyl-normorphine upon morphine. *J. Pharmacol. Exp. Ther.* 79:27, 1943.
14. Eckenhoff, J.E., Elder, J.D., and King, B.D. The effect of N-allyl-normorphine in treatment of opiate overdose. *Am. J. Med. Sci.* 222:115, 1951.
15. Wikler, A., Fraser, H.F., and Isbell, H. N-allylnormorphine: Effects of single doses and precipitation of acute abstinence syndromes during addiction to morphine, methadone or heroin in man (post-addicts). *J. Pharmacol. Exp. Ther.* 109:8, 1953.
16. Lasagna, L., and Beecher, H.K. The analgesic effectiveness of nalorphine and nalorphine-morphine combinations in man. *J. Pharmacol. Exp. Ther.* 112:356, 1954.
17. Fromherz, K., and Pellmont, B. Morphinantagonisten. *Experientia* 8:394, 1952.
18. Blumberg, H., Dayton, H.B., George, M., and Rapaport, D.N. N-allylnoroxymorphone: A potent narcotic antagonist. *Fed. Proc.* 20:311, 1961.
19. Jaffe, H.J., and Martin, W.R. Narcotic analgesics and antagonists. In R.S. Goodman and A. Gilman, eds., *The Pharmacological Basis of Therapeutics*, 5th ed. New York: Macmillan, 1975, p. 245.
20. Beckett, A.H., and Casy, A.F. Synthetic analgesics: Stereochemical considerations. *J. Pharm. Pharmacol.* 6:986, 1954.
21. Lewis, J.W., Bentley, K.W., and Cowan, A. Narcotic analgesics and antagonists. *Ann. Rev. Pharmacol.* 11:241, 1971.

22. Archer, S., Albertson, N.F., and Pierson, A.K. Structure–activity relationships in the opioid antagonists. In H.W. Kosterlitz, J.O.J. Collier, and J.E. Villarreal, eds., *Agonist and Antagonist Actions of Narcotic Analgesic Drugs*. Baltimore: University Park Press, 1973, p. 25.
23. Harris, L.S. Narcotic antagonists: Structure-activity relationships. In M.C. Braude et al., eds., *Narcotic Antagonists*. New York: Raven, 1974, p. 13.
24. Braude, M.C., et al., eds. *Narcotic Antagonists*. New York: Raven, 1974.
25. Jasinski, D.R., Martin, W.R., and Haertzen, C.A. The human pharmacology and abuse potential of N-allylnoroxymorphone (naloxone). *J. Pharmacol. Exp. Ther.* 157:420, 1967.
26. Martin, W.R., and Gorodetzky, C.W. Demonstration of tolerance to and physical dependence on N-allylnormorphone (nalorphine). *J. Pharmacol. Exp. Ther.* 150:437, 1965.
27. Mackenzie, A.I. Naloxone in alcohol intoxification. *Lancet* 1(8118):733, 1979.
28. Goldstein, A. The search for the opiate receptor. In *Pharmacology and the Future of Man. Proceedings of the Fifth International Congress on Pharmacology*, vol. 1. Basel: Karger, 1973.
29. Nutt, J.G., and Jasinski, D.R. Methadone-naloxone mixtures for use in methadone maintenance programs. I. An evaluation in man of their pharmacological feasibility. II. Demonstration of acute physical dependence. *Clin. Pharmacol. Ther.* 15:156, 1974.
30. Martin, W.R., Jasinski, D.R., and Mansky, P.A. Naltrexone, an antagonist for the treatment of heroin dependence. Effects in man. *Arch. Gen. Psychiatry* 28:784, 1973.
31. Weinstein, S.H., Pfeffer, M., and Schor, J. Metabolism and pharmacokinetics of naloxone. In M.C. Braude et al., eds., *Narcotic Antagonists*. New York: Raven, 1974, p. 525.
32. Zaks, A., et al. Naloxone treatment of opiate dependence. A progress report. *JAMA* 215:2108, 1971.
33. Keats, A.S., et al. Morphine antagonists in man. In *Minutes of the 21st Meeting of Committee on Drug Addiction and Narcotics*. Appendix 2. Washington, D.C.: NAS-NRC, 1960.
34. Gilbert, P.E., and Martin, W.R. The effects of morphine and nalorphine-like drugs in the nondependent, morphine-dependent and cyclazocine-dependent chronic spinal dog. *J. Pharmacol. Exp. Ther.* 198:66, 1976.
35. Egan, T.M., and North, R.A. Both mu and delta opiate receptors exist on the same neuron. *Science* 214:923, 1981.
36. Lord, J.A., et al. Endogenous opioid peptides: Multiple agonists and receptors. *Nature* 267:495, 1977.
37. Goldstein, A. Endorphins: Physiology and clinical implications. *Ann. N.Y. Acad. Sci.* 311:49, 1978.
38. Lowney, L.I., et al. Partial purification of an opiate receptor from mouse brain. *Science* 183:749, 1974.
39. Pert, C.B., and Snyder, S.H. Opiate receptor: Demonstration in nervous tissue. *Science* 179:1011, 1973. Also: Opiate receptor binding of antagonists and antagonists affected differentially by sodium. *Molec. Pharmacol.* 10:868, 1974.
40. Rosenfeld, G.C., Strada, S.J., and Robinson, C.A. Cyclic nucleotides and the central effects of opiates: An overview of current research. In H.H. Loh and D.H. Ross, eds., *Neurochemical Mechanisms of Opiates and Endorphines. Advances in Biochemical Psychopharmacology*. New York: Raven, 1979.
41. Ross, D.H., and Cardenas, H.L. Nerve cell calcium as a messenger for opiate and endorphin actions. In H.H. Loh and D.H. Ross, eds., *Neurochemical Mechanisms of Opiates and Endorphines. Advances in Biochemical Psychopharmacology*. New York: Raven, 1975.
42. Martin, W.R. Opioid antagonists. *Pharmacol. Rev.* 19:463, 1967.
43. Jacquet, Y.F. Opiate effects after adrenocorticotropin or beta-endorphin injection in the periaqueductal grey matter of rats. *Science* 201(4360):1032, 1978.
44. Jasinski, D.R., Martin, W.R., and Hoeldtke, R.D. Effect of short- and long-term administration of pentazocine in man. *Clin. Pharmacol. Ther.* 11:385, 1970.
45. Blumberg, H., Pachter, I.J., and Matossian, Z. 14-Hydroxydihydromorphinone derivatives. *U.S. Patent no. 3,332,950*, July 25, 1967.
46. Blumberg, H., and Dayton, H.B. Naloxone and related compounds. In H.W. Kosterlitz, H.O.J. Collier, and J.E. Villarreal, eds., *Agonist and Antagonist Actions of Narcotic Analgesic Drugs*. Baltimore: University Park Press, 1973, p. 110.
47. Vereby, K. The clinical pharmacology of naltrexone: Pharmacology and pharmacodynamics. In R.E. Willette and G. Barnett, eds., *Narcotic Antagonists: Naltrexone Pharmacochemistry and Sustained Release Preparations*. (NIDA Research Monograph 28) Washington, D.C.: NIDA, 1981, p. 147.
48. Vereby, K., et al. Naltrexone: Disposition, metabolism and effects after acute and chronic dos-

ing. *Clin. Pharmacol. Ther.* 20:315, 1976.

49. Cone, E.J. Human metabolite of naltrexone (N-cyclopropylmethylnoroxy-morphone) with a novel 6-isomorphine configuration. *Tetrahedron Lett.* 28:2607, 1973.
50. Chatterjie, N., and Inturrisi, C.E. Stereospecific synthesis of the 6β-hydroxy metabolites of naltrexone and naloxone. *J. Med. Chem.* 18:490, 1975.
51. Vereby, K., Chedekel, M.A., Mulé, S.J., and Rosenthal, D. Isolation and identification of a new metabolite of naltrexone in human blood and urine. *Res. Comm. Chem. Pathol. Pharmacol.* 12:67, 1975.
52. Cone, E.J., et al. The identification and measurement of two new metabolites of naltrexone in human urine. *Res. Comm. Chem. Pathol. Pharmacol.* 20:413, 1978.
53. Vereby, K., and Mulé, S.J. Naltrexone pharmacology, pharmacokinetics and metabolism: Current status. *Am. J. Drug Alcohol Abuse* 2:357, 1975.
54. Blumberg, H., and Ikeda, C. Comparison of naltrexone and β-naltrexol for narcotic antagonist action in rats and mice. *Fed. Proc.* 35:469, 1976.
55. Jasinski, D.R. Effects in man of partial morphine agonists. In H.W. Kosterlitz, H.O.J. Collier, and J.F. Villarreal, eds., *Agonist and Antagonist Actions of Narcotic Analgesic Drugs*. Baltimore: University Park Press, 1973, p. 94.
56. Waldron, V.D., Klimt, C.R., and Seibel, J.E. Methadone overdose treated with naloxone infusion. *JAMA* 225:53, 1973.
57. Blachly, P.H. Naloxone for diagnosis in methadone programs. *JAMA* 224:334, 1973.
58. Elliott, H.W., Nomof, N., and Parker, K.D. The use of naloxone in the pupil test for the detection of narcotic abuse. In *Proceedings of the Fourth National Conference on Methadone Treatment*. New York: National Association for the Prevention of Addiction to Narcotics, 1972, p. 35.
59. Fink, M., et al. Naloxone in heroin dependence. *Clin. Pharmacol. Ther.* 9:568, 1968.
60. Kurland, A.A., et al. Naloxone and the narcotic abuser: A low-dose maintenance program. *Int. J. Addict.* 8:127, 1973.
61. Olsen, J., and Kinel, F.A. A review of parenteral sustained-release naltrexone systems. In R.E. Willette and G. Barnett, eds., *Narcotic Antagonists: Naltrexone Pharmacochemistry and Sustained Release Preparations*. (NIDA Research Monograph 28) Washington, D.C.: 1981, p. 187.
62. Fink, M. Questions in cyclazocine therapy of opiate dependance. *Psychopharmacol. Bull.* 9:38, 1973.
63. Brodgen, R.N., Speight, T.M., and Avery, G.S. Pentazocine: A review of its pharmacological properties, therapeutic efficacy and dependence liability. *Drugs* 5:6, 1973.
64. Jaffe, J.H. Cyclazocine in the treatment of narcotic addiction. *Curr. Psychiat. Ther.* 7:147, 1967.
65. Wikler, A. Conditioning factors in opiate addiction and relapse. In D.M. Wilner and G.G. Kasselbaum, eds., *Narcotics*. New York: McGraw-Hill, 1965, p. 85.
66. Martin, W.R., et al. Tolerance to and physical dependence on morphine in rats. *Psychopharmacologia* 4:247, 1960.
67. Schecter, A. Consumer acceptance of drug abuse programs: A provider's view. *J. Psychedel. Drugs* 6:213, 1974.
68. Fraser, H.F., and Rosenberg, D.E. Comparative effects of (1) chronic administration of cyclazocine (ARC-II-C-3) (II) substitution of nalorphine for cyclazocine and (III) chronic administration of morphine. Pilot crossover study. *Int. J. Addict.* 1:50, 1966.
69. Freedman, A.M., et al. Clinical studies of cyclazocine narcotic addiction. *Am. J. Psychiatry* 124:1499, 1968.
70. Jaffe, J.H., and Brill, L. Cyclazocine: A long-acting narcotic antagonist: Its voluntary acceptance as a treatment modality by narcotics abusers. *Int. J. Addictions* 1:99, 1966.
71. Resnick, R., Fink, M., and Freedman, A.M. A cyclazocine typology in opiate dependence. *Am. J. Psychiatry* 126:1256, 1970.
72. Martin, W.R., and Sandquist, V.L. Long-acting narcotic antagonists. Presented to Committee on Problems of Drug Dependence. National Academy of Sciences–National Research Council, 1972.
73. Martin, W.R., and Sandquist, V.L. A sustained release depot for narcotic antagonists. *Arch. Gen. Psychiatry* 30:31, 1974.
74. Marks, P.H., Marks, C.G., Marks, T.A., and Schindler, A. Biodegradable drug delivery systems based on aliphatic polyesters: Application to contraceptives and narcotic antagonists. In R.E. Willette and G. Barnett, eds., *Narcotic Antagonists: Naltrexone Pharmacochemistry and Sustained Release Preparations*. (NIDA Research Monograph 28) Washington, D.C.: NIDA, 1981, p. 232.
75. Fink, M. Narcotic antagonists in opiate dependence. *Science* 169:1005, 1970.
76. Blumberg, H., and Dayton, H.B. Narcotic an-

tagonist studies with EN-1639A (N-cyclopropylnoroxymorphone hydrocholoride). Fifth International Congress on Pharmacology, *Abstracts of Volunteer Papers*, 1972, p. 23.

77. Stone-Washton, Resnick, R.B., and Washton, A.M. Naltrexone and psychotherapy. In *Problems of Drug Dependence, 1981, Proceedings of the 43rd Annual Scientific Meeting*, the Committee on Problems of Drug Dependence, Inc. (NIDA Research Monograph 41). Washington, D.C.: NIDA, 1982, p. 505.
78. Schecter, A.J., and Grossman, D.J. Naltrexone in a clinical setting, preliminary observations. Presented to the Committee on Problems of Drug Dependence. National Academy of Sciences. Washington, D.C.: National Research Council, 1974.
79. Berkowitz, B., and Spector, S. Evidence for active immunity to morphine in mice. *Science* 178:1290, 1972.
80. Hofmann, F.L. *A Handbook on Drug and Alcohol Abuse. The Biomedical Aspects*. New York: Oxford University Pr., 1975, p. 68.

## SUGGESTED READINGS

Bucher, K. Pathophysiology and pharmacology of cough. *Pharmacol. Rev.* 10:43, 1958.

Clouet, D.H., ed. *Narcotic Drugs: Biochemical Pharmacology*. New York: Plenum, 1971.

Dole, V.P. Biochemistry of addiction. *Ann. Rev. Biochem.* 39:821, 1970.

Domino, E.F., IX. Effects of narcotic analgesics on sensory input, activating system and motor output. *Res. Publ. Assoc. Res. Nerv. Ment. Dis.* 46:117, 1968.

Duggan, A.W. Narcotic antagonist—Problems in the interpretation of their effects in laboratory and clinical research. *Adv. Pain Research* 5:309, 1982.

Eckenhoff, J.E., and Oech, S.R. The effects of narcotics and antagonists upon respiration and circulation in man: A review. *Clin. Pharmacol. Ther.* 1:483, 1960.

Eddy, N.B., Halbach, H., and Braenden, O.J. Synthetic substances with morphine-like effect: Clinical experience, potency, side-effects, addiction liability. *Bull. WHO* 17:569, 1957.

Lim, R.K.S. A revised concept of the mechanism of analgesia and pain. In R.S. Knighton and P.R. Cumke, eds., *Pain*. Boston: Little, Brown, 1966, p. 117.

Martin, W.R. Analgesic and antipyretic drugs: Strong analgesics. *Physiolog. Pharmacol.* 1:275, 1963.

May, E.L., and Sargent, L.J. Morphine and its modifications. *Analgesics* 5:123, 1965.

Merck Sharp and Dohme Research Laboratories. Medical Literature Dept. *Codeine and Certain Other Analgesic and Antitussive Agents: A Review*. Rahway, N.J.: Merck, 1970.

Miller, R.R., Feingold, A., and Paxinos, J. Propoxyphene hydrochloride: A critical review. *JAMA* 213:996, 1970.

Mulé, S.J. Physiological disposition of narcotic agonists and antagonists. In D.H. Clouet, ed., *Narcotic Drugs: Biochemical Pharmacology*. New York: Plenum, 1971, p. 99.

Murphree, H.B. Clinical pharmacology of potent analgesics. *Clin. Pharmacol. Ther.* 3:473, 1962.

Musto, D.F. *The American Disease: Origins of Narcotic Control*. New Haven: Yale Univ. Press, 1973.

Reynolds, A.K., and Randall. *Morphine and Allied Drugs*. Toronto: Univ. of Toronto Press, 1957.

Salem, H., and Aviado, D.M., eds. *Antitussive Agents*, 3 vol. (International Encyclopedia of Pharmacology and Therapeutics, Section 27). Oxford: Pergamon, 1970.

Sapira, J.D. The narcotic addict as a medical patient. *Am. J. Med.* 45:555, 1968.

Scrafani, J.T., and Clouet, D.H. The metabolic disposition of narcotic analgesic drugs: Biotransformations. In D.H. Clouet, ed., *Narcotic Drugs: Biochemical Pharmacology*. New York: Plenum, 1971, p. 137.

Sloan, J.W. The effects of narcotic analgesic drugs on general metabolic systems: Corticosteroid hormones. In D.H. Clouet, ed., *Narcotic Drugs: Biochemical Pharmacology*. New York: Plenum, 1971, p. 262.

Soulairac, A., Cahn, J., and Charpentier, J., eds. *Pain*. New York: Academic, 1968.

Terry, C.E., and Pellens, M. *The Opium Problem*. New York: Committee on Drug Addictions with the Bureau of Social Hygiene, 1928.

Way, E.L. Distribution and metabolism of morphine and its surrogates. *Res. Publ. Assoc. Res. Nerv. Ment. Dis.* 46:13, 1968.

Way, E.L., and Adler, T.K. The pharmacologic implications of the fate of morphine and its surrogates. *Pharmacol. Rev.* 12:383, 1960.

Way, E.L., and Shen, F.H. Effects of narcotic analgesic drugs on specific systems: Catecholamines and 5-hydroxytryptamine. In D.H. Clouet, ed., *Narcotic Drugs: Biochemical Pharmacology*. New York: Plenum, 1971, p. 229.

Weinstock, M. Sites of action of narcotic analgesic

drugs: in peripheral tissues. In D.H. Clouet, ed., *Narcotic Drugs: Biochemical Pharmacology*. New York: Plenum, 1971, p. 394.

Wikler, A. *Opiates and Opiate Antagonists. A Review of Their Mechanisms in Relation to Clinical Problems*. (Public Health Monograph No. 52). Washington, D.C.: U.S. Government Printing Office, 1958.

Winter, C.A. The physiology and pharmacology of pain and its relief. In G. deStevens, ed., *Medicinal Chemistry* (Analgetics, vol. 5). New York: Academic, 1965, p. 10.

# Chapter 7

# Methadone and Other Narcotic Maintenance Drugs:

## PHARMACOLOGIC ISSUES, MYTHS, AND REALITIES

### A. INTRODUCTION[1]

Since the introduction of methadone maintenance to the armamentarium of treatment modalities for drug dependence of the opiate type, there has been tremendous misunderstanding concerning the merits of methadone, as well as its limitations and alleged evils and hazards.

An incredible attitudinal polarization also persists, to occupy the opposite ends of the full spectrum of confusion. And at these poles are the more vocal individuals, which may contribute to the persistence of the confusion.

Of particular concern is the fact that a great deal of this confusion exists within the army of people involved in treatment programs. It is certainly no surprise that with the rapid expansion of such programs, workers have been recruited from every possible source. It is to be expected that very few among these recruits will have had any specialized practical experience or training in drug dependence. However, to allow workers to continue merely to fill a slot, to assume responsible roles in treatment programs with no understanding of drug dependence in general, and even less understanding of methadone as an adjunct in treatment, is a tragic solution at best.

The lack of a rational and practical perspective toward methadone and its use in treatment includes even those persons charged with the responsibility for determining the relevant controls and guidelines. It is apparent that at least some of the various complicated regulations we must live with are the result of political compromise, rather than of a scientific and objective evaluation of the available data.

At all levels, it appears that the choice of an attitudinal position concerning methadone (as if we are supposed to choose a favorite team) is far too often based on emotional, moral, political, and philosophic grounds, than on objective evaluation and understanding of the drug-dependence problem and the utilization of methadone, including full recognition of its value, limitations, hazards, and how it can fit into, and enhance, other treatment approaches.

The purpose of this chapter is to establish a

rational perspective from which to view methadone as an adjunct in the treatment of opiate drug dependence in relation to the total problem, as well as its relationship to other treatment modalities. This task must include, of course, a discussion of the properties of the drug, along with an effort to deal with some of the extreme positions both for and against. Some of the more prevalent myths are discussed simply by stating exactly what methadone is, how it is similar to other opiate-like drugs, and how it differs from them. The chapter is not intended to promote a particular position or attitude, but to set forth an accurate description in such a manner as to encourage a realistic and objective understanding by physicians faced with the problem of heroin dependence. This will allow the reader to form an opinion on the basis of fact rather than on emotional reactions mixed with misunderstanding and inaccurate information. Any interpretation that this chapter is trying to sell methadone is unfortunate; the intent is to place it in an objective position in relation to other tools currently at our disposal.

## B. HISTORY

The pharmacologic profile of methadone is similar to that of morphine. Methadone came into clinical use after its synthesis by German chemists at the end of World War II. It has been utilized as a substitute for heroin because it is very similar to it. However, they do differ in that methadone is effective when taken orally (with an effect approximately equivalent to 45 percent of an intramuscular dose), and it has a longer duration of action than heroin.[3] These two properties are the basis for methadone's long-standing clinical use as a maintenance drug for opiate abusers as well as its use as a short-term detoxification agent.

Medical uses for methadone include reduction of pain as an analgesic, amelioration of withdrawal symptoms from chronic opiate abuse, and as a maintenance drug for the opiate abuser. Federal regulations still classify the use of the drug for maintenance as experimental and require that it only be taken in authorized research programs.

Today methadone plays a significant role in the street. It is used for self-imposed withdrawal to lose tolerance to heroin and thus reduce daily supply requirements and also for "mainlining" or oral usage to produce a "high." The number of addicts utilizing methadone has increased. The problem of street diversion into illicit channels is becoming uncontrollable and street deaths have been reported from overdoses of the drug. By 1971, some 10,000 heroin addicts were under treatment in New York City and Washington, D.C., and there were, as of January 1981, 83,370 patients being treated with methadone for maintenance and 3340 patients treated with methadone as a detoxification drug (according to information obtained from the Division of Methadone Monitoring, Food and Drug Administration).

## C. CHEMISTRY

The evaluation of structural-activity relationships for the synthetic compounds of the Methadone series have striking similarities in terms of analgesic properties, respiratory depressant action and dependance liability with their parent congener as well as with morphine.[3,4,5]

In terms of steric chemistry, the pseudopiperidine ring confers opioid activity and the resolution of the racemic mixture provides the l-methadone and d-methadone. Clinical evaluation reveals that the l-isomer is between 10–50 times more potent as a painkiller than is the d-form.

There is general consensus that drugs that resemble each other in some part of their molecular structure may be expected also to be similar in their chemical function. A good example of this is the drug, isomethadone, which is different from methadone only in the methyl group in the side chain (Figure 7–1), and retains opioid activity.

## D. PHARMACOLOGY[1-4]

The most important feature about methadone is that after 18 years since Dole began maintaining chronic opiate (heroin) abusers on chronic doses of methadone, it has become the most popular form of treatment, as evidenced by the approximate 90,000 patients in such programs.

The main pharmacological property which affords methadone such recognition is its so-called heroin "blocking" properties, which will be described later in more detail. Although, any narcotic could serve as an opioid maintenance substance, methadone has the advantages of being long-acting, effective orally with few side effects, and relatively inexpensive.

However, the general pharmacologic properties of methadone are similar to morphine in terms of opioid activity, smooth muscle, heart and circulatory actions, as well as respiratory actions.

### *Central Nervous System (CNS)*

Although the chemical structures of heroin, morphine, and methadone are quite different, their potencies as analgesics are similar. Approximately 2 mg. of methadone can substitute as a painkiller for 2 mg. of heroin and 4 mg. of morphine.[2,3] In non-tolerant adults, the lethal dose of methadone hydochloride is 75 mg.

Early literature by the Isbell group[6] or Martin and Associates[7] documents that although single doses of methadone produce less sedative effects than morphine at equivalent doses, chronic administration in some patients has induced severe sedation. The central nervous system effects of methadone include: 1) suppression of the release of gonadotropic hormones by the anterior pituitary, 2) hyperglycemia, 3) miosis, 4) respiratory depression, 5) antitussive effects, 6) hypothermia and 7) release of Anti-Diuretic Hormone, (ADH).

### *Actions on Smooth Muscle Target Organs*

Over the past decade clinicians have become aware of the side effects produced by methadone maintenance. To date, research has not been able to uncover significant evidence for cellular damage. Certain of these side effects are due to the effects of methadone on smooth muscle. Smooth muscle studies of the biliary tract, ureters, and uterus have been done in humans to determine methadone's extent of action.

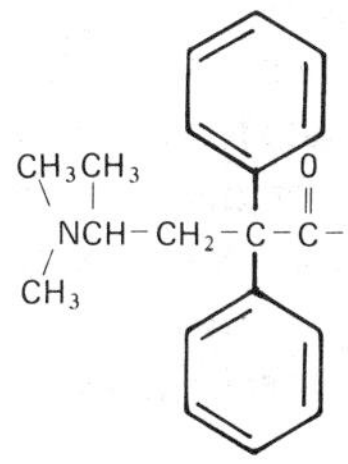

**Figure 7-1. Methadone (Amidon; Dolophine).**

### *Heart and Circulatory Effects*

Scrutiny of the literature reveals that methadone has insignificant cardiovascular actions. The only effects appearing are peripheral vasodilation and orthostatic hypotension. There are no Electrocardiogram (EEG) pattern changes, nor is there any interference on cardiovascular reflex activity.

## E. PHARMACODYNAMICS AND METABOLISM

The basic pharmacodynamic properties of a drug and its destruction in the body (metabolism) are important prerequisites for clinical acceptability and usefulness as a therapeutic agent. In this regard, methadone outweighs heroin as an opioid maintenance agent. The prime reasons for its clinical effectiveness include:

1) complete absorption from the gastrointestinal tract within 30 minutes;

2) maximum concentration peak occurs in four hours;

3) subcutaneous injection of methadone results in the reaching of plasma concentration within 10 minutes[8,9];

4) In nontolerant persons methadone's apparent mean half-life is about 15 hours[10,11];

5) Methadone binds firmly to plasma and tissue proteins and is slowly released from the extramuscular binding sites into the plasma[8,9];

6) Analgesic effects can be observed after one to two hours and continue until all the drug is released from the plasma and tissue proteins;

7) About 85 percent of the therapeutic methadone dose is bound to the plasma protein and subsequently accumulates in target organs;

8) The liver is the major site of biotransformation of methadone, and Pyrrolidine is a major metabolite resulting from N-demethylation and cyclization;

9) Excretion of both the changed and unchanged drug takes place in the urine and bile.

Additionally, an advantage of methadone is that it eliminates in most instances the need for heroin-dependent individuals to inject themselves frequently daily. The pharmacodynamic properties of methadone serve in the broadest sense to reduce the constant preoccupation of the addict to obtain his "fix."

## F. METHADONE DISPOSITION IN HUMANS[12,13]

Sensitive and specific basic liquid chromatographic techniques for measuring levels of methadone and its major metabolites in plasma, urine, and other body fluids and tissue extracts have been developed in several laboratories.[14–20] The interested reader is referred to the review by Kreek[13] for a complete description of the metabolism of methadone.

According to Kreek,

> The mild symptoms of opiate abstinence experienced by many patients following complete detoxification from methadone, which have persisted for long periods of time, may be related to suppression or alteration in negative feedback control of endogenous endorphin synthesis or release, and also may be related, in part, to a slow disappearance of all active drug and drug metabolites from tissue reservoirs.

Kreek also points out that the development of tolerance to and dependence on narcotic drugs may depend, in part, on the continued availability of a drug, or an active metabolite, on a chronic basis, to critical receptor sites. Along these lines, Misra et al.[21] found that significant amounts of methadone persist in the brain of both rats and dogs for up to three weeks. In addition, Harte et al.[22] reported that physiologically active amounts of unchanged methadone persist in multiple organs, including the brain, liver, intestine, and testes–vas deferens, for at least ten weeks after a single, radiolabeled dose.

The metabolic fate of methadone in humans has been studied, and several metabolites have been identified in urine and feces, using a variety of techniques, including solvent partition, thin-layer and column chromatography, gas chromatography, and mass spectrometry.[23–26]

The primary site for biotransformation of methadone is the liver, although the intestinal mucosa and lungs may also metabolize this drug. In humans, the major metabolic pathway of biotransformation of methadone is initial N-demethylation, followed by immediate cyclization of this unstable intermediate to form a pyrrolidine, the major metabolite found in urine and the major product from methadone excreted in human feces.[27] A second N-demethylation then may occur, to transform the pyrrolidine into pyrroline, a minor metabolite that has been measured in human urine.[28–30] Hydroxylated derivatives of both the pyrrolidine and pyrroline metabolites have been isolated from human urine. In humans on methadone maintenance treatment, the major and minor metabolite outpourings have been delineated (see Figures 7-2 and 7-3).

A recent paper by Vereby et al.[12] examines the pharmacokinetic parameters of methadone in humans.

> The biologic disposition of methadone in acute and during chronic administration was studied in 12 human volunteers. In the acute study, a biexponential methadone plasma level decay was observed. The acute primary half-life ($t½$) of 14.3 hr in combination with the acute secondary 5½ of 54.8 hr were longer than the single exponential chronic $t½$ of 22.2 hr, determined in the same subjects. The urinary and fecal excretion of methadone and its mono-N-demethylated metabolite increased from 22.2% in the acute of 62.0% in the chronic phase of the study. The urinary metabolite to methadone ratio tripled from the acute to the chronic phase. The pupillary effects of methadone monitored throughout 24 hr were nearly the same in magnitude in the acute and the chronic studies, whereas the plasma levels increased 3- to 8-fold following chronic methadone administration. These findings suggest that both dispositional and pharmacologic tolerance are involved in the development of tolerance following chronic administration of methadone.

Using studies to compare the disposition of the active l-isomer and inactive d-isomer, Kreek et al.[31] found that in methadone-maintained patients, the half-life for the l-isomer is 56 hours and for the inactive d-isomer it is 34 hours.

Information on methadone metabolism in a variety of normal and altered physiologic states, such as chronic liver disease, and with other drugs of abuse, such as alcohol, is urgently needed, and is being investigated with the aid of newly developed techniques.

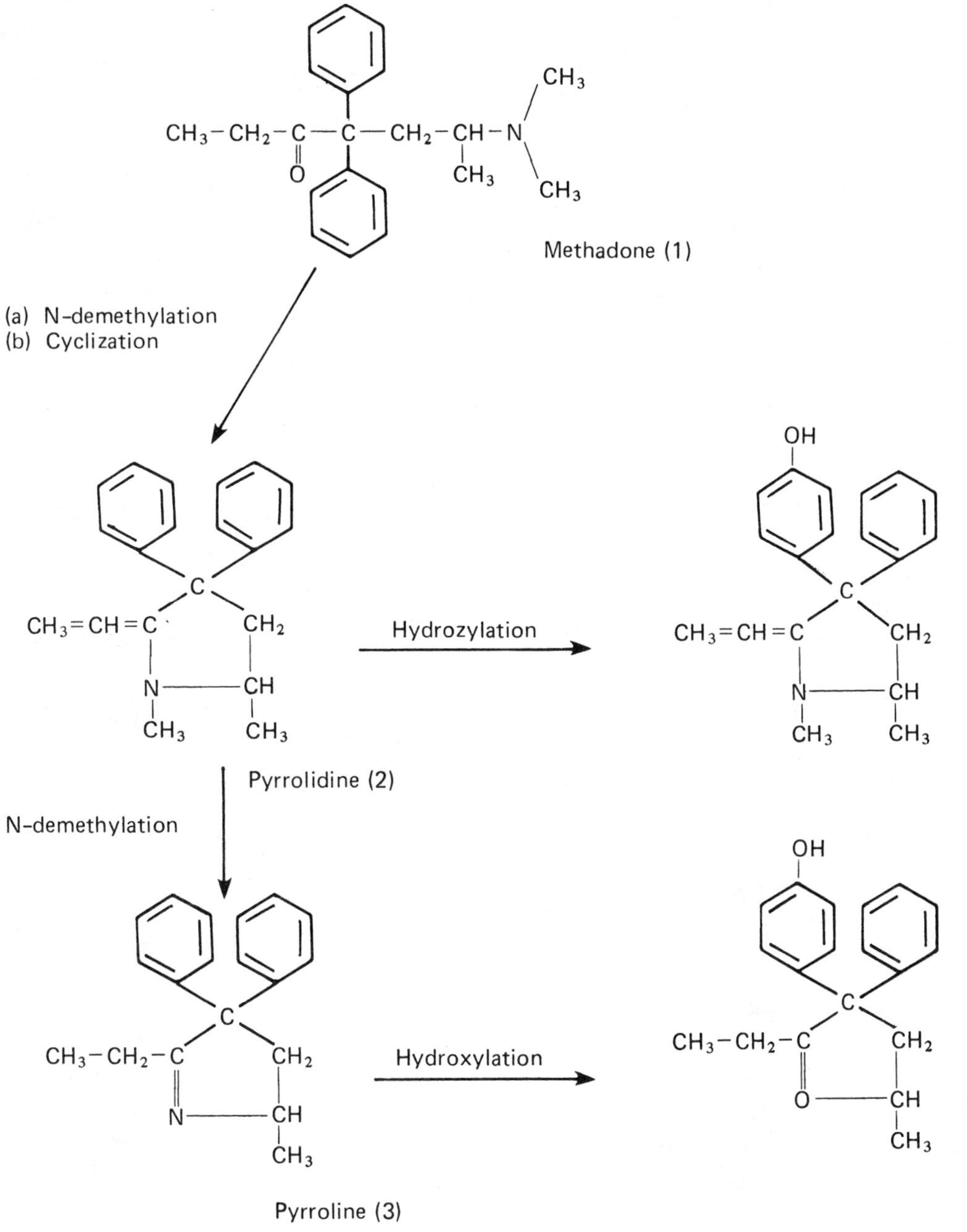

Methadone (1)

(a) N-demethylation
(b) Cyclization

Hydrozylation

Pyrrolidine (2)

N-demethylation

Hydroxylation

Pyrroline (3)

**Figure 7-2. Major pathway of di-methadone metabolism in humans. Compounds 1, 2, and 3 are major products excreted in human urine. (Adapted from Sullivan, H.R., and Due, S.L. *J. Med. Chem.* 16:910, 1973. With permission.)**

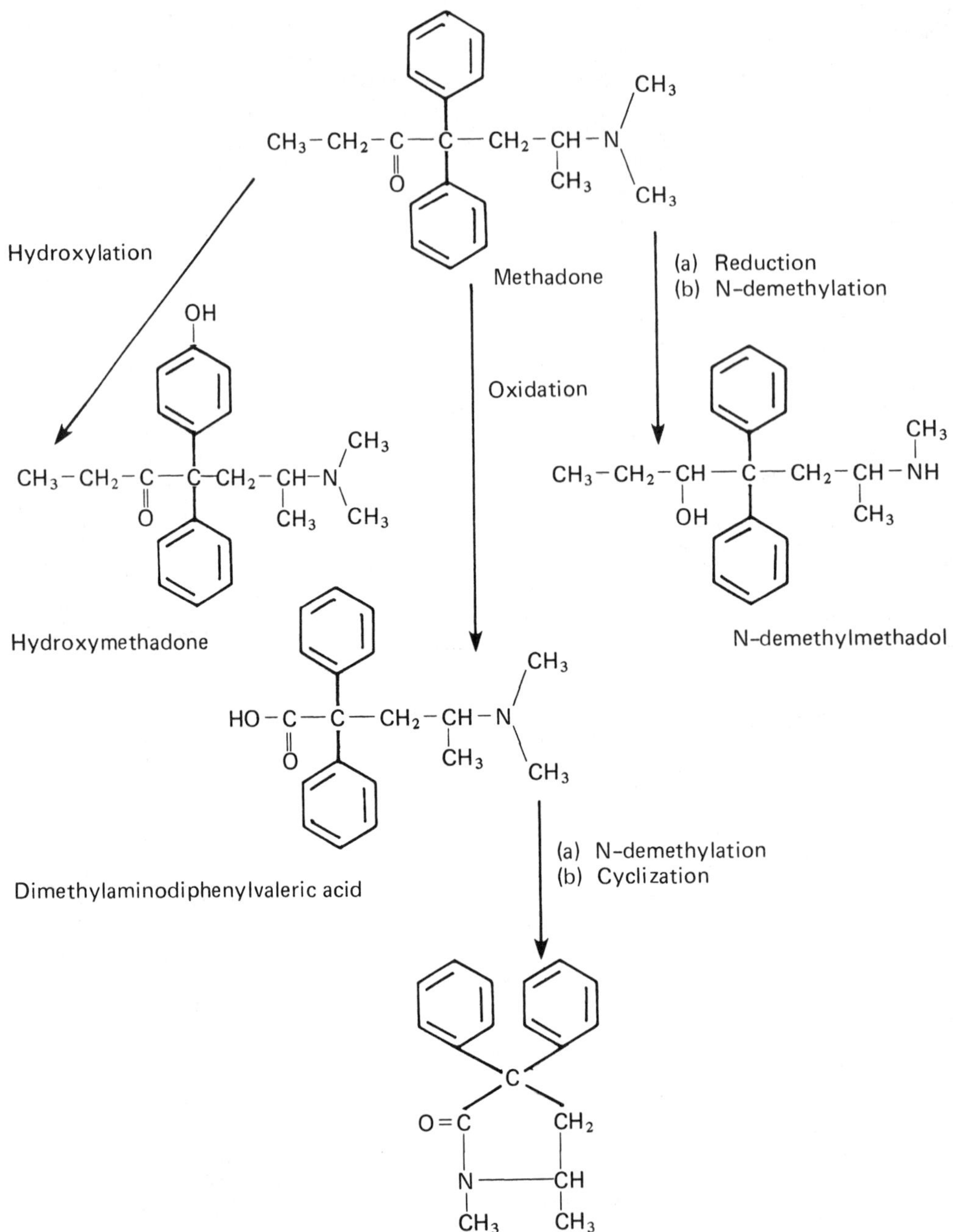


**Figure 7-3. Minor pathways of di-methadone metabolism in humans. (Adapted from Sullivan, H.R., and Due, S.L. *J. Med. Chem.* 16:910, 1973. With permission.)**

## G. TOXICITY AND PRECAUTIONS

While exerting their healing properties some drugs inevitably produce side effects that may or may not cause the individual discomfort. Some drugs exhibit acute side effects while other side effects are seen only after prolonged or chronic use of the drug. Side effects, however, will vary in severity depending on the rate at which tolerance develops and on the dose of the drug that is used. Undoubtedly upsetting to methadone-addicted patients are the acute side effects of delirium, transient hallucinations, and hemorrhagic urticaria, as well as pulmonary ventilation during drug overdose. Fortunately, these side effects are not often experienced but, as with morphine, they are more often observed in ambulatory patients than in bed-ridden patients. When a methadone patient is in a maintenance treatment program, tolerance to the drug is built up during the early weeks or months of treatment. Until tolerance is developed, narcotic side effects may be experienced by the patient. During this time undesirable chronic or prolonged side effects such as euphoria, drowsiness, and somnolence may also occur. This, however, is a consequence of too rapid an intake of methadone. Table 7-1 illustrates side effects observed in patients during the first six months of methadone maintenance treatment, and Table 7-2 shows side effects observed in patients during chronic methadone maintenance treatment.

Kreek[13] reported the following.

Abnormalities of sexual function and libido are more difficult to relate to a specific physiological effect of methadone treatment, since such problems are common in the general population and no adequate studies have been carried out to determine the prevalence of such complaints and documented problems in contrast to subjects of similar age, sex, ethnicity, social, economic and living conditions. Complaints of sexual dysfunction, such as decreased libido, inability to achieve or sustain an erection, or premature ejaculation, often come from maintenance patients who are known to have had children while in treatment. Conversely, some patients in maintenance treatment, with documented abnormalities of biochemical tests reflecting reproductive endocrine function, such as lowered serum testosterone level, have no clinical complaints of sexual dysfunction or decreases in libido. Sexual dysfunction may result from depression, fear of parenthood and from use of a wide variety of drugs of different types.

In both prospective and retrospective studies of the medical status of patients in chronic methadone treatment, there has been no evidence of toxicity of meth-

### TABLE 7-1

### Side Effects Observed in Patients During the First Six Months of Methadone Maintenance Treatment*

1. Primary narcotic effects
    - Euphoria ("high")
    - Drowsiness
    - Somnolence ("nodding")
2. Constipation
3. Excessive sweating
4. Insomnia, often accompanied by nightmares while sleeping
5. Interference with sexual function
6. Menstrual irregularities
7. Difficulty in urination—transient
8. Edema of lower extremities—transient
9. Joint pains and swelling—transient
10. Skin rash—transient
11. Upper gastrointestinal symptoms (pain, nausea, vomiting)
12. Bradycardia and hypotension

*Incidence not quantitated; occurrence not related to dose or rapidity of ascending to that dose; transient—occurrence in first few days, lasting for a very brief period only.

(Adapted from Dobbs, W.H., *JAMA* 218:1536-1541, 1971. With permission.)

adone for any organ system. In a prospective study in which patients were followed from time of admission until after 3 or more years of chronic methadone treatment, with each patient serving as his own control, significant changes of values were found for three tests only: polymorphonuclear leukocytes on differential count, which fell from elevated to normal levels; lymphocytes on differential count, which became increasingly elevated; and blood urea nitrogen levels, which fell from elevated to normal levels. Two of these three changes represent a return to normalcy. The rise in lymphocyte count remains unexplained, although large percentages of patients had abnormal liver function or serum protein test values, or both, at the time of admission, and these abnormalities persisted without significant change during 3 or more years of methadone-maintenance treatment. The only subgroup of patients in whom deterioration of liver function occurred during chronic treatment was those known to be abusing alcohol on a chronic basis.

Certain abnormalities during the first 12 months of methadone treatment have been observed by Kreek,[13] Cushman and Kreek,[32,33] Renault et al.,[34] Martin et al.,[35] Santen et al.,[36] Santiago et al.,[37] Mendelson et al.,[38] and Cicero et al.[39] (see Tables 7-3, 7-4, and 7-5).

Deaths attributable to methadone overdose itself have not occurred in methadone-maintained patients stabilized on usual clinic doses. However, it must be emphasized that methadone, in maintenance treatment doses, when accidentally or purposefully taken by a nontolerant or partially tolerant individual will cause a potentially lethal overdose syndrome within 30 minutes to six hours. If such an overdose is discovered while the person is still alive, it can be effectively reversed by prompt and proper treatment, including establishing an airway, sustaining respiration, establishing an intravenous line, and administering the specific narcotic antagonist, naloxone, intravenously.[40,41]

In treating a methadone overdose, since naloxone has only a two- to three-hour duration of action, whereas methadone has a 24- to 72-hour duration of action, naloxone must be readministered every two to three hours, as needed, and the patient must be kept under close observation in the hospital for up to 72 hours.[42]

**TABLE 7-2**

**Side Effects Observed in Patients During Chronic Methadone Maintenance Treatment**

| *Intermediate-Length Treatment (Six Months or More: <80 mg/day)** Percent | Symptoms and Signs | *Long-Term High-Dose Treatment (Three Years or More) 80–120 mg/day)†* Percent |
|---|---|---|
| 47 | Increased sweating | 48 |
| 57 | Constipation | 17 |
| | (initial laxative use, average eight months) | (59) |
| 26 | Libido abnormalities | 22 |
| — | Orgasm abnormalities | 14 |
| 23 | Sleep abnormalities (insomnia) | 16 |
| 19 | Appetite abnormalities | 4 |
| 25 | Nausea | — |
| 23 | Drowsiness | — |
| 21 | Nervousness—tenseness | — |
| 12 | Headaches | — |
| 11 | Body aches and pains | — |
| 10 | Chills | — |
| (?) | Weight gain | (??) |

*Adapted from Yaffe, G.J., Strenlinger, R.W., and Parwatikar, S. In *Proceedings of Fifth National Conference on Methadone Treatment* 1973, p. 509.

†Adapted from Kreek, M.J., *JAMA* 223:665, 1973.

Scrutiny of the literature[13] reveals there have been no indications of significant acute or any chronic physiologic effects of methadone on cardiovascular, renal, or other organ or functional systems during chronic treatment with methadone. After ten to 14 years of follow-up studies in adult patients, and five to seven years of follow-up studies in adolescent patients in chronic methadone treatment, no toxic or serious adverse effects due to the methadone itself have been documented, with the exception of one case of fatal constipation.[43,44] Thus the implications for treatment are that methadone (and, it is to be hoped, any long-lasting narcotic con-

## TABLE 7-3

### Endocrine and Respiratory Control Abnormalities Observed During First 12 Months of Methadone Treatment

1. Indirect evidence of release of antidiuretic hormone
2. Abnormal metapirone test of hypothalamic reserve (hypothalamic–pituitary–adrenocortical axis)
3. Abnormal plasma cortical response to stress (cold exposure) (hypothalamic-pituitary–adrenocortical axis)
4. Decreased FSH levels (hypothalamic–pituitary–gonadel axis)
5. Decreased LH levels (hypothalamic–pituitary–gonadel axis)
6. Abnormal positive feedback control by estrogen of LH release (hypothalamic-pituitary–gonadel axis)
7. Decreased sensitivity of CNS receptors to $CO_2$
8. Alveolar hypoventilation
9. Arterial hypercapnia

## TABLE 7-4

### Endocrine and Respiratory Control Abnormalities Observed During Chronic Methadone Treatment (12 Months or Longer in Treatment)

1. Decreased testosterone levels
2. Decreased seminal-fluid volume
3. Decreased sperm motility
4. Increased or decreased prolactin levels
5. Altered diurnal variation of prolactin levels
6. Increased thyroxine-binding globulin
7. Increased thyroxine levels
8. Increased triiodothyronine levels
9. Decreased sensitivity of CNS receptors to hypoxia

## TABLE 7-5

### Serum Protein and Immunologic Abnormalities Observed During Chronic Methadone Treatment

| | *Percent of Patients with Abnormalities Studied* |
|---|---|
| 1. Increased total serum protein | <30 |
| 2. Increased serum albumin | <20 |
| 3. Increased serum globulins | <30 |
| 4. Increased serum IgM | 30–70 |
| 5. Increased serum IgG | 30–50 |
| 6. Lymphocytosis | <20 |
| 7. Abnormal percent of B cell and T cell rosette formation in *vitro* | -0- |
| 8. Biologic false positive test for syphilis | <10 |
| 9. Increased thyroxine-binding globulin | <50 |

Fran Kreck, M.D. In R.I. Dupont et al., eds., *Handbook on Drug Abuse* (NIDA). Washington, D.C.: U.S. Government Printing Office, 1979, p. 57.)

gener) appears to be safe, even when used in high doses (80 to 120 mg/day) for long-term treatment of opiate addiction. Certainly chronic methadone administration has an important effect on the CNS where it acts to maintain physical dependence.

## H. ABUSE LIABILITY, ADDICTION, AND TOLERANCE

The use of methadone as a maintenance modality is still under the scrutiny of the FDA and is considered experimental. The overall rationale for its continued utilization is that it possesses cross-tolerance with heroin as well as with other common narcotics which prevents euphoria due to its blockading action. Another important factor is that it reduces the actual "craving" for heroin.

The major disadvantages are primarily due to its high abuse liability and tolerance.

Partial tolerance develops to the nauseant, miotic, respiratory depressant, anoretic and heart and circulatory actions. Martin in his extensive review of the literature[7] points out that tolerance to methadone occurs more gradually, in its depressant effects, compared to morphine because of the cumulative effects of the drug or its metabolites.

Certainly, physical dependence and euphoria occur with long-term illicit abuse of methadone. In fact, both the typical abstinence syndrome as well as euphoric effects have been noted following methadone abuse. In former narcotics "addicts" (dependent persons) euphoria occurs after subcutaneous administration of 10–20 mg. of methadone equivalent to that seen with morphine or other narcotics.

### 1. Medicinal Uses

Dolorphine (methadone), as it is known clinically, is used for coughs, pain, and detoxification of heroin-dependent persons, besides its popular use as a narcotic maintenance drug. Lasagna[45] has reported on the analgesic uses of methadone. Accordingly, he notes:

"In contrast to morphine, methadone and many of its congeners retain their effectiveness to a considerable degree when given daily."

Additionally, it has been noted by Beaver[46] that when methadone is given orally it is about one half as effective as the same dose administered intramuscularly.

*Addiction*

The use of methadone in the treatment of compulsive heroin users has revived interest in other methadone congeners, such as α-dl- and l-acetyl-methadol (LAAM).

The synthesis of LAAM and first investigations of its toxic and analgesic properties were carried out by Chen in 1948.[47] LAAM was found to have analgesic effects that were delayed in onset and had a long duration of action as compared with the d-isomer. This unique time–response characteristic has been attributed to its biotransformation via N-demethylation to two active metabolites, noracetylmethadol (N-LAAM) and dinoracetylmethadol (DN-LAAM).[48] The location of the demethylating enzyme in the liver accounts for the more rapid onset of action after oral, as compared with parenteral, administration. Clinical trials of its possible use as an analgesic in humans revealed that doses of 5 to 10 mg given orally or subcutaneously three to four times a day were effective and well tolerated; with this drug, constipation becomes troublesome with daily doses of about 30 mg.

Interest in LAAM as a long-term treatment agent for chronic addition did not emerge until the late 1960s. In a series of studies carried out on postaddicts at the Addiction Research Center in Lexington, Kentucky, Fraser and Isbell[49] examined the addiction liabilities and pharmacologic actions of LAAM. With subcutaneous injection of 10 to 30 mg, they noted no morphine-like effect for the first four to six hours; thereafter, very striking effects became apparent and persisted for as long as 48 to 72 hours.

Repeated administration of 15 mg of LAAM subcutaneously twice daily for three days led to cumulative toxicity, manifested by severe nausea and vomiting, confusion, respiratory depression, and altered consciousness, approaching coma.

In terms of liability potential, Fraser and Isbell[49] found that subcutaneous administration of LAAM resulted in inconsistent relief of morphine abstinence, but that a single oral dose of 30 to 60 mg, administered 28 hours after the last dose of morphine, completely abolished all symptoms of abstinence in patients who were stabilized on 400 mg of morphine daily. In addition, acute substitution of LAAM for morphine was adequate when 1 mg of LAAM orally was substituted for 6 mg of morphine. Sixty milligrams of LAAM were adequate in suppressing abstinence for up to 72 hours for patients stabilized on 60 mg of morphine four times daily. An abstinence syndrome similar in intensity and time course to that of abstinence from methadone appeared with abrupt discontinuance. Gradual reduction over seven days did not seem to alter the subsequent course and intensity of abstinence. In subjects physically dependent on a α-deli-acetylmethadol, opioid withdrawal symptoms are not perceived for 72 to 96 hours after the last oral dose, and subjects are entirely comfortable when given a single dose of the drug as infrequently as every 72 hours.[49,50] The relatively slow onset and protracted duration of action of this drug, which is probably inactive, are thought to be due, in part, to its conversion to active metabolites (noracetylmethadol and normethadol) that slowly are metabolized further or excreted.[51,52]

Investigations of the past decade have established LAAM as a safe and effective maintenance treatment agent for chronic opiate addiction. The interested reader should refer to a review by Ling and Blaine[53] and articles on the subject by Senay et al.,[54] Goldstein and Judson,[55] Savage et al.,[56] Ling et al.,[57] Blaine et al.,[59] and Lehmann.[60]

Perhaps the best argument for using LAAM in narcotic treatment programs is that its use may eliminate take-home methadone, or at least reduce it substantially. According to Ling and Blaine,[53]

> The above argument not only protects the community from the hazard of street methadone but also benefits the patients in ways that are less apparent but nonetheless quite important. For instance, victims of accidental poisoning are most often members of the patient's own family; eliminating take-home doses protects them from such risks. Eliminating take-homes also removes from the patient the pressure and temptation to sell or give away part of his/her medications. It also eliminates the possibility of theft or other losses of medication from his/her possession. From the clinician's standpoint, eliminating take-homes removes any incentive from a patient to obtain more drugs than she/he needs and makes dosage bargaining unnecessary. It also removes from the clinic routine the many games and tricks designed to cheat and defeat the urine-testing procedure upon which the granting of take-home privileges all too often rests. The clinician is freed from the dilemma of having to decide whether or not to give patients take-home methadone which may jeopardize the community and the patient or to deny this privilege and hamper rehabilitation.

In terms of its safety, evidence is clear that LAAM is as safe as methadone and can be used safely in long-term treatment of chronic heroin addicts. The incidence of side effects appears comparable for LAAM and methadone.

Although LAAM is addictive and tolerance develops with repeated use, there are reports[53] that in phase II studies, some patients were able to discontinue LAAM abruptly without undergoing withdrawal.

Since only a few have been treated with LAAM, there is no definite statement regarding its safety for females; its effect on the human fetus especially, remains unknown.

It should be pointed out that LAAM is available only to clinicians, under approved investigational protocols. No LAAM has been allowed to leave the clinic. Some believe that the lack of immediate quantification after dosing would make it less subject to street abuse and thus safer in that regard. The delayed time course makes it more dangerous until the drug-culture population becomes knowledgeable about this unique property of LAAM.

Like all opioids, the major problem with LAAM is acute overdose. Nevertheless there appears to be strong evidence that LAAM is effective as a maintenance drug and that it is acceptable to most opiate abusers and may be preferred by some.

## I. CLINICAL ASPECTS OF METHADONE MAINTENANCE TREATMENT

Now that we have reviewed the basic pharmacology of methadone, what do we know about the nature of the addictive process as it relates to realistic goals in treatment and methadone therapy? What follows is a brief conceptual view of the nature of addiction[1,51,61] so that we can better understand the myths, realities, and issues concerning methadone maintenance treatment.

### 1. Anatomy of a Fix[1]

Methadone maintenance has become the most widely used and effective modality in the treatment of narcotic addiction. In 1979, approximately 83,370 former heroin abusers were receiving methadone daily from authorized programs approved by the U.S. Food and Drug Administration (FDA). The intention here is to provide a basis for mutual understanding of how the addiction process might be perceived.

The purpose of Figure 7-4 is not to present a precise time–dosage–effect relationship. In all probability, it is scientifically inaccurate; however it has a practical application at a conceptual level to aid in the understanding of what is happening.

The illustration is based on an addict with a well-established tolerance threshold. The amount of heroin injected is in excess of his/her tolerance dose (the amount required to prevent withdrawal) to the extent that the addict experiences a full-blown high. He/she is sedated, nodding, somewhat immobilized, and totally oblivious to stress, strain, and discomfort, either internal or external, and really feels a direct and definite positive drug effect. The individual is "loaded."

As the most intense effects of the fix wane, the user moves into a state of well-being during which he/she is not really "feeling" the drug but is mildly high or mildly euphoric, to the point where the person can function well and may be able to work hard and efficiently (at least perceiving such labors to be efficient). It is during this state, which might last two to three hours, and up to perhaps six hours, that the addict would like to think he/she feels normal. This state is referred to as the "abnormal normality." It is this elusive state that many clients anticipate they will have and maintain while on methadone maintenance and may explain their frequent misconception of normality. It is an elusive state in that, in order to maintain it, narcotic dosage (methadone or heroin) constantly must be raised to keep the dose above the tolerance level, to some unknown point, probably many times what we consider a very high dose.

Moving on down the slope to the range of effect equal to the exact tolerance threshold with a range of perhaps 10 percent above and below the tolerance threshold is a state of temporary physiologic normality. He/she is in a state of full awareness internally and externally. It is this level of effect that is achieved and maintained for 24 hours or more in the patient who is stabilized on a fixed dose. One who is experiencing this level of methadone effect is, aside from having taken methadone, at one's particular level of normality. The problem not infrequently encountered in drug-dependent persons is that the state of full awareness, for many, may be uncomfortable and associated with anxiety. Both new and old methadone patients must understand that this level of effect is all they can expect from methadone and that, being in

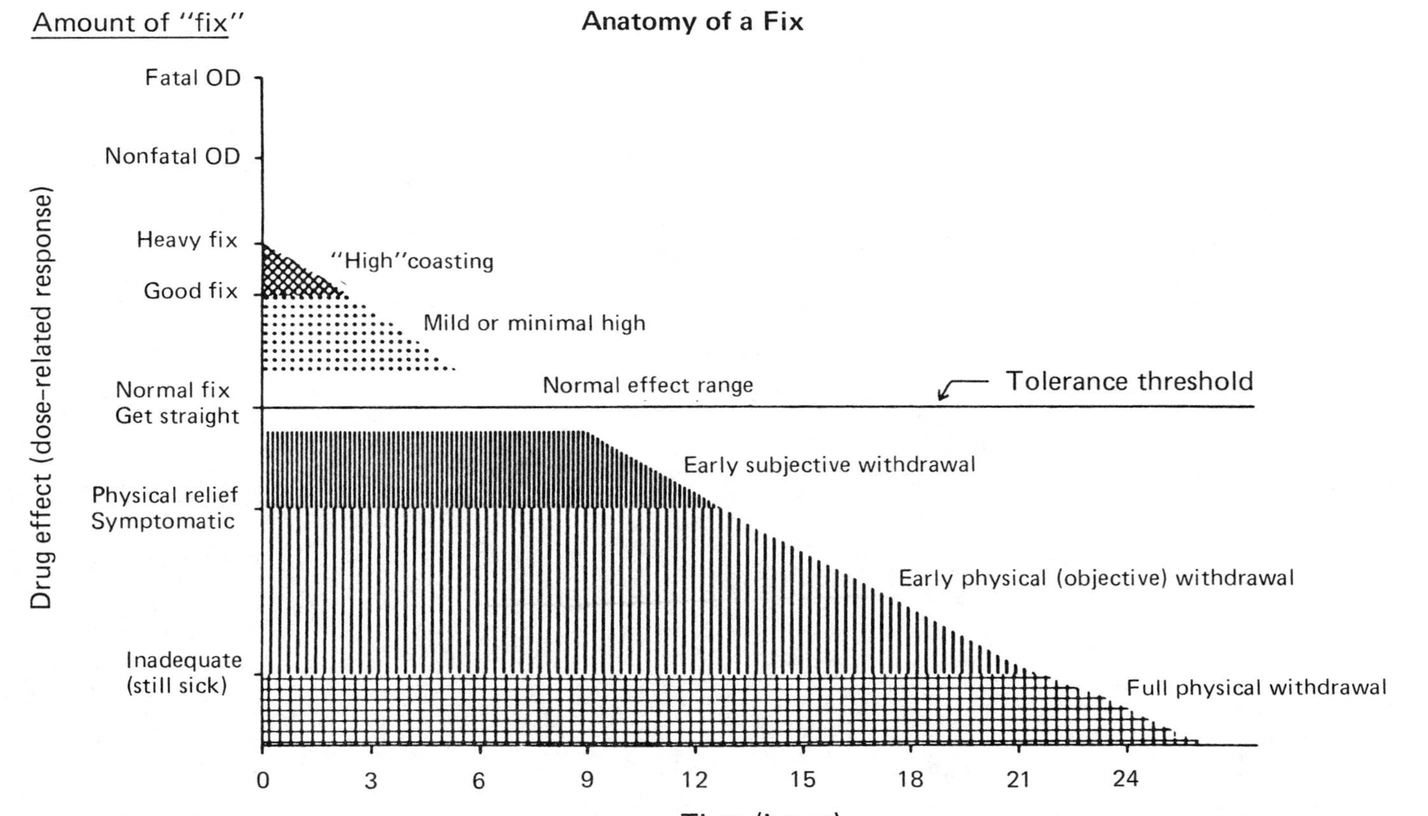


**Figure 7-4.** This illustrates the comparatively rapid deterioration of the effect of heroin with (in contrast to methadone) early onset of the withdrawal syndrome (methadone). The onset of early physical withdrawal is less than 24 hours, although the peak of withdrawal signs and symptoms may not occur until between 48 and 72 hours. The illustration does not indicate a repeat dose, which, in the case of the active opiate addict, would occur between eight and 16 hours (after the stage of physiologic normality starts and, if possible, before the onset of physical abstinence). The important point is that the repeated sequence may condition the addict to perceive himself/herself as getting sick with the return of full internal and external awareness; that is, while in a state of physiologic normality. ***Note:*** **(1) There is no intention to imply that the time–effect curve is scientifically accurate. It is of practical and illustrative value. (2) It should also be noted that in the case of the active opiate-dependent person, the higher the "tolerance threshold" (the bigger the habit), the more frequent the injections are, and the withdrawal symptoms start earlier and are more intense.**

a state of physiologic normality, they are indeed subject to all the various problems to which the general population is subject. These include anxiety, insomnia, headaches, colds, flu, mild depressions, and on and on. Applicants for methadone maintenance treatment programs who have the misconception that somehow they will be spared the normal stress of so-called normality while taking methadone are certain to be disappointed and likely will be constantly seeking increased doses or will resort to other chemical means to alter their state of consciousness. The individual who finds this state of physiologic and emotional normality uncomfortable or unbearable is not likely to do well on methadone.

It is important to distinguish between the normal level of anxiety and the onset of the anxiety associated with early withdrawal syndrome. However, it is perhaps asking too much that the patient be able to say which anxiety is attributable to being normal and which is attributable to early withdrawal. The patient long since has learned by a constantly reinforced conditioned response that anxiety means getting sick and is the signal to seek chemical relief by fixing again or ingesting more methadone. The reinforcing of the conditioned response continues during methadone treatment regardless of the cause of the anxiety. The anxious patient may report "drug hunger" and the physician may order an increase in the methadone dose. Even if the anxiety is not drug-dose related, the patient will experience relief of the anxiety if the dose increase is enough to feel and this, of course, will "prove" that the increase really was needed and that the cause of the anxiety was indeed an inadequate dose of methadone. Hence the problem of altering or changing this particular conditioned response is made more difficult. An essential part of the total therapy is to convince the patient that not all anxieties and other problems that occur are dose related, to seek and find other factors that induce anxiety states, and, most important, to begin to develop alternate means of dealing with and tolerating reasonable levels of anxiety.

As the narcotic effect continues to diminish, the area of subjective symptoms of wthdrawal becomes apparent, as illustrated in Figure 7-4. Anxiety is increased and other symptoms may appear, such as irritability, insomnia, and general malaise. The desire to fix is naturally increased as the feeling described as "drug hunger" becomes manifest. Drug hunger is probably nothing more than actual withdrawal and anticipated withdrawal, coupled with the learned conditioned response that a fix will make the symptoms disappear.

The next phase is characterized by increasing intensity of the subjective symptoms and the first appearance of physical withdrawal or objective signs. The first signs are rhinorrhea and lacrimation. Pupils are no longer constricted but have not yet begun to dilate. They are normal in size. As physical withdrawal increases, dilated pupils appear, along with piloerection and gastrointestinal disturbances. The physical signs continue until another fix or dose of narcotic is administered or, if untreated, continue to increase in severity, reaching a peak at about 48 to 72 hours, and then gradually decreasing over a period of days as the detoxification process takes place.

The entire process described in Figure 7-4 is for illustration purposes and does not exist in reality, in distinct delineated phases as the graph would suggest. The concept is useful, however, in explaining the process to patients and to new staff.

## 2. Management of Methadone Maintenance

The breakthrough use of methadone as a replacement for opioid dependence by Dole and Nysnander[63] provided the addict with a new lifestyle free of potentially illicit activities. Initially, heroin dependent patients received 20 to 30 mg. of methadone orally daily, which was gradually stepped up to 80 to 120 mg. daily.

As previously mentioned, the theoretical pharmacological principle, which was not clear in 1964, was that methadone, because of a similar pharmacologic response to heroin, would assist narcotic-dependent persons in their rehabilitation efforts by preventing withdrawal symptoms and blocking the euphoric actions of opiates. It has become well known since that time that opiate-like substances act in the brain through specific receptors, and methadone, like other opioid compounds, interact at these specific "opioid receptors." The belief, of not only Dole and Nyswander[64] but of other active clinicians in the drug-abuse field, is that, by "blocking" the pleasurable effects of heroin with methadone, abusers would be less likely to continue their abuse of narcotics but return to a "normal" drug-free state. The use of methadone as a "blocking" drug differs from utilizing heroin per se in that the former substance is used as an "antinarcotic agent," whereas the latter is used as a direct substitute for maintenance.[66,67]

According to Dole,[40] there are three states in an addict's life: 1) "straight" (feeling normal) 2) "high," and 3) "sick." The heroin abuser spends much of his time seeking the means to obtain his "fix" so that little time is spent being "straight," so, as Dole states it, "he's pretty much a lost soul."

The use of methadone therapy in long-term narcotic rehabilitation efforts should not be confused with the clinical application of narcotic antagonists (see Chapter 6). The narcotic antagonists actually "neutralize" heroin's effects. In contrast, methadone produces a "high" even in tolerant individuals, which seems to reduce the hunger or craving of other opiates.

In a ten-year survey by Dole and Nyswander[67] it was mentioned in a personal communication, that by 1972 there were 60,000 narcotic addicts in methadone maintenance programs; by 1976 there were 90,000, and approximately the same number in the 1980s.

Presently, in spite of increased costs of the program and reduced federal spending for social programs as an outcome of "Reaganomics," there has been an expanded and widespread adoption of this rehabilative modality. Today no one employs the high levels of methadone originally used in the initial study. Some programs use 40 mg. of methadone a day, which does not seem to work as well as 60 to 80 mg. or more a day.[68]

Over the past decade of treating "heroin abusers" with methadone, not only did the dosage regimen change, but the characteristics of the patients seen by the clinics did also. In 1974 there was an increased percentage of clients with a skilled or white-collar background, which is even more obvious today, in the so-called "year of the middle-class junkie."

This change has allowed greater liberalism in terms of "trust" in the clinic setting. In the long-term ambulatory period (about 1 year) the patient returns to the clinic daily, receives a liquid containing methadone, and is observed to drink it. Since on the street there is a tendency for methadone diversion, the patients who have been ascertained as acceptable receive up to several days' supply of medication. All patients' urine is tested for the presence of illicit drugs. The utilization of the methadone-diluted juice is a take-home medication designed to reduce clinic visits, enabling some to return to a "normal" lifestyle.

A third phase in the program paradigm is the stabilizing period which should result in a productive member of society. In this final phase of treatment a minimum of one dose of medication is taken in the program facility and one urine specimen is evaluated. In addition, the patient is counseled for guidance to develop job skills and is taught personal problem-solving methods.

In all phases, supportive services are readily available and are related to the needs of the individual patient. Only a few have been found to need little more than medical supervision. Most need substantial support, guidance, and assistance in developing job skills and in resolving personal problems.

As with most treatment modalities, there are distinct advantages and disadvantages.

*Advantages of Methadone Maintenance:*

1. Methadone maintenance reduces the need to engage in illegal practices to obtain the money for the habit. The abuser becomes less dependent upon self-injection many times a day with unsterile materials. The narcotic abuser does not have to deal with criminals to buy supplies or

to sell stolen merchandise, and is not as preoccupied with plans to procure a "fix."

2. Since controlled addiction to methadone is preferable to an uncontrolled addiction to heroin, methadone maintenance is a realistic mass treatment modality for the hundreds of thousands of heroin abusers.

3. Criminal activities will decrease as significant numbers of people enter methadone maintenance programs.

4. The methadone maintenance patient tends to engage in constructive activities, and becomes self-supporting in many instances, being capable of driving a car, operating heavy machinery, and performing complex psychomotor tasks.

5. Methadone maintenance programs are not expensive in comparison with other therapeutic efforts. Between $2000 and $4000 per patient per year is required to maintain a successful program.

*Disadvantages of Methadone Maintenance:*

1. The patient remains addicted to a narcotic, and may have to remain on methadone permanently.

2. The amount of methadone given for maintenance may be lethal to a nontolerant individual.

3. Diversion of methadone onto the black market by patients or staff members poses a problem, especially in poorly managed programs.

4. The heroin not utilized by methadone maintenance patients may be a source of supply for new addict populations.

5. Conclusive proof of long-term safety is not yet available.

6. The requirement to return to the clinic several times a week is an inconvenience, especially for the working patient. However, a longer acting methadone analog (1-α acetylmethadol) is now under study (as reviewed in this chapter).

### *b. Methadone Abstinence*

With today's world of inflation, the drug dealer is forced to significantly "cut" and dilute the percentage of heroin contained in a street "bag." The result is that some individuals who label themselves "addicts" are not at all very dependent on narcotics. Accordingly, it has become generally known that about 20% of program participants in a large city are not physically dependent and when tested in the clinic with narcotic antagonists show no response. Furthermore, another 15 to 20% are categorized as being only mildly dependent and are commonly referred to as "needle freaks." Hospitalization is usually required for the individual who is strongly addicted to narcotics and is experiencing moderate to severe withdrawal signs. This type of addiction requires methadone substitution. The initial dose is between 15 to 20 mg. of orally administered methadone. Sometimes, when necessary, the dose is repeated every 4 to 6 hours. After one and a half days of treatment, the daily methadone requirements are estimated by summing up the total number of milligrams administered during that period. Usually it takes ten days for detoxification to result in an almost symptom-free individual, during which time the daily calculated dose is reduced by 20% each day until the ten days are up. Mild forms of withdrawal symtomatology are treated on an ambulatory basis and diazepam is prescribed as a calming agent.

### *c. Stabilization on Methadone*

Those individuals who have been successfully detoxified by methadone continue, as in the short-term maintenance program, on an ambulatory basis, prior to their entry into a full-time methadone maintenance program. Usually 20 mg. of methadone is employed as an initial dosage per day. The patient is seen once daily, at which time the urine is checked.

### *d. Methadone and Alcohol Consumption*

There is evidence that some individuals maintained on methadone consume large amounts of alcohol as a possible substitute for their drug dependence.[69,70]

Over the past decade, numerous studies have focused on the possibility that alcohol and opiates share a common mechanism in terms of their pharmacologic actions.[71] It has been further postulated that the peptidyl opiate system may be involved in alcohol actions.[72,73] These theories have met with severe criticism[74–76] on the basis that acute effects of opiates and ethanol are dissimilar, the dependence phenomena are different, narcotic antagonists do not antagonize ethanol or precipitate withdrawal asymptoms in animals dependent on ethanol, the withdrawal symptoms of morphine are unlike those of ethanol, and there is no experimental evidence to link alcohol and opiate effects.

Numerous studies that support the view that both ethanol and opiates act at similar opioid receptors and mutually influence common biologic territories,[77–79] such as dependence,[80] cross-tolerance,[81] preference,[82,83,84] intoxication,[85] and withdrawal,[86,87] have appeared. More surprising are the reports, in humans, of naloxone-induced antagonism of acute ethanol intoxication,[88] and even reversal of ethanol-induced coma.[89]

If, indeed, ethanol and the opioid analog, methadone, acted on similar sites, it should follow that during methadone blockade[90] of opiate receptors, ethanol should not induce euphoria. This fact, if it is correct, should result in reduced ethanol consumption rather than an induction of alcohol ingestion as reported clinically by many investigators.[91]

How can this paradox be explained in terms of the common mechanism thesis?[92] In recent years, numerous studies have suggested the existence of several classes of opiate receptors. Martin and co-workers,[93,94] on the basis of pharmacologic evidence, concluded that there are three such classes (μ, κ, and σ). Lord et al.[95] discovered a difference between the receptors that predominate in guinea pig ileum and those in mouse vas deferens. They named them μ, or morphine preferring, and σ, or enkephalin preferring, respectively.

Blum's laboratory proposed a selective action for ethanol on the σ (peptide-preferring) receptor rather than on the μ (morphine-preferring) site, based on pharmacologic studies on the mouse vas deferens.[96] Most interesting is the work by Hiller et al.,[97] which fully supports this original suggestion. These investigations demonstrated unequivocably that the addition of ethanol or other aliphatic alcohols to rat brain membranes strongly inhibits the binding of enkephalins at concentrations at which little inhibition of opiate alkaloids is seen. The difficulty with this study is that at least 1 percent ethanol is required for an effect on σ receptor binding of its respective ligand and, to achieve the maximal effect, over 5 percent ethanol is required. These concentrations are considered high and not close to levels obtained under normal alcohol consumption in humans. Hiller et al.[97] postulate that the inhibitory effects of ethanol on σ receptor binding may be mediated through the membrane-fluidizing (making membranes rigid) effects of alcohol. Nevertheless, in support of these findings, Pfeiffer et al.[98] show that chronic ethanol imbibation interferes with σ- but not with μ-opiate receptors at more believable concentrations of ethanol.

The results suggest that σ receptors are considerably more sensitive to alcohols than μ receptors, and demonstrate that the opiate receptors can be affected by a reagent that is not a ligand for the receptor.

Thus, in terms of understanding the mechanism for enhanced alcohol consumption in humans maintained on methadone, the dualism theory of multiple opiate receptors is postulated. Since methadone is a synthetic analog similar to morphine, it strongly binds to μ receptors preferentially. During methadone blockade in humans, although typical morphine-like μ receptors are saturated, the σ receptors are open for occupancy. Since it has been established that ethanol binds preferentially to the enkephalin-preferring σ receptors,[97,98] euphoria could be achieved through σ receptor-membrane perturbation in spite of methadone blockade.

The opiate addict can still obtain a drug-induced feeling of well-being by utilizing ethanol and, in fact, probably better than with heroin or some other opioid.

Future research, in terms of these results, strongly supports the need to find σ receptor inhibitors. Certainly, the finding of such inhibitors would pave the way for the implementation of therapeutically useful compounds providing "true" opioid blockade as once postulated for both methadone[90] and narcotic antagonists.

### e. Pharmacological complications of Chronic Methadone Use

With long-term use of methadone the most problematic side reactions include constipation, alterations in sexual drive, and nausea. Unexpectedly, amenorrhic women return to normal menses, and this results in enhanced fertility. It has been observed that while under the influence of methadone maintenance many have conceived and normal infants have been born.

### f. Dangers[99,100]

The use of a new synthetic substitute, acetylmethadol, has a distinct advantage over methadone in that its effects last for as much as 96 hours. The drug has achieved some degree of success in the clinic since it can be given to patients three times a week, significantly reducing clinic visitation and the possibility of home methadone diversion. The use of acetyl-methadol also significantly reduces the possibility of narcotic poisoning in children from home methadone.[99,100]

### g. Methadone Diversion

The rechanneling of licit methadone into illicit traffic is referred to as methadone diversion. The method or channel of sale may be through the selling or giving of their methadone to others by clients, through sales by clinic staff, or through robberies or hijackings. Sales by doctors, as a result of the change in the laws to prohibit the prescribing of methadone except under special conditions, for the most part have been eliminated.

Methadone now appears on the street in two major forms. One is in a liquid, usually a synthetic orange juice such as Tang. The other is the 40-mg diskette. Both forms are used only in methadone programs and are said to be incapable of conversion to intravenous use. The diskette brings about $5 on the street and the liquid between $6 and $10. The amount of methadone in the latter varies according to the client's daily dose, which may be from 20 mg to 120 mg.

Walter et al.[101] found that in a small survey of 95 heroin abusers in Brooklyn, some 79 percent reported that methadone was available for purchase on the street. According to this study, when asked whether they had purchased any during the past six months, 56 percent responded "yes." In their neighborhood, the diskette form was seen exclusively. The average price of a diskette was $4. Methadone patients were the source of supply for 74 percent. The reasons given for purchase were: to prevent withdrawal sickness, 41 percent; to "clean up," 17 percent; to "boost" other drugs, 40 percent; to resell, 2 percent.

To determine the extent of the problem of methadone diversion, the National Institute on Drug Abuse funded a study through the Institute for Social Research at Fordham University. This study was performed in five cities: New York, St. Louis, Philadelphia, Miami, and San Juan, Puerto Rico. Some basic conclusions and recommendations of the survey, as summarized by Cohen,[102] are as follows:

1. Illicit methadone was widely reported as being available by the drug abusers. Information from enforcement officials confirmed this fact. A substantial proportion of addicts not in treatment use methadone every day. An even larger number said that they use it a few times a month. The reasons for methadone use varied from "to get high" to "to keep from getting sick."
2. The chief source of illicit methadone is the patient attending a methadone maintenance clinic.
3. Methadone has become an important new commodity in the illicit drug subculture.
4. At the time the study was done, enforcement officials were much more involved in heroin control

than in the problem of methadone diversion. When arrests for illicit methadone did occur, they were triggered by complaints about notorious treatment programs or by blatantly overdealing activities.

5. Treatment programs should monitor diversion activities more effectively. As a result of this study, there is sufficient reason to believe that a significant traffic in diverted methadone exists. Take-home privileges should be tightened for those who do not use their methadone as prescribed.

6. The use of a tracer substance in the methadone (a minute quantity of a vitamin, for example) is feasible for special situations. It is not recommended for universal use. From a tracer, police seizures can identify the source of the confiscated methadone.

Certainly methadone diversion can do harm and must be reduced to the lowest possible level.

Interestingly it appears that a significant number of methadone maintenance clients sell these take-home supplies to "street people," who say they use illegal methadone to keep from getting sick. With the revenue obtained, clients buy heroin to "shoot over," or cocaine, barbiturates, or amphetamines to "shoot around" their habits. Cheating on the program, manifested by "conning" the therapist, indicates not only a loss of respect and mutual openness between the client and therapist, but also a cynical attitude toward the rehabilitation process.

### *h. Realities*

*Methadone Versus Other Opiate-like Drugs:* Methadone is, a potent narcotic drug that possesses all of the properties of heroin. It is far simpler to explain how methadone differs from other opiates and opiate-like drugs than to describe it as an isolated substance. As for its practical use in the treatment of drug dependence, methadone has one important property—in appropriate dosage, it will prevent the onset of withdrawal for 24 hours or more.

Other properties often have been attributed to methadone; some of these are difficult to accept, including the so-called blockage effect and reduction of drug hunger, which, for some reason, has been separated from the simple property of prevention of withdrawal. Methadone differs from heroin in two ways. First, methadone is effective when taken orally, and second, the time required for the onset of withdrawal is much longer. These two characteristics are the essence of methadone maintenance. The need for multiple daily doses and frequent injections is thus eliminated, allowing for controlled, carefully supervised, daily ingestion of single doses of methadone and providing a minimum of disruption of daily routine.

The widespread use and acceptance of methadone should never tempt an individual to minimize its properties as a very potent, highly addictive, and dangerous substance. When used properly, with adequate supervision and skill, it has proved to be an unusually safe, nontoxic drug. In the hands of the nontolerant individual, however, routine maintenance doses can be extremely dangerous, if not fatal. Deaths resulting from the improper use of diverted street methadone or accidental ingestion by children or unsuspecting adults, although infrequent, have been reported in all parts of the United States.

As the quality and potency of heroin continue to decline, caution must be continually exercised to minimize dangerous side effects and reactions, as well as the increasing potential for introducing dependence in individuals who merely think they are dependent on extremely small amounts of heroin. Thus it is necessary to prove true current physiologic dependence to opiates before even short-term administration of methadone.

There is an abundance of information available as to the commonly reported side effects of methadone (Tables 7-1 and 7-2), and so any detailed discussion is unnecessary. It does appear that tolerance, in terms of specific side effects, may develop at different rates. This means that an individual taking a fixed daily dosage of methadone may experience certain undesirable side effects, such as constipation and impotence, far longer than that same individual would experience euphoria or other side effects. There is still a great deal to be learned about the rates at which tolerance develops in relation to specific effects and side effects of the drug.

To summarize the realities, the long-term stable administration of methadone after the development of maximum tolerance simply maintains a state of physiologic normality and prevents the onset of withdrawal. To expect anything more from methadone alone is to invite disappointment, frustration, and probably treatment failure.

Methadone, as an opiate-like narcotic, has full cross-tolerance to heroin and other opiates; hence it easily can be substituted for or considered interchangeable with other narcotics of the opiate and opiate-like family.

## *i. Myths*

*Methadone Mythology Concerning Blockade:* An entire book could be devoted to the exploration and explanation of the numerous myths that have enjoyed some level of persistent popularity. As with other myths, most are relatively harmless; however, a few could be considered dangerously misleading. It is hoped that many such myths have been dispelled by the material already presented; but some deserve special attention.

1. *Blockade.* The misleading and inaccurate term *blockade* was common in earlier writings about methadone, and is still somewhat popular today. The phenomenon described as blockage was based on reports of patients who found that, while they were on methadone maintenance, the use of heroin had no effect. Therefore, the practice of ''fixing on the side'' was abandoned in many cases. It is totally erroneous to assume that methadone in any way blocks or interferes with the action of other opiates. A patient maintained on a potent, high-dose methadone has acquired a very high tolerance threshold, when compared with average street heroin habits. The result is that many methadone maintenance patients whose dosage was in the neighborhood of 80 to 100 mg or more simply require large doses of heroin to experience euphoria. That is, through the use of methadone, such a high tolerance threshold has been developed as to require unusually large single doses of heroin to exceed the tolerance threshold and to produce a high. True blockage may be observed with the use of antagonists of the $\mu$- and $\sigma$-opiate receptor type, but not of methadone or narcotics. A comparison might be the hard-working drinker who gradually develops such a tolerance to alcohol as to be able to consume two fifths of bourbon daily while outwardly appearing sober. That this person neither would feel nor appear intoxicated from a glass of sherry does not mean that bourbon blocks the effect of sherry, but that a far greater quantity of the milder beverage would be required to produce intoxication.

2. *Dual addiction.* Far too frequently, opiate-addicted persons fail to seek treatment for fear of developing a different or new addiction to methadone. As previously stated, there is complete cross-tolerance and interchangeability of methadone with other opiates and opiate-like narcotics. Practical reassurance should be offered to the potential methadone patient by simply explaining that the patient is now dependent, and that the introduction of methadone will merely maintain that dependence and not introduce a new or different one. It is possible, however, to be dependent on more than one substance at the same time, such as opiates, barbiturates, and alcohol. In fact, Antabuse is being prescribed for some alcohol-dependent methadone maintenance patients.[103]

## *j. Issues*

To explore the issue of whether we say ''yes'' or ''no'' to methadone, as the basis of an introduction to this section, some of the major ideas in a paper by Ron Bayer,[104] presented at the Fourth National Conference on Methadone Treatment, are presented in the following.

From a radical perspective, dependence is seen as a social problem, not only because of the number of heroin users in our society (that is, a function of desperation), but primarily because it is a reflection of the depths of the American social crisis. Bluntly stated: there is a direct relationship between the racism which daily assaults the Black and Brown underclass of this society and the rate of dependency in America's ghettos: between the increasing alienation of the middle class youth from the institutions, symbols and values of an increasingly bureaucratized technocratic society and the rise of compulsive use on the campus: between the brutalizing and dehumanization existence of American soldiers in Southeast Asia and the reported rates of opiate use of returning GI's.

The mediations through which these social factors affect the individual are complex. But, what is a rather obvious fact, is that hundreds of thousands of Americans have found life so unbearable and the pain so deep that they have "chosen" a narcotized existence as preferable to the everyday life they must confront.

It is upon this analysis of social roots that the radical critique of methadone maintenance is based. *Three elements seem to characterize the radical position.* They are: 1) Methadone, like heroin, produces dependence; thus, it cannot be used successfully in combatting drug dependency and its consequences; 2) Governmental control over methadone clinics creates the possibility of subjecting former patients to extensive social control; and 3) While on methadone maintenance, many turn to "pills" and alcohol and thus its efficacy is questionable. Each of the above criticisms shall be dealt with successively.

The radical position has been expressed by Dr. Tom Levin, in an article entitled "New Myths About Drug Programs." He states: If one has a powerful anti-drug ideology and sees drugs as basically a way of cutting consciousness, breeding apathy and destroying social involvement and action, *then one cannot condone the use of any addictive drug, whether methadone or heroin.*[105]

The connection between the first and second parts of this statement is not at all clear and, indeed, there appears to be a non-sequitor. While heroin dependence does, in fact, cut consciousness and the possibilities of social involvement by blotting out social reality, this is not the case with methadone when administered in a medically regulated manner. Whether one accepts the Dole–Nyswander theory which suggests the necessity of life-long maintenance, or the modifications of that theory which see methadone as a transitional phase, leading eventually to freedom from drug dependence, at this point, methadone maintenance is clearly the most successful technique for meeting the *limited though vital* task of combatting the client's street problem, by accomplishing the task of blocking the heroin "hunger" which drives the addict into increasingly deeper levels of despair.

Moreover, by eliminating the narcotized state of mind, it provides the first condition for allowing the former patient to see society for what it is and it makes possible his involvement in the struggle for social change.

The fact that methadone, itself, produces dependence, seems largely irrelevant to the issue at hand. Not all such drugs have the same consequences for the user. Thus, to oppose methadone because of this, can only be understood in terms of an a-priori moralism.

The second general criticism, which radicals have made of methadone maintenance, is related to the potential in social control—implicit in a network of governmentally funded and regulated clinics, upon which clients will be dependent as a result of methadone. Indeed, a good deal of the literature has stressed that as a result of stabilization on methadone, the "maladaptive" behavior, which characterizes heroin users, will be eliminated, the end result of this process being "reintegration" into the fabric of society. By those who view "reintegration" as another euphemism for the "pacification" of those who are alienated from the current social order, the "promise" of methadone maintenance is viewed with considerable alarm. As Dr. Levin states, "Many Black community leaders are justifiably concerned about Black peoples' getting hooked on methadone with the state as the sole 'pusher' and 'supplier.' "[105]

Disregarding the quite obvious effort at linking heroin and methadone through the use of emotionally charged terms such as "hooked," "pusher," and "supplier," the issue here remains rather serious. As Dr. Robert Newman pointed out in his paper at the Third National Methadone Conference, there is the possibility that the public authorities who fund methadone programs might make efforts to control, through the threat of termination from maintenance, those who, by acting in a militant fashion, confront the representatives of our social system.[106] What is so interesting about this criticism is that it implicitly recognizes the value of methadone in combatting heroin dependence and its consequences. Indeed, it is premised upon the realization that those being maintained on methadone will begin to understand the nature of the society in which they live and will have both the inclination and capacity to act upon that new understanding.

It would seem, then, that though maintenance programs pose the potential threat of social control, the problem must be dealt with by assuring patients that they will not face the possibility of termination because of political involvement. Such guarantees can best be established through the creative involvement of community forces and patients in the control of programs. To reject methadone maintenance because of the possibility of social control is to doom many to a form of control (by heroin itself) which, it would seem, is all the more pernicious because it does not even permit the first steps toward collective action directed against social problems. In addition, it would doom other residents of the ghettos and other high incidence areas to terrorization by those who are driven by their dependence.

The third criticism that radicals have made of methadone maintenance relates to its efficacy as a treatment modality. With the increasing accuracy of reporting and the expansion of the scope of maintenance programs, it is becoming quite clear that the initial forecasts of success were far too sanguine. The drop-out and termination rates are higher than we were led to expect. Many were simply not ready to give up using heroin. In addition, those who are successfully "blockaded" in rather large numbers resort to the abuse of other drugs (notably barbiturates and amphetamines or alcohol), the choice of being "high" determined by availability and/or cultural factors. The language conventionally used to describe this process of substitution is instructive. Patients "cheat." They still seek "thrills and kicks." These assertions are posed in moralistic terms and focus upon the putative perversity and/or intractability of the patient. Most important, these terms are merely descriptive and not at all explanatory. The question of why patients continue to seek highs is not dealt with.

When radicals in the field confront this situation, they see a continuation of the desperate effort of patients to escape from the social reality that is the root cause. Life in the ghetto does not change after one is stabilized on methadone, nor does the emptiness of existence become altered. Thus, radicals question the value of methadone, which, while eliminating heroin dependence, turns many to alcohol and pill abuse. Here again we can see both the value as well as the limitations of methadone, for while maintenance accomplishes its task of ending the dependence upon heroin, it does not and cannot, by itself, come to grips with the reason people become compulsive users to begin with. To achieve this end, treatment programs must be created that provide people with both the insight to understand the source of their pain and the skills with which to combat the socioeconomic system that is at the root of so much of that pain.

It has been argued that the radical critique of methadone maintenance fails because it does not recognize the fact that, for many, methadone provides the first condition for personal and social liberation. Yet, by focusing on the social roots of compulsive use, the radical perspective is able to elucidate both the limitations of methadone treatment and of treatment in general, in dealing with the problems of dependence in American society.

Just as it is absurd to treat the illness of children in the ghettos without striking at the racism, poverty, and malnutrition that are responsible for that illness, there is something absurd about planning national campaigns against dependence without recognizing and striking out against its social roots. If we grasp this fact, then we must recognize that the ultimate solution is neither personal, moral, nor psychologic, but political, for it requires a fundamental transformation of our social order. In short, if we are committed to the elimination of dependence, we must be committed to the transformation of objective social reality so that men and women will no longer feel the need to nod their way through or overdose their way of life.

In another kind of response concerning methadone and medical ethics, Dr. James Maddux made the following remarks in a paper presented to the Fourth National Conference on Methadone Treatment.[107]

Physicians working on methadone maintenance programs often act as if empirical data and technical procedures represent their primary concerns, while ethical considerations represent something to be taken for granted and hardly worth discussing. Nevertheless, ethical choice underlies nearly everything the physician does in maintaining drug dependence with methadone. Emotionally charged arguments for and against methadone maintenance arise more from differences in value judgements than from differences in knowledge.

According to Maddux, the ethics of methadone maintenance must be considered in relation to the paramount ethical concern of the physician: the welfare of the patient. Divergence of opinion among physicians about methadone maintenance does not mean that some opinions are "moralistic" and others not; all opinions become equally ethical if they equally reflect concern with the welfare of the patient. But, among equally ethical physicians, differences may exist as to the weights given to the benefits and hazards of methadone maintenance.

The physician confronts four problems of ethics in methadone maintenance: (1) the benefits and hazards for the individual; (2) protection of human research subjects; (3) coercion to choose methadone maintenance; and (4) coercion to conform with methadone.

*Benefits and Hazards for the Individual:* Maintaining drug dependence with orally administered methadone frees the individual from the illegal hustle for heroin, from intravenous use of an illicit mixture of uncertain composition, and from the use of dirty needles. But these benefits have costs. Regularly administered methadone, as does morphine, probably produces profound and long-lasting changes in physiologic and psychologic equilibrium. Quite possibly, these changes become more severe and deeply imbedded with continued daily high-dose methadone. For the individual with the hope of overcoming drug dependence, methadone maintenance may reduce the probability of achieving an enduring abstinence. The hazard of permanent drug dependence as a consequence of methadone maintenance has not been adequately evaluated, as follow-up studies of abstinence have not been done. Whatever the long-term follow-up data may show, the physicians who today place patients on methadone maintenance make an ethical choice: they weigh the benefits and hazards, and then do what they consider good for their patients. (See section on advantages and disadvantages.)

*Protection of Human Research Subjects:* As long as the value of methadone maintenance is still being investigated, protection of the rights and welfare of human research subjects will remain an ethical requirement of the procedure. The welfare of the patient overlaps that of the human research subject in that both require estimation of risks and potential benefits, but for the research subject, informed voluntary consent becomes a special additional requirement. Yet physicians are confronted by the problem of accepting patients for methadone maintenance under legal coercion.

*Coercion to Choose Methadone Maintenance:* In 1969, Mrs. Albert D. Lasker was quoted as saying that judges should be able to sentence appropriate addicts to methadone as a public health measure.[108] In 1971, in San Antonio, Texas, a court convicted a heroin user of robbery by assault and then suspended the sentence on condition that the "defendent will immediately apply for and receive methadone treatment for his narcotic addiction. . . ." The ethical problem for the physician of compulsory methadone maintenance was discussed in 1970 by Newman,[108] who considered it a serious danger to methadone maintenance programs. In the same year, Dole[109] objected to the legal imposition of methadone maintenance, stating that "the rights of addicts must be respected." Since criminal sentences are imposed more for the protection of society than for the benefit of the individual, the physician who orders methadone for maintenance in response to a court order primarily serves society rather than the patient.

*Coercion to Conform with Methadone:* All methadone maintenance programs appear to set some behavioral standards for patients. The standards vary from the minimum performance necessary for participation in the program—for example, taking the methadone and providing information and urine specimens—to additional broad requirements that the individual become law-abiding, legitimately employed or a student, abstinent from illicit drugs, and use alcohol moderately, if at all. Failure to comply with the requirements leads to reduction or withholding of methadone, and, if the lack of compliance persists, to termination of methadone maintenance. In the Denver program for addicts under legal coercion, as reported by Starkey and Egan,[110] repeated positive urines can send an addict back to jail. Use of an illicit drug leads to loss of both methadone and liberty. Concern also has been expressed about the possible use of methadone to control the behavior of members of two minority groups, blacks and persons of Mexican background.

The physician who gives or withholds methadone to obtain ''socially desirable'' behavior primarily serves society. As noted before, the physician's ethic requires that the patient come first. Newman[106] also identified the problem of using methadone maintenance to obtain socially conforming behavior. Of course, society cannot survive without adherence by its members to established rules and, conceivably, society, through its courts, not only could order and dispense methadone for drug-dependent persons, but also could give or withhold the drug to obtain socially conforming behavior. Distribution of a pleasure-giving drug by government officials was a major feature of control of behavior in Huxley's *Brave New World.*[111] The political use of methadone may attract or repel us as individuals, but must not influence the physician's concern for the welfare of the patient.

Unconscious coercion to obtain socially or personally pleasing behavior could be reduced if physicians were to prescribe methadone primarily for a pharmacologic purposes; that is, to substitute a methadone dependence for a heroin dependence. Patients then would be free to use or not to use psychotherapy or other assistance, to work or not to work, and to steal or not to steal. Nevertheless a completely permissive and impersonal dispensing of methadone for its pharmacologic effects alone is not likely to be achieved under existing conditions, as limit setting is required, and personal interaction is always involved.

In his paper, Dr. Maddux made special comments to physicians working in methadone maintenance programs,[107] pointing out that the physician and others in a methadone maintenance program must not tolerate behavior harmful to the program, such as violence toward staff members or other patients, or illegal activity on the premises. While disruptive behavior may require withholding the methadone, the precise limits are not easily defined. How often can drunkenness at the outpatient office be overlooked, and how drunk must the individual become to be considered disruptive? What action should the staff members take if they believe that a methadone patient is selling heroin across the street from a dispensing facility? Should they take any special steps to prevent unemployed patients from, after getting their free methadone, going to a nearby bar, because their drinking probably will inhibit their job seeking? Should a physician permit a patient to use obscene language upon being denied a three-day supply of methadone to take home? What should the staff do about an employable patient who remains unemployed, perhaps to avoid paying a fee for the service? Wherever limits are defined, this introduces an unavoidable measure of control of behavior.

Finally, Dr. Maddux[107] believes that the complex of problems of political or personal coercion related to the giving or withholding of methadone could be eliminated by removal of legal controls on drugs. As already noted, removal of legal controls would also eliminate the problem of coerced choice of methadone maintenance. If controls were removed, individuals could freely choose to use methadone or morphine or heroin, while their behavior, like that of other people, would be regulated by the normal sanctions of society. The cost of such removal of legal controls would probably be a marked increase in drug dependence of the morphine type.

The physician in methadone maintenance confronts four ethical problems. First, the hazards and benefits must be evaluated, and then an ethical choice made that is for the patient's good. The potential for possible permanent drug dependence consequent to the methadone maintenance, however, has not been adequately evaluated. Second, as long as methadone maintenance continues in investigational status, the protection of human research subjects, primarily through informed voluntary consent, is required. Third, legal coercion of patients to choose methadone maintenance restricts voluntary choice and tends to serve society rather than the patient. Fourth, giving and withholding methadone to obtain socially desirable behavior also tends to serve society rather than the patient.

The problem of legally coerced choice of methadone maintenance could be avoided by accepting only patients free from legal pressure. The problem of influencing behavior by offering methadone as a reward could be reduced by dispensing methadone primarily for its pharmacologic effects. Both problems of coercion could be eliminated by the removal of legal controls on drugs, but at the cost of a probable marked increase in the prevalence of drug dependence.

*Politicization of Methadone*[112]: The nonmedical use of drugs has become a political concern. Drug abuse intervention has also become highly politicized. Methadone maintenance has become one of the recent victims of political rhetoric and promises.

Political leaders and spokespeople have taken pro and con positions on methadone maintenance. Oddly enough, relatively few public positions have been taken on individual counseling, group therapy, hypnotherapy, and the like. Perhaps not as odd is that equally few public statements have been made about the problems associated with the treatment of excessive alcohol intake generally, and specifically the use of Antabuse, or about smoking and its treatment. The U.S. public, upon which the political leader is dependent, is not overly concerned with the effects of the consumption of alcoholic beverages or the use of tobacco products, but is concerned about the nonmedical use of other drugs (in that they do not want to be affected by it).

This limited concern permits the politicization of methadone maintenance. Promises are made, depending upon the constituency, to expand or restrict the use of methadone, with the implication that whatever action is taken, the difficulties that concern the public automatically will be decreased, if not eliminated. We must remember that funding for drug intervention may have political preference, whereas drug action has none. We must also remind ourselves that there are no chemical solutions to human issues, although there are many necessary chemical tools and techniques. This central issue is quite simple. The sad reality is that the efficacy of methadone treatment, or its limitations, can never be fully realized as long as it is colored by political action and rhetoric. Individuals working in methadone treatment must be aware that they are entering a highly politicized arena and that their delivery of services cannot be apolitical.

*Critical Issues Concerning Methadone:* Many critical issues concerning methadone remain with us—in part, because we do not fully understand the etiology of drug use, the pharmacologic action of drugs in general, and of methadone specifically, or the process of effective treatment. The confusion resulting from these unresolved issues—which is then reinforced by the general anxiety and sense of helplessness about contemporary drug use, the pressure from the political arena, and the empire building of professionals and paraprofessionals—makes it difficult, but imperative, to delineate these issues. To do otherwise can only result in ritual activity rather than effective treatment.

Some critical issues that demand attention and have been discussed elsewhere[112] are presented herein:

1. *What is the most effective methadone treatment process?*

It is a system that develops and reinforces the highest level of functioning possible for a person in an acceptable, conventional life-style based on the person's skills, abilities, and needs, the intervention agent's skills and ability, and the general community's acceptance of the patient's new or renewed functional role.

2. *Who makes decisions about permitting the development or expansion of a methadone maintenance program?*

The decision should be based on the evaluated effectiveness of the process and not on political or budgetary expediency. The decision makers should include representatives of those being affected in whatever way by opiate-related behavior, rather than just by the treatment agent. Thus the patient and the general community must be involved. One must distinguish between the medical facets, other therapy facets, and more generic treatment facets in deciding upon the expansion of a program. A methadone treatment program is not equivalent to a medical program. A difficulty is that most of these decisions are not usually made by the knowledgable and concerned individual but by less informed bureaucrats.

3. *Which patients will benefit from methadone?*

From an empirical perspective, we do not know, in any predictive sense, and have little useful data on this issue.

4. *When is methadone treatment contraindicated?*

It is contraindicated, from the patient's perspective, based on available data, when it either is not helping (given the criteria of a given program) or when it is harmful; from the treatment agent's perspective, when the necessary conjunctive services or skills are too limited or are absent; and from the community's perspective, when the program is unacceptable to its value system, or when other community concerns take on higher priority and need public funding. When the factors for contraindication change, then the treatment once more may be indicated. This may necessitate changing the screening and treatment criteria for patients, developing the necessary levels of skills for staff and necessary conjunctive services, and dispelling the myths and stereotypes that a community may have about methadone treatment.

5. *Do side effects militate against an expanded use of methadone maintenance?*

Usually side effects are evaluated in terms of the number of patients reporting them and/or the extent to which they interfere with daily functioning. Whatever the source of these effects, or their extent, we must also consider the side effects for the treatment agent and the general community. The health of an individual and the community necessitates an accurate assessment not only of the status and effect of various side effects, but of their meaning as well.

6. *What is the relationship between methadone and pregnancy?*

To date, studies have indicated that females on methadone show normal menstruation, ovulation, conception, and pregnancy. There may be a tendency for babies to be smaller than average but as they grow, their physical and intellectual development should be normal. No congenital anomalies have been found.[113]

7. *What contemporary typologies of methadone maintenance patients have predictive value for success or failure?*

The lack of scientifically based, useful typologies in the field of drug abuse, in general, and so in the limited field of methadone maintenance, is one of the key factors that make it impossible, in a predictive sense, to determine what types of therapy, with what goal(s), are more or less desirable for a given individual at a given point in the treatment.

8. *What criteria should be utilized for screening patients for methadone maintenance?*

The criteria, as arbitrary as they may be, should be based on the ability of the patient to use the goal system and the conjunctive services of a given program. They should relate, in a pragmatic way, to the available skills and abilities of the program's treatment staff.

Program criteria are based on the pragmatic assumption that they serve to screen in individuals who will be helped by the available process and screen out those not helped by the process. Such issues as age, sex, length of drug use, arrests, and time served are, to date, unpragmatic, nonscientific issues that are colored by moral–ethical considerations. The FDA eligibility criteria includes (a) physical dependence on an opioid drug at least one year before admission, and (b) current physical dependence.

9. *Who is to decide which addicts should be included in or excluded from a methadone maintenance program?*

Such decisions should be made by individuals who clearly understand what this form of therapy can and cannot do, and have the ability and the power to develop a methadone treatment process that meets the health needs of the affected individuals and the community.

10. *What types of goal systems should be utilized in methadone maintenance?*

The same theoretic goal system that is developed for any treatment system should be used in methadone maintenance. The goals should be *meaningful, achievable,* and *acceptable* for the patient-to-be, and *acceptable* by the treatment agent and the community at large. If the goals are not personally meaningful, then they do not relate to a proposed level of functioning or life-style that can effectively challenge a drug-oriented life. If they are not achievable, it is unfair to expect the person to aspire to them, and to experience another built-in failure and a further sense of frustration. If they are not acceptable, for whatever reason, then treatment is not possible. At the present time, almost no drug treatment programs conceptualize treatment goals in this manner. Rather they use a homogeneous goal—abstinence—for a heterogeneous group, thereby reinforcing a high attrition and/or failure rate.

11. *What are the possible roles, during methadone maintenance, for the intervention agent, the patient, and the general community?*

The classic, or medical model, role assumes that intervention agents develop and carry out a series of therapies on a passive patient, for a passive community that funds the process.

A constituency model of care demands that each of the participants have an active but clearly delineated role in the entire process, from its inception to extramural evaluation. Decision making, extent and types of responsibilities, specific tasks, such as therapy, early case finding, prevention, and their associated roles are to be based on the strengths and weaknesses of the constituents and the needs of the affected and the general community, and are to change as the situation, conditions, and priorities change. This type of model assumes that a patient is not only the drug user, but the community as well; and that the use of a particular technique—methadone treatment—has relevance for the life-style of the community as well as of the client.

12. *What criteria are to be used to determine whether to use high- or low-dose treatment?*

The dose must be related to the patient's present, as well as achievable, state of functioning derived from baseline evaluation data. Unfortunately, more often than not, the dose is determined by a program's commitment to a specific dose philosophy. A specific philosophy, and specific dose, are certainly no replacement for a well-planned delivery-of-treatment system. It has been empirically suggested that "50 mg of methadone daily would totally prevent any effect of ordinary heroin doses and would significantly diminish the effects of quite large heroin doses."[114]

13. *What are the minimal conjunctive services that must be available for methadone maintenance patients?*

Given that methadone maintenance is a type of therapy that should be part of a treatment process hand-tailored to the needs and abilities of the patient, and the strengths and weaknesses of the treatment system and the community in which it occurs, the treatment system must include all those services that are necessary for increasing or maintaining the health of the individual, the system, and the community. This has to be determined empirically and must change over time.

The term *ancillary services* all too often means the minimum service that we can give the patient and still look good enough to be reimbursed.

14. *What criteria should be utilized for screening the staff of a methadone maintenance program?*

The primary criteria concern a staff member's ability to communicate hope to the patients, to point out alternatives to any given situation, to avoid stereotyping the drug user, not to be committed to only one treatment philosophy or one model of care, to be trained in the techniques that will be used.

The client has enough difficulties without having to adapt to saviors whose treatment philosophy is based on the notion that if the patient gets better, it is because of the worker's efforts. If the patient gets worse, it is because of the patient's lack of motivation.

15. *Who is to be given the role of maintaining continuity of care and of responsibility in a methadone maintenance program?*

The connotation of these concepts is that once treatment has been planned and begun, it will continue—until it is no longer serving any useful purpose. Someone has to take the responsibility for assessing ongoing changes in the patient and the system as they relate to needed changes in treatment, as well as monitoring a plan's effectiveness or seeing why it has not been carried out. These people must understand the treatment process and the various models for its delivery. They must have the respect of all who are involved in the process, be able to delegate responsibilities, and be willing and able to permit, if not to arrange for, other people to take the credit for successful intervention. This proposed *central case manager,* whether the case be a person, a system, an institution, or a community, is there to see that the methadone treatment system works, or that it is improved and corrected in order to make it work.

16. *What type of training is necessary for the staff of a methadone maintenance program?*

The minimal training must cover the purposes underlying the development of a program. These include issues relative to evaluation of the person's and system's strengths and weaknesses; goal systems that are meaningful, achievable, acceptable, and flexible; role definitions for all the constituents; and the understanding of various models of health and delivery of health services and their associated consequences. Training also must include the development or reinforcement of specific skills that are necessary for treatment to continue; systems for ongoing and effective evaluation; systems for appropriate referral; techniques for termination and their consequences; means of follow-up; and the communication of hope and a knowledge of achievable alternatives. Additional training should include nature of opioid dependence, etiology of opioid dependence, pharmacology of opioid drugs, effects of methadone, and counseling skills.

The training must be broadly based because the goal of treatment is broadly based: increased health and function for the individual, the system, and the general community. We need general advocates of health, not parochial advocates of a particular technique.

17. *What is the role of, and what are the issues related to, reevaluation in a methadone maintenance program?*

Meaningful reevaluation implies an ongoing assessment of the patient's strengths and weaknesses as they relate to a treatment plan; the availability and use of necessary community resources; the status of the selected goal(s); role achievement and meaning and its effect on the treatment process; the appropriateness of a specific methadone technique, with or without conjunctive services, for the patient; the status of a treatment agent's training and availability; the status of continuity of care and responsibility for a given patient and plan of action; and the need for referral and termination. Ongoing evaluation permits the reinforcement of what is effective and the changing of what is ineffective so that we can meet the needs of present or future intervention agents, political and community leaders, and the like.

18. *What is the relationship between follow-up and posttreatment in methadone maintenance?*

Follow-up is the secular term for the more parochial concept of Judgment Day. At some point after treatment, the process has to be evaluated in terms of results. The patient, the intervention agent, and the general community are entitled to know whether it was all worth it. There are various ways of assessing this: Have the crtieria that were used had predictive value? Have the goals been achieved? Has the delivery system worked smoothly? Is the process easily replicated? Must minor or major changes be made? Have the consequences of the process created more problems than the process was meant to cause? The final question is perhaps the most difficult to answer, because of its arbitrariness: Were the personal, systemic, and financial costs worth the effort, given other individual and community problems, needs, and priorities?

19. *What does prevention mean in methadone maintenance?*

Traditionally prevention (with regard to the nonmedical use of drugs) has meant eliminating the use of all but certain substances for medically or socially approved reasons. Transposed to methadone maintenance, this means helping the addict to use substances as medicine and to come to terms with using only certain substances (alcohol, cigarettes) for social rituals or recreation. The dilemma that this presents is that more often than not, the addict "knows" what should not be done—what is to be prevented—but may not know or may be confused about what should be aspired to, achieved, or reinforced.

What is at issue is whether a methadone program prepares a person for adaptation to a world of chemicals or to a world of people, in which the actions and reactions of people often will be less predictable than that of chemical action.

20. *What type of training and/or education about methadone treatment is necessary for the community, and who is to do it?*

The community should be made aware of the difference between a treatment process and the use of a particular technique; what results can be expected from each and what role they play in furthering a successful outcome or in preventing one.

The public should be made aware of the fact that communities have a vested interest, both economic and social, in drug abuse, and that no single technique will alter the pattern of recreational drug use until the community's economic and social priorities change. The community should be offered the opportunity to take an active role in the methadone program, instead of the single role of funding agent. In the process of doing this, it will learn what the gaps in necessary services are and whether the agreed-upon program is meeting the needs of the affected, as well as the general community.

Responsibility for this course of education should be given to individuals who not only have the skill to do this, but who are trained and committed to patient and community health, rather than spokespersons for only one of the constituents. Perhaps the central case manager would be able to take on this additional task.

21. *What relationship does the study of altered states of consciousness have to methadone maintenance?*

No relationship is obvious, and from a research perspective, it may prove to be irrelevant. Nevertheless the meaning of altered states of consciousness, drug-related or not, for the patient, staff, and the community should be seriously examined, given the present expanding interest in this field. Increased awareness of one's self, and meaningful and effective utilization of what is discovered through induced altered states of consciousness, may be a useful adjunct to achieving the goals of a methadone program.

According to Einstein and Burrell[112]:

> There are many more questions and issues that each of us can raise. At best, methadone can serve as one of many tools in helping compulsive narcotic users. It can't return the client to the mainstream of living, if he never lived there before. It cannot create drug freedom if a community's value system and life style are not based on this concept. We must keep in mind that there are no instant magic solutions—drugs or otherwise—for the problems of living. No drug, short- or long-acting, can create adequate coping mechanisms, maturation and realistic decision making. It takes a lifetime, and there are no shortcuts. Unfortunately, there are, all too often, many man-made barriers. We can help determine whether methadone treatment becomes a useful tool or another barrier.

## *Summary of the Issues*[115]

One cannot yet fully evaluate the effectiveness and impact of methadone maintenance upon compulsive narcotic use. Dole and colleagues[109,116] report that 80 percent of all patients who enter the program remain for at least two years; that of those who had previously been involved in crimes, 90 percent ended such activity; and that 75 percent of all patients retained in the program returned to productive lives. No other therapeutic modality used today can even approach these claims.

Critics of methadone maintenance generally fall into three categories. First are those who condemn the perpetuation of the addicted state and the long-term use of a narcotic agent for moral, sociologic, or psychologic reasons.[117–119] Others accept maintenance as valid therapy under highly controlled circumstances but fear that the easing of restrictions on distribution, to reach more addicts, may result in illicit diversion of methadone on a large scale, and thus the addition of another narcotic to illegal street traffic.[120,121] A third group perceives weaknesses within the program protocol.[122] Scrutiny of the Dole–Nyswander program indicates that approximately 20 percent of those on methadone maintenance have resorted to the use of such other agents as alcohol, barbiturates, and CNS stimulants, and that 14 percent had to be discharged as a consequence of psychotic, delinquent, or other provocative or disruptive forms of behavior. Maintenance (in its present form) does not appear to be a valid method for treating clients with such traits. Connor and Kremen[124] concluded that there should be a much more structured program of ongoing therapy, and a wider range of supportive services, after evaluating a group of patients on methadone and finding that they suffered from moodiness, loneliness, poor self-image, and conflict in sex identification, despite outward social productivity.[123,124]

External review committees will need to examine long-term results of methadone maintenance from the point of view of both the return of an individual to a rewarding and meaningful life and the relief of society from the burden of the user and any attendant crime. It appears that methadone maintenance has won a place in the therapeutic armamentarium for management of the opiate-dependent person who has failed or has been unresponsive to other forms of treatment.[125] Certainly programs are developing throughout the country at a rapid pace.[125] We do not see methadone maintenance as a panacea, but rather as one of a number of approaches, which have a rightful place in further investigations but none of which can reach a substantial number of the "hard-core" population or answer the question of how to prevent individuals from becoming users of narcotics.

Dole and Nyswander think that methadone maintenance will prove to be necessary for an indefinite period of time. In reviewing 350 patients withdrawn from methadone and returned to a narcotic-free state, they reported that most still felt a craving for heroin, even when successful adjustments had been made that led the patients to feel that they could live without drugs. Most sought readmission to the program and, if not taken back, started taking heroin again. These investigators[128] conclude that their experience definitely does not support the traditional assumption that drug hunger is a symptom of social and psychologic problems, but may be biological.

## *General Comments and Summary*[126,127]

Although much still remains unsaid, some of the practical and less scientific aspects of methadone and methadone treatment have been presented here. It should be established that, when used properly, methadone is a valuable tool in selected cases of drug dependence on opiate-like drugs. From a rational and realistic perspective toward methadone, it is clear that there is nothing magic about it. Methadone simply affords symptomatic relief and control of some of the symptoms of the process, thus allowing the patient time to effect other changes in life-style, to acquire new skills, and to develop more appropriate alternatives.

The concept of total rehabilitation or cure will always depend more on the effectiveness of supportive services and counseling skills than on the pharmacologic effects of methadone. As in other modalities of treatment, much depends on the level or motivation of the patient who allegedly wants to make changes. Motivation can be encouraged by convincing the patient that there is, realistically, an alternative to life-long drug dependence. The patient should select alternatives with the assistance of staff when possible. Forced behavior modification to ensure continued methadone supply is not only dangerous, but unethical and immoral. Minority groups have expressed concern about, as well as opposition to, the use of methadone maintenance, recognizing the potential for methadone to be used to impose social change or conformity, or to establish acceptable behavior and life-style. A certain amount of structure and regulation is essential to the effective operation of a treatment program; however, constraint should be exercised to avoid exceeding reasonable expectation, depriving the patient of self-determination. Compulsive opiate users for years have been aptly described as having a chronic and relapsing disorder. This very basic fact is often overlooked in highly judgmental programs and by those who shape policy and regulate just how, when, and where methadone is to be used, and for whom and for how long. To state that methadone maintenance treatment will not ordinarily exceed two years is about as rational as limiting the treatment of diabetes to two years, assuming that if in that period the body has not learned how to produce its own insulin again, or to get by without it, treatment should be discontinued. This is not meant to minimize or deny the ideal goal of total rehabilitation—a long and good life free from all forms of chemical dependence—but we must consider genetic predisposition as part of the disorder, thereby limiting a drug-free existence. To interview a new patient, say a man 30 years of age who has spent the first half of life getting messed up and the remainder being messed up, who has either been on heroin or in prison all of his adult life, and who has other functional disabilities, and tell him that we have two years in which to rebuild him into a new, whole, and healthy person, is being naive.

The disorder is medical, social, psychologic, genetic (in some), and behavioral, and its effects extend beyond the addict, family, and community. To focus all attention on the fact of fixing heroin is to see only one small facet of the total picture and the result is distorted and fuzzy thinking and treatment. Those persons involved in treatment programs will save themselves considerable frustration and serve their clients better by accepting the chronicity of the disorder, as well as their own limitations, in terms of being able to help or effect real change in a personality. Treatment in any modality should be considered a very-long-term process, measured in years, not weeks or months. The unlearning of conditioned responses and the learning of alternatives are extremely slow and uncertain procedures. People who do not wish to change are not likely to be altered by any form of therapy. Those who are highly motivated have a better prognosis. Still, the best prognosis for "cure" is poor, even in the best patients. But if we lower our sights and take a realistic approach, we must find some satisfaction in the comfort and symptomatic relief offered by the methadone maintenance treatment program and its supportive services. The patient, family, and community benefit if a significant degree of control is realized, even if the cure remains elusive. Workers in programs need to look deeper than a "clean" urine record and steady job and staying out of jail as measures of success in the treatment of patients.

Is the drug-dependent person who is able to maintain a drug-free state while living with discomfort, anxiety, irritability, impaired job function, erratic compensatory behavior, and insomnia, and is working and staying out of jail, better off than a methadone patient who is also working and staying out of jail, but relatively free of other symptoms? A possible goal of treatment is to allow a person to live a full and meaningful life, with a minimum of discomfort. This is far more important to the patient than being drug-free, that is, off methadone and other psychoactive drugs. How long should methadone treatment last? The answer is: As long as it benefits the patients and no better alternative is available.

Alcohol use among methadone maintenance patients is the subject of growing national interest and concern. It is not incredible that a significant percentage of methadone maintenance is associated with alcoholism; alcoholism in methadone maintenance programs reflects program failure, in the sense of being able to deal with the total pattern of drug dependence. Prior to being placed on methadone maintenance, the patient has already established a pattern of relying on certain drugs to self-medicate for the relief of anxiety and other symptoms. The user has spent most waking hours either in the pursuit of the next fix or in the enjoyment of the last.

When methadone is substituted for heroin, addicts may find they have a lot of free time. This time can be used constructively, or it may result in boredom and an increased awareness of the situation, thus provoking new anxiety and/or depression, as well as other symptoms.

As tolerance is acquired to methadone, no significant antianxiety effect is obtained, and small doses of street heroin not only are ineffective, but will be detected by urine screening. If additional self-medication is needed, the most likely drug is alcohol. It will not be detected by urine screening, is relatively inexpensive, and is legally and socially acceptable. (See section on methadone and alcohol consumption.)

These comments offer no solution to the alcohol problem, but simply serve to emphasize that the basic problem of drug dependence is the established pattern of reliance on drugs to cope with stress, and not an isolated problem based on the pharmacology of narcotics. We have only scratched the surface in the area of effective treatment and rehabilitation and are fortunate to have a useful drug such as methadone to afford symptomatic relief while continued efforts are made to reform and improve treatment approaches. Methadone deserves a place in the treatment of selected cases but should be offered in conjunction with a full range of other services, as well as alternative (nonnarcotic) modalities.

## J. PROPOXYPHENE

In October 1973, propoxyphene napsylate (Darvon-N) was administered to patients in Los Angeles for the purpose of finding an alternative and adjunct to methadone treatment. The initial results indicated that this agent could detoxify and maintain most individuals who are physically dependent upon heroin.

### 1. History

Inaba et al.[129] have reviewed the historic development of the use of Darvon-N as a maintenance tool.

Stimulated by the continued controversy surrounding methadone in the treatment of heroin dependence, much interest has been generated in the search for a substance that would retain methadone's beneficial effects while remaining free of its undesirable characteristics.

Tennant, of the University of California at Los Angeles, has demonstrated propoxyphene napsylate (Darvon-N) to be an effective substitute for both maintenance and detoxification therapy.[130,135–137] In a nine-month study, he noted specific advantages of propoxyphene napsylate (PN) over methadone for use in treatment. Of a total population of 372 patients, 230 were reported satisfactorily detoxified from heroin as inpatients, 50 were detoxified as outpatients, and 92 were maintained (for a period of greater than 21 days) on PN as outpatients. Initial daily dosages of PN ranged from 300 to 1600 mg, and although most were well above the recommended maximum daily human dose of 8 mg/kg, no toxicity was noted. It was concluded that PN not only demonstrated the full benefits of methadone therapy, but also produced minimal physical dependence, had no reports of impotence, induced an unpleasant euphoria (thus leading to negligible incidence of voluntary abuse), could not be injected, produced unpleasant effects when ingested simultaneously with other abused drugs, and had a low overdosage potential because of its slow absorption from the gastrointestinal tract—thus clearly establishing many clinical advantages over methadone therapy.

Cases of propoxyphene hydrochloride (PCl) abuse and true physical addiction,[138–142] along with many cases of PC overdosage and death,[143–146] have been reported in the medical literature in recent years. The potentially lethal consequences of propoxyphene, with intoxication frequently complicated by pulmonary edema, convulsions, and generalized CNS depression,[144] warrant further elucidation with regard to the water solubility of its two common clinical salts.

Convulsions appear to be particularly common with propoxyphene overdose (being noted much less frequently with other opioid-type drugs), thus severely complicating the course of therapy. Further, although narcotic antagonists such as naloxone (Narcan) are less effective in reversing the respiratory depressant effects of propoxyphene, they seem to be *less* effective as compared with their dramatic reversal of opiates, such as morphine or heroin.

Propoxyphene napsylate is only slightly soluble in water (1.5 mg/ml), whereas PCl is very water soluble (2 g/ml).[147] This lower water solubility of PN has been proposed to explain its slower absorption from the gastrointestinal tract and lower peak plasma levels. It is, therefore, hypothesized that the overdose potential of PN is much lower than that of PCl. Wolen et al.[148] have demonstrated that therapeutic oral doses of PCl (65 to 130 mg) and PN (100 to 200 mg) ingested with a given volume of water (180 ml) result in significantly slower absorption of PN into the plasma, although the peak plasma concentration of PN is not significantly affected. It is reasonable to assume, however, that if the dosage of PN were increased while the amount of water ingested remained the same, significantly lower peak plasma concentration of PN would result in comparison with that expected for PCI, because of the (demonstrated) lower water solubility of PN. It follows then that as a result of this crucial distinction in water solubility between the napsylate and hydrochloride salts of propoxyphene, PN may well have a lower overdose potential than PCl. Indeed, a 9-gram dose of PN has been survived with sequellae.[130,132–137]

### 2. Chemistry of Propoxyphene[3]

Of the four stereoisomers, only the alpha

racemate, known as propoxyphene, has analgesic activity. Its analgesic effect resides in the dextrorotary isomer, d-propoxyphene (dextropropoxyphene). However, levopropoxyphene seems to have some antitussive activity. As can be seen from the formula (Figure 7-5), it is related structurally to methadone.

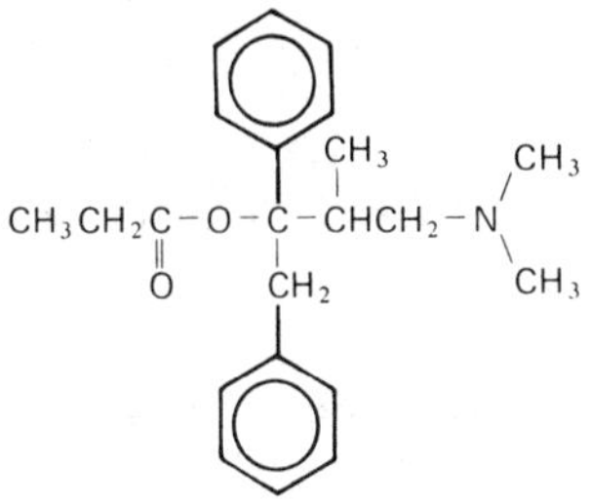

**Figure 7-5. Propoxyphene.**

## 3. Pharmacology

The pharmacological actions of propoxyphene are similar to codeine. This includes both its agonistic opioid activity as well as side reactions, such as nausea, drowsiness, reduced eating, and gastrointestinal disturbances. There is a question as to the actual pain-relieving qualities of this drug. Although some studies indicate that 32 mg. of propoxyphene provided no better pain-relief than a placebo, Beaver[46] reported that approximately 120 mg. was equivalent to 60 mg. of codeine as an analgesic, which makes it about half as effective as the latter drug. In comparison, aspirin is about ⅕th to ⅒th the potency of codeine. In this regard, a popular prescription analgesic combination is that which contains both propoxyphene and aspirin. Experimental evidence suggests that the combination is better than either agent alone.[45,46, 149,150] Darvon has no antipyretic action and therefore the combination is not suitable in arthritic conditions.

## 4. Pharmacokinetics and Metabolism

Both the oral as well as parenteral routes are readily absorbed. Although the two salts of propoxyphene are safe in average doses, it is well known that the water-soluble hydrochloride is absorbed more quickly than the water-insoluble napsylate. With these salts, peak concentration is reached within two hours after administration. The mean half-life of propoxyphene after parental (intravenous) administration is approximately one half of that observed for the oral route, reported to be 3½ hours. Following repeated administration every six hours a steady-state peak concentration is reached after two days.

The major pathway of biotransformation is N-demethylation. The pharmacodynamic and metabolic properties of propoxyphene varies greatly between patients.[151] In humans, rats, and dogs no propoxyphene has been shown to be excreted in urine.[152]

## 5. Side Reactions and Toxicity

There is ample evidence to show that the napsylate salt of propoxyphene is safer than the hydrochloride when high doses are taken. In chronic toxicity studies (two years) in animals, investigators reported that the napsylate salt produced no significant toxicity with daily doses of 50 mg./kg./day in the dog and 200 mg./kg./day in the rat. At these doses elevations of alkaline phosphatase, indicating a liver enlargement, was found which was similar to the tissue changes seen with chronic hepatitis. In both humans and animals, acute lethal doses also produce convulsions and respiratory depression.

Propoxyphene hydrochloride or its napsylate salt in usual therapeutic doses do not produce significant effects on the cardiovascular system. Tennant *et al*,[130] noted that toxic doses induce delusions, hallucinations and confusion; death is due to pulmonary edema. Naloxone but not nalorphine consistantly blocks the acute toxicity of propoxyphene. Other side effects include blurred vision, dizziness, drowsiness, nervousness, and feelings of detachment, as reported by subjects. Darvon-N on the street is known as "Yellow Footballs." It can be purchased for about one dollar a capsule. Its prime street use is diverted toward reducing a heroin "habit" or abolishing potential heroin abstinence effects. Since the drug is rather insoluble in water, the intravenous route will probably not become very popular.

### 6. Addiction Liability

Propxyphene (Darvon) was clinically introduced as a pain-killer over 25 years ago. Today it is recognized as the leading prescription analgesic in America. Darvon has only slight cross-dependence with other narcotic analgesics such as morphine. In fact, 800 mg. of the hydrochloride salt per day reduce the morphine abstinence syndrome. Propoxyphene produces its own addiction as noted by scientists[130,150] working with patients who were taking up to 800 mg. per day for two months, the withdrawal from which resulted in mild abstinence, i.e., withdrawal symptoms. Large oral doses up to 600 mg. induces a state of euphoria which is much less discernable than with morphine.

For over twenty years the drug has not been under strict narcotic controls. This led to a short period in the United States of serious intravenous use and dependence which lessened when stronger prescribing regulations appeared. Currently, the drug is not under strict narcotic control in the United States. Tennant[130] pointed out in an article on the complications of propoxyphene abuse:

"Administered intravenously, it is recognized as a narcotic; however, it is quite irritating when administered intravenously or subcutaneously, so that use by these routes results in severe damage to veins and soft tissues, which limits the time the drug can be used parenterally."

During 1973, Tennant reported a widespread abuse of the drug among American soldiers stationed in West Germany. He estimated that 15 to 20 percent of the 180,000 soldiers had used Darvon for nonmedical purposes, and reported 13 deaths due to overdose. Respiratory depression with pulmonary edema and convulsions were the commonly observed terminal events. Other complications included toxic psychotic reactions and inflammatory reactions at the site of the intravenous injection. Propoxyphene has a marked sclerosing effect upon veins of soft tissue. In this regard, propoxyphene dependence is supposed to be self-limiting because of sclerosis of the superficial veins over a period of weeks or months.

## K. CLINICAL, PHARMACOLOGIC, PHYSIOLOGIC, TOXICOLOGIC, AND SOCIOLOGIC ASPECTS OF PROPOXYPHENE NAPSYLATE

### 1. Pharmacologic Effects

To determine various pharmacologic effects of high-dose propoxyphene napsylate maintenance, 24 active patients who had taken the drug for 30 or more continuous days filled out a written questionnaire. A key finding was that the drug, in maintenance doses, has a variety of effects that may differ greatly among patients. A total of 71 percent reported that propoxyphene napsylate diminishes the desire to use heroin and suppresses withdrawal sickness. Only 25 percent felt the drug sedates or "calms nerves." Too much propoxyphene napsylate was reported to produce an unpleasant high or hallucinations by approximately 30 percent to 40 percent of patients.

Of particular interest is the physical dependence liability of propoxyphene napsylate. Of 16 patients who missed one day's dose of medication, 14 (88 percent) reported that withdrawal sickness would occur, whereas two (12 percent) reported no withdrawal sickness. The severity of withdrawal sickness, however, was reported by the majority (69 percent) to be much less than from heroin.

### 2. Effects on Physiologic and Social Functions

The written responses of 24 patients maintained for 30 or more days indicate that propoxyphene napsylate maintenance has little negative effect on physical or social functions. The majority reported that appetite, weight, sleep, and gastrointestinal function remained normal or were improved. There is little reported interference with work or driving. Of special importance is that only one of 19 males reported that the drug interfered with sexual relations. None of the five females in this group reported adverse effects on menstrual function (see Tables 7-6 and 7-7).

In the street, Darvon-N is called "yellow footballs." It sells for about a dollar a capsule on the black market. Much of its nonmedical use seems to be directed toward reducing a heroin habit or avoiding the withdrawal effects of heroin. Since Darvon-N is insoluble in water, parenteral injection probably never will be popular, although instances of addicts injecting suspended material is known. The use of Darvon-N for the treatment of opiate addiction represents a new use for an approved drug.

### *Interaction with Other Drugs*

In early clinical trials, several patients related that propoxyphene napsylate decreased the desire to use heroin and other psychoactive drugs. To obtain some measure of this phenomenon,

**TABLE 7-6**
**Pharmacologic Effects of Propoxyphene Napsylate (Darvon-N): Self-Reports of 24 Patients Maintained Over 30 Days**

| *Effect* | **Number of Patients** *On Heroin* | *On Darvon-N* |
|---|---|---|
| 1. Subjective moods and feelings | | |
| Depressed | 7 (29%) | 9 (38%) |
| Nervous | 4 (17%) | 11 (46%) |
| Sedated | 9 (38%) | 4 (17%) |
| Anxious | 7 (29%) | 9(38%) |
| High | 15 (63%) | 6 (25%) |
| Feel normal | 10 (42%) | 17 (71%) |
| 2. Treatment effects of Darvon-N | | |
| a. Takes away desire to use heroin | | 17 (71%) |
| b. Takes away withdrawal sickness | | 17 (71%) |
| c. Stimulates | | 7 (29%) |
| d. Sedates | | 6 (25%) |
| e. Calms nerves | | 6 (25%) |
| f. Feel high | | 5 (21%) |
| 3. Effects of too much Darvon-N | | |
| a. Unpleasant high | | 10 (42%) |
| b. Hallucinations | | 5 (33%) |
| c. Mouth numb | | 5 (21%) |
| d. LSD trip | | 4 (17%) |
| e. Ears ring | | 4 (17%) |
| f. Body "separating" | | 2 ( 8%) |
| g. Mouth dry | | 2 ( 8%) |
| 4. Events when dose missed for one day or more | | |
| a. Do not get withdrawal sickness | | 2 ( 8%) |
| b. Withdrawal sickness immediately | | 10 (42%) |
| c. Withdrawal sickness only after two to three days | | 4 (17%) |
| d. Have not missed | | 8 (33%) |
| 5. Severity of withdrawal sickness | | |
| a. No withdrawal sickness | | 2 (13%) |
| b. Much less than from heroin | | 11 (69%) |
| c. About the same as from heroin | | 2 (13%) |
| d. Worse than from heroin | | 1 ( 5%) |

(From Tennant, F.S., et al. *J. Psychedel. Drugs* 6(2), 1974. With permission.)

24 patients maintained over 30 days responded by written questionnaire regarding their consumption of cigarettes, alcohol, marihuana, and diazepam (Valium) while taking maintenance doses of propoxyphene napsylate. Approximately 20 to 30 percent of patients reported that they decreased or discontinued consumption of one or more of the drugs. The explanation for this is unknown.

Another interesting attribute of propoxyphene napsylate maintenance is that patients frequently report that heroin use results in adverse reactions—usually marked nausea and myalgia or hallucinations. Thirty-three percent of patients, however, reported that heroin use produces its normal euphoric effects.

Five out of 100 maintenance and 30 detoxification outpatients reported a seizure-like event that occurred within six hours following heroin use. The term ''seizure-like'' is used since we have been unable to document grand mal convulsion in these cases. None of these seizure-like events were observed by medical personnel and none were associated with tongue biting or

**TABLE 7-7**

**Effects of Propoxyphene Napsylate (Darvon-N) on Physiologic Functions: Self-Reports of 24 Patients maintained Over 30 Days**

| *Effect* | *Number of Patients* |
|---|---|
| 1. Appetite: | |
| Increased | 15 (63%) |
| Same | 8 (33%) |
| Decreased | 1 (14%) |
| 2. Weight change | |
| Gained | 10 (42%) |
| Same | 11 (46%) |
| Lost | 3 (12%) |
| 3. Sleeping pattern | |
| Sleeps six or more hours per night | 21 (88%) |
| Sleeps less than six hours per night | 3 (12%) |
| 4. Gastrointestinal distress | |
| Does not bother stomach | 18 (75%) |
| Nausea unless takes antacids with medication | 3 (12.5%) |
| Nauseated immediately after taking medication | 3 (12.5%) |
| Stomach always upset | 0 ( 0%) |
| 5. Number of bowel movements per day | |
| One | 1 ( 4%) |
| Two | 14 (59%) |
| Three | 8 (33%) |
| Four | 1 ( 4%) |
| 6. Bowel habits | |
| Constipated when started using Darvon-N, now normal | 13 (54%) |
| Normal when started Darvon-N and now normal | 9 (38%) |
| Normal when started Darvon-N and now constipated | 1 ( 4%) |
| Normal when started Darvon-N and now diarrhea | 1 ( 4%) |
| 7. Males—sexual function | |
| Could not have sexual relations when started; do now | 9 (38%) |
| Normal sex relations when started Darvon-N; still do | 9 (38%) |
| Normal sex relations when started Darvon-N; no longer do | 1 ( 4%) |
| 8. Females—menstrual function | |
| Did not have normal periods when started Darvon-N; now do | 1 ( 4%) |
| Had regular periods when started Darvon-N; still do | 4 (10%) |
| Had regular periods when started Darvon-N; no longer do | 0 ( 0%) |

(From Tennant, F.S., et al. *J. Psychedel. Drugs* 6(2), 1974. With permission.)

incontinence. Syncopy and marked tremor in each instance have been reported by nontrained observers. It is important to point out that all seizure-like events occurred within the first 22 days of treatment and four of the five cases occurred in patients administered initial, outpatient doses of 800 mg of propoxyphene napsylate in one single dose. Since beginning initial outpatient doses of 400 mg or less, only one seizure-like event has resulted. Low initial doses of propoxyphene napsylate and appropriate warning to the patient regarding heroin use appear to be the keys to prevention of these events.

## 3. Toxicologic Complications

Toxicologic monitoring for adverse effects of propoxyphene napsylate on hematologic, renal, cardiac, pulmonary, endocrine, and hepatic function have shown no such effects during short-term detoxification. Of particular interest has been possible toxicologic effects of high-dose maintenance on the liver. Doses of 40 to 110 times the human analgesic dose were administered to rats for 90 days and resulted in liver enlargement and fatty change.[153] Possible hepatotoxicity has been reported in humans.[154]

The toxicologic monitoring of 14 patients who had been maintained with high doses of propoxyphene napsylate over 90 days showed no significant alteration in transaminase, bilirubin, alkaline phosphatase, lactic acid dehydrogenase, urea nitrogen, glucose, uric acid, hematocrit, or white blood cell count.

The mean values for cholesterol and lymphocyte count increased over 90 days of high-dose propoxyphene napsylate maintenance, but the explanation for this is unknown. The toxicologic data in these 14 patients indicate that further studies should be conducted to determine possible long-term complications of the high-dose propoxyphene napsylate maintenance.

## 4. Methadone Detoxification

The severity of methadone detoxification with protracted abstinence is well known.[7,155] At least partially as a result of these difficulties, only a minority of methadone-dependent individuals are able to withdraw successfully and achieve a state of opiate abstinence.[92] Eight patients who were enrolled in a methadone treatment program have been successfully detoxified with propoxyphene napsylate. In all eight patients, the daily maintenance dose of methadone was abruptly discontinued and a maintenance dose of propoxyphene napsylate substituted. Abstinence symptoms from methadone withdrawal could be satisfactorily suppressed in all cases. Multiple daily doses of propoxyphene napsylate were required, however, during the first seven to ten days following methadone withdrawal.

List,[153] in Baltimore, Maryland, has successfully utilized propoxyphene napsylate in a different manner to assist methadone withdrawal. Rather than abrupt methadone withdrawal, propoxyphene napsylate, in doses of 200 to 600 mg per day, was concomitantly administered with methadone, as the dose of methadone was lowered over a several-week period from 40 to 0 mg per day.

## 5. Unresolved Issues

There are several unresolved issues, including the following.

1. Long-term toxicologic complications.
2. Effectiveness compared with methadone.
3. Whether split daily maintenance doses are more effective than single daily doses.
4. Ability of posttreatment patients to remain abstinent.

According to Tennant and associates,[130] not enough time has elapsed since the beginning of propoxyphene napsylate treatment adequately to determine medium-term and long-term abstinence rates following treatment. It is hoped that the mild, acute, and protracted abstinence seen following propoxyphene withdrawal will result in high rates of heroin abstinence.[156]

## 6. General Summary and Comments

By way of final comments on the usefulness of Darvon-N for maintenance therapy, Dr.

Barry Stimmel[157] made the following remarks in the *American Journal of Drug and Alcohol Abuse*.

> The use of propoxyphene napsylate (Darvon-N)[34,35] has been advocated in the treatment of heroin dependence. Darvon-N has been advertised as a nonnarcotic agent with minimal abuse potential, few side effects and great social acceptability, therefore, able to replace methadone in both detoxification and maintenance therapy. Unfortunately, such is not the case. Darvon-N (dextropropoxyphene) is an ester of methadone generically located within the methadone family, having a potency considerably less than that of morphine.[13] Similarly, abuse and physical dependence to Darvon has been amply documented.[158-160] Indeed, the practice of injecting crushed Darvon capsules has been well-known among certain groups, notably persons confined in institutions where Darvon was readily available via physicians' prescriptions for headaches.

When viewed in this light, the paper by Inaba and colleagues,[129] as previously discussed, is of special interest, according to Dr. Stimmel. This paper deals with the efficacy of Darvon-N as an agent in the treatment of heroin dependence. Unfortunately, of the original sample of 32 patients elected for Darvon-N therapy by the authors, only 22 were regarded as full participants in the study. The hazards of drawing conclusions on the basis of shrinking sample size have been lucidly discussed by Maddux and Bowden.[161] Nonetheless this study[129] does permit certain observations concerning the effectiveness of this agent. Of those individuals participating, 68 percent were considered to be using opiates when last seen at the clinic. Of 12 persons for whom follow-up was obtained, 50 percent reported withdrawal symptoms upon discontinuing the medication. Although the dosage utilized for the therapy was in excess of that recommended by the manufacturer, 82 percent of persons questioned revealed euphoria to some degree when injecting heroin, with 41 percent reporting no tolerance whatsoever to the euphoric effects of heroin. Side effects of the drug were considerable in 11 out of 23 persons, the most common complaint being a "spaced-out feeling." Euphoria as a primary effect was reported by nine participants.

These results, combined with relatively little research concerning the acute and chronic toxicity of this drug, suggest that as a therapeutic agent in detoxification or maintenance therapy, Darvon-N leaves much to be desired. The criteria for a successful maintenance agent are (1) the ability to retain persons in therapy, (2) the ability to prevent withdrawal, (3) the ability to prevent euphoria upon injection of illicit heroin, (4) continued abstinence from illicit opiate use, and (5) the freedom from untoward side effects. All appear to be wanting with this agent.

Even more important, however, from the public's point of view, is the misconception that has arisen concerning the preference for Darvon-N over methadone maintenance because of its "nonnarcotic" qualities. Darvon-N, as with all other agents utilized in maintenance, must have a narcotic property to be effective. All such drugs, even if used appropriately, under controlled conditions, will produce dependence, and if used inappropriately, will result in significant mood-altering effects.

For too long, drug dependence has been equated solely by the public with narcotic use. This is far from accurate. Indeed there are many dependence-producing drugs consumed by far greater numbers of persons than those dependent on narcotic agents.* Examples include the minor and major tranquilizers, alcohol, barbiturates, and nicotine. Furthermore, the physical and social effects of some of these agents can be more serious than those of properly administered narcotics, and the dependencies, at times, of equal severity. Yet these dependencies are not only condoned by society, but avidly "pushed" by the media.

Dependence on any pharmacologic agent is not optimal, yet may be necessary for an individual to function. What is important is that the agent utilized be presented to the public accurately so that the appropriate decisions as to effectiveness and acceptability can be made.

*Although the exact explanation for polydrug abuse, especially alcohol consumption in metabolic maintenance patients, is controversial,[162,163] it represents a potentially dangerous problem that requires additional scientific scrutiny as well as public awareness. However, there is some evidence that methadone may indeed have a positive influence on alcohol consumption in those individuals having alcohol problems in addition to their addiction to opiates. Dr. Dole, in evaluating over 100,000 cases, has not found any significant increase in alcohol abuse in methadone-maintained patients.[164,165] Dr. Dole also points out that there are not enough methadone maintenance programs and that there are still "addicts" or potential patients who need help but are not able to obtain methadone legally even as medicine for their disease. This fact, according to Dole, may be the reason for uncontrollable diversion of methadone in the street. What is really needed are more legally sanctioned methadone programs staffed by doctors who are well versed in the pharmacologic properties of methadone.

## REFERENCES


1. Payte, J.T. Methadone: Myth or reality. In K. Blum and A.H. Briggs, eds., *Drugs: Use or Abuse (a Manual)*. Sponsored by the U.S. Office of Drug Education, 1970.
2. Hofmann, F.G. *A Handbook on Drug and Alcohol Abuse: The Biomedical Aspects*. New York: Oxford University Press, 1975, p. 272.
3. Jaffe, J.H., and Martin, W.R. In L.S. Goodman and A. Gilman, eds., *Narcologic Analgesics and Antagonists: The Pharmacological Basis of Therapeutics*, 5th ed. New York: Macmillan, 1975, p. 245.
4. Goldstein, A., Arnow, L., and Kalman, S.M. *Principles of Drug Action: The Basis of Pharmacology*, 2nd ed. New York: Wiley, 1975.
5. Braenden, O.J., Eddy, N.B., and Halbach, H. Synthetic substances with morphine-like effect. Relationship between chemical structure and analgesic action. *Bull. Wld. Hlth. Org.* 13:937, 1955.
6. Isbell, H., et al., Liability of addiction to 6-dimethyl-amino-4-4-diphenyl-3-heptanone (methadone, "amidone" or "10820") in man. *Arch. Intern. Med.* 82:363,1948.
7. Martin, W.R., et al. Methadone—A re-evaluation. *Arch. Gen. Psychiat.* 28:286, 1973.
8. Misra, A.L., and Mule, S.J. Persistence of methadone-3H and metabolite in rat brain after a single injection and its implications on pharmacological tolerance. *Nature* 238:155, 1972.
9. Dole, V.P., and Kreek, M.J. Methadone plasma level: Sustained by a reservoir of drug in tissue. *Proc. Natl. Acad. Sci. U.S.A.* 70:10, 1973.
10. Inturrisi, C.E., and Verebely, K. The levels of methadone in the plasma in methadone maintenance. *Clin. Pharmacol. Ther.*, 13:633, 1972.
11. Inturrisi, C.E., and Verebely, K. Disposition of methadone in man after a single oral dose. *Clin. Pharmacol. Ther.* 13:923, 1972.
12. Vereby, K., et al. Methadone in man: Pharmacokinetic and excretion studies in acute and chronic treatment. *Clin. Pharmacol. Ther.* 182:180, 1975.
13. Kreek, M.J. Methadone in treatment: Physiological and pharmacological issues. In R.I. Dupont, A. Goldstein, and S. O'Donnell, eds., *Handbook on Drug Abuse*. Washington, D.C.: NIDA, U.S. Government Printing Office, 1979, p. 57.
14. Robinson, A.E., and Williams, F.M. The distribution of methadone in man. *J. Pharm. Pharmacol.* 23:353,1971.
15. Sullivan, H.R., and Blake, D.A. Quantitative determination of methadone concentrations in human blood, plasma and urine by gas chromatography. *Res. Comm. Chem. Pathol. Pharmacol.* 3:467, 1972.
16. Baselt, R.C., and Casarett, L.J. Urinary excretion of methadone in man. *Clin. Pharmacol. Ther.* 13:64, 1972.
17. Henderson, G.S., and Wilson, B.K. Excretion of methadone and metabolites in human sweat. *Res. Comm. Chem. Pathol. Pharmacol.* 5:1, 1973.
18. Horns, W.H., Rado, M., and Goldstein, A. Plasma levels and symptom complaints in patients maintained on daily dosage of methadone hydrochloride. *Clin. Pharmacol. Ther.* 17:636, 1975.
19. Lynn, R.K., et al. The secretion of methadone and its major metabolite in the gastric juice of humans: Comparison with blood and salivary concentrations. *Drug Metab. Dispos.* 4:504, 1976.
20. Bellward, G.D., et al. Methadone maintenance: Effect of urinary pH on renal clearance in chronic high and low doses. *Clin. Pharmacol. Ther.* 22:92, 1977.
21. Misra, A.L. et al., Physiological disposition and biotransformation of levo-methadone- ± -$^3$H in the dog. *J. Pharmacol. Exp. Ther.* 188:34, 1974.
22. Harte, E.H., Gutjahr, C.L., and Kreek, M.J. Long-term persistence of di-methadone in tissues. *Clin. Res.* 24:623A, 1976.
23. Kreek, M.J. et al. Rifampin-induced methadone withdrawal. *N. Engl. J. Med.* 294:1104, 1976.
24. Anggard, E. et al. Use of deuterium-labeled methadone to measure steady state pharmacokinetics during methadone maintenance treatment. In E.R. Klein and P.D. Klein, eds., *Proceedings of the Second International Conference on Stable Isotopes*. ERDA-CONF-751027. Springfield, Va.: National Technical Information, 1976, p. 117.

25. Pohland, A., Boaz, H.E., and Sullivan, H.R. Synthesis and identification of metabolites resulting from the biotransformation of DL-methadone in man and in the rat. *J. Med. Chem.* 14:194, 1971.
26. Sullivan, H.R., et al. Metabolism of d-methadone: Isolation and identification of analgesically active metabolites. *Life Sci.* 11:1093, 1972.
27. Bowen, D.V., Smit, A.L.C., and Kreek, M.J. Fecal excretion of methadone and its metabolites in man: Application of GC-MS. In N.R. Daily, ed., *Advances in Mass Spectrometry*, vol. 7-B. Philadelphia: B. Heyden, p. 1634.
28. Kreek, M.J. Medical safety, side effects and toxicity of methadone. In *Proceedings of the Fourth National Conference on Methadone Treatment*. New York: National Association for the Prevention of Addiction to Narcotics, 1972.
29. Kreek, M.J., et al. Fecal excretion of methadone and its metabolites: A major pathway of elimination in man. In J.H. Lowinson, ed., *Critical Concerns in the Field of Drug Abuse*. New York: Dekker, 1976, p. 1206.
30. Sullivan, H.R., Due, S.L., and McMahon, R.E. The identification of three new metabolites of methadone in man and in the rat. *J. Am. Chem. Soc.* 94:4050, 1972.
31. Kreek, M.J., Hachey, D.L., and Klein, P.D. Differences in disposition of di-, d- and l-methadone; Stable isotope studies in man. *Clin. Res.* 25:271A, 1977.
32. Cushman, P., Jr., and Kreek, M.J. Some endocrinologic observations in narcotic addicts. In E. Zimmermann and R. George, eds., *Narcotics and the Hypothalamus*. New York: Raven Press, 1974, p. 161.
33. Cushman, P., Jr., and Kreek, M.J. Methadone-maintained patients: Effects of methadone on plasma testosterone, FSH, LH and prolactin. *N.Y. State J. Med.* 74:1970, 1974.
34. Renault, P.F., et al. Altered plasma cortisol response in patients on methadone maintenance. *Clin. Pharmacol. Ther.* 13:269, 1972.
35. Martin, W.R., et al. Methadone—A re-evaluation. *Arch. Gen. Psychiatry* 28:286, 1973.
36. Santen, R.J., et al. Mechanism of action of narcotics in the production of menstrual dysfunction in women. *Fertil. Steril.* 26:538, 1975.
37. Santiago, T.V., Pugliese, A.C., and Edelman, N.H. Control of breathing during methadone addiction. *Am. J. Med.* 62:347, 1977.
38. Mendelson, J.H., Mendelson, J.E., and Patch, V.D. Plasma testosterone levels in heroin addiction and during methadone maintenance. *J. Pharmacol. Exp. Ther.* 192:211, 1975.
39. Cicero, T.J., et al. Effects of morphine and methadone on serum testosterone and lutenizing hormone levels and on the secondary sex organs of the male rat. *Endocrinology* 98:367, 1976.
40. Dole, V.P., et al. Methadone poisoning. Diagnosis and trement. *N.Y. State J. Med.* 71:541, 1971.
41. Gay, G.R., and Inaba, D.S. Treating acute heroin and methadone toxicity. *Anesth. Analg.* 55:607, 1976.
42. Kreek, M.J. Medical complications in methadone patients. *Ann. N.Y. Acad. Sci.* 311:110, 1978.
43. Rubenstein, R.B., and Wolff, W.I. Methadone ileus syndrome: Report of a fatal case. *Dis. Colon Rectum* 19:357, 1976.
44. Kreek, M.J. Medical safety and side effects of methadone in tolerant individuals. *JAMA* 223:665, 1973.
45. Lasagna, L. The clinical evaluation of morphine and its substitutes as analgesics. *Pharmacol. Rev.* 16:47, 1964.
46. Beaver, W.T. Mild analgesics: A review of their clinical pharmacology II. *Am. J. Med. Sci.* 251:576, 1966.
47. Chen, K.K. Pharmacology of methadone and related compounds. *Ann. N.Y. Acad. Sci.* 51:83, 1948.
48. Billings, R.E., McMahon, R.E., and Blake, D.A. l-acetylmethadol (LAM) treatment of opiate dependence: Plasma and urine levels of two pharmacologically active metabolites. *Life Sci.* 14:1437, 1974.
49. Fraser, H.F., and Isbell, H. Actions and addiction liabilities of alpha-acetylmethadols in man. *J. Pharmacol. Exp. Ther.* 105:458, 1952.
50. Jaffe, J.H., et al. Methadyl acetate vs. methadone: A double-blind study in heroin users. *JAMA* 222:437-442, 1972.
51. Way, E.L., and Adler, T.K. The pharmacologic implications of the rate of morphine and its surrogates. *Pharmacol Rev.* 12:383, 1960.
52. Way, E.L. *The Biological Disposition of Morphine and Its Surrogates*. Geneva: World Health Organization, 1962.
53. Ling, W., and Blaine, J.D. The use of LAAM in treatment. In A. Goldstein, and J. O'Donnell, eds., *Handbook on Drug Abuse*. Washington, D.C.: NIDA, U.S. Government Printing Office, 1979, p. 87.
54. Senay, E.C., et al. A 48-week study of meth-

adone, metadyl acetate and minimal services. In S. Fisher and A.M Freedman, eds., *Opiate Addiction: Origins and Treatment*. Washington, D.C.: Winston, 1974, p. 185.

55. Goldstein, A., and Judson, B. Three critical issues in the management of methadone programs: Critical issue 3: Can the community be protected against the hazards of take-home methadone? In P.G. Bourne, Ed., *Addiction*. New York: Academic Press, 1974, p. 140.
56. Savage, C., et al. Methadone/LAAM maintenance: A comparison study. *Compr. Psychiatry* 17:415, 1976.
57. Ling, W., Klett, C.J., and Gillis, R.D. A cooperative clinical study of methadyl acetate. I. Three-times-a-week regimen. *Arch. Gen. Psychiatry* 35:345, 1978.
58. Whysner, J.A., and Levine, G.L. Phase III clinical study of LAAM: Report of current status and analysis of early terminations. In R.C. Peterson, ed., *The International Challenge of Drug Abuse*. Washington, D.C.: NIDA Research Monograph 19. DHEW Publication (ADM) 78-654, Superintendent of Documents, U.S. Government Printing Office (in press).
59. Blaine, J.D., et al. Clinical use of LAAM. Paper presented at Conference on Recent Developments in Chemotherapy of Narcotic Addiction. Washington,D.C., November 1977.
60. Lehmann, W.X. The use of l-alpha-acetylmethadol (LAAM) as compared to methadone in the maintenance and detoxification of young heroin addicts. In J.D. Blaine and P.F. Renault, eds., *RX: 3 × 1 Week LAAM, Alternative to Methadone*. NIDA Research Monograph Series No. 8. Washington, D.C.: U.S. Government Printing Office, 1976, p. 82.
61. Lowinson, J.H., and Milman, R.B. Clinical aspects of methadone maintenance treatment. In R.I. Dupont, A. Goldstein, and J. O'Donnell, eds., *Handbook on Drug Abuse*. Washington, D.C.: NIDA, U.S. Governmental Printing Office, 1979, p. 49.
62. Hofmann, F.G. *A Handbook on Drug and Alcohol Abuse*. New York: Oxford University Press, 1975, p. 265.
63. Dole, V.P., and Nyswander, M. A medical treatment for diacetylmorphine (heroin) addiction. *JAMA* 193:646, 1965.
64. Dole, V.P., and Nyswander, M. Heroin addiction—A metabolic disease. *Arch. Intern. Med.* 120:19, 1967.
65. Dole, V.P., Nyswander, M., and Kreek, M.J. Narcotic blockade. *Arch. Intern. Med.* 118:304, 1966.
66. Dole, V.P., and Nyswander, M. The use of methadone for narcotic blockade. *Br. J. Addict.* 63:55, 1968.
67. Dole, V.P. and Nyswander, M.E., "Methadone Maintenance Treatment; a Ten-Year Perspective." *Journal of the American Medical Association*, 235:2117. 1976.
68. Manber, N.M., "Methadone." *Medical World News*, 22 (18):50. September 1, 1981.
69. Freedman, L.Z. Methadone and alcohol. *Ann. N.Y. Acad. Sci.* 273:624, 1976.
70. NIDA. The problem drinking addict. Services Research Report. DHEW publication no. ADM, 79:8937, 1979.
71. Blum, K., et al. In H. Rister and J. Crabbe, eds., *Alcohol Tolerance and Dependence*. Amsterdam: Elsevier, North Holland: Biomedical Press, 1980.
72. Blum, K., et al. Genotype dependent responses to ethanol and normorphine on vas deferens of inbred strains of mice. *Subst. Alcohol Actions Misuse* 1:459, 1980.
73. Vereby, K., and Blum, K. Alcohol euphoria: Possible mediation via endorphinergic mechanisms. *J. Psychedel. Drugs* 11:305, 1979.
74. Goldstein, A., and Judson, B.A. Alcohol dependence and opiate dependence: Lack of relationship in mice. *Science* 172:290, 1971.
75. Seevers, M.H. Morphine and ethanol physical dependence: A critique of a hypothesis. *Science* 170:1113, 1970.
76. Mendelson, J.H., and Mello, N.K. Basic mechanisms underlying physical dependence upon alcohol. *Ann. N.Y. Acad. Sci.* 311:69, 1978.
77. Blum, K., Hamilton, G.H., and Wallace, J.E. Alcohol and opiates: A review of common neurochemical and behavioral mechanisms. In K. Blum, ed., *Alcohol and Opiates: Neurochemical and Behavioral Mechanisms*. New York: Academic Press, 1977, p. 203.
78. Blum, K., et al. Naloxone antagonizes the action of low ethanol concentrations on mouse vas deferens. *Subst. Alcohol Actions Misuse* 1:327, 1980.
79. Pinsky, G., Labella, F.S., and Leybin, L.C. Proceedings of the National Drug Abuse Conference. In D.E. Smith, et al., eds., *A Multicultural View of Drug Abuse*. Boston: G.K. Hall, 1978.
80. Blum, K., et al. Naloxone-induced inhibition of ethanol dependence in mice. *Nature* 265:49, 1977.
81. Khanna, J.M., et al. Cross-tolerance between ethanol and morphine with respect to their hy-

pothermic effects. *Eur. J. Pharmacol.* 59:145, 1979.
82. Ross, D., Hartmann, R.J., and Geller, I. Ethanol preference in the hamster: Effects of morphine sulfate and naltrexone, a long-acting morphine antagonist. *Proc. West. Pharmacol. Soc.* 19:326, 1976.
83. Ho, A.K.S., Chen, C.A., and Morrison, J.M. Interactions of narcotics, narcotic antagonists and ethanol during acute, chronic and withdrawal states. *Ann. N.Y. Acad. Sci.* 281:297, 1976.
84. Altshuler, H.L., Feinhandler, D., and Aitken, C. The effects of opiate antagonist compounds on fixed-ratio operant responding in rats. *Fed. Proc.* 38:424, 1979.
85. Harris, R.A., and Erickson, C.K. Alteration of ethanol effects by opiate antagonists. In *Currents in Alcoholism*. New York: Grune & Stratton, 1979.
86. Blum, K., Wallace, J.E., Schwertner, H.A., and Eubanks, J.D. Morphine suppression of ethanol withdrawal in mice. *Experentia* 32:79, 1976.
87. Hong, J.S., Moschrowicz, E., Hunt, W.A., and Gillin, J.C. Reduction in cerebral methionine enkephalin content during the ethanol withdrawal syndrome. *Sub. Alcohol Actions Misuse* 2(4):233, 1981.
88. Jeffcoate, W., et al. Prevention of effects of alcohol intoxication by naloxone. *Lancet* 2:1157, 1979.
89. Mackenzie, A.I. Naloxone in alcohol intoxication. *Lancet* 1:7, 1979.
90. Goldstein, A. Heroin addiction and the role of methadone in its treatment. *Arch. Gen. Psychiatry* 26:291, 1972.
91. Goodwin, D.W., Davis, D.H., and Robins, L.N. Drinking amid abundant illicit drugs. The Vietnam case. *Arch. Gen. Psychiatry* 32:230, 1975.
92. Blum, K. In L. Manzo, ed., *International Cons. Neurotox. Proc. Ital. Soc. of Tox.* Oxford: Pergamon Press, 1980, p. 71.
93. Martin, W.R., et al. The effects of morphine- and nalorphine-like drugs in the non-dependent and morphine-dependent chronic spinal dog. *J. Pharmacol. Exp. Ther.* 197:517, 1976.
94. Gilbert, P.E., and Martin, W.R. The effects of morphine- and nalorphine-like drugs in the nondependent, morphine-dependent and cyclazocine-dependent chronic spinal dog. *J. Pharmacol. Exp. Ther.* 198:66, 1976.
95. Lord, J.A., et al. Endogenous opioid peptides: Multiple agonists and receptors. *Nature* 267:495, 1977.
96. Blum, K., et al. Genotype-dependent responses to ethanol and normorphine on vas deferens of inbred strains of mice. *Subs. Alcohol Action/Misuse* 1:459, 1980.
97. Hiller, J.M., Angel, L.M., and Simon, E.J. Multiple opiate receptors: Alcohol selectivity inhibits binding to delta receptors. *Science* 214:468, 1980.
98. Pfeiffer, A., Seizinger, B.R., and Herz, A. Chronic ethanol inhibition interferes with delta-, not with mu-opiate receptors. *Neuropharmacology* 20:1229, 1981.
99. McDonald, L.K., Maddux, J.F., and Blum, K. Fetal consequences of chronic methadone administration to pregnant rats: Methodological problems. *Cur. Therap. Res.* 17:308, 1975.
100. Jaffe, J.H., et al. Comparison of acetylmethadol and methadone in the treatment of long-term heroin users. A pilot study. *JAMA* 211:1831, 1970.
101. Walter, P.V., Sheridan, P.K., and Chambers, C.D. Methadone diversion: A study of illicit availability. In C.D. Chambers and L. Brill, eds., *Methadone: Experiences and Issues*. New York: Behavioral Publications, 1973, p. 171.
102. Cohen, S. *The Substance Abuse Problems*. New York: Haworth Press, 1981, p. 83.
103. Maddux, J.F., and Elliott, B., 3d. Problem drinkers among patients on methadone. *Am. J. Drug Alcohol Abuse* 2:245, 1975.
104. Bayer, R. The radical critique of methadone maintenance: A radical response. In *Proceedings of the Fourth National Conference on Methadone Treatment*. Washington, D.C.: National Institute of Mental Health, 1972, p. 359.
105. Levin, T. New myths about drug programs. *Social Policy* 32, 1971.
106. Newman, R.G. Methadone maintenance treatment: Special problems of government-controlled programs. In *Proceedings of the Third National Conference on Methadone Treatment*, p. 265.
107. Maddux, J.F. Methadone and medical ethics. In *Proceedings of the Fourth National Conference on Methadone Treatment*, 1970, p. 127.
108. Yuncker, B. Methadone: Can it get them off the hook? In B. Milbauer and G. Leinnand, eds., *Drugs*. New York: Washington Square Press, 1970, p. 140.
109. Dole, V.P. Planning for the treatment of 25,000 heroin addicts. In *Proceedings of the Third National Conference on Methadone Maintenance*. Washington, D.C.: Public Health Service Publication no. 2172, U.S. Government Printing Office, 1970, p. 121.
110. Starkey, G.H., and Egan, D.J. Combined treat-

ment of the criminal opiate addict by medical and law enforcement officials. In *Proceedings of the Third National Conference on Methadone Maintenance*. Public Health Service Publication no. 2172. Washington, D.C.: U.S. Government Printing Office, 1970, p. 108.

111. Huxley, A. *Brave New York*. New York: Harper & Row, 1972.
112. Einstein, S., and Burrell, C.D. The non-medical use of drugs: Contemporary intervention issues. Monograph sponsored by the Institute for the Study of Drug Addiction. Sandoc Wander, Inc., 1973.
113. Blinick, G., et al. Methadone in pregnancy. In *Proceedings of the Fourth National Conference on Methadone Treatment*. New York: Napan, 1972.
114. Goldstein, A. The pharmacologic basis of methadone treatment. In *Proceedings of the Fourth National Conference on Methadone Treatment*. New York: Napan, 1972.
115. Payte, J.T. The private physician in the future of methadone treatment. In *Proceedings of the Fourth National Conference on Methadone Treatment*. New York: Napan, 1972, p. 263.
116. Dole, V.P., et al. Methadone treatment of randomly selected criminal addicts. *N. Engl. J. Med.* 280:1372, 1969.
117. Frigel, H. Methadone maintenance for the treatment of addiction. *JAMA* 215:299, 1971.
118. Jonas, S. Methadone treatment of addicts. *N. Engl. J. Med.* 281:391, 1969.
119. Myerson, D.J. Methadone treatment of addicts. *N. Engl. J. Med.* 281:390, 1969.
120. Brill, H. Methadone maintenance: A problem in delivery of service. *JAMA* 215:1148, 1971.
121. Methadone: Cracks in the panacea. *Sci. News* 97:366, 1970.
122. Walsh, J. Methadone and heroin addiction: Rehabilitation without a "cure." *Science* 168:684, 1970.
123. Perkins, M.E., and Block, H.I. Survey of a methadone maintenance treatment program. *Am. J. Psychiatry* 126:33, 1970.
124. Connor, T., and Kremen, E. Methadone maintenance—Is it enough? *Br. J. Addict.* 66:53, 1971.
125. Dupont, R.L., and Katon, R. Development of a heroin-addiction treatment program. *JAMA* 216:1320, 1971.
126. Jaffe, J.H., Zaks, M., and Washington, E. Experience with the use of methadone in a multi-modality program for the treatment of narcotics users. *Br. J. Addict.* 4:481, 1969.
127. Ranzal, E. Mayor seeks $92 million for methadone. *N.Y. Times*, March 5, 1971.
128. Dole, V.P. Research on methadone maintenance treatment. *Int. J. Addict.* 5:359, 1970.
129. Inaba, D.S., Gay, G.R., and Whitehead, C.A. I got a yen for that Darvon-N. *Am. J. Drug Alcohol Abuse* 1:67, 1974.
130. Tennant, F.S., Jr., Russell, B.A., McMarns, A., and Cassas, M.K. Propoxyphene napsylate treatment of heroin and methadone dependence: One year's experience. *J. Psychedel. Drugs* 6:201, 1974.
131. Dole, V.P. Methadone maintenance treatment for 25,000 heroin addicts. *JAMA* 215:1131, 1971.
132. Senay, E.C., and Renault, P.F. Treatment methods for heroin addicts: A review. *J. Psychedel. Drugs* 3:47, 1971.
133. Newmeyer, J.A., Gay, G.R., Corn, R., and Smith, D.E. Methadone for kicking and for kicks. *Drug Forum* 1:383, 1972.
134. Aronow, R., Paul, S.D., and Woolley, P.V. Childhood poisoning—An unfortunate consequence of methadone availability. *JAMA* 219:321, 1972.
135. Abel, S. Darvon-N shows promise in heroin treatment. *The Journal*. Addict Research Foundation, Toronto, 2:1, 1973.
136. Tennant, F.S., Jr. Heroin detoxification with propoxyphene napsylate. In *Proceedings of the Committee on Problems of Drug Dependence*. Washington, D.C.: National Academy of Sciences, 1973, p. 614.
137. Tennant, F.S., Jr. Propoxyphene napsylate for heroin addiction. *JAMA* 266:1012, 1973.
138. Chambers, C.D., and Moffett, A.D. Five patterns of Darvon abuse. *Int. J. Addict.* 6:173, 1971.
139. Wolfe, R.C., Reidenberg, M., and Vispo, R.H. Propoxyphene (Darvon) addiction and withdrawal syndrome. *Ann. Intern. Med.* 70:773, 1969.
140. Tennant, F.S. Complications of propoxyphene abuse. *Arch. Intern. Med.* 132:191, 1973.
141. Javel, A.F., and Inaba, D.S. Beyond heroin? A case study of mixed pill addiction. *Drug Forum* 2:403, 1973.
142. Fier, M. Addiction to a massive dosage of Darvon: A case report. *J. Med. Soc. N.J.* 70:393, 1973.
143. Sturner, W.Q., and Garriott, J.C. Deaths involving propoxyphene—A study of 41 cases over a two-year period. *JAMA* 1125, 1973.
144. Young, D.J. Propoxyphene suicides—Report of nine cases. *Arch. Intern. Med.* 129:62, 1972.
145. Hunt, V. Treatment of dextropropoxyphene poisoning. *Br. Med. J.* 1:554, 1973.

146. Kersh, E.S. Treatment of propoxyphene overdosage with naloxone. *Chest.* 63:112, 1973.
147. Gruber, C.M., Stephens, V.C., and Terrill, P.M. Propoxyphene napsylate: Chemistry and experimental design. *Toxicol. Appl. Pharmacol.* 19:423, 1971.
148. Wolen, R.L., et al. Concentrations of propoxyphene in human plasma following oral, intramuscular and intravenous administration. *Toxicol. Appl. Pharmacol.* 19:480, 1971.
149. Merck, Sharp and Dohme Research Laboratories. Codeine and certain other analgesic and antitussive agents: A review. Merck and Co., Rahway, N.J., 1970.
150. Miller, R.R., Feingold, A., and Poxinos, J. Propoxyphene hydrochloride: A critical review. *JAMA* 213:996, 1970.
151. Wolen, R.L., Gruber, C.M., Jr., Kiplinger, G.F., and Scholz, N.E. Concentration of propoxyphene in human plasma following oral, intramuscular and intravenous administration. *Toxicol. Appl. Pharmacol.* 19:493, 1971.
152. McMahon, R.E., et al. The fate of radiocarbon labeled propoxyphene in rat, dog and human. *Toxic. Appl. Pharmacol.* 19:427, 1971.
153. List, N.D. Methadone detoxification using propoxyphene napsylate (Darvon-N). Presented before Eli Lilly and Company Symposium on Propoxyphene Napsylate Treatment of Opiate Dependence. Washington, D.C., November 19, 1973.
154. Emmerson, J.L., et al. Short-term toxicity of propoxyphene salts in rats and dogs. *Toxicol. Appl. Pharmacol.* 19:452, 1971.
155. Cushman, P., and Dole, V.P. Detoxification of rehabilitated methadone-maintained patients. *JAMA* 266:747, 1973.
156. Inaba, D.S., et al. ''I got a yen for that Darvon-N'': A pilot study on the use of propoxyphene napsylate in the treatment of heroin addiction. *Am. J. Drug Alcohol Abuse* 1:67, 1974.
157. Stimmel, B. The emperor's new clothes: The reality of Darvon-N. *Am. J. Drug Alcohol Abuse* 1:137, 1974.
158. Kane, F.J., Jr., and Norton, J.L. Addiction to propoxyphene. *JAMA* 211:300, 1970.
159. Salquero, C.H. et al. Propoxyphene dependence. *JAMA* 210:135, 1969.
160. Wolfe, R.C., Reidenberg, M., and Vispo, R.H. Propoxyphene (Darvon) addiction and withdrawal syndrome. *Ann. Intern. Med.* 70:773, 1969.
161. Maddux, J.F., and Bowden, C.L. Critique of success with methadone maintenance. *Am. J. Psychiatry* 129:440, 1972.
162. Blum, K., Briggs, A.H., and Delallo, A.L. On the mechanism of methadone-induced alcohol consumption in humans. *Sub. Alcohol Action/Misuse* 3:1, 1982.
163. Siegel, S. More on the ''paradox'' of opioid-induced alcohol consumption. *Sub. Alcohol Action/Misuse* 3(6):303, 1982.
164. Dole, V.P., Nyswander, M.E., Desjarlais, D., and Joseph, H. Performance-based rating on methadone maintenance programs. *N. Engl. J. Med.* 306(3):169, 1982.

Chapter 8

# Internal Opioids: A Look Into the Future

## A. INTRODUCTION

Alcoholism and the abuse of other psychoactive agents are considered the primary public health problem in the United States, with a cost in the billions.

Drug-seeking behavior, or, more specifically, the phenomenon of craving, is one of the most perplexing problems of human behavior. Abuse of nontherapeutic substances is so complex that one cannot ascribe simple solutions to overcome the dilemma of compulsive self-administration of a drug.

The neuropsychopharmacologist knows that although all central acting substances induce neurochemical changes, not all of these drugs are positive reinforcers with high abuse potential, such as antidepressants, but certainly most of the psychoactive drugs fall into the abuse liability category.

Although tremendous accomplishments have been achieved via both psychologic and sociologic approaches, it is basic biochemical research of substance abuse that ultimately will lead to the knowledge to understand the underlying mechanisms of the substance abuse phenomenology. The cost of basic research has been trivial when compared with its ultimate benefits to improve prevention and treatment and eliminate the disease.

In the title of this chapter, the idea of *a look into the future* is included. Certainly it is expected that some day, through the efforts of science, a clearer understanding of the universe will emerge. The true understanding of the creation of the universe is no small task for the scientist. There is nothing more difficult to imagine than the creation, in the sense in which it is normally taught in religious institutions. In 1935, Haslett[1] wrote: "It is not so much a matter of the violation of scientific law, which, after all, is outside the purview of most of us, but of the inherent inconceivableness of the sudden appearance of matter and energy out of nothing." In this regard, the prime question that we can contemplate relates to whether modern science can offer any help. Can it, through all its triumphs, explain the beginning; explain why matter and radiant energy are interchangeable? Can it explain why both matter and energy remain uncreatable and indestructible, except at each other's expense, and how people deal with themselves?

A second, and possibly more interesting, question is the relationship between human beings and the universe. Are people machines?

Can their actions be explained by the laws of physics and chemistry? How do human beings cope with their environment, as influenced by their inheritabilities? Atoms can be split, light from the most distant stars analyzed, and electricity harnessed, but the answers regarding the meaning of life and the intricate working of the mind and body become more difficult. The growing controversy over recombinant DNA research some day may provide at least some knowledge about the laws governing life. Until that time, the scientist can only guess or speculate on the future.

While we might accept not being able to deal with something as enormous as the universe, we have become even more frustrated in trying to deal with something as common and familiar and as small as the human brain.

Unlike the preceding chapters, in this one established dogma is replaced in some cases with speculations about the brain and its components, as they relate to pain, substance dependence, affective disorders, emotionality, elation, sexuality, and meditation.

## B. HISTORY OF ENDOGENOUS OPIOID PEPTIDES[2]

In 1975, after a deliberate search, two substances were discovered in pigs' brains that have the pharmacologic actions of morphine, heroin, and related opiates. These materials were small peptides consisting of a chain of five amino acids. As mentioned in Chapter 5, one has the sequence tyrosine–glycine–glycine– phenylalanine–methionine (methionine-enkephalin) and the other is very similar, differing only in that it contains leucine instead of methionine and is termed leucine-enkephalin. Following this finding, a 31-amino-acid peptide was discovered in the pituitary gland, and was called β-endorphin. Interestingly the first five amino acids of this peptide are identical to methionine-enkephalin and are considered to be its natural precursor, but this point is controversial.[3] These are not the only morphine-like peptides; others, such as dynorphins, have been identified. There is another peptide in the pituitary gland, probably more potent, and there is also a small heptapeptide in the brain that is very much like morphine in its chemical properties.

To assist the reader, the term *endorphin* is used in a generic sense to mean any morphine-like peptide. The specific term β-endorphin refers to the long pituitary peptide and the term enkephalin refers to the small brain peptides, both methionine-enkephalin and leucine-enkephalin.

The finding of ligands (something that binds to receptors or other macromolecules) in the brain with opiate-like activity has given an exciting new dimension to the research on brain function. The discovery of these opiate peptides has immense implications since these substances are involved with endogenous ligands for opioid receptors that are associated with known nerve tracts and a thorough knowledge of the nature of these nerve cells should facilitate the understanding of the basis of certain neurologic and behavioral disorders.

Looking back, prior to the discovery, the existence of an endogenous substance with opiate-like activity was suspected by many pharmacologists for the following reasons.

1. Morphine is known to affect the hypothalamus and pituitary in many ways, and these are manifested, for example, by the drug effects on temperature, libido, menstrual function, urine flow, adrenocotropin (ACTH), and growth hormone release.
2. An opiate analgesic-enhancing principle was reported to be extracted from the pituitary.[4]
3. During the past two decades (prior to 1980), a number of peptides in the hypothalamus have been isolated and found to have a regulatory role on the pituitary.
4. The existence of a native substance in the brain with opiate-like properties was suggested by the fact that electric stimulation of the brain in the region where morphine was established earlier to act selectively on the periaqueductal gray region resulted in analgesia that outlasted the period of stimulation.
5. Acupuncture analgesia is antagonized by naloxone.
6. The opiate receptors were identified and characterized.

Certainly it was no surprise when Hughes and associates[5] announced, late in 1975, that they had isolated two related pentapeptides from pig brain with potent opiate agonist activity; these were, as previously mentioned, methionine- and leucine-enkephalins. Of interest is that, in the same paper, the authors noted that the amino acid sequence of methonine-enkephalin corresponds to the amino acid residues 61–65 of a larger peptide, β-lipotropin (β-LPH). Li and associates,[6] in 1964, isolated this peptide from the pituitary of sheep; it was found to consist of 91 amino acids. Fragments of β-LPH were subsequently isolated, the most interesting to date being a 31-amino acid residue β-endorphin or β-LPH 61–91. In terms of opiate agonist-like activity. β-endorphin, known also as the C fragment (of β-LPH), is by far more potent and the most similar to morphine in its pharmacologic profile. Dynorphin is seen to be several orders of magnitude more potent than even β-endorphin in some tests (i.e., guinea pig ileum). However, Akil et al.[7] have demonstrated that a new fragment, *N-acetyl-beta-endorphin-27,* possesses no opiate activity and is found in high concentrations in the intermediate and posterior-pituitary of rats. Akil suggests that this substance is a prominent artifact in the measurement of biologically active β-endorphins.

## C. CHEMISTRY

Hughes[8] reported a material in mammalian brain extracts that acts like morphine to inhibit electrically induced contraction of smooth muscle. In the same year, Terenius and Wahlstrom[9] and Pasternak et al.[10] characterized a morphine-like substance in extracts of calf, rabbit, and rat brain. The compound was reported to have a molecular weight of approximately 1000 and to be inactivated by carboxypeptidase A and B, as well as leucine aminopeptidase, and, to a lesser extent, by chymotrypsin, but not by trypsin. Terenius and Wahlstrom, in the same study, provided evidence of the existence of a similar substance in human cerebrospinal fluid. Subsequently, Hughes et al.[5] isolated, characterized, and synthesized two naturally occurring pentapeptides present in pig brain: H-tyr-gly-gly-phe-met-OH (met-enkephalin) and H-tyr-gly-gly-phe-leu-OH (leu-enkephalin) in a ratio of approximately 6:1. Interestingly both peptides inhibited the field-stimulated guinea pig ileum and mouse vas deferens as morphine does. An essential feature of inhibition is that it is reversed by naloxone. In the receptor assay, met-enkephalin is about 20 times more potent than morphine and leu-enkephalin is somewhat less potent than the methionine analog. However, in other studies,[11] it appears that leu-enkephalin is more potent as an opiate agonist relative to met-enkephalin.

In 1964, Li and colleagues[6] first discovered and isolated β-LPH from sheep pituitary glands. β-LPH has also been discovered in highly purified form from bovine,[12] porcine,[13–15] rat,[16] and human[17–19] pituitaries and the compound's amino acid sequence has been proposed.[16–25]

Table 8-1 illustrates the amino acid composition of camel and human β-endorphin (β-EP).

In terms of structural activity and relationships, besides met-enkephalin and β-EP, other fragments of β-lipotropin (β-LPH), including B-LPH (61–77) and B-LPH (61–76), β LPH (61–77) and β-LPH (61–79) possess *in vitro* opiate activity.[21–24] According to Li,[25] β-LPH probably serves as the prohormone for these biologically active peptides. It is likely that enkephalins are derived from protein or large peptide precursors; however, the exact biosynthetic pathways are still unknown. Met-enkephalin and leu-enkephalin in striatrum,[18] adrenal medulla,[12] and sympathetic ganglia[16] were initially believed to be derived from β-endorphin (β-lipotropin 61–91) or from leu$^5$-β-endorphin (leu$^5$-β-endorphin 61–91). However, other polypeptides as possible precursor candidates are being actively studied.[26]

Among various fragments of β-LPH having opiate activity, only β-EP possesses potent analgesic activity by intravenous injection, and it is the most active fragment when administered directly into the brain. Synthetic β-EP[27] by intravenous injection is active in patients with severe pain, narcotic abstinence, schizophrenic behavior, and deep depression by intravenous injection.

## TABLE 8-1

## Amino Acid Composition of Camel and Human β-Endorphin

| Amino Acid | Camel Analysis | Camel Sequence | Human Analysis | Human Sequence |
|---|---|---|---|---|
| Lysine | 5.1 | 5 | 4.6 | 5 |
| Histidine | 0.9 | 1 | 0.0 | 0 |
| Asparagine | 2.0 | 2[a] | 2.2 | 2[a] |
| Threonine | 3.2 | 3 | 2.8 | 3 |
| Serine | 1.6 | 2 | 2.0 | 2 |
| Glutamine | 2.7 | 3[b] | 3.2 | 3[c] |
| Proline | 0.7 | 1 | 1.0 | 1 |
| Glycine | 3.2 | 3 | 2.7 | 3 |
| Alanine | 1.7 | 2 | 2.3 | 2 |
| Valine | 0.9 | 1 | 0.8 | 1 |
| Methionine | 0.6 | 1 | 0.8 | 1 |
| Leucine | 1.0[d] | 2 | 0.9[d] | 2 |
| Tyrosine | 2.0 | 2 | 1.9 | 2 |
| Phenylalanine | 0.9 | 1 | 1.6 | 2 |
| | 1.9 | 2 | 1.8 | 2 |

[a] Two asparagine residues.
[b] Sum of one glutamic acid and two glutamine residues.
[c] Sum of two glutamic acids and one glutamine residue.
[d] Hydrolysis (72 hours) revealed the presence of two residues.
(From Li, C.H. Chemistry of β-endorphin. In H. Loh and D. Ross, eds., *Neurochemical Mechanisms of Opiates and Endorphins.* New York; Raven Press, 1979, p. 148. With permission.)

## TABLE 8-2

## Distribution of Opioid Peptides in Brain and Pituitary Gland

| | *β-Endorphin* | *Enkephalin* |
|---|---|---|
| Pituitary | ng/mg Tissue | mU Enk-mg Tissue |
| Whole | 269.0 ± 20 (11) | 72.0 ± 4.0 (6) |
| Adenopypophysis | 128.0 ± 9 ( 3) | 3.7 ± 0.7 (3) |
| Neurohypophysis and pars intermedia | 1,500.0 ± 600 ( 3) | 740.0 ± 47.0 (3) |
| Pineal | 4.8 ± 0.8 (10) | 19.0 ± 2.0 (7) |
| Brain | ng/g Tissue | U Enk/g Tissue |
| Whole | 108 ± 8 (10) | 25.0 ± 2.0 (6) |
| Hypothalamus | 490 ± 30 ( 5) | 120.0 ± 7.0 (6) |
| Septum | 234 ± 34 ( 3) | 85.0 ± 7.0 (6) |
| Midbrain | 207 ± 15 ( 5) | 32.0 ± 1.0 (6) |
| Medulla and pons | 179 ± 5 ( 5) | 30.0 ± 4.0 (6) |
| Striatum | None ( 5) | 112.0 ± 11.0 (6) |
| Globus pallidus | | 566.0 ± 23.0 (4) |
| Hippocampus | None ( 5) | 13.0 ± 1.0 (6) |
| Cortex | None ( 5) | 15.0 ± 2.0 (6) |
| Cerebellum | None ( 5) | 5.0 ± 1.0 (6) |

Means and SEMS, number of animals in parentheses. One unit of immunoreactive enkephalin corresponds to 1 nonogram (ng) leu[5]-enkephalin or 30 ng met[5]-enkephalin. (From Rossier, J., and Bloom, F. Central neuropharmacology of endorphins. In H. Loh and D. Ross, eds., *Neurochemical Mechanisms of Opiates and Endorphins.* New York; Raven Press, 1979, p. 169. With permission.)

## D. SOME PHARMACOLOGIC ASPECTS OF INTERNAL OPIOIDS

### 1. Endorphins

The cellular localization of endorphins[27,28] in rat pituitary, as well as in mouse, kitten, pig, and frog pituitaries, utilizing immunocytochemical and radioimmunoassay techniques, indicates that endorphin (α-EP) and β-EP are found in every cell of the intermediate lobe and in isolated cells of the adenohypophysis, whereas α-EP and β-EP are not present in the neurohypophysis.[27,28] Of interest with the enkephalin radioimmunoassay, enkephalin-immunoreactive material is restricted to the intermediate lobe and posterior pituitary but is almost absent from adenohypophysis.[29]

Rossier and Bloom[30] report that significant amounts of β-EP were found within whole brain and in hypothalamus and midbrain. However, these researchers also observed that no β-EP component could be extracted from the enkephalin-rich corpus striatum (caudate–globus pallidus, putamen) or the cerebral, cerebellar, or hippocampal cortices.[31–34] (See Table 8-2.)

Evidence strongly suggests that β-EP and enkephalin are found in the brain within different neuronal systems. Hokfelt and co-workers[32,36] indicate that enkephalin-containing neurons are mainly short interneurons present in discrete regions throughout the central nervous system (CNS). In contrast, β-EP-reactive cells are restricted to the basal hypothalamus.

Table 8-3 summarizes select neuropharmacologic actions of the endorphins.

### 2. Enkephalins

The gross distribution of met$^5$- and leu$^5$-enkephalin in rat brain is shown in Table 8-4.

The results presented in Table 8-4 are consistent with most other reports of enkephalin distribution in the CNS.[38–40] It is of interest that in the pituitary, β-lipotropin and β-endorphin probably do not serve as precursors to the enkephalins as there appears to be virtually no met$^5$- or leu$^5$-enkephalin in this tissue.[41–43] So far, most evidence does not seem particularly to support the notion that β-endorphin is a precursor to met$^5$-enkephalin; however, this question is being investigated. There is the possibility that, for example, a molecule such as leu$^{65}$-β-lipotropin or leu$^5$-β-endorphin exists in the brain and acts as a precursor for leu$^5$-enkephalin. In this regard, some evidence also exists that β-lipotropin is itself not the ultimate precursor of β-endophin and possibly met$^5$-enkephalin. Mains et al.[44] suggested that a molecule of molecular weight 31,000 known as "$L_5$" ACTH may serve, in fact, as a precursor to both ACTH and β-lipotropin. Some have already speculated that the existence of such a molecule in the CNS may serve as a "common" source of all of the ACTH and β-lipotropin-related molecules.[45–48]

Table 8-5 summarizes select neurobiologic actions of the enkephalins.

Although peptidyl opiates were discovered less than a decade ago, one cannot help but be impressed by the exciting work already accomplished in this field. Not only did the hypothetic endogenous opiate prove to exist, but its chemical structure was totally unexpected and, in turn, was found to be related to a peptide hormone whose sequence had been known for several years and whose function was a complete mystery.

Opiate peptides already have been produced that are both stable and orally effective. Certainly such compounds will be shown increasingly to be important in the control of behavior.

#### *Opioid Peptide Breakdown Inhibitors*

In 1978 the first report was published showing the feasibility of using compounds that inhibit the breakdown of enkephalins *in vitro* as analgesic agents in mice. Little was known about brain enkephalnases, although some clues were already available as to their possible nature. Hughes reported that both carboxypentidase A and leucine aminopeptidase could hydrolyze metenkephalin *in vitro*. A search of the literature revealed only a few componds that inhibited these enzymes and could be used in animal studies. Among these were D-phenylalanine (DPA), d-leucine, and hydrocinnamic acid. As pre-

## TABLE 8-3

## Summary of Neuropharmacologic Effects of β-Endorphins (a Sampling)

| *Type of Action* | *Species* | *Citation (See References)* |
|---|---|---|
| 1. Akinesia | Rats | Jacquet and Marks, 1976 |
| | | Bloom et al., 1976 |
| 2. Analgesia | Rat | Jacquet and Marks, 1976 |
| | Mice | Bloom et al., 1976 |
| | Cats | Feldberg and Smyth, 1977 |
| | Humans | Tseng et al., 1976 |
| | | Roemer et al., 1977 |
| | | Loh et al., 1976(a) |
| | | Graf et al., 1976 |
| | | Meglio et al., 1977 |
| | | Fields, 1981 |
| 3. Antidepressant | Humans | Kline et al., 1977 |
| 4. Electrocortical | Rats | Nistico et al., 1981 |
| 5. Encephalomyelopathy | Humans | Kline et al., 1977 |
| 6. Estrous cycle | Rats | Barden et al., 1980 |
| 7. Feeding | Rats | Grandison and Guidotti, 1977 |
| 8. Growth hormone | Rats | Rivier et al., 1977 |
| | | Sarne et al., 1981 |
| 9. Heart rate | Dogs | Laubie and Schmitt, 1981 |
| 10. Hyperglycemia | Cats | Feldberg and Smyth, 1977 |
| 11. Hypothermia | Rats | Bloom et al., 1976 |
| 12. Immobilization response | Rats | Jacquet and Marks, 1976 |
| 13. Leutinizing hormone | | Bloom et al., 1976 |
| 14. Locomotion | Rats | Parivisi and Ellendorff, 1980 |
| 15. Locus caeruleus | | Shulz et al., 1981 |
| (inhibition) | Rats | Stinus et al., 1980 |
| 16. Naloxone—interaction | | |
| on neurons | | Strahlendorf et al., 1981 |
| | Rats | Henriksen et al., 1977 |
| 17. Neurotransmitters | | French et al., 1977 |
| | | Nicoll et al., 1977 |
| a. *Release* | | |
| ACH (I) | Guinea pigs (ileum) | Kosterlitz et al., 1977 |
| NE (I) | Rats (vas deferens) | Taube et al., 1976 |
| DA (I) | Rats (brain) | Loh et al., 1976(b) |
| 5HT (E) | Rats (brain) | Loh et al., 1976 |
| Pituitary—endorphin | Rats | Haracz et al., 1981 |
| b. *Turnover* | | |
| ACH (I) | Rats (nuclei of brain) | Moroni et al., 1977 |
| DA (I) | Rats (basol ganglia) | Izumi et al., 1977 |
| | | VanLoon et al., 1980 |
| 18. Obesity | Rats | Gurlow and Peters, 1981 |
| 19. Parasympathiolytic | Humans | Kline et al., 1977 |
| 20. Polyphosphionsitide | | |
| metabolism (brain) | Rats | Jolles et al., 1981 |
| 21. Prolactin | Rats | Dupont et al., 1977 |
| 22. Respiration | Cats | Florez et al., 1980 |
| 23. Retrograde amnesia | Rats | Izquierdo et al., 1980 |
| 24. Rigidity syndrome | Rats | Bloom et al., 1976 |
| | | Jacquet and Marks, 1976 |
| 25. Seizures | Rats | French et al., 1977 |
| 26. Thyroid hormone | Rats | Gambert, 1981 |
| 27. "Wet-dog" shakes | Rats | Bloom et al., 1976 |

I = inhibition; E = excitation.

**TABLE 8-4**

**Concentrations of Met⁵- and Leu⁵-Enkephalins in the Brains of Normal and Hypophysectomized Rats**

| Brain Region | Normal | | | Hypophysectomized | | |
|---|---|---|---|---|---|---|
| | *Met* | *Leu* | *M/L* | *Met* | *Leu* | *M/L* |
| Medulla | 2.6 ± 0.6 | 0.70 ± 0.06 | 3.71 | 2.2 ± 0.31 | 0.66 ± 0.08 | 3.33 |
| Cerebellum | 0.2 ± 0.03 | < 0.1 | — | 0.1 ± 0.10 | < 0.1 | — |
| Pons | 2.8 ± 0.4 | 0.55 ± 0.04 | 5.09 | 2.2 ± 0.42 | 0.51 ± 0.02 | 4.31 |
| Central gray | 4.8 ± 0.2 | 1.7 ± 0.09 | 2.82 | 5.1 ± 0.04 | 1.50 ± 0.07 | 3.40 |
| Midbrain | 1.2 ± 0.1 | 0.31 ± 0.04 | 3.57 | 1.0 ± 0.10 | 0.28 ± 0.03 | 3.57 |
| Hippocampus | 1.1 ± 0.08 | 0.17 ± 0.12 | 8.46 | 1.3 ± 0.10 | 0.17 ± 0.04 | 7.65 |
| Medial hypothalamus | 4.4 ± 0.3 | 0.60 ± 0.07 | 7.33 | 3.7 ± 0.27 | 0.53 ± 0.01 | 6.98 |
| Lateral hypothalamus | 1.9 ± 0.3 | 0.2210.02 | 8.64 | 1.4 ± 0.11 | 0.18 ± 0.01 | 7.78 |
| Thalamus | 2.0 ± 0.1 | 0.64 ± 0.03 | 3.13 | 2.3 ± 0.19 | 0.66 ± 0.02 | 3.48 |
| Amygdala | 3.3 ± 0.3 | 1.2 ± 0.07 | 2.75 | 3.3 ± 0.21 | 1.8 ± 0.09 | 1.83 |
| Globus pallidus | 29.5 ± 3.5 | 5.5 ± 0.10 | 5.36 | 31.5 ± 2.75 | 5.0 ± 0.35 | 6.30 |
| Caudate | 2.6 ± 0.4 | 0.53 ± 0.06 | 6.91 | 2.5 ± 0.16 | 0.75 ± 0.06 | 3.33 |
| Cortex | 0.81 ± 0.09 | 0.44 ± 0.04 | 1.82 | 1.0 ± 0.05 | 0.3710.04 | 2.70 |
| NPO | 0.95 ± 0.1 | 0.11 ± 0.01 | 8.64 | 0.79 ± 0.06 | 0.10 ± 0.02 | 7.9 |
| Septum | 1.95 ± 0.1 | 0.40 ± 0.02 | 4.75 | 1.8 ± 0.16 | 0.36 ± 0.03 | 4.86 |
| N. accumbens | 5.2 ± 0.4 | 1.1 ± 0.09 | 4.73 | 5.6 ± 0.04 | 0.91 ± 0.06 | 6.18 |

(From Miller, R.J., and Cuatrecasas, P. Neurobiology and neuropharmacology of the enkephalins. In H. Loh and D. Ross,, eds., *Neurochemical Mechanisms of Opiates and Endorphins,* New York; Raven Press, 1979, p. 189. With permission.).

dicted, these componds produced analgesia in mice and the analgesia was reversed by naloxone or prevented by prior administration of naloxone or naltrexone. Other compounds shown to inhibit enkephalin degradation *in vitro* are bacitracin, puromycin, and thiophan. (See Ehrenpreis, 1982.)

## E. COMMENTS AND SPECULATIONS ON POSSIBLE PHYSIOLOGIC RELEVANCE OF PEPTIDYL OPIATES

### 1. Stress

One possible role for the peptidyl opiates, especially the endorphins, may be as respondents to stress. For example, Akil et al.[49] demonstrated that naloxone was effective in reversing stress-induced analgesia. Furthermore, other related work implies that endorphins, as well as ACTH,[50] increase as a consequence of stressful stimuli. Guillemin et al.[51] and Rossier et al.[52] provided direct evidence that both β-EP and ACTH are secreted in equimolar amounts in response to different stressors. Of interest is the fact that since both ACTH and endorphins may share the same cellular storage sites in the pituitary,[53–55] their secretion may be commonly regulated. In this regard, a paper was published that showed that alcohol addicts have three times less β-EP and significantly more ACTH in their cerebrospinal fluid (CSF) than normal volunteers.[56] Most of these alcoholics tested complained of anxiety–depression.

### 2. Pain

We now know that the brain contains opiate receptors and there are opiate-like substances that occur naturally with these receptors. In addition, the intrinsic activity of the narcotic antagonist in various systems further supports the postulation of the existence of an endogenous compound. For example, it has been shown that naloxone (1) increases the acetylcholine release in the *in vitro* preparation of the isolated guinea pig ileum[57] (a standard opiate bioassay model); (2) enhances the nociceptive response in rats and mice[58]; and (3) reverses electroanalgesia in rats.[59] These results would suggest that the narcotic antagonist blocks the response to the naturally occurring opiate ligand.

Goldstein[60] believes that since naloxone, which blocks the opiate receptors, has little pharmacologic effect of its own, we may be able clearly to define the exact role of endorphins physiologically. It is possible that the endorphinergic systems are not tonically active (released at a constant rate to give a tonic influence) but function on a standby basis, being called into play only by circumstances that require their presence as a modulator.[61] Electric stimulation of the periaqueductal gray area (high in opiate receptors) produces analgesia, which is partially blocked by naloxone.[59] Acupuncture analgesia is also blocked to some degree by naloxone,[62] and there is some evidence that naloxone increases the sensitivity of mice to a noxious effect on a hot plate,[58] all of which are examples of support for a role for the endorphins in pain control. On the other hand, naloxone failed to alter the threshold of aversive stimulation at which rats escape from foot shock.[63]

With regard to pain and the role of the endogenous opiate, as suggested by Goldstein,[61] it seems improbable that a neural system should exist to antagonize acute pain that has important survival value, but possibly one of the functions of endorphins is to obtund chronic pain. Research in this area is continuing.

Certainly the area is an intriguing one, especially in light of the fact that reaction to pain differs among people and may be influenced by

**TABLE 8-5**

**Summary of Neurobiologic Effects of Enkephalins (a Sampling)**

| *Type of Action* | *Species* | *Citation (See References)* |
|---|---|---|
| 1. Abuse potential (self-administration) | | Belluzzi and Stein, 1977 |
| | Rats | Summer and Nayre, 1980 |
| 2. Acetaldehyde—interaction | Rats | Jhamandas and Elliott, 1980 |
| 3. Acetylcholine (release) | Rats | Jhamanadas and Sutak, 1980 |
| 4. Acetylcholine (turnover) | Rats | Herman and Kowalski, 1981 |
| 5. Acetyltransferase activity | Rats | Brandt et al., 1976(a) |
| 6. Adenylate cyclase (I) | NG-108-15 cells | Goldstein et al., 1977 |
| | | Brandt et al., 1976(b) |
| 7. Adenylate cyclase (E) | NG-108-15 cells | Lampert et al., 1976 |
| | | Schulz et al., 1981 |
| 8. Alcohol (consumption) | Rats | Blum et al., 1982 |
| | Hamsters | Hong et al., 1981 |
| 9. Alcohol (withdrawal) | Rats | Pfeiffer et al., 1981 |
| 10. Alcohol (opioid receptors) | Rats | Belluzzi et al., 1976 |
| 11. Analgesia | Mice | Buscher et al., 1976 |
| | Rats | Wei et al., 1978 |
| | | Pert, 1976 |
| | | Wei et al., 1978 |
| | | Szeckely et al., 1977 |
| | | Römer et al., 1977 |
| 12. Anterior pituitary hormones | Rats | Ferland et al., 1977 |
| 13. Antidiarrheal effects | | Lein et al., 1976 |
| 14. Convulsions | Mice | Miller et al., 1978 |
| 15. Cross-tolerance | Rats | Hong et al., 1980 |
| | Rats | Blasig and Herz, 1976 |
| | | Bhargava, 1977 |
| 16. Cyclic GMP | NG-108-15 cells | Lampert et al., 1976 |
| 17. Dependence development | NG-108-15 cells | Minneman and Iverson, et al., 1976 |
| 18. DOPA-potentiation | Rats | Wei and Loh, 1976 |
| 19. Dopamine synthesis | Mice | Plotnikoff et al., 1981 |
| 20. Electroencephalogram effects | Mice | Urwyier and Tabakoff, 1981 |
| | Rats | Baxter et al., 1977 |
| 21. Electrophysiologic effects | Rabbits | Aloisi et al., 1980 |
| | Rats | Frederickson and Norris, 1976 |

the "set" (psyche), inheritance, and environmental factors. In this regard, no one knows why Eskimo women are noted for their pain tolerance. Soldiers in battle are sometimes oblivious to their wounds until hours after the fighting. There are a few individuals who feel no pain at all and, as a result, continually risk injury. Others are in continual pain for obscure reasons.

In a rather popularized account, Schneck[64] has pointed out that:

> In general, men tend to be somewhat less sensitive to pain than women of the same age; older persons of each sex tend to be less sensitive than the young. A person's body is least sensitive to pain on the side controlled by the dominant side of the brain. Some ethnic groups show more pain sensitivity than others, but subtle appeals to pride during an experiment have sometimes—though not always—made such persons more tolerant of pain.

In looking at social pharmacology, an approach to the basic understanding of the variation in pain response among people is of interest. Let us consider applying the following formula.

$VP = VG + VE + VGE$. Then *BRP* (behavioral response to pain) = *G* (genetic variance) + *E* (environmental factors) + *GE* (interaction between genotype and environment).

Thus the facial expression of pain or the phen-

## TABLE 8-5

### Summary of Neurobiologic Effects of Enkephalins (a Sampling) (Continued)

| *Type of Action* | *Species* | *Citation (See References)* |
|---|---|---|
| 22. Epileptic phenomena | | McCarthy et al., 1977 |
| 23. GABA interaction | Rats | Urca et al., 1977 |
| 24. GABA transport | Rats | Sanwynok and Labella, 1981 |
| 25. Huntington's disease | Rabbits | Cupello and Hyden, 1981 |
| 26. Hypersensitivity | Humans | Emerson et al., 1980 |
| 27. Inhibitory pathways | Rats | Pert and Pert, 1977 |
| | Rats | Nicoll et al., 1980 |
| 28. Minor tranquilizers | Rats | Wuster et al., 1980 |
| | | Duke et al., 1980 |
| 29. Monoamine synthesis | Rats | Garcia-Sevilla et al., 1980 |
| | Rats | Lee et al., 1980 |
| 30. Neuronal activity (E) | Cats (brain) | Gent and Wolstencroft, 1976 |
| 31. Neuronal activity (I) | Rats (single | Hill et al., 1976 |
| | neurons) | Bradley et al., 1976 |
| | Cats (single | Sprick et al., 1981 |
| 32. Neurotransmitter release | neurons) | |
| Acetylcholine (I) | hippocampois | Waterfield et al., 1977 |
| Norepinephrine (I) | and neocortex) | Waterfield et al., 1977 |
| | | Miller and Cuatrecasa, 1979 |
| 33. Opiate receptors | Guinea pigs (ileum) | Audigier et al., 1977 |
| | Mice (vas deferens) | Simantov and Snyder, 1976 |
| 34. Opiate withdrawl | Rats | Catlin et al., 1978 |
| 35. Opioid activity | Rats | Beddell et al., 1977 |
| | | Chang et al., 1976 |
| | Humans | Day et al., 1976 |
| 36. Prostaglandins | Mice | Vincent et al., 1980 |
| 37. Purines (release) | Guinea pigs | Stone, 1981 |
| | Rats | |
| | Rats, mice | |
| 38. Spinal cord (E) | Cats | Duggan et al., 1976 |
| 39. Tolerance production | | Davies and Dray, 1976 |
| 40. Vasopressin | Rats | Pert et al., 1976 |
| | | Römer et al., 1977 |
| | Cats | Micevych and Elde, 1980 |

I = inhibition; E = excitation.

otype is influenced by a combination of factors that include genetic difference possibility in the amounts and ability to release endorphins and environmental factors; that is, previous experience, psychologic "set" and "setting," and the influence of all these factors on each other or their interaction. It is reasonable to suggest that an individual who has an inability to release adequate amounts of the opiate ligand for reasons that include reduced levels via synthesis impairment (either genetic or environmental, or both) will respond to pain more intensely than an individual who releases high amounts of the natural opiate in response to an acute nociceptive stimulation. Other speculations (not without experimentation) suggest that reduced function of the natural opiate may be the result of the presence of an endogenous substance with antagonist-like activity.

In this regard, direct demonstration of the existence of an endogenous antagonist-like factor has not been successful. However, there are many reports supporting the notion of the existence of such a factor. There are reports that blockade of opioid tolerance occurs with protein synthesis inhibitors[65] and numerous observations in the literature that ACTH and β-MSH (melanocyte-stimulating hormone) antagonize morphine effects.[66]

A list of possible antagonist candidates includes a brain hexapeptide (H-arg-tyr-gly-gly-phe-met-oh), thyrotropic-releasing hormone (TRH), and substance P.[67]

In terms of chemical relief of pain, the pharmaceutical industry has been charged with finding a nonaddictive, nontoxic pain killer. In 1979, Ehrenpreis and associates found that the amino acid phenylalanine was effective in treating patients with chronic pain. As previously mentioned, when the enkephalins are released in the brain in response to a painful stimulus, they are quickly broken down into inactive fragments by a carboxypeptidase enzyme or other enzymes. DL and D-phenylalanine inhibit the breakdown of the internal opiates (natural pain killers), thereby relieving pain. To date, clinical trials have been encouraging and no evidence of chronic toxicity has been observed, but additional research is underway.

### 3. Addiction (Psychologic and Physical Dependence)

Since endorphins interact at opiate receptors and (1) have been shown to produce profound analgesia; (2) produce dependence when administered to rodents; (3) are euphorogenic[24,79]; and (4) can alter opiate abstinence in animals[67] and humans,[24] they are strong candidates as biologic markers to explain the genetic propensity for substance addiction. In addition, the fact that opiates are primary reinforcers in operant self-administration paradigms suggests that endorphins may play a significant role in the central "reward system." Goldstein[61] and others[11,67] have speculated that a common pathway of certain addicting drugs (morphine, alcohol) could involve endorphin and opiate receptors. In simpler terms, it is possible that a preexisting genetic deficiency of endorphins in the brain could lead to drug dependence.

The question of a unified theory of addiction has been raised,[68,69] especially with regard to alcohol and opiate common *links*.[70] When alcohol is ingested, it has been found that a new class of compounds, termed isoquinolines, subsequently is produced. These isoquinolines, because of their ability to act on similar sites in the brain (opiate receptors), may function as the link between alcohol and opiates. The isoquinolines have been found to induce long-term drinking of alcohol in rodents.[71] This may be important when we consider the fact that certain mice (C57), which are genetically bred to drink alcohol, also tend to drink more morphine in solution compared with other mice (BDA) that do not drink alcohol or morphine in solution. In addition, animals that prefer alcohol are far less sensitive to its effects.[72] In contrast, an animal that does not like alcohol is far more sensitive to the effects. The human correlation of these findings may be that the body is attempting to adapt to the effects of alcohol by resisting dependence production and toxicity. Further work also indicates that alcohol-preferring animals may have a greater sensitivity to opiate receptor actions, as measured by the response of ethanol to induce inhibition of electrically stimulated contractions of the mouse vas deferens (naloxone blocks this inhibitory response), a typical opiate model, whereas alcohol-avoiding animals have a lower opiate receptor activity.[73] This is supportive of the notion that people may drink for the same reason a dependent person chooses to shoot heroin. Both substances, alcohol and opiates, may interact with similar brain receptors to cause euphoria. This is possibly the internal opiate site. Can we test such a hypothesis?

Opiate effects are not uniquely related to any of the known neurotransmitters,[61] although changes in content and turnover of several transmitters are associated with opiate actions and with tolerance and dependence. Accordingly, Goldstein[60] points out that the opiate receptors seem to subserve a general inhibitory function in various neuronal pathways, and that administration of an exogenous opiate might result in suppression of synthesis of endogenous opioids, by analogy to the effects of administering a pituitary hormone. This would suggest that administration of an opiate, by negative feedback as a result of saturation of the opiate (δ-endogenous peptidyl opiate) receptor, could cause a shutdown of endorphin production. (See Chapter 5 for a discussion of multiple opioid receptors.) In this regard, Blum and associates[74] found a significant reduction in basal ganglia amounts of enkephalin measured by an immunohistochemical method in hamsters, using 10 percent ethanol as a free-choice solution for over 12 months. These findings were further confirmed by others.[75] It is tempting to speculate that ethanol, or possibly a metabolite (isoquinoline), saturated opiate (endorphin) receptor sites and produced a negative feedback inhibition of enkephalin production. On the basis of these and other genetic studies,[76] Blum and associates[77] proposed the "psychogenetic theory of drug-seeking behavior." A detailed analysis of the proposed theory is presented in Chapter 10. Although there may be a number of other plausible explanations for this finding, future research along these lines may lead to a clearer understanding of the tolerance, physical dependence, and withdrawal from alcohol and opiates, as well as from other addictive agents.

## F. PEPTIDYL OPIATES IN PSYCHIATRY

Evidence that opiate-like peptides (endorphins) play a role in symptoms of some psychiatric illnesses and certain brain functions comes from two basic sources: direct pharmacologic testing of narcotic antagonists and endorphins in psychiatrically ill populations and studies of endorphin mediation of physiologic function, such as endorphin influences on pain regulation, pituitary function, and temperature regulation. In this regard, several reviews have discussed current evidence that opiate peptides may play a role in psychiatric illnesses.[78–80]

### *Schizophrenia*

Evidence from clinical studies suggests that opiates can be helpful in the treatment of some psychotic states. Further, the biochemical pharmacology of the opiates is quite similar, but not identical, to that of the antipsychotic drugs.[81] At present, there are clinical studies and data implicating endorphins as both agonists and antagonists in psychotic states.

In this regard, Kline et al.[82] reported transient improvement following intravenous administrations of synthetic α-endorphins to schizophrenic patients. In another study, a nonopiate peptide was cited as improving schizophrenic symptoms following daily intramuscular administration for about a week, in a small number of patients.[83] Although these investigations suggest that enhancing central endorphinergic transmission would be helpful in schizophrenia, there is also substantial research that suggests that a decrease in endorphins is therapeutic. For example, Terenius et al.[84] reported elevated endorphin levels in the CSF of psychotic patients as compared with healthy controls. Along the same lines, opiate antagonists have been studied for their potential effect in ameliorating schizophrenic symptoms.[85]

Human experiments on hemodialysis for the treatment of schizophrenia have been performed. Early studies claimed that an unknown peptide, βH-leu$^5$-endorphin, was present in the dialysate of those patients treated by Wagemaker and Cade.[86] In response to these claims, Lewis et al.[87] were unable to identify this compound in the dialysate from two well-diagnosed chronic schizophrenics.

The hypothesis that certain dopaminergic systems and other catecholamines may be phasically or tonically overactive in schizophrenia formed the basis of several excellent investigations, which have been reviewed by Sternberg et al.[88–90]

In this regard, Garcia-Sevilla et al.[91] showed opposite effects of the opiate, morphine, compared with the narcotic antagonists naloxone and naltrexone on the synthesis of dopamine in rat brain. In addition, they found that the effects of β-endorphin on rat brain biogenic amine synthesis are similar to those of morphine. The authors conclude that opiate receptors and their endogenous ligands are involved in the regulation of dopamine synthesis. These findings make it plausible that the endorphins play an important role in neurotransmitter regulation and neuropsychiatric disorders.

### *Depression*

The possibility that the internal opiates or opiate receptors may play a role in the affective disorder known as depression has been reviewed by Davis and Bunney.[92]

Early reports by workers in the field have been quite controversial. Although Fink et al.[93] reported that narcotic antagonists might be beneficial in depressive illnesses, other work by Terenius et al.[94] and Davis et al.[95] did not show any significant improvement of depressive illnesses utilizing narcotic antagonists. However, Kline and his colleagues[82] administered β-endorphin to a number of depressed patients in an open study and reported transient improvement in the mood of some subjects. In addition, Angrist and Gershon[96] administered β-endorphin to six depressed patients, precipitating mania or hypomania in four. Along similar lines, Meyerson and Terenius[97] have also reported elevations of CSF endorphins in depressed patients of the manic-depressive type.

### *Summary*

In summary, as pointed out by Davis and Bunney,[92] suggestive evidence exists linking endorphin to the schizophrenic syndrome. The basis for this speculation is that (1) narcotic antagonists appear to alternate some symptons (e.g., attentional performance is improved) and (2) CSF opiate binding substances are reported to be elevated in schizophrenic patients.

In terms of the relationship between opiate peptides (endorphins) and affective illness, little evidence is accumulating, although CSF endorphins appear elevated in some manic-depressive patients. Opioid effects of manic symptoms in humans have been reported by only a few research groups and no definitive conclusions can be made at this time.

### *Sexuality*

The possible role of endorphins in sexual activity has recently been studied. Meyerson and Terenius[97] reported that the percentage of male rats mounting receptive females decreased when the males received an intraventricular injection of 1 microgram of β-endorphin; the decrease in mounting activity was prevented by naltrexone, an opiate antagonist. This observation could have important clinical relevance since long-term users of narcotic analgesics frequently complain of frigidity and impotence.[98]

These studies prompted Gessa et al.[99] to investigate the possible role of endorphins in the regulation of sexual behavior. These researchers and others found that the intraventricular injection of D-ala$^2$-methionine-enkephalinamide, a synthetic analog of met-enkephalin that is resistant to enzymatic degradation, inhibits copulatory behavior in sexually vigorous male rats, and that this effect is prevented by naloxone. In addition, naloxone induced copulatory behavior in sexually inactive male rats. These findings strongly suggest that endorphins play an important role in the regulation of sexual behavior.

Social pharmacology would tell us that if endorphins play such a role, then individuals who possess high levels of endogenous opioids will probably be sexually inactive, whereas people with low levels should be highly sexual. It also points toward the possibility that, some day, instead of "turning on" to a sexual partner, one may indeed turn on to the flip of a switch of an electronic pleasure module properly placed for the immediate release of the natural high (endorphin).

The serious reader should refer to recent reviews on endorphinegic pharmacology.[100–102]

## G. SOCIAL PHARMACOLOGIC REMARKS

There is a basic need in human beings to achieve pleasure states and some think that drugs provide a means of getting there. For one person, it might be a couple of martinis on the rocks, whereas another might chew coca leaves. We do not know as yet how to curtail or control the abuse of various kinds of pleasure states—whether drinking, smoking marihuana, gambling, or watching television—but society is going to have to learn to deal with drugs and pleasure in ways other than by sheer emotional reaction. In this regard, a recommendation of the book by Dr. Joel Fort entitled *The Pleasure Seekers*[103] is in order. This account not only accurately documents drug abuse patterns and statistics as to amounts of different kinds of drugs consumed, but points out that people need pleasure and will actively seek it out.

This point may be debated by Dr. Norman Zinberg (personal communication), who does not believe that seeking pleasure is inborn, but is learned. Nevertheless, just the idea of pleasure, in its purest form, excites neurons, dilates blood vessels, speeds the heart, increases blood flow, make gastric acids flow, raises the pulse, opens up the pupils, increases saliva and all body juices, tingles the spine, depolarizes muscles, piloerects, and causes a bodily explosion that results in total loss of control and a euphoric glow or high.

As reviewed in this speculative chapter, the discovery of an opiate-like polypeptide raises interesting questions about the addictive process. For example, what happens chemically when a person has a natural deficiency of these potentially euphoria-producing endorphins? Can this deficiency drive some people into seeking another kind of euphorogenic-producing substance to make up for it? Are imbalances in the production of natural opiate-like endorphins responsible for certain "abnormal" behaviors that we label psychosis (schizophrenia, etc.) and are some people who are prone to addiction deficient in the natural opiate? The foregoing should provide insight into the notion of "pleasure as a natural entity," as far as possibly being mediated via naturally occurring substances is concerned.

This fact provides us with one of our most frustrating paradoxes. On the one hand, we seek fulfillment and satisfaction through the attainment of pleasure states—naturally or synthetically induced. On the other hand, human beings can easily overload their pleasure circuits through abuse, misuse, or simple miscalculation. Most of us travel through unchartered territories of pleasure, and there are many pitfalls hidden along the way. Society does not always condone pleasure if it is not a pleasure that is convenient to current social mores. It has long been speculated that when the guardians of the law interfere with the pursuit and enjoyment of some illegal pleasure, they themselves find pleasure in the process.

## H. SOCIAL–LEGAL IMPLICATIONS

If, indeed, we are pleasure seekers and our brain produces naturally occurring substances with potential euphorogenic properties, then it should follow that we seek out natural ways to "turn on." Many of us know people who always seem bored or unhappy or sad, and for whom nothing seems to turn them on, except when they use psychoactive chemicals to attain brief glimpses of paradise. These people turn on to the same phenomenon as the diver diving 100 feet into the depths of the sea, the skydiver speeding toward the ground, the daredevil jumping a motorcycle over a river, the soccer player scoring a goal, the batter hitting a home run, the quarterback throwing a winning pass, the mountain climber reaching the top, the boxer defeating an opponent by a knockout, the bank robber escaping from the scene of the crime, Eve biting into the forbidden fruit, the teenager kissing on the first date, and lovers finding each other after a long period of absence. In all these cases, the effect is characterized as pleasurable, filled with gratification of the senses or the mind.

Are there laws against deep-sea divers, skydivers, daredevils, soccer players, boxers, mountain climbers, or lovers? If not, then why are there laws against the user of psychoactive chemicals? Certainly there must be laws to protect society, and thus laws against bank robbers have their place, but how do we explain other laws that affect only consenting individuals? Are such laws valid?

For years, we have heard the cries of philosophers concerning the search for natural highs as a way of life, instead of seeking unnatural highs through psychoactive chemicals. Research on the subject some day might reveal that when we "meditate," we do indeed "medicate"—a statement projected on the potential of endorphins, as previously described. In other words, is the Nirvana of life endorphins? If endorphins are opiate-like in their pharmacologic actions, and if they are released during states of meditation, then meditators are getting high, just as those in the drug culture are, but they are using "natural" methods.

If this is true, then should not the state have an interest in making laws against a natural process such as meditation? If there were such a law, how would it be enforced?

At present, the legal authorities have a great interest in opiate use, or misuse, as a means for people to achieve pleasure. The law focuses on opiates because the people who utilize these substances are compelled to lie, cheat, steal, and prostitute themselves to obtain adequate supplies, and in doing so hurt other members of society. When other members of society are intimately affected, the state should make laws against this potential hazard. However, if heroin or other psychoactive agents were easily available at little or no cost to the seeker, the actual damage to other members of society would become very minimal, and thus there would be no compelling interest for the state and no laws would be necessary. The question is: Are people mature enough to survive without law and order?

## I. CONCLUSIONS

If drugs induce pleasure states, and if pleasure states are natural, then how responsible or guilty are these people when they turn to artificial forms of euphorogenic-producing substances? Are our laws really adequate for dealing with this human reality? Are we making laws against drugs or against nature (pleasure)? These are the kinds of questions that need to be explored seriously by the physician, by the legal profession, by the courts, and by the social pharmacologist.

Certainly the elucidation of the role of opioid peptides ultimately will unravel the mysteries of our brain. This will provide relief for one of our greatest frustrations. The accomplishment will be no small feat for humankind.

## REFERENCES

1. Haslett, A.W. *Unsolved Problems of Science*. New York: Macmillan, 1933, p. 17.
2. Goldstein, A. Endorphins: Physiology and clinical implications. *Ann. N.Y. Acad. Sci.* 311:49, 1978.
3. Yang, H.Y.T., and Costa, E. Estimating *in vivo* the turnover rate of brain enkephalins. In H.H. Loh and D.H. Ross, eds., *Neurochemical Mechanisms of Opiates and Endorphins*. New York: Raven Press, 1979.
4. Mayer, D.J., and Price, D.D. Central nervous system mechanisms of analgesia. *Pain* 2:379, 1976.
5. Hughes, J., et al. Identification of two related pentapeptides from the brain with potent opiate antagonistic activity. *Nature* 258:577, 1975.
6. Li, C.H., et al. Isolation and amino acid sequence of B-LPH from sheep pituitary glands. *Nature* 208:1093, 1965.
7. Akil, H., et al. A sensitive coupled HPLC/RIA technique for separation of endorphins: Multiple forms of beta-endorphin in rat pituitary

intermediate vs. anterior lobe. *Neuropeptides* 1:429, 1981.

8. Hughes, J. Isolation of an endogenous compound from the brain with pharmacological properties similar to morphine. *Brain Res.* 88:295, 1975.
9. Terenius, L., and Wahlstrom, A. Morphine-like ligand for opiate receptors in human CSF. *Life Sci.* 16:1759, 1975.
10. Pasternak, G.W., Goodman, R., and Snyder, S.H. An endogenous morphine-like factor in mammalian brain. *Life Sci.* 16:1765, 1975.
11. Blum, K. Alcohol and central nervous system peptides. *Subs. Alc. Actions/Misuse* 4:73, 1983.
12. Lohmar, P., and Li, C.H. Biological properties of ovine β-lipotropic hormone. *Endocrinology* 82:898, 1968.
13. Desranleau, R., Gilardeau, D., and Chretien, M. Radioimmunoassay of ovine beta-lipotropic hormone. *Endocrinology* 91:1004, 1972.
14. Iudaev, N.A., and Pankov, I.U.A. N-terminal 1-47 sequence of amino acid residues in the molecule of swing β-lipotropin. *Probl. Endocrinol.* 16:49, 1970.
15. Cseh, G., Graf, L., and Goth, E. Lipotropic hormone obtained from human pituitary gland. *FEBS Lett.* 2:42, 1968.
16. Rubenstein, M., et al. Isolation and characterization of the opioid peptides from rat pituitary: Beta-lipotropin. *Proc. Nat. Acad. Sci. U.S.A.* 74:3052, 1977.
17. Scott, A.P., and Lowry, P.J. Adrenocorticotrophic and melanocyte stimulating peptides in the human pituitary. *Biochem. J.* 139:593, 1974.
18. Chretien, M., et al. Purification and partial chemical characterization of human pituitary lipolytic hormone. *Can. J. Biochem.* 54:778, 1976.
19. Li, C.H., and Chung, D. Primary structure of human lipotrophin. *Nature* 260:622, 1976.
20. Li, C.H., and Chung, D. Isolation and structure of an untriakowtapeptide with opiate activity from camel pituitary glands. *Proc. Nat. Acad. Sci. U.S.A.* 73:1145, 1976.
21. Doneen, B.A., et al. Beta-endorphine: Structure-activity relationships in the guinea pig ileum and opiate receptor binding assays. *Biochem. Biophys. Res. Commun.* 74:656, 1977.
22. Graf, L., et al. Opioid agonist activity of beta-lipotropin fragments: A possible biological source of morphine-like substances in the pituitary. *FEBS Lett.* 64:181, 1976.
23. Graf, L., et al. Comparative study on analgesic effect of met 5-enkephalin and related lipotropin fragments. *Nature* 263:240, 1976.
24. Catlin, D.H., et al. Pharmacologic activity of beta-endorphin in man. *Commun. Psychopharmacol.* 1:493, 1977.
25. Li, C.H. Chemistry of beta-endorphin. In H.H. Loh and D.H. Ross, eds., *Neurochemical Mechanisms of Opiates and Endorphins.* New York: Raven Press, 1979.
26. Yang, H.-Y., et al. Detection of two endorphin-like peptides in nucleus caudatus. *Neuropharmacology* 17:433, 1978.
27. Bloom, F., et al. Endorphins are located in the intermediate and anterior lobes of the pituitary gland, not in the neurohypophysis. *Life Sci.* 20:43, 1977.
28. Bloom, F.E., et al. Beta-endorphin: Cellular localization, electrophysiological and behavioral effects. *Adv. Biochem. Psychopharmacol.* 18:89, 1978.
29. Rossier, J., et al. Regional dissociation of beta-endorphin and encephalin contents in rat brain and pituitary. *Proc. Natl. Acad. Sci. U.S.A.* 74:5162, 1977.
30. Rossier, J., and Bloom, F. Central neuropharmacology of endorphins. In H.H. Loh and D.H. Ross, eds., *Neurochemical Mechanisms of Opiates and Endorphins.* New York: Raven Press, 1979.
31. Elde, R., et al. Immunohistochemical studies using antibodies to leucine enkephalin: Initial observations on the nervous system of the rat. *Neuroscience* 1:349, 1976.
32. Hokfelt, T., et al. The distribution of enkephalin—Immunoreactive cell bodies in the rat central nervous system. *Neurosci. Lett.* 5:25, 1977.
33. Simantov, R., et al. Opioid peptide enkephalin: Immunohistochemical mapping in rat central nervous system. *Proc. Natl. Acad. Sci. U.S.A.* 74:2167, 1977.
34. Yang, H.Y., Hong, J.S., and Costa, E. Regional distribution of leu and met enkephalin in rat brain. *Neuropharmacology* 16:303, 1977.
35. Kuhar, M.J., and Uhl, G.R. Histochemical localization of opiate receptors and the enkephalins. In H.H. Loh and D.H. Ross, eds., *Neurochemical Mechanisms of Opiates and Endorphins.* New York: Raven Press, 1979.
36. Agarwal, N.S., et al. Synthesis of leucine-enkephalin derivatives: Structure and function studies. *Biochem. Biophys. Res. Commun.* 76:129, 1977.
37. Miller, R.J., and Cuatrecasas, P. Neurobiology and neuropharmacology of the enkephalins. In

H.H. Loh and D.H. Ross, eds., *Neurochemical Mechanisms of Opiates and Endorphins*. New York: Raven Press, 1979.

38. Schiller, P.W., Yam, C.F., and Lis, M. Evidence for topographical analogy between methionine-enkephaline and morphine derivatives. *Biochemistry* 16:1831, 1977.
39. Smith, J.W., et al. Enkephalins: Isolation, distribution and function. In H. Kosterlitz, ed., *Opiates and Endogenous Opioid Peptides*. Amsterdam: North-Holland, 1976, p. 57.
40. Wahlstrom, A., Johansson, L., and Terenius, L. Characterization of endorphins and endogenous morphine-like factors in human CSF and brain extracts. In H. Kosterlitz, ed., *Opiates and Endogenous Opioid Peptides*. Amsterdam: North-Holland, 1976, p. 41.
41. Cox, B.M., et al. A further characterization of morphine-like peptides (endorphins) from pituitary. *Brain Res.* 115:285, 1976.
42. Gentleman, S., et al. Pituitary endorphins. In H. Kosterlitz, ed., *Opiates and Endogenous Opioid Peptides*. Amsterdam: North-Holland, 1976, p. 27.
43. Simantov, R., Childers, S.R., and Snyder, S.H. Opioid peptides: Differentiation by radioimmunoassay and radioreceptor assay. *Brain Res.* 135:358, 1977.
44. Mains, R.E., Eipper, B.A., and Ling, N. Common precursor to corticotropins and endorphins. *Proc. Natl. Acad. Sci. U.S.A.* 74:3014, 1977.
45. Dube, D., and Pelleticer, L. Immunohistochemical localization of a α-MSH in the rat brain. *Proc. Endocrinol. Soc.* 319 (abs.) 1977.
46. Krieger, D.T., Liotta, A., and Brownstein, M.J. Presence of corticotropin in brain of normal and hypophysectomized rats. *Proc. Natl. Acad. Sci. U.S.A.* 74:648, 1977.
47. Krieger, D.T., et al. Presence of immunoassayable beta-lipotropin in bovine brain and spinal cord: Lack of concordance with ACTH concentrations. *Biochem. Biophys. Res. Commun.* 76:930, 1977.
48. LaBella, F., et al. Lipotropin: Localization by radioimmunoassay precursors in pituitary and brain. *Biochem. Biophys. Res. Commun.* 75:350, 1977.
49. Akil, H., et al. Stress induced increase in endogenous opiate peptides: Concurrent analgesia and its partial reversal of naloxone. In H.W. Kosterlitz, ed., *Opiates and Endogenous Opioid Peptides*. Amsterdam: North-Holland, 1976, p. 63.
50. Engeland, W.C., et al. Circadian patterns of stress-induced ACTH secretion are modified by corticosterone responses. *Endocrinology* 100:138, 1977.
51. Guillemin, R., et al. Beta-endorphin and adrenocorticotropin are selected concomitantly by the pituitary gland. *Science* 197:1367, 1977.
52. Rossier, J., et al. Foot-shock induced stress increases beta-endorphin levels in blood but not brain. *Nature* 270:618, 1977.
53. Bloom, F., et al. Endorphins are located in the intermediate and anterior lobes of the pituitary gland, not in the neurophypophysis. *Life Sci.* 20:43, 1977.
54. Pelletier, G., et al. Immunohistochemical localization of β-lipotropic hormone in the pituitary gland. *Endocrinology* 100:770, 1977.
55. Queen, G., Pinsky, C., and LaBella, F. Subcellular localization of endorphine activity in bovine pituitary and brain. *Biochem. Biophys. Res. Commun.* 72:1021, 1976.
56. Genazzini, A.R., et al. *Clin. Endocrinol. Metab.* (in press).
57. Waterfield, A.A., and Kosterlitz, H.W. Stereospecific increase by narcotic antagonists of evoked acetylcholine output in guinea-pig ileum. *Life Sci.* 16:1787, 1975.
58. Jacob, J.J., Tremblay, E.C., and Colombel, M.C. Enhancement of nociceptive reactions by naloxone in mice and rats. *Psychopharmacologia* 37:217, 1974.
59. Akil, H., et al. Enkephalin-like material elevated in ventricular cerebrospinal fluid of pain patients after analgesic focal stimulation. *Science* 201:463, 1978.
60. Goldstein, A. The opiate narcotics: Neurochemical mechanisms in analgesia and dependence. In *Proceedings of the International Narcotics Club Conference*, Airlie House, Virginia. New York: Pergamon Press, 1975.
61. Goldstein, A. Future research on opioid peptides (endorphins): A preview. In K. Blum, ed., *Alcohol and Opiates: Neurochemical and Behavioral Mechanisms*. New York: Academic Press, 1977, p. 397.
62. Pomeranz, B. Do endorphins mediate acupuncture analgesia? *Adv. Biochem. Psychopharmacol.* 18:351, 1978.
63. Goldstein, A., et al. On the role of endogenous opioid peptides: Failure of naloxone to influence shock escape threshold in the rat. *Life Sci.* 18:599, 1976.
64. Schneck, H.M., Jr. Chemistry of pain begins to emerge—*Science Times*. *N.Y. Times* May 1979.
65. Loh, H.H., Schen, F.H., and Way, E.L. In-

hibition of morphine tolerance and physical dependence development and brain serotonin synthesis by cycloheximide. *Biochem. Pharmacol.* 18:2711, 1969.

66. Zimmerman, E., and Krivoy, W. Antagonism between morphine and the polypeptides ACTH, ACTH 1-24 and beta-MSH in the nervous system. *Prog. Brain Res.* 39:383, 1973.
67. Loh, H., and Law, P.Y. Pharmacology of endogenous opiate-like peptides. In K. Blum, ed., *Alcohol and Opiates: Neurochemical and Behavioral Mechanisms*. New York: Academic Press, 1977, p. 321.
68. Blum, K., Hamilton, M.G., and Wallace, J.E. Alcohol and opiates—A review of common neurochemical and behavioral mechanisms. In K. Blum, ed., *Alcohol and Opiates: Neurochemical and Behavioral Mechanisms*. New York: Academic Press, 1977, p. 1977.
69. Davis, V.E., and Walsh, M.J. Alcohol, amines and alkaloids: a possible biochemical basis for alcohol addiction. *Science* 167:1005, 1970.
70. Blum, K., et al. Putative role of isoquinoline alkaloids in alcoholism: A link to opiates. *Alcoholism Clin. Exp. Res.* 2:113, 1978.
71. Myers, R.D. Tetrahydroisoquinolines in the brain: The basis of an animal model of alcoholism. *Alcoholism* (N.Y.) 2:145, 1978.
72. Elston, A.H., et al. Ethanol intoxication as a function of genotype dependent responses in three inbred mice strains. *Pharmacol. Biochem. Behav.* 16:13, 1982.
73. Blum, K., et al. Genotype dependent responses to ethanol and normorphine on vas deferens of inbred strains of mice. *Subst. Alcohol Actions Misuse* 1:459, 1980.
74. Blum, K., et al. Reduced leucine-enkephalin-like immunoreactive substance in hamster basal ganglia after long-term ethanol exposure. *Science* 216:1425, 1982.
75. Schultz, R., et al. Acute and chronic ethanol treatment changes endorphin levels in brain and pituitary. *Psychopharmacology* 68:221, 1980.
76. Blum, K., et al. Ethanol preference as a function of genotypic levels of whole brain enkephalin in mice. *Toxicol. Eur. Res.* 3:261, 1981.
77. Blum, K., et al. Psychogenetics of drug seeking behavior. *Subst. Alcohol Actions Misuse* 1:255, 1980.
78. Vereby, K., Volavka, J., and Clouet, D. Endorphins in psychiatry: An overview and a hypothesis. *Arch. Gen. Psychiatry* 35:877, 1978.
79. Stein, L. Reward transmitters: Catecholamines and opioid peptides. In M.A. Lipton, A. DiMascio, and K.F. Killam, eds., *A Review of Psychopharmacology: A Second Decade of Progress*. New York: Raven Press, 1978, p. 569.
80. Davis, G.C., Buchsbaum, M.S., and Bunney, W.E., Jr. Research in endorphins and schizophrenia. *Schizophr. Bull.* 5:244, 1979.
81. Carenzi, A., et al. Molecular mechanisms in the actions of morphine viminol (Rz) on rat striatum. *J. Pharmacol. Exp. Ther.* 194:311, 1975.
82. Kline, N.S., et al. Beta-endorphin-induced changes in schizophrenic and depressed patients. *Arch. Gen. Psychiatry* 34:1111, 1977.
83. Verhoeven, W.M., et al. (Des-tyr[1])-gamma-endorphin in schizophrenia. *Lancet* 1:1046, 1978.
84. Terenius, L., Wahlstron, A., and Johansson, L. In E. Usdin, W.E. Burney, Jr., and N.S. Kline, eds., *Endorphins in Mental Health Research*. New York: Macmillan, 1979, p. 553.
85. Watson, S.J., et al. Effects of naloxone on schizophrenia: Reduction in hallucinations in a subpopulation of subjects. *Science* 201:73, 1978.
86. Wagemaker, H., Jr., and Cade, R. The use of hemodialysis in chronic schizophrenia. *Am. J. Psychiatry* 134:684, 1977.
87. Lewis, R.V., et al. On beta H-Leu 5-endorphin and schizophrenia. *Arch. Gen. Psychiatry* 36:237, 1979.
88. Sternberg, D.E., et al. The effect of pimozide on CSF norepinephrine in schizophrenia. *Am. J. Psychiatry* 138:1045, 1981.
89. Carlsson, A. Does dopamine have a role in schizophrenia? *Biol. Psychiatry* 13:3, 1978.
90. Volavka, J., Davis, L.G., and Ehrlich, Y.H. Endorphins, dopamine and schizophrenia. *Schizophr. Bull.* 5:227, 1979.
91. Garcia-Sevilla, J.A., Magnusson, T., and Carlsson, A. Effects of enkephalins and two enzyme resistant analogues on monoamine synthesis and metabolism in rat brain. *Naunyn-Schmiedeberg's Arch. Pharmacol.* 310:211, 1980.
92. Davis, G.C., and Bunney, W.E., Jr. Psychopathology and endorphins. *Adv. Biochem. Psychopharmacol.* 22:455, 1980.
93. Fink, M., et al. Clinical antidepressant activity of cyclazocine a narcotic antagonist. *Clin. Pharmacol. Ther.* 11:41, 1970.
94. Terenius, L., et al. Increased CSF levels of endorphins in chronic psychosis. *Neurosci. Lett.* 3:157, 1976.
95. Davis, G.C., et al. Intravenous naloxone administration in schizophrenia and affective

illness. *Science* 197:74, 1977.
96. Angrist, B.M., and Gershon, S. The phenomenology of experimentally-induced amphetamine psychosis: Preliminary observations. *Biol. Psychiatry* 2:95, 1970.
97. Meyerson, B.J., and Terenius, L. Beta-endorphin and male sexual behavior. *Eur. J. Pharmacol.* 42:191, 1977.
98. Hollister, L.E. The mystique of social drugs and sex. In M. Sandler and G.L. Gessa, eds., *Sexual Behavior: Pharmacology and Biochemistry*. New York: Raven Press, 1975, p. 85.
99. Gessa, G.L., Paglietto, E., and Quarahtotti, B.P. Induction of copulatory behavior in sexually inactive rats by naloxone. *Science* 204:203, 1979.
100. Cox, B.M., and Baizman, E.R. Physiological functions of endorphins. In J.B. Malick, and M.S.R. Bell, eds., *Endorphins*. New York: Marcel Dekker, 1982, p. 113.
101. Malick, J., and Goldstein, J.M. Animal pharmacology and endorphins. In J.B. Malick, and M.S.R. Bell, eds., *Endorphins*. New York: Marcel Dekker, 1982.
102. Terenius, L. Clinical aspects. In J.B. Malick, and M.S.R. Bell, eds., *Endorphins*. New York: Marcel Dekker, 1982.
103. Fort, J. *The Pleasure Seekers: The Drug Crisis. Youth and Society*. Indianapolis: Bobbs-Merrill, 1965.

## Monographs and Reviews

Ehrenpreis, S. D-phenylalamine and other enkephalinase inhibitors as pharmacological agents: Implications for some important application. *Subs. Alc. Actions/Misuse* 3:231, 1982.
Morley, J.S. Chemistry of opioid peptides. *Br. Med. Bull.* 39(1):5, 1983.

## Table 8-3 References

Barden, N., et al. *Brain Res.* 204:441, 1980.
Bloom, F.E., et al. *Science* 194:630, 1976.
Dupont, A., et al. *Proc. Natl. Acad. Sci. U.S.A.* 74:358, 1977.
Feldberg, W., and Smyth, D.G. *J. Physiol. (Lond.)* 265:25p, 1977.
Fields, H.L. *Adv. Biochem. Psychopharmacol.* 28:199, 1981.
Florez, J., Mediavilla, A., and Pazos, A. *Brain Res.* 199:197, 1980.
French, E.D., et al. *Neurosci. Abst.* 3:291, 1977.
Gambert, S.R. *Neuroendocrinology* 32:114, 1981.
Graf, I., et al. *FEBS Lett.* 64:181, 1976.
Grandison, L., and Guidotti, A. *Neuropharmacology* 16:533, 1977.
Gunson, M.W., and Peters, R.H. *Am. J. Physiol.* 241:R-173, 1981.
Haracz, J.L., et al. *Neuroendocrinology* 33:170, 1981.
Henriksen, S.J., Bloom, F.E., Ling, N., and Guilemin, R. *Neurosci. Abst.* 3:293, 1977.
Izquierdo, I., et al. *Psychopharmacology* 70:173, 1980.
Izumi, K., et al. *Life Sci.* 20:1149, 1977.
Jacquet, Y.F., and Marks, N. *Science* 194:632, 1976.
Jolles, J., Bar, P.R., and Gispen, W.H. *Brain Res.* 224:315, 1981.
Kline, N.S., et al. *Arch. Gen. Psychiatry* 34:1111, 1977.
Kosterlitz, H.W., et al. In C.W.M. Cowan and J.A. Ferrendelli, eds., *Society for Neuroscience Symposia*, vol. II. Rockville, Md.: Society for Neuroscience, 1977, p. 291.
Laubie, M., and Schmitt, H. *Eur. J. Pharmacol.* 71:401, 1981.
Loh, H.H., et al. *Proc. Natl. Acad. Sci., U.S.A.* 73:2895, 1976(a).
Loh, H.H., et al. *Nature* 264:567, 1976.
Meglio, M., et al. *Proc. Natl. Acad. Sci., U.S.A.* 74:774, 1977.
Moroni, F., Cheney, D.L., and Costa, E. *Nature* 267:267, 1977.
Nicoll, R.A., et al. *Proc. Natl. Acad. Sci., U.S.A.* 74:2584, 1977.
Nistico, G., et al. *J. Med.* 12:463, 1981.
Parvizi, N., and Ellendorff, F. *Nature* 286(5775):812, 1980.
Rivier, C., et al. *Endocrinology* 100:238, 1977.
Roemer, D., et al. *Nature* 268:547, 1977.
Sarne, Y., Gil-Ad, I., and Laron, Z. *Life Sci.* 28:681, 1981.
Schulz, R., et al. *Nature* 294:757, 1981.
Stinus, L., et al. *Proc. Natl. Acad. Sci., U.S.A.* 77:2323, 1980.
Strahlendorf, H.H., Strahlendorf, J.C., and Barnes, C.D. *Prog. Clin. Biol. Res.* 68:161, 1981.
Taube, H.D., et al. *Eur. J. Pharmacol.* 38:377, 1976.
Tseng, L.-F., Loh, H.H., and Li, C.H. *Nature* 263:239, 1976.
VanLoon, L.R., et al. *Can. J. Physiol. Pharmacol.* 58:436, 1980.

## Table 8-5 References

Aloisi, F., Scotti, De Carolis, A., and Longo, V. *Pharmacol. Res. Commun.* 12:467, 1980.
Audigier, Y., Malfroy-Camine, B., and Schwarz, J.C. *Eur. J. Pharmacol.* 41:247, 1977.
Baxter, M.G., Fallenfant, R.L., Miller, A.A., and Sethna, D.M. *Br. J. Pharmacol.* 59:523p, 1977.
Beddell, C.R., et al. *Br. J. Pharmacol.* 61:351, 1977.
Belluzzi, J.D., et al. *Nature* 260:625, 1976.
Belluzzi, J.D., and Stein, L. *Nature* 266:556, 1977.
Bhargava, H.N. *Eur. J. Pharmacol.* 41:81, 1977.
Blasig, J., and Herz, A. *Naunyn-Schmiedeberg's Arch. Pharmacol.* 294:297, 1976.
Blum, K., et al. *Science* 216:1425, 1982.
Bradley, P.B., et al. *Nature* 261:425, 1976.
Brandt, M., et al. *FEBS Letts.* 68:38, 1976(a).
Brandt, M., et al. *Nature* 262:311, 1976(b).
Buscher, H.H., et al. *Nature* 261:423, 1976.
Catlin, D.H., et al. In *Advances in Biochemical Psychopharmacology*. New York: Raven Press, 1978.
Chang, J.-K., et al. *Life Sci.* 18:1473, 1976.
Cupello, A., and Hyden, H. *J. Neurosci. Res.* 6:579, 1981.
Davies, J., and Dray, A. *Nature* 262:603, 1976.
Day, A.R., et al. *Res. Commun. Chem. Pathol. Pharmacol.* 14:597, 1976.
Duggan, A.W., Hall, J.A., and Headley, P.R. *Nature* 264:456, 1976.
Duke, T., Wurster, M., and Herz, A. *Life Sci.* 10:26:771, 1980.
Emerson, P.C., et al. *Brain Res.* 13:199:147, 1980.
Ferland, L., et al. *Eur. J. Pharmacol.* 43:89, 1977.
Frederickson, R.C.A., and Norris, F.H. *Science* 194:440, 1976.
Garcia-Sevilla, J.A., Magnusson, T., and Carlsson, A. *Naunun-Schmiedeberg's Arch. Pharmacol.* 310:203, 1980.

Gent, J.P., and Wolstencroft, J.H. *Nature* 201:426, 1976.

Goldstein, A., et al. *Nature* 265:362, 1977.

Herman, Z.S., and Kowalski, J. *Acta Physiol. Pol.* 32:233, 1981.

Hill, R.G., Pepper, C.M., and Mitchell, J.F. *Nature* 262:604, 1976.

Hong, J.S., et al. *Adv. Biochem. Psychopharmacol.* 22:385, 1980.

Hong, J.S., et al., *Subs. Alcohol Action/Misuse* 2(4):233, 1981.

Hong, J.S., and Schmid, R. *Brain Res.* 2:205, 415, 1981.

Jhamandas, K., and Elliot, J. *Br. J. Pharmacol.* 71:211, 1980.

Jhamandas, K., and Sutak, M. *Br. J. Pharmacol.* 71:201, 1980.

Lampert, A., Nirenberg, M., and Klee, W.A. *Proc. Natl. Acad. Sci. U.S.A.* 73:3165, 1976.

Lee, H.K., Dunwiddie, T., and Hoffer, S. *Brain Res.* 184:331, 1980.

Lein, E.L., et al. *Life Sci.* 19:837, 1976.

McCarthy, P.S., Walker, R.J., and Woodruff, G.N. *J. Physiol.* 1977.

Micevych, P., and Elde, R. *J. Comp. Neurol.* 190:135, 1980.

Miller, R.J., and Cuatrecasas, P. In *Neurochemical Mechanisms of Opiates and Endorphins*. New York: Raven Press, 1979.

Miller, R.J., et al. In *Biological Council Symposium on Centrally Acting Peptides*. 1978, pp. 195-214.

Minneman, K., and Iversen, L.L. *Nature* 262:313, 1976.

Nicoll, R.A., Alser, B.E., and Jahr, C.E. *Nature* 287:22, 1980.

Pert, A. In H. Kosterlitz, ed., *Opiates and Endogenous Opioid Peptides*. Amsterdam: North-Holland, 1976, p. 87.

Pert, A., and Pert, C. *Nature* 265:645, 1977.

Pert, C.B., Pert, A., and Tallman, J. *Proc. Natl. Acad. Sci. U.S.A.* 73:2226, 1976.

Pfeiffer, A., Seizingh, B.R., and Here, A. *Neuropharmacology* 20:1229, 1981.

Plotnikoff, N.P., et al. *Life Sci.* 18:28:2277, 1981.

Römer, D., et al. *Nature* 268:547, 1977.

Sawynok, J., and LaBella, F.S. *Eur. J. Pharmacol.* 12:70:103, 1981.

Schulz, R., et al. *Nature* 24:294, 757-759, 1981.

Simantov, R., and Snyder, S.H. *Proc. Natl. Acad. Sci. U.S.A.* 73:2515, 1976.

Sprick, U., Oitzl, M.S., Ornstein, K., and Huston, J.P. *Brain Res.* 210:243, 1981.

Stone, T.W. *Br. J. Pharmacol.* 74:171, 1981.

Summer, M.C., and Nayee, R.J. *FEBS Lett.* 113:99, 1980.

Szekely, J., et al. *Eur. J. Pharmacol.* 43:292, 1977.

Urwyler, S., and Tabahoff, B. *Life Sci.* 28:2277, 1981.

Urca, G., et al. *Science* 197:83, 1977.

Vincent, J.E., Zijlstra, F.J., and Dzolijic, M.R. *Adv. Prostaglandin Thromboxane Res.* 8:1217, 1980.

Waterfield, A.A., et al. *Eur. J. Pharmacol.* 43:107, 1977.

Wei, E., and Loh, H.H. *Science* 193:1262, 1976.

Wei, E.T., et al. *Life Sci.*, 1978.

Wuster, M., Duka, T., and Herz, A. *Neuropharmacology* 19:501, 1980.

Chapter 9

# CNS Depressants: Sedative-Hypnotics (Barbiturates and Nonbarbiturates)

It is the purpose of this chapter to review available information on central nervous system (CNS) depressants, including their pharmacology, prevalence, abuse potential, and treatment.

This discussion is limited to the barbiturates and the nonbarbiturate sedative-hypnotics. Alcohol, one of the most widely used of the CNS depressants, presents a problem of such magnitude and is so unique in nature that it requires independent attention. Similarly the antianxiety drugs, such as diazepam and chlorodiazepoxide types, are included in a separate chapter.

## A. INTRODUCTION

The depressants discussed here include the barbiturates, glutethimide, and methaqualone.

Overuse of barbiturates is America's hidden drug problem, perhaps comparable in scope to the hidden opiate dependence around the turn of the century. Medical supervision of the use of these drugs too often has been lax, resulting in abundant availability of barbiturates within the medical distribution system. In 1970, barbiturates (and the considerably lesser used barbiturate substitutes) accounted for over 25 percent of the total prescriptions issued for psychoactive drugs. Only the minor tranquilizers, with 38.8 percent, were higher. Forty million barbiturate prescriptions were issued in 1971—22 million of them refills of old prescriptions.

According to a survey conducted by the National Institute of Drug Abuse, in 1979, for psychotherapeutics (which include stimulants, sedatives, tranquilizers, and analgesics), the highest prevalence and current use rates are reported by young adults. These 18–25-year-olds report the most nonmedical experience with stimulants (18.2 percent), followed by sedatives (17.0 percent), tranquilizers (15.8 percent), and analgesics (11.8 percent). They report current use for each of these as follows: stimulants, 3.5 percent; sedatives, 2.8 percent; tranquilizers, 2.1 percent; analgesics, 10 percent. Among youths and older adults, prevalence rates for these substances are about 6 percent, with current use about 1 percent.

It is noteworthy that from 1977 to 1979, lifetime prevalence and current use rates show no significant changes for youths, young adults, or older adults.

Drugs that induce a ready sleep are hypnotic. For centuries, the only such drugs known were alcohol, opium, and belladonna (deadly nightshade). The hypnotic-type drugs are general CNS depressants, depressing both the CNS and a wide range of cellular functions in many vital organ systems. In small doses, hypnotics have a sedative effect with a tendency to produce drowsiness or apathy; with an overdose, they are anesthetic, and ultimately fatal. In prescribed dosage, they usually induce sleep. These drugs do not relieve pain, but may augment the pain-killing action of other drugs, such as morphine and aspirin. The hypnotic drugs are primarily abused by the adult community. Many people who have lost the habit of sleep without the assistance of drugs become very dependent on them. They should be avoided during early months of pregnancy, and children seldom need them.[1]

Because of the enormous amount of information available concerning the biosocial aspects of sedative-hypnotics, a brief summary is presented here to assist the less serious reader.

## 1. Barbiturates

The barbiturates refer to any of the derivatives of barbituric acid (malonylurea). More than 2500 barbiturates have been synthesized but, although approximately 50 of these have been approved for clinical use, only about a dozen are widely used. These drugs, however, are the most common, and perhaps the most valuable, CNS depressants utilized in medicine today.

The traditional method of classifying the barbiturates is based upon their relative duration of action. The ultrashort-acting barbiturates, which include sodium methohexital (Brevital), sodium thiamylal (Surital), and sodium thiopental (Pentothal), are employed primarily as intravenous anesthetics, often in conjunction with nitrous oxide or other inhalational agents. The short- to intermediate-acting barbiturates are used primarily as sedative-hypnotic agents; they include amobarbital (Amytal), sodium butabarbital (Butisol), sodium pentobarbital (Nembutal), secobarbital (Seconal), and vinbarbital (Delvinal). Phenobarbital (Luminal), mephobarbital (Mebaral), and metharbital (Gemonil) are long-acting barbiturates and are used as sedative-hypnotics and as agents in the emergency treatment of convulsions.

While it must be kept in mind that the action of these drugs upon the CNS depends on the particular barbiturate, the dosage, the route of administration, the state of the CNS at the time of administration, and the degree of tolerance that may exist, it is possible to present some general information about the pharmacology and effects of the barbiturates.

Although they may be injected, oral administration is the safest and most common method of introducing barbiturates into the body. These drugs are absorbed rapidly from the stomach and, since there is no impenetrable barrier to their diffusion, they enter the bloodstream and tend to be distributed rather uniformly throughout the body. The further distribution and concentration of the barbiturates in various tissues and organs are largely dependent upon lipid solubility and protein binding. Thus fat depots and protein-rich organ tissues accumulate the highest concentrations of the barbiturates. Great variations exist among the different barbiturate compounds. The highly lipid-soluble and protein-bound drugs, such as thiopental, are absorbed more readily by the brain and other organs, and thus are of quicker onset and shorter duration of action.

Whereas peripheral structures will not be directly affected until significantly higher dose levels are attained, the CNS is exquisitely sensitive to the depressant effects of the barbiturates and will exhibit physiologic responses at sedative-hypnotic dosages. The barbiturates produce a general reduction in CNS activity at sedative doses, leading to drowsiness and muscular incoordination. In some instances, however, certain individuals have experienced anxiety and excitement rather than sedation following the administration of low doses of barbiturates. In hyperkinetic children, for example, both barbiturates and amphetamines produce effects opposite to those found in the normal population. Thus, whereas barbiturates produce excitability in these children, amphetamines are used to calm the hyperactive child. The aftereffects of barbiturate-induced sleep may include drowsiness, hangover, headache, overt excitement, and decrements in motor performance, which may last for several hours.

Although the ultrashort-acting barbiturates are administered intravenously to induce anesthesia for surgery, they do not (nor do other barbiturates) relieve pain. In fact, in the presence of severe pain, the barbiturates are often incapable of producing sedation or sleep. In small doses, they may cause hyperalgesia, an increase in the reaction to painful stimuli.

Barbiturates can exert a depressant effect on the respiratory, renal, hepatic, cardiovascular, and other biologic systems, but these effects are not significant until doses well above therapeutic levels are reached. The toxic state produced by these drugs is discussed later.

The psychologic effects observed following the ingestion of the barbiturates are remarkably similar to those produced by alcohol. As with all psychoactive drugs, the set (the personality and emotional state of the user) and the setting (the environment in which the drug is taken) greatly affect the outcome of the drug experience. Thus one individual may find a pleasant, serene, and relaxed enjoyment, whereas another may feel hostile and aggressive. While low doses produce variable effects, moderate doses commonly reduce reaction time, impair mental functioning and memory, and result in slurred speech, a loss of inhibitions, a reduction in emotional control, and other effects resembling alcohol intoxication.

### *Medical Uses*

These drugs depress the CNS and are prescribed in small doses to reduce restlessness and emotional tension, and to induce sleep. Some are valuable in the treatment of certain types of epilepsy.

### *Abuse*

Continued excessive dosages of barbiturates result in slurring of speech, staggering, loss of balance and falling, faulty judgment, quick temper, and a quarrelsome disposition. Overdoses, particularly when taken in conjunction with alcohol, result in unconsciousness and death, unless the user receives proper medical treatment.

The appearance of drunkenness without an alcoholic breath may indicate excessive use of depressant drugs. However, an unsteady gait and speech problems may also be signs of neurologic disorders.

### *Physical Dependence and Tolerance*

A marked degree of both physical dependence and tolerance develops to all the barbiturates. The upper limit to the tolerance is not high, and a slight increase in dosage can precipitate toxic symptoms.

### *Effects of Abuse*

For almost eight decades, since the introduction of barbiturates, hundreds of barbituric acid derivatives have been studied and dozens have been approved for nocturnal hypnosis and daytime sedation.

Dr. Carlton Turner of the White House Office of Drug Abuse Policy, in a personal communication, has evaluated the risk/benefit ratio of barbiturates. Although there is little objection to prescribing small doses for the hypnotic-inducing actions of short-acting barbiturates, there is little justification for their use in the condition of insomnia. As an anti-convulsant and an inexpensive anti-stress agent, phenobarbital is still medicinally useful.

Therapeutic doses of barbiturates may cause unwanted side reactions, which include a) reduced mental activity b) slowed speech, and c) sedation. Higher doses induce more profound effects, which include a) positive Rombert sign b) diplopia c) nystagmus d) respiratory depression e) decreased total REM sleep, and f) intermittent porphyia.

Unlike opiates, the respiratory actions of

barbiturates are not consistently blocked by nalorphine or levallorphan.

Although there is no social hazard for barbiturate abuse, it is the leading drug used to commit suicide.

### *Abstinence*

Compared to opiate-induced withdrawal symptoms, the abstinence syndrome which develops following abrupt removal of the barbiturates in a chronic abuser is much more dangerous. Effects observed during the barbiturate abstinence syndrome include a) insomnia b) tremulousness c) weakness d) cramps e) vomiting e) hyperthermia f) confusion g) chronic blink reflex, and h) low blood pressure. There are cases whereby delayed convulsions and death have occurred. Alcohol is similar to the barbiturates particularly with regard to resultant delirium tremens. Short-acting barbiturates, when abused, could lead to convulsions after the second and third day of abstinence, whereas the long-acting barbiturates might induce convulsions between the third and eighth day of abstinence.[2]

Barbiturates are sometimes combined with other drugs to achieve unique "highs." Generally, if delayed convulsions are observed, the astute clinician immediately suspects the presence of barbiturates and takes appropriate measures.

During hospital stays of patients, especially adults, detailed histories should uncover possible barbiturate use, illicit or licit. Urine testing of heroin dependent individuals should assist in the identification of additional barbiturate abuse. Along with the above testing, barbiturate tolerance should also be evaluated. To accomplish this aim, Goth[3] has described the methodology usually employed:

"An ordinary therapeutic dose of pentobarbital is administered and the patient is observed for clinical signs of drug effect. . . . Additional increments of pentobarbital are administered until drug effect is evident . . . subsequent doses are tapered over the ensuing seven to 14 days."

### *Barbiturate Poisoning and Toxicity*

The licit use of barbiturates presents a public health problem for a variety of reasons.

In 1975, more than a thousand people succeeded in employing barbiturates to induce their demise. The barbiturates, as previously mentioned, are the most frequent chemical agents used to commit suicide. Medical examiners are well acquainted with accidental deaths due to sublethal combinations of barbiturates and alcohol.

There are no age barriers to barbiturate use and abuse. From grammar school, to the "funk" crowd, to the overworked businessperson, to the bored housewife, to the elderly, there is a visible problem with barbiturates—alone or in combination with other drugs—as a drug of abuse. Interestingly, the geriatric crowd is at higher risk in terms of idiosyncratic effects. In fact, many older citizens exhibit idiosyncratic excitement instead of depression with licit barbiturate use.

Acute use of barbiturates may induce violent behavior, and overdosage will cause death due to respiratory paralysis. Unlike other addicting drugs, there is no pure antagonist to barbiturate poisoning. Even if overdosage does not result in death, other serious complications must be monitored such as cyanosis of skin, slowed respiration, hypothermia, reduced reflexes, coma, circulatory impairment, and hypostatic pneumonia.

Sometimes patients with marginal pulmonary edema may become apneic when full doses of barbiturates are used for their insomnia. In this condition, porphyria barbiturates are contraindicated because they produce toxic paralysis.[4]

### *Slang Terms*

Barbiturates are known to drug abusers as "barbs," "candy," "goofballs," "sleeping pills," and "peanuts." Specific types are often named for their color or shape.

Pentobarbital sodium in solid yellow capsule form, for example, is known by abusers as "yellow jackets" or "nembies" (after a trade name of this drug). Secobarbital sodium in red capsule form is called "reds," "pinks," "red birds," "red devils," and "seggy" (after trade names). Amobarbital sodium, combined with secobarbital sodium, in red and blue capsule form, is known as "rainbows," "red and blues," and "double trouble." (For a complete list, see Table 9-2.)

## 2. CNS Depressants Other Than Barbiturates

Nonbarbiturate drugs are classified as sedative-hypnotic drugs. They are used therapeutically to induce sleep. Although there are a variety of chemical structures and pharmacologic properties that are exclusive to these drugs, they are in some ways similar to barbiturates in their activity. Therefore what is known about the barbiturates is also representative of the hypnotics. No significant advantages are offered by the hypnotics over the barbiturates and statements to the contrary have no clear foundation. Drugs included in the nonbarbiturate sedative-hypnotic group are chloral hydrate (Noctec, Somnos); bromide (Bromo-Seltzer, Nervine, Sleep-Eze, Sominex); ethchlorvynol (Placidyl); paraldehyde (cyclic ether); glutethimide (Doriden) and methyprylon (Noludar) "piperidinedione derivatives"; methaqualone (Quaalude, Sopor); fluthenazine (Prolixin); carbamates (urethane and related drugs, including alcohol).

The oral doses used to induce sleep vary—chloral hydrate, 0.5 to 1.0 gram; ethchlorvynol, 100 to 200 mg and 500 mg for hypnotic levels; paraldehyde, 4 to 8 milliliters; glutethimide, 500 mg; methyprylon, 200 to 400 mg; and the standard hypnotic dose for methaqualone is 150 to 300 mg.

Chloral hydrate (1832) is the oldest of the nonbarbiturates. It is advantageous because it suppresses the rapid-eye-movement (REM) phase during sleep. However, its popularity has decreased with the introduction of the barbiturates.

Some of the more widely known over-the-counter preparations of bromide include Bromo-Seltzer, Nervine, Sleep-Eze, and Sominex. Bromide was first used in 1857 in the treatment of epilepsy. It has a half-life of 12 days and is therefore excreted slowly from the kidneys. Ethchlorvydol has two main characteristics. It is fast acting and has a fast absorption rate. It is a tertiary alcohol that reaches peak blood levels within 1 to 1½ hours and disappears within three hours.

Currently paraldehyde is mainly used in institutions. It is also rapidly absorbed and reaches brain peak levels within 30 minutes. It is excreted through the lungs and a large portion of it is metabolized in the liver.

Glutethimide and methyprylon are similar to secobarbital in their actions. However, glutethimide is useful in motion sickness and exhibits anticholinergic actions.

Methaqualone includes Quaaludes, which are among the most popular of the illicit drugs among the young people in the United States. It is one of the most potent members of the quinozoline series of nonbarbiturate sedative-hypnotic compounds. It has a rapid absorption rate in the gastrointestinal tract, and its duration of action is longer than either Tuinal (amobarbital/secobarbital combination) or chloral hydrate. Unlike the other drugs of its kind, it acts centrally on the brain and does not depress the brain reticular system or medulla.

Some of the risks of using hypnotics other than for therapeutic purposes are quite apparent. Chloral hydrate may produce unconciousness if taken in combination with alcohol (Mickey Finn, knockout drops). Bromides may accumulate in the body if taken daily for a period of weeks. Chronic bromide intoxication (bromism) includes impaired memory, drowsiness, dizziness, irritability, dermatitis (skin rash), and gastrointestinal distress. Delirium, hallucinations, mania, or coma may occur in severe cases. Paraldehyde has significant effects upon the respiratory and cardiovascular systems after therapeutic doses are surpassed. At high concentrations, it inhibits the release of acetylcholine from the nerve endings and may lead to muscle weakness and fatigue. Doriden, Quaalude, and Prolixin accumulate in the body fat and thus are harder to expel from the system. The stored compound further complicates toxicity. Doriden is highly toxic. The only nonbarbiturates that rarely have any side effects include the piperidine derivatives, glutethimide and methyprylon. The nonbarbiturates are useful in producing sleep, however, precautionary measures must be taken when surpassing therapeutic levels.

## B. HISTORY[5]

### 1. Overview

The term barbiturates is used to refer to any derivative of malonylurea. The sedatives or barbiturates are derivatives of barbituric acid, first synthesized in Germany in 1862. There are several stories with regard to the naming of *barbituric acid*. Some believe, for example, that it was so named because it was first obtained from uric acid (by Von Baeyer) on St. Barbara's Day.[6] Others say that the new compound was named in honor of a Munich waitress.[7] Barbital (Veronal), the first barbiturate to be used clinically, was introduced into medicine in Germany in 1903 by Fischer and Von Mering. Most of the 2500 barbiturates that have been synthesized enjoy excellent CNS depressant properties, even though the parent compound was not such a depressant. The second barbiturate to receive wide acclaim was phenobarbital, introduced in 1912 under the trade name Luminal. This compound is still very widely used, and is probably the best in its class. Since phenobarbital, which was clinically used for hypnotic purposes, has a very long duration of action with the production of a "hangover" effect, a search for hypnotics with a shorter duration of action resulted in the development of, among others, amobarbital (1923), pentobarbital (1930), and secobarbital (1930). The development of the ultrashort-acting barbiturates, such as thiopental (1935), and trisubstituted barbiturates (hexobarbital in 1936), paved the way for modern intravenous anesthesia.

Anxiety and insomnia, two of the most common human afflictions, were treated during the 19th century with opiates, bromide salts, chloral hydrate (introduced in 1869), paraldehyde (1882), and alcohol. Because the opiates were known to produce physical dependence, the bromides carried the risk of chronic bromide poisoning, and chloral hydrate and paraldehyde (their potential for dependence unknown) had an objectionable taste and smell, alcohol became the prescribed depressant drug of choice. But the search for a better drug continued, because "pledged teetotalers" refused to use alcohol, and many other patients either did not like its taste and smell or tended to take more than prescribed.

By the 1920s, an estimated billion grains of barbiturates were taken in the United States alone. Evidence increasingly accumulated during the 1930s and 1940s indicating that barbiturates (especially the short-acting types), when misused, posed many of the same problems as alcohol with regard to the dependency syndrome. But the parallel between the effects of these two CNS depressants was not confirmed until almost a half century after the introduction of barbital.

The campaign against nonmedical use began with 1942 and 1945 articles in *Hygeia* (now *Today's Health*), an American Medical Association publication designed for the lay public. Other magazines followed suit, including *Collier's*, with a 1949 article called "Thrill Pills Can Ruin You." States began passing laws against nonprescription barbiturates, arrests made newspaper headlines, black market barbiturates became profitable, and "thrill pills" and "goofballs" became popularized. At first, the illicit users were mostly adults, many of whom would never have otherwise taken a sedative or sleeping pill.

Because the barbiturates came under frequent attack, efforts were revived in the 1940s to find additional drugs to compete for the flourishing market for depressants. Glutethimide, ethchlorvynol, and methyprylon appeared on the market in 1954 and 1955. Their manufacturers urged physicians to prescribe them precisely because they were nonbarbiturates. It was found, however, that the same potential for abuse existed with these drugs, as well as with a second class of drugs introduced in the mid-1950s, the minor tranquilizers.

The abuse of barbiturates and other sedative-hypnotics has been reviewed by Smith et al.[8] Part of the following information presented in this overview of barbiturates and other sedative-hypnotics is adapted from the book *Barbiturates: Their Use, Misuse and Abuse* by Wesson and Smith.[9]

## 2. Epidemiology and Depressant Usage

Various estimating techniques are used in determining the epidemiology of CNS depressant usage. These include surveys of subpopulations such as adults, students, and cross sections of the general population; statistics on production and prescription of depressants; data on drug-related deaths and hospital admissions; and law enforcement statistics, including figures for arrests and confiscations.

If all use of CNS depressants were legal, valid and reliable statistics on the number of types of users, trends in patterns of use, and the various effects on users would be fairly easy to obtain, as they are for tobacco. Official data provide knowledge of widespread illicit use, but this information, in turn, is reason for a reluctant attitude toward obtaining further data. Agencies fail to employ precise and consistent categories in collecting and presenting data from year to year. Statistics are affected by alterations in the drug laws, changes in the practices of enforcement agencies, and changes in the characteristics of the drug users and the drug market. Discussions of prevalence, therefore, are based on available, rather than complete, data.

Studies of the late 1960s and early 1970s reveal widespread use of both sedative-hypnotic drugs (barbiturate and nonbarbiturate) and tranquilizers, with the latter being slightly more popular. Fort[10] estimates the number of users of prescription CNS depressants at between 20 and 25 million. Approximately 300 tons of barbiturates alone are consumed in the United States annually.

In a survey of California adults,[11] 30 percent had used either prescription or nonprescription sedative-hypnotics and tranquilizers at one time or another, and frequent use was reported by 7 percent for sedative-hypnotics and 10 percent for tranquilizers. Among frequent users, the most significant subgroup variables are age, sex, and marital status. Sedative-hypnotic use increases with age and occurs most often among those 60 and over, while the frequent use of tranquilizers is greater among those between 30 and 60. Almost twice as many women as men are frequent users (but, in overall depressant usage, this discrepancy is diminished because of the greater use of alcohol by men), and persons who are separated or divorced report frequent use more often than single or married persons. Studies of barbiturate use alone[12] indicate that whites, persons from the middle socioeconomic classes, and persons with higher educations are more likely to be regular users of barbiturates.

The use of CNS depressants has become much more common among younger people. According to an extensive 1969 study of college students,[1] 24 percent have used sedative-hypnotics and 19 percent had used tranquilizers, but among those who had used both types of drugs, tranquilizer use was greater at a ratio of four to one. Motivations cited by these students were relief of tension by both types of users, reduction of sexuality by sedative-hypnotic users, and avoidance of panic by tranquilizer users.

Physicians, especially general practitioners, remain the major source of CNS depressants for all age groups, but among minors, parents are a significant source as well. It is common to find the use of depressants at the fourth and fifth grade level; as far back as May 1972, a survey of the Los Angeles city schools showed barbiturates to be the leading school drug problem, ahead of both marihuana and alcohol.

There appears to be a decline, however, in the utilization of physicians to obtain prescriptions for CNS depressants. Within a cross section surveyed,[13] 27 percent of the prescription drugs (including stimulants) that were used were obtained illicitly. Nonmedical sources (including over-the-counter) were used more by those under 30 and more by men than women, but those drugs obtained medically were used on a more continuing basis. The CNS depressants are widely used in response to emotional needs and, according to Mellinger,[13] the growing tendency to avoid the physician as source indicates a difference in attitude between physicians and patients as to whether emotional distress can be considered disabling—that is, is it "dys-ease" or disease?

Fort[10] estimates that 500,000 of the millions of users of CNS depressants can be considered abusers; that is, use that is nonspecific, excessive in amount or duration of time used, serving to obscure real causes while treating symptoms, or not being beneficial. An estimated 50 percent of all barbiturates manufactured are of the short- to intermediate-acting variety that are particularly subject to abuse.

By 1971, barbiturates reportedly had taken a dominant place in the use of drugs as intoxicants.[14] Chronic intoxication is seen most often in the 30- to 50-year age range, while teenagers and young adults are more involved in patterns of episodic intoxication. Although oral use of CNS depressants greatly predominates, these authors also report the existence of "barb freaks," or the intravenous barbiturate use among young adults "who have a strong commitment to the illegal drug culture. . . . Barbiturates are injected primarily for the 'rush' effect . . . experienced immediately after injection."

Some 50 percent of all narcotic-dependent persons also abuse CNS depressants, with approximately 30 percent of them dependent on both narcotics and depressants.[15]

Simultaneous abuse of barbiturates and amphetamines is also common,[16] and the combination is said to produce more elevation of mood than either drug type alone. This combination occurs in at least two other known abuse patterns. One is an alternating cycle of sedation and stimulation—using stimulants to overcome a drowsy hangover, and by evening using depressants to ward off insomnia. Barbiturates are also used by the "speed freak" to produce sleep after several days of continuous amphetamine injection.

The Drug Enforcement Administration, formerly known as the Bureau of Narcotics and Drugs (BNDD), historically reported in 1971 that 17 percent of those arrested for serious crimes in six major U.S. cities were current barbiturate users. According to arrest figures from Los Angeles County,[17] seizures of barbiturates rose 2000 percent in the preceding five years, more than for any other drug, and the data also showed that no community was exempt from the problem. Of all the traffic accidents involving drugged individuals between 1970 and 1972 in another southern California county, 40 percent involved secobarbital.

Secobarbital (reds, red devils, red birds) is the compound most frequently seized from the illicit traffic in CNS depressants, with phenobarbital (bennies) second, pentobarbital (yellow bullets, yellow jackets) third, and secobarbital/amobarbital combinations (rainbows, tooies, double trouble) fourth. Secobarbital also accounts for a disproportionate number of toxicology cases.

Estimates of deaths per year attributed to prescription CNS depressants range as high as 10,000 and the most commonly used estimate of barbiturate-caused deaths is over 3000 annually. Barbiturate overdosage is currently one of the major methods of committing suicide, and will probably remain so because of their easy availability. Blum[1] reports that 70 percent of those students admitting to suicide attempts via ingestion were CNS depressant users.

A major danger associated with CNS depressant use is that combined use with alcohol potentiates the action of both. Accidental overdosage can occur under these circumstances, as well as when sleeping pills are left by the bedside and an already sedated and confused person ingests a lethal dose. Prescription CNS depressants presently account for over 50 percent of all accidental drug poisonings, with nonbarbiturate sedative-hypnotics being the major cause, barbiturates second, and tranquilizers third.[18]

The discreditation of the barbiturates had its most recent effect in the popularity of the nonbarbiturate sedative-hypnotic methaqualone. Originally introduced in 1951 as an antimalarial agent, its greater usefulness as a sedative-hypnotic brought it to the United States via England in 1965 as a barbiturate substitute.

Manufacturers' claims—now discredited—that methaqualone was superior to other CNS depressants in the quantity and quality of sleep produced encouraged widespread manufacture, prescription, and distribution of the drug. A marked increase in use had begun by 1969, and by 1972, private physicians, teachers, hospitals and clinics, "street people," drug manufacturers, and BNDD all confirmed the sudden illicit use of "soapers."[19] This drug enjoys the highest popularity among white suburban teenagers, who sometimes have reported that it is more available than marihuana. Although the William H. Rorer Company, manufacturer of Quaalude, claimed to have put strict controls on the drug, free advertising samples have been widely distributed to physicians. Methaqualone was introduced as a prescription drug, but it was not included on the 1971 list of controlled substances and, in May 1972, BNDD reported more than 275 incidents of poisonings, overdoses, and suicide attempts during the previous year, resulting in 16 deaths.

As previously mentioned, the NIDA survey of 1979 revealed that sedative use did not significantly change in terms of prevelance rates from 1977 to 1979.

## C. CHEMISTRY

The main chemical ingredients in the synthesis of barbiturates and hypnotics are urea and organic acids. Their combination results in monoureides and diureides. The parent compound in the barbiturate series is malonic acid or malonylurea, or barbituric acid, which is made from urea and malonic acid. The parent compound of thiopental (Pentothal), which is a series of ultrashort-acting barbiturate intravenous anesthetics, is made by combining thiourea and malonic acid, called thiobarbituric acid. The structural formulas of urea, malonic acid, and barbituric acid are shown in Figure 9-1.

Synthesizing different types of barbiturates usually requires changing the molecule either at position 5, or replacing a hydrogen in the ring. Thus phenobarbital becomes ethylphenylbarbituric acid, or mephobarbital (Mebaral), if either a change is made at the fifth position, or an additional methyl group is attached to the nitrogen atom, respectively.

### 1. Classification

Barbiturates are used therapeutically as "sedative-hypnotic barbiturates," or "anesthetic barbiturates."[20] Phenobarbiturate, a sedative-hypnotic barbiturate, has a slow absorption rate, and is more useful for maintaining sedation than either secobarbital or pentobarbital. However, the duration of action for promoting sleep has been overemphasized. The recommendation of barbiturates on the basis of whether they are ultrashort, short, intermediate, or long-acting barbiturates, is not strongly supported.[21] Well-controlled clinical studies are not available to determine barbiturate effectiveness, in terms of duration of action. Secobarbital, pentobarbital, and phenobarbital, in 100-mg doses, were found to be equally effective in inducing sleep in patients with chronic diseases.[22] Phenobarbital had no more noticeable hangover effects than either secobarbital or pentobarbital. The various ultrashort-, short-, intermediate-, and long-acting barbiturates are indicated in Tables 9-1, and 9-2.[9]

## D. ABSORPTION, DISTRIBUTION, EXCRETION, METABOLISM, AND CUMULATION

### 1. Absorption[23]

Barbiturates are well absorbed from the stomach, but the short-acting barbiturates absorb

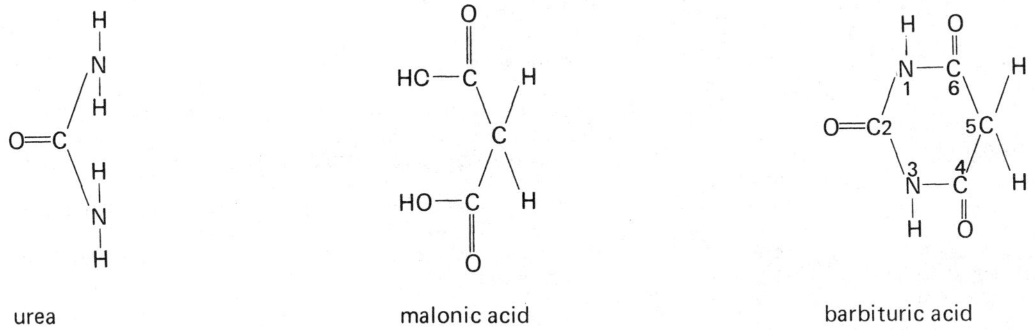

urea

malonic acid

barbituric acid

**Figure 9-1**

more readily than the longer acting ones. Alcohol enhances absorption and produces an additive sedative-hypnotic effect. The sodium salts of barbiturates can be injected intramuscularly or intravenously, though the solutions, including those prepared by pharmaceutical companies specifically for injection, are very alkaline.

Several studies in animals have indicated that rectal administration of certain barbiturates is more efficient than oral administration.

## 2. Distribution[24,25]

The barbiturates are widely distributed in fats and penetrate into the CNS and the fetus. Studies on the distribution of the barbiturates in the CNS have not revealed selective localization in any particular area.

Barbiturates are distributed throughout the body and cross the placental barrier within a few minutes after injection. The concentration

**TABLE 9-1**

**Classification, Structure, and Dosage of Commonly Used Barbiturates**

| *Name* | *Substituents in Postion 5* | *Hypnotic Dose, grams* | *Duration of Action* |
|---|---|---|---|
| Thiopental* (Pentothal) | Ethyl, l-methylbutyl | | Ultrashort (intravenous anesthetics) |
| Thiamylal* (Surital) | Allyl, l-methylbutyl | | |
| Hexobarbital† (Evipal) | Methyl, cyclohexenyl | | |
| Secobarbital (Seconal) | Allyl, l-methylbutyl | 0.1–0.2 | Short |
| Pentobarbital (Nembutal) | Ethyl, l-methylbutyl | 0.1 | |
| Butabarbital (Butisol) | Ethyl, sec-butyl | 0.1–0.2 | Intermediate |
| Amobarbital (Amytal) | Ethyl, isoamyl | 0.05–0.2 | |
| Vinbarbital (Delvinal) | Ethyl, l-methyl-l-butenyl | 0.1–0.2 | |
| | Ethyl, phenyl | | |
| Phenobarbital (Luminal) | Ethyl, phenyl | 0.1–0.2 | Long |
| Mephobarbital† (Mebaral) | Ethyl, ethyl | 0.1–0.2 | |
| Barbital (Veronal) | | 0.3–0.5 | |

* Thiobarbiturate.

† A $CH_3$ group is attached to the nitrogen atom.

(From Goth, A. *Medical Pharmacology,* 12th ed., St. Louis: C.V. Mosby, 1981. With permission.)

**TABLE 9-2**

**Short-Acting Barbiturates: Trade and "Street" Names**

| *Generic Name* | *Trade Name (Manufacturer)* | *Street Names* |
|---|---|---|
| Amobarbital | Amytal (Lilly) | Blue angels, blue dolls, bluebirds, blue heavens, blue bullets, blues, blue devils, blue tips |
| Pentobarbital | Nembutal (Abbott) | Nebbies, yellow dolls, nembies, yellow jackets, yellows, yellow bullets |
| Secobarbital | Seconal (Lilly) | F-40's, red devils, Mexican reds, red dolls, M & M's, red lillies, R.D.'s, reds, red birds, seccies, red bullets, seggies |
| Equal parts of secobarbital and amobarbital | Tuinal (Lilly) | Double trouble, toosies, gorilla pills, trees, rainbows, tuies, reds and blues |

From Smith, D.E., and Wesson, D. R. Diagnosis and treatment of adverse reactions to sedative-hypnotics. DHEW Publication No. (ADM), 75-144, 1974.

in fetal blood approaches that of maternal venous blood.

### 3. Metabolism and Excretion[23,26]

In the body, most barbiturates are transformed by the liver into inactive metabolites. Barbiturates not metabolized by the liver are excreted unchanged in the urine. Phenobarbital is dependent mainly on renal excretion for the termination of its pharmacologic action and 65 to 90 percent of the total amount taken appears in the urine unaltered. The other barbiturates are seen in negligible quantities in the urine.

The ultrashort action of the barbiturates listed in Table 9-1 is not the result of their metabolic destruction but of redistribution throughout body tissues. This has been studied most carefully in the case of thiopental. Only about 0.3 percent of an administered dose is excreted unchanged in the urine. The rate of metabolism is 10 to 15 percent of the dose per hour, which is much too slow to account for the brief duration of action of this compound. The rapid emergence from sleep after a single administration of an anesthetic dose of thiopental depends upon a shift of the drug from the brain to other tissues. The rate at which various tissues take up thiopental is determined by the rate of blood flow. The brain, kidneys, and heart obtain maximum concentration 30 seconds after intravenous administration. Muscle and skin require 15 to 30 minutes to become saturated with thiopental, and several hours are needed for fat deposits to become saturated. Therefore, after a dose is administered, the high concentration achieved rapidly in the brain is redistributed to the muscles, skin, and fat. This produces a drop in the effective concentration in the brain and accounts for the observed ultrashort action.

### 4. Factors That Interfere with Barbiturate Pharmacodynamics[27]

The following factors have been observed to interfere with barbiturate intoxication, excretion, and metabolism.

1) The presence of food stuff in the stomach significantly alters the intoxicating properties of most barbiturates. Doses of barbiturates, when consumed one and a half hours after a breakfast, induced mild intoxication compared to severe intoxication when the barbiturate was taken before breakfast.

2) The barbiturates are metabolized in the liver where no unchanged barbiturates appear in the urine. The kidney and liver may intensify the pharmacological actions of the barbiturates by interfering with their metabolism and excretion. Mixed-function oxidases located in the microsomes of liver cells are responsible for biotransformation and the subsequent production of a polar alcohol, ketone, phenol, or carboxylic acid. Additionally, nephrotic diseases tend to prolong the halflife of barbiturates excreted in the urine. The toxicity of barbiturates is increased in uremia.

3) Certain central nervous system active drugs which are hepatic microsomal enzyme inhibitors, such as SKF-525 (trasentine) and MAO inhibitors, prolong barbiturate actions.

## E. MECHANISMS OF ACTION[28]

It was once thought that barbiturates cause their profound effects by interfering with cellular intermediary metabolism which ultimately affects tissue oxygenation, mitochrondial respiration and cellular excitability. Although it was thought that a common site of action was not applicable to barbiturate induced central depression, it was suggested that excitability in each tissue is depressed by an effect on cellular membranes which might act via a common pathway.

Barbiturates depress the activity of all excitable tissue. However, not all tissues are equally affected by the same amounts. For example, sedative and hypnotic doses may not significantly change or alter the normal functioning of skeletal, smooth, or heart muscle.

Olsen[28] reviewed the mechanism and sites of action for CNS depressants. Interesting evidence supports a role for the major inhibitory neurotransmitter, $\gamma$-aminobutyric acid (GABA), in the action of many CNS depressant and excitatory drugs. *In vitro* interactions between barbiturates, benzodiazepines, and GABA receptors are consistent with physiologic observations that some of the actions of all of these drugs converge at the level of the GABA receptor–ionophore complex in mammalian brain. The GABA receptors, although sometimes coupled to barbiturate receptors, are considered to be distinct both in characteristics and in distribution in the brain. Furthermore considerable numbers of barbiturate receptors coupled to benzodiazepine receptors, but not to GABA receptors, exist in some brain regions, especially cerebellum. Research is underway in an attempt to identify and isolate natural endogenous ligands for the barbiturate receptor, as well as the benzodiazepine receptor. Modulation of the postsynaptic GABA receptor–chloride ionophore complex appears to mediate many of the sedative, anxiolytic, anticonvulsant, and muscle relaxant actions of sedative-hypnotics and benzodiazepines. The fact that biochemical investigations have demonstrated the presence of two specific receptor sites, one for the barbiturates and one for the benzodiazepines, and then coupled to the GABA-receptor–ionophore, certainly provides information on the molecular mechanism of action of these abusable substances.

In the section that follows, attention first is devoted to the actions of the drugs at a cellular level, and then their effects on the CNS and other organ systems are considered.

## F. PHARMACOLOGIC PROPERTIES

The barbiturates are readily absorbed when taken by mouth, are widely distributed in fats and penetrate into the CNS and the fetus, and are metabolized in the liver and excreted in the urine.[29] The interrelationships of these factors determine the delay in onset, the potency, and the duration of action, and are affected by liver or kidney disease, obesity, dependency, the stability or vitality of the patient, and the dosage. The major action of these drugs is the same: depression of the CNS, which causes sedation and hypnosis.

At first, the barbiturates produce relaxation, lassitude, and a reduction in tension. However, once dependent, the user tends to become slovenly. Rapid shifts of mood, usually associated with irritability, are manifested. Judgment and the ability to concentrate are strikingly impaired, for both intellectual and motor functions. A chronic user of barbiturates develops slurred, incoherent speech, tremors, and a staggering gait.

**TABLE 9-3**

**Effects of Barbiturates on Drug Activity**

| *Drug or Drug Class* | *Altered Drug Effect* | *Cause* |
|---|---|---|
| Phenothiazines | Decreased tranquilizer effect | Enzyme induction |
| Tricyclic antidepressants | Decreased antidepressant effect | Enzyme induction |
| Anticoagulants | Decreased anticoagulant effect | Enzume induction |
| Corticosteroids | Decreased steroid effect | Enzyme induction |
| Quinidine | Decreased quinidine effect | Enzyme induction |
| Tetracyclines | Decreased antibiotic effect | Enzyme induction |
| Phenytoin | Decreased anticonvulsant effect | Enzyme induction |
| Digitoxin | Decreased cardiac effect | Enzyme induction |
| Alcohol | Decreased sedative effect during chronic alcohol intake | Enzyme induction |
| Alcohol | Increased CNS depression during acute alcohol intoxication | Reciprocal, potentiation, or additive action |

(From Cohen, S. *The Substance Abuse Problems.* New York: Haworth Press, 1981, p. 123. With permission.)

## G. EFFECTS OF BARBITURATES ON ORGAN SYSTEMS[29]

Since the barbiturates affect most organ systems, only a brief description is presented here to familiarize the reader with a broad idea of their actions.

The primary action of the barbiturates is on nervous tissue. The consequences of this primary action are manifested as (1) hypnosis and anesthesia, (2) anticonvulsant effects, and (3) miscellaneous effects such as analgesia, autonomic nervous system actions, and respiratory effects. A summarization of these effects is discussed in the following and illustrated in Table 9-4.

### 1. General Brain Effects

The central nervous system consists of all the nerve cell bodies and fibers, called neurones, that compose the brain and spinal cord. The human brain alone contains approximately 12 billion neurones and the number of possible interconnections is so vast and complex that the physiology, biochemistry, pathology, and consequently the pharmacology, of the CNS are not completely understood.

The CNS depressants affect the central nervous system in such a manner as to inhibit or impair the transmission of neurologic signals. As a result, these drugs act to "depress" a wide range of physiologic and cellular functions in many vital organ systems. The action of CNS depressants should be distinguished from the psychologic state of "depression," which is a mood characterized by feelings of hopelessness, worthlessness, inferiority, and guilt.

While individual drugs differ in their potency and maximal effects, the CNS depressants produce effects along a continuum that defines deeper levels of unconsciousness:

Antianxiety ➧ Sedation ➧ Hypnosis ➧ Anesthesia ➧ Coma ➧ Death

where

*Sedation* = state of decreased responsiveness to stimuli without producing sleep

*Hypnosis* = altered state of consciousness, sometimes resembling sleep

*Anesthesia* = state of loss of sensation

*Coma* = state of consciousness from which the patient cannot be aroused, even by powerful stimulation

The barbiturates produce either sedation or hypnosis, depending on the dosage levels—hence the term *sedative-hypnotic*.

### 2. Effects on Sleep and Dreaming

The barbiturates, although they are used for the induction of sleep, decrease the amount of sleep time spent in dreaming. A certain amount of evidence suggests that humans have to dream at least three to six times each night to be psychologically healthy during their waking hours.

According to Ray,[30] "When an individual who has been using barbiturates regularly as a sleeping pill suddenly stops using them, he may overdream or even have nightmares."

**TABLE 9-4**

**Effects of Barbiturates on Organ Systems**

| *Organ System* | *Typical Action* | *Direction and Comments* |
|---|---|---|
| CNS | Neuronal activity (sedative-hypnosis) | Depression |
| | Sleep | Induce |
| | Dreaming | Reduce |
| | Respiration | Depress |
| Cardiovascular | Blood pressure | Slightly reduce |
| Gastrointestinal tract | Gastrointestinal upset | Secondary to depression, and slight |
| Kidney | Urine function | Depress only following anesthetic doses |
| Liver | Liver damage (jaundice) | Induce |
| | Drug-metabolizing enzymes | Induce |
| Body temperature | —hypothermia | Large doses depress |

### 3. Respiration

Barbiturates are potent respiratory depressants.

### 4. Heart and Circulatory Effects

The cardiovascular system is not significantly affected by the administration of normal oral sedative or hypnotic doses. Because of their sedative effect, they may induce a slight decrease in blood pressure. However, these drugs do not have specific blood-pressure-lowering properties.

### 5. Gastrointestinal and Urogenital System

In humans, the barbiturates, when used properly for their sedative action, have no significant direct effect on the gastrointestinal tract. However, the distressing gastrointestinal symptoms reported for barbiturates probably are secondary to depression of the CNS. In the doses required to produce deep anesthesia, the barbiturates suppress urine function. In the dose levels commonly employed, however, there is no evidence that the barbiturates have any direct action on the kidneys. The effects of barbiturates on sexual function and dysfunction are clearly described in Chapter 20 of this book.

### 6. Hepatic Actions

Jaundice may occur with doses large enough to produce acute intoxication. Additional liver damage may be produced if there is preexisting liver disease. It is important to note that barbiturates play a definite role in altering the metabolism of other drugs, such as alcohol.

### 7. Body Temperature

Body temperature after normal sedative doses is not significantly altered; however, larger doses greatly decrease body temperature.

**TABLE 9-5**

**Classification of Barbiturates by Duration of Pharmacologic Effects**

| *Ultrashort Acting ¼ to 3 Hours* | *Short Acting, 3 to 6 Hours* | *Intermediate Acting, 6 to 12 Hours* | *Long Acting, 12 to 24 Hours* |
|---|---|---|---|
| Thiopental (Pentothal) | Amobarbital (Amytal) | Butabarbital (Butisol) | Phenobarbital* (Luminal) |
| | Pentobarbital (Nembutal) | | |
| | Secobarbital (Seconal) | | |

**Primary Medical Uses**

A. Ultrashort acting
   1. Anesthetic induction
B. Short acting
   1. Hypnotic
   2. Sedative (preoperative)
   3. Injected for rapid seizure control
C. Intermediate acting
   1. Daytime sedative
D. Long acting
   1. Control of epilepsy
   2. Daytime sedative
   3. Treatment of sedative-hypnotic withdrawal

* Most commonly used as the generic product.

From Smith, D.E., and Wesson, D. Diagnosis and treatment of adverse reactions to sedative-hypnotics. DHEW Publication No. (ADM), 75-144, 1974.

## H. DURATION OF ACTION

In general, the duration of action of the barbiturates depends upon the compound employed, dose, route, and the state of the individual taking the drug. However, in hypnotic doses, the long-acting barbiturates such as phenobarbital last from 12 to 24 hours. The short-acting barbiturates, such as secobarbital, produce a CNS depression of three to eight hours' duration.[31]

Table 9-5 gives the generic and trade names of the most widely medically prescribed barbiturates in the United States, divided according to their pharmacologic duration of action.

## I. ROUTE OF ADMINISTRATION AND DOSAGE

In humans, the barbiturates can be administered orally, rectally, intravenously, or intramuscularly. The barbiturates are well absorbed from the entire gastrointestinal tract. Dosages usually range from 60 to 100 mg several times a day. Illicit users take up to several thousand milligrams daily. Since tolerance develops, the dependent user may take from 20 to 60 tablets or capsules a day.[2]

## J. NEUROHORMONAL EFFECTS

Studies in experimental animals have demonstrated that barbiturates alter the brain concentrations of several chemical substances that may function as hormones or nerve impulse transmitters. In the rat, anesthetic doses almost double the normal concentration of acetylcholine, and sedative doses produce a smaller but definite effect.[27] The subnormal release of brain acetylcholine could be responsible for the central nervous system's induced depression. The barbiturates also have a marked action on the brain norepinephrine. Work in rats has indicated that doses that are sedative completely prevent the stress-induced release of norepinephrine in the brain stem. Other substances considered as possible neurotransmitters in the CNS, such as serotonin and γ-aminobutyric acid (GABA), are not significantly affected by barbiturates, even at high doses. The barbiturates also affect the liberation of the pituitary hormones, such as inhibiting the release of corticotropin and stimulating the release of the antidiuretic hormone.[23]

## K. Variables that Affect Action

In earlier chapters we discussed the various factors such as psychological set and sociological setting which could influence the behavioral effects of psychomimetic drugs. Here we specifically will point out important factors which will either enhance or attenuate the pharmacological actions of the barbiturates.

Factors which could interfere with the metabolism of excretion of barbiturates have been discussed earlier.

Generally, it is known that when barbiturates are taken at the same time with stimulants, the latter drug class will tend to oppose the action of the former class of drugs. Unlike the antidotal action as seen with nalorphine and morphine, the stimulant and barbiturate antagonism is not as specific and is much weaker in observed antagonism, especially in severe prolonged barbiturate anesthesia. A list of the drugs which could antagonize the action of barbiturates is as follows: 1) bemeigride (β, β-methylethylglutarimide; Megimide); 2) picrotoxin; 3) caffeine 4) strychnine 5) pentylenetetrazol.

Another important factor which could result in the shortening of barbiturate action is the status of the pH or the urine.

Alkalinization of the urine significantly enhances the excretion of phenobarbital but, because of a higher PK value, this factor probably would not influence the excretion of the short-acting and intermediate-acting sedative drugs.

## L. BARBITURATE-DRUG INTERACTION: DRUGS THAT INTENSIFY ACTION

Barbiturates are known as central nervous system depressants or "downers." The effects of stimulants or "uppers" to oppose the barbiturate actions is somewhat as expected. Today there is literature which points towards a specific brain receptor as the site of action of barbiturates. Thus, other drugs which impinge on this receptor site (Benzodiazepine-GABA complex) would be expected to intensify barbiturate actions. These psychotropics include 1) alcohol 2) phenothiazine tranquilizers 3) antianxiety drugs, and 4) reserpine.

Table 9–3 refers to a variety of drugs which could also accelerate the depressant action of barbiturates by virtue of their ability to stimulate metabolism of many drugs by enzyme induction in liver microsomes. Phenobarbital is a good example.

## M. TOXICITY

### 1. Acute Toxicity

The wide use of the barbiturates provides for their involvement in accidental intoxication and in suicide attempts. It is of interest that in the United States these drugs account for about 15 percent of all poisonings and for far more deaths than any other form of poison (solid or liquid). In Copenhagen, approximately 1100 patients are treated for barbiturate intoxication each year.

Accidental suicide with barbiturates is termed *automatism*. This is defined as a state of drug-induced confusion in which the patient forgets having taken the medication and ingests more of it. Ray[30] has stated that "after the regular sleeping dose has been taken, the individual may doze briefly and then awaken slightly sedated. In this condition, he may be confused about whether he has taken his medication and may then take a second dose or even more—sometimes a fatal amount."

Fatality in the addict by "automatism" has been the subject of great controversy since there is a very wide difference between the usual hypnotic dose and toxic doses of barbiturates. However, the concept provides a convenient mechanism for protecting patients and their families from the social stigma attached to suicide. Barbiturates are the single most frequently used class of drugs for suicide and account for about one fifth of all suicides.

### 2. Effects of Intoxication[23]

Intoxication with barbiturates is qualitatively similar to being drunk on alcohol and, at present, it is the short-acting barbiturates—secobarbital, pentobarbital, and amobarbital—that primarily are used to produce intoxication, and thus have the highest abuse potential.

The exact effects of barbiturate intoxication may vary from time to time, even with the same individual. The expectations of the user have a marked influence on the drug effect. The 100 mg of secobarbital taken with the expectation of sleep in a suitable sleeping environment usually will induce sleep. The same amount of secobarbital taken with the expectation of "having a good time" in a stimulating environment may produce a state of "excitement" or "disinhibition euphoria." For example, personnel of medical facilities at rock concerts report dealing with drug overdose crises precipitated by the ingestion of 300 to 400 mg or more of secobarbital in conjunction with alcohol. But it is not uncommon for individuals in such stimulating environments to ingest two capsules (200 mg) of secobarbital and achieve a state of intoxication similar to an alcohol high.

A state of disinhibition euphoria is not necessarily synonymous with intoxication. An intoxicated individual may or may not experience disinhibition euphoria. Individuals intoxicated with phenobarbital commonly have unsteady gait, slurred speech, sustained vertical and horizontal nystagmus, and poor judgment, but their subjective state frequently is reported to be unpleasant or "dysphoric." Furthermore the perception of intoxication with any drug as being pleasant is, in part, a learned response, and is influenced greatly by expectation and environment.

It is this disinhibition, euphoria-producing property that makes barbiturates and certain other sedative-hypnotics appealing as intoxicants. Smith et al.[8] estimated the ability of barbiturates and other sedative-hypnotics to produce a disinhibition europhoria state. Table 9-6 illustrates that, in most cases, disinhibition occurs at dosages above those commonly prescribed.

Barbiturate blood levels correlating with various behavioral changes can be seen in Table 9-7. There is appreciable individual variation and the intoxicating level overlaps with the common therapeutic range.

Intoxication produces a reduction in the ability to make accurate judgments and markedly impairs motor coordination. The ability of barbiturates and other sedative-hypnotics to produce intoxication is compared in Table 9-8.

There is not sufficient data that could adequately describe the exact mechanism of action for the phenomenon of barbiturate-induced intoxication. However, it is known that intoxicating effects, according to Hofmann[33], could last from four to five hours when the total daily intake an addict ingests is 2000 mg. If the drug of choice is the short-acting barbiturate (seco-

**TABLE 9-6**

**Clinical Estimates of Ability of Intoxicants to Produce Disinhibition Euphoria**

| *Generic Name* | *Common Trade Name* | *Estimated Ability to Produce Disinhibition Euphoria at an Intoxicating Dose* |
|---|---|---|
| Alcohol | Many brand names | + + + + |
| Amobarbital | Amytal | + + + + |
| Butabarbital | Butisol | + + |
| Chloral hydrate | Aquachloral Supprettes | + + |
| | Felsules | |
| | Kessodrate | |
| | Noctec | |
| | Rectules | |
| | Somnos | |
| Chlordiazepoxide hydrochloride | Libritabs | + + |
| | Librium | |
| Diazepam | Valium | + + + |
| Flurazepam hydrochloride | Dalmane | + |
| Glutethimide | Doriden | + + + |
| Meprobamate | Equanil | + + + |
| | Kello-Bamate | |
| | Meprospan | |
| | Meprotabs | |
| | Miltown | |
| | SK-Bamate | |
| Methaqualone | Optimil | + + + + |
| | Parest | |
| | Quaalude | |
| | Somnafac | |
| | Sopor | |
| Methyprylon | Noludar | + + + |
| Pentobarbital | Nembutal | + + + + |
| Phenobarbital | Eskabarb | + |
| | Luminal | |
| | Solfoton | |
| | Stental | |
| Secobarbital | Seco-8 | + + + + |
| | Seconal | |
| Secobarbital and amobarbital | Tuinal | + + + + |

Note: Table based on author's clinical estimation of propensity to produce disinhibition euphoria. ( + = small tendency to produce disinhibition euphoria to + + + = a high tendency.) Dosages required to produce inhibition are typically larger than those commonly prescribed and are usually associated with intoxication.

(From Smith, D.E., Wesson, D.R., and Seymour, R.B. The abuse of barbiturates and other sedative-hypnotics. In R.T. Dupont, A. Goldstein, and J. O'Donnell, eds., *Handbook on Drug Abuse.* Washington, D.C.: NIDA, U.S. Government Printing Office, 1979, p. 235.)

barbital), then three or four doses must be taken during the course of the day. Isbell and associates[34], evaluating the intoxicating properties of a series of barbiturates in humans, discovered that these drugs accumulate and that, as the day goes on, there is an increase in the intensity of the intoxicating state. They noted that the severity of neurologic disturbances was minimal in the morning, and became most intense in the late evening.

## 3. Termination of Action

Barbituates are inactivated and metabolized in the liver. There are three processes in the regulation of barbiturate action: 1) physical redistribution, 2) metabolic degradation, and 3) renal excretion.

Working together, these three distinct processes all reduce the overall concentration of the barbiturate at its central site of action. Redistribution is the process whereby the drug moves from the brain to other tissues.

Inactivation or metabolic degradation is the result of the mixed-function oxidases located in the endoplasmic reticulum (''microsomes'') of liver cells. Hepatic activity transforms lipid-soluble drugs into more polar derivatives (alcohol, ketone, phenol, or carboxylic acid) that can be excreted by renal mechanisms. Except for barbital, all barbiturates are excreted in the urine and feces in the metabolized changed form. The metabolites would appear in the urine in the free or glucuronide form.

**TABLE 9-7**

**Barbiturate Blood Levels with Expected Behavioral Changes in a Nontolerant Individual**

| *Barbiturate* | *Blood Barbiturate Level, in μ/ml* | *Behavioral Changes* |
|---|---|---|
| Pentobarbital | 0.5–3.0 | Therapeutic range: sedated, calm, relaxed, and easily aroused |
| | 2 | Appreciably impaired for purposes of tasks requiring alertness, unimpaired judgment, and reaction time |
| | 10–15 | Comatose |
| | 15–40 | Usual lethal levels |
| Secobarbital | 0.5–5.0 | Therapeutic range: sedated, calm, relaxed, and easily aroused |
| | 2 | Appreciably impaired for purposes of tasks requiring alertness, unimpaired judgment, and reaction time |
| | 10–15 | Comatose |
| | 15–40 | Usual lethal level |
| | 15–40 | Usual lethal level. |
| Amobarbital | 2–10 | Therapeutic range: sedated, calm, relaxed, and easily aroused |
| | 3 | Appreciably impaired for purposes of tasks requiring alertness, unimpaired judgment, and reaction time |
| | 30–40 | Comatose |
| | 40–80 | Usual lethal levels |
| Butabarbital | 3–25 | Therapeutic range: sedated, calm, relaxed, and easily aroused |
| | 5 | Appreciably impaired for purposes of tasks requiring alertness, unimpaired judgment, and reaction time |
| | 40–60 | Comatose |
| | 60–100 | Usual lethal levels |
| Phenobarbital | 5–40 | Therapeutic range: sedated, calm, relaxed, and easily aroused |
| | 10 | Appreciably impaired for purposes of tasks requiring alertness, unimpaired judgment, and reaction time |
| | 50–80 | Comatose |
| | 100–200 | Usual lethal levels |

(From Smith, D.E., and Wesson, D. Diagnosis and treatment of adverse reactions to sedative-hypnotics. DHEW Publication No. (ADM) 75-144, 1974.)

## N. OTHER DRUGS AND BARBITURATES

The interaction of barbiturates and amphetamines is well known. Illicit users of amphetamine (speed) rely on barbiturates (''downers'') to terminate the so-called ''speed run.''

Barbiturates do not mix well with alcohol. The number of accidental deaths from the combination of these two agents seems to be growing each year. According to Dr. Louria,[35] ''Although not entirely proved, the evidence suggests that even moderate doses of barbiturates, combined with a few alcoholic drinks, can cause death.'' (See Chapter 19 for greater detail.)

## O. THERAPEUTIC USES (LEGITIMATE USE)

The choice of a barbiturate for a specific application is usually determined by the duration of action that is needed. The duration of action of the barbiturates ranges from ten to 15 minutes for the intravenous type and a day or more for the long-acting oral types, such as barbital. Generally the barbiturates may be employed for almost any condition in which nonspecific depression of the CNS is desirable. These drugs control convulsion, reduce or prevent vomiting, provide sedation, produce hypnosis, lower blood pressure in anxious patients, control epilepsy, and induce sleep.

**TABLE 9-8**

**Estimated Ability to Produce Disinhibition Euphoria of Some Common Intoxicants**

| *Generic Name* | *Common Trade Name* | *Estimated Ability to Produce Disinhibition Euphoria* |
|---|---|---|
| Alcohol | Many brand names | + + + + |
| Amobarbital | Amytal | + + + + |
| Butabarbital | Butisol | + + |
| Chloral hydrate | Aquachloral Supprettes | + + |
| | Felsules | |
| | Kessodrate | |
| | Noctec | |
| | Rectules | |
| | Somnos | |
| Chlordiazepoxide hydrochloride | Libritabs | + + |
| | Librium | |
| Diazepam | Valium | + + + |
| Flurazepam hydrochloride | Dalmane | + |
| Glutehimide | Doriden | + + + |
| Meprobamate | Equanil | + + + |
| | Kello-Bamate | |
| | Meprospan | |
| | Miltown | |
| | SK-Bamate | |
| Methaqualone | Optimil | + + + + |
| | Parest | |
| | Quaalude | |
| | Somnafac | |
| | Sopor | |
| Methyprylon | Noludar | + + + |
| Pentobarbital | Nembutal | + + + + |
| Phenobarbital | Eskabarb | + |
| | Luminal | |
| | Solfoton | |
| | Stental | |
| Secobarbital | Seco-8 | + + + + |
| | Seconal | |
| Secobarbital and amobarbital | Tuinal | + + + + |

Note: Table based on a scale from + = small tendency to produce disinhibition euphoria to + + + + = high tendency in street abuse pattersn.

[From Smith, D.E., and Wesson, D. Diagnosis and treatment of adverse reactions to sedative-hypnotics. DHEW Publication No. (ADM) 75-144, 1974.]

## 1. Sleep and Sleeping Pills

Generally the major legitimate use for the sedative-hypnotics is for the disorder known as insomnia and they are prescribed in the form of sleeping pills.

The biologic rhythm of waking and sleep is a powerful one, but it can be disturbed by many factors—physical, mental, and environmental. The disorder called insomnia is a subjective condition in which the patient complains of chronic insufficient or poor sleep, along with fatigue or even drowsiness during waking hours.

Interestingly certain drugs that are prescribed for or taken by an individual cause insomnia. These drugs include amphetamines and sympathominetic agents, such as ephedrine or methylphenidate (Ritalin), which can be found in cold remedies, coffee, cola drinks, LSD, and other hallucinogens, except cannabis; and, in certain cases, the actual withdrawal from CNS depressants induces insomnia.

Sleeping pills are the treatment of choice for the short-term cure of insomnia. Cohen[36] suggests that if you understand the real cause of the insomnia, then its treatment may not always include sleeping pills. Table 9-9 outlines causes of this sleep disorder.

According to Cohen,[36]

> The casual overprescribing of barbiturate and nonbarbiturate hypnosedatives can produce a number of undesirable effects. When used rationally, these are valuable agents, but they have some built-in hazards that require a thoughtful approach to the problem of the insomniac. The barbiturates are a popular manner

**TABLE 9-9**

**The Sleep Disorders**

1. Insomnia (hyposomnia)
   1. Physiologic hyposomnia of the aged
   2. Pseudoinsomnia (sleep neurosis)
   3. Primary (idiopathic)
   4. Secondary, as a result of—
      Physical factors:
      a. Pain while lying prone or supine
      b. Itching
      c. Angina decubitus
      d. Sleep apnea
      e. Hypermetabolic states as hyperthyroidism and hypoglycemia
      f. Pregnancy
      g. Restless legs syndrome
      h. Impending delirium tremens
         Nocturia
      Situational:
      a. Discomfort due to bed, noise, heat, humidity, etc.
      b. Sleeping pill withdrawal
      c. Stimulant ingestion
      Psychologic:
      a. Depression
      b. Tension states and worry
      c. Mania
      d. Paranoid states
II. Hypersomnia (excessive sleep pattersn)
   1. Idiopathic
   2. Narcolepsy with or without cataplexy
   3. Daytime sedative or tranquilizer use
III. Dyssomnia (abnormal sleep patterns)
   1. Somnambulism
   2. Night terrors
   3. Excessive bruxism and snoring
   4. Enuresis

(From Cohen, S. *The Substance Abuse Problems.* New York: Haworth Press, 1981, p. 116. With permission.)

of attempting or achieving suicide, particularly in females. Since insomnia is often associated with depression, providing large quantities of these drugs makes self-destruction easy. Even the practice of giving no more than a week's supply is no guarantee that the determined patient will not save up sufficient supplies to acquire a lethal amount. Psychological autopsies of some suicides have revealed that they had obtained sleeping prescriptions from a number of doctors prior to their death. As little as ten 100 mg secobarbital or pentobarbital capsules might be deadly in a non-tolerant person, and even fewer are needed when they are combined with other CNS depressants. The tranquilizers have a much more favorable ratio between the effective dose and the lethal dose.

Consensus of the literature demonstrates that insomniacs on hypnotics for many months or years sleep no better than insomniacs not receiving medication. Certainly the removal of a patient from moderate or large amounts of sleeping medication should proceed gradually, by reducing a dosage unit every few days, to decrease the severity of REM rebound, which, paradoxically, will induce insomnia.

Cohen[36] further points out, in discussing sleeping pills as a common drug of abuse, that:

Hypnosedatives are the favored drugs of abuse by the aging adult. Usually, they are legally obtained, but the directions on the bottle are disregarded and larger than ordinary amounts are consumed. This happens over time as one capsule becomes ineffective, then two, then more. Eventually, very large amounts of these drugs are ingested in the pursuit of sleep and the person has become physically and psychologically dependent on his medication.

A second form of abuse is the consumption of sleeping pills as daytime sedatives. This develops in individuals with high anxiety levels. A calming effect occurs, but tolerance development soon requires additional amounts. One or two dozen sleeping capsules may be consumed every 24 hours. These people are in a precarious position: a sudden increase of a few more capsules may produce poisoning; on the other hand, a sudden drop in their daily intake may provoke the delirium tremens.

A third type of problem resides in the presence of these agents in the home. Young people have been known to explore the medicine cabinet for mind-altering substances to sample. Medically prescribed sedatives can initiate drug-taking practices, which are later continued with black market "sleepers."

## P. CHRONIC TOXICITY

In a previous section of this chapter, the pharmacology of barbiturates was described. The information that follows reviews the chronic toxicity not only of the barbiturates, but also of nonbarbiturate hypnotics and alcohol (to a lesser degree). The reader who requires greater detail concerning this matter is referred to the manual on *Diagnosis and Treatment of Adverse Reactions to Sedative-Hypnotics*.[23]

The pharmacology of nonbarbiturates follows this discussion on tolerance, effects of abuse, and treatment.

### 1. Tolerance to Barbiturates and Other CNS Depressants[3]

The CNS depressants have all been shown to be capable of producing both tolerance and, if used chronically, physical dependence. Several mechanisms are involved in the development of tolerance to these agents. The barbiturates —chloral hydrate, glutethimide, methyprylon, and meprobamate—stimulate the production of metabolic enzymes in the liver, which inactivate these drugs. Adaptation of nervous tissue to the presence of the CNS depressants also occurs. As the individual becomes experienced as to the effects produced by these drugs, a certain amount of psychologic control can be exerted. Acquired tolerance disappears almost completely after one or two weeks of abstinence.

Because of the similarity in action of these substances, one CNS depressant is often substituted for another. Thus, for example, if one develops a dependence on one CNS depressant, the physical or psychologic demands associated with the dependence may be met by using another depressant drug; that is, a cross-dependence develops. In a similar manner, if tolerance has developed to the use of a barbiturate, resistance to the effects of other CNS depressants (including alcohol) will be observed (cross-tolerance). Because of this cross-tolerance, withdrawal symptoms from dependence upon one CNS depressant may be prevented or diminished by administration of another. This property is exploited therapeutically in the management of

CNS depression or alcohol withdrawal, as well as nonmedically when supplies of the drug of preference are unavailable.

According to Smith and Wesson,[23] psychologic dependence refers to a strong *need* to experience the drug effect repeatedly, even in the absence of physical dependence. Physical dependence refers to the establishment of objective signs of withdrawal that occur after the drug is abruptly stopped. Tolerance refers to the adaptation of the body to the drug in such a manner that larger doses are required to produce the original effects. Table 9-10 compares estimates of these parameters of commonly used intoxicants. With barbiturates, tolerance of two types develops. *Drug-disposition tolerance* develops from activation of drug-metabolizing enzyme systems in the liver capable of more rapidly destroying barbiturates. *Pharmacodynamic tolerance* is caused by the adaptation of the CNS to the presence of the drug. Unlike tolerance to opiates, barbiturate tolerance does not significantly increase the lethal dose. Therefore, as the individual increases the dose to maintain the same level of intoxication, the margin between the intoxicating dose and the fatal dose becomes smaller. This is illustrated in Figure 9-2.

That a moderate amount of tolerance can be developed to the depressant actions of barbiturates is beyond doubt.[37] Tolerance to the effect of barbiturates on temperature, blood pressure, pulse, and respiratory rate, however, did not develop in human volunteers who received 0.4 gram for 90 days. Singh[38] has shown that the thyroid gland is involved in the development of tolerance to pentobarbital and thiopental.

Investigations[39,40] involving the repeated administration of therapeutic or somewhat larger doses of pentobarbital, secobarbital, or phenobarbital have shown that tolerance to the sedative and hypnotic actions is practically complete within a few weeks.

## 2. Abuse Potential and Effects of Abuse[3]

It is perhaps not surprising that the CNS depressants, which produce psychologic and physical effects nearly identical to those of alcohol, should have gained widespread acceptance and desirability as substances for nonmedical use. Some individuals are prone to overuse any drug that will lessen their worries or anxieties. The prime purpose of their drug usage is to maintain an anxiety-free state.

These individuals are generally 30 to 50 years old and are likely to be introduced to barbiturates by physicians who prescribe them as "mild tranquilizers" or "sleeping pills." Most of these individuals have no identification with youthful drug-using subcultures. However, they find that barbiturates make coping with life easier and, as tolerance to the tranquilizing and sedative effects develops, they increase their dose—often without their physician's knowledge. It is this tendency to escalate dosage against medical advice that distinguishes these individuals from those who advantageously use sedative to reduce excessive anxiety or stress. Because they may see several physicians, none of whom may be aware that the patient is abusing the barbiturate prescribed, these individuals' drug abuse may go unidentified for some time, until confusion, irritability, decreased ability to work, and episodes of acute intoxication with slurred speech and staggering gait finally draw attention to their drug usage.

**TABLE 9-10**

**Parameters of Dependence and Tolerance of Some Common Intoxicants**

| *Drug* | *Tolerance* | *Psychologic Dependence* | *Physical Dependence* |
|---|---|---|---|
| Alcohol | + | + + + | + + + |
| Barbiturates | + + | + + + | + + + |
| Heroin | + + + | + + + + | + + + + |
| Marihuana | + | + + | 0 |

Note: + = slight to + + + + = marked.
From Smith, D.E., and Wesson, D. Diagnosis and treatment of adverse reaction to sedative-hypnotics. DHEW Publication No. (ADM) 75-144, 1974.

An episodic abuse pattern is seen most commonly in teenagers and young adults. Sufficient amounts of barbiturates (100 to 200 mg) are taken orally to produce a "high" or disinhibition intoxication in much the same manner as others use alcohol. Sometimes the sedatives are combined with alcohol.

Barbiturate capsules can be dissolved in water and injected primarily for the "rush" effect—a warm, drowsy feeling experienced immediately after injection. The intravenous use is by far the most hazardous in that the user is exposed to the dangers of nonmedical needle use, as well as of an accidental overdose, resulting in respiratory arrest and death. Intravenous barbiturate users are known as "barb freaks" in the drug-abusing subculture and occupy a low status in that culture. They may become so engrossed in their drug use that they neglect basic hygiene and nutrition.

Barbiturates are used in conjunction with stimulants to "come down" after abuse of amphetamines. Heroin addicts may supplement heroin with barbiturates when the supply of heroin is low, or unknowingly inject barbiturates because a dealer "cuts" the heroin with them.[41]

The potential for abuse of the CNS depressants is quite high, especially if doses exceeding therapeutic levels are taken. The patterns of abuse, as with alcohol, are varied and may range from periodic episodes of gross intoxication (acute) in an effort to achieve a state of well-

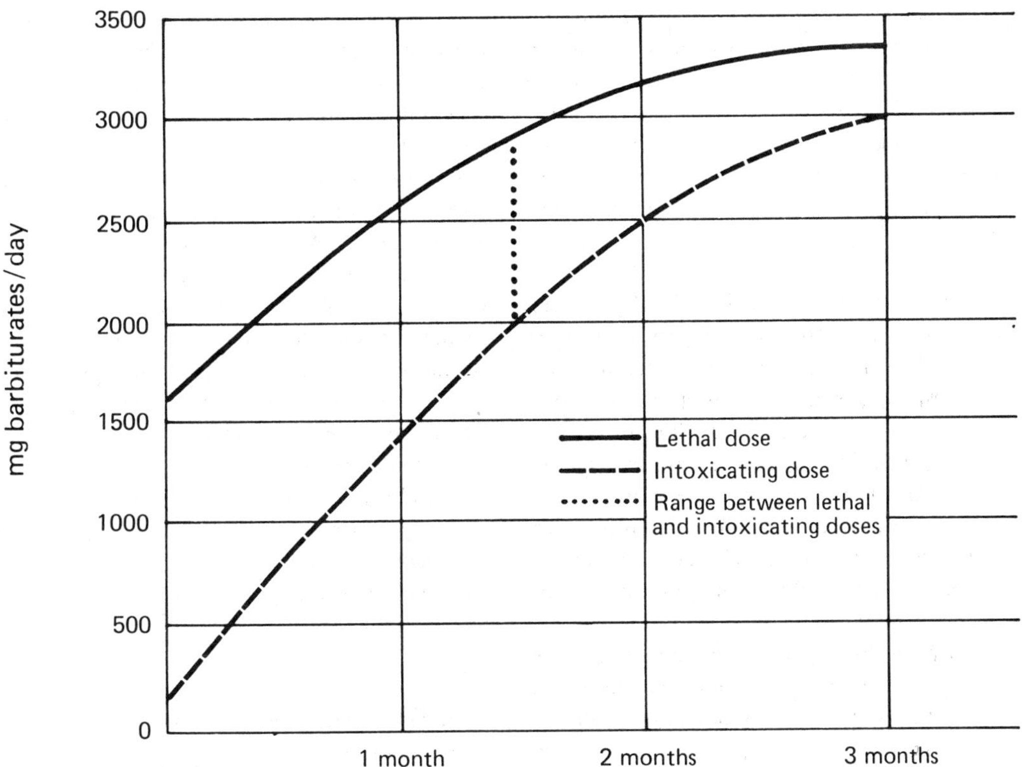


**Figure 9-2. Relative relationships between lethal and intoxicating levels of short-acting barbiturates as tolerance develops. Dosages are approximate due to individual differences in drug tolerance and use patterns. [From Smith, D.E., and Wesson, D. Diagnosis and treatment of adverse reactions to sedative-hypnotics. DHEW Publication No. (ADM) 75-144, 1974.]**

being to prolonged, compulsive, daily use (chronic). The chronic abuse of the CNS depressants is characterized by psychologic dependence and, if it is not terminated, will eventually lead to physical dependence.

As previously noted, the CNS is exquisitely sensitive to the effects of the CNS depressants at therapeutic doses and few, if any, effects are seen on other physiologic functions. At higher doses or following prolonged abuse, however, a variety of effects are manifested, the symptoms of which are detailed here.

The symptoms of acute and chronic intoxication with CNS depressants resemble those of intoxication with alcohol, and include sluggishness, difficulty in thinking, slowness of comprehension, poor memory, faulty judgment, shortened attention span, emotional instability, and exaggeration of basic personality traits. Irritability, quarrelsomeness, and moroseness are common. There may be laughing or crying without provocation, untidiness in personal habits, hostile and paranoid ideas, and suicidal tendencies. Overt signs may include slurred speech, staggering gait, nystagmus (involuntary eye movements), and tremor of the hands.

Chronic intoxication with CNS depressants results in the development of tolerance in which there is a loss of sensitivity to the general effects of the drug unless larger doses are taken. However, while tolerance may develop to the sedative and intoxicating effects, the lethal dose level appears to be unaltered. The chronic user thus is no less susceptible to fatal overdose than the neophyte drug taker. The development of tolerance is very gradual and is not as marked or as rapid as with the opiates.

Following prolonged chronic intoxication of one or more months, physical dependence may occur. The abrupt cessation or marked decrease in drug intake will result in a characteristic abstinence syndrome, termed the general depressant withdrawal syndrome. The severity of the symptoms is determined, in part, by the dose level attained before the drug use was discontinued, although the duration of use may also play a significant role. The general depressant withdrawal syndrome may initially be evidenced by a reduction in intoxication and an apparent improvement in condition, but within 24 hours, minor withdrawal phenomena are observable. These can include anxiety, apprehension, agitation, anorexia (loss of appetite), nausea, vomiting, excessive sweating, tachycardia (increased heart rate), hyperactive reflexes, insomnia, abdominal cramps, tremulousness, and muscle twitches. Orthostatic hypotension is characteristic and the individual may faint upon standing or sitting up suddenly. The symptoms usually peak during the second and third days of abstinence from the short-acting barbiturates and meprobamate; however, peak effects may not be reached until the seventh or eighth day with the long-acting barbiturates and chlordiazepoxide. It is during this peak period that the major withdrawl phenomena, if they are to develop, usually emerge. Generalized convulsions can occur marked by seizures indistinguishable from those seen in grand mal epilepsy. The number of seizures varies from a single one to status epilepticus (continuous seizures). More than half of these individuals experiencing convulsions go on to develop delirium. Mild delirium may be characterized by mounting anxiety leading to visual hallucinations. As the delirium becomes more severe, sensory clouding and disorientation result in a psychotic state identical to the delirium tremens of the alcohol withdrawal syndrome. Agitation and elevated body temperature can lead to exhaustion and cardiovascular collapse, which has resulted in death.

It should be emphasized that the full range of withdrawal effects only appears subsequent to heavy, chronic use. Regular use of ordinary therapeutic doses does not usually cause significant tolerance or physical dependence (see Figure 9-3 on page 198.)

## 3. Overdose and Emergency Treatment[3]

Nearly 5000 deaths each year are associated with barbiturates and the barbiturate overdose represents a potential major medical emergency with life-threatening implications.[42] This life-threatening emergency cannot be treated definitively by nonmedical personnel.

The majority of patients who are treated for an overdose of sedative-hypnotics are acutely intoxicated or in coma following the ingestion of a single large dose; however, they are not physically dependent. Unless the sedative-hypnotic has been used daily for more than a month in an amount equivalent to 400 to 600 mg of short-acting barbiturates, a severe withdrawal syndrome will not develop.

The lethal dose of the barbiturates and other CNS depressants cannot be ascertained with any accuracy. A general rule is that if more than ten times the full hypnotic dose of a drug is ingested at one time, severe poisoning is likely to result. Many factors, including potency, route of administration, and the biochemical composition of the individual, affect the actual dosage at which death will occur. One dangerous aspect of CNS depressant abuse is the synergistic effect these drugs possess when taken in combination with each other or with alcohol. Relatively safe amounts of CNS depressants are potentiated to produce effects far greater than expected. These combinations are often lethal.

The toxic or poisoned state induced by barbiturate overdose is characterized by coma and a general shock syndrome (e.g., weak, rapid pulse, low blood pressure, and cold, sweaty skin), and may result in death as the result of respiratory arrest, cardiovascular collapse, or kidney failure. Because the overdose of nonbarbiturate depressants presents a similar syndrome, the drug (or drugs) involved cannot be readily identified by physical examination. Friends of the victim or the presence of tablets or capsules or of empty prescription vials may provide helpful clues. Although an accurate determination may be made by various laboratory methods, the overdose crisis situation requires immediate medical attention. For this reason, it is generally advisable to treat symptoms as they appear.

The comatose individual will display a level of reflex activity correlating to the intensity of CNS depression. The pupils may be pinpointed (maximally dilated, in the case of glutethimide) but reactive to light. However, late in the course of CNS depressant poisoning, the pupils may show paralytic dilatation. Respiration may be either slow or rapid and shallow, perhaps resulting in hypoxia (lack of oxygen) and respiratory acidosis. Respiratory complications, including pulmonary edema and bronchial pneumonia, are not uncommon. The ratio of cardiovascular to respiratory depression may be higher with a nonbarbiturate sedative-hypnotic overdose.

While debate continues as to the most efficacious treatment technique for CNS depressant overdose, certain lifesaving procedures are basic to all of them. Emergency management is directed primarily toward maintenance of vital cardiopulmonary functions. The establishment of an unobstructed airway is critical, and, if respiration is depressed and oxygenation is inadequate, mechanical ventilation and administration of oxygen are initiated. To prevent death from circulatory collapse, transfusion of whole blood, plasma, or plasma expanders is begun, thereby elevating the blood pressure. Vasopressor drugs may be added to these fluids if shock symptoms persist, although it has been recommended that, in the case of barbiturate poisoning, this action need not be taken. In these cases, the volume of infusion fluid can be increased in an effort to reduce shock. Once cardiopulmonary stability is achieved, additional treatment procedures are undertaken.

If there is evidence that the drug was ingested within a period of four to 12 hours before hospital admission, gastric lavage (the emptying of stomach contents) may be attempted to prevent further drug absorption. It has been found, however, that very little drug is effectively removed. Although hemodialysis and renal dialysis are efficient methods for eliminating the presence of the drugs in the body, they are of questionable lifesaving value, except in the occurrence of renal failure. Hemodialysis is more effective in removing long-acting than short-acting compounds.

## 4. Use of Pharmacologic Agents in the Overdose Treatment of CNS Depressants

The role of various pharmacologic agents in the treatment of CNS depressant overdose is particularly controversial. Some clinicians espouse the use of stimulants or analeptics (e.g., methylphenidate, pentylenetetrazol, nikethamide, caffeine) to reverse CNS depression, or vasopressors to elevate blood pressure, or diuretics to promote urinary excretion. Others, however, contend that the presence of these substances may mask symptoms and place additional stress on an already taxed physiologic system. Current treatment practices reflect the latter point of view.

## 5. Sedative-Hypnotic Overdose in the Methadone Maintenance Client[23]

It is becoming apparent that increasing numbers of methadone maintenance clients are taking barbiturates or other sedative-hypnotics. Thus methadone programs should anticipate the growing problem of sedative-hypnotic overdose in their methadone maintenance clients.

There is no cross-tolerance between sedative-hypnotics and narcotics (including methadone), but there is with alcohol. If a sedative-hypnotic overdose is suspected in an individual who is being maintained on methadone and a reliable and accurate history (drug or drugs ingested, time and method of ingestion, existing medical complications) cannot be obtained, the recommendation is the use of a narcotic antagonist to counteract any respiratory depression that may be caused by the methadone. Smith and Wesson prefer to use naloxone (Narcan), as it is a pure narcotic antagonist with little agonist effect. This will determine whether methadone is contributing to the patient's respiratory depression. Then, if the respiratory depression continues or worsens, it is treated as for a pure sedative-hypnotic overdose. At this point, it is important to caution the attending physician about making an assumption that what is being treated is now pure sedative-hypnotic overdosage. Recent work by Blum and associates,[43] Ross,[44] and Ho and associates[45] points to the possibility that naloxone may not be so specific only for narcotics, but may block the pharmacologic actions of alcohol as well. This gains even greater importance as many methadone-maintained patients also abuse alcohol.[46] (Refer to Chapter 7.)

As a way of illustrating the treatment protocol of acute barbiturate and other sedative-hypnotic overdose, a diagram developed by Smith and Wesson[23] is presented in Figure 9-4.

## 6. Treatment of Chronic Abuse[3]

Our discussion has dealt with the essential emergency lifesaving procedures in a CNS depressant overdose. The concern in such situations centers on helping the patient through the immediate crisis brought about by overdose. Another dimension to treatment of a CNS depressant abuse involves the treatment of the chronic abuser. In cases of chronic dependence on depressants, the individual must first undergo withdrawal.

Once a patient has been diagnosed as physically dependent on CNS depressants, the most immediate concern becomes the management of withdrawal. The procedure for withdrawal is analogous to that for withdrawal from opiates. After a determination has been made as to the amount of drug the person has been taking, gradual withdrawal is begun. Pentobarbital, a short-acting barbiturate, and phenobarbital, a long-acting one, are two of the more commonly used withdrawal agents. The drug on which the patient is dependent can also be used. The process involves gradually decreasing the dosage level until the individual finally no longer needs the drug to ward off withdrawal symptoms. If withdrawal symptoms appear, further decreases in the dosage level should be halted and the dosage maintained at that level until the symptoms disappear. The withdrawal process usually requires two to three weeks.

There are clear similarities between withdrawal from barbiturates and nonbarbiturate sedative-hypnotic drugs; hence the term *general depressant withdrawal syndrome* has been used in referring to withdrawal symptoms. Withdrawal after chronic use of depressant drugs can be extremely hazardous, depending on the rate of excretion of the drug. Abrupt withdrawal can cause severe convulsions, anxiety, hallucination, disorientation, delirium, coma, and death. When the patient enters the delirium phase, even administration of large dosages of barbiturates often fails to provide immediate relief. During the delirium, the patient may experience exhaustion and cardiovascular collapse. In view of these reactions, abrupt withdrawal (or "cold turkey") from both barbiturates and nonbarbiturate depressant drugs is to be guarded against.

Because of the life-threatening complications that can arise during the withdrawal phase, it is generally agreed that close supervision is needed, preferably on an inpatient basis. But although it is easier to maintain the necessary control in a hospital setting, outpatient withdrawal is possible and probably useful in reaching people who otherwise would not receive treatment. Wesson et al.[47] describe such a program in which they used outreach workers to maintain daily contact with patients in treatment in order to achieve necessary supervision. Their clients were people who refused to submit to conventional hospitalization.

Dependence on CNS depressants, as with other forms of drug dependence, is usually a chronic relapsing disorder. Many abusers follow a pattern of withdrawal, followed by a reversion to dependence. This situation often implies some form of underlying psychopathology, a problem more difficult to resolve than physical withdrawal.

Continuing treatment of the attendant psychologic problems of the patient is essential. Individual supportive counseling is important, since a major problem is the inability of the person to cope with stressful situations. Continued contact with the patient over a prolonged period will usually be required. In some cases, there is a need for counseling or therapy for one or more members of the patient's family. In other cases, supportive therapy for the patient over a long period of time may be necessary.

Specialized treatment programs for CNS depressant abusers unfortunately are rare. Treatment is usually arranged on an individual case basis, taking into consideration the pattern of the abuse cycle and the particular needs of each patient.

## 7. Specific Treatment of Physical Dependence of the Barbiturate Type[23]

As previously stated, the majority of the barbiturate and other sedative-hypnotic overdose victims who come into an emergency room are not physically dependent upon barbiturates, primarily because drug combinations have become so popular and this class of drugs is such a favorite suicide technique. As a consequence, drug detoxification aftercare may not be the appropriate referral, but rather psychiatric evaluation and treatment to ascertain the underlying reasons for the overdose. In suicidal cases particularly, this may be the appropriate management for this patient.

The drug program that deals with barbiturates and other sedative-hypnotic drug abuses must be broad in spectrum and flexible in nature, capable of coping with a range of problems from the acute medical crisis produced by overdose to detoxification of the dependent individual. This should include appropriate aftercare techniques, when indicated, and effective psychiatric evaluation and treatment for those disturbed patients who enter into the drug scene not because of compulsive involvement with the drug itself, but because of a wide variety of underlying psychologic problems.

## 8. Strategies for Withdrawal from Sedative-Hypnotic Drugs[23]

The medical aspects of barbiturate withdrawal are described in an excellent monograph, *The Barbiturate Withdrawal Syndrome: A Clinical and Electroencephalographic Study*.[48] The barbiturate withdrawal syndrome was experimentally studied in humans by Isbell et al.[49] Hollister et al.[50] reported an experimental study of chlordiazepoxide (Librium), and in another work,[51] an experimental study of diazepam (Valium). Clinical case reports include Swartzburg et al.,[52] methaqualone; Flemenbaum and Gumby,[53] ethchlorvynol (Placidyl); and Swanson and Okada,[54] meprobamate.

The sedative withdrawal syndrome can be conceptualized as a spectrum of signs and symptoms occurring after the sedative is stopped. Symptoms do not follow a specific sequence, but can include anxiety, tremors, nightmares, insomnia, anorexia, nausea, vomiting, postural hypotension, seizures, delirium, and hyperpraxia. The syndrome is similar for all sedative-hypnotics; however, the time course depends upon the particular drug involved. With pentobarbital, secobarbital, meprobamate, and methaqualone, withdrawal symptoms may begin 12 to 24 hours after the last dose, and peak in intensity between 24 and 72 hours. The withdrawal reactions to phenobarbital, diazepam, and chlodiazepoxide develop more slowly and peak on the fifth to eighth day.

During the first one to five days of untreated sedative-hypnotic withdrawal, the electroencephalogram may show a paroxysmal burst of high-voltage, low-frequency activity, which precedes the development of seizures. The withdrawal delirium may include disorientation to time, place, and situation, as well as visual and auditory hallucinations. The delirium generally follows a period of insomnia. Some individuals may have only delirium, others may have only seizures, and some may have both delirium and convulsion.

Once a diagnosis of physical dependence on sedative-hypnotics is established, treatment for withdrawal becomes crucial. Because of the severity and even life-threatening nature of sedative-hypnotic withdrawal, close medical supervision is necessary. Withdrawal from barbiturates and other sedative-hypnotics generally should be accomplished in a hospital.

The basic principle is to withdraw the individual slowly from sedative-hypnotic drugs. Careful monitoring of signs and symptoms is of utmost importance to assure a slow, graded withdrawal. Adequate observation must be maintained to avoid the danger of seizures that may arise from too rapid a withdrawal. Treatment may be designed in accordance with either of two strategies: slow withdrawal of the addicting agent or substitution of a long-acting barbiturate and subsequent withdrawal of the substitute agent.

### *Withdrawal of the Addicting Agent*

Traditionally withdrawal from barbiturates is done with the addicting agent at dosages that produce mild toxicity. Generally, withdrawal should proceed at no greater than 100 mg of secobarbital or pentobarbital per day. Recent data from sleep research laboratories appear to indicate that even at this rate of withdrawal, rebound of dreaming intensity (suppressed with physical-dependence-producing amounts of hypnotics) is sufficient to produce sleep disturbances and withdrawal rates should be much slower.

### *Substitution Technique*

The rationale for substitution withdrawal is much the same as for substituting methadone for heroin. The longer acting agent permits a withdrawal with fewer fluctuations in blood levels throughout the day, thereby allowing for the safe utilization of smaller doses. Smith and Wesson[23] prefer to substitute phenobarbital for the short-acting barbiturates or other sedative-hypnotic drugs, and then withdraw the phenobarbital. For example, withdrawal from glutethimide, using phenobarbital, was reported by Vestal and Rumack.[55] Table 9-11 lists the equivalent of phenobarbital used to withdraw patients from the barbiturates and a variety of other sedative-hypnotics.

The safety factor for phenobarbital is greater than for the shorter acting barbiturates. Fatal amounts of phenobarbital are several times greater than toxic doses and signs of toxicity produced by phenobarbital (such as sustained nystagmus, slurred speech, and ataxia) are easy to observe.

It usually takes two days to transfer the individual from short-acting barbiturates to phenobarbital.

The dosage of phenobarbital is calculated by substituting one *sedative dose* (30 mg) of phenobarbital for each *hypnotic dose* (100 mg) of the short-acting barbiturate the patient reports using. In spite of the fact that many addicts exaggerate the magnitude of their addiction, Smith and Wesson[23] have found the patient's history to be the best guide to initiation of withdrawal. If the extent of the addiction has been grossly overstated, toxic symptoms will occur during the first day or so of treatment. This problem is easily managed by omitting one or more doses of phenobarbital and recalculating the daily dose.

Some clinicians use a pentobarbital challenge to help establish the degree of the barbiturate tolerance and dependence when they initially see the patient. With this technique, 200 mg of a short-acting barbiturate, such as pentobarbital, are injected intramuscularly and the patient is observed for toxicity to gauge the true tolerance. With the phenobarbital substitution technique, Smith and Wesson[23] have found this diagnostic test to be unnecessary in most cases.

Should signs of withdrawal occur, such as anxiety, sleep disturbances, orthostatic hypotension, hyperreflexia, muscle twitches, or stomach cramps, 200 mg of phenobarbital are given intrasmucularly and the total daily amount increased by 25 percent. If the patient shows signs of phenobarbital toxicity (sustained nystagmus, slurred speech, staggering gait), the daily dosage is divided in half and withdrawal proceeds.

The phenobarbital substitution technique may be used with short-acting sedative-hypnotics other than barbiturates. There is no reason to substitute, however, with the benzodiazepines, as their duration of action is similar to that of phenobarbital.

## Q. MIXED DRUG AND SEDATIVE-HYPNOTIC DEPENDENCE

If there is a mixed addiction, such as alcohol–barbiturate dependence, the phenobarbital schedule must be modified to reflect the alcohol–sedative cross-tolerance.[56] The phenobarbital equivalents are shown in Table 9-12. The phenobarbital equivalence to the alcohol is added to the phenobarbital equivalence for the other sedative-hypnotic in determining the total initial daily dose.

People may abuse both sedative-hypnotics and heroin concurrently in sufficient amounts to develop physical dependence on both; for example, individuals on methadone maintenance can develop sedative-hypnotic dependence.

Since withdrawal symptoms from opiates and barbiturates are similar, the clinical picture is difficult to assess if both drugs are withdrawn at the same time. Generally it is preferable to withdraw the sedative-hypnotic first while preventing opiate withdrawal by using methadone to maintain the patient. After the patient is barbiturate-free, the methadone is withdrawn gradually, using the standard detoxification technique.

It is estimated that as many as two thirds of heroin users take barbiturates because they think that barbiturates prolong the heroin high. Treatment for heroin addicts who use barbiturates generally consists of administering barbiturates

**TABLE 9-11**

**Phenobarbital Withdrawal Equivalents for Common Sedative-Hypnotics Equal to 30 mg Phenobarbital***

| *Drug* | *Daily Dosages Equivalent to 30 mg Phenobarbital in Management of Withdrawal* |
|---|---|
| Amobarbital | 100 |
| Butabarbital | 60 |
| Pentobarbital | 100 |
| Secobarbital | 100 |
| Chloral hydrate | 500 |
| Ethchlorvynol (Placidyl) | 350 |
| Glutethimide (Doriden) | 250 |
| Meprobamate (Equanil, Miltown) | 400 |
| Methaqualone (Quaalude, Sopor, etc.) | 300 |
| Methyprylon (Noludar) | 100 |
| Chlordiazepoxide (Librium) | 100 |
| Clorazepate (Tranxene) | 50 |
| Diazepam (Valium) | 50 |
| Flurazepam (Dalmane) | 30 |
| Oxazepam (Serax) | 100 |

* Withdrawal equivalence is not the same as therapeutic dose equivalency.

(From Smith, D.E., Wesson, D.R., and Seymour, R.B. The abuse of barbiturates and other sedative-hypnotics. In R.I. Dupont, A. Goldstein, and A. O'Donnell, eds., *Handbook on Drug Abuse.* Washington, D.C.: NIDA, U.S. Government Printing Office, 1979, p. 238.)

in gradually decreasing doses over a period of one to four weeks.

The following abstract concerning the abuse of barbiturates by heroin users clearly expresses the problems.[56]

The history, motivation, patterns and withdrawal attempts of dual abusers of drugs (heroin and barbiturates) were studied for purposes of effectively planning a preventive and medical care program. The population studied comprised 30 heroin addicts (16 men, 14 women) who admitted barbiturate abuse as well. The addicts reported that they used barbiturates to potentiate the action of heroin, reduce awareness of heroin withdrawal symptoms, and alleviate personality and interpersonal relationship problems. Most of the sample started abusing heroin before abusing barbiturates. Providing they could obtain sufficient heroin for their needs, only 33 percent felt they could continue to use barbiturates. The barbiturate capsule of choice was Tuinal (equal parts of amobarbital and secobarbital), which is freely available on the illicit market. Dual abusers employed the same illegal methods to obtain funds as did heroin addicts. In contrast to the heroin addict, however, the work capacity of the dual abuser was minimal. With respect to withdrawal, half of the sample had, at one time, withdrawn from barbiturates alone. Barbiturate abuse is considerably more dangerous to the addict than heroin abuse, particularly with regard to withdrawal and lethal dose.

## R. SEDATIVE-HYPNOTIC DETOXIFICATION METHODS

There are two major methods of detoxifying the barbiturate-dependent patient: (1) gradual withdrawal of the addicting agent on a short-acting barbiturate[49] and (2) the substitution of long-acting phenobarbital for the addicting agent and gradual withdrawal of the substitute drug.[57–59] Either method uses the principle of stepwise withdrawal. Abruptly discontinuing sedative-hypnotics in an individual who is physically dependent upon them is poor medical practice, and has resulted in death,[60] as well as malpractice suits.[61] A third major method advocates the use of short-acting barbiturates.[62]

## S. PHARMACOLOGIC CONSIDERATIONS OF OTHER CNS DEPRESSANTS[23]

### 1. Tranquilizers as Sedative-Hypnotics

In addition to the barbiturates, a great number of compounds that possess a wide variety of chemical and pharmacologic properties nonetheless share the ability to produce a general reversible depression of the CNS. The varying terminology applied to some of these drugs has created much confusion. Depending on the context in which they are used, they may be called "antianxiety" agents, "sedative-hypnotics," "minor tranquilizers," or "hypnotics." The term *minor tranquilizer,* although commonly applied, has contributed to the misunderstanding. Drs. Klein and Davis[62] state:

The irretrievably ingrained term "minor tranquilizer" is most unfortunate for it implies that these

**TABLE 9-12**

**Alcohol/Phenobarbital Withdrawal Equivalents**

| *Average Daily Quantity of Alcohol (80 Proof) Consumed for More than One Month* | *Phenobarbital Equivalent* |
|---|---|
| 1 ounce (30 cc) | 15 mg |
| 1 pint (480 cc) | 240 mg |
| 1 fifth (4/5 quart) (760 cc) | 380 mg |
| 1 quart (960 cc) | 480 mg |

(From Smith, D.E., Wesson, D.R., and Seymour, R.B. The abuse of barbiturates and other sedative-hypnotics. In R.I. Dupont, A. Goldstein, and J. O'Donnel, eds., *Handbook on Drug Abuse.* NIDA, U.S. Government Printing Office, Washington, D.C.: 1979, p. 239.)

agents act like major tranquilizers but to a lesser degree; one might expect large doses of the minor tranquilizers to have approximately the same clinical effects as small doses of the major tranquilizers and to be effective in the same range of clinical conditions. Actually, this is not the case: the minor tranquilizers more closely resemble sedative-hypnotic drugs such as the benzodiazepines than the major tranquilizers, such as the phenothiazines.

In general, abuse of tranquilizers is not common with young people, but is more or less restricted to middle-class, middle-aged Americans who use or abuse them alone or in combination with alcohol. A detailed discussion of antianxiety and antipsychotic drugs is presented in Chapter 13.

Tranquilizers, in the early 1950s, were defined as drugs that calm the mind without significantly disturbing the patient's normal functioning. The tranquilizers are divided into two categories. Major tranquilizers are used in the treatment of major psychiatric disorders, such as schizophrenia, and the minor tranquilizers, most commony referred to as antianxiety agents, are used in the neurotic or anxious patient and tend to be employed in the treatment of less severe mental disorders.[63]

*Major tranquilizers*
Reserpine
Chlorpromazine (Thorazine)
Trifluoperazine (Stelazine)
Promazine (Sparine)
Thioridazine (Mellaril)
Prochlorperazine (Compazine)
Haloperidol (Haldol)

*Minor tranquilizers*
Chlordiazepoxide (Librium)
Diazepam (Valium)

It is interesting to note that the major and minor tranquilizers are not usually sold on the illicit market. Much of their abuse is attributable to what is generally termed ''legal physician prescription writing abuse.''

Overdose with the minor tranquilizers is rare. However, tolerance to and dependence on them can develop. Although not very common, clinically induced dependence has occurred.[64,65] High-dose regimens on minor tranquilizers produce convulsions upon withdrawal from the drug.

The major tranquilizers are not addictive and it is very difficult to use them to commit suicide, even though a few deaths have been reported to have followed ingestion of high doses. These drugs, however, may precipitate suicidal tendencies in depressed patients. One of the most common side effects with the major tranquilizers is the development of extrapyramidal symptoms, including facial and other abnormal movements of the head and neck, to the usual symptoms reported in Parkinson's syndrome, which has been identified as ''tremor at rest, rigidity, and shuffling walk.''

The phenothiazines, prototype for the major tranquilizers, are metabolized very slowly from the body.[66] In fact, some investigators have identified the breakdown products of chlorpromazine (Thorazine) in the urine several months after termination of medication. Since the breakdown of these drugs is slow, and since people who are on this form of medication may ingest other drugs, it is possible that untoward side effects may result from drug interaction. A very common form of adverse drug interaction is between phenothiazines and alcohol. From tests involving over 4000 mice, it was found that, when given together with alcohol, Thorazine increased the sleeping time response from 1.2 to 5.0 hours.[67] Drinking alcohol and taking Thorazine or other psychotropic drugs thus may be detrimental in driving a car. Lockett and Milner[68] suggest that it is generally inadvisable to combine alcohol and Thorazine or other psychotropic drugs. Some sudden deaths (including those declared to be the result of drowning, traffic accidents, and ''natural'' or ''unknown'' causes) could be caused by the interaction of a psychotropic agent and alcohol.

## 2. Benzodiazepines[23]

A chemical class of drugs known as the benzodiazepines—chlordiazepoxide (Librium), clorazepate (Tranxene), diazepam (Valium), oxazepam (Serax)—have found wide acceptance as antianxiety compounds. Flurazepam (Dalmane), also a benzodiazepine, is marketed for the treatment of insomnia. Although cases

**TABLE 9-13**
**Some Commonly Prescribed Benzodiazepines**

| *Generic Name* | *Trade Name (Manufacturer)* | *Usual Dosage* |
|---|---|---|
| | *Used Primarily as Sedatives or Antianxiety Agents* | |
| Chlordiazepoxide | Libritabs (Roche) | |
| | Librium (Roche) | 5.0–25 mg t.i.d. |
| Clorazepate | Tranxene (Abbott) | 2.5–15 mg, t.i.d. |
| Diazepam | Valium (Roche) | 2.0–10 mg, t.i.d. |
| Oxazepam | Serax (Wyeth) | 10.0–30 mg, t.i.d. |
| | *Used Primarily as Hypnotics* | |
| Flurazepam | Dalmane (Roche) | 15–30 mg at bedtime |

From Smith, D.E., and Wesson, D. Diagnosis and treatment of adverse reactions to sedative-hypnotics. DHEW Publication No. (ADM) 75-144, 1974.

### *a. Chlordiazepoxide Hydrochloride*

| *Brand Name (Manufacturer)* | *Dosage Form (mg)* |
|---|---|
| Libritabs (Roche) | 5, 10, and 25; tablets |
| Librium (Roche) | 5, 10, and 25; capsules |
| Librium Injectable (Roche) | 100 mg/2 ml; sterile solution for parenteral administration |

### *b.Clorazepate Dipotassium*

| *Brand Name (Manufacturer)* | *Dosage Form (mg)* |
|---|---|
| Tranxene (Abbott) | 3.75, 7.5, and 15; capsules |

### *c. Diazepam*

| *Brand Name (Manufacturer)* | *Dosage Form (mg)* |
|---|---|
| Valium (Roche) | 2, 5, and 10; tablets |
| Valium Injectable (Roche) | 2 ml (5 mg/ml); ampules<br>10 ml (5 mg/ml); vials |

### *d. Flurazepam Hydrochloride*

| *Brand Name (Manufacturer)* | *Dosage Form (mg)* |
|---|---|
| Dalmane (Roche) | 15 and 30; capsules |

### *e. Oxazepam*

| *Brand Name (Manufacturer)* | *Dosage Form (mg)* |
|---|---|
| Serax (Wyeth) | 10, 25, and 30; capsules<br>15; tablets |

(From Smith, D. E., and Wesson, D. Diagnosis and treatment of adverse reaction to sedative-hypnotics. DHEW Publication No. (ADM) 75-144, 1974. With permission.)

## TABLE 9-13
## Some Commonly Prescribed Benzodiazepines (Continued)

### Other Sedative-Hypnotics

#### *a. Chloral Hydrate*

| *Brand Name (Manufacturer)* | *Dosage Form (mg)* |
|---|---|
| Aquachloral Supprettes (Webster) | 300, 600, and 900; rectal suppositories |
| Felsules (Fellows Medical) | 250, 500, and 1000; capsules |
| Kessodrate (McKesson) | 250 and 500; capsules |
| Noctec (Squibb) | 500 mg/5 cc; syrup<br>250 and 500; capsules |
| Rectules (Fellows Medical) | 500 mg/5 cc; syrup |
| Somnos (Merck Sharp and Dohme) | 650 and 1300; rectal suppositories<br>250, 500, and 1000; capsules<br>500 mg/5 cc; elixir |

#### *b. Ethchlorvynol*

| *Brand Name (Manufacturer)* | *Dosage Form (mg)* |
|---|---|
| Placidyl (Abbott) | 100, 200, 500, and 750; capsules |

#### *c. Glutethimide*

| *Brand Name (Manufacturer)* | *Dosage Form (mg)* |
|---|---|
| Doriden (USV Pharmaceutical*) | 125, 250, and 500; tablets<br>500; capsules |

* Prior to January 1972, Doriden was manufactured by Ciba.

#### *d. Meprobamate*

| *Brand Name (Manufacturer)* | *Dosage Form (mg)* |
|---|---|
| Equanil (Wyeth) | 200 and 400; tablets<br>400; capsules<br>200/5 cc; suspension |
| Kesso-Bamate Tablets (McKesson) | 200 and 400; tablets |
| Meprospan (Wallace) | 200; sustained release capsules |
| Meprospan-400 (Wallace) | 400; sustained release capsules |
| Meprotabs (Wallace) | 400; tablets |
| SK-Bamate (Smith Kline and French) | 200 and 400; tablets<br>200 and 400; tablets |

#### *e. Methyprylon*

| *Brand Name (Manufacturer)* | *Dosage Form (mg)* |
|---|---|
| Noludar (Roche) | 50 and 200; tablets |
| Noludar-300 (Roche) | 300; capsules |

(From Smith, D.E., and Wesson, D. Diagnosis and treatment of adverse reaction to sedative-hypnotics. DHEW Publication No. (ADM) 75-144, 1974. With permission.)

of abuse of these compounds do occur, their abuse potential appears to be less than that of the barbiturates, meprobamate, or hypnotics such as ethchlorvynol (Placidyl) and methyprylon (Noludar). The physical-dependence-producing dose of any of the benzodiazepines is at least five times greater than the usually prescribed therapeutic dose. These drugs also are much safer from an overdose standpoint. Deaths from overdose, when these compounds are the only drugs ingested, are exceedingly rare. Most often deaths that occur are combination overdoses involving other drugs and alcohol. Table 9-13 lists some commonly used benzodiazepines, along with the usual clinically prescribed dosage range. The upper dose listed sometimes is exceeded in severe cases.

It should be noted that drug abuse patterns in a given population vary according to myriad factors. For example, methaqualone abuse now is very much in fashion. It is important to realize that we should not neglect a thorough understanding of the (currently) more obscure sedative-hypnotics. Today's overlooked sedative-hypnotic may be tomorrow's popular drug of abuse.

### *a. Chlordiazepoxide*

Chlordiazepoxide hydrochloride also is available in combination as Librax (Roche): capsules containing 5 mg of chlordiazepoxide hydrochloride and 2.5 mg of clidinium bromide.

*Metabolism and Excretion:* Chlordiazepoxide is almost completely metabolized in the liver. It is excreted slowly in the urine, 1 to 2 percent appearing unchanged and 3 to 6 percent appearing as a conjugate. Excretion of measurable amounts continues for several days following discontinuation of the drug.

*Detection:* Following oral administration, several hours are needed for peak blood levels to be reached. The half-life of the drug is 24 hours. When the drug is discontinued, plasma levels decline slowly over a period of several days.

*Toxicity:* While patients have survived doses of from 0.2 to 2.25 grams, the lethal dose has not been established in humans.

*Overdose Management:* See Figure 9-4. Immediate gastric lavage and general supportive measures are indicated. Intravenous fluids should be administered and an adequate airway main-

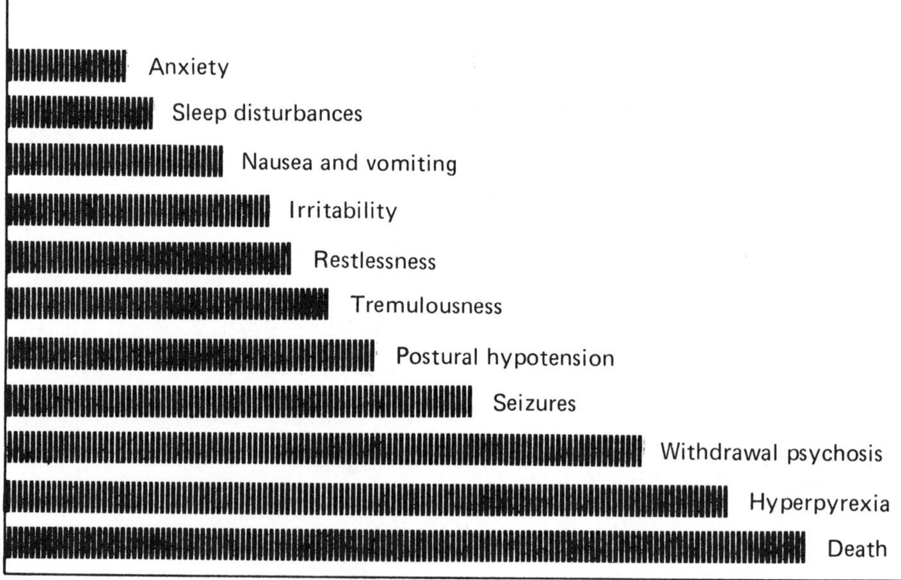


**Figure 9-3. The spectrum of barbiturate withdrawal signs and symptoms. [From Smith, D.E., and Wesson, D. Diagnosis and treatment of adverse reactions to sedative-hypnotics. DHEW Publication No. (ADM) 75-144, 1974.]**

tained. Dialysis is of limited value. If excitation occurs, barbiturates should *not* be given.

*Dependence-Producing Dose:* Ten of 11 patients who received 300 to 600 mg per day of chlordiazepoxide for 60 to 180 days experienced clear withdrawal symptoms following discontinuation of the drug.[50]

*Phenobarbital Equivalent:* Phenobarbital substitution for withdrawal generally offers no pharmacologic advantage over slow withdrawal of the addicting agent.

### *b. Clorazepate*

Clorazepate dipotassium is a member of the benzodiazepine family, marketed primarily as an antianxiety agent. Because of its recent introduction, cases of abuse have not been reported. There is no reason to believe that abuse potential for clorazepate is substantially different than for the other benzodiazepines.

*Metabolism and Excretion:* Clorazepate is completely metabolized in the liver. It is excreted primarily in the urine as the metabolites nordiazepam, oxazepam, and parahydroxy-nordiazepam. Some 4 to 5 percent of a single dose is excreted in six hours, 7 percent in 12 hours, and 14 to 15 percent in 24 hours. Approximately 80 percent is recovered in the urine and feces within ten days following ingestion.

*Detection:* Following oral administration of clorazepate, its primary metabolite, nordiazepam, quickly appears in the bloodstream, with peak levels at about one hour. Plasma half-life is approximately one day.

*Toxicity:* The lethal dose has not been established in humans. Prolonged administration of 120 mg daily in a single oral dose was without toxic effects and abrupt cessation of the drug did not produce serious signs and symptoms.

*Overdose Management:* See Figure 9-4. Immediate gastric lavage and general supportive measures are indicated. Intravenous fluids should be administered and an adequate airway maintained. Dialysis is of limited value. If excitation occurs, barbiturates should *not* be given.

*Dependence-Producing Dose:* Dependence-producing dosage in humans has not been determined. Based on a comparison with equipotent dosages of diazepam (Valium), the dosage sufficient to produce withdrawal seizures is *estimated* to be 150 to 180 mg, taken daily for one month.

*Phenobarbital Equivalent:* Phenobarbital substitution for withdrawal generally offers no pharmacologic advantage over slow withdrawal of the addicting agent.

### *c. Diazepam*

*Metabolism and Excretion:* Following a single dose, a portion is excreted rapidly and the remainder slowly in the urine.

*Detection:* Part of the drug is excreted quickly, having a half-life of from seven to ten hours. The remainder, with a half-life of from two to eight days, is excreted slowly. Seventy percent of the metabolites can be found in the urine, 10 percent as the N-demethylated derivative, 10 percent as the 3-hydroxylated compound, and 33 percent as oxazepam.

*Toxicity:* The lethal dose has not been determined in humans.

*Overdose Management:* See Figure 9-4. Immediate gastric lavage and general supportive measures are indicated. Intravenous fluids should be administered and an adequate airway maintained. Dialysis is of limited value. If excitation occurs, barbiturates should *not* be given.

*Dependence-Producing Dose:* This dosage is 80 to 120 mg daily for 42 days.

### *d. Flurazepam*

*Metabolism and Excretion:* Flurazepam is rapidly absorbed from the gastrointestinal tract and rapidly metabolized.

*Detection:* From studies in rats, it is indicated that the drug is widely distributed throughout body tissues with no excessive accumulation of drug or metabolite in any one tissue.

*Toxicity:* The lethal dose has not been determined in humans.

*Overdose Management:* See Figure 9-4. Immediate gastric lavage and general supportive measures are indicated. Intravenous fluids should be administered and an adequate airway maintained. Dialysis is of limited value. If excitation occurs, barbiturates should *not* be given.

*Dependence-Producing Dose:* Dependence-producing dosage in humans has not been determined. Based on a comparison with equipotent dosages of diazepam (Valium), the dosage sufficient to produce withdrawal seizures is estimated to be 100 to 150 mg, taken daily for one month.

*Phenobarbital Equivalent:* Phenobarbital substitution for withdrawal generally offers no pharmacologic advantage over slow withdrawal of the addicting agent.

### *e. Oxazepam*

*Metabolism and Excretion:* Oxazepam is excreted in the urine as the glucoronide conjugate.

*Detection:* After oral administration, the drug reaches peak plasma levels in four hours.

*Toxicity:* The lethal dose has not been determined in humans.

*Overdose Management:* See Figure 9-4. Immediate gastric lavage and general supportive

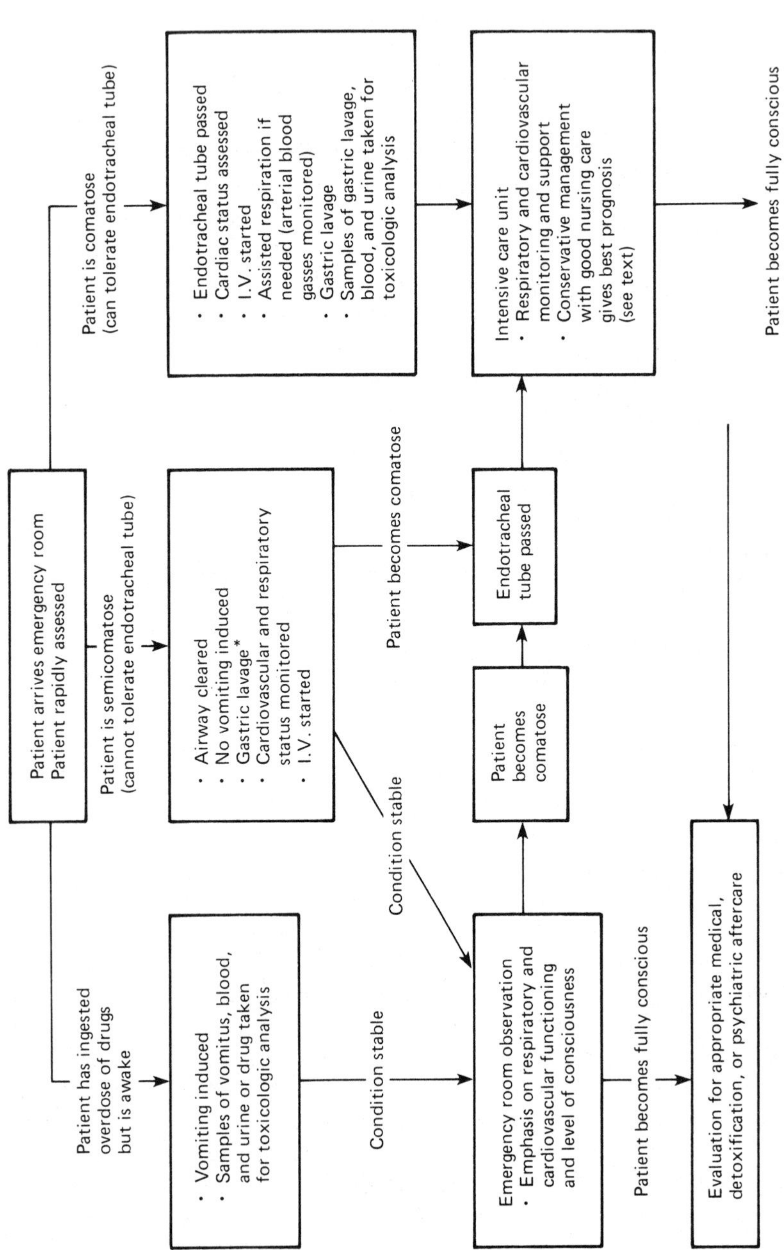


**Figure 9-4. Barbiturate and other sedative-hypnotic overdose acute treatment diagram. [Pros and cons of gastric lavage in semicomatose patients are discussed by Smith, D.E., and Wesson, D. Diagnosis and treatment of adverse reactions to sedative-hypnotics. DHEW Publication No. (ADM) 75-144, 1974, p. 32.]**

measures are indicated. Intravenous fluids should be administered and an adequate airway maintained. Dialysis is of limited value. If excitation occurs, barbiturates should *not* be given.

*Dependence-Producing Dose:* This is unknown.

*Phenobarbital Equivalent:* Phenobarbital substitution for withdrawal generally offers no pharmacologic advantage over slow withdrawal of the addicting agent.

## 3. Other Sedative-Hypnotics

### *a. Chloral Hydrate*

Chloral hydrate also is available as Beta-chlor (Mead Johnson): tablets containing 870 mg of chloral betaine (equivalent to 500 mg of chloral hydrate).

*Metabolism and Excretion:* Chloral hydrate is metabolized to trichlorethanol in the liver and other tissues, including whole blood. It does not appear in the urine as such. The fraction of the total dose that is excreted in metabolized form as trichlorethanol, urochloralic acid, and trichloracetic acid is quite variable and there may be other routes of disposal. Some fraction of urochloralic acid is concentrated and excreted in the bile.

*Detection:* The drug and its metabolites are readily diffused throughout the body. Significant amounts of chloral hydrate in the blood are not detectable following oral administration but its presence in cerebrospinal fluid, milk, amniotic fluid, and fetal blood has been reported.

*Toxicity:* The toxic oral dose of chloral hydrate for adults is approximately 10 grams, although death has been reported from as little as 4 grams and some individuals have survived after ingesting as much as 30 grams.

*Overdose Management:* See Figure 9-4. Immediate gastric lavage and general supportive measures are indicated.

*Dependence-Producing Dose:* Habitual use may result in tolerance, physical dependence, and addiction. It is reported that some addicts have taken as much as 12 grams nightly. Sudden withdrawal of the drug may result in delirium. The exact dependence-producing dosage is not known.

*Phenobarbital Equivalent:* Thirty milligrams of phenobarbital equal 250 mg of chloral hydrate.

### *b. Ethchlorvynol*

*Metabolism and Excretion:* Ethchlorvynol is completely metabolized.

*Detection:* Maximum blood levels are reached one to one and a half hours after oral ingestion. This falls rapidly and the drug is no longer detectable in the blood three hours following administration.

*Toxicity:* Patients have recovered after ingesting oral doses of from 7.5 to 60 grams. Deaths have occurred following single doses ranging from 7.0 to 49.5 grams.

*Overdose Management:* See Figure 9-4. General supportive measures and immediate gastric lavage are indicated. An adequate airway should be maintained. Peritoneal dialysis or hemodialysis may be of value. The value of analeptics is controversial and may aggravate the condition of comatose patients.

*Dependence-Producing Dose:* Dosage is 1 to 1.5 grams per day.

*Phenobarbital Equivalent:* Thirty milligrams of phenobarbital equal 200 mg of ethchlorvynol.

### *c. Glutethimide*

*Metabolism and Excretion:* Glutethimide is entirely metabolized. A large part of the metabolic products are eliminated in the bile into the intestine. Excretion of the drug or its metabolites in the urine is minimal.

*Detection:* Although glutethimide is rapidly converted in the body, its metabolites tend to be captured in the hepatic circulation. Thus excretion of these metabolites in the urine is very slow.

*Toxicity:* The lethal dose is between 10 and 20 grams. Patients have recovered after ingesting as much as 35 grams and have died after ingestion of as little as 7.75 grams.

*Overdose Management:* See Figure 9-4. Immediate gastric lavage, general supportive measures, and monitoring of vital signs are indicated. An adequate airway should be maintained. Hemodialysis is not of value. Patients tend to show fluctuations in levels of intoxication unless sufficient amounts of activated charcoal are in the intestine to inhibit reabsorption. Convulsions and muscular spasms may occur. Pupillary dilation (and occasional pupillary assymetry) occur. Paralytic ileus and atony of the bladder are common.

*Dependence-Producing Dose:* The dose sufficient to produce withdrawal convulsions is *estimated* to be 1.5 to 3 grams daily for a month (estimate based on clinical data).

*Phenobarbital Equivalent:* Thirty milligrams of phenobarbital equal 125 mg of glutethimide.

### *d. Meprobamate*

Meprobamate is also available in combination as:

Bamadex Sequels (Lederle): 300 mg meprobamate plus 15 mg dextroamphetamine sulfate, sustained-release capsules.
Deprol (Wallace): 400 mg meprobamate plus 1 mg benactyzine hydrochloride, tablets
Milpath-200 (Wallace): 200 mg meprobamate plus 25 mg tridihexethyl chloride, tablets
Milpath-400 (Wallace): 400 mg meprobamate plus 25 mg tridihexethyl chloride, tablets
Milprem-200 (Wallace): 200 mg meprobamate plus 0.45 mg conjugated estrogens, tablets
Milprem-400 (Wallace): 400 mg meprobamate plus 0.45 mg conjugated estrogens, tablets
Miltrate-10 (Wallace): 200 mg meprobamate plus 10 mg pentaerythritol tetranitrate, tablets
PMB-200 (Ayerst): 200 mg meprobamate plus 0.4 mg conjugated estrogens (equine), tablets
PMB-400 (Ayerst): 400 mg meprobamate plus 0.4 mg conjugated estrogens (equine), tablets
Pathibamate-200 (Lederle): 200 mg meprobamate plus 25 mg tridihexethyl chloride, tablets
Pathibamate-400 (Lederle): 400 mg meprobamate plus 25 mg tridahexethyl chloride, tablets

*Metabolism and Excretion:* Meprobamate is metabolized in the liver and excreted by the kidney.

*Detection:* The drug is readily absorbed from the intestinal tract and reaches a peak concentration in the blood one or two hours after ingestion. This peak declines slowly over a period of ten hours or more. Meprobamate is relatively uniformly distributed throughout the body. About 10 percent of the unchanged drug can be found in the urine within 24 hours after ingestion. Most of the remainder is excreted in the urine as an oxidated derivative, hydroxymeprobamate, and as a glucoronide. Meprobamate may be detected in body fluids by two methods: colorimetric and gas chromatography.

*Toxicity:* Death has resulted from the ingestion of as little as 12 grams. Patients have survived after ingestion of as much as 40 grams.

*Overdose Management:* See Figure 9-4. Immediate gastric lavage and general supportive measures are indicated. Diuresis, osmotic (mannitol) diuresis, peritoneal dialysis, and hemodialysis may be of value. Careful monitoring of urinary output is necessary and caution should be taken to avoid overhydration. Should severe hypotension develop, pressor amines should be used parenterally to restore blood pressure to normal levels. Relapse and death, after initial recovery, have been attributed to incomplete gastric emptying and delaying absorption.

*Dependence-Producing Dose:* A dose of 2400 to 3200 mg per day for 270 days is sufficient to produce withdrawal seizures.

*Phenobarbital Equivalent:* Thirty milligrams of phenobarbital equal 400 mg of meprobamate.

### *e. Methyprylon*

*Methyprylon* is another drug classified under the hypnotics. One hundred milligrams are as potent as 30 mg of phenobarbital. Methyprylon is almost completely metabilized and is excreted in the urine as glucoronides and as unconjugated metabolites. Three percent of oral doses of methyprylon remains unchanged in the urine. Although death has been observed from the use of 6 grams of methyprylon, some patients have survived more than 20 grams of the drug. Not only is the lethal dose still unknown but it is also unclear whether 3 grams of methyprylon are sufficient to produce a physical dependence. Overdose treatment requires a general supportive measure, immediate gastric lavage, intravenous fluids, and cleared airways. Analeptics are believed to be of little or no value and their side effects may be hazardous. Hemodialysis may be beneficial.

## 4. Methaqualone (Quaalude)

In the following, special emphasis is given to *methaqualone* because of its popularity for abuse.

Methaqualone is a synthetic organic chemical unrelated structurally to the barbiturates. Its hypnotic activity was discovered in connection with the search for antimalarials.[69] The drug, which does not seem to be better than other somnifacients (sleeping pills), has been available since 1960.

Cohen[70] points out that, in 1965, even though the abuse of methaqualone in Japan and England was known, the drug was placed in schedule V (minimal abuse potential), whereas equivalent agents such as the barbiturates were in schedule III (moderate abuse potential). Almost 15 years later, the drug was placed in schedule II (high abuse potential). In its second report, the National Commission on Marihuana and Dangerous Drugs recommended its inclusion in schedule II.

For the most part, the social cost of the nonbarbiturate sedatives is significantly lower than that of other CNS depressants. However, there is one important exception—methaqualone—which is not even classified as a controlled substance and, therefore, is subject only to a minimal level of control. The risk potential of metaqualone is roughly equivalent to that of the short-acting barbiturates. Moreover, recent evidence indicates that illicit use of this too easily obtained substance is increasingly common among adolescents and has become a significant problem in a number of locations. Since, unlike the barbiturates, methaqualone does not have large-scale medical uses, the Commission recommends that it be placed in Schedule II, along with the amphetamines.

Methaqualone is, according to Daniel Zwendling of *The Washington Post*, the hottest selling sedative-hypnotic. Evidence for his statement about the drug includes the facts that (1) one of the streets in Miami was called "Quaalude Alley" during the Presidential Convention of 1972; (2) there is enough Quaalude to "pave the streets of Columbus"; (3) quantities of the drug are supposed to have been stolen from manufacturers, truckers, and wholesalers; and (4) physicians who use it believe that it is safe, causes no hangover, and is not addicting.

Some of the information on methaqualone concerns its effect in humans. Although it has been associated with a placebo effect, methaqualone is just as potent as a pentobarbital and phenobarbital and is effective as a sleeping pill. It is used therapeutically for patients who do not respond adequately to other hypnotics. About 150 mg of methaqualone is comparable to 200 mg of cyclobarbital and 75 mg is equivalent to 30 mg of phenobarbital.[65] It appears to be inferior to chloral hydrate (500 mg) in its sleep induction and frequency of sleep disturbance. About 5 percent of methaqualone patients experience mild side effects, including headache, dizziness, drowsiness, anorexia, nausea and vomiting, dryness of the mouth, diarrhea, tachycardia, and skin rashes.[71]

Methaqualone has a rapid gastrointestinal tract absorption rate and is metabolized in the liver. There is a component breakdown before it is excreted in the bile and urine. Reabsorption in the intestines occurs before it is eliminated in the urine.

Acute and chronic toxicity from methaqualone use does occur. This is evident (particularly from the use of Mandrax, a mixture of 250 mg of methaqualone and 25 mg of diphehydramine HCL) by the convulsions, and eventually coma, that take place after the ingestion of large doses of the drug. Overdose from methaqualone is treated by immediate gastric lavage. Spontaneous vomiting is common. General supportive measures and an adequate airway should be maintained. Extreme and prolonged convulsions may call for dialysis treatment.

Lung edema has been observed, but the mortality rate from severe poisoning is unknown. Although death from the ingestion of 8 grams of methaqualone has taken place, patients have survived up to 22 grams of the drug. Physical dependence develops from the chronic use of methaqualone and the use of at least 7.5 grams daily. According to clinical studies, 2 grams of methaqualone used for one month are sufficient to produce withdrawal seizures.

Quaaludes, as they are commonly called in the streets, are often abused, especially by the young. They are usually mixed with alcohol in an effort to achieve a euphoria similar to that of a depressant drug or a "downer." Water pipes are also used to dissolve the Quaaludes so that they can be smoked in combination with marihuana. Pharmaceutical companies distribute methaqualone as Melsedine and Mandrax. It has been found as an illegally repackaged product. Methaqualone is also available in combination as Biphetamine-T 12½ (Pennwalt)—capsules containing 6.25 mg of amphetamines and dextroamphetamine plus 40 mg of methaqualone; and Biphetamine-T 20 (Pennwalt)—capsules containing 10 mg each of amphetamine and dextroamphetamine plus 40 mg of methaqualone.

Misconceptions regarding the use of methaqualone include enhanced sexual performance, safe use as a downer (since it is not a barbiturate), nonaddiction, and a safe "luding out" experience. Actually, although the drug disinhibits ego control and therefore makes it easier to permit sexual activities, it may in fact impair sexual functions. As mentioned previously, death from methaqualone has occurred from its combined use with alcohol. Its use also produces a physical dependence, tolerance, withdrawal, and a psychologic dependence. The addictive effects of "luding out" or the use of methaqualone and alcohol is indeed dangerous.

## T. OTHER CONSIDERATIONS

### 1. Neonatal Physical Dependence on Barbiturates

Individuals involved in drug abuse treatment programs encounter a wide variety of situations. While the problem of neonatal physical dependence on barbiturates cannot be explored in detail in this book, the subject deserves some mention.

It has long been known that barbiturates cross the placental barrier, thereby creating the theoretic possibility of physical dependence in the neonate. Reports of neonatal physical dependence on barbiturates have appeared in the medical literature. Because many female barbiturate abusers are of childbearing age, are often lax about practicing birth control, and may have life-styles that can lead to pregnancy, the possibility of the birth of an infant who is physically dependent upon barbiturates must be considered.

The onset of barbiturate withdrawal symptoms in the neonate may occur after the infant has left the hospital (median onset of symptoms—seven days). The functional immaturity of the liver and kidneys in the newborn may be a factor in the slow onset of withdrawal symptoms. The signs and symptoms of heroin and barbiturate withdrawal in children and adults are contrasted in Table 9-14.

*Treatment of Neonatal Barbiturate Withdrawal*[73–75]*:* As soon as the diagnosis of neonatal barbiturate withdrawal is established, treatment with phenobarbital should be started. Because of the gastrointestinal problems involved, initial therapy should be intramuscular. An initial dose of 10 to 12 mg/kg body weight is given and slowly tapered off over a period of at least one month.

## U. GLOSSARY OF DRUG TERMS RELATING TO SEDATIVE-HYPNOTICS

| | |
|---|---|
| Barb freak | Intravenous barbiturate user |
| Barbs | Barbiturates |
| Blue angels | Amytal (amobarbital) capsules |
| Bluebirds | Amytal (amobarbital) capsules |
| Blue bullets | Amytal (amobarbital) capsules |
| Blue devils | Amytal (amobarbital) capsules |
| Blue dolls | Amytal (amobarbital) capsules |
| Blue heavens | Amytal (amobarbital) capsules |

| | |
|---|---|
| Blues | Amytal (amobarbital) capsules |
| Blue tips | Amytal (amobarbital) capsules |
| Candy | Barbiturates—any drug you like |
| Chlorals | Chloral hydrate |
| Christmas trees | Dexamyl Spansule capsules (dextroamphetamine sulfate and amobarbital) |
| Cibas | Doriden (glutethimide) |
| Corals | Chloral hydrate capsules |
| Double trouble | Tuinal (sodium secobarbital and sodium amobarbital) capsules |
| Down | Barbiturates; any sedative drug; also a depressed state, sometimes related to the absence of drugs |
| Downer | c. 1919/soft drug users: same as "down" |
| Downs | Barbiturates; anyone or anything that puts you uptight |
| F-40's | Seconal Sodium (sodium secobarbital) capsules |
| Goofballs | Barbiturates |
| Goofers | Barbiturates; also Doriden (glutethimide) |
| Goofing | To be under the influence of a barbiturate; just hanging out |
| Gorilla pills | c. 1950/soft drug users: Tuinal (sodium secobarbital and sodium amobarbital) capsules |
| Hearts | Amphetamines; Dexamyl (dextroamphetamine sulfate and amobarbital) tablets |
| Idiot pills | Barbiturates |
| Jelly beans | Chloral hydrate capsules |
| Knockout drops | Chloral hydrate and alcohol |
| Luding out | Taking methaqualone in combination with alcohol |
| Mandrakes | Mandrax (methaqualone and diphenydramine) capsules |
| Mexican reds | Seconal Sodium (sodium secobarbital) capsules |
| Mickey Finn | Chloral hydrate and alcohol |
| M & M's | Seconal Sodium (sodium secobarbital) capsules |
| Nebbies | Nembutal Sodium (sodium pentobarbital) capsules |
| Peanuts | Barbiturates |
| Peter | Chloral hydrate |
| Phennies | Phenobarbital tablets |

**TABLE 9-14**

**Withdrawal Signs and Symptoms**

| | *Adult* | *Child* |
|---|---|---|
| Heroin | Anxiety<br>Runny nose<br>Dilated pupils<br>Cramps<br>Diarrhea, vomiting<br>Shaking chills<br>Profuse sweating<br>Sleep disturbances<br>Aches and pains | Irritability<br>Disturbed sleep<br>Hyperactivity<br>Tremulousness<br>Vomiting<br>Poor food intake<br>Diarrhea<br>Fever<br>High-pitched cry<br>Major seizures<br>Hyperreflexia |
| Barbiturates | Anxiety<br>Sleep disturbances<br>Irritability<br>Restlessness<br>Postural hypotension<br>Delirium<br>Major motor seizures<br>Hyperpyrexia | Restlessness<br>Disturbed sleep<br>High-pitched cry<br>Tremors<br>Hyperreflexia<br>Hyperphagia<br>Vomiting<br>Diarrhea |

(From Smith, D.E., and Wesson, D. Diagnosis and treatment of adverse reaction to sedative-hypnotics. DHEW Publication No. (ADM) 75-144, 1974. With permission.)

| | |
|---|---|
| Pillhead | Habitual user of barbiturates or amphetamines |
| Pink ladies | Barbiturates |
| Pinks | Seconal Sodium (sodium secobarbital) capsules cut with Darvon (propoxyphene hydrochloride) and strychnine |
| Quacks | Quaalude (methaqualone) tablets |
| Rainbows | Tuinal (sodium secobarbital and sodium amobarbital) capsules |
| Red bullets | Seconal Sodium (sodium secobarbital) capsules |
| Red devils | c. 1950/soft drug users: Seconal Sodium (sodium secobarbital) capsules |
| Red dolls | Seconal Sodium (sodium secobarbital) capsules |
| Red lillies | Seconal Sodium (sodium secobarbital) capsules |
| Reds | Seconal Sodium (sodium secobarbital) capsules |
| Reds and blues | Tuinal (sodium secobarbital and sodium amobarbital) capsules |
| Seccies | Seconal Sodium (sodium secobarbital) capsules |
| Seggies | Seconal Sodium (sodium secobarbital) capsules |
| Sleepers | Downers; barbiturates; CNS depressants |
| Soapers | Sopor (methaqualone) tablets |
| Softballs | Downers; barbiturates; CNS depressants |
| Sopors | Sopor (methaqualone) tablets |
| Stumblers | Downers; barbiturates; CNS depressants |
| Tootsies | Tuinal (sodium secobarbital and sodium amobarbital) capsules |
| Trees | Tuinal (sodium secobarbital and sodium amobarbital) capsules |
| Tuies | Tuinal (sodium secobarbital and sodium amobarbital) capsules |
| Wallbanger | Someone intoxicated and uncoordinated on downers (barbiturates) |
| Yellow bullets | Nembutal Sodium (sodium pentobarbital) capsules |
| Yellow dolls | Nembutal Sodium (sodium pentobarbital) capsules |
| Yellow jackets | Nembutal Sodium (sodium pentobarbital) capsules |
| Yellows | Nembutal Sodium (sodium pentobarbital) capsules |

## V. GENERAL COMMENTS

The barbiturates in the past have been primarily misused or abused by the older community, such as the overanxious housewife, the stressed businessman, the bored movie star, the "street walker." Most of them also used alcohol along with barbiturates. Some of these people died because the combination of alcohol and barbiturates brought on a fatal "down." Much of the abuse has come from legal prescription writing. However, we cannot blame all of the abuse on physicians and pharmacists. The pharmaceutical companies, large producers of the hypnotics, have been the subject of much controversy in recent years. Some believe that they overproduce these drugs, and that truck loads of barbiturates are confiscated off U.S. streets, shipped to Mexico, and brought back to the United States through the underground market. The reader should refer to the book by Silverman and Lee, *Pills, Profits and Politics*.[76]

Nevertheless abuse of hypnotic drugs exceeds heroin abuse and is potentially more dangerous than with heroin. Of greater interest is that today there is an increase of abuse in the young community. "Speed freaks" use the downers to come off of a "speed run." Some young people like to mix barbiturates or Quaaludes with wine, whiskey, or marihuana. It is also interesting that on the West Coast "red devils" contain 2.5 percent amphetamine.

Some barbiturates have dubious medical benefits and their misuse or abuse carry both public health and pharmacologic problems. Public officials have considered prohibiting their legal

**TABLE 9-15**

**Observed Rank Order Sedative-Hypnotic Abuse***

| *Type* | *Example* | *Common Name/Trade Name* | *Estimated Ability to Produce Euphoria*† |
|---|---|---|---|
| Alcohol | Ethyl alcohol | Booze, whiskey, etc. | +4 |
| Short- and intermediate-acting barbiturates | 1. Secobarbital | Seconal/reds | +4 |
| | 2. Amobarbital | Amytal/blue angels | +4 |
| | 3. Phenobarbital | Nembutal/yellow jackets | +4 |
| | 4. Equal parts 1 and 2 | Tuinal/rainbows | +4 |
| Quinazolones and azepams | 1. Methaqualone | Quaalude, sopors, Q's, etc. | +4 |
| | 2. Chlordiazeporide | Librium | +2 |
| | 3. Diazepam | Valium | +3 |
| | 4. Oxazepam | Serax | +3 |
| Propanediols and piperidinediones | 1. Meprobamate | Equanil, Miltown | +3 |
| | 2. Glutethemide | Doriden | +3 |
| | 3. Methyprylon | Noludar | +3 |
| Other alcohols | Chloral hydrate | Nortec | +2 |
| Intermediate- and long-acting barbiturates | 1. Butabarbital | Butisol | +2 |
| | 2. Phenobarbital | Luminal | +1 |

*Table prepared by Drs. Feinglass and Blum (1975).
† Scores obtained from Drs. Smith and Wesson, DHEW Publication No. (ADM) 75-144 (1974).

medical use. There are alternatives, such as the "antianxiety" agents, chloral hydrate, or other so-called safer nonbarbiturate sedative-hypnotics. Until the ideal hypnotic is discovered, however, one that has a wide safety margin, is effective, does not produce tolerance or physical dependence, and results in no hangover, educational efforts should continue to remind both physicians and lay people of the possible dangers and side effects involved.

The United States is really moving into the downer scene, and thus barbiturates and other hypnotic (downer) drugs are in. (See Table 9-15.)

## REFERENCES


1. Blum, R.H., et al. *Students and Drugs*. San Francisco: Jossey-Bass, 1969.
2. Goth, A. *Medical Pharmacology*, 7th ed. St. Louis: C.V. Mosby, 1974, p. 245.
3. *CNS Depressants, Technical Metabolism*. Papers no. 1, NIDA, DHEW Publication No. (ADM) 75, 1974.
4. Dimijiam, G.G., and Radelat, F.A. Evaluation and treatment of the suspected drug user in the emergency room. *Arch. Intern. Med.* 125:162, 1970.
5. Smith, D.E., Wesson, D., and Blum, K. Downers: CNS depressants. In K. Blum and A.H. Briggs, eds., *Introduction to Social Pharmacology* (in preparation).
6. Ray, O.S. In O.S. Ray, ed., *Drugs, Society and Human Behavior*. St. Louis: C.V. Mosby, 1972, p. 173.
7. Maynert, E.W. In J.R. DiPalma, ed., *Drills Pharmacology in Medicine*. New York: McGraw-Hill, 1971, p. 250.
8. Smith, D.E., Wesson, D.R., and Seymour, R.B. The abuse of barbiturates and other sedative-hypnotics. In R.I. Dupont, A. Goldstein, and J.O. Donnell, eds., *Handbook on Drug Abuse*. Washington, D.C.: NIDA, U.S. Government Printing Office, 1979, p. 233.
9. Wesson, D.R., and Smith, D.E. *Barbiturates: Their Use, Misuse and Abuse*. New York: Human Sciences Press, 1977.
10. Fort, J. *The Pleasure Seekers: The Drug Crisis, Youth and Society*. Indianapolis: Bobbs-Merrill, 1969, pp. 161–168, 181–182.
11. Manheimer, D.I., Mellinger, G.D., and Balter, M.B. Psychotherapeutic drug. Use among adults in California. *Calif. Med.* 109:445, 1968.
12. Chambers, C.D., Brill, L., and Inciardi, J.A. Barbiturate use, misuse and abuse. *J. Drug Issues* 2:15, 1972.
13. Mellinger, G.D. The psychotherapeutic drug scene in San Francisco. In P.H. Blachly, ed., *Drug Abuse: Data and Debate*. Springfield, Ill.: CC Thomas, 1970, pp. 226–240.
14. Wesson, D.R., and Smith, D.E. The downer hearings: A current perspective on the politics of barbiturates in America. *J. Psychedel. Drugs* 5:45, 1972.
15. Chambers, D.C., and Brill, L. The treatment of non-narcotic abusers. In L. Brill and L. Lieberman, eds., *Major Modalities in the Treatment of Drug Abuse*. New York: Behavioral Publications, 1972.
16. Jaffe, J.H. Drug addiction and drug abuse. In I.S. Goodman and A. Gilman, eds., *The Pharmacological Basis of Therapeutics*, 4th ed. New York: Macmillan, 1970, pp. 276–313.
17. Busch, J.P. Statement to the hearings before the Subcommittee to Investigate Juvenile Delinquency of the Committee on the Judiciary, U.S. Senate. U.S. Government Printing Office, Washington, D.C., 1972, pp. 581–592.
18. Simmons, H.E. Statement to the hearings before the Subcommittee to Investigate Juvenile Delinquency of the Committee on the Judiciary, U.S. Senate. U.S. Government Printing Office, Washington, D.C., 1972, pp. 363–368.
19. Zito, T. Sopors: Downs as a drug fad. Hearings before the Subcommittee to Investigate Juvenile Delinquency of the Committee on the Judiciary, U.S. Senate. U.S. Government Printing Office, Washington, D.C., 1972, pp. 1532–1533.
20. Mark, L.C. Archaic classification of barbiturates: Commentary. *Clin. Pharmacol. Ther.* 10:287, 1969.
21. Mark, L.C. Metabolism of barbiturates in man. *Clin. Pharmacol. Ther.* 4:504, 1963.
22. Lasagna, L. A study of hypnotic drugs in patients with chronic diseases: Comparative efficacy of placebo, methyprylon (Noludar), meprobamate (Miltown, Equanil), pentobarbital, phenobarbital; secobarbital. *J. Chronic Dis.* 3:122, 1956.
23. Smith, D.E., and Wesson, D. Diagnosis and treatment of adverse reactions to sedative-hypnotics. DHEW Publication No. (ADM)75–144, 1974.
24. Maynert, E.W. In J.R. DiPalma, ed., *Drills Pharmacology in Medicine*. New York: McGraw-Hill, 1971, pp. 261–264.
25. Butler, T.C. The rate of penetration of barbituric acid derivatives into the brain. *J. Pharmacol. Exp. Ther.* 100:219, 1950.

26. Waddell, W.J., and Butler, T.C. The distribution and excretion of phenobarbital. *J. Clin. Invest.* 36:1217, 1957.
27. Maynert, E.W. In J.R. DiPalma, ed., *Drills Pharmacology in Medicine.* New York: McGraw-Hill, 1971, p. 256.
28. Olsen, R.W. Drug interactions at the GABA receptor-ionophore complex. *Ann. Rev. Pharmacol. Toxicol.* 22:245, 1982.
29. Harvey, S.C. Hypnotics and sedatives: The barbiturates. In L.S. Goodman and A. Gilman, eds., *The Pharmacological Basis of Therapeutics.* New York: Macmillan, 1975, p. 124.
30. Ray, O.S. (Editor). In *Drugs, Society and Human Behavior.* St. Louis: C.V. Mosby, 1972, pp. 151–177.
31. Graham, J.D.P. *Pharmacology for Medical Students.* London: Oxford University Press, 1966, p. 38.
32. Hedner, P., and Revup, C. The effect of pentobarbital and ether anesthesia on the control of corticotropin in the pituitary glands of three animals species. *Acta Pharmacol. Toxicol.* 16:228, 1960.
33. Hofmann, F.G. Generalized depressants of the central nervous system. In *A Handbook on Drugs and Alcohol Abuse: The Biomedical Aspects.* London: Oxford University Press, 1975, pp. 95–128.
34. Isbell, H., Altschul, S., Kornetsky, C.H., et al. Chronic barbiturate intoxication. *Arch. Neurol. Psychiatr.* 64:1, 1950.
35. Louria, D. *Nightmare Drugs.* New York: Pocket Books, 1966, p. 26.
36. Cohen, S. *The Substance Abuse Problems.* New York: Haworth Press, 1981, p. 115.
37. Remmer, H. Tolerance to barbiturates by increased breakdown. In S. Steinberg, ed., *Scientific Basis of Drug Dependence.* New York: Grune & Stratton, 1969.
38. Singh, J.M. Factors affecting the development of tolerance to pentobarbital and thiopental. In S.M. Singh,, L.H. Miller, and H. Lal, eds., *Drug Addiction.* Mount Kisco, N.Y.: Futura, 1972.
39. Belleville, R.E., and Fraser, H.F. Tolerance to some effects of barbiturates. *J. Pharmacol. Exp. Therap.* 120:469, 1958.
40. Butler, T.C., Mahattee, C., and Waddell, W.J. Phenobarbital: Studies of elimination, accumulation, tolerance and dosage schedules. *Handbook Pharmacol. Exp. Therap.* III:425, 1954.
41. Hamburger, E. Barbiturate use in narcotic addicts. *JAMA* 189:366, 1964.
42. Dupont, R. *AMA News*, Dec. 12, 1977.
43. Blum, K., Wallace, J.E., Eubanks, J.D., and Schwertner, H.A. Effects of Naloxone on ethanol withdrawal, preference and narcosis. *Pharmacologist* 17:124, 1975.
44. Ross, D.H., Medina, M.A., and Cardenas, H.L. Morphine and ethanol: Selective depletion of regional brain calcium. *Science* 186:63, 1974.
45. Ho, A.K.S., Tsai, C.S., Chew, R.C.A., and Braude, M.C. Drug interaction between alcohol and narcotic agents in rats and mice. *Pharmacologist* 17:125, 1975.
46. Bihari, B. Alcoholism and methadone maintenance. *Am. J. Drug Alcohol Abuse* 1179, 1975.
47. Wesson, D.R., Gay, G.R., and Smith, D.E. Clinical political issues on barbiturate use and abuse. *Contemp. Drug Prob.* 453, 1972.
48. Wulff, M.H. The barbiturate withdrawal syndrome: A clinical and electroencephalographic study. *Electroenceph. Clin. Neurophysiol.* 14(suppl), 1959.
49. Isbell, H., et al. Chronic barbiturate intoxication: An experimental study. *Arch. Neurol. Psychiatr.* 64:1, 1950.
50. Hollister, L.E., Motzenbecker, F.P., and Degan, R.O. Withdrawal reactions from chlordiazepoxide. *Psychopharmacologia* 2:63, 1961.
51. Hollister, L.E., et al. Diazepam in newly admitted schizophrenics. *Dis. Nerv. Syst.* 24:746, 1963.
52. Swartzburg, M., Lieb, J., and Schwartz, A.H. Methaqualone withdrawal. *Arch. Gen. Psychiatr.* 29:46, 1973.
53. Flemenbaum, A., and Gumby, B. Ethchlorvynol (Placidyl) abuse and withdrawal. *Dis. Nerv. Syst.* 32:188, 1971.
54. Swanson, L.A., and Okada, T. Death after withdrawal of meprobamate. *JAMA* 184:780, 1963.
55. Vestal, R., and Rumack, B. Glutethimide dependence: Phenobarbital treatment. *Ann. Intern. Med.* 80:670, 1974.
56. Cumberlidge, M.C. *Canad. Med. Assoc. J.* 98:1045, 1968.
57. Smith, D.E., and Wesson, D.R. A new method for treatment of barbiturate dependence. *JAMA* 213:294, 1970.
58. Smith, D.E., and Wesson, D.R. A phenobarbital technique for withdrawal of barbiturate abuse. *Arch. Gen. Psychiatr.* 24:56, 1971.
59. Smith, D.E., Wesson, D.R., and Dammann, G. Treatment of the polydrug abuser. In *Proceedings of the National Drug Abuse Conference.* New York: Dekker, 1978.
60. Fraser, H.F., et al. Fatal termination of barbiturate abstinence syndrome in man. *J. Pharmacol. Exp. Ther.* 106:387, 1952.

61. American Medical Association. Failure to diagnose barbiturate intoxication. *Citation* 24:22, 1971.
62. Klein, D.F., and Davis, J.M. In *Diagnosis and Drug Treatment of Psychiatric Disorders*. Baltimore: Williams & Wilkins, 1969, p. 342.
63. Jarvik, M. Drugs used in the treatment of psychiatric disorders. In L. Goodman and A. Gilman, eds., *The Pharmacological Basis of Therapeutics*, 4th ed. New York: Macmillan, 1970, chap. 12.
64. American Medical Association. Dependence on barbiturates and other sedative drugs. *JAMA* 193:673, 1965.
65. Dimijiam, G.G. Contemporary drug abuse. In A. Goth, ed., *Medical Pharmacology*, 7th ed. St. Louis: C.V. Mosby, 1974, p. 299.
66. Maynert, E.W. In J.R. DiPalma, ed., *Drills Pharmacology in Medicine*. New York: McGraw-Hill, 1971, p. 242.
67. Milner, G. *Drugs and Driving*. Basel: S. Karger, 1971, p. 38.
68. Lockett, M.F., and Milner, G. Combining the antidepressant drugs. *Br. Med. J.* 1:921, 1965.
69. Harvey, C.S. Hypnotics and sedatives. In A.G. Gilman, L.S. Goodman, and A. Gilman, eds., *The Phenomenological Basis of Therapeutics*, 6th ed. New York: Macmillan, 1980, p. 367.
70. Cohen, S. *The Substance Abuse Problems*. New York: Haworth Press, 1981, p. 125.
71. *Physicians Desk Reference*. Oradell, N.J.: Albert B. Miller, p. 1139.
72. Cohen, S. *The Substance Abuse Problems*. New York: Haworth Press, 1981, p. 128.
73. Bleyer, W.A., and Marshall, R.E. Barbiturate withdrawal syndrome in a passively addicted infant. *JAMA* 221:185, 1972.
74. Freeman, J.M. Neonatal seizures—Diagnosis and management. *J. Pediatr.* 77:701, 1970.
75. Desmond, M.M., et al. Maternal barbiturate utilization and neonatal withdrawal symptomatology. *Pediatrics* 80:190, 1972.
76. Silverman, M., and Lee, P.R. *Pills, Profit and Politics*. Berkeley: University of California Press, 1974.

Chapter 10

# Solvent and Aerosol Inhalants ("Glue Sniffing")

## A. INTRODUCTION

Watson[1] points out that it has been many thousands of years since people first experimented with the naturally occurring substances in the environment in an attempt to relieve pain, overcome anxiety, or alter psychologic states. One technique for introducing chemicals into the body is through the inhalation of volatile substances. The efficiency of the pulmonary absorption of gases and volatile liquids has been known since prehistoric times. The large surface area of the lungs provides easy access and ensures a rapid onset of sensation. In addition to gases and volatile fluids, smoke, snuff, and nonvolatile solutions in aerosol sprays can produce systemic effects through their absorption along the airway.

Another advantage of respiratory tract absorption as compared with the gastrointestinal route is that the material is delivered directly to the target organ without passing through the liver with its detoxifying enzyme systems. Obviously effects upon the brain, for example, are more rapid and more intense than by oral administration. Many volatile substances have been exploited through the ages and no century can boast an immunity from their misuse or abuse. An example of ancient abuse is that of the Greeks at Delphi. To invoke the gift of prophecy, an old woman known as the Pythoness would be seated on a tripod placed over a vent in a rock from which carbon dioxide emanated. This induced a trancelike state during which the act of divination occurred. When the carbon dioxide vent gave out, sacred laurel leaves were scorched in a copper bowl and inhaled by the Pythoness. A sufficient concentration of carbon dioxide was achieved to reproduce the trance and the prophetic experience.[2]

Although inhalants are only abused sporadically, they still pose a problem that affects both children and adults. Like most other CNS depressants, inhalants develop a tolerance, impair judgment, distort reality perception, and in high concentration produce anesthesia and subsequent death. No physical dependence has been reported. Symptoms include exhilaration, lightheadedness, and hallucinations. Transient ataxia, slurred speech, diplopia, vomiting, coma, and even a fatal case due to aplastic anemia have been attributed to glue sniffing.[3] In this discussion, the focus will be on gases and highly volatile organic compounds, not on liquids sprayed into the nasopharynx (where droplet transport is required), or marihuana, which must be smoked before it is inhaled. The category includes the most commonly abused inhalants or household agents such as model airplane glue, plastic cements, gasoline, brake and lighter fluid, paint and lacquer thinners, varnish removers, cleaning fluids (spot remover), and nail polish remover. The chemical composition includes volatile aliphatics, and aromatic hydrocarbons, such as benzene, toluene, xylene, carbon tetrachloride, chloroform, acetone, amyl acetate, trichloroethane, naphtha, ethyl alcohol, and isopropyl alcohol. The inhalation of tetrachloride or chloroform has been reported to cause toxic damage to the liver, kidneys, and myocardium, which may result in hepatic or renal failure or cardiac arrythmias with severe hypotension, along with a mild poisoning, resulting in temporary oliguria and lasting only a few days. Hepatic or renal failure, bone marrow suppression, and encephalopathy are reported after high exposure to toluene.[4] Taken in place of gasoline, carbon tetrachloride was responsible for the near death of a drug abuser.[5]

The nonmedical abuse of inhalants is indeed unfortunate. The extreme danger of inhalant abuse is described in the ''sudden sniffing death'' syndrome.[6] After rapid inhalation of volatile hydrocarbons or fluorocarbons, the individual gets an urge to run, but immediately thereafter falls and dies. This is caused by the cardiac arrythmia burden resulting from the stress from exercise and hypercapnia. Aerosol sprays containing fluoroalkanes (once known as inert gases), toluene, and airplane glue have been shown to sensitize the hearts of mice to asphyxia-induced A-V block.[7] Fluoroalkane gases show additional asphyxia-induced sinus bradycardia, and ventricular T-wave depression.[8] Inhalation of fluorinated hydrocarbons (trichloromonofluoromethane and dichlorodifluoromethane), in the absence of hypoxia, and in closely monitored normal arterial oxygen tension, $CO_2$ tension, p-serum $CO_2$ level, and base excess, produce fatal cardiac arrythmias in dogs.[9]

The sought-after euphoria of inhalants is manifested by the use of nitrous oxide (laughing gas) or amyl nitrate. Amyl nitrate is a clear, strong-smelling liquid that produces immediate (60-second trip) light-headedness or dizziness. It reportedly heightens sexual intercourse experiences when partners inhale the amyl nitrate during climatic periods. Other names for amyl nitrate, which is neither a household nor an anesthetic agent, are ''snappers,'' ''poppers,'' and ''whiffenpoppers.'' It is made in absorbent fabric ampules called ''vaprorols'' or ''pearl,'' which are responsible for providing the absorbent surface required for rapid volatilization. In addition to the nonorganic compounds of nitrous oxide, other commonly abused inhalants include diethyl ether, cyclopropane, trichloroethylene (Trilene), and halothane (Flurothane). With regard to the toxic effects of solvent abuse, if inhalation is not interrupted, coma and death may result.[10–12] The development of a definite tolerance has been reported.[13] Physical dependence is not known to develop.

## B. HISTORY

The first inhalants to be utilized as intoxicants were anesthetic agents. Such inebriants include chloroform, ether, and nitrous oxide. These inhalants were used for their intoxicating properties even before their anesthetic properties were discovered. At Cambridge University, chloroform parties were popular until its toxicity was realized. Ether was used at Harvard and other schools. Now considered a simple oral anesthetic, it once was regarded as a means for expanding the consciousness with the power to evoke mystic or religious experience much like that of LSD. Nitrous oxide, or laughing gas, was even more popular, and became the fashionable thing to use on college campuses and at parties. For 25 cents, or less, one also could obtain nitrous oxide at country fairs and side shows. When the practice of inhaling glue and other solvents for their effects began is difficult to determine historically.

Though drug abuse via the route of alveolar absorption dates back to the nitrous oxide and ether ''jags'' commonly indulged in shortly after the discovery of the euphoric and hallucinogenic properties of these anesthetic agents, contemporary abuse of volatile substances was first recorded in the literature in 1951 in a description of gasoline sniffing by two boys.[14] In subsequent years, increasing numbers of reports have appeared of many youths, and some adults, sniffing such fluids as model cement, lighter fluid, lacquer thinner, and cleaning solutions,[15] and, more recently, the propellant gases of aerosol products.[16]

These products contain not only a conventional solvent, but also one of the freons, a chlorinated, fluorinated substituted methane or ethane derivative. In addition, of course, each has an ingredient that provides its specific commercial activity. Initially glass chillers and vegetable nonstick frying sprays were used. It seems that, at some time, almost every type of aerosol has been inhaled. A partial list would include cold weather car starters, air sanitizers, window cleaners, furniture polishes, insecticides, disinfectants, various spray medications, deodorants, hair sprays, and antiperspirants. And recently, clear lacquers and gold and bronze sprays have become increasingly popular.[17] The first published reports on the voluntary inhalation of plastic cement fumes appeared in 1960.[18] Since that time, there have been scattered reports, and in recent years, there has been what appears to be a marked increase in the sniffing of inhalants.

In the early 1960s, the problem became acute, and a number of deaths were reported. The Hobby Industry of America and other concerned industries gradually acted to remove the two most toxic solvents, benzene and carbon tetrachloride, from those commercially available products most apt to be sniffed or inadvertently inhaled in large amounts. Today few products (and none of those generally used by sniffers) contain either of these compounds. As an added safeguard, the federal government has banned the inclusion of carbon tetrachloride in any product sold to the public.

Although young people appear most likely to abuse inhalants, undoubtedly for fun-seeking purposes, adults cannot be excluded as likely abusers. Most of the concrete data indicate that most inhalant abusers are young people reported by juvenile authorities. New York reported an estimated 1173 cases of glue sniffing in 1965, and Chicago and Los Angeles found 507 and 651 reported cases respectively.[15] An exact representative figure for inhalant abuse cannot be ascertained, but evidence of its rise warrants immediate concern. As mentioned earlier, solvent intoxication is a menacing problem that has been on the increase since the early 1960s. However, the short duration of its effects and its low death rate mask the need for medical attention. No hard evidence can be provided by law enforcement sources regarding the magnitude of the problem. It appears that the United States has more of a problem with this type of drug abuse than other countries. Scandinavia reports inhalation of toluene containing lacquer thinner, and Canada reports a brief epidemic with nail polish remover.[15] No serious problem is reported by Great Britain.[19]

Efforts to control the potential widespread abuse of solvents or aerosols and glue sniffing are manifested in several ways. California, Illinois, Maryland, New Jersey, New York, and Rhode Island and 26 cities have enacted statutes in an effort to control solvent inhalation, and as a result, many cities now restrict glue sales to minors. Plastic cement is not sold without the purchase of model kits in New York City, Detroit, San Antonio, and Minneapolis. This regulation, of course, does not prevent the would-be user from buying the whole kit for the sake of the glue. With the introduction of cocktail glass chillers in 1967, another inhalant became popular and available as aerosol gas propellant. The fluorinated hydrocarbons contained in this and similar products are responsible for producing the "high" as well as the potential for death. Fortunately, the Inter-Industry Committee on Aerosol Use (Aerosol Education Bureau, 300 East 44 Street, New York, N.Y. 10017) is available to inform the public on the fatal risk of aerosol sniffing. However, legislative restriction on the sale of aerosols or the identity requirements of nonfood products still do not exist. Another means to help control solvent abuse was provided by the Testor Corporation in 1969. As the largest manufacturer of plastic cement, this corporation not only found a way to make the product safer, but also shared its innovative idea with other manufacturers of hazardous and volatile solvents. With the addition of an oil of mustard called allyl isothiocyonate, the plastic cement is now irritating (much like horseradish) to the nasal passages of the abuser who sniffs it directly, but is safe for the ordinary model builder who does not deliberately abuse it.

In the broad sense, glue sniffing also pertains to inhaling other substances that contain aromatic hydrocarbons, such as gasoline, paint thinners, lacquer thinners, cigarette lighter fluids, marking pencils, and spray paints. In many cases, the material is squeezed into paper or plastic bags, and these bags are placed over the nose and mouth. Inhalation is continued until the desired sensation is achieved, or until the solvent has evaporated. The use of these bags has led to death in at least 40 instances.

Most studies indicate that glue sniffing is primarily a teenager problem.[18] The usual age is from 9 to 16 years, with an average age of 13 years. There is a very heavy predominance of boys involved. Most studies in the past indicated that these children were in the lower socioeconomic group, had definite underlying emotional problems, and came from deprived homes. A high percentage of the families had no father, and there also was a high percentage of alcoholism in one parent. More recent evidence, however, indicates that glue sniffing is no longer confined to the lower socioeconomic bracket.

It should not be assumed that the marketed products are simple solutions of one or a small number of solvents. Prockop[20] analyzed a lacquer thinner and could identify 11 solvents. In addition, small amounts of unidentifiable impurities were found. It also cannot be presumed that any of the commercial formulations will remain constant. They change, often without notice, when improvements are made, or when some of the constituents increase in price or are in short supply.

A special group of volatile substances requires mention. Ampules of amyl nitrite (poppers or snappers) are used medically to dilate coronary arteries during an episode of angina pectoris. Apparently cerebral arteries are also dilated, rapidly producing a diffusion of blood to the brain. As the perception of time is slowed, adults have used these solvents for recreational purposes almost exclusively, to prolong and intensify the subjective effects of orgasm.

Advertisements for other products, including Toilet Water, Locker Room, Vaporole, Rush, Kick, Bullet, and Joc Aroma, have appeared in underground newspapers and magazines devoted to recreational drug use. These items contain isobutyl nitrite, isobutyl alcohol, and isopentyl nitrite. In a study of 85 cocaine snorters, it was found that 7 percent of them had used at least one of these products in 1975. Twelve months later, 19 percent were found to be inhaling these "orgasm extenders."

The use of volatile substances for purposes of intoxication appears to be worldwide. Countries that have expressed special concern include the United States, Canada, Mexico, a number of Central and South American nations, and many in Europe and Africa. Reports from Japan and Sweden have described "thinner" problems among juveniles. Even the Australian aborigines[21] and the Indians of arctic Manitoba[22] are not exempt from the practice.

## C. CLASSIFICATION AND PREPARATIONS USED

A list of the more common solvents that have been abused is given in Table 10-1.

An individual intent on abusing a drug can always find a way to reach the desired euphoric state. Evidence of this is provided by the long list of diversified solvent and aerosol products that are frequently abused. Among these products are gasoline, cleaning solutions, lighter fluids, paint and lacquer thinners, household and plastic model cements and glues, cocktail glass chillers, spray deodorants, foot powders, spot removers, furniture polish, and nonstick frying pan sprays. A "high" is the main objective for the abuser. Most of the products listed are used because of their chemical composition, which may include such substances as aliphatic hydrocarbons and gasoline, aromatic hydrocarbons, halogenated hydrocarbons, ketone, ester, alcohol, and glycerols. All of these organic compounds have the capacity to depress the CNS, and to do much more. The overall effect is similar to a general volatile anesthetic. Solvents like trichloroethylene are not only anesthetics, but also are used as industrial solvents. This gives some idea of the potential and concentration of these organic compounds. Perhaps this is why some solvents such as toluene become much more popular than other solvents. They do not seem to be as irritating or to have as unpleasant an odor as other solvents, but more important for the abuser, they vaporize quickly to produce a "good" high. Other popular products and their active chemical ingredients include plastic model cement, which usually contains toluene; lighter fluids containing naphtha; cleaning solutions and aerosol products, which contain halogenated hydrocarbons; and nail polish remover, where acetone is implicated. Aerosol may be propelled by carbon dioxide, nitrous oxide, or other relatively inert compressed gases as well as fluorocarbons. Although well-established facts concerning the hazards of abusing inhalants are available, legislative efforts are needed to provide information on containers with different types of propellant. Food and insecticide products are required by law to list their contents and the same should be required of other products whose potential damage is evident.

Table 10-2 lists the ingredients of commercial products commonly involved in volatile solvent sniffing.

## D. EXTENT OF THE PROBLEM AND PATTERNS OF USE

Cohen[23] points out that the deliberate use of industrial solvents for purposes of intoxication is a surprising leisure-time activity of the past quarter century. Inhalant abuse toxicity is unlike that encountered in industrial plants. For example, in industry the exposure is in low concentrations over a long period. In contrast, juvenile inhalant abuse is brisk, intermittent, of a remarkably high concentration of the hydrocarbons—hundreds of times the permitted maximum limits.

School surveys that do not specifically inquire into solvent abuse, do not include grade and junior high schools, and do not sample dropout populations will underreport the prevalence of solvent inhalation. These drugs are often the

**TABLE 10-1**

**A Classification of Abused Solvents**

1. Aliphatic and aromatic hydrocarbons:
   Hexane
   Naphtha
   Petroleum distillates
   Gasoline
   Benzene
   Xylene
   Toluene
2. Trichloroethylene
   1, 1, 1, trichloroethane (methylchloroform)
   Carbon tetrachloride
   Ethylene dichloride
   Methylene chloride
   Chloroform
   Halothane
   Freons:
   Trichlorofluoromethane (FC11)
   Dichlorodifluoromethane (FC114)
   Cryoflurane
   Dichlorotetrafluoromethane (FC12)
3. Aliphatic nitrites:
   Amyl nitrite
   Isobutyl nitrite
4. Ketones:
   Acetone
   Cyclohexanone
   Methyl ethyl ketone
   Methyl isobutyl ketone
   Methyl butyl ketone
   Methyl amyl ketone
5. Esters:
   Ethyl acetate
   Amyl acetate
   Butyl acetate
6. Alcohols:
   Methyl alcohol
   Isopropyl alcohol
7. Glycols:
   Methyl cellulose acetate
   Ethylene gylcol
8. Ethers
9. Gases:
   Nitrous oxide

(From Cohen, S. Inhalant abuse: An overview of the problem. In C. W. Sharp and M. L. Brehm, eds., *Review of Inhalants: Euphoria to Dysfunction.* NIDA Research Monograph No. 15. Washington, D.C.: U.S. Government Printing Office, 1977, p. 5.)

first nonmedically used psychoactive agents, sometimes antedating tobacco and alcohol. Solvent usage tends to decrease with increasing age, one of the few substances showing this pattern in adolescents. The fact that the abuse of solvents occurs at an early age, and that they may be the first of the culturally unacceptable agents to be employed, suggests that they may serve as an introduction to a career of drug dependence.

Cohen[24] further suggests that since it is young children who tend to become involved with solvent sniffing, issues regarding their physical and emotional maturation arise. According to Cohen:

> It is well known that growing tissues are more sensitive to toxic products than mature cells. Thus cellular damage can occur in pubescents at concentrations not as likely to cause impairment in older persons. It is also during these formative years that techniques of coping with life stress are learned. If, instead of dealing with the daily frustrations and problems, a youngster dissolves them in solvent fumes, then the techniques for coping with life's difficulties are never learned, and he or she may remain emotionally immature, perhaps for a lifetime.

In a 1976 survey, which attempted to discern why young people are willing to inhale concentrations 50 or 100 times greater than the maximum allowable concentration in industry, the following justifications (see also Table 10-3) were elicited.

1. Peer group influences.
2. Cost effectiveness.
3. Easy availability.
4. Convenient packaging. "You can put a supply in your pocket, and nobody can tell."
5. Mood elevation. "I like the high."
6. The course of the intoxication. "It's a quicker drunk."
7. The legal issue. "It's not illegal to buy it."
8. They don't last too long. Depending on the dose, the inebriation is over in minutes, or one can sniff all day long and stay stoned.
9. The hangover is not as bad as from alcohol. Headache seems to be the most common postintoxication complaint.

**TABLE 10-2**

**Types of Commercial Products Commonly Involved in Volatile Solvent Sniffing**

| *Brand* | *Solvent* |
|---|---|
| Glues: | |
| Black Magic adhesive | Naphtha |
| Bond's Rubber Cement | Petroleum distillates |
| Dupont "Duco" household cement | Ethyl acetate, methyl ethyl ketone |
| Dupont Plastic Cement | Toluol (toluene) |
| Testor's Plastic Cement | Toluol |
| Testor's Specific Formula Plastic Cement | Methylisobutylketone, methyl cellosolve acetate |
| Lacquer and paint removers: | |
| Baldwin's "Benzine" | Naphtha |
| Baldwin's Lacquer Thinner | Toluol |
| Bulldog Paint and Lacquer Remover | Methylene chloride, methanol |
| Bulldog Paint Brush Cleaner | Toluol, acetone, methanol |
| Red Devil Paint and Varnish Remover | Benzol, acetone, methanol |
| Nail polish removers: | |
| Cutex | Acetone |
| Revlon | Acetone |
| Cleaning fluids and spot removers: | |
| AFTA | Trichlorethylene, petroleum distillates |
| Carbona | Trichloroethylene, 1, 1, 1-trichloroethane |
| K2R | Perchloroethylene |
| Lighter fluid: | |
| Ronsonal | Naphtha |

(From Hofman, F. G. *Handbook of Drug and Alcohol Abuse.* New York: Oxford University Press, 1974, p. 132. With permission.)

Today, in the era of the '80's, with great technological advancements in mass communication and electronic media, our youth's imaginations are captive early on. It is not surprising that many of our children are highly advanced for their age. The child today wants, at a very early age, to experience everything that he or she visualizes as being the "real thing"—the real thing as seen on television or the big screen. A boy of 7 or 8, learning about drugs, sex and break-dancing, soon becomes a "high risk" child and may turn to solvent sniffing for a cheap, albeit distorted, glimpse of paradise. According to Clinger and Johnson,[15] the most volatile solvent sniffers are boys between the ages of 10 and 15. The majority of inhalers are 7 or 8 years old. In terms of solvent abuse, boys usually outnumber girls ten to one in published data. Usually in their midteens, the children consider solvent sniffing a childish way of "getting kicks."

This notion seems unusually critical. It is noteworthy that most of the very young, 7 through 13, are not usually able to get the drugs, except for alcohol, that older teenagers are using. To obtain a similar experience, the resort to substances that are cheaper and readily available to them—volatile substances. Thus the very young primarily follow the lead of their elders, and use what they can get. For some who are indeed troubled, the risk of death increases with the extent to which they abuse the chemical substances. Also, since a great deal of drug use is associated with urban poverty, such youths enter the drug-taking cycle early, and are at a higher risk for death and show a strong potential for drug use and abuse.

A young person who has used inhalants will not necessarily turn to harder drugs. Some young people will undoubtedly experience harder drugs but engaging in this type of drug abuse depends to a great extent on personal and often emotional levels. The social and physical environment of the individual will help establish reliable data. A young person growing up without proper parental and social support and exposed to the drug pusher is more likely to be caught up in drug use than the young person who has a proper upbringing, is emotionally nurtured, and is unexposed to the drug culture. The important point to recognize is that given a hint that a young person has resorted to intoxicating substances for whatever reason, immediate steps should be taken to correct the situation.

Rich man, poor man, beggar man, thief—all have had their fling at experimenting with solvent-sniffing, as with other types of drug use and abuse. Although the focus for abuse prevention has been primarily in the cities and suburbs, rural areas have also dabbled with this "casual, experimental" form of intoxication.

**TABLE 10-3**

**Preferred Substances and Stated Reason for Preference, by Site**

| *Site* | *Favored Product* | *Reason for Use, Comment* |
|---|---|---|
| New York | Plastic cement, amyl nitrite (Locker Room) | "Gives longest high." |
| Miami | Transgo transmission fluid | "Made in the area—good high." |
| Louisville | Spray paint (Toohey's Gold) | "Gives longest high—made in the area." |
| Los Angeles | Clear plastic spray paint, glue, Pam | No reason given. |
| Houston | Spray shoeshine (Texas Shoeshine), paint | Shoeshine made in area. |
| Albuquerque | Spray paint (5-Star Gold) | "Gives longest high." |
| Sandoval Pueblos | Gasoline, spray paint, spray acrylic | No reason given. |
| Denver | Clear plastic spray | "Gives longest high." |

(From NIDA Research Monograph No. 15, Sharp, C. W., and Brehm, M. L. (Editors) *Review of Inhalants: Euphoria to Dysfunction.* Washington, D.C.: U.S. Government Printing Office, 1977, p. 27.)

Solvent-sniffing assumes the same dimension of psychic significance as does occasional marihuana smoking. Unfortunately, while solvent-sniffing offers a convenient and inexpensive escape hatch from unpleasant reality, the spray of halogenated hydrocarbons also threatens the user with a considerable risk to life (see below).

Juvenile chronic sniffers have been studied in depth by a number of sociologic and psychologic observers.[15,25,26] Poor academic performance and sub-par societal adjustments are common to most of the subjects studied, although solvent abuse is not thought to be a factor of inadequate intellectual capacity. Truancy and delinquency, as well as dysfunctional family lives, were also common hallmarks of the backgrounds of these subjects. Parental absenteeism in addition to alcoholism was not infrequent with one or both parents.

Certainly the price that some inhalant abusers pay in the form of physical and psychologic impairment is well documented. We should not be overcritical about this group of abusers, however. The costs to the medical and social services and to the criminal justice system are visible, but they are not excessively high at present. On a cautionary note, those in the immediate vicinity of solvent-intoxicated persons may be at risk because of their unpredictably bizarre, impulse-ridden behavior.

## E. SOCIAL COSTS AND TRENDS

Cannabis, tobacco, alcohol, and the sedative-hypnotics are more widely abused. There is a compelling interest in society to be concerned about the abuse of solvent inhalants and aerosols. The youthfulness of the population involved is a matter of apprehension, both in their added vulnerability to toxic chemicals and in their future tendencies to be overinvolved in recreational drug-using practices.

The morbidity and mortality from acute cardiac arrest, asphyxiation, accidents, and organ failures are sufficiently numerous to cause concern. Particularly disquieting are the preliminary findings by Berry et al.[27] that indicate a wide range of neuropsychologic impairments in a group of chronic solvent abusers. If these dysfunctions were established in further studies, it could have serious implications regarding the treatability of such individuals and their capacity to acquire the information and values that would enable them to be productive citizens.

Cohen,[24] in discussing trends, makes three salient points:

1. Consistent with the increased involvement of females with all drugs of abuse, the male–female ratio for solvents is decreasing. There are greater numbers of users in the 21- to 30-year-old age group than previously reported.
2. In the past few years, aerosols have become more popular as intoxicating agents, and these carry hazards beyond those accruing to the solvent itself. Among them are the inhalation of additional toxic ingredients (copper, insecticide, oil) and the cardiac arrhythmic properties of the propellant freons.
3. In connection with gasoline, another development might also have a favorable impact. Now that it has become more expensive, more locks are seen on gasoline tanks. If locking gasoline tanks becomes fairly universal, a reduction in this form of sniffing should occur.

Watson[1] proposes that most children and young people never will experiment, at any time, in any circumstances, with substances containing solvents. Furthermore those who do will regard it more as a passing phase, rather than as long-term abuse that could lead to damage or death.

## F. METHODS OF ADMINISTRATION

Inhalation of solvents or aerosols or glue sniffing, besides having toxic effects, can also lead to death by suffocation. Using paper or plastic bags is a common technique for inhaling intoxicating substances. Because the plastic is nonporous, and the seal between the mouth and bag is tight, little ambient air enters the respiratory tract. A partial vacuum may result, leading to hypoxia and a stuporous state where the abuser cannot remove the plastic bag from the face. Suffocation by plastic is the leading cause of death among volatile-solvent sniffers, where toxic effects of halogenated hydrocarbons in some aerosol propellant and cleaning solutions produce cardiac arrest.

The manner in which an inhalant is administered depends largely upon the kind of inhalant being abused—whether a semiliquid material such as glues or cements, or a liquid solvent such as gasoline, or an aerosol propellant gas. Most glues and cements are inhaled by placing from a third of a tube to five tubes of the glue into the bottom of the paper bag, then using either the mouth or nose, or both, to inhale the substance. A gauze or cotton cloth may be saturated with the liquid solvent to achieve the desired euphoria. The saturated cloth may then be held in the hands and placed over the mouth and nose, or placed into a bag and inhaled. Beer or wine may be consumed to prolong the effect.

In aerosol inhalation, the abuser may use a bag or a balloon to reach a "high." Some even spray the aerosol directly into the mouth without prefiltering, although most aerosol sniffers separate the propellant from the other contents. This can be done in several ways. Inverting the gas can will allow the gas to evacuate separately. To prefilter the gas, one allows it to pass through a washcloth or rag, or the aerosol can be sprayed into the sides of the bag so that only the gaseous contents are inhaled.

To intensify the "high," the abuser will increase the solvent concentration or engage in techniques that prolong the euphoric state. Increasing the solvent concentration may be done by warming the solvent in the hands or over a radiator or hot plate. This may result in vapor concentration 50 times the maximum allowed industrial concentration (which for toluene is 200 parts per million). Up to 3.6 mg of toluene has been recovered from 100 ml of air from such a glue-containing bag. Sometimes the sniffer will continue to inhale the toxic substance until unconciousness is reached. Unconsciousness helps to avoid respiratory depression, hypoxia, and death.

Certain characteristics are observed in the inhalant abuser. Most will tend to seek isolated areas where the obvious odor of solvents is undetected. Either alone or in groups of three to ten persons, usually of the same sex, the abusers may use abandoned buildings, roof tops, basements, school lavoratories, or locker rooms as a place in which to get high. There may also be rags, handkerchiefs, balloons, or plastic and paper bags containing dried films of solvent-containing products. In the case of the beginning glue sniffer, a white powdery ring may be visable around the mouth or breath odor may be noticed. Northern cities are found to have fewer glue sniffers, and this may be due to the cold climate, which is both physically uncomfortable and is not as conducive to solvent evaporation.

## G. PHYSICAL AND CHEMICAL PROPERTIES OF VOLATILE SOLVENTS

The volatile solvents are often used in combinations that vary from region to region and from manufacturer to manufacturer. Couri[28] tabulated occurrences and properties of commonly available compounds. Most of these compounds are liquids at room temperature and inhaled toxicity is dependent upon their physical properties. A selected group of mixtures of commonly available compounds is presented in Table 10-4 according to chemical class.

Table 10-5 includes physical and chemical properties of various volatile agents. These data may be utilized in this manner to determine the relative toxicity of absorption that would occur from humans exposed to these vapors.

## H. ABSORPTION, METABOLISM, AND EXCRETION

All the inhalants are rapidly absorbed in the lungs and have a rapid onset of action. These substances are metabolized in the liver and excreted in the urine combined with other substances or excreted unchanged by the lungs and kidneys. The absorption of these compounds through alveolar membranes and into tissues is enhanced by their organic solubility and decreased, in general, by their water solubility.

## TABLE 10-4
## Occurrences of Volatile Substances

| *Compounds* | *Antifreeze* | *Gasoline* | *Paint Thinner* | *Degreasers* | *Windshield Washers* | *Adhesives and Rubber Cement* | *Model Cements* | *Aerosol Sprays* | *Spray Shoe Polish* | *Room Odorants* | *Foam Dispensers* |
|---|---|---|---|---|---|---|---|---|---|---|---|
| Alcohols | | | | | | | | | | | |
| Methanol | X | | X | | X | | | | | | |
| Ethanol | | | X | | | | X | X | | | |
| Isopropanol | X | | X | X | | | X | X | X | | |
| Esters | | | | | | | | | | | |
| Ethyl acetate | | | X | | | | | | | | |
| n-Propyl acetate | | | X | | | | | | | | |
| n-Butyl acetate | | | | X | | | | | | | |
| Ketones | | | | | | | X | | | | |
| Acetone | | | X | | | | | | | | |
| Methyl ethyl ketone | | | X | X | | | | | | | |
| Methyl butyl ketone | | | X | | | | | | | | |
| Aromatic hydrocarbons | | | | | | X | | | | | |
| Benzene | | X | | X | | X | X | X | X | | |
| Toluene | | X | X | X | | X | X | X | | | |
| Xylene | | X | X | X | | X | X | | | | |
| Styrene | | | | | | X | | | | | |
| Naphthalene | | X | X | | | | | | | | |
| Aliphatic hydrocarbons | | | | | | X | X | | | | |
| n-Hexane | | X | | | | X | | | | | |
| n-Heptane | | X | X | | | | | | | | |
| Anesthetics | | | | | | | | | | | |
| Methylene chloride | | | X | X | | | | | | | |
| Trichloroethylene | | | | X | | | | | | | |
| Tetrachloroethylene | | | | X | | | | X | | | X |
| Nitrous oxide | | | | | | | | | | | |
| "Freons" | | | | | | | | | | X | |
| Aliphatic nitrite | | | | | | | | | | | |
| Isoamyl nitrite | | | | | | | | | | | |

(From Couri, D. In C. W. Sharp and M. L. Brehm, eds., *Review of Inhalants: Euphoria to Dysfunction.* NIDA Research Monograph, No. 14. Washington, D.C.: U.S. Government Printing Office, 1977, p. 100.)

## TABLE 10-5
## Properties of Volatile Solvents

| *Compound* | *Molecular Weight* | *Boiling Point °C, 760 mm Hg* | *Solubility* g/100 ml Water, 25 C* | *Vapor Pressure, mm Hg., 25 C* |
|---|---|---|---|---|
| Alcohols | | | | |
| Methanol | 32 | 65 | — | 160 |
| Ethanol | 46 | 78 | — | 50 |
| Isopropanol | 60 | 82 | — | 44 |
| Esters | | | | |
| Methyl acetate | 74 | 57 | 32.0 | 235 |
| Ethyl acetate | 88 | 77 | 8.6 | 100 |
| n-Propyl acetate | 102 | 102 | 1.9 | 35 |
| n-Butyl acetate | 116 | 125 | 1.0 | 1.5 |
| Methyl formate | 60 | 32 | 30.0 | 600 |
| Ethyl formate | 74 | 54 | 11.8 | 200 |
| Ketones | | | | |
| Acetone | 58 | 56 | — | 226 |
| Methyl ethyl ketone | 72 | 80 | 25.6 | 100 |
| Methyl propyl ketone | 86 | 86 | 5.5 | 16 |
| Methyl butyl ketone | 100 | 128 | 1.6 | 3.8 |
| Methyl Hexyl ketone | 128 | 173 | 0.1 | 1.2 |
| Di-isobutyl ketone | 142 | 142 | VSS | 2.4 |
| Methyl amyl ketone | 114 | 114 | 0.4 | 1.6 |
| Aromatic hydrocarbons | | | | |
| Benzene | 78 | 80 | VSS | 76 |
| Toluene | 92 | 111 | VSS | 36.1 |
| Xylenes | 106 | 141 | I | 10 |
| Styrene | 104 | 145 | I | 6.5 |
| Naphthalene | 128 | 211 | I | 0.1 |
| Aliphatic hydrocarbons | | | | |
| n-Pentane | 72 | 36 | I | 409 |
| n-Hexane | 86 | 68 | I | 103 |
| n-Heptane | 100 | 100 | I | 41 |
| n-Octane | 114 | 114 | I | 10.2 |
| Aliphatic nitrite | | | | |
| Isoamyl nitrite | 117 | 97-99 | I | 0.11 |
| Anesthetic agents | | | | |
| Nitrous oxide | 30 | 89 | NA | Gas |
| Chloroform | 119 | 61 | — | 200 |
| Diethyl ether | 74 | 35 | — | 439 |
| Halothane | 197 | 50 | — | 240 |
| Ethyl chloride | 67 | 12 | NA | Gas |
| Trichloroethylene | 131 | 87 | — | 77 |

*All compounds listed in this table are miscible at all proportions in organic solvents.
— = Miscible at all proportions.
VSS = Very slightly soluble.
I = Insoluble.
NA = Not applicable.
(From Couri, D. In C. W. Sharp and M. L. Brehm, eds., *Review of Inhalants: Euphoria to Dysfunction.* NIDA Research Monograph, No. 15. Washington, D.C.: U.S. Government Printing Office, 1977, p. 101.)

# I. PHARMACOLOGY AND TOXICOLOGY

## 1. Toxic Products Involved

The primary toxic agents of inhalant solvents are toluene, acetone, and aliphatic acetates. The toxic products involved in solvent sniffing are listed in Table 10-2.

As far as plastic cements are concerned, toluene is the toxic ingredient. There is a fairly large volume of evidence obtained from animal studies and industrial poisonings on the effects of toluene and similar compounds.[29,30] It is difficult, however, to compare these because of the different way in which the materials are used. That is, in industrial toxicology, animals or humans are exposed to relatively low concentrations of the agents over long periods of time. In glue sniffing, the patients are exposed to high concentrations over very short periods of time. It is best to start with what is known about glue sniffing and then add some details about what is known of the toxic ingredients.

## 2. General Toxicity and Deaths

The toxicity of inhalants varies greatly with the specific substance. The causes of fatalities are not clear; most seem to involve cardiac arrhythmias. Many coroners and forensic toxicologists, however, do not believe that there is a major physiologic hazard related to inhalant use, yet these same individuals admit that they do not carefully evaluate whether inhalants may be the potential cause in some deaths.

Sharp and Brehm[31] point out that unless a can, rag, or other evidence is found nearby, the examiner may not suspect solvent overdose. It has also been observed that unless alveolar air is appropriately sampled, the level of the more insoluble substances (such as freons) may be undetected. Appropriate evaluation of the incidence of this hazard, especially in communities where the prevalence of use is high, would assist greatly in defining the extent of deaths related to inhalant use. Records would need to be examined thoroughly to evaluate whether some deaths listed as "cause unknown" might be attributable to inhalants. Even then it might be very difficult to obtain this information, even if the examiners are aware of the difficulties and are prepared ahead of time to obtain the needed data, because some people do not want to identify the deceased as an inhalant abuser.

Although many clinics are set up to analyze for many drugs of abuse, few are equipped to measure solvents, especially mixtures. Therefore validation by the type of inhalant used is unlikely and the data must come from in-depth personal interviews. This latter method is much less reliable when the subject knows that the data will be made available to authorities. Also, even when the interviewer has the confidence of the subject, the inhalant user usually has poor recall, especially of the substance used, beyond a week or two. This may be the effect of brain damage resulting from inhalation or of a general lack of desire to know exactly what was used. Multiple-drug use also complicates the approach to the problem.

There were 15 deaths recorded in the literature through 1968 that were related, either directly or indirectly, to solvent sniffing.[8] Eight of these were apparently due to suffocation by plastic bags. Two deaths were possibly the result of intoxication from the solvent itself, and a few apparently were suicides under the influence (patients who feel they can fly and jump off buildings or who walk in the midst of traffic in the belief that they cannot be injured). In 1970, Bass reported 110 cases of sudden deaths as a result of sniffing.[32] Fifty-nine cases were due to aerosols, eight to toluene, and 43 to other products, including one to benzene, two to trichlorethane, and three to gasoline. Acute deaths may be due to heart problems. Inhalation of glue or toluene in mice can produce fatal heart block when oxygen is lacking.[33] In addition, serious abnormal heart rhythms can be produced in monkeys by their inhalation of aerosol propellants.[10]

Inhalation of volatile material from a plastic bag (a common practice) can result in hypoxia as well as an extremely high concentration of vapor. Aerosol propellants containing fluorinated hydrocarbons produce cardiac arrhythmias and ischemia increases sensitivity to fluorocarbon-induced arrhythmias as illustrated in Table 10-6 compiled by Aviado.[34]

Chlorinated solvents, such as trichloroethylene, depress myocardial contractility, and sympathetic activity is thereby increased reflexly. Ketones can produce pulmonary hypertension. Peripheral neuropathies and progressive, fatal neurologic deterioration have followed the so-called "huffing" of lacquer thinner. In 1977, Sharp and Brehm,[35] in studying inhalers of aerosol paints, found indications of long-lasting brain damage. Similar reports on brain damage have also appeared in the literature.[36]

## 3. Acute Actions

### *Central Nervous System*

Some of the effects of inhaling aerosol solvents or glue sniffing include physical and mental symptoms similar to those seen with alcohol. Inhalant intoxication involves initial stimulation, which is followed by CNS depression. The high lasts 30 to 40 minutes or up to one to two hours, depending on the amount and length of inhalation. The individual experiences a sense of euphoria, excitement, slurred speech, and ringing in the ears. On occasion, delusions and visual hallucinations, mental confusion, bizarre behavior, and blackouts may occur. Acting out impulsive actions, such as trying to fly, may have serious consequences. Patients may also experience loss of memory during acute intoxication. Some of the characteristics of inhalant intoxication include unpleasant breath odor, increased salivation, nausea, vomiting, anorexia (loss of appetite), and local irritation to the eyes and mucous membranes. There is a tolerance development. A person can start with one tube per day, then go up to five to six tubes per day to achieve the same results. Psychologically, there is a craving for glue, and the patient will often do other drugs to compensate for the loss of the euphoric feelings of glue sniffing.

Withdrawal from inhalants may lead to a delirium tremens-like syndrome that includes in-

**TABLE 10-6**

**Inhalational Toxicity of Fluorinated Hydrocarbons,* Percent**

| | *Trichlorofluoromethane ($CCl_3F$) FC 11* | *Dichlorodifluoromethane ($CCl_2F_2$) FC 12* | *Dichlorotetrafluoroethane ($CClF_2CClF_2$) FC 114* |
|---|---|---|---|
| Cardiac arrhythmia | | | |
| Dog heart sensitized to epinephrine | 0.3 | 5.0 | 5.0 |
| Monkey heart spontaneous arrhythmia | 2.5 | 10.0 | 10.0 |
| Monkey heart tachycardia | 2.5 | 10.0 | 10.0 |
| Myocardial contractility | | | |
| Monkey heart depression | 2.5 | 10.0 | 10.0 |
| Dog heart depression | 0.5 | 10.0 | 2.5 |
| Hemodynamic parameters | | | |
| Dog cardiac output reduced | 1.0 | 10.0 | 10.0 |
| Dog total systemic vascular resistance increased | 2.5 | 20.0 | 5.0 |
| Airway resistance | | | |
| Dog bronchospasm | (absent) | (absent) | 10.0 |
| Monkey bronchospasm | (absent) | 10.0 | 20.0 |
| Rat bronchospasm | 2.5 | (absent) | 15.0 |
| Mouse bronchospasm | 1.0 | 2.0 | 2.0 |

*(From Aviado, D. Toxicity of aerosol propellants, in the respiratory and circulatory systems: Proposed classification. *Toxicology* 3:321, 1975. With permission.)

creased irritability, tremors, sleeping difficulties, and hallucinations. This is not a common occurrence with glue sniffing.[37]

Some reports on glue sniffing have found reversible changes shown in electroencephalograms, and transient changes in the urine (increased protein and pus cells) that clear up after abstinence from glue sniffing. Additional information reveals that there is no certainty concerning the possibility of permanent brain damage from glue sniffing, except in cases where anoxia has occurred. No direct evidence of cerebellar degeneration caused by glue sniffing exists at this time.[38] The results of a study to test the psychologic effects on individuals who sniff glue found no difference, based on the control group, in the person's ability to maintain attention or to concentrate on problems during distraction.[39]

## 4. Chronic Effects

The potential toxicity effect on the CNS, liver, and kidneys is difficult to assess since the information and literature are based on projected studies in humans chronically exposed in industry and on experimental animals exposed to low concentrations over long periods of time. The maximum allowable concentration of toluene for industrial operations as set by the American Conference of Governmental and Industrial Hygiene is 200 parts per million. The concentration achieved by inhalation from bags has been measured, and is approximately 50 times greater than this concentration. Thus 3.6 mg of toluene can be recovered from 100 ml of air in the bag. No one seems to have studied the long-term effects of periodic exposure to these high concentrations, except in small groups of chronic glue sniffers. It must be pointed out that these are uncontrolled studies, the results of which are difficult to evaluate. It appears, however, that the following is known.

### *a. Blood Effects*

In glue sniffing, there are probably no toxic effects in the blood. One case of an aplastic anemia in a chronic glue sniffer recently was reported in the literature. Earlier reports of bone marrow toxicity as a result of glue sniffing or toluene are not valid because 15 to 20 years ago, most toluene products were contaminated by a high percentage of benzene, a compound known to produce bone marrow abnormalities.

### *b. Kidneys*

In some studies, transient protein, blood, and pus cells have been found in the urine of glue sniffers, but this is of doubtful significance. Abnormal renal function tests have not been seen.

### *c. Liver*

The results of liver studies have been variable. Some studies report no abnormalities. Others have had some increase in the size of the liver, but no abnormal function tests. Furthermore, in 17 to 30 patients studied, liver abnormalities were indicated by high-alkaline phosphatase test or by liver biopsy. The injury was minimal, but was still present three or four weeks after the last sniffing episode. Complete recovery was expected if the sniffing was stopped.

### *d. Central Nervous System*

Except for transient electroencephalographic changes, there is no good evidence that chronic brain damage occurs. One case of cerebellar degeneration was noted previously.[35,36]

### *e. Chromosomes*

One study found that there was a chromosomal abnormality rate of 6 percent in a mixed group of solvent sniffers, as compared with 2 percent in controls. This included 35 gaps, 13 breaks, and two complex chromosomes. In the control group, no breaks or complex chromosomes were found. What these chromosomal abnormalities mean in terms of future abnormalities in the patients or abnormalities in offspring is not known at present.

### 5. Exposure and Clinical Effects

Inhalant abuse describes a pattern of behavior that involves the voluntary inhalation of gases or vapors in order to achieve a modified state of consciousness. Usually the intent is to achieve a state of euphoria or high. The response induced by inhalation is dose-related and cumulative over short periods of time. The desired alteration is attained by high concentrations of gas or vapor in air within one to two minutes, whereas lower concentrations may require five to ten minutes to achieve the desired effects. Depending on the amount consumed, an "altered state" may persist for a few minutes to several hours. Generally the effects may become excessive, leading to CNS dysfunction, depression, sedation, coma, with poor control of dose, and, as previously discussed, death due to respiratory depression or major cardiac arrhythmias. Certainly, depending upon the administration technique, a hazard exists for reduction of oxygen content of inhaled air with anoxia leading to unconsciousness and death from respiratory failure. Table 10-7, as compiled by Comstock and Comstock,[40] summarizes published reports concerning the circumstances of exposure and the clinical effects.

## J. OTHER DRUGS

There is little evidence that glue sniffing itself leads to the use of other drugs.[37] Many teenagers try sniffing for kicks once or twice and never become chronic users. The chronic users appear to have a different type of emotional makeup. If glue sniffers go on to other drugs later, it is most likely that their basic underlying difficulties are responsible for the drug abuse, rather than exposure to any particular agent.

### 1. Effects of Other Agents

To complete this survey, some of the effects observed with other agents that are inhaled are discussed briefly.

#### *a. Benzene*

Benzene is widely used as a commercial solvent and may be a contaminant of commercial xylene, toluene, and other solvents. In addition to acute intoxications such as that with toluene, benzene is toxic to the bone marrow, and can produce a fatal aplastic anemia and leukemias. It can also produce degeneration of the seminiferous tubules of the testes and so affect sperm formation.[30]

#### *b. Gasoline and Petroleum Naphthas*

These have acute effects on the CNS similar to toluene, but produce more severe depression and excitation. Both convulsions and fatal respiratory depression are more common. There have been heart arrhythmias, anemia, leukopenia, liver and kidney damage through long exposure, and severe bone marrow depression.

#### *c. Acetone*

Acetone acts like ethyl alcohol on the CNS, but it is a more severe depressant. There is one case reported of possible liver and kidney damage from sniffing liquid cleaner containing acetone (other products were present).

#### *d. Aliphatic Acetates (Methyl, Ethyl, Butyl, Amyl)*

All are CNS depressants with more marked effect as the molecular weight of the compound increases. They are all irritants to the respiratory passages and can cause renal, hepatic, and bone marrow damage.

#### *e. Testor Model Cements*

Allylisothiocyanates (volatile oil of mustard) was added to glue to produce a pungent, irritating odor.

## TABLE 10-7

## Summary of Clinical Syndromes of Selected Cases from the Literature*

| | Neurologic/CNS Effects | | |
|---|---|---|---|
| *Chemical Compound/Product* | *Clinical Effects* | *Diagnostic/Pathologic Findings* | *Other Effects* |
| **N-hexane products** | | | |
| *Yamamura, 1969*<br>Author presents a study checking 1667 workers in Japanese industries with exposure to n-hexane. | Quadriplegia, muscle weakness dysesthesia, muscle atrophy, hypesthesia | Polyneuropathy, axonal degeneration | |
| *Herskowitz et al., 1971*<br>A report of three cabinet workers who developed neuropathy while exposed to n-hexane. | Muscle weakness, hypesthesia, areflexia | Neuropathy, increased number of neurofilaments, axonal degeneration | |
| *Gonzalez and Downey, 1972*<br>Case history of 20-year-old male with 15-month history of glue sniffing (80 percent n-hexane) who presented with progressive polyneuropathy. Improvement occurred two to six months after admission. | Muscle weakness, hypesthesia, paresthesia, muscle atrophy | Polyneuropathy, neurogenic atrophy | |
| *Goto et al., 1974*<br>Report of four cases primarily motor polyneuropathy caused by inhalation of an adhesive agent. Weakness and sensory impairment developed in seven to 30 months with symptom progression noted after cessation of activity. Glue also contained toluene | Muscle weakness, muscular atrophy, flaccid quadriplegia, hypesthesia, areflexia, foot and wrist drop | Polyneuropathy, axonal degeneration, neurogenic atrophy, decreased nerve conduction rates | |
| *Shirabe et al., 1974*<br>Report of two patients involved in glue sniffing: one for a three-year period, one for two years plus. Glue first used contained small amounts of n-hexane (0–30 percent n-hexane, 70–100 percent toluene). | Paresthesia, flaccid paralysis of extremities, muscular atrophy, hypesthesia | Polyneuropathy, axonal degeneration, denervation atrophy | |
| *Korobkin et al., 1975*<br>Case report of 29-year-old male with five-year history of contact cement inhalation. Several months prior to symptom onset, patient changed to brand containing n-hexane. Improvement followed avoidance of n-hexane exposure. | Muscle weakness, paresthesia, muscle atrophy of distal extremities | Peripheral neuropathy, axonal abnormalities, decreased nerve conduction rates | |

## TABLE 10-7

## Summary of Clinical Syndromes of Selected Cases from the Literature* (Continued)

### Neurologic/CNS Effects

| *Chemical Compound/Product* | *Clinical Effects* | *Diagnostic/Pathologic Findings* | *Other Effects* |
|---|---|---|---|
| *Paulson and Waylonis, 1976* Authors review situation in a small plant using n-hexane in which at least eight of 50 employees (in 25-year period) developed mild neuropathy. Four patient summaries are presented. | Muscle weakness, hyporeflexia | Polyneuropathy | |
| *Towfighi et al., 1976* Report of two cases exhibiting chronic glue sniffing behavior. Both patients initially used glues containing no n-hexane (part 1, five years on hexane, part 2, ten years on hexane) and experienced good health. Both changed to brand containing n-hexane with onset of symptoms appearing in one to two months. | Paresthesia, muscle weakness, atrophy of distal extremities, areflexia | Neuropathy, neurogenic-atrophy, axonal swelling, decreased nerve conduction rate | |
| **Toluene products** | | | |
| *Grabski, 1961* Author presents case of irreversible cerebellar degeneration following continuous pattern of toluene sniffing lasting several years. | Ataxia, intention tremor, posterior column signs, adiadochokinesis | Cerebellar degeneration | Hepatomegaly |
| *Massengale et al., 1963* Summary of 27 children chronically habituated to inhalation of cement vapors. Toluene was major component of glue used. Two detailed case histories are presented. | | | Microscopic hematuria |
| *Satran and Dodson, 1963* Summary of patient presenting with ten-year history of toluene inhalation who presented because of loss of consciousness. No systemic abnormalities were found. | | | |
| *Knox and Nelson, 1966* This paper discusses the report and conclusion of Grabski, 1961. | Ataxia, nystagmus tremor, diffuse EEG, Babinski's reflex | Permanent encephalopathy, corticobulbar damage, diffuse cerebral atrophy, corticospinal damage | |

## TABLE 10-7

## Summary of Clinical Syndromes of Selected Cases from the Literature* (Continued)

### Neurologic/CNS Effects

| *Chemical Compound/Product* | *Clinical Effects* | *Diagnostic/Pathologic Findings* | *Other Effects* |
|---|---|---|---|
| *O'Brien et al., 1971*<br>Case history of 19-year-old male with six-year history of glue sniffing. Presentation followed six-hour sniffing of a liquid cleaner. | | | Jaundice, hepatocellular damage; anuria, hematuria, proteinuria |
| *Taher et al., 1974*<br>Two case histories are presented: one patient with a three-year history of glue sniffing, with a one-year history of toluene sniffing, other patient with five-to-six-day history of sniffing paint (60.4 percent toluene). | Muscle weakness, flaccid quadriplegia, areflexia | | Renal tubular acidosis |
| *Kelly, 1975*<br>Presentation of case history of 19-year-old female with one-year history of paint sniffing. Toluene was common in all brands she sniffed. | Intention tremors, impossible tandem gait, ataxia | Cerebellar dysfunction | |
| **Glue sniffing, general** | | | |
| *Blaser and Massengale, 1962*<br>An overview of glue sniffing among children. The authors note that in a two-year period in Denver, 130 (average age 13) were arrested for glue sniffing. Six detailed case histories are presented. | | | |
| *Merry and Zachariadis, 1962*<br>Case history of 20-year-old man presenting with an 18-month history of glue sniffing. Presentation was precipitated by the inhalation of six tubes of cement glue, which resulted in a semicomatose state. | | | |
| *Powars, 1965*<br>Paper describes five adolescents (all with sickle cell disease) who developed hematologic disorders associated with glue sniffing. | Wallerian degeneration, neuronal death | | Septicemia; aplastic anemia, reticulocytopenia, hypoplasic pancytopenia |
| **Gasoline products** | | | |
| *Easson, 1962*<br>Two cases of gasoline inhalation in children (ages 11 and 14) are presented in which a degree of physical tolerance is indicated. | Borderline EEG | | |

## TABLE 10-7

## Summary of Clinical Syndromes of Selected Cases from the Literature* (Continued)

### Neurologic/CNS Effects

| *Chemical Compound/Product* | *Clinical Effects* | *Diagnostic/Pathologic Findings* | *Other Effects* |
|---|---|---|---|
| *Tolan and Linql, 1964*<br>Two cases of adolescents with history of gasoline inhalation are presented. | Model psychosis | | |
| *Karani, 1966*<br>A case report of a 20-year-old mechanic with a three-year history of gasoline consumption and inhalation. Author attributes diagnosis to triorthocresyl phosphate component of gasoline. | Muscle weakness, moderate–severe areflexia, bilateral foot drop, bilateral claw deformity, muscle atrophy, paresthesia | Peripheral neuritis, neurogenic muscular atrophy | |
| *Law and Nelson, 1968*<br>Report of a 41-year-old female presenting with eight-month history of leaded gasoline sniffing (three to four hours a day) exhibiting a chronic psychosis. | Ataxia, tremor, psychotic behavior, recent memory impairment | Lead encephalopathy | Anemia |
| *Carroll and Abel, 1973*<br>Case report of chronic gasoline inhalation (six years) in a 14-year-old male. | Choreiform movements, diffuse EEG delerium | Diffuse encephalopathy | Mild liver congestion |
| **Aerosol products**<br>*Bass, 1970*<br>The author discusses the incidence of sudden sniffing deaths (without plastic bag suffocation) in the 1960s. Details of five case histories are presented. In four of the five cases autopsies were performed that showed no anatomic cause of death. Death occurred after sniffing followed by some stressful situation, such as exercise. | | | |
| *Treffert, 1974*<br>The author discusses sudden sniffing death problem and the mechanism of death. | | | Hypercapnia; severe cardiac arrthythmia, ventricular fibrillation |
| *Wenzl et al., 1974*<br>Discussion of four teenagers who sniffed PAM. | | | Acute renal tubular necrosis, proteinuria, uremia; azotemia |

## TABLE 10-7

## Summary of Clinical Syndromes of Selected Cases from the Literature* (Continued)

### Neurologic/CNS Effects

| *Chemical Compound/Product* | *Clinical Effects* | *Diagnostic/Pathologic Findings* | *Other Effects* |
|---|---|---|---|
| *Kamm, 1975*<br>Report of a 16-year-old male who inhaled Arid Extra Dry deodorant. Death followed immediately after inhalation. | Cerebral edema | | Pulmonary edema, mild to moderate pulmonary vascular congestion, ventricular fibrillation |
| *Poklis, 1975*<br>Report of case history of adolescent death due to aerosol propellant inhalation. | | | Pulmonary and laryngeal edema at autopsy |
| *Standefer, 1975*<br>Case history of 13-year-old male who died following inhalation of fluorocarbons F11 and F12 in cooking spray. | | | Lung congestion, cardiac arrhythmia |
| *Wilde, 1975*<br>Discussion of inhalation of spray paints with particular reference to those that contain metals (zinc and copper). | Stepping gait | | Systemic absorption of metals |
| *Carlton, 1976*<br>Discussion of 12 cases of death due to fluorocarbon inhalation from 1971 to 1975. Postmortems are nonspecific; excitation precedes death. | Anesthetic | | |
| *Crawford, 1976*<br>Report of the death of an adolescent following inhalation of fluorocarbons. | | | Cardiac arrhythmia |
| **Lacquer thinner** | | | |
| *Prockop et al., 1974*<br>Seven cases of severe peripheral neuropathy are reported as seen in seven males (ages 17–22 years) with history of chronic inhalation of lacquer thinner. Syndrome progression was predominately motor. | Muscle weakness, hypalgesia, hypesthesia, decreased nerve conduction, acute denervation paralysis, paresthesia | "Huffer's" neuropathy, neurogenic muscular atrophy, corticobulbar neuropathy | Respiratory distress, diminished vital capacity |
| *Oh and Kim, 1976*<br>Summary of findings in case of 20-year-old male with two-year history of "huffing" lacquer thinner. | Muscle weakness, hyperesthesia, moderate areflexia, decreased nerve conduction | Peripheral neuropathy, giant axonal swelling | |

## TABLE 10-7

### Summary of Clinical Syndromes of Selected Cases from the Literature* (Continued)

#### Neurologic/CNS Effects

| *Chemical Compound/Product* | *Clinical Effects* | *Diagnostic/Pathologic Findings* | *Other Effects* |
|---|---|---|---|
| **Lighter fluid** | | | |
| *Ackerly and Gibson, 1964* Summary of 12 cases of lighter fluid inhalation among children in the San Antonio, Texas, area. Duration of involvement ranged from limited to continuously for three years. | Minimal EEG abnormality | Convulsive disorder | |
| **Chloroform** | | | |
| *Storms, 1973* Case report of a 10-year-old male who participated in a "chloroform party" at which large amounts of chloroform were inhaled. | Coma | Severe hepatic damage | |
| **Trichloroethylene** | | | |
| *Mitchell and Parson-Smith, 1969* Case description of 33-year-old male who worked as a metal degreaser, which involved lowering a basket containing metal into warm trichloroethylene. | Loss of taste, vertigo, analgesia in all divisions of RT trigeminal nerve | Neuropathy | |
| *Seage and Burns, 1971* Report of male with history of cardiac disease who drank alcohol following inhalation of trichloroethylene. | | | Pulmonary edema |
| *Hayden et al., 1976* The authors cite three sources of inhalation of cleaning fluids that contained trichloroethylene. | Vertigo, trigeminal analgesic, decreased visual field | Neuropathy | Jaundice, centrilobular necrosis, hepatomegaly; anuria, hematuria, oliguria, proteinuria (tubular necrosis) |
| **Trichloroethane** | | | |
| *Travers, 1974* Case report of an 18-year-old male seaman who collapsed on ship; 24 hours later, death occurred. Evidence in his bunk indicated he had been sniffing the substance. | Cerebral edema | | Hematuria; ventricular fibrillation, tachycardia, cardiac arrest |
| *Cuberan et al., 1976* Case report of a 20-year-old mechanic who inhaled trichloroethane in an episode that led to his death. Autopsy showed no anatomic cause of death. | | | Ventricular fibrillation |

## TABLE 10-7

### Summary of Clinical Syndromes of Selected Cases from the Literature* (Continued)

**Neurologic/CNS Effects**

| *Chemical Compound/Product* | *Clinical Effects* | *Diagnostic/Pathologic Findings* | *Other Effects* |
|---|---|---|---|
| **Benzene** | | | |
| *Vigliani and Saita, 1964* A review of the history of benzene exposure resulting in leukemia, plus six case reports from personal observations in which all worked with benzene. | | | Epistaxis, hemocytoblastic leukemia; mucosanguineous diarrhea |
| *Forni and Moreo, 1967* Case report of a 38-year-old female who worked for 22 years as a cable cleaner using solvents containing benzene. | | | Hyporegenerative anemia, leukemia |
| *Winek and Collom, 1971* Case report of 18-year-old male who died following inhalation of reagent-grade benzene. Boy was found with his head inside a plastic bag. | Cerebral edema | | |
| *Aksoy et al., 1972* Four case histories are reported in which shoemakers using benzene-containing adhesives developed acute leukemia. | | | Pancytopenia; aplastic anemia, acute myeloblastic leukemia, thrombocythemia |
| *Aksoy et al., 1974* Two case reports of leukemia following exposure to benzene are discussed with particular reference to the familial factors in this case. | | | Acute lymphoblastic leukemia, acute myeloblastic leukemia |
| *Hayden et al., 1976* The authors enumerate several sources of principally industrial exposure resulting in hematologic damage. | | | Erythroleukemia pancytopenia, thrombocytopenia, myeloid metoplasia, aplastic anemia |

*Although the inhalants described are listed by categories of major or identified constituent, the physiologic effects may not be associated solely with this agent or may be due to an action of this and other agents present in the commercial mixture.
(From Comstock, E. G., and Comstock, B. S. NIDA Research Monograph, No. 15. C. W. Sharp and M. L. Brehman, eds., Washington,, D.C.: U.S. Government Printing Office, 1977, pp. 57–65.)

### *f. Carbon Tetrachloride and Chlorinated Hydrocarbons (Trichlorethane)*

These are capable of producing liver and kidney damage and can result in cardiac arrhythmias (ventricular fibrillation).

### *g. Trichlorethylene*

This is used in paints, lacquers, and adhesives as a useful solvent for degreasing metals, and for dry cleaning and fat extraction. Medically it is limited to anesthesia and analgesics. Two of the most commonly used products are Carbona cleaning fluid [44 percent trichlorethylene (TCE), 56 percent petroleum distillate] and Carbona number 10 special spot remover (40 percent TCE, 10 percent trichloroethane, 50 percent petroleum distillate).

The effects include CNS depression preceded by mild excitation or euphoria, postrecovery headache, and acute organic cerebral and cerebellar dysfunction with EEG abnormalities. Fourteen cases of cardiac arrhythmias with ventricular tachycardia and fibrillation, cardiac failure with pulmonary edema, renal damage (rare, but probably tubular necrosis), and hepatic damage (acute toxic hepatitis with centrilobular necrosis) have been reported.

### *h. Aerosol Propellants (Fluoroalkane Gases—Freons)*

These can produce fatal heart arrhythmias when inhaled in large amounts. Forty-nine sudden deaths have been reported in youths who inhaled aerosol propellants to "turn on."[32] These gases can produce fatal arrhythmias in mice, rats, and dogs, and serious arrhythmias in monkeys.[33,41]

The most recent inhalants that have been subject to abuse are spray paints. These contain a variety of aliphatic and aromatic hydrocarbons, including toluene. They are sprayed either into a plastic bag or directly through a tube.

### *i. Alcohols*

Data show that alcoholic substances are not strong volatile solvents and are therefore much more effective when taken orally. Inhaled alcohols, including butyl, methyl, and isopropyl alcohol, are similar to ethyl alcohol in their metabolism and toxicology. Some of the generalized characteristics and effects of inhaling alcohols are as follows: Isopropyl alcohol may cause either CNS depression or elevation, or both. Methyl alcohol may cause blindness, although no reported cases have been found. None of the alcohols are known to cause liver, kidney, or blood disorders from inhalation.

### *j. Glycols*

Severe consequences, including permanent brain damage, are results of the abuse of glycol compounds. Fortunately abuse of glycol as an inhalant is not widespread, and this is probably because it is highly irritating to the mucous membrane. Used in antifreeze solutions, ethylene glycol causes liver and renal impairment and may produce permanent brain damage, providing enough oxalic acid is accumulated. Its injestion may result in prolonged oliguria, secondary to tissue degeneration, and crystal deposits in the kidney.[42] Acute poisoning may result in pulmonary edema. The presence of calcium oxalate crystals, albuminuria, hematuria, and cysts is shown by urinalysis after constant exposure to ethylene glycol vapors. No crystals have been found in the urine of the glycol sniffer.

Methyl cellulose acetate, a solvent used in some liquid plastic cements, produces significant liver and kidney damage.

### *k. Naphtha*

There is only one article which has appeared in the scientific literature reporting abuse of lighter fluid (naptha). From this study, naptha abuse seems to result in abnormal blood cell count and electroencephalogram. No major organic problems were observed with its abuse.

### *l. Other Solvents*

There are undoubtedly a great number of other intoxicating substances that are potentially hazardous as inhalants. The lack of conclusive data regarding the potential for organic damage from other solvents does not eliminate the possible risks for their abuse, since toxic effects may be deduced from toxicology and industrial studies previously done. Benzene has been implicated in a single well-documented fatal case of a 16-year-old boy who died after inhaling rubber cement containing benzene.[18] Respiratory depression caused his death, but cerebral and pulmonary edema, plus congestion of the spleen, liver, stomach, and duodenum, were also found. There have been some cases of nail polish remover (acetone) sniffing reported, but no physical or laboratory data are available.[19]

## K. HABITUAL USE OF VOLATILE SOLVENTS

### 1. Psychologic Dependence

Becoming psychologically dependent on inhalants or glue sniffing is as prevalent as any other form of drug abuse. Many users are known to rely heavily on their favorite product or brand to obtain their high and are unwilling to substitute another product unless theirs is unavailable. A large-scale compulsive user reportedly inhaled up to 25 tubes of glue (21 cubic centimeters each) daily.[16]

### 2. Tolerance

The chronic abuser is much more likely to require greater doses of inhalants, and much more rapidly, than the individual who has had little exposure to lower vapor concentration of inhalants or solvents. This increased requirement is due to the development of tolerance to the effects on the CNS. Two separate examples indicate that tolerance does develop in inhalant abuse. After taking unspecified amounts of model cement, a user built up his tolerance only three months after inhaling the intoxicating substance once weekly. Another user needed eight tubes of glue instead of one tube, three years after he initiated his usage.[16] It is not certain whether an individual develops a tolerance to gasoline. It is difficult to observe tolerance development because the gasoline sniffer usually sniffs from a large, open container such as a tank, barrel, or a one-gallon tin and it is hard to ascertain whether, over a period of time, an increased dose is needed to achieve the same result.

There appears to be cross-tolerance and cross-dependence between barbiturates and chloroform.[43]

### 3. Physical Dependence

Physical dependence on inhalants has not been well documented. Some reports indicate the abuser's discomfort, with fine tremors, irritability, and anxiety. However, little data are available on physiologic dependence.

## L. SUMMARY

The acute manifestations of toxicity are obviously dangerous. Deaths from acute exposure do occur. In addition, during the inebriated state, a young person may either inflict self-injury, or, being accident prone, injure others. There are many reported cases of misdemeanors performed while under the influence of glue. As far as long-term toxic effects are concerned (other than chromosomal abnormalities and psychic dependence), there is no good substantial evidence of chronic organ toxicity as far as toluene is concerned. Chronic brain damage, when it occurs, is probably secondary to lack of oxygen, most likely from the use of plastic bags.

Dr. Hofmann[14] summarized his excellent chapter on solvent inhalants in the following manner:

> In summary, we feel that the practice of voluntary volatile solvent inhalantion bears a significant potential for mortality, even though the number of deaths seem exceedingly low relative to the number of youths who are probably involved in the practice. The halogenated hydrocarbons that appear in cleaning solutions and some aerosol sprays are the most dan-

gerous agents. There seems to be a considerably greater safety factor when most other agents, and toluene, in particular, are used. Deaths implicating these latter substances typically entail plastic bag suffocation, rather than the toxic effects of the chemical agent itself.

The intentional inhaling of commercial solvents is a practice of adolescents and young adults. Precise statistical information is difficult to obtain. Peer group influences appear to be a powerful factor in the initiation and perpetuation of volatile solvent abuse. Other contributory factors in sustaining the practice are social, familial, and intrapsychic disruption.

There is no specific treatment for the inhalant abuser. However, community education and the judicious supply of early information to both school children and their parents about the volatile hydrocarbons may be worthy preventive efforts. The development of research programs to study epidemiologic information (high-risk populations) and long-term animal studies mimicking the human abuse situation could be helpful. Finally the establishment of a few special-study solvent-abuse clinics is desirable from treatment, training, and research viewpoints.

## REFERENCES


1. Watson, J.M. Solvent abuse by children and young adults: A review. *Br. J. Addict.* 75:27, 1980.
2. Cohen, S. *The Beyond Within: The LSD Story.* New York: Atheneum, 1967.
3. Powars, D. Aplastic anemia secondary to glue sniffing. *N. Engl. J. Med.* 273:700, 1965.
4. Knox, J.W., and Nelson, J.R. Permanent encephalopathy from toluene inhalation. *N. Engl. J. Med.* 275:1494, 1966.
5. Durden, W.D., Jr., and Chipman, D.W. Gasoline sniffing complicated by acute carbon tetrachloride poisoning. *Arch. Intern. Med.* 119:371, 1967.
6. Bass, M. Sudden sniffing death. *JAMA* 212:2075, 1970.
7. Flowers, N.C., and Horan, L.G. Nonanoxic aerosol arrhythmias. *JAMA*219:33, 1972.
8. Taylor, G.J., and Harris, W.S. Cardiac toxicity of aerosol propellants. *JAMA* 214:81, 1970.
9. Taylor, G.J., and Harris, W.S. Glue sniffing causes heart block in mice. *Science* 170:866, 1970.
10. Ackerly, W.C., and Gibson, G. Lighter fluid "sniffing." *Am. J. Psychiatry* 120:1056, 1964.
11. Easson, W.M. Gasoline addiction in children. *Pediatrics* 29:250, 1962.
12. Winck, C.L. Collom, W.D., and Wecht, C.H. Fatal benzene exposure by gluesniffing. *Lancet* 1:683, 1967.
13. Massengale, O.N., et al. Physical and psychologic factors in glue sniffing. *N. Engl. J. Med.* 269:1340, 1963.
14. Hofmann, F.G. *A Handbook on Drug and Alcohol Abuse: The Biomedical Aspects.* New York: Oxford University Press, 1975, p. 129.
15. Clinger, O.W., and Johnson, N.A. Purposeful inhalation of gasoline vapors. *Psychiat. Q.* 25:557, 1951.
16. Press, E., and Done, A.K. Solvent sniffing. Physiologic effects and community control measures for intoxication from the intentional inhalation of organic solvents. I. *Pediatrics* 39:451, 1967.
17. Gellman, V. Glue-sniffing among Winnipeg school children. *Can. Med. Assoc.* 98:411, 1968.
18. Brewer, W.R., Picchioni, A.L., and Chin, L. Hazards of intentional inhalation of plastic cement fumes. *Ariz. Med.* 17:747, 1960.
19. Glaser, H.H., and Massengale, O.N. Glue sniffing in children: Deliberate inhalation of vaporized plastic cements. *JAMA* 181:300, 1962.
20. Prockop, L.D., Alt, M., and Tison, J. "Huffer's" neuropathy. *JAMA* 229:1083, 1974.
21. Norcombe, B., et al. A hunger for stimuli. The psychosocial background of petrol inhalation. *Br. J. Med. Psychol.* 43(4):367, 1970.
22. Boecks, R., and Coodin, F. An epidemic of gasoline sniffing. Presented at the First International Symposium on the Deliberate Inhalation of Industrial Solvents, Mexico City, 1976.
23. Cohen, S. Inhalant abuse. In *The Substance Abuse Problems.* New York: Haworth Press, 1981, p. 46.
24. Cohen, S. Inhalant abuse: An overview of the problem. In C.W. Sharp and M.L. Brehm, eds., *Review of Inhalants, Euphoria to Dysfunction.* NIDA Research Monograph No. 15. Washington, D.C.: U.S. Government Printing Office, 1977.
25. Massengale, O.N., et al. Physical and psychological factors in glue sniffing. *N. Engl. J. Med.* 269:1340, 1963.
26. Brozovsky, M., and Winkler, E.G. Glue sniffing in children and adolescents. *N.Y. J. Med.* 65:1984, 1965.

27. Berry, G., et al. Neuropsychological assessment of chronic inhalant abusers: A preliminary report. Presented at the First International Symposium on Voluntary Inhalation of Industrial Solvents, Mexico City, 1976.
28. Couri, D. Introduction: Preclinical pharmacology and toxicology. In W. Sharp and M.L. Brehm, eds., *Review of Inhalants: Euphoria to Dysfunction*. NIDA Research Monograph No. 15. Washington, D.C.: U.S. Government Printing Office, 1977, p. 98.
29. Gerarde, H.W. Toxicologic studies on hydrocarbons. IX. Influence of dose on the metabolism of mono-n-alkyl derivatives of benzene. *Toxicol. Appl. Pharmacol.* 9:185, 1966.
30. Lewis, P.W., and Patterson, D. Acute and chronic effects on voluntary inhalation of certain commercial volatile solvents by juveniles. *J. Drug Issues* 162, 1974.
31. Sharp C.W., and Brehm, M.L. Approaches to the problem. In C.W. Sharp and M.L. Brehm, eds., *Review of Inhalants: Euphoria to Dysfunction*. NIDA Research Monograph No. 15. Washington, D.C.: U.S. Government Printing Office, 1977, p. 226.
32. Medical News. Glue sniffing may alter chromosomes. Other solvents also implicated. *JAMA* 207:1441, 1969.
33. Winek, C.L., Wecht, C.H., and Collom, W.D. Toluene fatality from glue sniffing. *Pa. Med.* 71:81, 1968.
34. Aviado, D. Toxicity of aerosol propellants in the respiratory and circulatory systems: Proposed classification. *Toxicology* 3:321, 1975.
35. Sharp C.W., and Brehm, M.L. (Editors) *Review of Inhalants: Euphoria to Dysfunction*. NIDA Research Monograph No. 15. Washington, D.C.: U.S. Government Printing Office, 1977, pp. 77–553.
36. Sharp C.W., and Carroll, C.T. (Editors) *Voluntary Inhalation of Industrial Solvents*. NIDA No. (Adm). Washington, D.C.: U.S. Government Printing Office, 1978, pp. 75–77.
37. Todd, J. "Sniffing": and addiction. *Br. Med. J.* 4:255, 1968.
38. Grabski, D.A. Toluene sniffing producing cerebellar degeneration. *Am. J. Psychiatry* 118:461, 1961.
39. Dodds, J.B., et al. A comparison of the cognitive functioning of the glue sniffers and non-sniffers. *J. Pediatr.* 64:565, 1964.
40. Comstock, E.G., and Comstock, B.S. Medical evaluation of inhalant abuser. In C.W. Sharp and M.L. Brehm, eds., *Review of Inhalants: Euphoria to Dysfunction*. NIDA Research Monograph No. 15. Washington, D.C.: U.S. Government Printing Office, 1977, p. 54.
41. Baerg, R., and Kimberg, D.V. Centrilobular hepatic necrosis and acute renal failures in "solvent sniffers." *Ann. Intern. Med.* 73:713, 1970.
42. Collins, M.J., et al. Recovery after prolonged oliguria due to ethylene glycol intoxication. *Arch. Intern. Med.* 125:1059, 1970.
43. Jaffe, J.H. Drug addiction and drug abuse. In A.G. Gilman, I.S. Goodman, and A. Gilman, eds., *The Pharmacological Basis of Therapeutics*, 6th ed. New York: Macmillan, 1980, p. 569.

Chapter 11

# Alcohol: The World's Most Devastating Drug

## A. INTRODUCTION

Alcoholism is a treatable progressive illness that may be defined as the excessive use of alcohol to the extent that it causes continuing adverse effects on the individual, the family, and the community. Certainly there is no single cause of alcoholism; rather it develops from a complicated interaction of genetic, physiologic, psychologic, and environmental factors.

Alcoholism ranks with heart disease and mental illness as one of the major U.S. health problems. The National Institute on Alcohol Abuse and Alcoholism (NIAAA) estimates that there are 11 million alcoholic individuals and problem drinkers in the United States. A 1977 national study of the economic effects of alcohol-related problems estimated a cost to society of more than $42.75 billion. Today it is over $120 billion.

Even more devastating are the social costs that involve family life with the emergence of marital problems and poor child-rearing practice when an alcoholic individual attempts to maintain a family and deal with alcohol abuse at the same time. Poor job performance or absence, divorce, child neglect or abuse, heavy financial debts, and other problems may cause the alcoholic to drink even more heavily or to desert the family.

The NIAAA estimates that alcohol-related problems are the cause of more than 85,000 deaths in the United States annually. More than 70 percent of the adult population in the United States (approximately 100 million people) use alcoholic beverages. And it is estimated that one out of every ten drinkers is a problem drinker and nearly half of all alcoholics in the United States are women.

In a national survey on drug abuse,[1] young adults (95.3 percent) and older adults (91.5 percent) report greater experience with alcoholic beverages than do youth (70.3 percent). Current drinking is highest in the 18- to 25-year-old group, with 75.9 percent reporting use as compared with 61.3 percent of older adults and 37.2 percent of youths. Current use of alcohol is related to chronologic age. Drinking is lowest among those aged 12 to 13 years (20 percent); it rises to 36 percent in the 14- to 15-year-old group, and increases to 55 percent among those who are 16 to 17 years old. Among those aged 18 to 21 years, the rate jumps to 75 percent, and for those 22 to 25 years old, it is 78 percent. The rate falls to 70 percent among those 26 to 34 years old and to 58 percent for those 35 years of age and older. Maximum consumption in any one day reaches highest levels for young adults: 24.8 percent of all young adults report having five to ten drinks (older adults, 11.1 percent; youth, 8.7 percent) and 9.6 percent say they have had as many as 11 drinks on any one day over the period of a month (older adults only 3.1 percent and youth, 2.1 percent). Interestingly, current drinkers are more likely than those who are not current drinkers to have used psychotherapeutic pills, marihuana, and ''stronger'' drugs (hallucinogens, cocaine, heroin). The report indicates that, although this holds true for all three age groups, it is most pronounced among young adults and least pronounced among older adults.

Although people have used alcohol since the dawn of history, a clear reason for its use is not known. It has little therapeutic value and is a socially abused drug. With the introduction of distillation by the Arabs in the Middle Ages, alchemists believed that alcohol was the answer to all of their ailments. The word ''whiskey,'' or, in Gaelic, *usquebaugh,* meaning ''water of life,'' became widely known. Beer and wines are among the oldest fermented alcoholic beverages reported.

Alcoholism is the country's oldest drug problem or ''its first drug scene,'' and one from which we may learn something about drug abuse generally. Medical progress has led to the recognition of vitamin B complex deficiency in alcoholism and the mortality rate in severe alcoholism due to delirium tremens (DTs) has been reduced by an understanding of the causative factors, the availability of new tranquilizing drugs, and better biochemical management of the hospitalized patient. Progress in the social realm can be seen in the repeal of Prohibition and the formation of Alcoholics Anonymous. Today not only is alcoholism being accepted as a public health problem, but, more important, it is gradually being accepted as an illness concomitant with the implied possibility of cure or improvement. As a result of this more positive viewpoint, more public funds gradually are being allocated for research, which, it is hoped, will lead to the cure and prevention of alcoholism.[2]

Medical and lay authorities are paying increased attention to the use and abuse of the drug, ethyl alcohol ($C_2H_5OH$). Employers are trying to identify and treat personnel who have alcohol-related problems. The judicial and penal systems are making special efforts with alcoholics. The medical profession, slow to regard the alcoholic as anything more than a nuisance, is beginning to recognize the complex abnormalities induced by excess alcohol consumption. It is especially important, in light of these abnormalities, that we establish precise diagnostic criteria and apply rigorous scientific methods to our therapeutic approaches.

## 1. Definition of Addiction[3]

Since alcoholism is an addictive disorder, let us consider the general pharmacologic definition of addiction. There are three major aspects to this definition: psychologic dependency, withdrawal, and tolerance. Psychologic dependency, the most important factor, involves compulsive use of and craving for a drug—the feature of addiction that is least understood and most important to treat. The other two factors in addiction are physical dependency (which includes withdrawal), manifested by a series of physiologic events when the drug is discontinued, and tolerance, which occurs when continued use of the drug is necessary for normal function or, looked at in another way, when increasing doses of that drug are required to produce a given effect. Alcohol meets these criteria for addiction because psychologic dependency, withdrawal, and tolerance are clearly present in patients who abuse the drug. When patients are detoxified, two of the three factors of addiction—withdrawal and tolerance—are quickly reversed, but little has been done to modify a patient's psychologic dependence and resultant behavior in any lasting way. It also should be recognized that normal individuals can be made physically dependent on alcohol, but are not alcoholics unless they exhibit the behavioral abnormalities that determine abuse. In viewing alcohol abuse in this light, it is worthy to note that one of the prime differences between alcohol and other drugs of abuse, especially those in the narcotic class, is the relative risk of addictive behavior. Many individuals consume alcoholic beverages, but relatively few (approximately 10 percent) develop psychologic and physical dependency on the drug. With narcotic drugs, the risk of physical and psychologic addiction is greater.

Alcoholism is an illness characterized by:

1. Preoccupation with alcohol and loss of control over its consumption such as usually lead to intoxication once drinking is begun.
2. Chronicity.
3. Progression.
4. Tendency toward relapse.

In 1960, Doctor E. M. Jellinek* characterized five types of alcohol addiction:

1. Alpha alcoholism. Drinking is heavy, but there is no loss of control, nor are there any withdrawal symptoms. This is problem drinking characterized by recurring dependence to relieve emotional and bodily pain.
2. Beta alcoholism. This includes complications such as polyneuropathy, gastritis, and cirrhosis of the liver. There is no physical dependence, nor are there any withdrawal symptoms.
3. Gamma alcoholism. This is characterized by increased tissue tolerance to alcohol. There are craving and withdrawal symptoms if deprivation occurs. Temporary abstinence is possible. This is what Alcoholics Anonymous recognizes as alcoholism.
4. Delta alcoholism. This is the same as gamma alcoholism, except that there is an inability to abstain from drinking.
5. Epsilon alcoholism. This involves periodic bouts with alcoholism. The "weekend drunk" and explosive drinking are characteristic of this type of alcoholism. In the course of these periodic bouts, tissue damage or acute illness may result.

## 2. Criteria for Diagnosis of Alcoholism[3]

The evaluation of the efficacy of any therapeutic approach depends upon exact criteria for diagnosis. In the past, some physicians have defined the alcoholic as one who drinks more than the physician does. This humorous definition suggests that a key problem in managing alcoholic patients is that there are no specific physical findings or laboratory tests for diagnosing their condition. Since the physician may depend on subjective clinical criteria rather than objective scientific fact to diagnose alcoholism, it is commonly identified too late for treatment to be of value. Recognizing the importance of establishing precise criteria for the diagnosis of alcoholism, the National Council on Alcoholism (NCA) established a committee to prepare such criteria.

Given the relationship of addiction to behavior and physical dependency, we should examine in detail the criteria proposed by the NCA. Although not absolute, these criteria form a starting point for diagnosis. They are divided into three diagnostic levels. Level 1 is classic, definitive, and obligatorily associated with alcoholism. Level 2 is probable or frequently indicative of an association with alcoholism; that is, an individual who satisfies these criteria is under strong suspicion for alcoholism, but other corroborative evidence is necessary. Level 3 is a potential for or possible association with alcoholism. At this level, the manifestations are common in many individuals but are not in themselves a strong indication for the existence of alcoholism. Although these criteria may arouse suspicion, further evidence is needed for a certain diagnosis.

In addition to the three diagnostic levels, the criteria also have been divided into "major" and "minor" on the basis of physiologic and clinical as well as behavioral, psychologic, and attitudinal changes.

Those criteria that are classic and definitive for an association with alcoholism in a physiologic and clinical sense include signs of physical dependence—manifested by a withdrawal syndrome including tremor, hallucinosis, seizures, and delirium tremens (Table 11-1). Although the degree of tolerance is less than that to other drugs such as narcotics, definitive diagnostic criteria (level 1) include a blood alcohol level of more than 150 mg% without gross evidence of intoxication. In addition, the consumption of one fifth of a gallon of whiskey, 1.7 quarts of fortified wine, 2.9 quarts of table wine, or 23 12-ounce bottles of beer by a 180-pound person in one day also forms a definitive (level 1) diagnosis of alcoholism. Alcoholic hepatitis and alcoholic cerebral degeneration are clinically definitive criteria for alcoholism. Psychologically a definitive diagnosis of alcoholism includes drinking despite a strong medical contraindication known to the patient or despite an identified social contraindication (job loss or marriage disruption because of drinking, arrest for intoxication or driving while intoxicated). Minor definitive (level 1) diagnostic criteria include a blood alcohol level at any time of more than 300 mg%, a level of more than 100 mg% in a routine examination, or "blatant indiscriminate use of alcohol."

Diagnostic level 2—that is, probable or frequently associated with alcoholism—includes alcoholic "blackout" periods, fatty degeneration of the liver in the absence of other known cases, Laennec's cirrhosis, Wernicke–Korsakoff syndrome, a cerebral degeneration in the absence of Alzheimer's disease or arteriosclerosis, peripheral neuropathy, alcoholic myopathy, and alcoholic cardiomyopathy (Table 11-2). A final probable diagnostic criterion includes a patient's subjective complaint of losing control of alcohol consumption.

It is of special interest that a physican often treats peptic ulcer disease, uncontrolled diabetes, cardiac arrhythmias, or transient hyperuricemia, any of which could be an early reflection of alcoholism. To apply the foregoing criteria, the physican must have a high index of suspicion. In the natural history of the illness, the physician is most likely to come into contact with the potential alcoholic because of problems on the job, especially Monday morning absenteeism, or medical conditions that seem refractory or difficult to manage. It is also important to note that the earlier the diagnosis of the illness is made and accepted, the more remedial the treatment may be.

Those people with the most major criteria for the diagnosis of alcoholism, most visible to society and in county hospitals, account for less than 5 percent of the total number of people who abuse the drug. The treatment applicable to these alcoholic patients is not the same as that used if the disease is detected early.

The NCA criteria for alcoholism have engendered much debate. Contemporary researchers and leaders in the field are not as "hung up" on a differential diagnosis in the classic manner. Other approaches are focusing on the understanding of motives for and styles of drinking; that is, the interaction between personality and drinking and their relationship to treatment.

## TABLE 11-1

### Criteria for Diagnosis of Alcoholism: Classic, Definite, Obligatory

**Major**

*Physiologic*

1. Physical dependency, withdrawal syndrome (gross tremor, hallucinations, seizures—DTs).
2. Tolerance:
   Blood level = 150 mg% without intoxication
   One-fifth whiskey, 1.7 quarts fortified wine, 2.9 quarts table wine, or 23 12-ounce bottles of beer per day in a 180-pound individual

*Clinical*

1. Alcoholic hepatitis.
2. Alcoholic cerebellar degeneration.

*Behavioral, psychologic, attitudinal*

1. Drinking despite strong medical contraindication known to patient.
2. Drinking despite strong social contraindication known to patient.

**Minor**

Blood alcohol level at any time more than 300 mg%.
Blatant indiscriminate use of alcohol.

(From Becker, C. E., Roe, L. R., and Scott, R. A. *Alcohol as a Drug: A Curriculum on Pharmacology and Toxicology*. New York: Medcom Press, 1974. With permission.)

## 3. Suggested Predisposing Factors

In addition to applying the criteria cited, we should recognize the epidemiologic and sociologic factors that indicate a high risk for developing alcoholism. Although not all experts agree, there is a consensus that these factors include either a family history of alcoholism or a family history of complete abstinence from alcohol. Other factors may be a history of alcoholism or of complete abstinence from alcohol in a sibling, an upbringing in a broken home or in one with parental discord, being the last child or among the younger children in a large family, or a family history of severe depression. Another factor may be heavy cigarette smoking. There is some evidence that certain cultural groups, especially the Irish and Scandinavians, have a higher incidence of alcoholism than other groups, such as Jews, Chinese, and Italians. The epidemiologic and sociologic studies on which these cultural differences are based are not enough; however, we do place great weight on them.

## 4. Incidence of Alcoholism

Alcohol is the most abused drug in the United States, and the problem is increasing.

A 1979 national survey indicates that 15 percent of adult male drinkers and 3 percent of adult female drinkers are drinking at levels that indicate a substantial risk for the development of either alcoholism or serious problem drinking. If we consider only alcohol-dependence behaviors and characteristics, then 5 percent of male and 2 percent of female drinkers are experiencing symptoms that indicate a substantial risk of alcoholism or serious problem drinking; and on the basis of only adverse social consequences, 9 percent of male and 5 percent of female drinkers are at substantial risk in this regard.

## 5. Effects of Abuse

The effects of alcohol abuse include a continous CNS depression that leads to many phys-

**TABLE 11-2**

**Criteria for Diagnosis of Alcoholism: Probable, Frequently Indicative**

**Major**

*Physiologic*

1. Alcoholic "blackout" periods.

*Clinical*

1. Fatty liver.
2. Laennec's cirrhosis.
3. Pancreatitis without cholelithiasis.
4. Chronic gastritis.
5. Wernicke–Korsakoff syndrome.
6. Cerebral degeneration.
7. Peripheral neuropathy.
8. Alcoholic myopathy.
9. Alcoholic cardiomyopathy.

*Behavioral*

1. Loss of control (subjective).

**Minor**

Odor of alcohol at time of medical appointment.
Surreptitious drinking.
Morning drinking.
Repeated conscious attempts at abstinence.
Skid row social behavior.

(From Becker, C. E., Roe, L. R., and Scott, R. A. *Alcohol as a Drug: A Curriculum on Pharmacology, Neurology, and Toxicology.* New York: Medcom Press, 1974. With permission.)

ical and psychologic complications. Ethanol, the most commonly abused alcohol, decreases mental judgment and impairs motor coordination even when used in small amounts. Drinking alcohol gives a false sense of control or improved performance and also diminishes feelings of inhibition. Alcohol causes cirrhosis of the liver, fatty metamorphosis, peripheral polyneuropathy, alcoholic gastritis, Korsakoff's psychosis, Wernicke's encephalopathy, and the complications of portal hypotension. It is believed that ethanol is directly incriminated in the pathogenesis of alcoholic fatty liver.[4] The gain in weight observed from drinking alcohol causes a nutritional deficiency because ethanol supplies calories that maintain body weight and decrease appetite. Taking alcohol and barbiturates at the same time strengthens the effects of CNS depressants and heightens the sensitivity to barbiturates.[5] Ethanol consumption seems to slow down the hepatic metabolism of other drugs, and in chronic amounts, leads to hypertrophy of hepatic smooth endoplasmic reticulum and active drug metabolism. This may partly explain the tolerance of alcoholics, when sober, to drugs such as barbiturates.

After getting into fights while drunk, many opiate dependent individuals remember turning to heroin. Follow-up studies on these alcohol-to-opiate converts reveals that such uncontrolled "violence" disappeared.

### 6. Withdrawal Syndrome

Alcohol withdrawal in chronic alcoholism may result in death. The effects of chronic alcohol withdrawal occur within a few hours and may last up to five to seven days. Experiencing of tremulousness, weakness, anxiety, intestinal cramps, and hyperreflexia within 12 hours precedes acute visual hallucinations. "Delirium tremens" with gross tremulousness occurs in conjunction with confusion, disorientation, and delusional thinking, which are part of the acute brain syndrome seen in alcoholism. Major convulsive seizures ("rum fits") are seen more often in barbiturate withdrawal than alcohol withdrawal.

## B. HISTORY AND NATURE OF ALCOHOL

The use of alcohol can be traced back to the Neolithic age. Beer and berry wine were known and used about 6400 B.C., and grape wine was consumed in 300 to 400 B.C. The oldest alcoholic beverage known, however, is a product made from honey, called mead. Some authorities believe that it appeared in the Paleolithic age about 8000 B.C. Thus alcohol use has been around for a long time; even the American Indians were drinking beer and wine at the time they met their first white visitors.

In 1518 Cortez in Mexico first discovered the recreational use of a native alcoholic beverage (pulque) which was obtained from the fermentation of aqua cactus. This beverage had a 6 percent alcohol content. Today fermentation still forms the chemical basis for all alcoholic products. Simply, fermentation takes place when yeast acts on sugar in the presence of water. Chemically $C_6H_{12}O_6$ (glucose) and $H_2O$ (water) is transformed into $C_2H_6O$ (ethyl alcohol) and $CO_2$ (carbon dioxide). Wine, for example, is made from grapes, which contain sugar; thus the addition of yeast, water and crushed grapes begins the fermentation process. Cereal grains, which contain starch (a sugar parent), can also be utilized to obtain alcoholic beverages such as beer.

Japanese saki, made from rice, is between 12 and 16 percent alcohol, whereas mead, which comes primarily from Denmark and Great Britain, has an alcoholic content of about 10 percent.

Distillation is used whenever a high content of alcohol is desired as in various fine liquors and whiskeys. The process of distillation involves heating the alcohol solution and collecting the resultant vapors, which are condensed by cooling to form a liquid again. All this can be accomplished, since alcohol has a lower boiling point than water and there is a higher percentage of alcohol in the distillate (the condensed liquid) than there was in the original source.

The term "alcohol," which in Arabic means "finely divided spirit," probably was first coined in about 800 A.D., when the process of distillation was discovered. However, the Italians, in about the 10th century, were the ones to introduce fine distilled wine for medicinal purposes. It was not until the 13th century that a French professor from Montpellier University referred to these distilled spirits as "aqua vitae," or "water of life." Brandewijn, which means "burnt wine," was coined by the Dutch in the 17th century.

Table wines today contain up to 20 percent alcohol. All of the "hard liquors" are made from a mash composed of a starch grain and malted barley to which yeast is added. In his chapter on alcohol, Dr. Oakley Ray[6] had the following to say about whiskey:

> The name "whiskey" comes from the Irish Gaelic equivalent of aqua vitae and was already commonplace around 1500. The distillation of whiskey in America started on a large scale toward the end of the eighteenth century and was the basis for the first major political-social drug problem in this country. The chief product of the area just west of the Appalachian Mountains, western Pennsylvania, western Virginia, and eastern Kentucky was grain.

Other famous distillates include scotch, from fermented malted barley; rum is the distillate from fermented molasses, a byproduct of sugar cane and the pure alcohol distillate called "little water," better known as Russian vodka.

What happens to alcohol once it enters the body? How does it interact with other drugs? Does alcohol in different forms produce different reactions—and if so, why?

In this chapter, consideration is given to the chemistry, absorption, distribution, elimination, kinetics, and metabolism of alcohol, as well as to the genetic and environmental factors affecting the metabolism. Alcohol–drug interactions are discussed extensively, since such interactions contribute significantly to the clinical morbidity of acute alcohol abuse. Finally, the effects of alcohol on the body's metabolic economy and its role in nutrition and nutritional disease are briefly summarized.

## C. THE CHEMICAL COMPOSITION OF ALCOHOLIC BEVERAGES[7]

In all the major alcoholic beverages—beers, table wines, cocktail or dessert wines, liqueurs or cordials, and distilled spirits—the chief ingredient is identical: ethyl alcohol, known also as ethanol, or simply as alcohol. The concentration is usually about 4 percent by volume in beers, 12 percent in table wines, 20 percent in cocktail or dessert wines, 22 to 50 percent in liqueurs, and 40 to 50 percent (80 to 100 proof) in distilled spirits (See Table 11-3).

In addition, these beverages contain a variety of other chemical constituents. Some come from the original grains, grapes, or other fruits. Others are produced during the chemical processes of fermentation or during distillation or storage. Others may be added as flavoring or coloring.

Modern investigations have shown that many of these nonalcoholic substances do more than contribute to color, flavor, aroma, or palatability. Some actually may have a direct effect on the body; others apparently affect the rate at which alcohol is absorbed into the blood and the rate at which it is oxidized or metabolized in the tissues.[8]

The critical factor in analyzing the effects of drinking is not the amount of alcohol that is drunk or that reaches the stomach, but the amount that enters the bloodstream and the speed at which it is metabolized.[8,9] Only after the alcohol has been absorbed from the digestive tract into the blood and carried to the brain and other tissues, do its most important physiologic and psychologic effects become apparent.

Studies at such institutions as Yale University,[10,11] Stanford University, the Institute of Nutrition in Rome,[12] and the Karolinska Institute in Stockholm[10] have demonstrated that beers, wines, and distilled spirits may vary markedly in the rate at which the alcohol they contain is absorbed into the blood. In general, the higher the concentration of the alcohol, the more rapid is its absorption, and the higher the concentration of nonalcoholic components, the slower is its absorption.

### 1. The Congeners

The use of the term *congeners*, at one time the name for the various nonethyl alcohol substances in alcoholic beverages, has often been misleading. Strictly defined, congener means "of the same kind," and thus would seem to apply only to such other alcohols as methyl, propyl, and isopropyl alcohol. But such beverages as beers and wines also contain many organic acids, aldehydes, ketones, esters, minerals, salts, sugars, antibacterial compounds, amino acids, and vitamins that clearly are not alcohols but nonetheless are called congeners.

The notion that all congeners are toxic, unhealthy, or otherwise undesirable is invalid since some of the nonalcoholic substances—such as the salts, sugars, amino acids, and vitamins—are useful nutritionally.

### 2. The Fusel Oils

Certain components of alcoholic beverages, especially some of the higher alcohols known as fusel oils, are relatively more toxic than ethyl alcohol. But these usually occur in such low concentrations that they pose no clinically significant hazard.[8]

Contrary to the popular belief that fusel oils are found primarily in new, raw, or unaged whiskey, and similar spirits, and cause most of the objectionable taste and aroma of such beverages, chemical analysis has shown that their concentration actually increases with aging.[13]

### 3. The Value of Chemical Data

The rapidly growing knowledge of the chemical composition of the various alcoholic beverages has obvious importance to the beverage industry in controlling the taste, aroma, and appearance of its products. It also has value to scientists engaged in investigating allergic reactions to these beverages, their effects, clinical applications, and hazards.

In summary, the oldest alcoholic drinks were fermented beverages of relatively low alcoholic content (beers and wines). The alchemists, at the dawn of history, believed that alcohol was the long-sought elixir of life and was the remedy for practically all diseases. It is now recognized that the therapeutic value of alcohol is much more limited than its social value.

## D. PHARMACOKINETICS AND METABOLISM OF ALCOHOL AND ALCOHOLIC BEVERAGES IN THE BODY

The quantity of alcohol consumed will have varying effects on the body, however, there is a complexity of other factors that are important in determining the effect of wine, beer, and distilled spirits. Plain alcohol, for example, has different actions on the body than do alcoholic beverages. It is for this reason that pure ethanol is discussed separately, followed by a discussion of the alcoholic beverages. Once the alcohol is in the body, it is handled similarly, at least with regard to its pharmacologic effects; thus only pure ethanol is discussed when dealing with effects on organ systems.

**TABLE 11-3**

**Alcoholic Beverages**

| | | |
|---|---|---|
| Whiskey | = | 50% ethyl alcohol (volume) |
| Wine | = | 11–20% ethyl alcohol (volume) |
| Beer | = | 4.5% ethyl alcohol (volume) |

(From Becker, C. E., Roe, L. R., and Scott, R. A. *Alcohol as a Drug: A Curriculum on Pharmacology and Toxicology*. New York: Medcom Press, 1974. Modified with permission.)

## 1. Absorption of Ethanol[3] and Alcoholic Beverages[7]

Alcohol is rapidly absorbed from the stomach, small intestine, and colon. Vaporized alcohol can be absorbed through the lungs and fatal intoxication has occurred as a result of its inhalation. Many factors modify the rate of absorption of alcohol from the stomach, such as the volume, character, and dilution of the alcoholic beverage. The presence of food, the time it takes to ingest the drink, and individual peculiarities are major influences on the rate at which the stomach empties. Depending upon these factors, complete absorption may require from two to six hours or more. Most foods in the stomach tend to retard absorption, milk being especially efficacious in this respect. Beer exerts a retarding action, like that of food. On the other hand, absorption from the small intestine is extremely rapid and complete, and is independent of both the concentration of alcohol and the presence of food.

Certain amino acids such as glycine have been found to delay absorption of alcohol from the gastrointestinal tract.

Ethyl alcohol consists of a hydroxyl group attached to a two-carbon hydrocarbon chain. It is moderately polar; it forms hydrogen bonds readily; like water, it exhibits intermolecular association and has a high rate of hydrogen ion conductance in an electric field; it is infinitely soluble in water. These properties help us to understand the *in vivo* phenomena of absorption, distribution, excretion, and metabolism. It is generally agreed that ethyl alcohol is absorbed across the biologic membranes of the gastrointestinal tract by simple diffusion, and it has been shown that the rate of alcohol absorption *in vivo* is affected by alcohol concentration, regional blood flow, and the absorbing surface. Evidence suggests that there is rapid absorption from the

**TABLE 11-4**

**Metric Conversion of Common Quantities of Alcoholic Beverages**

*Standard U.S. volumes*
- 1-oz shot = 30 cc = 30 g
- 2-oz shot = 60 cc = 60 g
- 1 pt = 16 1-oz shots = 480 cc
- Tenth = ½ bottle = 12.8 oz = 380 cc
- Fifth = ⅘ of 1 qt = 25.6 oz = 768 cc
- 1 qt = 32 1-oz shots = 960 cc
- Magnum = 2 fifths = 1510 cc

*French volumes (red wine)*
- ½ bottle = 12.68 oz = 375 cc
- Bottle = 25.36 oz = 750 cc
- Magnum = 2 bottles = 50.71 oz = 1500 cc
- Marie Jeanne = 84.53 oz = 2500 cc
- Double magnum = 4 bottles = 101.42 oz = 3000 cc
- Jeroboam = 6 bottles = 152.16 oz = 4500 cc
- Imperial = 8 bottles = 202.85 oz = 6000 cc

*Champagne*
- Split = ¼ bottle = 6.76 oz = 200 cc
- Pint = ½ bottle = 13.52 oz = 400 cc
- Quart = 1 bottle = 27.05 oz = 800 cc
- Magnum = 2 bottles = 54.09 oz = 1600 cc
- Jeroboam = 4 bottles = 108.19 oz = 3200 cc
- Rehoboam = 6 bottles = 162.28 oz = 4800 cc
- Methuselah = 8 bottles = 216.37 oz = 6400 cc
- Salmanazar = 12 bottles = 324.46 oz = 9600 cc
- Balthazar = 16 bottles = 432.74 oz. = 12,800 cc
- Nebuchadnezzar = 20 bottles = 540.93 oz = 16,000 cc

(From Becker, C. E., Roe, L. R., and Scott, R. A. *Alcohol as a Drug: A Curriculum on Pharmacology and Toxicology.* New York: Medcom Press, 1974. With permission.)

duodenum and jejunum; slower absorption from the stomach, ileum, and colon; and minimal absorption from the mouth. Because of this differential in diffusion rate, it is obvious that the rapidity of absorption in the human subject depends upon the rate at which alcohol passes from the stomach to the duodenum.

Under ordinary conditions, the alcohol in any beverage is absorbed relatively quickly—some through the stomach, but most through the small intestine—and then distributed generally throughout the body. The absorption can be markedly influenced by a number of factors.[7–9]

1. Alcohol concentration. The greater the alcohol concentration of the beverage (up to a maximum of about 40 percent, or 80 proof, the more rapidly the alcohol is absorbed and the higher is the resulting peak blood alcohol concentration. With identical amounts of alcohol swallowed, the highest blood alcohol levels are produced by undiluted distilled spirits, and the lowest by esters.

2. Other chemicals in the beverage. The greater the amount of nonalcoholic chemicals in the beverage, the more slowly the alcohol is absorbed. For this reason, too, the alcohol in distilled spirits—especially vodka and gin—is absorbed most rapidly and that in table wines and beers most slowly.

3. Presence of food in the stomach. Eating with drinking has a notable effect on the absorption of alcohol, especially when alcohol is consumed in the form of distilled spirits or wine. When alcoholic beverages are taken with a substantial meal, peak blood alcohol concentrations may be reduced by as much as 50 percent.

4. Speed of drinking. The more rapidly the beverage is ingested, the higher will be the peak blood alcohol concentrations. Thus these levels are lower when the beverage is sipped or taken in divided amounts than when it is gulped or taken in a single dose.

5. Emptying time of the stomach. In a number of clinical conditions, such as that marked by the "dumping syndrome," the stomach empties more rapidly than is normal, and alcohol seems to be absorbed more quickly. Emptying time may be either slowed or speeded by fear, anger, stress, nausea, and the condition of the stomach tissues.

6. Body weight. The greater the body weight of an individual, the lower will be the blood alcohol concentration resulting from ingestion of a standard amount of alcohol. The blood alcohol level produced in a 180-pound man consuming 4 ounces of distilled spirits, for example, will generally be substantially lower than that occurring when the same amount is taken by a 130-pound man in the same length of time.

## 2. Distribution[3]

Once absorption has occurred, distribution takes place rapidly, since alcohol diffuses readily across capillary walls. This rapid diffusion has been well studied in the lung and brain, and can be anticipated to occur across all other capillary surfaces in the body as well. Since ethanol also rapidly diffuses across cell membranes, allowing prompt equilibration of intra- and extracellular concentrations, it is obvious that only a limited number of anatomic and physiologic parameters can affect the rate of ethanol equilibration between the intravascular space and any tissue mass. These factors are the total surface area of the capillaries within the tissue mass, the average intercapillary distance between those capillaries, and the fraction of the cardiac output that perfuses the tissue mass per unit time. Thus, after intravenous bolus infusion of ethanol, the brain and kidney equilibrate with the circulating blood concentration in less than ten minutes, while skeletal muscle requires more than an hour. When ethyl alcohol is ingested by mouth, distribution parameters are somewhat more complex, since with decreasing absorption, tissues with the greatest perfusion (i.e., those with the greatest vascularity and the highest percentage of cardiac output) will rapidly lose the capillary–tissue concentration difference and begin to give up alcohol.

If static tissue concentrations are determined, the ethyl alcohol concentration in any tissue will be proportional to the water content of that tissue, because the lipid–water partition coefficient of ethanol is quite low. Thus tissues with a high lipid content, such as the brain, will have a lower alcohol concentration (milligrams per gram of tissue), while tissues or body fluids with a high water content, such as the testes, cerebrospinal fluid, and urine, will contain a high alcohol concentration. Recall that ethanol diffuses readily from blood to alveolar air. Since analysis of expired air is relatively easy using the Breathalyzer® and gas chromatographic methods, many studies have been carried out to establish the blood–breath partition coefficient of ethanol and to validate blood alcohol values estimated from breath analysis. In general, the concentration of alcohol in expired air is lower than in blood; the discrepancy is particularly greater at higher blood levels of alcohol.

## 3. Elimination[3]

Ethyl alcohol is eliminated from the body by excretion via breath, urine, and sweat, and by metabolism, primarily in the liver, but in other tissues as well. The rate of elimination is the sum of the rates of these phenomena. Excretion follows first-order kinetics (fixed percentage per unit time) since the excretion of alcohol is based almost entirely on diffusion and is therefore proportionate to the blood alcohol concentration. Thus the longer the blood alcohol concentration remains high, the greater will be the proportion of the dose excreted rather than metabolized. Nevertheless the total amount of alcohol excreted via breath, sweat, and urine is usually 5 percent or less of an administered dose, although, if the combination of very high blood levels and forced diuresis pertains, up to 10 percent may be excreted. Therefore most of an ingested dose of alcohol must be removed from the body by metabolism. In a 70-kg man, the rate of metabolism approximates 8 g/hr; a cocktail made with 2 ounces of 86 proof bourbon contains 26 grams of alcohol.

## 4. Metabolism of Alcohol in the Body[14]

The enzyme primarily responsible for the metabolism of ethanol is alcohol dehydrogenase, which is found almost exclusively in the liver. This enzyme converts ethanol to alcetaldehyde, the enzyme aldehyde dehydrogenase, then catalyzes the oxidation of acetaldehyde in the presence of nicotinamide adenosine dinucleotide (NAD) and coenzyme A to acetyl CoA as follows:

$$\text{(1)}\quad \underset{\text{(Ethanol)}}{C_2H_5OH} + NAD^+ \xrightarrow[\text{Dehydrogenase}]{\text{Alcohol}} NAD.H + H^+ + \underset{\text{(Acetaldehyde)}}{CH_3CHO}$$

$$\text{(2)}\quad \underset{\text{(Acetaldehyde)}}{CH_3\,CHO} + NAD^+ + HS-CoA \xrightarrow[\text{Dehydrogenase}]{\text{Aldehyde}} NAD.H + H + \underset{\text{(Acetyl CoA)}}{CH_3Co-S-CoA}$$

Another enzyme responsible for the metabolism of alcohol is catalase, which is found in the microsomes of the cell. It appears that catalase (peroxidase) is not a rate-limiting step in ethanol metabolism. In fact, some investigators, such as Lieber and Rubin,[4,5] believe that another system referred to as the microsomal ethanol oxidizing system (MEOS) may be very important in the metabolism of alcohol in the body.

About 98 percent of the alcohol that is absorbed is completely oxidized to $CO_2$ and water. The metabolism of alcohol differs from that of most other substances in that the rate of oxidation is a linear function of time and is only moderately increased by raising the concentration in the blood. The amount oxidized per unit time is roughly proportional to body weight, and probably to liver weight, and, in the adult, the average rate at which 100 percent ethanol can be metabolized is about 10 ml per hour (8 grams). The relatively slow and constant rate of metabolism places a definite limit on the amount of alcohol that can be consumed over a given period of time. The energy released per gram of ethanol is about 7 kilocalories.

Various dietary, hormonal, and pharmacologic factors have been reported to alter the metabolism of alcohol. For example, starvation decreases, insulin increases, and thyroxin has no significant effect on alcohol metabolism.

### 5. Alcohol Kinetics

Research has demonstrated that the rate of alcohol metabolism, like that of alcohol absorption, may be influenced by a number of factors. A Massachusetts General Hospital study has shown that both alcoholic and nonalcoholic subjects maintained on good diets can moderately increase their rate of alcohol metabolism if they consume substantial amounts over a long period of time. In general, it appears that the rate of alcohol metabolism may have a small influence on behavioral tolerance to alcohol, but that no significant differences in ability to oxidize alcohol differentiate the alcoholic from the nonalcoholic.[15] At the Karolinska Institute in Stockholm, it has been reported that normal drinkers can metabolize on the average approximately 7 grams per hour of pure alcohol; 8 grams in the form of whiskey; 9 grams in the form of dessert wines; 12 grams in the form of table wines; and 9 to 11 grams in the form of beer.[9]

Considerable effort has been devoted to a search for some method that can effectively speed the rate of alcohol metabolism and thus be useful in the treatment of intoxication. Particular interest has been expressed in the administration of insulin, tri-iodothyronine, fructose, and other agents, although none has yet been found to make any clinically significant difference in the rate of alcohol metabolism.[16]

## E. PHARMACOLOGY OF ALCOHOL

Ethyl alcohol is a clear liquid with a fiery taste, is miscible with water, and is inflammable in concentrations over 50 percent. It has been used throughout the years as an important solvent for drugs, as a topical antiseptic and irritant, and for its systemic actions. Ethyl alcohol has a wide range of actions on most systems of the body.

### 1. Acute Actions

#### *a. General Brain Effects*

The main pharmacologic effect of alcohol is to depress the CNS over a wide range of doses. It is commonly thought that alcohol may elicit stimulation in humans through the depression of inhibitions. This concept has been generally accepted since it was first proposed by Schmeidelberg in 1902. (However, the concept of alcohol-induced depression is being actively researched and no definitive conclusions have been reached as yet.) Like the barbiturates and other general anesthetics, alcohol depresses, first, the reticular activating system (RAS), which integrates the activity of all other parts of the nervous system. Release of the cortex from the integrating action of the reticular activating system leads to disruption of both motor and thought processes.

The result of depression of these regulators is to release repressed feeling, hence the widespread social use of alcohol and the false idea concerning its stimulatory properties. The drinker may become too euphoric to recognize muscular incoordination, a lengthened reaction time, and loss of visual acuity and behavioral inhibitions. An early sign of the depressant action is dilation of the pupils with sluggish light reflex, nystagmus, and reddening of the conjunctiva. A sign of severe intoxication is the occurrence of double vision.

Although some types of achievement may be facilitated by the release of inhibitions, the performance of most tasks is impaired. The power of muscular coordination is affected at an early stage and tremor and difficulty in performing certain tasks that require skill and concentration are noted long before the production of slurred speech, sagging facial muscles, and staggering gait. Reflexes are diminished only slowly, but ultimately may be more or less extinguished as coma deepens and death from respiratory and cardiovascular failure approaches.

It is important to note that tasks involving complicated mental problems are decreased; habitual tasks requiring less skill, thought, and attention are less markedly affected.

In general, the effects of alcohol on the CNS are proportional to the concentration of alcohol in the blood. Unlike the volatile anesthetics, the margin of safety between surgical anesthesia and death is very low.

It is impossible to state the specific amounts of alcoholic beverages that will give specific concentrations of alcohol in the blood. In general, it has been found that a 155-pound moderate drinker rapidly consuming 90 proof whiskey on an empty stomach will probably have a peak blood alcohol level of 0.05 percent—0.05 gram per 100 cc of blood—with 3 ounces, 0.10 with 6 ounces, 0.20 with 12 ounces, and 0.30 with 15 ounces.[17]

The blood alcohol level may be slightly higher if the drink is gin or vodka rather than whiskey, or if the drinker weighs much less than 155 pounds. The level will be lower if the beverage is beer or wine, if the drinking is spaced over a prolonged period, if the drinker weighs more than 155 pounds, or if solid foods are eaten at the same time.

These levels have important legal implications. In most parts of the United States, and in some countries in Europe, an individual legally is presumed to be sober and able to operate a motor vehicle with a blood alcohol level of 0.15 percent or less, whereas one with a level of 0.15 or more is legally intoxicated or "under the influence."

### *b. Special Brain Effects*[7]

The most notable and dramatic effects of alcohol are those on behavior attributed to the action of alcohol on the brain. These are related not necessarily to the amount of alcohol drunk, but to the concentration in the blood. Very low blood alcohol levels usually produce mild sedation, relaxation, or tranquility. Slightly higher levels may produce behavioral changes that seem to suggest stimulation of the brain—garrulousness, aggressiveness, and excessive activity—but that may result from depression of the brain centers that normally inhibit or restrain such behavior. At still higher levels, greater depression of the brain occurs, producing incoordination, confusion, disorientation, stupor anesthesia, coma, and death.

Because of the variations among individuals, it is not possible to give the exact concentrations at which these changes occur. For most people, however, it is usually accepted that blood alcohol levels up to 0.05 percent will induce some sedation or tranquility; 0.05 to 0.15 may produce lack of coordination; at about 0.15 to 0.20, intoxication is obvious; 0.30 or 0.40 may produce unconsciousness; and levels of 0.50 or more may be fatal.

Earlier investigators proposed that these actions of alcohol resulted from direct effects on relevant parts of the brain—first the cerebral cortex, the most highly developed portion of the brain, depressing critical faculties and reasoning powers, and producing the behavior pattern characteristic of drunkenness. With larger doses, it was believed, alcohol would directly depress successively lower levels of the brain, eventually striking vital centers of the medulla, such as the one that controls respiration.

Later observations, however, have led investigators to suggest that alcohol may act from the start upon a regulatory structure, which in turn modifies the activity of the cortex and other parts of the nervous system. This regulatory structure is the reticular formation, the so-called master switchboard or activating system of the brain. Even under the influence of low blood alcohol concentrations, it has been found that the reticular formation not only affects brain function, but also serves as an intermediary in producing the sensation of warmth, flushing of the skin, relaxation of muscles, reduction of blood pressure in peripheral vessels, stimulation of gastric secretion, and increased peristalsis—all typical reactions to alcohol.[15]

It has not been clearly established whether

there is a threshold below which alcohol has no detectable influence on reflex responses, reaction time, and various complex skills. When the blood level reaches 0.03 or 0.04 percent, it is generally agreed that changes are evident.[19]

At very low blood alcohol levels, such simple reflex responses as the knee jerk seem to be more rapid. At levels above 0.03 or 0.04, reflex responses, reaction-time responses, and performances in such activities as automobile driving and many kinds of athletics generally change for the worse. Significantly, as drinking impairs performance, a driver's judgment often deteriorates, and the driver believes that he or she is driving even better. A British investigator has found that, for motorists, the added risk is small and probably not significant up to about 0.05. Above that level, the risk increases sharply.

Levels of consumption have impact on other functions as well, including respiration and brain wave activity.

While it is indicated that human respiration may be initially accelerated by alcohol when ingested in moderation, there is a high likelihood of depression of respiration, even to the point of lethality, when induced by large doses (400 mg or more). The same depressive activity can be seen in the retardation of brain wave rhythms observed throughout EEG, deteriorating in direct/obverse ratio to the increase of alcohol consumption. Alcohol withdrawal may impact the EEG with dysrhythmic spikes and abnormal patterns that have not yet been demonstrated as reliable predictors of potential convulsive behavior.

The suppression of convulsions in laboratory animals has been achieved through alcohol in quantities large enough to induce general depression of the central nervous system. On the other hand, convulsions as a symptom of second stage withdrawal in some alcoholics may begin as early as 12 hours after the beginning of abstinence, and can range in severity from minor to epilectic and lethal in nature. In fact, ethanol has been shown to bring on convulsions in humans, and is contraindicated in the treatment of epilepsy.

There has been little or no success to date in efforts to reveal a metabolic base for the effects of alcohol on the central nervous system. An unsuccessful search for brain alcohol and aldehyde dehydogenase enzymes and the artifactual presence of acetaldehyde following alcohol consumption are prime examples. Hence, the question of alcohol's impact on intermediate metabolites and tissue oxygenation remains unresolved at this time.

### *c. Body Temperature*

The primary effect of ethyl alcohol with regard to body temperature is that it lowers it, but it may instead (or also) lead to general failure to thermoregulate well. Thus in a hotter than normal environment ethanol might lead to fever. After the ingestion of alcohol, there is a feeling of warmth because alcohol induces dilation of the peripheral blood vessels (enhanced cutaneous flow) and gastric flow. Increased sweating may also occur. Heat thus is lost more rapidly and the internal temperature consequently falls. The action of alcohol in lowering body temperature is greater when the environmental temperature is low or when mechanisms for dissipating heat are disturbed, as during fever. The taking of alcoholic beverages to keep warm in cold weather is obviously irrational, and may be dangerous if the conservation of body heat is essential. Under these conditions, blood is needed in the central parts of the body and heat loss must be diminished.

### *d. Heart and Circulatory System*

While cardiovascular effects of alcohol are minor in practically every instance, there are certain circumstances that can lead quickly to lethal consequences.[98] Cutaneous vasodilation caused by moderate doses of alcohol can prevent the reflex cutaneous vasoconstriction required in response to cold, and an intoxicated individual will succumb more rapidly to hypothermia—despite popular myths to the contrary about the efficacy of St. Bernard dogs and their casks of cognac for stranded travelers in the frozen Alps. Another myth exaggerates the beneficial use of alcohol as a vasodilator for coronary circulation. The action of alcohol on blood vessels has been demonstrated as insignificant, and there is little, if any, support for the prescription of moderate doses of alcohol daily for angina patients. It is thought that vitamin deficiency and malnutrition are more likely culprits for cardiovascular abnormalities than is the direct effect of alcohol found to be deleterious to the cardiovascular system.

### *e. Gastrointestinal and Urogenital System*

Alcohol's impact as an irritant inducing gastrointestinal responses is well documented.[98] Inflammation of the GI tract, gastritis, diahhrea, vomiting, hemorrhaging and ulceration are but a few of the potential results of alcohol usage and abuse. Prolonged intoxication can shut down the motor and secretory activities of the entire GI tract. On the other hand, alcohol may stimulate gastric secretions through sensory excitation, and can also encourage secretion of hydrochloric acid (HCL), a less than desirable phenomenon for peptic ulcer sufferers.

Alcohol usually exerts a diuretic effect through the ingestion of large amounts of other fluids, as well as by inhibition of anti-diuretic hormone from the posterior pituitary.

In alcoholic patients, it has been shown that, on initiation of drinking, aldosterone levels rise, then fall to abnormally low levels, and then return to approximately normal values with continued drinking. This, of course, would have a profound influence on salt and water metabolism in the alcoholic subject.

But while salt and water have been basic necessities for centuries of human survival, alcohol is one of the world's oldest alleged aphrodisiacs, and a popular ingredient of our sexual drives and needs. There is no denying that aggressive sexual behavior often follows quickly on the heels of alcohol consumption. Even moderate ingestion can help in the lowering of inhibitions and the loosening of societal restraints. Shakespeare's oft-quoted phrase is still relevant today, however, noting that ''[alcohol] . . . provokes the desire, but it takes away the performance.'' See Chapter 20 for additional information on this subject.

### *f. The Liver*

There is a wide range of liver dysfunctions that can be found in alcoholics, from the mildest form of ''fatty liver'' to the most severe form of cirrhosis. Speculation abounds as to the relative significance of genetics, vitamin and nutritional deficiencies, environmental factors, and the sheer amount of alcohol abuse itself. Fat may accumulate in the livers of normal individuals following moderate consumption of alcohol. Teenagers may develop severely advanced cirrhosis. Necrosis of liver cells and accompanying inflammation may become significant with continued heavy drinking, and is a condition that is called alcoholic hepatitis—a serious, sometimes deadly condition. Nonetheless, the complications of cirrhosis are found in only about 10 percent of all alcoholics, and is by no means limited to alcoholics. However, when cirrhosis does occur in the alcoholic, it is usually found after many years of heavy drinking habits.

### *g. Performance (Skeletal Muscle)*

Performance may be increased in the short term with low to moderate consumption of alcohol, as a result of lower perceived fatigue levels. However, the larger the doses of alcohol, the less muscular work that is performed, primarily as a result of CNS depression springing from the increased alcohol intake.

### *h. Hormonal Effects*

The moderate consumption of alcohol prompts stimulation of adrenal medulla or postganglionic nerve endings which results in increased urinary excretion of catecholamines. During early intoxication stages, the pupillary dilation, transient hyperglycemia and slight increase of blood pressure which follow, may be partially attributable to this catecholamine phenomenon.

### *i. Deficiency Diseases*

In the past, alcohol has been held responsible for a wide variety of diseases often seen in heavy drinkers, including "gin-drinker's heart," "beer-drinker's heart," "wine-drinker's stomach," irritations of the mucous membranes of the mouth, Wernicke's disease, Korsakoff's disease, and "alcoholic pellagra." Physicians generally believe these conditions are caused mainly by nutritional deficiencies.[23,24]

### *j. Resistance to Infection*

The lowered resistance of alcoholics to pneumonia and other infectious diseases has long been known, and is usually attributed to malnutrition. Research at Cornell University has shown that lowered resistance may also occur in well-nourished heavy drinkers, and appears to result from a direct interference with immunity mechanisms. With blood alcohol levels of 0.15 to 0.25 percent, produced by intravenous administration of alcohol, the inhibition of white blood cell mobilization was found to be as intense as that found in states of severe shock.[25]

### *k. Gout*[7]

An old tradition is the belief that port wine is the cause of gout. A nationwide study conducted by a group of investigators at the University of California has shown, however, that more than 60 percent of all gouty patients had never drunk wine in any form before the onset of their disease. In patients whose gouty attacks seem to be precipitated by ingestion of alcohol, physicians have often noted that such factors as mental stress, infection, cessation of physical exercise, or ingestion of purine-rich foods were also involved.

### *l. The Hangover*[7]

The hangover is a common, unpleasant, but rarely dangerous aftereffect of overindulgence affecting the moderate drinker who occasionally takes too much, as well as the excessive drinker after a prolonged drinking bout. The exact mechanism is unknown. The symptoms are most severe many hours after the peak of the drinking bout, when little or no alcohol can be detected in the body.[26] Although hangover has been blamed on mixing drinks, it can be produced by any alcoholic beverage alone, or by pure alcohol. There is inadequate evidence to support beliefs that it is caused by vitamin deficiencies, dehydration, fusel oils, or any other nonalcoholic component.

No satisfactory specific treatment for hangover is known, and there is no scientific evidence to support such popular remedies as coffee, raw egg, oysters, chili peppers, steak sauce, "alkalizers," vitamin preparations, or such drugs as barbiturates, thyroid, amphetamine, and insulin. For general treatment, physicians usually prescribe aspirin, bed rest, and ingestion of solid foods as soon as possible.

### *m. Effects on Longevity*[7]

There is little evidence to demonstrate whether or not drinking has an appreciable effect on longevity. Frequently cited are the findings of Raymond Pearl, who reported the shortest life expectancy for heavy drinkers, a somewhat higher expectancy for abstainers, and the highest for moderate drinkers.[27]

## F. NEUROPHYSIOLOGIC EFFECTS OF ALCOHOL

It is known that the CNS is more markedly affected by alcohol than is any other system of the body. However, not all areas of the brain are affected equally. In fact, the cortex does not seem to be the part of the brain that is most sensitive to the action of alcohol. As previously mentioned, electrophysiologic studies[28] suggest that alcohol, like other general anesthetics, exerts its first depressant action upon a more primitive part of the brain, namely, the reticular activating system. The basic neurologic and physiologic effects of alcohol have been reviewed by Kalant[28] and Mardones[29] and, more recently, by Majchrowicz and Noble.[30]

### 1. Membrane-Receptor Effects of Alcohol

At high concentrations, ethanol is capable of disorganizing neuronal membrane structure.[31] Chronic ethanol administration to animals has been found to produce changes in the conformation of membrane-bound proteins.[32] Chin and Goldstein[33] showed, by a sensitive electron paramagnetic resonance (EPR) technique, that low concentrations of ethanol increased the fluidity of mouse erythrocyte and synaptosomal plasma membranes. Additionally, in other studies, the same authors reported that tolerance to ethanol developed to this effect.[33] Of great interest was the finding that ethanol altered the lipid composition of neuronal membranes.[34,35] Although ethanol could directly modify the characteristics of activities of membrane-bound proteins, it has also been demonstrated that membrane microenvironment is a critical regulator of the function of enzymes embedded in cell membranes.[36-38] In this regard, it has been suggested by Hoffman et al.[39] that adaptive modifications of neuronal membrane lipids after ethanol treatment could be expected to result in the observed conformational changes of the membrane-bound proteins.

Numerous studies[40] on the effects of ethanol on neurotransmitter function have already been reviewed. According to the consensus of the literature, the interaction of ethanol with neuronal membranes may also account in part for its diverse effects on neurotransmitter turnover and release. Since neurotransmitter receptors in the CNS have been demonstrated to respond to decreases or increases in the availability of their particular transmitters with adaptive changes that lead to altered sensitivity to these transmitters,[41,42] it might be postulated that ethanol exposure would secondarily alter receptor function. In this regard, the existence of a direct correlation between receptor interaction and alcohol membrane partition coefficients is plausible. There are studies that support[43] and that refute[44] this view.

Work by Tabakoff and coresearchers showed that ethanol could alter the receptor microenvironment. Chronic administration of ethanol to mice, for example, resulted in abnormal function of striated dopamine (DA) receptors, possibly as a result of ethanol-induced modification of neuronal membrane structure.[45,46] Specifically Hoffman et al.[39] report that the membrane-bound enzyme ($Na^+ - K^+$) ATPase, obtained from ethanol-withdrawn animals, displays an altered transition temperature and resistance to the effects of ethanol on enzyme activity. These changes also suggest compensatory alterations in neuronal membrane properties. Additional support is derived from the work of Rangaraj and Kalant,[47] similarly demonstrating that norepinephrine can alter the inhibitory effects of ethanol on ($NA^+ - K^+$)ATPase activity of rat neuronal membranes. These findings, therefore, suggest that the norepinephrine–ethanol interaction is a direct action on the membrane, probably mediated by an α-receptor modified perturbation of the membrane microenvironment of the enzyme.

## 2. Brain-Neurotransmitter Receptor/Effector Coupling Effects of Ethanol

Central nervous system actions of ethanol may reflect alterations in the properties of one or more neurotransmitter receptor/effector systems. Prolonged treatment of rats with ethanol has been reported to result in changes in the cortical sensitivity to norepinephrine as measured by cyclic AMP accumulation.[48] Banerjee et al.[49] reported that administration of ethanol for 60 days resulted in a decrease in the density of β-adrenergic receptors in whole rat brain while receptor density was increased after 48 and 72 hours of withdrawal. It is of great interest that these changes were not associated with changes in the affinity of the receptor for the radioligand [$^3$H]-dihydroalprenolol.

Early studies[50] revealed that dopamine, when administered in conjunction with ethanol, prolonged ethanol-induced narcosis in mice. In 1974, Hunt and Majchrowicz[51] demonstrated that both acute and chronic administration of ethanol have a biphasic effect on dopamine turnover with no alterations in dopamine content. Along these lines, Blum et al.[52] demonstrated that ethanol-induced withdrawal convulsions in mice could be significantly suppressed by low concentrations of dopamine injections. Tabakoff et al.[45] reported a reduction in the effect of dopaminergic agonists on locomotor activity and body temperature during withdrawal following chronic ethanol treatment. These investigators also demonstrated that dopamine-stimulated adenylate cyclase activity in the striatum was reduced in mice withdrawn from ethanol for 24 hours.[53,54] Conversely Engel and Liljequist[55] and Liljequist[56] showed that rats treated with ethanol for five to nine months displayed an increase in locomotor activity after the bilateral application of dopamine into the nucleus accumbens or striatum, suggesting that an increased sensitivity to dopamine occurs following ethanol administration.

Although Rabin and Molinoff[57] found altered norepinephrine sensitivity in animals chronically treated and withdrawn from ethanol, no change in cyclic AMP accumulation in cortical slices was observed with either α-adrenergic or β-adrenergic receptor stimulation. Furthermore no difference in dopamine-stimulated adenylate cyclase activity was observed in either ethanol-treated mice or in animals withdrawn from ethanol for 24 hours.[57] It is possible, however, that a decrease in dopamine-stimulated adenylate cyclase occurs only in severely withdrawing mice, as suggested by Tabakoff (personal communication).

It is known that ethanol administration also induces changes in central cholinergic systems. The acute administration of ethanol depresses both the *in vivo*[58,59] and *in vitro* release of acetylcholine.[60]

Chronic ethanol administration reduces the content of acetylcholine in the hippocampus[61] and cortex[62] and eliminates the depressant action of ethanol on the *in vitro* release of acetylcholine.[60] In addition, both ethanol-induced electroencephalographic synchrony[63] and ethanol-induced sleep time[64] are antagonized by the acetylcholinesterase inhibitor physostigmine.

Although neurotransmitter turnover may change with acute and chronic ethanol administration, and neurotransmitter precursor amines may influence ethanol intoxication, dependence, and withdrawal, studies designed to determine direct effects on numerous receptor sites reveal no apparent significant alterations.[65]

In the Hunt et al.[65] investigations, ethanol did not alter [$^3$H]-haloperidol binding to study dopaminergic receptors, or [$^3$H]-3-quinuclidinyl benzilate (QNB) binding to study muscarinic cholinergic receptors.

In spite of these negative observations, recently Davis and Ticku[44] demonstrated that ethanol enhanced [$^3$H]-diazepam binding at the benzodiazepine-γ-aminobutyric acid receptor-ionophore complex. The rank order of enhancement of [$^3$H]-diazepam binding with various alcohols (ethanol > methanol > isopropyl alcohol > propanol-l or t-butyl alcohol) did not agree with their partition coefficients. These results suggest that ethanol, like pentobarbital, enhances [$^3$H]-diazepam binding at the benzodiazepine-γ-aminobutyric acid (GABA) receptor-ionophore complex. This interaction will result in facilitation of GABAergic transmission and may be responsible for some of the central effects of alcohol, such as antianxiety, muscle relaxation, and sedation. In addition, these results by Davis and Ticku[44] may also explain the synergistic effects observed with alcohol and diazepam *in vivo* and the use of antianxiety drugs as agents of choice during alcohol withdrawal.

The cited literature reveals that acute and chronic administration of ethanol can affect neurotransmitter function, but it must be emphasized that neurotransmitter systems should not be examined in isolation. Studies on the neurophysiology and biochemistry of brain neurotransmitter receptor-coupling mechanisms are necessary to understand adequately the mechanisms that mediate ethanol-induced neurologic and behavioral decrements.

## 3. The Cyclic Nucleotide "Model" of Alcohol Tolerance and Dependence

Cyclic nucleotides seem to function in the brain as mediators or "second messengers" of first messages communicated by such agents as neurotransmitters, hormones, and "local modulators."[66–69] Recently Siggins[70] commented on cyclic nucleotides in the development of alcohol tolerance and dependence, and the interested reader is strongly urged to review this paper.

According to Siggins, the "homeostatic" modulations of the norepinephrine adenylate cyclase systems with alterations of functional norepinephrine levels, suggested by biochemical[71] and electrophysiologic experiments, present a hypothetical model for alcohol tolerance and dependence. Siggins proposes an interaction between the neurotransmitters, norepinephrine and acetylcholine, and alcohol.

It is known that norepinephrine normally inhibits, and acetylcholine excites, pyramidal neurons to the extent that norepinephrine can prevent and acetylcholine can augment, or even trigger, epileptiform activity.[72] These responses are thought to be mediated by cyclic AMP and cyclic GMP respectively.[73]

Alcohol in this system could cause an increased release of norepinephrine.[74,75] With continued alcohol administration, the norepinephrine –receptor–adenylate cyclase system would respond by down-regulation to adjust to the increased local norepinephrine, while converse changes might occur in the acetylcholine-guanylate cyclase system. Abrupt removal of alcohol treatment would then find the diminished norepinephrine–adenylate cyclase system incapable of dampening the enhanced excitatory acetylcholine system, with the result that seizures develop. Similar sequelae could apply to the cerebral cortex with the production of motor convulsions.

The Siggins model seems to agree with pharmacologic studies indicating that decreases in brain norepinephrine exacerbate the convulsions following alcohol withdrawal.[76] Furthermore intraventricular administration of dibutyryl cyclic GMP increases the severity of alcohol withdrawal symptoms in mice, while dibutyryl cyclic AMP administration decreases the symptoms.[70]

Although this proposal seems logical, it may be an oversimplification in that it does not involve other systems such as the peptidyl opiates, substance P, and other biologically active brain endogenous substances.

## 4. Neuropathologic Actions of Alcohol

Certainly ethanol produces alterations of the electrophysiologic pattern in the brain.[77] The response is complex, for example, using extracellular recordings of single neurons, iontophoretic and micropressure application of ethanol-depressed cerebellar Purkinje cells in a concentration-dependent manner. The depressions appear to be nonspecific, and local anesthetic-like in nature, however, since they are often accompanied by a reduction in spike size with broadening of the spike duration. In accord with this interpretation, and in contrast to previous reports,[78] Siggins and French[77] found that the inhibitions of activity produced by either iontophoretic GABA or norepinephrine were antagonized nonspecifically by direct application of alcohol to Purkinje cells.

In spite of the complex nature of the electrophysiologic properties of ethanol, a variety of neuropathologic[79,80] and neuropsychologic[81] alterations have been observed and delineated in chronic alcoholics. Initially this observed brain damage and the resulting impairment in learning and memory were attributed to malnutrition, especially thiamine deficiency,[82] rather than to the direct neurotoxic effects of ethanol. Nevertheless both neuropathologic[83] and neuropsychologic[84] deficits have been observed in long-term alcoholic patients with no history of malnutrition.

Furthermore Walker and Hunter[85] reported that long-term ethanol exposure results in a residual impairment in the acquisition of a variety of behavioral tasks. Other work by Riley and Walker[86] demonstrated that four months of ethanol consumption by mature mice resulted in a 50 to 60 percent loss of dendritic spines on hippocampal pyramidal cells and dentate gyrus granule cells. Interpretation of the cited study strongly suggests that long-term ethanol consumption, in the absence of malnutrition, produces neuronal loss in the CNS. Additionally it is plausible that the residual learning and memory deficits induced by long-term ethanol consumption in animals[87] and humans[88] may be related in part to hippocampal damage; or, as suggested by Victor et al.[80] for alcoholic Korsakoff patients, the dorsomedial thalamus is correlated with impaired memory.

Although it is clear that prolonged ethanol consumption can have neuropathologic consequences despite good nutrition, the exact mechanism by which it does so remains unclear. Speculations include:

1. Ethanol or a metabolite would be directly neurotoxic.
2. It could exert its effect by inhibiting neuronal protein synthesis.
3. It could do so by altering cerebral blood flow, resulting in chronic ischemia.[89]

Further research in which quantitative behavioral neurohistologic, neurophysiologic data are obtained in ethanol-dependent and nutritionally controlled animals and humans should help to clarify the relationships among the behavioral neuropathologic consequences of alcohol abuse.

## 5. Biogenic Amines and Alcohol[90–93]

Many recent papers describe the ability of alcohol to shift the metabolism of serotonin *in vitro* and *in vivo* from the "normal" 5-hydroxylindoleacetic acid (5HIAA) end product to the neutrals, 5-hydroxyindoleacetaldehyde and 5-hydroxytryptophol. Of course, an analogous alteration in the metabolism of catecholamines can also occur as a result of alcohol treatment. Recently both tryptophols and 3,4-dihydroxyphenylethanol have been found to augment the actions of alcohol. This finding, coupled with the observation that p-chlorophenylalanine (a serotonin depletor) and α-methylparatyrosine (a catecholamine depletor) alter alcohol preference in rodents, raises new speculations about a possible relationship between alcoholism and serotonin and/or catecholamine metabolism.

It has been postulated that norepinephrine and serotonin (and possibly acetylcholine and γ-aminobutyric acid) serve as the neurotransmitters in the CNS. Norepinephrine mediates alertness and increased psychomotor activity, and serotonin mediates drowsiness and decreased psychomotor activity. It has been shown that acutely intoxicated alcoholics have higher urinary levels of epinephrine and norepinephrine than nonintoxicated alcoholics. However, during convalescence, the higher levels decrease and do not rise in response to an alcohol challenge. Study of the withdrawal syndrome is also of interest. Urinary catecholamine excretion is highest in patients with delirium tremens and is elevated in clinically less severe forms of withdrawal; the degree of clinical severity correlates well with the urinary and plasma concentrations of catecholamines. The increased urinary and plasma levels seem to be associated with the general adrenergic hyperactivity observed in withdrawing patients. It has even been suggested that alcoholics may have a congenitally impaired sympathetic nervous system that is normalized by ethanol ingestion and worsened by withdrawal.

Although studies of the effect of ethyl alcohol on the synthesis of catecholamines are scanty, it has been demonstrated that ethanol alters the biotransformation of norepinephrine predominantly to glycol rather than to vanillylmandelic acid. Alcohol also has a multiplicity of effects on the economy of catecholamines in the CNS. It has been suggested that the behavioral effects of ethyl alcohol might be related to the fact that ethanol blocks the neuronal membrane reuptake of norepinephrine, which, in turn, prolongs the action of the norepinephrine released onto receptor sites and thus possibly induces euphoria. It has also been demonstrated that both exogenous norepinephrine and epinephrine potentiate ethanol-induced sleep.

The circulating level of serotonin is increased in nonalcoholic patients with carcinoid tumors who have ingested alcohol. Whether this is mediated by release from tissues or decreased uptake of circulating serotonin is unclear, although it may be related to the increased number of platelets present. In alcoholics, the level of serotonin in the cerebrospinal fluid is not increased, nor is the platelet level. However, ethanol does induce a much greater than normal increase in urinary excretion of tryptamine in alcoholics. Not only are serotonin levels within normal limits in the cerebrospinal fluid of alcoholics, but 5-hydroxyindoleacetic acid levels are also normal. It has been reported, however, that urinary levels of 5-hydroxyindoleacetic acid are low in chronic alcoholics followed over a long period of time. It has been suggested that this reflects decreased serotonin biosynthesis, since both monoamine oxidase and tryptophol dehydrogenase are within normal limits. In general, tryptophan metabolism in alcoholics has proved difficult to study and the results have been conflicting.

There are reports that alcohol in humans activates the enzyme tryptophan pyrolase, and thus increases the metabolic breakdown of tryptophan, thereby reducing its biologic concentrations.[94,95]

Ethanol appears to block the uptake of serotonin by the neuronal membrane and storage granule and to decrease the efflux of 5-hydroxyindoleacetic acid and 5-hydroxytryptamine. There are data that suggest that this effect may be responsible for the behavioral changes induced by ethyl alcohol, since an ethanol-like intoxication can be induced by the administration of tryptophan or serotonin. At this point, it is interesting to note that p-chlorphenylalanine, which inhibits synthesis of serotonin in the brain, reduces preference for ethanol; α-methyl-p-tyrosine, which depletes brain serotonin, has a similar but much less marked effect. Opposite effects have been reported by other investigators.

Understanding of the metabolism of biogenic amines in the alcoholic has recently become of increasing importance, since it has been suggested that addictive alkaloid derivatives are formed by the interaction of biogenic amines and the acetaldehyde derived from the metabolism of ethanol. Acetaldehyde inhibits competitively the aldehyde dehydrogenase that is normally responsible for the oxidation of the aldehyde derivative of 5-hydroxytryptamine to 5-hydroxyindoleacetic acid. As a consequence, the intermediate indole aldehyde is shifted to a reductive pathway, forming the alcohol 5-hydroxytryptophol in increased concentrations. This alcohol is soporific in mice, and the effect is potentiated by ethanol.[96] The metabolism of other biologically active amines follows an analogous process. It has been demonstrated extensively *in vitro* that aldehydes condense with certain phenolic amines to form tetrahydroisoquinolines. *In vitro*, the benzyl tetrahydroisoquinoline condensing from dopamine plus the aldehyde derived from dopamine oxidative deamination form the alkaloid tetrahydropapaveroline. The process is enhanced by ethanol and acetaldehyde. This alkaloid has marked pharmacologic activity, particularly β-adrenergic agonist activity. It is postulated that, since the structure of tetrahydropapaveroline closely resembles that of morphine, which is highly addictive, it might form the molecular basis for ethanol addiction. Another similar compound, tetrahydro-β-carboline, the condensation product of aldehyde and certain tryptophan derivatives, has also been postulated to play a similar role. Much more data will have to be collected before these possibilities can be considered anything other than interesting postulations.

A more detailed review of this important area of research is presented later in this chapter.

## G. ACUTE TOXICITY

### 1. Lethal Doses of Alcohol in Humans and Animals

In laboratory animals and in humans, doses of alcohol that produce blood levels greater than 400 mg/100 ml may be fatal. Lethal blood levels of alcohol range from 420 mg/100 ml in humans to 930 mg/100 ml in the rat. It is clear that ethanol is not a highly toxic substance, if we consider the amount consumed and the few who die directly of it. But it is a contributory factor in many cases of death, especially when it is combined with other drugs, such as barbiturates.

### 2. Factors that Modify Alcohol Toxicity

These factors include the following.

a. Age. In preschool children, the lethal dose of ethanol is about 3 g/kg, less than one half of that in adults.

b. Deaths from doses of alcohol. Less than 4 g/kg have resulted in death in patients with adrenal insufficiency.

c. Toxic reactions to alcohol may occur in persons exposed to chlorinated hydrocarbons. Solvent inhalation will augment the behavioral actions of ethanol.

d. Depressants such as barbiturates, meprobamate, and other psychotropic agents augment the actions of alcohol. The impairment of muscular coordination and judgment is very much enhanced in a person who has taken chlorpromazine prior to alcohol. Synergy of ethanol and other agents such as levodopa, serotonin, alcohol-like metabolites (tryptophols and 3,4-dihydroxy-phenylethanol), γ-aminoxybutyric acid (GABA), and glycine have also been reported. Stimulants such as amphetamine may antaganize the effects of moderate doses of alcohol—but speed or amphetamine actually will increase the toxicity of mean lethal doses.

In discussing the pharmacology of ethyl alcohol, Dr. J. D. P. Graham[97] had this to say: "The cruder manifestations of love, hate, greed, or aggression are more rapidly ventilated than normal which is doubtless of prophylactic value psychologically, but also causes much antisocial behavior and traumatic experience. . . ."

### 3. Intoxication[3]

The relationships between the ingestion of alcohol, the blood ethyl alcohol concentration, and the clinical signs and symptoms of intoxication are variable and depend to a large extent on the rate of ingestion, the alterations in absorption, metabolism and excretion, and the chronicity of exposure.

To reiterate certain already discussed facts and to present other pertinent information, alcohol is fully absorbed within 30 minutes to two hours, depending upon the beverage consumed and the concomitant food intake. Once absorbed, 90 percent of the alcohol is oxidized in the liver by hepatic alcohol dehydrogenase. In the adult, the capacity to metabolize alcohol is limited to approximately 7 g/hr (1 gram = 1 ml of 100 percent ethyl alcohol); metabolism and minimal excretion yield a linear decline in the blood alcohol level at an average rate of 15 mg of body weight per hour. The clinical effect of a given blood alcohol level can be summarized roughly as follows: A blood alcohol concentration of 20 mg% to 99 mg% is associated with muscular incoordination, impaired sensory function, and changes in mood, personality, and behavior (Table 11-5 and 11-6). A concentration of 100 mg% to 199 mg% is associated with marked mental impairment, incoordination, a prolonged reaction time, and ataxia, while a

## TABLE 11-5

### Approximate Alcohol Consumption to Achieve a Blood Alcohol Level of 100 Mg% (Legal Definition of Intoxication)

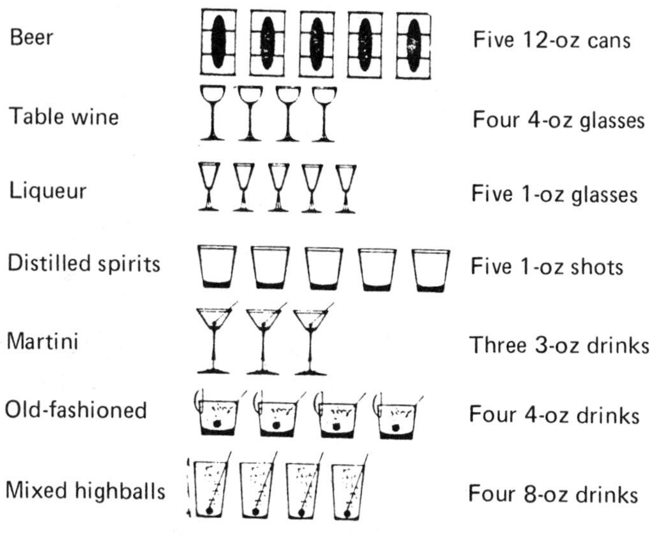

| | |
|---|---|
| Beer | Five 12-oz cans |
| Table wine | Four 4-oz glasses |
| Liqueur | Five 1-oz glasses |
| Distilled spirits | Five 1-oz shots |
| Martini | Three 3-oz drinks |
| Old-fashioned | Four 4-oz drinks |
| Mixed highballs | Four 8-oz drinks |

Drunk within 1 hr by 80-kg person

(From Becker, C. E., Roe, L. R., and Scott, R. A. *Alcohol as a Drug: A Curriculum on Pharmacology and Toxicology*. New York: Medcom Press, 1974. With permission.)

## TABLE 11-6

### Blood Alcohol Levels and Behavioral Effects

| *Blood Alcohol Level, Percent* | *Ray* Behavior* | *Bogen† Behavior* |
|---|---|---|
| 0.03 | —— | Individual is dull and dignified |
| 0.05 | Lowered alertness; usually good feeling | Individual is dashing and debonair |
| 0.10 | Slowed reaction times: less caution | Individual may become dangerous and devilish |
| 0.15 | Large, consistent increases in reaction time | —— |
| 0.20 | Marked depression in sensory and motor capability: decidedly intoxicated | Individual is likely to be dizzy and disturbing |
| 0.25 | Severe motor disturbance, staggering; sensory perceptions greatly impaired, "smashed" | Individual may be disgusting and disheveled |
| 0.30 | Semistupor | Individual is delirious and disorientated, and surely drunk |
| 0.35 | Surgical anesthesia: about the $LD_1$ minimal level, causing death | Individual is dead drunk |
| 0.40 | About the $LD_{50}$ | —— |
| 0.60 | —— | The chances are that the person is dead |

*Ray, O. *Drugs, Society, and Human Behavior*, C. V. Mosby, St. Louis, 1972, p. 88.

†Bogen, E. Human toxicology of alcohol. In H. Emerson, editor. *Alcohol and Man*. Macmillan, New York, 1932, pp. 126–152.

concentration of 200 mg% to 200 mg% superimposes nausea, vomiting, diplopia, and marked ataxia on the clinical condition. With a blood concentration of 300 mg% to 399 mg%, hypothermia, severe dysarthria amnesia, and stage 1 anesthesia develop; finally, with a concentration of 400 mg% to 700 mg%, coma, respiratory failure, and death occur. A rough approximation of the blood alcohol level can be estimated by assuming that 10 ounces of 100 proof whiskey (50 percent ethyl alcohol by volume) raises the blood level of a 70-kg adult by about 25 mg%.

## 4. Tolerance

The extent of tolerance developed to alcohol is not clearly defined. Only an approximation can be made at this time. It is usually said that tolerance developed to generalized depressant drugs is due to a prolonged use and high doses of the drug. However, no systematic studies have been done in humans.[98]

### *a. Genetic or Inherent "Tolerance"*

Different individuals are affected differently after drinking the same amounts of alcohol. Some can "hold" their liquor better than others. In an experimental study of simulated severe chronic alcoholism, no clear correlation was observed between the amount of alcohol consumed and the degree of drunkenness displayed by the various subjects, even in the early part of the experiment.[99] One subject, who had not previously been an alcoholic, was able to consume an average of 450 ml of 95 percent alcohol daily for 79 consecutive days without appearing more than mildly intoxicated. He appeared markedly intoxicated only when his intake was increased to between 600 and 700 ml/day.

### *b. Metabolic Tolerance*[98]

Some people are described as being "able to hold their liquor." Translated into medical terms, it means these individuals are able to process alcohol through their bodies in a metabolizing process that is simply more efficient than others. Isbell and his associates simulated chronic severe alcoholism in an important study, obtaining evidence to support the concept of metabolic tolerance to alcohol.[99]

The drinking days of Isbell's subjects included hourly dosage from 6 a.m. to 11 p.m., capping off each day with a triple dose at midnight and at 3 a.m. Blood alcohol concentrations were increased gradually to between 150 and 250 mg/100 ml. At that level, intoxication was evident, guaranteed by a daily consumption of 400 ml. of 95% alcohol. Maintaining intake levels, the subjects' alcohol blood levels dropped gradually to nearly zero within 10 days and the signs of intoxication vanished. Metabolism rate of the subjects had climbed to an estimated average rate of 455 ml./day. It was not possible to increase their intake by even so small an amount as 3 to 65 ml. at 2-hour intervals without again spurring blood alcohol concentrations higher and once more generating intoxicating behavior. The maximum metabolic tolerance had been achieved.

However, it has been demonstrated that once alcohol consumption stops, metabolic tolerance quickly disappears. Another study showed that when control subjects and "currently abstinent alcoholics" were administered the same dosage containing radioactive carbon dioxide, the rates of elimination were virtually the same for both groups of subjects.

Mendelson has found that transitory metabolic tolerance to alcohol is often designated as the result of "induction or accelerated biosynthesis of the enzyme . . . alcohol dehydrogenase." Indications are that not only is the enzyme a limiting factor in the initial rate of alcohol metabolism achieved, but also at work in the equation is the rate of regeneration that hepatic tissue can achieve in producing the required oxidized form of NAD from its reduced state, as well as the rate at which carbon dioxide may be converted from acetate.

### c. *Pharmacodynamic or Tissue Tolerance*

A popular hypothesis regarding the response or tolerance of the body to alcohol involves adaptive cellular changes. Though no hard evidence supports this conclusion, authorities believe that after long-term exposure to a drug, the magnitude of the evoked response gradually diminishes as a result of adaptive changes in the responding cells. Current studies on ethanol by Cappell include tolerance, treatment of abuse, and other fundamental issues.[104] Another area of investigation on the pharmacodynamic tolerance to the effects of severe alcoholism include a study by Isbell and colleagues in which brain waves (EEG) were determined in connection with alcohol. After one week of alcohol consumption, a slow EEG pattern, an increased occipital alpha percentage, a slowing of alpha frequency, and an increase in percentage of waves of frequencies of 4 to 6 cycles per second were observed.[99] The results occurred after individuals consumed 266 to 489 ml of 95 percent alcohol daily for 87 days. After 200 mg/100 ml or higher, and as the period of drinking increased, the slowing of the EEG pattern was less evident.

### d. *Cross-tolerance*

Alcoholics display cross-tolerance to other CNS depressant drugs, but the mechanism responsible for this is not understood. Animal studies have found a cross-tolerance between ethanol and opiates.[105] Data also show that alcoholics may exhibit cross-tolerance to the effects of sedative and hypnotic drugs and general anesthetic agents. This is viewed by some as being pharmacodynamic in nature, or a reflection of metabolic tolerance. In humans, according to a recent study, alcohol can affect induction of hepatic microsomal drug metabolizing enzymes of the type responsible for the degradation of barbiturates and other drugs.[101] This conclusion does not explain the tolerance to general anesthetic agents as they are metabolized to a negligible degree.

## 5. Treatment of Alcohol Overdose

Coma attributable to alcohol usually occurs in the young, first-exposure patient. It can also happen with adult patients, particularly binge drinkers who drink enormous quantities of alcohol rapidly. A mixture of drugs commonly abused will be found in association with the use of alcohol that results in coma. It is important to obtain a blood alcohol level and drug screen. There is usually a strong odor of alcohol about the patient. Respiratory depression can occur.

Because of the high incidence of pathologic consequences of alcoholism, the physician should always look for other problems or causes of coma in the patient with alcohol odor. In particular, one should check for the following.

1. Hypoglycemia.
2. Subdural hematoma.
3. Trauma, including skull fracture.
4. Septicemic meningitis.
5. Cardiac arrhythmia (ventricular fibrillation is a common cause of death; these patients should have cardiac monitoring).
6. Wernicke's encephalopathy.
7. Hepatic coma.
8. Diabetic acidosis.
9. Severe infectious process.

Treatment of alcohol overdose involves the following procedures.

1. Nasogastric lavage should be performed within one hour of ingestion to remove any unabsorbed alcohol.
2. Thiamine, 100 mg, should be given I.M. Glucose should be infused intravenously, as these patients may be hypoglycemic.
3. In the alcoholic presenting with coma, the probability of pneumonia is high. A chest film and careful examination of the lungs thus are indicated.
4. The use of 10 or 40 percent fructose solutions to speed the metabolism of alcohol must be regarded as experimental as present. The danger of producing hyperuricemia or lactic acidosis is associated with the use of these fructose solutions.

## H. CHRONIC TOXICITY

### 1. Alcohol Dependence

The repeated use of alcohol results in the development of tolerance; thus larger doses must be taken to attain the characteristic effects. Investigators have shown that "tissue tolerance" develops in chronic alcoholics. Goldberg showed, in a number of tests in humans, that alcohol, at a given blood level, produced less impairment of performance in heavy drinkers than in abstainers. Alcohol is toxic by itself, and the lack of dietary essentials in the alcoholic, such as the vitamin B complex, leads to kidney disease and to deterioration of mental faculties and predisposes an individual to psychotic episodes if the alcohol is withdrawn. The acute psychosis is termed delirium tremens (DTs). It is characterized by hallucinations and extreme fear, and is clear evidence of alcohol dependence in the patient: DTs do not occur in the social drinker. It is of interest to note that the occurrence of such an episode may prove fatal. It is also of interest that, although there is tolerance to the inebriating effects of alcohol, there is no tolerance to its lethal dose.

### 2. Abstinence Syndrome

It is now fairly well known that we can develop an addiction to alcohol just as we do to any other general depressant drug. This is known as physical dependence and is usually followed by withdrawal symptoms. Withdrawal effects depend upon individual variations. An estimation of the degree of physical dependence that will develop to alcohol is based upon the amount of alcohol consumed, the physical and mental condition of a person, and the severity of withdrawal symptoms. The extent of physical dependence determines whether complete recovery will occur within five to seven days.[106] If complete recovery is not possible, and in severe alcoholism, a state resembling schizophrenia may occur, and convulsive seizures and delirium tremens may result in the death of the alcoholic.[99]

Although it is not certain how much alcohol must be taken and for what length of time before withdrawal symptoms are experienced, it is well known that a "hangover" does occur almost immediately after a considerable amount of alcohol has been consumed.[106] An individual can also experience tremulousness called "the shakes." Some studies found psychotic delirium manifestations in persons who consumed 400 to 500 ml of alcohol per day for 48 or more days.[99] The symptoms associated with severe alcoholism may or may not be exhibited as withdrawal symptoms. There are inevitably variations caused by a multiplicity of factors. However, withdrawal symptoms may be assumed to manifest themselves according to the degree or duration of alcohol intoxication.

There are three chronologic stages in the development of alcohol withdrawal symptoms.[107] The first stage includes symptoms that appear within a few hours after taking 100 mg/100 ml alcohol. They include tremulousness, weakness, profuse perspiration, anxiety (commonly known as the "jitters"), headache, anorexia, nausea, abdominal cramps, retching, and vomiting. The patient may have a flushed face, and become restless, agitated, hyperreflexive, and startle easily, but generally remains alert. Craving for alcohol or a sedative drug is observed. The tremors may become generalized and marked. The EEG pattern at this time may be mildly dysrhythmic, with random spikes and brief episodes of high-voltage slow waves appearing.[109] The degree of abnormality of the EEG pattern, however, does not appear to be a reliable prognostic sign of whether convulsions will occur. Acute alcoholic hallucinosis ("seeing or hearing things") is experienced even with the eyes closed and the patient may lose insight. Usually considered an early sign of delirium tremens, acute alcohol hallucinosis may manifest itself throughout the abstinence period.

The second stage of the alcohol withdrawal syndrome is seen infrequently and in a small number of patients. These symptoms include convulsive seizures, or more commonly the "rum fit." Convulsive seizures may be fatal if they reach the epileptic stage where there is one seizure following another. Seizures are usually of the grand mal type and may begin as early as 12 hours after abstinence, but more often they appear during the second or third day. More data are needed to determine the accurate incidence of convulsive seizures that occur in patients undergoing withdrawal from alcohol. One observation included 13 percent convulsive seizures in 272 alcoholics.[109]

Delirium tremens, commonly known as the "horrors," are experienced and may last for three to four days during the third stage of the withdrawal syndrome.[108] Auditory, visual, and tactile hallucinations occur with a loss of insight. The patient cannot sleep and is severely agitated, extremely disoriented, restless, and almost continuously active. Fever, profuse perspiration (to the extent of marked dehydration), and tachycardia can be observed. Severe and bizarre delusions may occur. As with most generalized depressant drugs, delusion and hallucinations also occur in severe alcoholism withdrawal. In some cases they may be terrifying in nature. At this stage, the individual is agitated and can become self-destructive or a risk to others. In most cases of narcotic withdrawal, treatment can be facilitated with other drugs. In alcoholism, once delirium tremens develops, it is difficult to treat with a safe dose of drugs. Death attributed to delirium tremens is caused by hyperthermia, peripheral vascular collapse, or self-incurred injury. An estimated 37 percent death rate is reported due to delirium and 10 percent are commonly observed.[108]

More studies are required to combat the rise and severe consequences of alcoholism. There are many serious questions regarding delirium tremens as there is doubt that alcohol is the sole culprit in its development. It is thought that alcohol might act as an accomplice in the development of DTs in persons who were already predisposed to it because of some other ailment. "In alcoholics who have abstained from alcohol for several months, delirium tremens may occur following operation trauma or severe illness. During the attacks of delirium tremens, the body may be alcohol free."[108] Injury, surgical procedures, and intercurrent infection are believed to develop DTs although there is doubt as to whether the alcoholic can maintain the same amount of alcohol intake during this time. Was the duration of abstinence established by evidence other than the alcoholic's own statements, which are notoriously unreliable, or did abuse of such generalized depressants as barbiturates occur during the abstinence period? Numerous questions remain under investigation.

A detailed discussion concerning treatment approaches to alcohol withdrawal appears later in this chapter.

## 3. Minor and Major Abstinence Syndromes

According to Becker and associates,[3] there are both minor and major phases to the abstinence syndrome.

The treatment of alcohol withdrawal is complicated by the variability in the clinical course of each patient (Figure 11-1). Whereas most patients experience only minor symptoms, others who, when first examined, appear indistinguishable in terms of agitation and tremor, develop delirium tremens for reasons we cannot explain. Thus it is worthwhile to separate the withdrawal syndrome into two parts, minor and major.

The minor symptoms tend to occur early in the course of withdrawal, starting within eight hours of the last drink and being manifested most commonly as "shakes" in the morning. If the patient can drink on arising, these quickly abate, but if the gastritis that commonly terminates a drinking binge prevents the ingestion of alcohol in sufficient quantities, other, more serious symptoms ensue. Hallucinations, like withdrawal seizures, tend to occur within 24 hours after cessation of drinking and may be, as outlined, of almost any type. After 36 hours, seizures are infrequent, but hallucinations, instead of clearing, may become more severe, with increasing agitation and prominent autonomic signs such as tachycardia, fever, sweating, and marked tremulousness.

Whereas the hallucinations that occur early after withdrawal are intermittent and associated in general with a clear sensorium, and often with some insight into their illusory nature, those that persist are often accompanied by profound disorientation and commonly, though not always, by agitation. It is a misconception that the hallucinatory experiences so prominent in this major abstinence syndrome, which we call delirium tremens, are always frightening. Many patients observed, as far as can be inferred from listening to them, engage in casual conversation with friends or perform their daily work. The delirium, marked by ceaseless activity, may last from several days to a week and commonly terminates rather abruptly.

But it would be a mistake to maintain that things are always so clearly delineated. In fact, the two syndromes, minor and major, often merge imperceptibly and, in some patients, an atypical delusional–hallucinatory state develops in which agitation may or may not be present, but a fixed or varying delusional system is established. Such patients may be paranoid, certain that "they" are going to "get" them, and may be terrified for several days despite the apparent lack of hallucinatory experience. Others may be well oriented, engage in rational conversation, and yet hallucinate intermittently or have a peculiar delusional scheme. According to Becker and associates,[3] one such patient, quite intelligent, had the notion that a well-known state senator, a childhood friend, was limbless and confined in a bag under her pillow. She was convinced that they were both in the water, and implored the ward staff to help this man to prevent him from drowning. This concerned her for 24 hours and then gradually was mentioned less frequently; several days later, she could look back upon the experience with insight and humor, though insisting that at the time it had seemed totally real to her. Another patient believed that he had come to the hospital to star in a Candid Camera sequence and calmly maintained this delusion for several days. He expressed some irritation that the camera crew had not yet arrived, and hallucinated on and off during the period, all with no insight into his real reason for being in the hospital, yet without any indication of agitation, fear, or paranoia.

From the foregoing examples, it should be clear that the spectrum of behavior during acute abstinence from alcohol is indeed wide. A frequent question concerns its time course. How long can this delusional–hallucinatory state persist, and how long after cessation of drinking

**Phases of alcohol withdrawal**

SYMPTOMS AND SIGNS

| Mild tremor | Severe tremor |
|---|---|
| Mild increase blood pressure pulse, heart rate, and temperature | Marked increase blood pressure pulse, heart rate, and temperature |
| Hallucinations intermittent | Hallucinations persistent |
| Rum fits | Rare rum fits |
| Mild sleep disorders | Marked sleep disorders |
| Mild disorientation | Marked disorientation |
| Minor medical complications | Major life-threatening complications frequent |

8–10 hours — 48 hours — 4-6 days

Time after cessation of alcohol

**Figure 11-1. The Spectrum of the alcohol withdrawal syndrome Taken from: Becker, et al., Medcom Press, New York, 1974.** With permission can it occur? Firm answers are difficult to find, but some experiences suggest that it may last as long as a month, then clear, and it is known from the work of others than chronic auditory hallucinations in alcoholics may persist indefinitely. With regard to latency, data are even more sketchy, largely because it is hard for patients to be precise as to how much alcohol they consumed daily before entering the hospital. Since the abstinence syndrome seems to depend upon the rate of fall of blood ethanol levels, rather than on the absolute levels themselves, it is quite possible for a patient to have withdrawal symptoms even though an attempt has been made to resume drinking. The result is that data, using the time of the "last drink" before symptoms occur, may not really indicate the actual course of withdrawal. As a corollary, minor or major withdrawal symptoms have been observed three to four days after admission to the hospital. It may well be true that sedative drugs given for apparent "nervousness" or for insomnia may delay the onset and reduce the severity of frank abstinence symptoms. The other problem is that many patients are reluctant to report hallucinations, and only objective signs such as seizures, agitated behavior, and marked tachycardia are noted by the medical or nursing staff. At any rate, the implications for therapy are obvious. Strict criteria regarding time course or latency of onset are not to be relied on to make the diagnosis of withdrawal abnormalities; if the diagnostic criteria are overly rigid, many patients will be mistakenly diagnosed as having functional psychosis and, in all probability, will be treated incorrectly with phenothiazines or other potentially hazardous therapy. The functional psychosis diagnosis may be retained for life and cause untold harm.

## 4. Treatment of Alcohol Withdrawal

As previously stated, alcohol withdrawal can produce a variety of clinical syndromes, from a mild hyperadrenergic state to hallucinosis and delirium. Many classification systems have evolved for the alcohol withdrawal syndrome. The terminology can be confusing, but what is clear is that there are mild and severe types of alcohol withdrawal, and that some characteristics of withdrawal, such as rum fits and alcoholic hallucinosis, may be associated with either the mild or the severe form (see Figure 11-1).

While many sedative-hypnotic drugs have been utilized to treat the common abstinence syndrome, the benzodiazepines, chlordiazepoxide, and diazepam are currently in widest use. The benzodiazepines have the advantage of being cross-tolerant with alcohol, and their long half-life is usually an advantage. Chlordiazepoxide (Librium) is the most widely used, and is recommended for patients without severe and overt liver disease.

For mild to moderate withdrawal, an initial test dose of 50 to 100 mg of chlordiazepoxide is given orally (P.O.) and the patient is observed two to four hours later. If the symptoms and signs of withdrawal are not ameliorated or are progressing, the dose is repeated. In most patients, an initial divided dose of from 50 to 200 mg in the first 24-hour period usually provides mild sedation, decreases the tremulousness, and eases the bothersome symptoms of alcohol withdrawal. Occasionally doses as high as 400 to 600 mg of chlordiazepoxide are necessary in the first 24 hours in severely tremulous and agitated patients. Because of the long half-life of this drug, subsequent daily doses can be reduced rapidly, usually by 50 to 100 mg a day. Thus the usual pharmacotherapy for the alcohol withdrawal syndrome can be accomplished in three to six days. Benzodiazepines, particularly those with long half-lives, should be used with caution in elderly patients since such patients show increased sensitivity to the sedative effects of these drugs and also metabolize them more slowly. Severe hepatic disease can also complicate benzodiazepine therapy.

In patients with decompensating liver disease, lorazepam (Ativan) and oxazepam (Serax), both short-acting benzodiazepines, may be preferable. Lorazepam can be given 1 to 2 mg P.O. every six to eight hours and oxazepam 15 to 30 mg P.O. every six to eight hours.

In treating patients with delirium tremens, intravenous diazepam, 10 mg initially, followed by 5 mg every five minutes until a calming effect is achieved, has proved effective. Intramuscular absorption of diazepam is less reliable. Patients may be switched from parenteral diazepam to oral diazepam or chlordiazepoxide as soon as they are able to tolerate oral medication. In addition to the benzodiazepines, haloperidol, 2 to 4 mg intramuscularly every two to six hours as necessary, can be used as a supplement to diazepam to control the agitation, and is also helpful in controlling some of the behaviors secondary to hallucinations.

Together with these medications, the patient also may require physical restraints. Careful monitoring of electrolyte balance and cardiac status is indicated. Particular attention should be given to the treatment of hypokalemia and hypomagnesemia as well as to appropriate fluid and electrolyte replacement. Patients with DTs frequently have a coincident infectious disease, usually pneumonitis, which must be vigorously treated. The mortality rate rises sharply when DTs are accompanied by pneumonia, pancreatitis, or severe hepatitis.

Although the severe forms of alcohol withdrawal require hospitalization, and are a medical emergency, the mild syndrome need not be treated in a hospital setting. There are now a number of community-based detoxification centers that provide alcohol withdrawal treatment. Some employ pharmacologic agents to aid in the detoxification. Others, called social setting or nonmedical detoxification centers, afford psychologic and social support, usually in a homelike atmosphere designed to accomplish withdrawal without the use of pharmacologic agents. These social-setting programs have been very effective in the treatment of the mild, self-limited form of alcohol withdrawal.

Detoxification from alcohol is not the treatment of alcoholism. It does provide an opportunity, however, to engage the alcoholic in the early stages of treatment. Every effort should be made to couple alcohol detoxification with referral to or the provision of continuing care for the chronic disease of alcoholism.

## I. BIOMEDICAL CONSEQUENCES OF ALCOHOL USE AND ABUSE

Alcohol-related mortality from selected causes—such as alcoholic psychosis—appears to be remaining relatively constant in the United States[110] while cirrhosis mortality rates have declined each year since reaching a peak in 1973. Cirrhosis mortality rates are disproportionately high among black Americans, with seven major cities accounting for half of such deaths (Baltimore, Chicago, Detroit, Los Angeles, New York, Philadelphia, and Washington). In these cities, rates among black males aged 25 to 34 are as much as ten times higher than for white males of the same age. For all ages, the cirrhosis mortality rate for black Americans is nearly twice that for white Americans.[110]

In the sample studied, the actual mortality rate for alcoholics proved 2.5 times greater than expected four years after their admission to a treatment program.[111] Mortality rates are also higher for younger alcoholics than for older ones. More than half of the deaths in the sample were related to alcohol. While alcohol-related morbidity data are limited in scope and quality, the National Center for Health Statistics' Hospital Discharge Survey (HDS) indicates that alcoholism discharges increased from 1975 to 1977 and that rates of utilization have increased more sharply for males than for females. The HDS probably underestimates, perhaps seriously for some diagnoses, the occurrence of alcohol-related events that result in hospitalization. American society still tends to stigmatize alcohol-related difficulties, so patients may minimize or conceal the involvement of alcohol in their disease or injury. Furthermore, even if physicians are aware that alcohol is involved, they may be reluctant to report it in a hospital discharge record.

At least 2.5 percent of all discharges from short-stay hospitals in 1975 were directly linked to alcohol-related causes. Of these, most had first-listed diagnoses of "alcoholism"; other first-list diagnoses included liver cirrhosis, alcoholic psychosis, neuroses, symptomatic and chronic ischemic heart disease, gastritis, duodenitis, pancreatitis, diabetes, pneumonia and other respiratory diseases, esophageal varices, vitamin deficiencies, and trauma and other injuries. In Veterans Administration hospitals, the proportion of alcohol-related discharges to all discharges was much higher.[110] For example, 17 percent of all discharges were associated with alcoholism as a primary or secondary diagnosis. Between 1970 and 1977, the number of alcohol discharges from VA hospitals nearly doubled.

Major consequences of alcohol use and abuse, which include cardiovascular effects, endocrine actions, brain dysfunction, behavioral deficits, Wernicke–Korsakoff syndrome, cancer risk, and teratogenic effects, are discussed briefly here.

### 1. Cardiovascular Effects

#### *a. Heart Rate*

It has long been known that in healthy humans, alcohol doses equivalent to two to five ordinary drinks (30 to 75 ml of alcohol) produce slightly increased heart rate, blood pressure (systolic more than diastolic), and cardiac output. Blood pressure elevations in persons who use large amounts of alcohol may be due primarily to alcohol withdrawal rather than to direct alcohol action.[112] In severe intoxication, the nervous system is believed to predominate in contributing to low blood pressure, slow heart rate, and, ultimately, death from cardiac standstill.[113]

#### *b. Coronary Circulation*

Studies of the effects of alcohol on the blood supply to the heart muscle (the coronary circulation) are inconsistent. Some experiments show acute impairment of heart muscle contractile force with a concomitant increase in coronary blood flow.[114,115] Other studies suggest that acute alcohol ingestion decreases coronary blood flow,[116,117] and still others suggest that it has no effect.[118,119] Studies of humans with coronary disease who consumed alcohol suggested no benefit, or possibly even worsening, of impaired coronary blood flow during exercise.[120,121]

#### *c. Heart Pumping Action*

Persons with a long history of substantial alcohol intake and without clinical evidence of heart disease often have abnormally functioning heart muscles, which many consider to represent preclinical heart muscle disease. Men may be more susceptible than women to these effects.

Some chronic heavy users of alcohol show increased heart weight, dilatation of all heart chambers, scarring of heart muscle, and clots adhering to the inside linings of the chambers. Alcohol-induced abnormalities in heart muscle detected by microscopic or other histochemical techniques are not specific enough to distinguish heart muscle diseases in users of large amounts of alcohol from cardiomyopathy in other persons.

As previously mentioned, Leiber and associates[122] found that when animals were supplied with all essential nutrients and fed large amounts of alcohol, toxicity to the heart muscle was not related to associated nutritional deficiency, but to alcohol itself.

#### *d. Alcoholic Cardiomyopathy*

Many investigators have seen an association between chronic substantial alcohol use and heart muscle failure. Long-term use of substantial quantities of alcohol has been found in a large proportion of patients with unexplained heart disease, or "cardiomyopathy," who constitute 2 to 3 percent of patients hospitalized for heart disease. Alexander[123] reported that 80 percent of patients hospitalized for cardiomyopathy were heavy drinkers, compared with 28 percent of patients with other diseases. Several well-documented case reports indicate a relationship between alcohol intake and cardiomyopathy.[124,125]

There is circumstantial evidence relating drinking to heart rhythm disturbances. Brief drinking sprees in apparently healthy individuals can result in premature beats and paroxysmal atrial arrhythmias, especially atrial fibrillation, a phenomenon named "holiday syndrome."[126] More serious arrhythmias are believed to be related to acute alcohol use.[127,128] Among the earliest clinical features of alcoholic cardiomyopathy are nonspecific and often minor electrocardiographic (ECG) changes and rhythm disturbances. The prevalence of alcoholic cardiomyopathy and its likelihood of progression to chronic myocardial disease is not known.

It is presumed to affect a small and possibly high-risk group.[129]

Congestive heart failure, chronic rhythm disturbances, conduction abnormalities on the ECG, and high incidence of embolic complications are characteristic of the chronically weakened and dilated heart. Although some patients show partial regression, many progress inexorably despite abstinence from alcohol and optimal medical therapy. However, abstinence produces a good recovery rate in early disease and can result in a marked degree of recovery even with advanced disease.[124,125,130]

It has been established that 80 grams of ethanol a day (equivalent to six standard drinks) over a period of years is necessary to produce cardiomyopathy,[131] making it unlikely that only people with a drinking problem are at risk of permanent cardiac damage.[129]

### *e. Alcohol and Hypertension*

There is strong epidemiologic evidence that regular use of large amounts of alcohol is associated with a substantially higher prevalence of hypertension. The largest study showed a statistically strong association between blood pressure and known drinking habits of 83,947 men and women of three races.[132] The association between alcohol use and blood pressure could be influenced, at least in part, by such factors as psychosocial stress, by a common hereditary predilection for both alcohol use and hypertension, or by alcohol withdrawal, which is associated with increased heart rate and blood pressure in some heavy drinkers.[112]

A physiologic mechanism for the association between alcohol consumption and blood pressure elevation has not been established. Nevertheless there has been speculation that chronic corticosteroid excess[133,134] or action through the renin-angiotensin hormone system[135] may be involved. The possibility of direct association between alcohol consumption and blood pressure is strong enough to lead some health practitioners to advise hypertensive patients who take three or more drinks a day to cut down.[129]

### *f. Coronary Atherosclerosis*

Studies have shown a significantly lower hospitalization incidence for coronary disease among drinkers than among nondrinkers. They indicate that the largest difference in heart attack risk is between nondrinkers and those who have one or two drinks daily.[136]

Although most of the population studies suggest that drinkers suffer fewer major coronary events, caution in interpreting the reports on the presumably beneficial effects of moderate alcohol intake is clearly warranted. Encouraging the use of alcohol to reduce the likelihood of occurrence or recurrence of heart disease must be questioned because potential benefits appear to be outweighed by the attendant risks associated with increasing alcohol consumption.[137–140] These risks include adverse effects on the cardiovascular system such as hypertension, stroke, and alcoholic cardiomyopathy, as well as other health and social hazards.

### *g. High-Density Lipoprotein-Cholesterol*

Alcohol raises high-density lipoprotein-cholesterol (HDL-C) levels in blood. Studies have shown that elevated HDL-C is inversely related to coronary atherosclerotic disease and may play a protective role by aiding in removal of cholesterol from the body by retarding the formation of atherosclerotic plaques.[141,142] The effect of alcohol in raising HDL-C levels is generally proportional to the amount of alcohol taken.[143] Alcohol-induced HDL-C levels decrease within weeks if drinking is stopped.[144] There is evidence that the site of action of alcohol's influence on HDL-C is the liver. In some very heavy drinkers with acute or severe liver disease, however, HDL-C levels may be very low, presumably as a consequence of hepatic injury.[145] The possibly beneficial effects of moderate alcohol on HDL-C, therefore, must be separated from the deleterious effects of excessive alcohol use on the liver and its secondary effects on lipoprotein metabolism.

### *h. Stroke and Angina Pectoris*

A positive correlation between drinking and stroke incidence has been reported with a stronger relationship for hemorrhagic than for thrombotic stroke.[137] This is partly explained by the association of both drinking and stroke with hypertension; bleeding tendency due to alcohol also has been implicated.[146]

Alcohol has been reported to be one of the pharmacologic agents that can induce an unusual form of angina pectoris, known as Prinzmetal variant angina, but the association has not been widely observed. Myocardial infarctions have been reported among alcoholics with no evidence of atherosclerosis or thrombotic occlusion.[147]

### *i. Alcohol and the Endocrine System*

Numerous studies have shown that acutely or chronically administered alcohol lowers serum testosterone levels in males of all species, including humans. Many alcoholics manifest sexual impotence, loss of libido, and clinical symptoms of hypogonadism, including breast enlargement, loss of facial hair, and testicular atrophy as a result of diminished testosterone levels.

It is well documented that testosterone clearance is enhanced in chronic alcoholic humans and animals, primarily as the result of the induction of liver enzymes, which are responsible for the degradation of testosterone.[147-149] Prolonged administration of alcohol in male animals and humans causes their estrogen levels to rise,[150] and this correlates with an increase in the liver conversion of androgens.[150] It is probable that the signs of ''feminization'' in male chronic alcoholics are attributable to the simultaneous reduction in androgens and increase in estrogens.[151]

Considerable evidence suggests that alcohol administration also depresses testosterone synthesis in the testes. The effect of acute alcohol ingestion has recently been found to be biphasic: low doses increase testosterone levels and high doses depress them.[152-154] Serum testosterone levels are low in chronic alcoholics and it appears that repeated and persistent alcohol use ultimately causes irreversible damage to the structural and biochemical architecture of the testes.[155-160]

Evidence indicates that reduced synthesis of testosterone in the testes is not due to a fall in lutenizing hormone (LH) levels. Several investigators have found that alcohol can still produce a precipitous fall in serum testosterone even when human chorionic gonadotropin is administered to raise LH levels.[154,161,162] Thus reduced testosterone synthesis appears to be the result of direct toxic action on the testes. Recent studies show that the toxic agent may be acetaldehyde, the metabolic product of ethanol, rather than ethanol itself.[161-165]

## J. ALCOHOL AND THE NERVOUS SYSTEM

### 1. Brain Damage

There are still well-described organic brain syndromes associated with alcoholism, including dementia (general loss of cognitive or mental abilities), specific loss of recent memory, and, to a lesser extent, loss of remote memory. Approximately 10 percent of alcoholics may suffer from chronic brain syndrome,[166] a condition usually considered irreversible. A large number of alcoholics fall into the intermediate stage of brain damage,[167] in which acute brain syndrome symptoms are absent and cognitive changes that may be present are not sufficient to diagnose chronic brain syndrome. The condition is considered reversible, though there are questions as to whether recovery is complete.

Atrophy (loss of brain cells) has been considered for many years to be one of the major consequences of alcoholism. Parsons[166] concluded that in any given sample of alcoholics, the proportion of individuals with brain atrophy will range from 50 to 100 percent.

Computer-assisted tomography (CAT scan) has recently been applied to show signs of brain atrophy in alcoholics, including enlargement of the brain ventricles and widening of sulci.[168-174] Limited data suggest that female alcoholics appear to have the same incidence of brain atrophy as males.[173] Heavy social drinking also appears to be associated with definite cortical sulcal widening (40 percent), widened third ventricles (36 percent), and elevated ventricle/brain ratios.

Blood flow measurements, which indicate the

degree of functional activity and level of metabolism in various parts of the brain,[175,176] have shown lower cerebral blood flow in alcoholics, which seems linearly related to increasing age: the older the alcoholic, the lower is the cerebral blood flow.

## 2. Behavioral and Neuropsychologic Dysfunction

Alcoholics in treatment programs typically range from average to slightly above average in both verbal and performance intelligence; however, performance on certain visual–spatial and perceptual–motor tests is significantly lower in alcoholics as compared with controls. Studies show consistent evidence of mild impairment of adaptive abilities and general decrement in neuropsychologic functioning in alcoholics.[177] Males[178] and females[179] manifest the same pattern of neuropsychologic deficit. It is evident that intermediate-stage alcoholics who do not have clinically diagnosable brain disorders have a mild but still insignificant neuropsychologic impairment.

Parker and Noble[180] found that age and the amount of alcohol drunk interact: the older the social drinker and the more alcohol consumed per occasion, the poorer is the performance. Female alcoholics who previously had been moderate social drinkers had significantly poorer memory scores than light social drinkers, and the effects of a single acute dose of alcohol were greater in the moderate social drinkers than in the light social drinkers.[181]

Brain damage from chronic alcohol abuse has generally been thought to be irreversible, and improvements in the behavior of abstinent alcoholics were attributed to undamaged brain structures taking on the functions of damaged structures.

Different abilities appear to recover at different rates, however. Verbal deficits seem to disappear after about two or three weeks of abstinence. Similar improvement is seen in pure sensory and motor capacities. More complex abilities, such as short-term memory and visual–spatial learning, show somewhat less improvement within a month. Even more complex nonverbal abstracting ability and perceptual –motor abilities remain impaired, especially in some patients. Older patients with a longer period of alcohol abuse show the least improvement.

Six studies examined various aspects of cognitive reversibility over periods of one to six months.[182–186] Four of the six studies yielded evidence of significant improvement. In two studies that included a control group, the data suggest that, for some areas, the alcoholics remain impaired relative to the controls. Six additional studies examined reversibility over periods of one year or longer[187–192]; again four of the six studies indicated improvement, especially in abstracting and visual–perceptual motor abilities. It appears that a wide range of cognitive abilities of alcoholics is at least partly reversible, but that the deficits that remain a year or longer may be permanent.[193]

## 3. Wernicke–Korsakoff Syndrome

The Wernicke–Korsakoff syndrome represents an extreme on the continuum of cognitive impairment resulting from alcohol-induced brain damage. If not treated with large doses of thiamine (vitamin B), a patient with a Wernicke encephalopathy is in danger of fatal midbrain hemorrhage. After two or three weeks of thiamine treatment, the ophthalmic problems, ataxia, and confusional state disappear or improve greatly. Very few Wernicke patients whose etiology involves alcohol abuse completely recover. The neurotoxic effects of alcohol that can result from years of heavy consumption have been implicated in alcoholic Korsakoff patients. The most striking and persistent features of these patients are severe amnesia, confabulation, and remarkable personality alterations. The memory disorder involves difficulty both in learning new information and in recalling public and personal events from the recent past.

It is possible that the amnesic syndrome in the Korsakoff stage may result from an interaction of thiamine deficiency and the direct neurotoxic effects of alcohol.[194]

## 4. Cancer Risk

Although the mechanism is unknown, heavy alcohol consumption has been related to an increased risk of cancer at various sites in the human body, particularly the mouth, pharynx, and larynx.[195] There is a less striking positive association with alcohol and cancers of the esophagus, stomach, colon, liver, breast, thyroid gland, and malignant melanoma. The relative odds are usually higher in females, who also have an elevated risk of rectal cancer. Upper digestive tract cancers were found to occur with greater frequency in men, blacks, lower socioeconomic groups, and with increasing urbanization and increasing age (35 to 70 years).

Alcoholic patients with cancer have a poorer chance of survival and a greater chance of developing another primary tumor than do other patients with the same cancer.[196] The carcinogenic property of an alcoholic beverage may reside in other constituents or congeners of the beverage, not in the ethanol molecule itself. Tuyns[197] suggests that ethanol may enhance the action of carcinogenic substances such as polycyclic hydrocarbons, nitrosamines, and fusel oil, found in some foods and beverages. Recently n-nitrosodimethylamine (NDMA), a suspected carcinogen, has been detected in some brands of scotch, whiskey, and beer.[198]

## 5. Teratogenic Effects

Adverse effects on fetal development as a result of heavy drinking by the pregnant woman have been of medical concern for more than 250 years. The first modern reports appeared independently in French in 1968[199] and in English in 1973.[200] These reports have stimulated both clinical and basic scientific research over the past decade. Numerous studies of animal fetuses exposed to alcohol *in utero* have documented an increased frequency of resorptions, stillbirths, decreased litter size, decreased weight at birth, and anomalies similar to those seen in humans.[201] Current medical concern has been stimulated by the recognition of a specific pattern of dysmorphology called the fetal alcohol syndrome (FAS).[202] On the basis of 245 affected individuals, Clarren and Smith[202] have recommended that the diagnosis of FAS be made only when the patient has signs in each of three categories: (1) adverse CNS effects, marked by microcephaly, abnormal neuronal and glial migration, developmental delay, and persistent mental retardation; (2) prenatal and postnatal growth retardation; and (3) typical dysmorphologic features, particularly of the midfacial area. Associated features include abnormalities of the eyes, ears, and mouth; heart murmurs, particularly associated with septal defects; genitourinary anomalies; hemangiomas (birthmarks); and musculoskeletal anomalies such as hernias.

According to Sokol et al.,[203] from animal studies in which nutritional variables can be controlled and from the weight or other observations in humans, it is reasonable to conclude that alcohol is embryotoxic and teratogenic. It is noteworthy that estimates of FAS usually range from one in 600 to one in 1500 live births. Estimates as high as one in 50 births have been made for some American Indian reservations. Virtually all infants diagnosed as having FAS have been born to chronic alcoholics who drank heavily throughout pregnancy. In some cases, functional disturbances have been demonstrated in some neonates who show no morphologic anomalies. These disturbances include alterations in sleep episodes[204] and/or encephalographic polygraphic activity.[205,206]

Kaminski et al.[207] reviewed information from more than 9000 pregnancies; they report that women who consume more than 40 ml (1.5 ounces) of absolute alcohol have a higher risk of stillbirth. Offspring born to heavier drinkers have lower average birth weights.

Women who drink heavily may be different from other women in a number of ways that might adversely alter outcome, including cigarette smoking, age, parity, and trimester or registration.[207–209] Sokol reports that alcohol and nicotine together compound the risk for adverse outcome: for cigarette smoking, the risk was seen to be 1.8; for alcohol abuse, 2.4; and for cigarette smoking and alcohol abuse together, 3.9.[209] It was observed that women do not drink in consistent patterns. Those who reported that they consume five or more drinks on some occasions, and at least 45 drinks a month, were classified as heavy drinkers. Moderate drinkers were those who reported drinking less than once a month, never having five or more drinks on one occasion, or not drinking at all. Heavy drinkers have a 2.5-fold increase in the FAS risk factor as well as in absorption rate.

The possibility that moderate and social

drinking have adverse effects on fetal outcome has also been explored.[210] In one analysis,[211] the children of women who consumed one or more ounces of absolute alcohol per day just prior to or during pregnancy, or who experienced one or more episodes of heavy drinking during this period, were compared with children of light drinking and abstaining mothers. Of 163 infants examined, 11 infants with clinical features of abnormal growth and morphogenesis were found, nine from the index group and only two from the controls. Two of the nine in the index group were diagnosed as FAS; however, their mothers were alcoholics.

In another study,[212] a statistically significant decrease in infant birth weight of 91 grams was obtained for women who reported averaging 1 ounce of absolute alcohol per day for the pre-pregnancy period. The same amount ingested in late pregnancy was associated with a decrease in infant birth weight of 160 grams. The associations were independent of such variables as smoking, maternal age, height, parity, gestation age, and sex of the child. One study[213] reported that spontaneous abortion was positively associated with consumption of 1 ounce of absolute alcohol twice a week. Another study[214] reported an increased risk for second-trimester spontaneous abortion at the level of one to two drinks (0.5 to 1 ounce of absolute alcohol) a day. Both studies controlled for variables, including smoking.

Dr. Sokol[216] discussed the important and relevant question: "Does moderate drinking by pregnant women endanger the fetus?" He said:

> With over 800 papers concerning the effects of alcohol on pregnancy having been published in the last decade, it is clear that alcohol, in heavy doses, is both embryotoxic and teratogenic. Effects similar to those seen in the human, including growth retardation and congenital anomalies, can be elicited both *in vitro* and *in vivo* in several animal species. The question remains, however, as to whether there may be a safe level of drinking during human pregnancy. In my opinion, the best evidence in the literature indicates that although a spectrum of adverse effects of alcohol can be observed in the heaviest drinking approximately five percent of women, it is not clear that any important adverse effects are observed for the other 95 percent, those who drink "moderately" or "occasionally." Nonetheless, it is important to point out that we are unsure as to exactly how to define "moderate" and that there may be critical periods during pregnancy, for example, in the first trimester, when high blood alcohol levels, even for the short period of a single episode of binge drinking, may be deleterious. On these bases, our clinical approach to what to tell the patient about drinking during pregnancy is as follows:
>
> > We try to identify patients who have alcohol problems and to work with those patients either on attaining abstinence or, at least, on keeping their alcohol intake as low as possible. We tell all of our patients that, if they cut down on their drinking or don't drink at all during pregnancy, they can help themselves have a healthier baby. We reassure patients, however, that an occasional drink, say a glass of wine with dinner on the weekend, is unlikely to have adverse effect and that they should not worry about this level of alcohol intake. The woman who takes an occasional drink on a weekend is not a problem. The woman who admits to having a drink or two every day, however, may be a problem. While this may seem to us to be "moderate" drinking, the patient may actually be considerably underreporting her alcohol intake; she may be drinking much more than this. Moreover, this level and frequency of intake is distinctly unusual in the young woman in the reproductive age range.
>
> In short, from the clinical point of view, an occasional drink is not a problem. Heavier drinking which appears "moderate" when you take your history, may, because of underreporting, present heavy drinking and constitute a significant fetal risk.

The exact mechanisms of FAS are unknown. However, animal studies have been conducted. For example, Chernoff[215] and Randall and coworkers[217] observed defects in mice similar to those reported in FAS patients: cardiac anomalies, hydronephrosis, limb defects, and microphthalmia. Similar findings have been reported in beagles.[218]

Alcohol abuse is also associated with a number of nutrient deficiencies, including the vitamins thiamine, folate, and pyridoxine, and minerals such as zinc. In turn, deficiencies of such agents for even brief periods during pregnancy have been reported to be associated with teratogenesis.[209] It is possible, therefore, that the embryotoxic and teratogenic effects of alcohol abuse in pregnancy may be the result of nutritional deficiencies.

Alcohol consumption during lactation and the consequent effects on nursing infants is also an area of concern. Heavy alcohol consumption is known to decrease milk ejection.[219] Coupled with the impaired sucking ability noted in some offspring of heavy alcohol consumers,[202] this might contribute to nutritional deprivation in the infant. Alcohol also readily enters the breast milk, thereby providing alcohol to the nursing infant, attributed as the cause of a pseudo-Cushing's syndrome in infants.[220]

Many important questions remain: What are the dose–response relationships for FAS and other adverse outcomes associated with maternal alcohol consumption? What are the degrees of interindividual variability with respect to dose–response relationships? What are the vulnerable periods for susceptibility to alcohol-associated birth defects and anomalies? What are the effects of different patterns of consumption? What biologic characteristics of the mothers and fathers contribute to an increased risk of FAS or other alcohol-related damage in children?

As stated earlier, in Goteborg, Sweden,[221] an incidence of one in 600 births for definite FAS with an equal number of probable FAS cases has been reported. A similar incidence was reported in the north of France.[222] It has been reported in the literature that FAS is one of the leading causes of birth defects frequently associated with mental retardation.[202]

## K. CAUSES OF ALCOHOLISM[6]

Over the past decades, many different factors have been suggested as the cause of alcoholism. None has yet been accepted as the single causative agent. However, causes of alcoholism are usually sorted into three groups: biologic, physiologic, and sociocultural.

### 1. Biologic

Much effort has been exerted to find chemicals in specific beverages that might be responsible for alcohol addiction, or physiologic, nutritional, metabolic, or genetic defects that could explain excessive drinking. To date, these attempts have not succeeded. It has been impossible to produce clear-cut alcohol addiction by any practical means in experimental animals.[15]

Although alcoholism occurs frequently in the children of alcoholics, and thus may seem to have some hereditary basis,[223] it also occurs in children of devout abstainers.[224] Anne Roe[225] and Jellinek[226] have observed that children of alcoholics can be protected if they are reared away from their parents. This has added to the belief that alcoholism is related more to environment than to genetic factors (see the section on psychogenetic theory).

It has been suggested that alcoholism is caused by vitamin deficiencies or hormone imbalances. For example, much research by Dr. Roger Williams[227] and his associates at the University of Texas has demonstrated that increased alcohol intake in experimental animals may be induced by such deficiencies, but his findings have not been found applicable in human beings. Most of the nutritional and hormonal deficiencies observed in far-advanced alcoholics appear to be results rather than causes of excessive drinking.[15]

Allergy has been blamed for some cases of alcoholism, but there is no proof that alcoholics are generally allergic to alcohol itself or to other components of alcoholic beverages.

Although it is frequently said that alcoholics are unable to metabolize alcohol as rapidly as normal individuals, recent research has indicated that many actually metabolize it more rapidly when they are drinking heavily.[15] Whether alcoholics metabolize alcohol in a different manner—perhaps through different enzymatic processes—is not known.

It is suggested periodically that addiction may be due to certain nonalcoholic components in beer, wine, whiskey, rum, and brandy. Investigations have shown, however, that alcoholism also occurs in users of alcoholic beverages very low in these components, such as brandy in Sweden and Finland, and vodka in Russia, Poland, and the United States.[8]

Although alcoholism would be impossible without alcohol, alcohol can no more be considered its sole cause than marriage can be considered the sole cause of divorce, or the tubercle bacillus the sole cause of tuberculosis.

If addiction were caused entirely or even largely by overexposure to alcohol, the highest rates of alcoholism logically would be expected among groups with the highest per capita intake of alcohol. No such general relationship can be found. Although a high alcohol intake with a high rate of alcoholism has been reported in France,[228] a high intake but a low rate of alcoholism has been reported in Italy and Greece[229] and a relatively low intake but a high alcoholism rate in the United States[8] and Sweden.[230]

Even though research to date has not indicated any chemical, physiologic, or genetic factor as a cause of alcoholism, the possibility that such a physical factor exists cannot be ruled out, and further investigations are essential. In the section of this chapter dealing with modern theories on the etiology of alcoholism, chemical and genetic factors are more definitely characterized.

#### *a. Genetic*

The controversy over whether or not alcoholism is a genetic disease has existed for more than 30 years. For an even longer period, both popular and medical opinions have held that alcoholism is a disease, whether heritable or not, and this belief has fostered extensive clinical and experimental work, reviewed in part here.

For much of the early 20th century, investigators suggested that alcoholism was the clinical manifestation of a genetically determined allergy, a form of anaphylaxis. Although the idea was widely accepted by influential lay groups dealing with alcoholism, by midcentury a more sophisticated understanding of immunologic disease and a fruitless search for antialcohol antibodies had obviated support for the theory. Another subsequently discarded theory was based upon a postulated heritable enzyme deficit that resulted in an impaired ability to utilize one or more nutritional elements in the diet, thus requiring substitution of alcohol to meet nutritional needs. The clinical observations that led to this theory were made primarily in vitamin-deficient experimental animals in which increased caloric requirements in the deficiency state resulted in an increased ingestion of alcohol that could be mitigated by adding other carbohydrate sources to the diet. In general, it has not been demonstrated that the nutritional deficiencies observed in alcoholics are the cause and not simply the consequence of alcohol abuse.

Nevertheless it has been generally recognized that some individuals and ethnic groups—for example, American Indians and Canadian Eskimos—seem to be more prone to alcoholism, whereas others—such as American Jews—seem to be spared this disease. In the cases of the Indians and Eskimos, a marked decrease in the clearance rate of alcohol from the blood has been observed. The decreased clearance rate has been shown to be due to differences in the activity of liver alcohol dehydrogenase. Individual differences in the isoenzymes of alcohol dehydrogenase have been observed as well. It has also been proposed, although admittedly there is little support, that a microsomal enzyme system may be important in the metabolism of ethanol in humans, and that its activity may differ among individuals with the ancitipated effect on metabolic rates. Regardless of the enzymatic mechanisms, there is a growing body of data that confirms the fact that different people metabolize ethyl alcohol at different rates, quite possibly on a genetic basis. Few would also deny the clinical evidence that there is individual and probably ethnic variability in the physiologic response to alcohol. Nevertheless, although such work suggests a genetic determinant for alcoholism, it is far from conclusive.

An area of ongoing research that may help to elucidate this problem deals with the investigation of alcohol dehydrogenase in the eye. In the eye, alcohol dehydrogenase converts retinol to retinaldehyde, and when the enzyme is supplied with excess substrate (ethanol) in the chronic alcoholic, the relative deficiency thus produced may lead to amblyopia alcoholica. More important, its concentration in the eye may vary from one ethnic group to another. Therefore the fact that American Indians take longer to adapt to the dark than other groups may be viewed as additional supportive evidence of a deficiency of alcohol dehydrogenase in these people. This deficiency, in turn, also may cause the slower metabolic elimination of alcohol in Indians.

Animal studies have been carried out in an attempt to demonstrate genetic transmission of alcohol preference. An inbred strain of mice, which consumed 10 percent ethanol as two thirds of their daily fluid intake, was developed from outbred mice that preferred only alcohol. This supports the idea of genetic transmission. However, spontaneous preference for alcohol among experimental animals is not striking, and often, after a preference for alcohol is developed, it is lost when other choices are offered.

A person might inherit a susceptibility to the acute intoxicating effects of alcohol so that small quantities produce loss of control over one's subsequent intake. Along these lines, intoxication, dependence, and tolerance generally can be developed by force-feeding animals. In addition, rodents have been selectively bred for sensitivity to alcohol. For example, long-sleep and short-sleep mice have been developed at the Institute for Behavior Genetics in Colorado. Least affected and most affected rats have been obtained via selective breeding at Rutgers University Center for Alcohol Studies, and tolerant and nontolerant rats have been developed in Finland. Explanations for these inborn genetic differences include: (1) Ethanol is broken down in a series of metabolic reactions. People, perhaps even rats, differ in the rate of enzymatic degradation. A genetically determined, impaired ability to catabolize ingested alcohol would be associated with a poor ability to "hold" one's liquor. (2) The brain cells of different people may have an inherited, variable ability to adapt to high or chronic levels of alcohol.

Considerable effort has gone into the evaluation of human subjects in an attempt to obtain relevant data supporting the genetic transmission of an alcoholic tendency. Many studies have repeatedly shown that family members of alcoholics have a greater risk of alcoholism than do individuals whose families are free of alcohol abuse. While it is impossible to separate the effects of environment from those of inheritance in these studies, the finding seems valid. In a partially successful attempt to obviate the effect of environmental factors, twin studies have been employed. Although all these studies suffer from the same methodologic defects—namely, difficulty in diagnosing alcoholism and in determining zygosity—they all tend to demonstrate a higher concordance among monozygotic than dizygotic twins with respect to drinking behavior, frequency of drinking, amount consumed, and attitudes regarding alcohol consumption. Critics of the studies have been quick to point out, however, that environmental influences are not identical for monozygotic and dizygotic twins, and consequently a genetic factor cannot be clearly established as responsible for the concordance.

A more successful attempt to preclude the effect of environmental factors has been made by using adoption and half-sibling study techniques. Most of these studies have suggested that heredity is more important than environment in the etiology of alcoholism. Unfortunately all of the studies were relatively small. A recent, well-formulated adoption study,[231,232] using adequate adopted control groups, has demonstrated a significantly increased incidence of alcoholism and alcohol-related problems in the progeny of alcoholic patients. One of the biologic parents of each person in the study group had borne the "hospital" diagnosis of alcoholism. The parents of the progeny in the control group did not bear that diagnosis. Although the authors believe that their study indicates genetic factors in alcoholism, they are quick to point out that environmental factors still cannot be excluded completely.

Studies of families of alcoholics, however, always show higher rates among relatives than in the general population, quoted as about 4 percent for men and 0.5 to 1 percent in women. Sons of alcoholic parents have rates as high as 25 to 50 percent, while the rate for daughters is 3 to 7 percent. Shuckit et al.[233] believe that genetic factors do play a role in the transmission of an alcoholism potential to the children.

In a Danish twin study, 25 percent of nonidentical twins and 65 percent of identical twins who had at least one alcoholic parent become alcoholics whether they were reared by alcoholic parents or by nonalcoholic foster parents.

In summary, no study or series of studies has shown that heredity is more important than or separable from environment in the etiology of alcohol abuse. Nevertheless some metabolic studies and several twin, half-sib, and adoption studies have suggested that genetic factors are indeed active in the predisposition toward alcoholism. It remains quite possible that complex polygenic inheritance may account, at least in part, for a predisposition to alcohol abuse, whether it be via inherited metabolic differences or inherited personality differences.

## 2. Psychologic Factors

It is believed by some people that alcoholics are psychologically "different," that they possess a number of traits which, in common, make up the "alcoholic personality." There is, however, no agreement on the identity of these traits, or on whether they may be the cause for or the results of excessive drinking.

Psychologists and psychiatrists have described alcoholics as neurotic, maladjusted, unable to relate effectively to others, sexually and emotionally immature, isolated, dependent, unable to withstand frustration or tension, poorly integrated, and marked by deep feelings of sinfulness and unworthiness. Some have suggested that alcoholism is a disastrous attempt at the self-cure of an unseen inner conflict, and might well be called "suicide by inches."[234]

Freud and others proposed that excessive drinking may represent attempts to repress unconscious homosexual instincts, and thus the "two-fisted, he-man" drinker is in reality drinking heavily to cover his underlying homosexual drives.[235] Still others have attributed alcoholism to an unconscious need to dominate, or an attempt to escape from guilt feelings, or an inability to give or accept tenderness or love.[236] Many researchers have accumulated data to demonstrate that alcoholics often come from broken or unhappy homes and underwent serious emotional deprivation during their childhood.[237] But many of these same qualities and experiences have been observed in men and women who are not alcoholics, but who may be suffering from bizarre phobias or a wide assortment of mental ailments from mild neuroses to severe psychoses, or who may even be leading reasonably normal lives.

If there is an actual "alcoholic personality," or a "prealcoholic personality," its specifications are poorly defined and often contradictory, and seem to apply broadly to all mental illness. Knowledge of the role played by psychologic factors in alcoholics also awaits further research. However, it is the strong contention of most scientists today that the disease known as alcoholism is determined very strongly by both biogenetic and environmental elements.

## 3. Sociocultural Factors

Sociologic studies have been aimed at determining why alcoholism is widespread in some national and cultural groups but rare in others.[238]

Those with the highest reported cases of alcoholics are classed as high-incidence group. They include particularly the northern French, Americans (especially the Irish-Americans, but not the Irish in Ireland), Swedes, Swiss, Poles, and northern Russians.

By contrast, the relatively low-incidence groups include the Italians, some Chinese groups, Orthodox Jews, Greeks, Portuguese, Spaniards, and the southern French.

Differences among some of these cultural groups are reflected in the composition of groups of alcoholics studied in the United States. In one group analyzed in New York City where available figures indicate that roughly 10 percent of the total population is Irish, 15 percent is Italian, and 25 percent is Jewish, 40 percent of the alcoholics were Irish, 1 percent Italian, and none Jewish.[239] In an extensive California study, in an area with large proportions of Irish, Italian, and Jewish inhabitants, 21 percent of the alcoholics were Irish, 2 percent were Italian, and 0.6 percent were Jewish.[240]

It does not seem likely that genetics can adequately explain these variations. Various investigators have reported that alcoholism is decreasing among Irish-Americans and Swedish-Americans, but rising among second- and third-generation Italian-Americans.[241] Some workers claim that the rate may be rising among Italians in Italy, especially in Rome and other major cities, apparently paralleling the rise in personal income. A slight but distinct rise has been noted among Jews, particularly as they tend to change from Orthodox to Reform attitudes.[242,243]

Similar studies have shown that low rates of alcoholism exhibited by some groups cannot all be attributed to abstinence. Most Mormons and Moslems, for example, do not drink because of religious beliefs, and their alcoholism rates are low. But other groups (especially the Italians, Greeks, Chinese, and Jews) contain very high percentages of drinkers, and many of them use alcohol abundantly. For example, the per capita alcohol consumption in Italy is rated second only to that in France, but the rate of alcoholism among Italians is relatively low.

In a study published by the American Medical Association in its manual on alcoholism, Dr. Selden D. Bacon of Rutgers University compares two U.S. groups as follows:

*For the Orthodox Jews:* The social functions of drinking are strikingly clear. Drinking is to draw the family together, to cement the bonds of larger group membership, to activate the relationship between man and deity. This is understood by the participants. The rules and procedures of drinking are about as ritualized as those of a university football game or a church service. Violations of the rules, or violations of propriety while drinking, are quickly and severely penalized.

The custom is learned from infancy; it is instilled at the time that basic moral attitudes are learned and is taught by prestigeful members of the group (parents, rabbis, elders). The custom is closely entwined with family and religious constellations. No great emotional feeling about drinking as such are particularly noticeable; there have never been experiences with prohibition; there are no abstinence movements; there is no dionysiac cult or worship in drinking. Members of this group sneer at other groups that exhibit drunkenness. . . . All members of this society drink, they do so hundreds of times every year; they use beer, wine, and distilled spirits. . . . Alcoholism is practically unknown.

*For the Anglo-Saxon Protestant Group:* The social functions of drinking are rather vaguely and somewhat defensively described; they concern drawing people—both family members and also complete strangers—together, often for purposes of "fun," often to allow relaxation from (rather than, as in the preceding case, closer adherence to) moral norms. The rules and procedures are on occasion rather specific, but also show enormous variability so that a given individual may follow one set of rules with his family, another with business or professional associates, and a third on holiday occasions, and show even different patterns when away from the home town. Sanctions for violations are extremely irregular, ranging from accepting laughter to violent physical attack. . . . The custom is generally learned between the ages of 15 and 20. Sometimes the learning stems not from parents, ministers, physicians, elders and teachers, but from other adolescents. There is great emotional feeling about the problem on the mass level as well as by individuals. Activating the custom, especially by the young, is often attended with feelings of guilt, hostility and exhibitionism, and may occur as a secretive practice insofar as parents or employers or elders are concerned. . . . Perhaps three-quarters of the males over 15 years of age and perhaps over one-half of the females over 15 years of age use alcoholic beverages, there being not too much use of wine, relatively greater use of beer by men and use of distilled spirits. . . . Alcoholism is not rare in this group. Perhaps 3 to 7 of every 100 users of alcohol are alcoholics.

The full significance of such ambivalent feelings as a cause of alcoholism is yet to be determined. It may be at least hypothesized, however, that they play a significant role.

In general, research has shown that for groups that use alcohol to a significant degree, the lowest incidence of alcoholism is associated with certain habits and attitudes:

1. The children are exposed to alcohol early in life, within a strong family or religious group. Whatever the beverage, it is served in very diluted form and in small quantities, with consequent low blood alcohol levels.

2. The beverages commonly, although not invariably, used by the groups are those containing relatively large amounts of nonalcoholic components, which also give low blood alcoholc levels.

3. The beverage is considered mainly as a food and usually consumed with meals, again with consequent low blood alcohol levels.

4. Parents present a constant example of moderate drinking.

5. No moral importance is attached to drinking. It is considered neither a virtue nor a sin.

6. Drinking is not viewed as a proof of adulthood or virility.

7. Abstinence is socially acceptable. It is no more rude or ungracious to decline a drink than to decline a piece of bread.

8. Excessive drinking or intoxication is not socially acceptable. It is not considered stylish, comical, or tolerable.

9. Finally, and perhaps most important, there is wide and usually complete agreement among members of the group on what might be called the ground rules of drinking.

Cohen[244] points out that a subgroup under stress will find that large numbers of its members resort to drinking themselves into oblivion as the only way out. Alcoholic overindulgence actually has obliterated major segments of key people in a subculture.

It has been estimated that 100 million Americans consume alcoholic beverages, and approximately ten million of these are identified as alcoholics. Thus 10 percent of our population is faced with the devastation of this drug. Certainly the human burden of these people to themselves, their families, and the rest of the population is immense. These statistics strongly suggest that alcoholism is the most important drug problem from a public health point of view.

## 4. Modern Theories on the Etiology of Alcoholism

### *a. Addiction: A Unified Concept*

The widespread use of opiates and ethanol in modern society has led to intensive scientific investigations into the mechanisms of action of these two diverse classes of drugs. Although it is well known that excessive use of one drug is often associated with concurrent use of the other,[245] only recently has there been an effort devoted to establishing common underlying biochemical mechanisms. This is not surprising, as it is difficult to envisage the biochemical, physiologic, or metabolic pathways that complex phenanthrene-type alkaloids would have in common with a simple 2-carbon molecule. Nevertheless scrutiny of the literature points toward possible common mechanisms for certain actions of these two classes of addictive substances.

The basis for this research was a hypothesis proposed by Davis and Walsh[246] in a provocative 1970 paper in which they suggested that tetrahydroisoquinolines, alkaloid condensation products formed as a consequence of ethanol metabolism, might be involved in alcoholism. Battersby[246] pointed out that benzyl-isoquinoline alkaloids are requisite intermediates in the biosynthesis of morphine in the poppy plant *Papaver somniferum*. The possible biogenesis of these alkaloids in mammalian tissues stimulated the speculation that common biochemical mechanisms might exist between opiates and ethanol. In the same year, Cohen and Collins[247] proposed that simple tetrahydroisoquinolines (TIQs) such as those produced by condensation of catecholamines with acetaldehyde may contribute to the acute and chronic effects of ethanol intoxication. We subsequently suggested the "link" hypothesis (Figure 11-2), which states that TIQs formed following ethanol ingestion can function as opiates and thus serve as the biochemical "link" between alcohol and opiates.[248]

These theories have met with severe criticism[249,250] on the basis that the acute effects of opiates and ethanol are dissimilar, the dependence phenomena are different, narcotic antagonists do not antagonize ethanol or precipitate withdrawal symptoms in animals dependent on ethanol, the withdrawal symptoms of morphine are unlike those of ethanol, and there is no experimental evidence to link the isoquinolines with ethanol.

Although the isoquinoline question has not been resolved, numerous experiments in the past decade have substantiated the contention that common mechanisms exist for ethanol and opiates. Naloxone has been found to diminish ethanol narcosis[251] and dependence development.[252] Blum et al.[253] observed that morphine

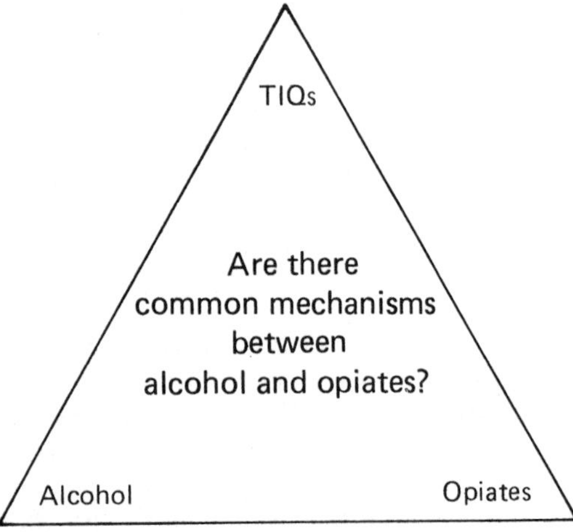


**Figure 11-2. "Link" Hypothesis Schematic. Taken from Blum et.al. in: Alcohol Tolerance and Dependence, Rigter, Crabbe (Eds.). Elsevier/North Holland Biomedical Press, p. 372, 1980.** With permission

can inhibit ethanol withdrawal convulsions in mice. Ross et al.[254] have reported a decrease in voluntary ethanol consumption following naloxone administration in the hamster. Altshuler et al.[255] have observed that naloxone alters ethanol consumption in monkeys trained to autoadminister ethanol, resulting in an extinction curve. Ho et al.[256] have reported a decrease in voluntary ethanol consumption in alcohol-preferring mice following morphine, methadone, or levorphanol administration, but no change in alcohol consumption after treatment with dextrophan, the inactive isomer of levorphanol. Acutely morphine, ethanol, and salsolinol have been found to cause a decrease in brain calcium in specific regions.[257,258] Interestingly naloxone blocks the calcium-depleting action of these agents, which would further support the possibility of similar or associated sites of action for both ethanol and opiates.

More surprising is that, in humans, there are reports of naloxone-induced antagonism of acute ethanol intoxication[259] and reversal of ethanol-induced coma, which may be due to direct delta receptor interaction.[260]

In addition to the number of reports that link the effect of ethanol action with opioids,[261] ethanol has been shown to alter such neuronal functions as synthesis, release, and degradation of certain neurotransmitters.[262,263]

In consideration of the possible involvement of the peptidyl opiate system in the actions of ethanol, and possibly in alcohol-seeking behavior, in general, certain pertinent facts are presented here.

### *b. Involvement of Peptidyl Opiates in the Actions of Alcohol*

Ethanol has been described as effectively interferring with the synthesis of brain peptides.[264] The peptidyl opiates, β-endorphin and enkephalins, being putative neurotransmitters, neuromodulators, or hormones,[265] have been shown to have altered concentrations upon acute and chronic treatment with various drugs.[266,267]

In terms of opiate receptor physiology, Pinsky et al.[268] have observed a shift in opiate receptor affinity utilizing a radioreceptor assay with rat brain homogenates after the addition of ethanol or acetaldehyde. These researchers found that these substances increased 3 H-morphine binding, but decreased naloxone binding. Interestingly salsolinol and tetrahydropaperoline, by-products of ethanol metabolism, as previously mentioned, have been found to have a weak but stereospecific interaction at opiate receptors.[269]

Since the discovery of endogenous opiates, it has become apparent that exogenous opiates such as morphine, codeine, and heroin simply

**TABLE 11-7**

**Percentage of 10th and 12th Graders by Volume of Drinking from 1978 National Survey of Drinking Groups**

| *Group* | *Drinking Pattern* | *Percentage* |
|---|---|---|
| Abstainers | Don't drink or drink less often than once a year | 25.0 |
| Infrequent drinkers | Drink once a month at most and drink small (one drink or less) amounts per typical drinking occasion | 7.6 |
| Light drinkers | Drink once a month at most and drink medium (two to four drinks) amounts per typical drinking occasion, or drink no more than three to four times a month and drink small amounts per typical occasion | 18.8 |
| Moderate drinkers | Drink at least once a week and small amounts per typical drinking occasion, three to four times a month and medium amounts per typical drinking occasion, or no more than once a month and large (five or more drinks) amounts per typical drinking occasion | 16.6 |
| Moderate/heavier drinkers | Drink at least once a week and medium amounts per typical drinking occasion, or three to four times a month and large amounts per typical drinking occasion | 17.3 |
| Heavier drinkers | Drink at least once a week and large amounts per typical drinking occasion | 14.8 |

Note: Percentages are based on "weighted" observations. A drink is equivalent to 12 fluid ounces of beer, 4 fluid ounces of wine, or 1 fluid ounce of distilled spirits. (From Rachal et al., Report to NIAAA, 1980.)

mimic the actions of compounds found in the body. This situation is comparable to that of exogenous substances such as nicotine and muscarine, which stimulate the receptors of acetylcholine. As with other receptor populations, it is suggested that multiple types of opiate (β-endorphin/enkephalin) receptors exist and that a wide range of functions may be mediated by their stimulation.[270] Accordingly those actions of ethanol that are blocked by narcotic antagonists, and therefore may be common or associated with exogenous opiates, may include:

1. Competition for opiate receptors by tetrahydroisoquinolines.
2. The stimulation of enkephalin release by ethanol, similar to the proposed actions of general anesthetics.
3. Postsynaptic membrane perturbation due to membrane fluidization induced by ethanol that results in increased opiate receptor stimulation.

Since opiates occupy the receptor sites for endogenous ligands, the question of whether chronic treatment with opiates will alter enkephalin content in the brain has been raised. Kosterlitz and Hughes[271] have proposed that a reduction in enkephalin release might be involved in the development of tolerance and dependence to opiates. By using radioimmunoassay, a number of laboratories have studied the effects of chronic morphine treatment on enkephalin levels in either whole brain or brain regions known to be high in enkephalins.[272–274] The consensus of opinion is that chronic morphine treatment does not change levels of met- or leu-enkephalin. Shani et al.,[274] however, did observe a fall in brain enkephalin in rats that received a single morphine pellet implant and were sacrificed three days later. In five other morphine regimens, they saw no change, which is in agreement with the other investigators. Höllt et al.[275] found a decrease in pituitary β-endorphin in animals treated chronically with morphine for one month and an increase in plasma β-endorphin with a precipitatory dose of naloxone in rats that were morphine tolerant/dependent. Interestingly they observed a rise in plasma β-endorphin coupled with a decrease in anterior pituitary lobe β-endorphin in morphine-dependent rats acutely withdrawn from naloxone. It should be noted that in rats made dependent on a shorter ten-day morphine regimen, Höllt et al.[275] saw no significant changes in β-endorphine levels. Ungar et al.[276] have reported an interesting experiment with rats injected with progressively decreasing doses of morphine. Brain extracts from these animals were subjected to electrophoretic fractionation and found to exhibit either opiate agonist or antagonist properties. Antagonist properties were assayed *in vivo* against morphine in mice, and *in vitro* against normorphine or synthetic endorphins in the mouse vas deferens. They found that fractions containing agonist-like activity had increased by 137 percent on day 12 of morphine treatment, but had fallen to 27 percent of the normal level on the 18th day. Antagonist activity was undetectable in untreated rat brains, but increased gradually during the first 12 days of morphine treatment, and declined thereafter.

The agonist-like activity observed by Ungar et al.[276] was presumably due to endogenous opiates; the identity of those substances with antagonist properties is not known. Whatever interpretation is placed on Ungar's work, it is obvious that chronic morphine receptor stimulation may have a marked effect on the physiology of enkephalinergic systems. Pinsky et al.[268] studied the effects of chronic alcohol treatment on enkephalin binding in rats. In rats treated with ethanol for 15 days, they observed a decrease in enkephalin activity. It should be noted, however, that they measured enkephalins indirectly via an opiate receptor binding technique. A report by Schulz[277] indicates that chronic treatment with ethanol decreases methionine-enkephalin levels in striatum, medulla, pons, and midbrain, or β-endorphin in the intermediate/posterior lobe of the rat pituitary. Certainly these studies suggest possible involvement of the peptidyl opiate system in the actions of ethanol.

### *c. The Psychogenetic Theory of Alcohol-Seeking Behavior*

The question of genetic versus environmental factors in the development of alcoholism has long been debated. McClearn and Rodgers[278] observed a substantial difference in preference for voluntary alcohol consumption among various mouse strains. Among the strains studied were mice of the C57 strain, which were found to prefer alcohol over water, and of the DBA strain, which prefer water over alcohol. We have observed differences between the two strains with respect to vas deferens responsibility to alcohol[279] and the induction of psychomotor impairment by alcohol.[280] Differences between the two strains can also be seen with respect to responses to morphine analgesia and running activity.[281] Since these differences are genetically determined, it is possible that a genetic marker reflecting an individual's preference and susceptibility to ethanol may be identified.

There is increasing evidence from both animals and humans that seems to support the possibility that both ethanol and narcotic drugs may induce euphoria via the endorphinergic system.[282] On the basis of the evidence that ethanol or a by-product of alcohol ingestion—that is, isoquinolines—interacts at opiate-mediated sites,[269] and the possibility that alcohol- and opiate-seeking behavior is a function of endogenous peptidyl opiate levels,[283] Blum and associates[284] proposed the "psychogenetic theory of drug-seeking behavior." In terms of alcohol- and opiate-seeking behavior, the psychogenetic theory proposes that individuals prone to such behavior possess a genetic deficiency of the peptidyl opiate system. In addition, continued utilization of either alcohol or opiates may be due, in part, to the possibility that long-term exposure to these drugs results in significant reduction of endogenous peptidyl opiates (type III).

A simple mathematical representation of the components of the theory is as follows:

$$\mathbf{DSB = G_{DIO} + E}$$

where *DSB* is drug-seeking behavior, $G_{DIC}$ is genetic deficiency of the internal opiate, anu *E* is environment.

Our laboratory has devoted considerable energy to the study of ethanol and, based on some experimental evidence, a model for typing alcoholics has been proposed as depicted in Figure 11-3.

Preliminary evidence for support of type I is derived from our findings that a negative correlation (0.56 = correlation coefficient) exists between mouse whole-brain methionine-enkephalin levels and genotype-linked ethanol preference.[285,286] Currently there is even some experimental support for the type II alcohol[287]; further sociologic data are warranted, however.

Since opiates occupy or alter the receptor sites for endogenous ligands, the question has been raised as to whether chronic treatment with opiates—or ethanol—will alter enkephalin content in the brain. In this regard, our findings of a marked reduction of basal ganglia leucine-enkephalin in hamsters drinking ethanol for a 12-month period are in full agreement with the studies by Pinsky et al.[268] and Schulz,[277] and further suggest possible opiate occupancy by ethanol as a metabolite. Interpretation of these results tends to support, in part, the negative feedback theory for agonist (opiatelike) -induced inhibition of neuronal enkephalin synthesis as proposed by Goldstein,[288] and is certainly supportive of type III alcoholics as proposed. Alternatively the ethanol-induced reduction of basal ganglia enkephalin-like material simply may be caused by the direct neurotoxic effects of ethanol[289] and warrants further investigation.

**Alcoholism—reclassification**

Type I

$AD = G_{DIO} + E$

Type II

$AD = G_{NIO} + E$

Type III

$AD = G_{NIO} + E + A_{DIO}$

AD = Alcohol desire
DIO = Deficiency of internal opiate
A = Alcohol
G = Genetic
E = Environment
NIO = Normal internal opiate

**Figure II-3. Schematic of "Psychogenetic Theory of Alcohol Seeking Behavior." Taken from Blum et.al., Substance and Alcohol Actions/Misuse. Pergamon Press, New York, Vol. 1:3, p. 255, 1980.** With permission

At least the psychogenetic theory of alcohol-seeking behavior serves as a useful model for research directions in pursuit of the underlying mechanisms involved in the phenomenology of such behavior. Certainly future research may include clinical development of nontoxic agents that will enhance the functional activity of brain peptidyl opiates via alteration of synthesis, release, turnover, or receptor interaction.[290]

## L. PATTERNS OF ALCOHOL CONSUMPTION

Viewed in historic perspective, U.S. drinking practices appear dynamic rather than static, characterized by shifts in the types of beverages consumed as well as by increases and decreases in the volume of consumption.

Two major sources are used to estimate alcoholic beverage consumption: apparent consumption (derived from official reports of states, tax-paid withdrawal records, and, in some cases, reports of sales by the beverage industry); and self-reported consumption (derived from individual responses to surveys).

In the United States, apparent consumption now averages about 1 ounce of ethanol (approximately two drinks) each day for each person 14 years of age and older. Averages, however, can be misleading. Since approximately one third of the U.S. adult population aged 18 years and older reports abstaining from alcoholic beverages,[291] average daily consumption for those who do drink is higher—1.5 ounces of ethanol (three drinks). But a small proportion of adults drink far more than the average, whereas the majority of adults drink less. The former group—approximately 11 percent of the population—consumes about half of all beverages sold.[292]

It is clear that Americans today are drinking more beer than wine or distilled spirits. They consume nearly as much ethanol from beer (49 percent) as from wine (12 percent) and distilled spirits (39 percent) combined.[292]

Although apparent consumption on a national level continued to rise during the 1970s, the rate of increase slowed considerably. In contrast to a 25 percent increase for the 1960s, the rate of increase in apparent consumption of ethanol for the 1970s slowed to 8 percent. Apparent consumption rates, however, are sensitive to assumptions concerning the ethanol content of various beverages (see Figure 11-3).

Between 1970 and 1978, apparent per capita consumption increased or was constant in all but five states—Alaska, Connecticut, Delaware, New Jersey, and New York—and the District of Columbia. Nevada has now surpassed Washington, D.C., as the nation's leader in apparent per capita consumption.

Most southern states showed large increases in apparent per capita consumption, although these increases are still lower than in other regions. Increases of more than 20 percent were also seen in half of the western states. Apparent consumption of ethanol from beer increased or remained at the same level in every state. Ethanol consumption from wine also increased in most states, and increased 19 percent for the nation as a whole. Consumption of ethanol from distilled spirits increased in 27 states, but decreased by 4 percent in the United States as a whole.

In terms of recent trends, the data do not reveal any striking changes in self-reported consumption by adults between 1971 and 1979. For adolescents, comparisons of data for 1974 and 1978 do not show substantial changes in either the percentage of adolescents who report drinking or the volume of drinking. The percentages of reported heavier drinking for 1974 and 1978 were virtually identical; comparisons of male and female adolescents for 1974 and 1978 suggest that male adolescent drinking is becoming similar to female drinking rather than the reverse. The 1978 data show an increase of 7 percent of males reporting abstinence. However, males continue to outnumber females in the heavier drinking group by a substantial margin.

## M. TREATMENT OF ALCOHOLISM[7]

The alcoholic who needs or seeks help faces at the outset a number of vital questions. Should the search for help begin with a relative or a well-meaning family friend? With the family physician, a psychiatrist, or a worker from Alcoholics Anonymous? With a member of the clergy or a social worker? Is a self-cure possible?

Should the alcoholic be treated at home, in a sanitarium, or in a hospital? Should he/she try to taper off gradually or stop all drinking immediately? Should the alcoholic look to drugs or psychotherapy? Will the treatment require a day, a month, a year, or longer? What are the chances of recovery?

Many of the answers will be dictated by the alcoholic's personal prejudices, fears, finances, and pressures by the family. Other answers will be influenced subtly but powerfully by community attitudes toward alcohol and the alcoholic. Some may be influenced by knowledge of the advances in alcoholism therapy—knowledge on the alcoholic's own part, and on the part of the therapist.

In any effective state or local alcoholism treatment program, it is clearly essential that alcoholics and their relatives—as well as physicians, members of the clergy, probation officers, personnel workers, social workers, and various social agencies—be provided with sound, up-to-date information on the types of treatment available in their communities, the precise locations where such therapy can be obtained, the probable costs, and the possible results.

On a national basis, the number of persons receiving treatment for alcoholism and problem drinking appears to have increased from an estimated 1,584,000 in 1976 to 1,712,000 in 1977. The State Alcoholism Profile Information System (SAPIS) indicates that 1,058,000 people (77 percent male and 15 percent female) were admitted to alcoholism treatment programs funded by NIAAA and state agencies in that year. Of those admissions for whom age was reported, 54 percent were 21 to 44; 35 percent were 45 to 65; 5 percent were 18 to 20; 3 percent

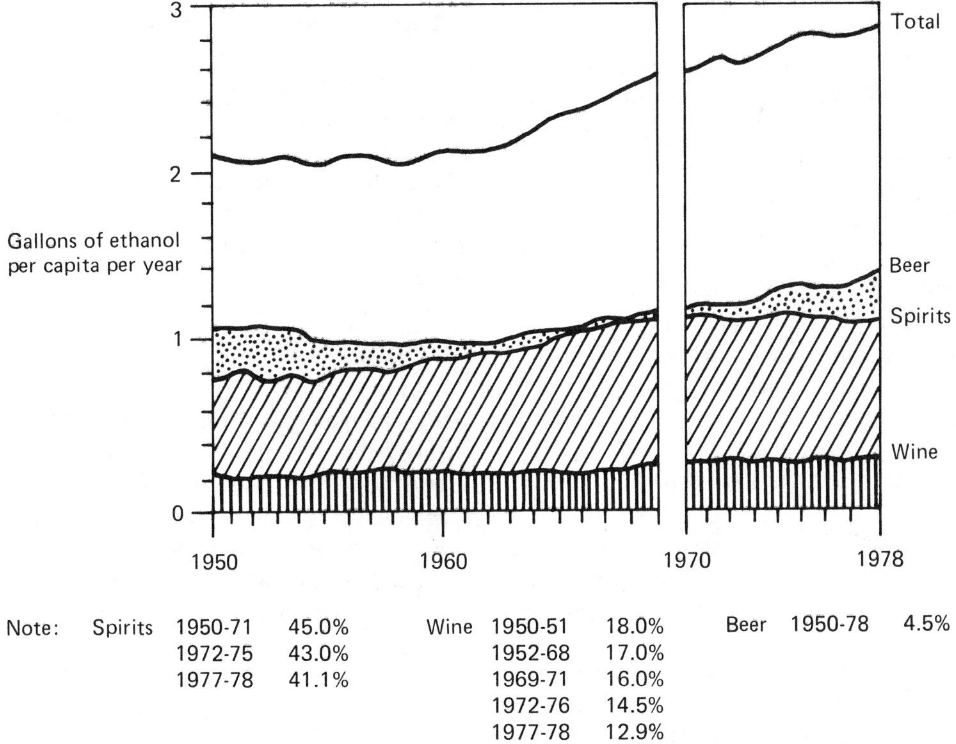


**Figure 11-4. Apparent U.S. consumption of alcoholic beverages in gallons of ethanol per capita of the drinking-age population. 1950-1978. Taken from Malin et al., Report to NIAAA, 1980.**

were over 65; and fewer than 3 percent were under 18.

Approximately 85 percent of alcoholics and problem drinkers, however, are not receiving formal treatment services: some eight million of the nation's alcoholics and problem drinkers were not receiving services in 1977.

## 1. Preliminary Treatment

Some alcoholics will begin treatment during a stage of temporary sobriety, and others during the throes of a severe hangover or during acute intoxication. For many, it will be during the drying-out or withdrawal stage, marked by such conditions as delirium tremens. In some cases of acute intoxication, and in most with severe withdrawal symptoms, competent medical management directed by a physician is essential. Without such care, the patient may die.[293]

Treatment of withdrawal symptoms formerly was based largely on such alcohol substitutes as chloral hydrate and paraldehyde. But in the past 15 years, these drugs have been replaced in part by new synthetic tranquilizers such as reserpine, chlorpromazine, meprobamate, promazine hydrochloride, and chlordiazepoxide. The impact of these tranquilizing drugs on the treatment of the acute alcoholic stage has been described by some clinicians as revolutionary.[294] With appropriate use of tranquilizers and other therapeutic aids, and especially the control of fluid and electrolyte balance, most patients recover promptly from delirium, hallucinations, and tremors, and are ready to start other forms of treatment.

## 2. Extent of the Problem

No one can state with accuracy the number of alcoholics in the United States, although estimates range from eight to 14 million. It is possible that these figures are very conservative. The total consumption of alcohol is increasing as indicated by continuing expansion of the liquor industry and per capita consumption; however, without reliable statistics, one cannot assume that this necessarily reflects an increase in alcoholism.

## 3. Treatment Approaches

### *a. Alcoholics Anonymous*[295]

Alcoholics Anonymous (AA) has probably been the most successful approach to the rehabilitation of the alcoholic. At first, these groups were not well received by the scientific community. An AA meeting is usually a very warm and friendly gathering of people trying to help each other solve their drinking problems. One of the primary reasons why AA succeeds may be the fact that its members must admit or actually "confess" publicly to their "alcologs" (their personal history of alcoholic problems) and that they cannot control their alcohol intake.

Alcoholics Anonymous is not a total treatment, but part of the treatment approach. The patient, along with the drinking problem, may have physical ailments or other mental problems. Some AA members become so excited about the program that they become "anti everything" except AA, including medications, doctors, and religion.

Important auxilliary family groups include Al-Anon and Al-Ateen. Al-Anon is composed of family members of the alcoholic, and Al-Ateen consists of teenage children of alcoholics. Al-Anon and Al-Ateen, which are autonomous of AA, have enabled the family to understand alcoholism better. Through Al-Anon, formally started in 1949, today there are more than 2000 groups.

### *b. Psychotherapy*

Psychotherapy is defined as the mental treatment of illness. It may be used on an individual, group, or family basis, and could include such techniques as verbal communication, medication, and hypnosis. Through psychotherapy, the alcoholic may learn to adjust more comfortably to the environment.

### *c. Group Therapy*

Group therapy may be the most effective type of psychotherapy available for alcoholics. This type of therapy is usually nonthreatening, yet challenging enough so that they can find support, and discuss their fears, anger, guilt, and feelings of inferiority and worthlessness, while learning how to cope with their feelings and to find alternative ways to solve their drinking problems. Many alcoholics prefer this type of therapy over AA meetings because it gives them the chance to relate interpersonally with other alcoholics rather than listen to alcologs.

#### *d. Family Therapy*

Some investigators have suggested that other members of the alcoholic's family may be responsible, in part, for the patient's drinking. It is estimated that for each alcoholic, there are at least two people in the alcoholic's family, including children, who are affected. It is generally believed, although not fully documented, that alcoholics are very destructive to the personalities of other family members.

It is for these reasons that family therapy, group therapy, Al-Anon, and Al-Ateen are so vital. They allow understanding, a new perspective on the situation, and even self-insights to develop family relationships, rather than family destruction. In a more formal sense, family therapy is aimed at examining and attempting to shift the destructive ways family members relate, so that new avenues of relating become possible. It has been stated that about 20 percent of the time the alcoholic family member is the wife and not the husband.

#### *e. Psychodrama*

Psychodrama was developed by Moreno.[296] It is another adjunct to psychotherapy. This form of therapy enables patients to project themselves into other people's roles to obtain a better understanding of themselves and others. In this way, patients may be able to deal better with inner conflicts as they spontaneously arise. Psychodrama may be advantageous since it allows the rest of the group to act as a sounding board for the "actors," and also involves the patients, who can observe themselves through television video replay.

#### *f. Psychoanalysis*

Psychoanalysis, a specific type of psychotherapy, is devised to investigate a patient's mental processes. The techniques utilized in this form of therapy include dream interpretation, free association, and the interpretation of the transference between patient and therapist. It is helpful in understanding the underlying conflicts and problems, and in assisting the patient to gain insight. However, this approach alone has not been successful in the treatment of alcoholism.

#### *g. Religion*

Religion provides the alcoholic a way in which to gain acceptance by his/herself and by loved ones. However, it has not been very successful in rehabilitating patients and probably has done little to curtail drinking. In fact, most patients find more acceptance in AA than in structured religion. It also has been suggested that, through AA, one attains a better understanding of one's self and one's relationship to God.

#### *h. Halfway Houses*

Halfway houses provide the alcoholic with time to make the transition back to society. During this transition, the halfway house furnishes a place to live comfortably with people with similar problems. In most cases, it supplies counseling, when necessary, concerning job, family, and friends. With time, patients reobtain a sense of self-respect because they now can pay their own way by working and can communicate meaningfully with others.

## N. DRUGS AND DETERRENCE OF ALCOHOL CONSUMPTION[297]

### 1. Aldehyde, Dehydrogenase Inhibitors

Disulfiram, first advocated as a therapeutic

aid in alcoholism by Danish workers in 1948, continues to occupy a role as an adjunct to psychotherapy and behavior therapy. At the very least, disulfiram appears to be a good test of the motivation of the patient for sobriety. That disulfiram acts by blocking aldehyde dehydrogenase, causing a toxic elevation of circulating acetaldehyde when alcohol is consumed, continues to be generally accepted as its primary mechanism of action. Whether such blockade solely accounts for the clinical manifestations of the disulfiram–alcohol interaction has been questioned. On the basis of studies in rabbits, it has been suggested that an unidentified acetaldehyde metabolite may be responsible for the hypotension. Since disulfiram is deposited in the fat of the body and not in the body's water, it is excreted from the body slowly. Once treatment is begun, one-half tablet a day or two or three tablets twice a week are given. Most doctors feel disulfiram is contraindicated during pregnancy because of possible danger to the fetus, and in patients with psychosis and even heart disease (due to its β-hydroxylase inhibiting properties).

Disulfiram (Antabuse) interferes with the breakdown of acetaldehyde, causing elevations of acetaldehyde in the blood sufficient to produce nausea, flushing, dysphoria, dyspnea, hypertension, and syncope. Heart failure, and in rare instances death, are possible. Antabuse is used by many clinicians, but its efficacy has not been established on a scientific basis.

Patients starting Antabuse therapy need to be free of alcohol for 12 hours. The dose and frequency of administration vary from clinician to clinician, but the usual procedure is to give a 500-mg loading dose for five days followed by a daily maintenance dose of 250 mg. Some clinicians prescribe it three times a week, but most prescribe it for daily use. If patients on Antabuse drink any alcohol, they are apt to have a reaction. Even the alcohol in aftershave lotion absorbed through the skin can cause a reaction in very sensitive people. A thorough indoctrination concerning the many foods and products containing alcohol is required before starting this drug. From practical experience, the most common inadvertent ingestion of alcohol occurs with medications in elixir form. Usually alcoholics taking disulfiram who cannot maintain sobriety will stop the drug for a few days before they resume drinking. Most who resume drinking after stopping Antabuse for seven to ten days will experience no adverse reaction. To be on the safe side, patients are advised to wait for at least 14 days. If they drink while taking Antabuse, they will have a reaction that is dependent on both the dose of Antabuse and the alcohol. This Antabuse–alcohol reaction is symptomatic, for example, treatment of shock by ordinary measures; inhalation of 95 percent oxygen and 5 percent carbon dioxide, is thought to be useful by some clinicians. Ascorbic acid has also been used.

Use of Antabuse in severe end-stage alcoholics can be dangerous, and if there is evidence that the alcoholic is unable to stop the use of alcohol, the clinician should attempt to control the situation by other means.

Antabuse should be used with caution in patients with major medical problems such as diabetes, cerebral damage, epilepsy, and renal problems, and is contraindicated in patients who are allergic to the drug, are psychotic, or have severe coronary artery disease. Antabuse itself, in some individuals, may cause mild sedation, confusion, and carbon disulfide poisoning. The clinician should monitor the patient taking Antabuse for neurologic problems secondary to carbon disulfide poisoning, as carbon disulfide is one of the major metabolites of disulfiram. There are a few cases in which Antabuse is thought to have caused hepatotoxicity. Antabuse also potentiates the effects of certain drugs, for example, phenytoin coumarin derivatives, and isoniazid, and is relatively contraindicated when these drugs are used. It is not an innocuous drug, and its chronic use should be carefully monitored. Antabuse should be prescribed only with the patient's full knowledge and consent.

For many patients, Antabuse provides insurance against the impulse to drink and can free energy for other pursuits. It is compatible with other forms of alcoholism treatment and has particular usefulness for the difficult-to-treat binge-drinking alcoholics.

While many thousands of alcoholics have been helped by taking Antabuse, those who do best are those with the best prognosis initially. The degree of its effectiveness, therefore, is still a matter of some scientific debate. Nonetheless many physicians feel that Antabuse is a unique and important contribution to the recovery of their alcoholic patients. It is not a cure, however, but merely affords a crutch, a way to fortify a sincere desire to stop drinking. The rationale for its use is that patients know they must avoid alcohol for at least three to four days after taking disulfiram or they will elicit the acetaldehyde syndrome. In this regard, they also must learn to avoid disguised forms of alcohol such as sauces, fermented vinegar, cough syrup, and even aftershave lotions and backrubs.

The following are other aldehyde dehydrogenase inhibitors that may result in an Antabuse-like reaction when patients who are taking them consume alcohol.

Calcium carbimide
Antidiabetic sulfonylureas
N-butyraldoxime
Tolazoline
Phenformin
Nitroduran
Phenylbutazone
Metronidazole

## 2. Miscellaneous Drugs—$NAD^+$ (DPN)

The coenzyme nicotinamide adenosine dinucleotide ($NAD^+$) was believed greatly to reduce the craving for alcohol. Other compounds that can serve *in vivo* as a source of $NAD^+$, such as pyruvate and fructose, have been reported to enhance the rate of disappearance of alcohol from blood.

## 3. Drugs Reported to Alter the Taste of Alcohol

Metronidazole and potassium thiocyanate (rhodanate of potassium) are said to alter the taste of alcohol. An extract from *Adiantum capillus veneris*, purportedly containing flavaspidic acid as the active principle, has also been reported to cause aversion to the taste of alcohol in humans.

## 4. Drugs Reported to Decrease Alcohol Preference in Rodents

Among these drugs are the following.
Metronidazole
Disulfiram
Sulfonylureas
Butyraldoxime
Alanine
Fructose
Amphetamine
Alloxan
Enkephalinase inhibitors
Opiates
Narcotic antagonists
Glutamine
Estrogens
Methionine-enkephaline
Methadone (in some reports but may increase consumption in others).

## 5. Other Drugs

Tranquilizers, particularly the benzodiazepines, Librium and Valium, have been used to treat the anxiety symptoms of recovering sober alcoholics or as an adjunct to an effort to assist the individual regain some moderate drinking behavior. Clinical experience with these drugs as a "substitute" for alcohol has been disappointing. More often than not, alcohol is used excessively along with drugs, thus increasing the risk of intoxication and lethal overdose. Experience with addiction shows that once control is lost with alcohol, it is often lost with other sedative-hypnotics. Only in very exceptional situations is their use recommended as a substitute for alcohol or as an adjunct to alcoholism treatment.

Tricyclic antidepressants and lithium have a specialized and sometimes beneficial effect in the sober recovering alcoholic who has depressive or manic symptoms. Caution should be exercised with tricyclics because, if the patient continues to drink excessively, the combination of alcohol and tricyclics greatly enhances the risk of harmful overdose reactions (see Chapter 19).

## O. PREVENTION

Prevention may prove most successful in at least four areas:

1. *Identification of the alcoholic-prone individual* will obviously lead to the possible curtailment of alcoholism in humans.

2. *Education* of society concerning the various aspects of alcoholism will produce an environment in which the alcoholic will be accepted, rather than demoralized. This education must begin with the young, but "scare techniques," such as showing a person dying from alcoholism, might do little to discourage the abuse of alcohol. It has already been reported that there is little alcoholism in those ethnic groups and societies where alcohol is specifically used in a ritualistic manner with meals or religious ceremonies.

3. *Community mental health* planning or organization could play a very vital role in preventing alcoholism in the United States. Outlets for frustration, hostility, anxiety, and depression, all part of the alcoholic personality trait, could be afforded through various well-executed community health programs.

4. *Scientists actively engaged in research* on the acute and chronic effects of alcohol in the body have provided important information that may have a direct bearing on the etiology and possible cure for alcoholism. However, there are several general areas that need to be further investigated. These include (a) the etiology of ethanol dependence; (b) the question of why some people depend on alcohol and others do not; (c) an alcohol substitute; (d) a long-acting substance that would make alcohol unpalatable, but is not dangerous; (e) a reclassification of alcoholic beverages according to their ingredients so that the purchaser would know all the pharmacologically active agents present in addition to ethanol; (f) a substance to decrease existing intoxication in an individual rapidly; and (g) a form of treatment that will prevent relapse of the individual into alcoholism.

## P. MEDICAL USES OF ALCOHOL

The medical uses of alcohol include:

1. As a solvent for many nonpolar drugs.
2. As a coolant.
3. As a rubefacient rubbed on the skin to prevent decubitus ulcers; it decreases sweating.
4. As a skin disinfectant—70 percent by weight.
5. In injections for the relief of pain.
6. As an antipyretic.
7. For head colds—"to be instituted at the first inkling of a cold, namely, to hang one's hat on the bedpost, drink from a bottle of good whiskey until two hats appear, and then get into bed and stay there."
8. For inhalation in acute pulmonary edema. Alcohol has been employed through inhalation as an antifoaming agent in the treatment of paroxysmal attacks of acute pulmonary edema secondary to heart failure.

## Q. SOCIAL IMPLICATIONS OF ALCOHOL ABUSE[298]

Alcoholism and alcohol abuse have an impact on almost every aspect of U.S. society.

### 1. Accidents

In the United States, traffic accidents are the major cause of violent death and a significant factor in serious injury. Between 35 and 64 percent of the drivers in fatal accidents and 6 to 25 percent of the drivers in nonfatal accidents had been drinking prior to the accident.[299] Motor vehicle crashes caused by alcohol abuse cost U.S. society $5.14 billion a year.[300]

Traffic accident studies show that the probability of crash involvement increases as blood alcohol content increases, and that men under 24 and over 65 are at greater general risk.

There are indications that the range of alcohol involvement in fatal motorcycle accidents is 40 to 50 percent, and 3 to 6 percent in nonfatal accidents. Evidence also indicates a higher rate of alcohol involvement in single-vehicle motorcycle accidents and fatalities.[301]

Research has consistently shown that between 45 and 60 percent of all fatal crashes involving a young driver are alcohol-related. The probability of alcohol involvement increases with the severity of the crash; for all traffic crashes, young drivers are considerably more likely to have been drinking than older drivers.[302] Traffic accidents are the leading cause of death among youths, and no other factor is as predictably associated with fatal traffic accidents as is alcohol.[303]

Alcohol as a factor in traffic crashes and driving-related consequences is an area of concern regarding special population groups other than youth, including native Americans,[304] Hispanic Americans,[305] and Asian Americans.[306]

Alcohol also appears to play a significant role in nontraffic accidents. In a study of high school students,[307] 36 percent of regular drinkers reported two or more accidental injuries in the previous year serious enough to interfere with daily activities, whereas 8 percent of nondrinkers had such accidents. Occupational accidents affect a significant portion of the working population, and alcohol may play a role.[308]

### *The Problem-Drinking Driver*

In 1978, NIAAA's 18 specialized problem-drinking driver programs served 15,798 persons, and 28 percent of all intakes in all program categories were related to driving while intoxicated. Drinking-driver program clients were most often male (86 percent), aged 35, white (71 percent), divorced or separated (52 percent), employed (88 percent), referred by the courts for the driving-while-intoxicated offense (49 percent), and were referred by AA during treatment (65 percent). For 73 percent, this was the first referral for formal treatment, and 95 percent received group treatment outpatient services. In follow-up data obtained 180 days after intake, abstinence increased from 8 percent to 46 percent; employment increased only slightly, but days worked and average monthly income increased.

Another special problem with single-vehicle accidents in particular and with alcohol is suicide. One estimate suggests that 10 to 15 percent of single-vehicle accidents are suicidal in intent.[309]

With the exception of motor vehicle accidents, falls account for more accidental deaths than any other cause and for over 60 percent of injuries. In a 1978 study,[310] almost 50 percent of those who died from falls had been drinking, and other studies have shown that alcoholics are at greater risk for falls that result in death than is the general population.

Alcohol also appears to be involved in fires and burns. One study[311] found that 52 percent of adult fire deaths involved alcohol.[299] Another study observed that alcoholics were ten times as likely to die in a fire as were members of a comparison population.[312] Alcohol lowers oxidation in the cells, increasing the risk of being overcome by smoke inhalation. Alcohol is involved in nearly three times as many deaths from cigarette-caused fires as in deaths in fires resulting from other causes.

Alcohol is also reported to play a significant contributory role in drownings. Haberman and Baden[310] found that 68 percent of drowning victims had been drinking; Hudson[313] found that 50 percent had been drinking. In recreational contexts, higher consumption of alcohol may lead to poor judgment, faulty coordination, and lack of attention. Swimmers may take more risks, and the "warming" effect of alcohol may encourage people to stay in cold water too long. Alcohol also can depress the swallowing and breathing reflexes.

## 2. Crimes

Event-based control studies of criminal behavior have not been made, but general observations indicate that alcohol is present in a large proportion of criminal events. Studies show that problem drinkers are more likely than other offenders to have been drinking at the time of the crime.[314,315] Moreover alcoholics and problem drinkers observed in treatment samples have criminal records far greater than normal. It is not clear, however, whether drinking alcohol leads to criminal behavior or whether involvement in criminal behavior leads to drinking.[316, 317]

For the possible explanation of alcohol-related crimes, the reader is referred to the works of Aarens et al.,[318] Pernanen,[319] Mark and Ervin,[320] and Tinklenberg.[321]

### 3. Suicide

Alcoholics are at particularly high risk for suicide. One study reports the risk of suicide among alcoholics to be 30 times greater than in the general population. Recent interpersonal loss may be a predictor of suicide among alcoholics.[322] Studies also have indicated that many alcoholic suicide victims were suffering from ill health or other problems. A possible connection between suicide and alcohol's mood-changing properties has been suggested; between 15 and 64 percent of suicide attempters and up to 80 percent of suicide victims had been drinking at the time of the event. Among problem drinkers, these proportions range from 1 to 33 percent for attempters and 2 to 48 percent for suicide victims. Research also shows that alcoholics who committed suicide had a history of more suicide attempts than nonalcoholics and alcoholic suicide attempters more closely resemble actual suicides than do nonalcoholic attempters. Among alcoholic women, the number of suicide attempts exceeds that for the female population as a whole,[323–325] and the rate of completed suicides among female alcoholics is 23 times the population rate.[326]

### 4. Special Populations

In the fourth special report to the United States Congress, certain special groups were identified as "high-risk" populations. These include the elderly,[327] native Americans,[328] native Alaskans,[329] Hispanic Americans,[330] black Americans,[331] Asian Americans,[307] women,[332] and adolescents.[333]

## R. SOCIAL IMPLICATIONS OF DRIVING WHILE INTOXICATED

It is a well-known fact that the excessive use of beverage alcohol causes a terrible loss of lives, injuries, and traumatic suffering of others, not to mention the economic losses. Most of this loss occurs on the U.S. highways.

Consider that more fatal injuries result from traffic accidents each year than from homicides and suicides combined.

Interestingly, although many young Americans lost their lives during the Vietnam conflict, many more lost their lives during those same years in domestic accidents. Cohen[334] suggests that it is incomprehensible why so few people become upset about the 45,000 or so who are killed and the hundreds of thousands who are injured in motor vehicle accidents each year. More than a third of these injuries and a half of the deaths are alcohol-related. Along similar lines, Congressman Michael D. Barnes (D–Md.)[335] has said that drunk driving is the most frequently committed violent crime in the United States today.

Over the past decade, more than one quarter of a million Americans have been killed in alcohol-related crashes on our roads, at a cost to Americans of $24 billion in 1981 alone. Barnes further points out that "while we lose 70 citizens in alcohol-related crashes every day, only one of every 2000 drunk drivers is caught and the chance of conviction is slim."

In a national study, it was reported that 45 percent of high school students drink in cars, 23 percent drive after drinking, and 59 percent of boys and 42 percent of girls have had drinking problems. In various studies, 18 to 51 percent of drivers involved in multivehicle fatalities had a blood alcohol concentration of 0.1 percent or higher. This finding is more evident in the one-vehicle accident where as many as 41 to 72 percent of the drivers had blood alcohol levels in the 0.1 percent range or higher.

In response to these facts, legislatures across the nation have encouraged new laws to deter "drunk driving." Generally these laws encourage state legislation to set up enforcement, establish a 0.10 blood alcohol level as uniform in statewide tracking systems to detect drunk drivers, and provide for suspension or revocation of licenses of drunk drivers by administrative action.

Other groups also have encouraged "harsh" or stronger penalties for "drunk drivers." Doris Aiken of Schenectady, New York, president of RID (Remove Intoxicated Drivers), suggests that random road blocks be instituted by all states; that on-line statewide record-keeping systems be set up and made accessible to police, the courts, and the public; and that there be immediate suspension of licenses for those with blood alcohol content over 0.10 percent. Additionally MADD (Mothers Against Drunk Drivers) chapters (77 as of the summer of 1983) have been established in many states and have also encouraged governmental concern for and public awareness of the drunk driver issue.

## S. GENERAL COMMENTS

In spite of the long history of alcoholism, the world has witnessed few serious medicinal/chemical approaches to the deterrence of alcohol consumption.

Time is needed to change society's negative bias toward alcoholism and the alcoholic so that a rich person shall not be treated as an eccentric drinker while the poor alcoholic is treated as a drunk. Time is required also for the public to accept all the humanistic implications of the disease concept of alcoholism while realizing that alcohol is one of the first drugs that people abused, and that it is still being abused today.

Alcoholism is a disease, not something evil. And the basic question we must ask is what to do with an individual who happens to have its symptoms. How do we begin to instruct this individual to obtain counseling, and where does the family structure come in? How do individuals who are prone to alcoholism get the proper care and the guidance to impel them to present themselves to Alcoholics Anonymous, or to seek some viable alternative? In dealing with any drug dependency, it is the individual, of course, who has to make the decision to stop abusing the drug. What are the roles of others, not only friends and family, but everyone who comes into contact with the alcoholic? If we motivate an individual to seek help from an organization such as AA, we have accomplished something.

Today it is known that we can treat the alcoholic who is experiencing withdrawal symptoms with tranquilizers such as Librium and Valium and can try to deter further drinking by giving Antabuse. Although punishment is not the answer, Antabuse has its place just as methadone has its place for the heroin-dependent individual; however, we need to develop other innovative treatment modalities.

How do we define alcoholism? Why do people drink alcohol, and what is the biochemical basis for alcoholism? At present, we as scientists cannot tell the public that the reason people become alcoholics is because of A, B, and C, and so let us treat A, B, and C with the following drugs so that we can prevent such individuals from ever having a drinking problem. But we are getting closer to understanding alcoholism. Some believe that the environment induces the first drink, and then many possibilities may occur that will maintain drinking. A person may be genetically prone to alcoholism as discussed in this chapter. Or, as suggested by data presented by Dr. David Lester, people possessing certain blood types may be prone to alcoholism. It is also possible that some individuals, because of heredity, may have a biochemical abnormality that needs alcohol to establish normality, and provides a basis for its chronic consumption. It is also possible that there is no genetic or biochemical proneness to alcoholism but that the individual's mental state induces the desire to drink on a chronic basis. The alcohol itself then alters the biochemistry of the brain, and even after the desire is gone, the individual must now continue alcohol consumption. This is the basis for the psychogenetic theory.

A novel definition of alcoholism is that it is a "trap" (*t* for its treatment, *r* for rehabilitation, *a* for abstinence, and *p* for prevention, all elements necessary in the possible eradication of the disease). Alcohol consumption has become a trap to at least ten million Americans, and it is the most devastating drug of abuse known. However, it is noteworthy that not all who imbibe this drug become hopelessly dependent on it. For example, connoisseurs of wine may be said to have a habit; they miss the presence of their drug, which they use as a part of a ritual. They thus are "dependent" on alcohol, but in all likelihood neither the quantity nor timing, nor the occasion for intake, nor the appropriate behavior during the drug state or that following it is out of control. Their habit does not impair their social, occupational, or personal competencies, which are maintained whether or not the drug is available. Nor do they seek other drugs as substitutes or to self-medicate either the mild withdrawal symptoms or other effects of alcohol.[333]

With the stresses of everyday life, this controlled habitual intake could become increasingly compelled and central to behavior. Whether or not these persons are "drunkards," they are at that juncture of being significantly "drug dependent" and may or may not show psychosocial disruptions. There are persons for whom the daily intake of a dose of alcohol (or marihuana) may be requisite for them to "feel right" and to accomplish organized activities, just as there are some for whom a nocturnal sedative seems critical to efficient daytime functioning. Such people, however, may require more alcohol more frequently—and (withdrawal risks aside) some or many segments of their lives may be affected.

With or without the existence of a significant daily habit, we know of compulsive flights—"episodic dependence"—with binges of excess during drug taking that may occur with severe toxic or social and behavioral consequences. Other drug-related tragedies may have nothing to do with drug dependence, but with a single, isolated occasion of excess intake and loss of personal controls. Still others constantly use excessive amounts of alcohol, but only episodically show a breakdown in functioning.

Dr. Daniel Freedman, a noted researcher, points out that for many alcohol is central to their existence, and abstinence—if it occurs—is seen only after immense suffering. For these abstinent people, it is important to appreciate the precariousness of their dependence and of the lure to return to their habit. Once established, a habit is never forgotten, and this fact ought to be kept in mind as a consequence of drug dependency. When possible, ex-alcoholics wisely avoid other sedative antianxiety agents, which they tend to use as they used alcohol.

Ewing and Rouse,[336] in discussing social policy concerning alcohol, suggest that a more moderate approach relative to the total elimination of alcohol is legal control over the alcohol industry and drinking behavior. This includes legal regulations of the kinds of alcohol consumed, its costs, its methods of distribution, the time and place of drinking, and the availability of alcohol to drinkers according to age, sex, or other socioeconomic characteristics. These authors[336] point out that the underlying assumption is that drinking is a privilege, like driving, and if abused, the privilege can be withdrawn.

Some researchers have suggested that society's goal should not be the prevention, but rather the minimization of alcohol damage.[337] For example, the 1920 liquor law of Finland stated that minimization of alcohol damage was the primary goal of that country's alcohol policies. Braun[338] suggests that areas of damage include health, life span, crime rate, public order, work performance, family life, and traffic safety.

## T. CONCLUSIONS

Alcoholism is a biologic "inheritable" disease. Most researchers agree that, although genetics is of ever-increasing importance in studies of alcoholism and drug addiction, environmental influences remain of paramount significance in any cause–effect equation. But one cannot look at either environment or genetics as *the* force that determines tendencies toward alcoholism. Either focus, taken exclusively, is an oversimplification that is a disservice to our search for solutions.

In terms of prevention, we must consider Huxley's view that euphoriants are a necessary evil. This being the case, modern legal, medical, and social approaches to the elimination of alcoholism and other substance abuse must recognize that society needs free access to the beneficial use of euphorigens in therapeutic medicine and psychiatry. Furthermore, if additional research into the biogenetics of alcoholism bears fruit, it might be possible to predict biologic predisposition to alcoholism by testing for either differential blood or urine chemistries, or possibly for natural endorphin levels. The future of alcoholism prevention might look brighter if a "dip stick" for internal opiates or other chemical components were developed. We could then implement programs to analyze these substances in urine of newborn infants.

Certainly the biologic angle is only one aspect of prevention. Labeling alcoholic beverages may be a step in the right direction. Consideration must be given to more stringent regulations covering advertising on television, and to more thorough education concerning alcohol and alcohol-related problems—not only for children, but for adults as well. We could use a Surgeon General's report on alcohol that could have the same impact on reducing problems that the report on cigarettes has had. Finally higher taxes on beverage alcohol might help to reduce consumption and, at the same time, create a special fund for treatment and research.

Heredity or environment? It is not an either/or proposition. It takes both heredity and environment to produce an alcoholic. It will take not only alertness to hereditary predisposition but also modifications in the environment to minimize the risk of future alcohol abuse.

There is a growing controversy over the widely published "controlled drinking" studies done by alcoholism researchers Mark and Linda Sobell. The Sobells' work sought to show that subjects in their studies successfully learned how to drink "socially" and, as a result of that learning, proceeded to carry on normal productive lives. However, a study by Mary Pendery and associates published in *Science*[339] showed that follow-up studies yielded "horrible outcomes" for virtually all of the subjects. On the basis of her follow-up, Dr. Pendery has waged a crusade to wipe out the influence that the Sobells have had, not only on the intensely emotional control versus abstention war, but also on the educational processes of students in psychologic disciplines—the students for whom the Sobell studies are models. Some authorities commend Dr. Pendery's research, which drew attention to the paucity of data on controlled drinking, while others are appalled. Nevertheless what really matters is that, on the basis of the Pendery studies, patients should be cautioned as to the potential dangers of the "controlled drinking" approach for the former alcohol abuser.

Of utmost importance is that society must view the alcoholic as being basically the victim of a human compulsive disorder similar to other disorders in this category, including smoking, other drugs, obesity, sexual promiscuity, and gambling. Society must also realize that the addictive behavior of the alcoholic is the result of a disease and that through research a potential "cure" is possible.

In this chapter we have explored many important aspects of the entire phenomenology of alcohol abuse and alcoholism. Certainly, though we are not yet able to provide a so-called "cure" for this devastating disease, America is becoming more aware of its sociologic implications. In that regard, a 1982 Congressional research study stated that the social and economic costs of alcoholism are staggering and may cost the nation as much as $120 billion a year. The Office of Technology Assessment, a highly respected nonpartisan research arm of Congress, performed the study at the request of the Senate Finance Committee's Subcommittee on Health.

The study said that alcoholism constitutes a vast syndrome of medical, economic, psychologic, and social problems. From 10 million to 15 million Americans are either alcoholic or have serious problems directly related to the abuse of alcohol. Up to 35 million more individuals are estimated to be affected indirectly. According to the study, alcoholism and alcohol abuse have been implicated in one half of all automobile accidents, half of all homicides, and one quarter of all suicides, and are responsible for 15 percent of the nation's total health care costs as well as being a major factor in 40 percent of all problems brought to family courts.

However, do these statistics really have impact on public awareness of the problem? In terms of the future, are we dealing with the after-sobering problems of former alcohol abusers? With all due respect to alcohol treatment approaches, for which claims of upward of 50 to 70 percent success rates have been reported, are these so-called abstainers really "addiction-free"? Follow-up studies reveal that most of these individuals switch their addiction from alcohol to tobacco, coffee, and sugar. Additionally, support services for reentry into society are inappropriate to meet the educational as well as psychologic and physical needs of these individuals. Sequelae, which are the result of chronic alcoholism, include vitamin deficiency, alcohol dementia, Korsakoff's syndrome, cirrhosis, and lack of self-esteem, and must be adequately assessed in the recovering alcoholic. The alcoholics must accept the fact that their fight against alcohol abuse is just one struggle and that there are many other "addictions" out there. They must realize that the fact that they have successfully kicked one habit does not mean that they can easily defend themselves against all others.

## REFERENCES


1. National Survey on Drug Abuse: Main Findings. NIDA. (ADM), 80–976. U.S. Government Printing Office, Washington, D.C., 1980, p. 23.
2. Blum, K., and Ryback, R. Alcohol: the first drug scene. In K. Blum and A.H. Briggs, eds., *Drugs—Use or Misuse*. Manual sponsored by the U.S. Office of Drug Education. San Antonio, Texas, 1970.
3. Becker, C.E., Roe, L.R., and Scott, R.A. *Alcohol as a Drug: A Curriculum on Pharmacology, Neurology, and Toxicology*. New York: Medcom Press, 1974, p. 1.
4. Lieber, C.S. Liver adaptation and injury in alcoholism. *N. Engl. J. Med.* 288:356, 1973.
5. Rubin, E., and Lieber, C.S. Alcoholism, alcohol, and drugs. *Science* 172:1097, 1971.
6. Ray, O.S. (Editor) *Alcohol in Drugs, Society, and Human Behavior*. St. Louis: C.V. Mosby, 1972, pp. 78–94.
7. National Institute of Mental Health. *Alcohol and Alcoholism*. Publication no. 5011. U.S. Department of Health, Education and Welfare, 1969.
8. Leake, C.D., and Silverman, M. *Alcoholic Beverages in Clinical Medicine*. Chicago: Year Book Medical Publishers, 1966.
9. Goldberg, L. The metabolism of alcohol. In S.P. Lucia, ed., *Alcohol and Civilization*. New York: McGraw-Hill, 1963.
10. Greenberg, L.A. Alcohol and emotional behavior. In S.P. Lucia, ed., *Alcohol and Civilization*. New York: McGraw-Hill, 1963.
11. Haggard, H.W., Greenberg, L.A., and Lolli, G. The absorption of alcohol with special reference to its influence on the concentration of alcohol appearing in the blood. *Q. J. Stud. Alcohol* 1:684, 1941.
12. Lolli, G., and Meschieri, L. Mental and physical efficiency after wine and ethanol solutions ingested on an empty and on a full stomach. *Q. J. Stud. Alcohol* 25:535, 1964.
13. Liebmann, A.J., and Scherl, B. Changes in whiskey while maturing. *Ind. Eng. Chem.* 41:534, 1949.
14. Von Warthburg, J.P. In I.B. Kissin and I.I. Begletter, (Editors), *The Biology of Alcoholism*. New York: Plenum Press, 1971, pp. 63–91.
15. Mendelson, J., and LaDou, J. Experimentally induced chronic intoxication and withdrawal in alcoholics: Part 2. Psychophysiological findings. *Q. J. Stud. Alcohol* (suppl.) 2:14, 1964.
16. Krantz, J.C., Jr., and Carr, C.J. *The Pharmacologic Principles of Medical Practice*, 6th ed. Baltimore: Williams & Wilkins, 1964.
17. Todd, F. *Teaching About Alcohol*. New York: McGraw-Hill, 1964.
18. Kalant, H. Some recent physiological and biochemical investigations on alcohol and alcoholism. *Q. J. Stud. Alcohol* 23:52, 1962.
19. Bjerver, K., and Goldberg, L. Effect of alcohol ingestion on driving ability. Results of practical road tests and laboratory experiments. *Q. J. Stud. Alcohol* 11:1, 1950.
20. Lieber, C.S., and DeCarli, L.M. An experimental model of alcohol feeding and liver injury in the baboon. *J. Med. Primatol.* 3:153, 1974.
21. Blum, K., et al. Ethanol narcosis in mice. serotonergic involvement. *Experientia* 30:1053, 1974.
22. McGivern, R.F., et al. Antagonism of tertiary butanol by ACTH4-10, naloxone and dexamethasone. *Subst. Alcohol Actions Misuse* 3:121, 1982.
23. Strauss, M.B. The etiology of "alcoholic" polyneuritis. *Am. J. Med. Sci.* 189:378, 1935.
24. Victor, M. Alcohol and nutritional diseases of the nervous system. *JAMA* 167:65, 1958.
25. Brayton, R.G., Stokes, P.S., and Louria, D.B. The effects of alcohol on host defenses. *Clin. Res.* 12:453, 1964.
26. Golberg, L. Alcohol, tranquilizers, and hangover. *Q. J. Stud. Alcohol* (suppl. 1):37, 1961.
27. Pearl, R. *Alcohol and Longevity*. New York: Knopf, 1926.
28. Kalant, H. Some recent physiological and biochemical investigations on alcohol and alco-

holism. *Q. J. Stud. Alcohol* 23:52, 1962.
29. Mardones, J. The alcohols. In W.S. Root and F.G. Hoffmann, eds., *Physiological Pharmacology*, vol. 1. New York: Academic Press, 1963.
30. Majchrowicz, E., and Noble, E.P. *Biochemistry and Pharmacology of Ethanol*. New York: Plenum Press, 1979.
31. Seeman, P. The membrane actions of anesthetics and tranquilizers. *Pharmacol. Rev.* 24:583, 1972.
32. Gruber, B., et al. Ethanol-induced conformational changes in rat brain microsomal membranes. *Biochem. Pharmacol.* 26:2181, 1977.
33. Chin, J.H., and Goldstein, D.B. Drug tolerance in biomembranes. A spin label study of the effects of ethanol. *Science* 196:684, 1977.
34. Chin, J.H., Parsons, L.M., and Goldstein, D.B. Increased cholesterol content of erythrocyte and brain membranes in ethanol tolerant mice. *Biochim. Biophys. Acta* 513:358, 1978.
35. Littleton, J.M., John, G.R., and Grieve, S.J. Alterations in phospholipid composition in ethanol tolerance and dependence. *Alcoholism* 3:50, 1979.
36. Charnock, J.S., et al. Activation energy and phospholipid requirements of membrane-bound adenosine triphosphatases. *Arch. Biochem. Biophys.* 159:393, 1973.
37. Farias, R.N., et al. Regulation of allosteric membrane-bound enzymes through changes in membrane lipid composition. *Biochim. Biophys. Acta* 415:231, 1975.
38. DeKruyff, B., et al. Influence of fatty acid and sterol composition on the lipid phase transition and activity of membrane-bound enzymes in *Acholeplasma laidlawii*. *Biochim. Biophys. Acta*. 330:259, 1973.
39. Hoffman, P.L., et al. Receptor and membrane function in the alcohol tolerant/dependent animal. *Adv. Exp. Med. Biol.* 132:761, 1980.
40. Tabakoff, B. Neurochemical aspects of ethanol dependence. In K. Blum, ed., *Alcohol and Opiates. Neurochemical and Behavioral Mechanisms*. New York: Academic Press, 1977.
41. Creese, I., Burt, D.P., and Snyder, S.H. Dopamine receptor binding enhancement accompanies lesion-induced behavioral supersensitivity. *Science*, 197:596, 1977.
42. Sporn, J.R., et al. Beta-adrenergic receptor involvement in 6-hydroxydopamine-induced supersensitivity in rat cerebral cortex. *Science* 194:624, 1976.
43. Hiller, J.M., Angel, L.M., and Simon, E.J. Multiple opiate receptors. Alcohol selectively inhibits binding to delta receptors. *Science* 214:468, 1981.
44. Davis, W.C., and Ticku, M.K. Ethanol enhances |3H|-diazepam binding at the benzodiazepine-gamma-aminobutyric acid receptor-ionophore complex. *Mol. Pharmacol.* 20:287, 1981.
45. Tabakoff, B., Hoffman, P.L., and Ritzmann, R.F. Dopamine receptor function after chronic ingestion of ethanol. *Life Sic.* 23:643, 1978.
46. Tabakoff, B., and Hoffman, P.L. Alterations in receptors controlling dopamine synthesis after chronic ethanol ingestion. *J. Neurochem.* 31:1223, 1978.
47. Rangaraj, N., and Kalant, H. Alpha-adrenoreceptor mediated alteration of ethanol effects on ($Na^+ - K^+$) ATPase of rat neuronal membranes. *Can. J. Physiol. Pharmacol.* 58(11):1342, 1980.
48. French, S.W, et al. Noradrenergic sensitivity of the cerebral cortex after chronic ethanol ingestion and withdrawal. *J. Pharmacol. Exp. Ther.* 194:319, 1975.
49. Banerjee, S.P., Sharma, V.K., and Khanna, J.M. Alterations in beta-adrenergic receptor binding during ethanol withdrawal. *Nature* 276:407, 1978.
50. Blum, K., et al. L-DOPA: Effect on ethanol narcosis and brain biogenic amines in mice. *Nature* 242:407, 1973.
51. Hunt, W.A., and Majchrowicz, E. Alterations in the turnover of brain norepinephrine and dopamine in alcohol-dependent rats. *J. Neurochem.* 23:549, 1974.
52. Blum, K., et al. Suppression of ethanol withdrawal by dopamine. *Experientia* 32:493, 1976.
53. Hoffman, P., and Tabakoff, B. Alterations in dopamine receptor sensitivity by chronic ethanol treatment. *Nature* 268:551, 1977.
54. Tabakoff, B., and Hoffman, P.L. Development of functional dependence on ethanol in dopaminergic systems. *J. Pharmacol. Exp. Ther.* 208:216, 1979.
55. Engel, J., and Liljequist, S. The effect of long-term ethanol treatment on the sensitivity of the dopamine receptors in the nucleus accumbens. *Psychopharmacology* 49:253, 1976.
56. Liljequist, S. Effects of dependence-producing drugs on neurotransmitters and neuronal excitability. In V. Neuhoff, ed., *Proceedings European Society on Neurochemistry*. New York: Verlag Chemie, 1978, pp. 359–373.
57. Rabin, R., and Molinoff, P.B Brain neurotransmitter receptor systems in alcohol treated mice and in mice genetically selected for differences in sensitivity to alcohol. *Adv. Exp. Med. Biol.* 132:787, 1980.

58. Phillis, J.W., and Thamandas, K. The effects of chlorpromazine and ethanol on *in vivo* release of acetylcholine from the cerebral cortex. *Comp. Gen. Pharmacol.* 2:306, 1971.
59. Erickson, C.K., and Graham, D.T. Alterations of cortical and reticular acetylcholine release by ethanol *in vivo*. *J. Pharmacol. Exp. Ther.* 185:583, 1973.
60. Kalant, H., and Grose, W. Effects of ethanol and pentobarbital on release of acetylcholine from cerebral cortex slices. *J. Pharmacol. Exp. Ther.* 158:385, 1969.
61. Hunt, W.A., and Dalton, T.K. Regional brain acetylcholine levels in rats acutely treated with ethanol or rendered ethanol-dependent. *Brain Res.* 109:628, 1976.
62. Rawat, A.K. Developmental changes in the brain levels of neurotransmitters as influenced by maternal ethanol consumption in the rat. *J. Neurochem.* 28:1175, 1977.
63. Erickson, C.K., and Chai, K.J. Cholinergic modification of ethanol-induced electroencephalographic synchrony in the rat. *Neuropharmacology* 15:39, 1976.
64. Erickson, C.K., and Burnam, W.L. Cholinergic alteration of ethanol-induced sleep and death in mice. *Agents Actions* 2:8, 1971.
65. Hunt, W.A., et al. Alterations in neurotransmitter activity after acute and chronic ethanol treatment studies of transmitter interactions. *Alcoholism* 3:359, 1979.
66. Daly, J. *Cyclic Nucleotides in the Nervous System*. New York: Plenum Press, 1977.
67. Bloom, F.E. The role of cyclic nucleotides in central synaptic function. *Rev. Physiol. Biochem. Pharmacol.* 74:1, 1975.
68. Siggins, G.R., et al. Purine and pyrimidine-mononucleotides depolarise neurones of explanted amphibian sympathetic ganglism. *Nature* 270:263, 1977.
69. Siggins, G.R. Electrophysiologic assessment of mononucleotides and nucleotides as first and second messengers in the neural system. In A. Kalin, V.M. Tweeyson, and H.J. Vogel, eds. *Neuronal Information Transfer*. New York: Academic Press, 1978.
70. Siggins, G.R. Cyclic nucleotides in the development of alcohol tolerance and dependence: A commentary. *Drug Alcohol Depend.* 4:307, 1979.
71. French, S.W., et al. Adrenergic subsensitivity of the rat brain during chronic ethanol ingestion. *Res. Commun. Chem. Pathol. Pharmacol.* 9:575, 1974.
72. Segal, M., and Bloom, F.E. The action of norepinephrine in the rat hippocampus. II. Activation of the input pathway. *Brain Res.* 72:99, 1974.
73. Hoffer, B., et al. Electrophysiology and cytology of hippocampal formation transplants in the anterior chamber of the Ege II cholinergic mechanisms. *Brain Res.* 119:107, 1977.
74. Ungerstedt, U. Postsynaptic supersensitivity after 6-hydroxydopamine induced degeneration of the nigro-striatal dopamine system. *Acta Physiol. Scand. (Suppl.)* 367:69, 1971.
75. Kuriyama, K., et al. Alterations of cerebral protein kinase activity following ethanol administration. *Biochem. Pharmacol.* 25:2541, 1976.
76. Blum, K., and Wallace, J.E. Effects of catecholamine synthesis inhibitions on ethanol-induced withdrawal symptoms in mice. *Br. J. Pharmacol.* 51:109, 1974.
77. Siggins, G.R., and French, E. Central neurons are depressed by iontophoretic and micropressure application of ethanol and tetrahydropaveroline. *Drug Alcohol Depend.* 4:239, 1979.
78. Lake, N.J., Yarbrough, G.G., and Phillis, J.W. Effects of ethanol on cerebral cortical neurons: Interactions with some putative transmitters. *J. Pharm. Pharmacol.* 25:582, 1973.
79. Courville, C.B. *Effects of Alcohol on the Nervous System of Man*. Los Angeles: San Lucas Press, 1966.
80. Victor, M., Adams, R.D., and Collins, G.H. *The Wernicke–Korsakoff Syndrone*. Philadelphia: Davis, 1971.
81. Butters, N., and Cermak, L.S. Some analyses of amnesic syndromes in brain-damaged patients. In K.H. Pribram and R.L. Isaacson, eds., *The Hippocampus*, vol. 2. New York: Plenum Press, 1975, p. 377.
82. Victor, M., and Adams, R.D. On the etiology of the alcoholic neurologic diseases with special reference to the role of nutrition. *Am. J. Nutr.* 9:379, 1961.
83. Freund, G. Chronic central nervous system toxicity of alcohol. *Ann. Rev. Pharmacol.* 13:217, 1973.
84. Jones, B., and Parsons, O.A. Impaired abstracting ability in chronic alcoholics. *Arch. Gen. Psychiatry*, 24:71, 1971.
85. Walker, D.W., and Hunter, B.E. Short-term memory impairment following chronic alcohol consumption in rats. *Neuropsychologia* 16:545, 1978.
86. Riley, J.N., and Walker, D.W. Morphological alternations in hippocampus after long-term alcohol consumption in mice. *Science* 201:646, 1978.
87. Walker, D.W., et al. Neuronal loss in hippo-

campus induced by prolonged ethanol consumption in rats. *Science* 209:711, 1980.
88. Talland, G.A. *Deranged Memory*. New York: Academic Press, 1965.
89. Goldman, H., et al. Alcohol and regional blood flow in brains of rats. *Proc. Soc. Exp. Biol. Med.* 144:983, 1973.
90. Feilstein, A. Effects of ethanol on neurohumoral amine metabolism. In B. Kissin and H. Begleiter, eds., *The Biology of Alcoholism*. New York: Plenum Press, 1971, pp. 127–149.
91. Blum, K., et al. Effects of catecholamine synthesis inhibition of ethanol narcosis in mice. *Curr. Ther. Res.* 14:324, 1972.
92. Blum, K., et al. Soporific action of ethanol in mice: Possible role of biogenic amines. *Pharmacol. Biochem. Behav.* 1:271, May–June, 1973.
93. Liljequist, S. Changes in the sensitivity of dopamine receptors in the nucleus accumbens and in the striatum induced by chronic ethanol administration. *Acta Pharmacol. Toxicol.* 43:19, 1978.
94. Branchey, L., and Leiber, C. Activation of tryptophan pyrrolase after chronic alcohol administration. *Subst. Alcohol Action/Misuse* 3(4):225, 1982.
95. Hjorth, M., Bille, M., and Smith, D.F. Serum tryptophan levels in alcoholics. *Drug Alcohol Depend.* 7:157, 1981.
96. Blum, K., et al. Synergy of ethanol and alcohol-like metabolites: Tryptophol and 3.4 dihydroxyphenylethanol. *Pharmacology* 9:294, 1973.
97. Graham, J.D.P. *Pharmacology for Medical Students*. London: Oxford University Press, 1966, p. 36.
98. Hoffman, F.G. *A Handbook on Drug and Alcohol Abuse: The Biomedical Aspects*. New York: Oxford University Press, 1975, p. 95.
99. Isbell, H., et al. An experimental study of the etiology of "rum fits" and delirium tremens. *Q.J. Stud. Alcohol* 16:1, 1965.
100. Mendelson, J.H. Ethanol-1-$C^{11}$ metabolism in alcoholics and nonalcoholics. *Science* 159:319, 1968.
101. Rubin, E., and Lieber, C.S. Hepatic microsomal enzymes in man and rat: Induction and inhibition by ethanol. *Science* 162:690, 1968.
102. Lieber, C.S. Metabolic effects of ethanol on the liver and other digestive organs. *Clin. Gastroenterol.* 10:315, 1981.
103. Khanna, J.M., and Israel, Y. Ethanol metabolism. *Int. Rev. Physiol.* 21:275, 1980.
104. Cappell, H. Tolerance to ethanol and treatment of its abuse, some fundamental issues. *Addict. Behav.* 6:152, 1981.
105. Mayer, J.M., Khanna, J.M., and Kalant, H. A role for calcium in the acute and chronic actions of ethanol in vitro. *Eur. J. Pharmacol.* 68:223, 1980.
106. Jaffe, J.H. Drug addiction and drug abuse. In L. Goodman and A. Gilman, eds., *The Pharmacologic Basis of Therapeutics*, 4th ed. New York: Macmillan, 1970, p. 276.
107. Victor, M., and Adams, R.D. The effects of alcohol on the nervous system. *Res. Pub. Assoc. Nerv. Ment. Dis.* 32:526, 1953.
108. Criteria Committee. National Council on Alcoholism. Criteria for the diagnosis of alcoholism. *Ann. Intern. Med.* 77:249, 1972.
109. Harney, R.B., and Harger, R.N. The alcohols. In J.R. DiPalma, ed., *Drill's Pharmacology in Medicine*, 3rd ed. New York: McGraw-Hill, 1965, p. 210.
110. Malin, H., et al. An epidemiologic perspective on alcohol use and abuse in the United States. Report to NIAAA, 1980.
111. Polich, J.M., Armor, D.J., and Braiker, H.B. *The Course of Alcoholism: Four Years After Treatment*. Santa Monica, Calif.: Rand Corp., 1980.
112. Wallace, R. Alcohol consumption and hypertension. Presented at 20th Annual Conference on Cardiovascular Epidemiology. San Diego, 1980.
113. Eliaser, M., and Giansiracusa, F.J. The heart and alcohol. *Calif. Med.* 84:234, 1956.
114. Mendoza, L.C., et al. The effect of intravenous ethyl alcohol on the coronary circulation and myocardial contractility of the human and canine heart. *J. Clin. Pharmacol.* 11:165, 1971.
115. Regan, T.J., Levinson, G.E. Oldewurtel, H.A., et al. Ventricular function in noncardiacs with alcoholic fatty liver: Role of ethanol in the production of cardiomyopathy. *J. Clin. Invest.* 48:397, 1969.
116. Regan, T.J., Korexenidis, G., Moschos, C.B., et al. The acute metabolic and hemo-dynamic responses of the left ventricle to ethanol. *J. Clin. Invest.* 45:270, 1966.
117. Webb, W.R., and Degerli, I.U. Ethyl alcohol and the cardiovascular system. *JAMA* 191:77/1055, 1965.
118. Schmitthenner, J.E., Hafkenschiel, J.H., Forte, I., et al. Does alcohol increase coronary blood flow and cardiac work? (abstract). *Circulation* 18:778, 1958.
119. Wendt, V.E., Stock, T.B., Hayden, R.O., et al. The hemodynamics and cardiac metabolism in the cardiomyopathies. *Med. Clin. N. Am.* 46:1445, 1962.

120. Orlando, J., et al. Effect of ethanol on angina pectoris. *Ann. Intern. Med.* 84:652, 1976.
121. Russek, H.I., Naegele, C.F, and Regan, F.D. Alcohol in the treatment of angina pectoris. *JAMA* 143:355, 1950.
122. Leiber, L. *Medical Disorders of Alcoholism.* Philadelphia: W.B. Saunders, 1982.
123. Alexander, C.S. Idiopathic heart disease. Analysis of 100 cases, with special reference to chronic alcoholism. *Am. J. Med.* 41:213, 1966.
124. Schwartz, L., Sample, K.A., and Wigle, D.E. Severe alcoholic cardiomyopathy reversed with abstention from alcohol. *Am. J. Cardiol.* 36:963, 1975.
125. Demakis, J.C., et al. The natural course of alcoholic cardiomyopathy. *Ann. Intern. Med.* 80:293, 1974.
126. Ettinger, P.O., et al. Arrhythmias and the ''Holiday Heart'': Alcohol-associated cardiac rhythm disorders. *Am. Heart J.* 95:555, 1978.
127. Singer, K., and Lundberg, W.B. Ventricular arrhythmias associated with the ingestion of alcohol. *Ann. Intern. Med.* 77:247, 1972.
128. Greenspon, A.J., et al. Provocation of ventricular tachycardia after consumption of alcohol. *N. Engl. J. Med.* 301:1049, 1979.
129. Klatsky, A. The relationship of alcohol and the cardiovascular system. Report to NIAAA, 1980.
130. Reeves, W.C., Nanda, N.C., and Gramiak, R. Echocardiography in chronic alcoholics following prolonged periods of abstinence. *Am. Heart J.* 95:578, 1978.
131. Regan, T.J., and Ettinger, P.O. Alcohol and the heart. In J.W. Hurst, ed., *The Heart: Update.* New York: McGraw-Hill, 1979, pp. 259–274.
132. Klatsky, A.L., et al. Alcohol consumption and blood pressure; Kaiser-Permanente Multiphasic Health Examination data. *N. Engl. J. Med.* 296:1194, 1977.
133. Rees, L.H., et al. Alcohol-induced pseudo-Cushing's syndrome. *Lancet* 1:726, 1977.
134. Smals, A., and Kloppenborg, P. Alcohol induced pseudo-Cushing's syndrome (letter). *Lancet* 1:1369, 1977.
135. Linkola, J. Alcohol and hypertension (letter). *N. Engl. J. Med.* 300:680, 1979.
136. Klatsky, A. The Kaiser-Permanente experience. Presented at 20th Annual Conference on Cardiovascular Epidemiology, San Diego, 1980.
137. Blackwelder, W.C., et al. Alcohol and mortality: The Honolulu heart study. *Am. J. Med.* 68:164, 1980.
138. Castelli, W.P., et al. Alcohol and blood lipids: The cooperative lipoprotein phenotyping study. *Lancet* 2:153, 1977.
139. Knochel, J.P., et al. The muscle cell in chronic alcoholism: The possible role of phosphate depletion in alcoholic myopathy. *Ann. N.Y. Acad. Sci.* 252:274, 1975.
140. Kozarevic, D., et al. Frequency of alcohol consumption and morbidity and mortality: The Yugoslavia cardiovascular disease study. *Lancet* 1:613, 1980.
141. Castelli, W. The Framingham experience: Presented at 20th Annual Conference on Cardiovascular Epidemiology, San Diego, 1980.
142. Goldbourt, U., and Medalie, J.H. High density lipoprotein cholesterol and incidence of coronary heart disease—the Israeli Ischemic Heart Disease Study. *Am. J. Epidemiol.* 109:296, 1979.
143. Hulley, S. Alcohol and HDL in selected populations. Presented at 20th Annual Conference on Cardiovascular Epidemiology, San Diego, 1980.
144 Kuller, L. Relationship between alcohol intake and high density lipoprotein cholesterol. Presented at 20th Annual Conference on Cardiovascular Epidemiology, San Diego, 1980.
145. Sabesin, S.M., Ragland, J.B., and Freeman, M.R. Lipoprotein disturbances in liver disease. In H. Popper and F. Schaffner, eds., *Progress in Liver Diseases*, vol. 6. New York: Grune & Stratton, 1979, pp. 243–262.
146. Kajan, A. The Hawaiian experience. Presented at 20th Annual Conference on Cardiovascular Epidemiology, San Diego, 1980.
147. Bode, C., Martini, G.A., and Bode, J.C. Effect of alcohol on microsomal cortisol 4en-5 alpha-reductase in the liver of rats fed on a standard or low protein diet. *Horm. Metab. Res.* 10:62, 1978.
148. Gordon, G.G., et al. The effect of alcohol (ethanol) administration on sex hormone metabolism in normal men. *N. Engl. J. Med.* 295:793, 1976.
149. Rubin, E., et al. Prolonged ethanol consumption increases testosterone metabolism in the liver. *Science* 191:563. 1976.
150. Gordon, G.G., et al. The effect of alcohol ingestion on hepatic aromatase activity and plasma steroid hormone in the rat. *Metabolism* 28:20, 1979.
151. Cicero, T. Alcohol effects on the endocrine system. Report to NIAAA, 1980.1
152. Cicero, T.J., Bell, R.D., and Badger, T.M. Multiple effects of ethanol on the hypothalamic-pituitary-gonadal axis in the male. *Adv. Exp. Med. Biol.* 126:463, 1980.
153. Cicero, T.J., Bernstein, D., and Badger, T.M.

Effects of acute alcohol administration on reproductive endocrinology in the male rat. *Alcoholism* 2:249, 1978.
154. Cicero, T.J. Meyer, E.R., and Bell, R.D. Effects of ethanol on the hypothalamic-pituitary-luteinizing hormone axis and testicular steroidogenesis. *J. Pharmacol. Exp. Ther.* 208:210, 1979.
155. Baker, H., et al. Study of the endocrine manifestations of hepatic cirrhosis. *Q. J. Med.* 45:145, 1976.
156. Lester, R., and Van Thiel, D.H. Gonadal function in chronic alcoholic men. *Adv. Exp. Med. Biol.* 85A:399, 1977.
157. Symons, A.M., and Marks, V. The effects of alcohol on weight gain and the hypothalamic-pituitary-gonadotrophin axis in the maturing male rat. *Biochem. Pharmacol.* 24:955, 1975.
158. Van Thiel, D.H., and Lester, R. Alcoholism: Its effect on hypothalamic-pituitary-gonadal function. *Gastroenterology* 71:318, 1976.
159. Van Thiel, D.H., et al. Alcohol-induced testicular atrophy. An experimental model for hypogonadism occurring in chronic alcoholic men. *Gastroenterology* 69:326, 1975.
160. Wright, J.W., et al. Abnormal hypothalamic-pituitary-gonadal function in chronic alcoholics. *Br. J. Addict.* 71:211, 1976.
161. Ellingboe, J., and Varanelli, C.C. Ethanol inhibits testosterone biosynthesis by direct action on leydig cells. *Res. Commun. Chem. Pathol. Pharmacol.* 24:87, 1979.
162. Gordon, G.G., Southren, A.L., and Lieber, C.S. Hypogonadism and feminization in the male: A triple effect of alcohol. *Alcoholism* 3:210, 1979.
163. Cicero, T.J., Newman, K., and Meyer, E.R. Ethanol-induced inhibition of testicular steroidogenesis in male rats. Mechanisms of action. *Life Sci.* 28:1871, 1981.
164. Cicero, T.J., Bell, R.D., and Meyer, E.R. Direct effects of ethanol and acetaldehyde on testicular steroidogenesis (abstract). *Fed. Proc.* 38:428, 1979.
165. Cobb, C.F., et al. Acetaldehyde and ethanol are testicular toxins (abstract). *Gastroenterology* 75(4):958, 1978.
166. Parsons, O.A., Neuropsychological deficits in alcoholics: Facts and fancies. *Alcoholism* 1:51, 1977.
167. Smith, J.W. Neurological disorders in alcoholism. In N.J. Estes and M.H. Heineman, eds., *Alcoholism: Development, Consequences, and Interventions*. St. Louis: C.V. Mosby, 1977, pp. 109–128.
168. Berman, H., et al. Computed tomography of the brain and neuropsychological assessment of male alcoholic patients and a random sample from the general male population. *Acta Psychiatr. Scand.* 286, 1980.
169. Cala, L.A., et al. Brain atrophy and intellectual impairment in heavy drinkers—A clinical, psychometric and computerized tomography study. *Aust. N.Z. J. Med.* 8:147, 1978.
170. Carlen, P.L., et al. Reversible cerebral atrophy in recently abstinent chronic alcoholics measured by computed tomography scans. *Science* 200:1076, 1978.
171. Epstein, P.S., et al. Alcoholism and cerebral atrophy. *Alcoholism* 1:61, 1977.
172. Hill, S.Y., et al. A comparison of alcoholics and heroin abusers. Computerized transaxial tomography and neuropsychological functioning. In M. Galanter, ed., *Currents in Alcoholism*, vol. 5. New York: Grune & Stratton, 1979, pp. 187–205.
173. Lee, K., et al. Alcohol-induced brain damage and liver damage in young males. *Lancet* 2:759, 1979.
174. Ron, M.A., Acker, W., and Lishman, W.A. Dementia in chronic alcoholism: A clinical psychological and computerized axial tomographic study. *Biolog. Psychiatry Today*, 1979.
175. Lassen, N.A., et al. Brain function and blood flow. *Sci. Am.* 239:62, 1978.
176. Risberg, J. Regional cerebral blood flow measurements by 133 Xe-inhalation: Methodology and applications in neuropsychology and psychiatry. *Brain Lang.* 9:9, 1980.
177. Chmielewski, C., and Golden, C.J. Alcoholism and brain damage: An investigation using the Luria-Nebraska Neuropsychological Battery. *Int. J. Neurosci.* 10:99, 1980.
178. Schau, E.J., and O'Leary, M.R. Adaptive abilities of hospitalized alcoholics and matched controls. The brain–age quotient. *J. Stud. Alcohol* 38:403, 1977.
179. Silberstein, J.A., and Parsons, O.A. Neuropsychological impairment in female alcoholics. In M. Galanter, ed., *Currents in Alcoholism*, vol. 7. New York: Grune & Stratton, 1980, pp. 481–495.
180. Parker, E.S., and Noble, P.E. Alcohol and the aging process in social drinkers. *J. Stud. Alcohol* 41:170, 1980.
181. Jones, M.K., and Jones, B.M. The relationship of age and drinking habits to the effects of alcohol on memory in women. *J. Stud. Alcohol* 41:179, 1980.
182. Carlen, P.L., and Wilkinson, D.A. Alcoholic brain damage and reversible deficits. *Acta Psychiatr. Scand. (Suppl.)* 286:89, 1980.

183. Guthrie, A., and Elliot, W.A. The nature and reversibility of cerebral impairment in alcoholism: Treatment implications. *J. Stud. Alcohol* 41:147, 1980.
184. Jenkins, R.L., and Parsons, O.A. Recovery of cognitive abilities in male alcoholics. In M. Galanter, ed., *Currents in Alcoholism*, vol. 7. New York: Grune & Stratton, 1980, pp. 229–237.
185. Kish, G.B., Hagen, J.M., Woody, M.M., and Harvey, H.M. Alcoholics' recovery from cerebral impairment as a function of duration of abstinence. *J. Clin. Psychol.* 36:584, 1980.
186. Page, R.D., and Schaub, L.H. Intellectual functioning in alcoholics during six months' abstinence. *J. Stud. Alcohol* 38:1240, 1977.
187. Grant, I., Adams, K., and Reed, R. Normal neuropsychological abilities of alcoholic men in their late thirties. *Am. J. Psychiatry* 136:1263, 1979.
188. Berglund, M., et al. Cerebral dysfunction in alcoholism and presenile dementia. A comparison of two groups of patients with similar reduction of cerebral blood flow. *Acta Psychiatr. Scand.* 55:391, 1977.
189. Hill, S.Y., and Mikhael, M. Computed tomography scans of alcoholics: Cerebral atrophy? *Science* 204:1237, 1979.
190. Long, J.A., and McLachlan, J.F.C. Abstract reasoning and perceptual motor efficiency in alcoholics: Impairments and reversibility. *Q.J. Stud. Alcohol* 35:1220, 1974.
191. O'Leary, M.R., et al. Assessment of cognitive recovery in alcoholics by use of the trail-making test. *J. Clin. Psychol.* 33:579, 1977.
192. Schau, E.J., O'Leary, M.R., and Chaney, E.F. Reversibility of cognitive deficit in alcoholics. *J. Stud. Alcohol* 41:733, 1980.
193. Parsons, O., and Leber, W. Alcohol, cognitive dysfunction, and brain damage. Report to NIAAA, 1980.
194. Butters, N. The Wernicke-Korsakoff syndrome. Report to NIAAA, 1980.
195. Williams, R.R., and Horn, J.W. Association of cancer sites with tobacco and alcohol consumption and socioeconomic status of patients: Interview study from the Third National Cancer Survey. *J. Natl. Cancer Inst.* 58:525, 1977.
196. Schottenfeld, D. Alcohol as a co-factor in the etiology of cancer. *Cancer* 43:1962, 1979.
197. Tuyns, A.J. Alcohol and cancer. *Alcohol Health Res. World* 2:20, 1978.
198. Broad, W.J. Carcinogens in scotch. *Science* 205:768, 1979.
199. Lemoine, P., et al. Les enfants de parents alcoholiques: Anomalies observées à propos de 127 cas. *Quest Med.* 477, 1968.
200. Jones, K.L., et al. Pattern of malformation in offspring of chronic alcoholic mothers. *Lancet* 1:1267, 1973.
201. Randall, C.L., Taylor, W.J., and Walker, D.W. Ethanol-induced malformations in mice. *Alcoholism* 1:219, 1977.
202. Clarren, S.K., and Smith, D.W. The fetal alcohol syndrome. *N. Engl. J. Med.* 298:1063, 1978.
203. Sokol, R.J., Miller, S.I., and Reed, G. Alcohol abuse during pregnancy: An epidemiologic study. *Alcoholism (N.Y.)* 4:135, 1980.
204. Rosett, H.L., et al. Effects of maternal drinking on neonate state regulation. *Dev. Med. Child Neurol.* 21:464, 1979.
205. Landesman-Dwyer, S., Miller, S.I., and Reed, G. Naturalistic observations of newborns: Effects of maternal alcohol intake. *Alcoholism* 2:171, 1978.
206. Havlicek, V. EEG frequency spectrum characteristics of sleep states in infants of alcoholic mothers. *Neoropaediatrie* 8:360, 1977.
207. Kaminski, M., et al. Alcohol consumption in pregnant women and the outcome of pregnancy. *Alcoholism* 2:155, 1978.
208. Rosett, H.L., et al. Reduction of alcohol consumption during pregnancy with benefits to the newborn. *Alcoholism* 4:178, 1980.
209. Sokol, R.J., Miller, S.I., and Reed, G. Alcohol abuse during pregnancy: An epidemiologic study. *Alcoholism (N.Y.)* 4:135, 1980.
210. Rosett, H.L. Clinical pharmacology of the fetal alcohol syndrome. In H. Majchrowicz and E. Noble, eds., *Biochemistry and Pharmocology of Ethanol*, vol. 2. New York: Plenum Press, 1979, pp. 485–509.
211. Hanson, J.W., et al. The effects of moderate alcohol consumption during pregnancy on fetal growth and morphogenesis. *J. Pediatr.* 92:457, 1978.
212. Little, R.E. Moderate alcohol use during pregnancy and decreased infant birthweight. *Am. J. Public Health* 67:1154, 1977.
213. Kline, J., et al. Drinking during pregnancy and spontaneous abortion. *Lancet* 2:176, 1980.
214. Harlap, S., and Shiono, P.H. Alcohol, smoking and incidence of spontaneous abortions in the first and second trimester. *Lancet* 26:173, 1980.
215. Chernoff, G.F. The fetal alcohol syndrome in mice: An animal model. *Teratology* 15:223, 1977.
216. Sokol, R.J. Alcohol and pregnancy: A clinical

perspective for laboratory research. *Subs. Alcohol Action/Misuse* 3:183, 1982.

217. Randall, C.L., and Taylor, W.J. Prenatal ethanol exposure in mice: Teratogenic effects. *Teratology* 19:305, 1979.
218. Ellis, F.W., and Pick, I.R. An animal model of the fetal alcohol syndrome in beagles. *Alcoholism (N.Y.)* 4:123, 1980.
219. Cobo, E., and Wuintero, C.A. Milk ejecting and antidiuretic activities under neurohypophyseal inhibition with alcohol and water overload. *Am. J. Obstet. Gynecol.* 105:877, 1969.
220. Binkiewicz, A., et al. Pseudo-Cushing syndrome caused by alcohol in breast milk. *J. Pediatr.* 93:965, 1978.
221. Olegard, R., et al. Effects on the child of alcohol abuse during pregnancy. *Acta Paediatr. Scand.* (suppl.) 1275:112, 1979.
222. Dehaene, P., et al. Le syndrome d'alcoolisme foetal dans le mond de la france. *Rev. Alcoolisme* 23:145, 1977.
223. Partanen, J., Bruun, K., and Markkanen, T. *Inheritance of Drinking Behavior.* Finnish Foundation for Alcohol Studies, Helsinki, 1966.
224. Bleuler, M. Familial and personal background of chronic alcoholics. In O. Diethelm, ed., *Etiology of Chronic Alcoholism.* Springfield, Ill.: C.C. Thomas, 1955.
225. Roe, A. Children of alcoholic parents raised in foster homes. In Yale University Center of Alcohol Studies. *Alcohol, Science, and Society. Q.J. Stud. Alcohol* 1954.
226. Jellinek, E.M. Heredity of the alcoholic. In Yale University Center of Alcohol Studies: *Alcohol, Science, and Society. Q.J. Stud. Alcohol*, 1954.
227. Williams, R.J. *Alcoholism: The Nutritional Approach.* Austin: University of Texas Press, 1959.
228. Sadoun, R., Lolli, G., and Silverman, M. *Drinking in French Culture.* New Brunswick, N.J.: Rutgers Center of Alcohol Studies, 1965.
229. Borkenstein, R.F. Handling the drinking driver. In *Alcohol and Road Traffic.* London: British Medical Association, 1963.
230. Swedish Temperance Education Board. *The Alcohol Question in Sweden.* Swedish Temperance Education Board (Central forbundet for Nykterhetsundervisning). Stockholm, 1960.
231. Goodwin, D.W., Crane, J.B., and Guze, S.B. Alcoholic "blackouts": A review and clinical study of 100 alcoholics. *Am. J. Psychiatry* 126:191, 1969.
232. Goodwin, D.W., et al. Alcohol problems in adoptees raised apart from alcoholic biological parents. *Arch. Gen. Psychiatry* 28:238, 1973.
233. Shuckit, M.A., Goodwin, D.A., and Winokur, G. A study of alcoholism in half siblings. *Am. J. Psychiatry* 128:1132, 1972.
234. Menninger, K.A. *Man Against Himself.* New York: Harcourt, Brace, 1938.
235. Chafetz, M.E. Practical and theoretical considerations in the psychotherapy of alcoholism. *Q. J. Stud. Alcohol* 20:281, 1959.
236. Lolli, G. *Social Drinking.* Cleveland: World, 1960.
237. Maddox, G.L. Childhood and alcohol: Some roots of pathological drinking behavior. In *Community Factors in Alcohol Education.* Montpelier, Vt., 1962.
238. Jellinek, E.M. Cited in *Alcoholism and Drug Addiction Research Foundation, Toronto, Twelfth Annual Report.* Appendix II:82, 1962.
239. Lolli, G., Schesler, E., and Golder, G.M. Choice of alcoholic beverage among 105 alcoholics in New York. *Q. J. Stud. Alcohol* 21:475, 1960.
240. Terry, J., Lolli, G., and Golder, G. Choice of alcoholic beverage among 531 alcoholics in California. *Q. J. Stud. Alcohol* 18:417, 1957.
241. Ullman, A.D. Attitudes and drinking customs. In *Mental Health Aspects of Alcohol Education.* U.S. Public Health Service, 1958.
242. Snyder, C.R. *Alcohol and the Jews.* New Brunswick, N.J.: Rutgers Center of Alcohol Studies 1958.
243. Ullman, A.D. Attitudes and drinking customs. In *Mental Health Aspects of Alcohol Education.* U.S. Public Health Service, 1958.
244. Cohen, G. *The Substance Abuse Problems.* New York: Haworth Press, 1981, p. 193.
245. Blum, K., Hamilton, M.G., and Wallace, J.E. Alcohol and opiates: A review of common neurochemical and behavioral mechanisms. In K. Blum, ed., *Alcohol and Opiates: Neurochemical and Behavioral Mechanisms.* New York: Academic Press, 1977.
246. Battersby, A.R. Alkaloid biosynthesis. *Q. Rev.* 25:255, 1961.
247. Cohen, G., and Collins, M. Alkaloids from catecholamines in adrenal tissues: Possible role in alcoholism. *Science* 167:1749, 1970.
248. Blum, K., et al. Putative role of isoquinoline alkaloids in alcoholism: A link to opiates. *Alcoholism* 2:113, 1978.
249. Goldstein, A., and Judson, B.A. Alcohol dependence and opiate dependence: Lack of relationship in mice. *Science* 172:290, 1971.
250. Seevers, M.H. Morphine and ethanol depend-

ence: A critique of a hypothesis. *Science* 170:1113, 1970.

251. Blum, K. Neurochemical and behavioral considerations on the relationship between ethanol and opiate dependence. In J.H. Lowinson, ed., *Proceedings of the National Drug Abuse Conference*. New York: Marcel Dekker, 1976, pp. 114–1150.
252. Blum, K., et al. Naloxone-induced inhibition of ethanol dependence in mice. *Nature* 265:49, 1977.
253. Blum, K., et al. Morphine suppression of ethanol withdrawal in mice. *Experientia* 32:79, 1976.
254. Ross, D.H., Hartmann, R.J., and Geller, I. Ethanol preference in the hamster: Effects of morphine sulfate and naltrexone, a long-acting morphine antagonist. *Proc. Western Pharmacol. Soc.* 19:326, 1976.
255. Altshuler, H.L., Feinhandler, D., and Aitken, C. The effects of opiate antagonist compounds on fixed-ratio operant responding in rats. *Fed. Proc.* 38:424, 1979.
256. Ho, A.K.S., Chen, R.C.A., and Morrison, J.M. Opiate-ethanol interaction studies. In K. Blum, ed., *Alcohol and Opiates: Neurochemical and Behavioral Mechanisms*. New York: Academic Press, 1977, pp. 189–202.
257. Ross, D.H., Medina, M.A., and Cardenas, H.L. Morphine and ethanol: Selective depletion of regional brain calcium. *Science* 186:63, 1974.
258. Ross, D.H. Inhibition of high affinity calcium binding by salsolinol. *Alcoholism* 2:139, 1978.
259. Jeffcoate, W.J., et al. Prevention of effects of alcohol intoxication by naloxone. *Lancet* 2:1157, 1979.
260. Mackenzie, A.I. Naloxone in alcohol intoxication (letter). *Lancet* 1:733, 1979.
261. Blum, K., et al. In H. Rigter and J. Crabbe, eds., *Alcohol Tolerance and Dependence*. Amsterdam: Elsevier-North Holland, 1980.
262. Kalant, H. Biochemical aspects of tolerance to, and physical dependence on, central depressants. In V. Neuhoff, ed., *Proceedings European Society of Neurochemistry*. New York: Verlag Chemie, 1978, pp. 317–331.
263. Seizinger, B.R., et al. Differential effects of acute and chronic ethanol treatment on particular opioid peptide systems in discrete regions of rat brain and pituitary. *Pharmacol. Biochem. Behav.* (in press).
264. Ehrenpreis, S., et al. Further studies on the analgesic activity of D-phenylalanine (DPA) in mice and humans. In E. Leong Way, ed., *Endogenous and Exogenous Opiate Agonists and Antagonists*. New York: Pergamon Press, 1980, pp. 379–382.
265. Beaumont, A., and Hughes, J. Biology of opioid peptides. *Ann. Rev. Pharmacol. Toxicol.* 19:245, 1979.
266. Hollt, V., et al. Beta-endorphin-like immunoreactivity in plasma, pituitaries, and hypothalamus of rats following treatment with opiates. *Life Sci.* 23:1057, 1978.
267. Przewlocki, R., et al. Long-term morphine treatment decreases endorphin levels in rat brain and pituitary. *Brain Res.* 174(2):357, 1979.
268. Pinsky, C., LaBella, F.S., and Leybin, L. Alcohol and opiate narcotic dependencies: Possible interrelatedness via central endorphin:opiate receptor system. In I.A. Schecter, ed., *Drug Dependence and Alcoholism*, vol. 1. New York: Plenum Press, 1981, pp. 1107–1128.
269. Greenwald, J.E., et al. Salsolinol and tetrahydropapaveroline bind opiate receptors in the rat brain. *Fed. Proc.* 38:379, 1979.
270. Goldstein, A. Future research on opioid peptides (endorphins): A preview. In K. Blum, ed., *Alcohol and Opiates: Neurochemical and Behavioral Mechanisms*. New York: Academic Press, 1977, pp. 397–403.
271. Kosterlitz, H.W., and Hughes, J. Some thoughts on the significance of enkephalin, the endogenous ligand. *Life Sci.* 17:91, 1975.
272. Childers, S.R., Simantov, R., and Snyder, S.H. Enkephalin radioimmunoassay and radioreceptor assay in morphine dependent rats. *Eur. J. Pharmacol.* 46:289, 197.
273. Wesche, D., et al. Radioimmunoassay of enkephalins. Regional distribution in rat brain after morphine treatment and hypophysectomy. *Naunyn Schmiedberg's Arch. Pharmacol.* 301:79, 1977.
274. Shani, J., et al. Enkephalin levels in rat brain after various regimens of morphine administration. *Neurosci. Lett.* 12:319, 1979.
275. Höllt, V., Przewlocki, R., and Herz, A. Beta-endorphin-like immunoreactivity in plasma, pituitaries and hypothalamus of rats following treatment with opiates. *Life Sci.* 23:1057, 1978.
276. Ungar, G., et al. Brain peptides with opiate antagonist action: Their possible role in tolerance and dependence. *Psychoneuroendocrinology* 2:1, 1977.
277. Schulz, R. Control of endorphin/receptor-interaction. *Naunyn-Schmiedebergs Arch. Pharmacol.* 308(Suppl):R4, 1979.
278. McClearn, G.E., and Rodgers, D.A. Differences in alcohol preference among inbred strains of mice. *Q. J. Stud. Alcohol* 20:691,

1959.
279. Blum, K., et al. Genotype dependent responses to ethanol and normorphine on vas deferens of inbred strains of mice. *Subst. Alcohol Actions/Misuse* 1:459, 1980.
280. Elston, S.F., et al. Ethanol intoxication as a function of genotype dependent responses. *Pharmacol. Biochem. Behav.* 16:13, 1982.
281. Castellano, C., and Oliverio, A. A genetic analysis of morphine-induced running and analgesia in the mouse. *Psychopharmacologia* 41:197, 1975.
282. Verebey, K., and Blum, K. Alcohol euphoria: Possible mediation via endophinergic mechanisms. *J. Psychedel. Drugs* 11:305, 1979.
283. Ho, W.K.K., Wen, H.L., and Ling, N. Beta-endorphin-like immunoreactivity in the plasma of heroin addicts and normal subjects. *Neuropharmacology* 19:117, 1980.
284. Blum, K., et al. Psychogenetics of drug seeking behavior. *Subs. Alcohol Actions/Misuse* 1:255, 1980.
285. Blum, K. Alcohol and central nervous system peptides. In International Symposium on the Psychology of Alcoholism. *Subst. Alcohol Action/Misuse* (in press).
286. Blum, K., et al. Whole brain methionine-enkephalin of ethanol-avoiding and ethanol-preferring C57BL mice. *Experientia* 38:1469, 1982.
287. Masserman, J.H., and Yum, K.S. An analysis of the influence of alcohol on experimental neurosis in cats. *Psychosom. Med.* 8:36, 1946.
288. Goldstein, A. Endorphins: Physiology and clinical implications. *Ann. N.Y. Acad. Sci.* 311:49, 1978.
289. Golden, C.J., et al. Difference in brain densities between chronic alcoholics and normal control patients. *Science* 211:508, 1981.
290. Ho, A.K.S., and Rossi, N. Suppression of ethanol consumption by MET-enkephalin in rats. *J. Pharm. Pharmacol.* 34:118, 1982.
291. Clark, W.B., and Midanik, L. Alcohol use and alcohol problems among U.S. adults: Results of the 1979 national survey. Report to NIAAA, 1980.
292. *Alcohol Health and Research World, Patterns of Alcohol Consumption.* U.S. Government Printing Office, Washington, D.C. 1981.
293. Lolli, G. Alcoholism, 1941–51: a survey of activities in research, education and therapy. V. The treatment of alcohol addiction. *Q. J. Stud. Alcohol* 13:461, 1952.
294. Block, M.A. Medical treatment of alcoholism. In *American Medical Association: A Manual on Alcoholism.*
295. *Alcoholics Anonymous Comes of Age.* New York: Alcoholics Anonymous, 1957.
296. Moreno, J.L. *Who Shall Survive?* Washington, D.C.: Nervous and Mental Disease Publishing Co., 1934, p. 435.
297. Weissman, A., and Koe, B.K. Drugs and deterrence of alcohol consumption. IN C.K. Cain, ed., *Annual Reports in Medicinal Chemistry.* New York: Academic Press, 1969, pp. 245–258.
298. *Alcohol Health and Research World, Social Implications of Alcohol Abuse.* U.S. Government Printing Office, Washington, D.C., 1981.
299. Roizen, J. Estimating alcohol involvement in serious events. Report to NIAA, 1980.
300. Berry, R.E., Jr., et al. The economic costs of alcohol abuse and alcoholism—1975. Report to NIAAA, 1977.
301. Quane, R.P. Motorcycle riding and alcohol—A problem? *J. Traffic Safety Educ.* 26(1):14, 1978.
302. Douglass, R.L. Youth, alcohol, and traffic accidents. Report to NIAAA, 1980.
303. Comptroller General of the United States. *Request to Congress on the Drinking Driver Problem—What Can Be Done About It?* Washington, D.C.: U.S. General Accounting Office, 1979.
304. Pollack, S. *Drinking Driver and Traffic Safety Project. First Annual Report* (microfiche.) NTIS No. PB-188-971. Los Angeles: University of California, Public Systems Research Institute, 1969.
305. Hall, D.C., Chacker, K., and Poland, B. *Review of the Problem: Drinking Behavior Literature Associated with the Spanish Speaking Population,* vol. 3. Menlo Park, Calif.: Stanford Research Institute, 1977.
306. Kitano, H.L. Asian American drinking patterns. Report to NIAAA, 1980.
307. Suchman, E.A. Accidents and social deviance. *J. Health Soc. Behav.* 2:4, 1970.
308. Mannello, T.A. and Seaman, F.J. *Prevalence, Costs and Handling of Drinking Problems on Seven Railroads.* Washington, D.C.: U.S. Dept. of Transportation. Federal Railroad Administration, 1979.
309. Schmidt, C.W., Jr. Suicide by vehicular crash. *Am. J. Psychiatry* 134:175, 1977.
310. Haberman, P.W., and Baden, M.M. *Alcohol, Other Drugs and Violent Death.* New York: Oxford University Press, 1978.
311. Halpen, B.M. A fire fatality study. *Fire J.* 5:11, 1975.
312. Schmidt, W., and deLint, J. Cause of death of alcoholics. *Q. J. Stud. Alcohol* 33(1):171, 1972.

313. Hudson, P. Alcohol and recreation-related deaths. *Nat. Safety Congr. Trans.* 27:13, 1976.
314. California Department of Public Health, Division of Alcoholic Rehabilitation. *Criminal Offenders and Drinking Involvement: A Preliminary Analysis.* Publication no. 3. Sacramento, Calif.: Department of Public Health.
315. Mayfield, D. Alcoholism. Alcohol intoxication and assaultive behavior. Presented at 30th International Congress on Alcoholism and Drug Dependence. Amsterdam, 1972.
316. Goodwin, D.W., Crane, J.B., and Guze, S.B. Felons who drink: An 8-year follow-up. *Q. J. Stud. Alcohol* 32:136, 1971.
317. Roizen, J., and Schneberk, D. Alcohol and crime. Report to NIAAA, 1977.
318. Aarens, M., et al. *Alcohol, Casualties and Crime.* Report no. C-18. Berkeley: University of California, Social Research Group, 1977.
319. Pernanen, K. Alcohol and crimes of violence. In F. Kissin and H. Begleiter, eds., *Social Aspects of Alcoholism. The Biology of Alcoholism*, vol. 2. New York: Plenum Press, 1976, pp. 351–444.
320. Mark, V.M., and Ervin, F. *Violence and the Brain.* New York: Harper & Row, 1970.
321. Tinklenberg, J.R. Alcohol and violence. In P.G. Bourne and R. Fox, eds., *Alcoholism: Progress in Research and Treatment.* New York: Academic Press, 1973.
322. Murphy, G.E., et al. Suicide and alcoholism. *Arch. Gen. Psychiatry* 36:65, 1979.
323. Curlee, J. A comparison of male and female patients at an alcoholism treatment center. *J. Psychol.* 74:239, 1970.
324. Rathod, N.H., and Thompson, I.G. Women alcoholics: A clinical study. *Q.J. Stud. Alcohol* 32:45, 1971.
325. Rimmer, J., et al. Alcoholism. II. Sex, socioeconomic status and race in two hospitalized samples. *Q. J. Stud. Alcohol* 32:942, 1971.
326. Adelstein, A. Alcoholism and mortality. *Pop. Trends* 7:1977.
327. Gomberg, E.S. The female alcoholic. In R.E. Tarter and A.A. Sugarman, eds., *Alcoholism: Interdisciplinary Approaches to an Enduring Problem.* Reading, Mass.: Addison-Wesley, 1977, pp. 603–636.
328. Andre, J.M., and Ghachu, S. *Suicide Occurrence in an American Indian Community of the Southwest.* Albuquerque, N. Mex.: Indian Health Service, 1975.
329. Kraus, R. Patterns of mental illness, alcohol abuse and drug abuse among Alaska natives. Report to the Alaska Federation of Natives, 1977.
330. Hyman, M.M., Helrich, A.R., and Besson, G. Ascertaining police bias in arrests for drunken driving. *Q. J. Stud. Alcohol* 33:148, 1972.
331. Keller, A.Z. Liver cirrhosis, tobacco, alcohol and cancer among blacks. *Natl. Med. Assoc.* 70:575, 1978.
332. Sandmaier, M. *The Invisible Alcoholics.* New York: McGraw-Hill, 1980.
333. Braucht, N.G. Problem drunking among adolescents. A review and analysis of psychosocial research. Report to NIAAA, 1980.
334. Cohen, S. The one vehicle accident. *Drug Abuse Alcohol, Newslett.* April 1981.
335. Culhan, C. Drunk driving a violent crime. *U.S. J. Drug Alcohol Depend.* 2, May, 1982.
336. Ewing, J.A., and Rouse, B.A. *Drinking—Alcohol in American Society—Issues and Current Research.* Chicago: Nelson-Hall, 1978, p. 377.
337. Room, R. Minimizing alcohol problems. *Alcohol Health Res. World* 12, 1974.
338. Braun, K. The minimization of alcohol damage. *Drinking Drug Prac. Surveyor* 8:47, 1973.
339. Pendery, M.L., Maltzman, I.M., and West, L.J. Controlled drinking by alcoholics? New findings and a reevaluation of a major affirmative study. *Science* 217(4555):169, 1982.

## GENERAL READING

### Articles

Begleiter, H. Porjesz, B., and Chou, C.L. Auditory brain stem potentials in chronic alcoholics. *Science* 211:1064, 1981.

Blum, K. Alcohol and central nervous peptides. *Subs. Alcohol Action/Misuse* in press.

Elmasian, R., et al. P3 amplitude differentiates subjects with and without family history of alcoholism. *Abstr. Soc. Neurosci.* 7:158, 1981.

Ryback, R. Biochemical and hematological definition of alcoholism. *Subs. Alcohol Action/Misuse*, in press.

Segal, S. More on the "paradox" of opioid-induced alcohol consumption. *Subs. Alcohol Action/Misuse* 3(6):303, 1982.

Streissguth, A.P. Alcohol and pregnancy: An overview and an update. *Subs. Alcohol Action/Misuse*, in press.

CHAPTER 12

# Central Nervous System Stimulants ("The Uppers")

The biomedical aspects of amphetamine, cocaine, and other stimulants with regard to their use, misuse, and abuse will be explored. The medicolegal, treatment, and preventative aspects will be reviewed only briefly, along with special problems of abuse. The reader may consult the reviews by Ellinwood and Kilbey,[1] Hofmann,[2] Smith and Wesson,[3] and Blum et al.[4]

## A. INTRODUCTION: GENERAL

The stimulants are mind-altering drugs that excite the entire nervous system. Natural stimulants have been used for centuries. Long before the conquistadores, Andean Indians used the juices of cocoa leaves to enhance physical endurance; East Africans utilized the leaves of the kat plant for similar reasons. Ever since the discovery of the "New World," the social stimulants nicotine and caffeine have been a part of European culture.[5]

Synthetic stimulant use began in 1927 with the introduction of amphetamines into clinical medicine. Since 1963, extensive use of illegal intravenous stimulants has developed in the United States and in Sweden, where the favored drugs are methedrine and phenmetrazine (Preludin) respectively. In both countries, overprescription by physicians has contributed significantly to the widespread problem of stimulant drug use. A survey reveals that other sources include the theft of medicinal stimulants, which are grossly overproduced, and undergroup manufacture of the chemicals.[6,7]

Table 12-1 lists some commonly encountered stimulants, but many others exist.[8]

Years of research and the world literature show that stimulant abuse is not confined to students as some might think but also includes other segments of the population. The most likely occupational group to be represented is the medical profession; housewives are next, and those who work at night follow. According to Griffith,[9] "Addiction to amphetamine also occurs . . . direct observations of amphetamine addicts now make it clear that amphetamine addiction is more widespread, more incapacitating, more dangerous, and socially disrupting than narcotic addiction."

The use and abuse of stimulants have come of age. It is time we realize that stimulant abuse in our society warrants a full-scale attack by: (1) developing "antagonists" that reverse the effects of drug overdose; (2) defining and controlling the legitimate uses of stimulants; and

(3) effecting a means of helping this segment of our drug-dependent population find a purpose in existence beyond the temporary solace found in drugs.

In terms of incidence, the 1979 National Drug Abuse Survey[10] found that stimulant nonmedical experience is significantly greater among young adults than among youths or older adults. About one in five young adults (18.2 percent) report using stimulants for nonmedical reasons compared with about one in 29 youths (3.4 percent) and one in 17 older adults (5.8 percent). Prevalence rates did not change significantly between 1977 and 1979.

For simplicity, amphetamines will be discussed as the prototype drug classified as a stimulant. Other stimulants, excluding cocaine, will be treated only briefly.

## 1. Amphetamines[2,11,12]

Amphetamine is phenylisopropylamine, the racemic mixture being benzedrine and the d-isoner being dexedrine; methamphetamine (Methedrine, Desoxyn) and phenmetrazine (Preludin) are two variants of the amphetamine structure.

The amphetamines are related both chemically and pharmacologically to the naturally occurring substances in the body, epinephrine and norepinephrine. These latter compounds are sometimes called sympathomimetic amines, pressure amines, or catecholamines. These drugs have a variety of effects in the body such as increasing heart rate, elevating blood pressure, and dilating pupils. Many of them also exert various stimulating effects on the central nervous system. These compounds are responsible for what physiologists call the fight–flight response.

The most markedly consistent CNS effect is the production of a wakeful state. This effect is used therapeutically in the treatment of some rare diseases such as narcolepsy (inability to remain awake), and for the improvement of performance and endurance by offsetting fatigue and sleepiness. Another CNS effect of amphet-

**TABLE 12-1**

**Commonly Abused Stimulants**

| *Drug* | *Trade Name* | *Slang* |
|---|---|---|
| Amphetamine | Benzedrine | Bennies, splash, peaches |
| Dextroamphetamine | Dexedrine | Diet pills, dexies, oranges, co-pilots, uppers |
| Methamphetamine | Methedrine Desoxyn | Meth, speed, water, crystal |
| Phenmetrazine | Preludin | |
| Methylphenidate | Ritalin | |
| Dextroamphetamine + amphetamine | Diphetamine | Footballs |
| Dextroamphetamine + amobarbital | Dexamyl | |
| Dextroamphetamine + aspirin | Daprisal | |
| Cocaine | | Coke, "c", flake, speedball, (when mixed with heroin) |
| Strychnine | None | None |
| Caffeine | Coffee, tea, cola | No-Doz |
| Nicotine | Tobacco | None |

| *Race* | *Age* | *Sex* | *Prior Treatment* |
|---|---|---|---|
| White: 71% | 18–20: 4% | Male: 67% | None: 73% |
| Black: 19% | 21–25: 24% | Female: 33% | One: 14% |
| Latino: 8% | 26–30: 35% | | Two or more: 13% |
| Asian: 1% | 31–44: 33% | | |
| Indian: 1% | 45+: 4% | | |

Median age = 29.2

From Project Speed Syllabus, 1971. (With permission)

amines is the inhibition of appetite, the basis for the most frequent medical use of amphetamines—the treatment of obesity.

Because of the sense of increased energy, self-confidence, well-being, and even euphoria, the drugs have a high abuse potential. In the past there was considerable controversy as to the seriousness of this problem, but recent experience with high doses of intravenous amphetamines indicates that their abuse poses a real danger to both society and the individual.

Some of the slang names for these drugs are uppers, pep pills, wake-ups, bennies, cartwheels, crystals, speed, meth, and dexies.

Hofmann,[2] in discussing violence and drug abuse, points out that

> In any layman's listing of the evils of drug abuse, one is likely to encounter the specter of the drug-crazed criminal, an individual made not only irrational by drugs but also impelled to commit vicious acts of violence. Like many bits of folklore, this concept has a foundation in fact; it seems to have arisen in the period from 1890 to 1915 and was derived most probably from accounts of behavior during the paranoid psychotic state cocaine can produce. Unfortunately, many lay people mistakenly regard violent behavior as a typical concomitant of all forms of drug abuse, yet it is a frequent consequence of the psychotoxic effects of large doses of all central nervous system stimulants.

Amphetamines were not the first stimulants to be imbibed for recreational reasons. That honor goes to cocaine, a local anesthetic drug capable of producing marked CNS excitation, which was the first agent with stimulant properties to be subjected to widespread abuse in the United States—a practice that probably began in the 1890s. However, by the late 1930s, scattered reports began to appear concerning the abuse of amphetamine, a stimulant that was both cheaper and more readily available than cocaine. The 1950s saw more alarming reports about the increasing magnitude of the problem of amphetamine abuse in this and other countries, and in 1958, Connell's authoritative monograph[13] on amphetamine psychosis was published. Connell emphasized that this form of toxic psychosis was not as rare as was generally supposed at that time. Until the 1960s, abusers of amphetamines typically took the drugs by mouth, but the problem escalated with the growing popularity of intravenous amphetamine usage.[14] The frightening and tragic figure of the "speed freak" came clearly into focus during this period.

There are many facets of amphetamine pharmacology and biochemistry, with concomitant psychological effects. In the '60s, many college students used pill forms of prescription-type amphetamines to produce overt brain stimulation, which allowed the individual to stay up all night and study for exams. Others who used amphetamines were truck drivers, employing the stimulants during cross-country runs, as well as horse trainers and athletes. Now, at a time when the socioeconomic milieu is possibly not quite right for many—when the threat of nuclear holocaust is quite real; when 1.8 trillion of American taxpayers' dollars are spent for military superiority (not for parity)—some individuals may look to drugs such as amphetamines for escape or to give them that extra lift. It all sounds so simple: relief of depression with an "upper." As usual, nothing is that simple, and the use—especially misuse—of amphetamines often produces harmful effects.

Many students soon find out the hard way that fatigue eventually sets in and blocks coherent thought at inopportune times, such as during the examination itself. As a result of using large amounts of amphetamines, the subject may experience irrational behavior and reduced mental acuity.

A peculiar phenomenon observed among amphetamine users is a condition of repetitive acts, described as being "hung up."

Long-term as well as short-term amphetamine abuse may result in psychosis. This is characterized by visual and auditory hallucinations and paranoid delusions. Griffith and associates[16] note that discontinuation of the drug results in a return to normal sensorium in a few days.

The fearful ideation that "meth is death" and "speed kills" reflects the belief that following large doses of methamphetamine, brain damage will ensue. In most cases, a prolonged acute brain syndrome follows abstinence.

Strong tolerance develops for the use and abuse of especially parenteral administration of methamphetamine. A total 24-hour dose of methamphetamine, estimated at over 10 grams has been observed. The intravenous effects of methamphetamine is similar to cocaine, except for the longer duration of amphetamines.

There is intracranial hemorrhage associated with high-dose abuse of amphetamines including mydriasis, elevation of blood pressure, and hyperreflexia.[17]

Amphetamines for medical purposes are available by prescription under a variety of trade names. They are also manufactured in clandestine laboratories and sold through illicit channels as crystalline powder, as tablets, and in a variety of liquid forms.

Among other sympathomimetic agents that are chemically related to the amphetamines and are commonly abused are ephedrine, phenmetrazine (Preludin), mephentermine (Wyamine and Dristan inhalers), and methylphenidate (Ritalin). These drugs all produce central stimulation much like that of the amphetamines, though generally less marked. As with the amphetamines, physical dependence is not known to develop.

## 2. Methylphenidate

Chemically, methylphenidate is a distant relative of the amphetamines. It is prescribed for the treatment of mild depression in adults and excessive excitability in children. Its misuse produces approximately the same consequences as does the abuse of the amphetamines.

## 3. Phenmetrazine

Like methylphenidate, phenmetrazine is related chemically to the amphetamines, and its abuse produces similar effects. Medically, it is used to reduce the appetite.

## 4. Cocaine[18]

Cocaine has now become the most popular drug of abuse in America. It is not a narcotic, however. It is erroneously classified with narcotic drugs (see drug schedules, Chapter 21). Cocaine is a CNS stimulant and a local anesthetic. In its rawest form it occurs naturally in the leaves of the coca plant, *Erythroxylon coca*, and in other species of Erythroxylon, which is indigenous to Peru and Bolivia. The leaves have been chewed by Indians for centuries to increase endurance, and as an aphrodisiac.

### *a. Tolerance and Physical Dependence*

Neither physical dependence nor tolerance is known to develop to the prolonged use of cocaine. It is possible that heightened responsiveness actually develops in some cases.[19]

### *b. Abuse*[18]

As described by Dimijian,[18] ''Euphoric excitement, often of orgastic proportions, is rapidly produced, even when cocaine is sniffed nasally (''snorted'' or ''horned'').''

The pharmacological and behavioral profile of cocaine even in experienced individuals cannot be distinguished from methamphetamine, especially when intravenously injected.

The toxic syndrome associated with cocaine is likewise indistinguishable from the amphetamine-induced syndrome. There are differences in duration of action. Intravenously administered cocaine lasts only a few minutes, while the actions of methamphetamine may persist for hours.

After using cocaine, the user is inclined to overestimate his/her capabilities; there are grandiose feelings; and strong sexual desires ensue, which in some cases lead to spontaneous ejaculation. College campus surveys reveal that, for some, cocaine is a substitute for a sexual partner; hence the names ''Charlie'' and ''girl.''

The toxic syndrome of acute high-dose cocaine includes pupillary dilatation, tachycardia, violence, hyperpyrexia, tremors, and sweating. Individuals taking cocaine may become paranoid and impulsive and may experience marked repetitious/compulsive behavior. ''Snorters'' of cocaine may experience perforation of the nasal septum.

The ''coming down'' phase of binges of cocaine abuse can be quite difficult and very uncomfortable. Sometimes it has been known that users may resort to opiates to reduce the need for cocaine. Usually, depression follows the euphoric state of cocaine abuse which may lead to death by respiratory failure.

A withdrawal syndrome is known to occur following discontinuation of cocaine. The associated symptoms of cocaine abstinence include hyperphagia, paranoia, marked fatigue, irritability, hypersomnia, and depression.[18]

Cocaine is absorbed topically from mucous membranes, and a common practice is its use during coitus to prolong erection in the male by direct application to the glans penis via a local anesthetic action.

Cocaine is not a good antidepressant despite its similarity in terms of mechanism of action with other antidepressants.

The cocaine abuser may feel a strong psychologic dependence on the drug although physical dependence does not develop. When use is stopped, there may be a feeling of depression, and hallucinations may persist. In serious cases, a drug psychosis resembling paranoid psychosis develops. In addition, violent behavior may follow the use of amphetamines as a result of unpredictable mood changes and overreaction to normal stimuli.

## B. HISTORY

### 1. General[20]

For centuries, societies have used various drugs as stimulants. Cocoa leaves have been used by the Andean Indians to provide a sense of well-being and endurance, as have the leaves of the kat plant in East Africa. An extract from the cocoa plant (cocaine) has been used as a stimulant, and we are all familiar with the mild stimulant, caffeine. Among the synthetic stimulants, amphetamine was first prepared in 1887, and methamphetamine in 1919. In 1927, the psychopharmacologic effects of amphetamines were first described, and from the 1930s to the 1950s they were used extensively for medicinal purposes. The first type of abuse to appear was oral ingestion of inhalers sold without prescription for relief of nasal congestion. In Japan abuse of I.V. amphetamines began after World War II, and involved as many as 500,000 people with 50,000 cases of amphetamine psychosis. Medically, amphetamines are still used in the treatment of some rare diseases such as narcolepsy and in the treatment of hyperactive children, but their most extensive use is for the treatment of obesity. In the late 1950s and early 1960s, the compound was considered a useful and relatively safe agent, although some toxic effects and some tendencies to produce drug dependence were noted. In 1963, the American Medical Association (AMA) Council on Drugs, although recognizing the abuse potential of amphetamines, stated that their compulsive use was a small problem at the time. In the past several years, however, it appears that amphetamine misuse has skyrocketed, to the point where it now constitutes one of the most dangerous forms of drug abuse in the United States. This abuse has been particularly related to the recent, prevalent use of amphetamines intravenously in high doses. Although, as pointed out, amphetamines may be of some use in the therapy of narcolepsy and hyperkinetic or hyperactive children, and are employed in the treatment of obesity, their medical value is far outweighed by the potential for abuse.

However, despite all the evidence of major abuse, actions to control amphetamines were hampered by the concepts of "addicting" versus "habituating" drugs. Addicting drugs were defined as those creating physical dependence and causing an abstinence syndrome when stopped. With habituating drugs physical dependence did not develop but only a mild psychic compulsion to continue the drug. Addicting drugs were regarded as extremely dangerous and habituating drugs as relatively harmless, and amphetamines were considered in the latter category. In 1964, the Expert Committee on Addiction Producing Drugs of the World Health Organization, which recognized that the terms addiction and habituation had clouded the issues, recommended that they be replaced by "drug dependence." This was defined as a state of psychic and/or physical dependence on a drug, arising from chronic or periodic administration. The characteristics of drug dependence vary with the agent involved, and must be described individually for each type of drug dependence. The risk of each type has to be evaluated separately.

### 2. The Stimulant Abuse Problem in America

The indiscriminate abuse of psychoactive drugs among Americans has been considered an epidemic problem for over 25 years. Explanations of the origin of drug problems, including amphetamine abuse, are based on both sociologic and political observations peculiar to America (i.e., Vietnamese War and racial inequality) but fail to account for similar abuse in Sweden, Japan, and Great Britain. Thus other, more explicit explanations are necessary to understand the phenomenology of stimulant abuse.

In 1971, Edison[20] reviewed the medical evidence indicating that stimulants are only somewhat effective in the management of obesity and in mild depression. Today, the only reasons for the medical use of stimulants seem to be in the management of narcoleptics, epileptics receiving phenobarbital, and hyperkinetic young people. Interestingly, the number of prescriptions for amphetamines for patients falling into these three categories is miniscule compared with the past use of amphetamines.

The problem of diversion of stimulant drugs reached great proportions in the early to late 1960s.[22–24] In fact, in 1968, according to the FDA, nearly half of the 8 to 10 billion doses of stimulant drugs produced by the U.S. pharmaceutical industry was diverted into channels of illegal usage. In this regard, Kramer et al.[21] point out that amphetamine abuse in the 1960s may be due to the ease with which distributors of illicit drugs could obtain substantial amounts of bulk or individual dosage forms of amphetamine. It is well known that ''basement chemists''[25] provide most of the ''speed'' bought on the street for intravenous injection.

Another major reason for widespread amphetamine abuse in the United States is the acclaimed ''gratifying'' effects of ''uppers.'' Additionally adults who achieve relaxation or pleasure through the use of such ''downers'' as alcohol, tranquilizers, sedatives, and sleeping pills may believe that an ''upper'' is a requisite to ''get going'' in the morning and keep up with business pressures. The prevalent reasons for adolescent amphetamine usage or abuse is that intravenous administration results in kicks, action, and instant pleasure. People who use stimulants such as amphetamines believe that the drug is an antidote for emotional malaise or will pleasurable states.[2]

### 3. History of the User[8]

The profiles of intravenous amphetamine users are quite similar. They have tried amphetamines orally, have liked them or not, have used other drugs to varying degrees, and have associated with various drug-using groups. The first intravenous use of amphetamine is considered a fantastic experience that differs from the effects of oral amphetamines, not only quantitatively, but also qualitatively. In the beginning, use of the drug is intermittent, injections being taken once or a very few times over a day or two. Days or weeks may pass between sprees. Gradually the sprees become longer, the intervening periods shorter; doses become greater, and injections more frequent. After a period of several months, a pattern is reached in which the user, now called a ''speed freak,'' injects the drug in high doses many times a day, and remains awake continuously for three to six days, gradually becoming more tense, tremulous, and paranoid as the run progresses. The runs are interrupted by bouts of very profound sleep called ''crashing,'' which last a day or two. Shortly after the user wakes from the crash, the drug is again injected and a new run starts. The periods of continuous wakefulness may be prolonged to weeks if the user attempts to sleep even as little as an hour a day.

## C. CHEMISTRY AND PREPARATIONS OF CNS STIMULANTS[8]

The chemistry of drugs that act as CNS stimulants is so diverse as to defy generalization.

Forty years ago when the drug was manufactured in two chemical forms, the l- and d-

Structural formulas of representative CNS stimulants are as follows:

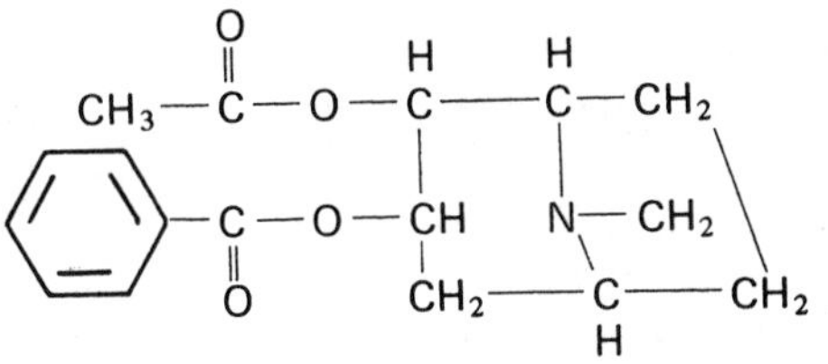

cocaine

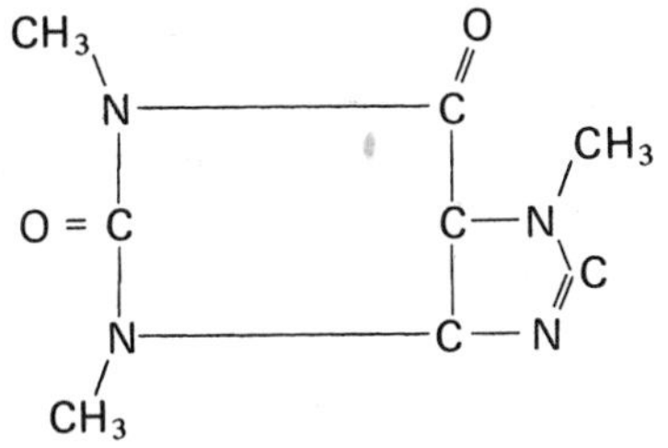

caffeine

OR

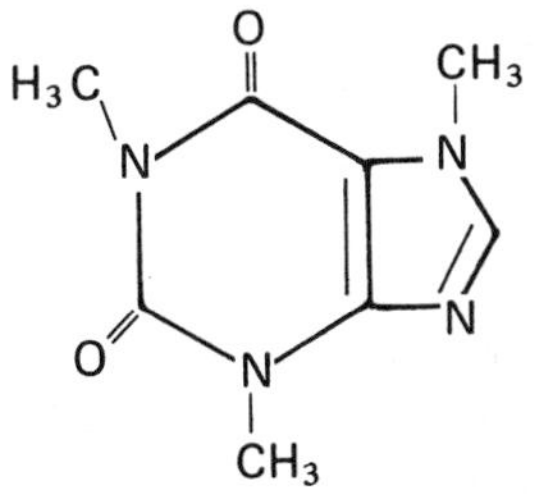

**Natural CNS stimulants**

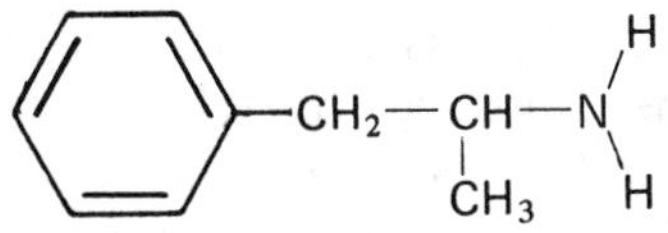

amphetamine
(methylphenethylamine)

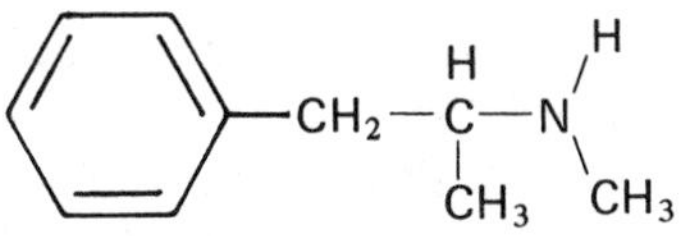

methamphetamine
(dimethylphenethylamine)

**Synthetic CNS stimulents**

isomers of amphetamine, the world was not familiar with the potential abuse liability of these medically useful drugs. The racemic mixture of amphetamine was first synthesized in 1927. Benzedrine was the first commercially available product and was popular as a nasal decongestant. Since the 1930s this has also become very popular as an inexpensive and easily available euphoriant. By the 1940s the central stimulant properties of amphetamine products had taken their place among other analeptics.

Although there is no pharmacological profile difference between the two isomers of amphetamine on a weight basis, the dextroamphetamine (Dexedrine) is the more potent form relative to the l-isomer.

The myth "meth is death" is not far from the truth. Methamphetamine ("speed," "crystal," and methedrine) is usually the drug of choice for the chronic amphetamine abuser (the injection-type). Methamphetamine is more potent as a CNS stimulant but less potent in terms of blood pressure effects relative to amphetamines. Commercially available names of methamphetamine used in the clinic to treat underlying depression in drug abusers[25] include syndrox, norodin, eroxine, semoxydrine, desoxyn, desyphed, dexoval and ampheddroxyn.

Ready availability, low cost, and wide publicity have been the prominent factors in worldwide abuse of stimulants. Phenmetrazine (Preludin), popular in Sweden, is only episodically abused in the United States. "Purple hearts," tablets of Dexamyl or Drinamyl (a dextroamphetamine barbiturate mixture) was the compound that initiated the "speed scene" in Great Britain. Other drugs, such as methylphenidate (Ritalin), pipradol (Meratran), and mephentermine (Wyamine, once a component of Dristan inhalers), are rarely abused.

## D. INCIDENCE AND USE[12,28]

Amphetamines have enjoyed widespread use since the 1930s but have been notoriously abused, at least as far as public awareness is concerned, only in the past 20 years.

There are five basic types of amphetamine abuse.[12] 1) sporadic use of average amounts 2) average oral doses used indefinitely 3) large oral doses 4) large inhaled or injected doses and 5) in combination with other drugs.

A complete description of each type is found in the work of Cohen[12]. The first type involves students and truck drivers, among others, looking for a quick stimulant to postpone the need for sleep. The second type includes those that believe the amphetamines will reduce weight and fatigue as well as depression. These people may be secret addicts. The third type includes tolerant abusers whose intake levels are at a dosage of 50–150 mg. daily. The fourth type includes individuals who relish the amphetamine "high," and discover that "snorting" or injecting the substance intravenously provides a faster and more intensive "flash." Another technique is "balling" the material, i.e., instilling it into the vagina prior to intercourse. During a "speed run," 1,000 mg. may be injected intravenously in a single dose, and over a 24-hour period as much as 5,000 mg. could be injected. This is the "speed freak."

The fifth type is one who combines usually cocaine or amphetamine with heroin or barbiturates. This combination is termed the "speedball." When the "speed" scene becomes too exhausting, some users convert exclusively to heroin. The drug has been used to enhance and prolong the effects of heroin and LSD, and as "uppers" has been used to reduce the overall actions of "downers," such as barbiturates. In adolescents amphetamines have been used with marihuana as well as with other agents.[21]

Several million Americans are involved with oral abuse of stimulants. A large number is involved with the "run" in which large doses of speed are injected intravenously at intervals for as long as six to twelve days.[12] Intravenous usage may initially entail 20 to 40 mg.-doses three to four times a day.

The oral abuser of amphetamines rarely exceeds 1000 to 2000 mg., whereas a speed freak's intravenous usage may reach 30,000 mg. or more with only a two-hour interval between injections.

In evaluating studies[14,21,31,32] concerned with amphetamine abuse, four possible factors were cited to explain the rapid progression to severe patterns of abuse. They are (1) the characteristic hedonistic life-style of a high percentage of abusers; (2) the pharmacologic effects of the drug compatible with the "action" and "kicks," described as prime motives for amphetamine abuse; (3) high psychologic dependence liability; (4) high degree of tolerance.

There is similarity between the narcotic abuser and the speed freak in that both require almost full-time involvement in acquiring their next "fixes." Steady employment is impossible and thus money is usually obtained by criminal means.[14] The pattern of abuse for the speed freak is so intense that overt attempts at self-destruction may occur at any time. Once a "run" ceases, the speed freak "crashes" or "falls out," either spontaneously falling asleep or seeking a "downer" or barbiturate to aid in the is ravenously hungry, lethargic, and sometimes emotionally depressed. There have been numerous studies involving amphetamines and other anorectics. Data from these studies indicate that, although there was a remarkable drop in 1970 from over 20 million to 5 million prescriptions per year for amphetamines, there has been little change in the prescription level since 1973. Prescription of other anorectics has risen from approximately 8 million to 14 million prescriptions per year.[33]

There are two questions pertinent to stimulant misuse:

1. Does prescription of stimulant anorectics to individuals over a short (or alternatively, a chronic) period of time lead to a substantial pool of misuse recruits through introduction to the euphoric and energizing effects of these drugs?
2. What is the level of diversion of legal amphetamines and anorectics into channels where they will be abused?

Approximately 25 percent of amphetamines

mentioned in the DAWN System emergency room report come from legal prescriptions, with 75 percent are attributed to other sources (e.g., street buys or treats).[33]

The exact amount of amphetamines diverted by means of poor medical practice or actual malpractice is not known but it is thought to be high. Furthermore, in 1976 at least 5 million dosage units of amphetamines were stolen from pharmacies and their suppliers as well as from physicians.[34] However, only 2 percent of anorectics seized in drug arrests come from legitimate domestic manufacturers; the overwhelming number have been identified as clandestinely manufactured, and indicate that illegal manufacturers are certainly capable of taking up slack induced by enforcement controls.[35]

Current levels of nonmedical use of prescription stimulants are greater than those for prescription sedatives or prescription tranquilizers, according to a NIDA survey conducted in 1975–1976. Among young adults, nonmedical use of stimulants is second only to marihuana use.[36] Anorectic stimulants are second only to sedatives and marihuana as the primary drug of abuse for admissions to NIDA-monitored rural drug programs.[37] In 1974, Robins reported that amphetamines were second only to marihuana in misuse by both veterans and nonveterans interviewed.[37] In addition, the maladjustment correlation for amphetamines is higher than for a number of other drugs, including heroin, barbiturates, various sedatives and cocaine.

## E. PHARMACOKINETICS AND METABOLISM*[38]*

Stimulants, like amphetamines, are noncatecholamines that release catecholamines (i.e., norepinephrine) from tissue stores. With usual doses of oral dextroamphetamines the effects occur within 1 to 1½ hours, whereas the effects of intravenous administration appear within minutes. Amphetamine and its derivatives are metabolized by the liver, and excreted as unchanged and/or metabolic products in the kidneys.

Amphetamines are clinically effective when given orally. The processes involved in biotransformation of this non-catecholamine include p-hydroxylation, N-demethylation, deamination, and conjugation in the liver. A substantial fraction of amphetamine is excreted in the urine unchanged. The pH dictates the urinary excretion of amphetamine. The pka of amphetamine is 9.9. Thus, the percentage of non-ionized drug increases in alkaline urine, and the drug is readily absorbed by the renal tubules; at pH 8.0 only 2 to 3 percent is excreted. Since 80% of the drug is excreted in acidic urine, amphetamine effects are more prolonged in patients with alkaline urines. Amphetamine poisoning could be controlled by acidification of the urine by the administration of ammonium chloride.

Patients treated with monoamine oxidase inhibitors (MAO) should not take amphetamines or injest foods that contain tyramine, such as certain cheeses. These noncatecholamines provoke the release of catecholamines (norepinephrine) and thus the actions of the neurotransmitter (norepinephrine) can be potentiated by the MAO inhibitors, substances known to inhibit neurotrasmitter metabolism[40]

## F. PHARMACOLOGIC AND TOXICOLOGIC PROPERTIES*[40]*

### 1. Heart and Circulatory System, Smooth Muscles, and Metabolic Effects

In humans and animals, oral amphetamine can raise both systolic and diastolic blood pressure, reflexly slow the heart rate, and induce cardiac arrhymias. With therapeutic doses, cerebral blood flow changes very little and cardiac output is not enhanced. It is noteworthy that, unlike the central actions of amphetamines, the l-isomer is slightly more potent than the d-isomer in its cardiovascular actions.

Amphetamines relax the bronchial muscle and markedly contract the urinary bladder sphincter. The gastrointestinal effects of amphetamines are unpredictable. The response of the human uterus varies, but usually there is an increase in tone.

Amphetamine increases the plasma concentration of free fatty acids but does not modify carbohydrate utilization or respiratory quotient or affect the concentration of blood glucose or lactate. Therapeutic doses cause either no change, or a slight increase or decrease (10 to 15 percent) in the metabolic rate in humans while large doses of amphetamine increase oxygen consumption in animals. Some patients show a rise in body temperature though not a significant one. The calorigenic action may be due to restlessness caused by the drug.

## 2. General Brain Effects

Amphetamines produce stimulation of the central nervous system and may provoke tremor, restlessness, anorexia, insomnia, agitation, and increased motor activity. The d-isomer (dextroamphetamine) is three to four times as potent as the l-isomer, and stimulates the respiratory center, counteracts CNS depressant drugs, exerts cortical stimulation, and possibly stimulates the reticular activating system. An important factor in the clinical use of amphetamines for control of epilepsy is dulling the maximal electric shock seizure discharge.

Amphetamines have an effect on fatigue and sleep. Rapid-eye-movement (REM) sleep is reduced to about 10 percent, less than half the normal proportion of total sleeping time. When the drug is discontinued after long use, total sleep increases, and REM sleep is prolonged. Smith[40] and Oswald[41] suggest that the pattern of sleep may take as long as two months to return to normal.

The psychic effect depends upon the dose, mental state, and personality of the individual. The results of oral doses of 10–30 mg include wakefulness, alertness, a decrease in sense of fatigue, and elevation of mood with increased initiative, confidence, often elation and euphoria, and an increase in motor and speech activity. Thus the drug has been used in certain professions when alertness is necessary, such as the space program. Athletes have also used the drug to improve their physical performance; however, the effects vary in this aspect.

The amphetamines cause a rise in performance of simple tasks (verbal and aythmetic), but not in more complex tasks such as solving calculus problems. They do not improve intelligence performance, or raise intelligence scores. Their effect on learning is difficult to determine. There is some evidence that judgment may be impaired.

In humans, oral amphetamines cause a rise in blood pressure. There may be a reflex slowing of heart rate, but cardiac arrhythmias may occur.

Prolonged use in large doses is almost always followed by mental depression and fatigue. Many individuals experience headaches, palpitations, dizziness, agitation, confusion, dysphoria, apprehension, or delirium. The amphetamines and similar drugs do depress the appetite. This is probably related both to reduction of food intake and to an effect that cannot be accounted for by a caloric basis alone. However, people rapidly develop an increasing tolerance to the drug with continued administration, so that many of the CNS effects, including appetite suppression, disappear, necessitating increased amounts of the drugs.

## 3. Specific Brain Effects

### *a. The Flash and Euphoria*

A few seconds following the intravenous dose, there is a sudden intense generalized sensation. It is difficult to describe exactly, but the user calls it ecstatic, likening it to a sexual orgasm in which the feeling is localized in the abdomen (some say speed is sex). This so-called flash changes in intensity and quality, according to the purity of the material. The euphoria experienced comes from the sense of well-being in which individuals feel that they have marked ability, are invulnerable, no longer are bored, and are able to talk rapidly and for long periods.

Tolerance does develop both to the flash and euphoria, and thus leads to the need for increasing doses of the drug. The desire to reexperience the flash and euphoria and to avoid the fatigue and depression of the coming-down period leads the user to increase not only the dose, but the frequency of injection as well. It is this that leads to the other ill effects of the drug.

#### *b. Anorexia*

Moderate doses of the amphetamines have, in many cases, been used for weight reduction, but large-dose amphetamine abuse may produce very severe and profound anorexia. After the crash, the user usually becomes extremely hungry, but in general, because of lack of desire for food during the spree period, undernutrition and malnutrition result.

#### *c. Insomnia*

During the early stages of abuse, the user tends to remain awake for a day or two at a time. Gradually these periods become longer so that runs may last from three to six days. The sleep deprivation itself can produce difficulties in performing complex tasks, as well as hallucinations and other phenomena. However, it is felt that a combination of sleep deprivation and the drug effect contributes to the difficulties since all of these effects can be produced in short periods of time if the dose of the drug is large.

#### *d. Paranoia*

A paranoid psychosis (a severe behavior disorder in which people have delusions that others are plotting against them) can be seen with either a single large dose or long-term moderate doses of amphetamines. Recent evidence suggests that, although there may be individual differences in sensitivity to the psychosis or severe behavior disorder produced by amphetamines, anyone given a large enough dose for a long enough time will probably become psychotic. Griffith, Cavenaugh, and Oates gave amphetamines to four subjects in high doses (120–220 mg per day for 24–120 hours). Each had previously self-administered large amounts of the drug without experiencing psychosis. They all were diagnosed as having moderate personality disorders. All four subjects developed frank paranoid psychoses, which were reversible when the drug was stopped. Generally, paranoia does not start in the first few months of high-dose intravenous use of amphetamines. When it does, it is usually mild, and most amphetamine users are aware that they will sooner or later experience paranoia, and can usually discount it. Thus the ideas of pursuit and the visual illusions usually will not be acted upon because users are aware that these are drug-induced. However, when the drug is very intense, or toward the end of the long run, even this intellectual awareness may fail and the user may respond to the delusional system. Once an amphetamine user has experienced a psychosis, it will readily return, even after a prolonged period of abstinence.

#### *e. Analgesia*

Amphetamines have only a small analgesic action in both humans and experimental animals, which is of no therapeutic value.

#### *f. EEG*

Brain waves are increased by amphetamine. In humans, the drug causes a shift of the resting

EEG through the higher frequencies to a smaller degree than that occurring during attention. It depresses the amplitude and duration of large delta waves that are present during sleep after prolonged insomnia and in narcolepsy.

Amphetamines abolish both the seizure and the abnormal EEG discharge seen in children with disorders such as dysrhythmia (petit mal and typical three-per-second spike and dome). This is caused by the effect on alertness and activity. Amphetamines also help control behavioral disorders and abnormal EEGs (of children with at least 6 cycle-per-second rhythm).

#### *g. Respiration*

When respiration is depressed by psychotropic agents, amphetamines may stimulate respiration. However, in a normal person, the respiratory rate or minute volume is not appreciably stimulated with usual doses of amphetamine. In animals, the respiratory center is stimulated by amphetamine and the rate and depth of respiration increased.

#### *h. Violence*

From most evidence, it would appear that the amphetamines set up conditions in which violent behavior is likely to occur. Thus the paranoid psychosis and the hyperactivity may combine to induce precipitous and assaultive behavior. The mood of the user may change abruptly from very friendly to furiously hostile. The role that the use of other drugs in conjunction with amphetamines plays in this aggressive behavior is not known. It appears that the barbiturates, however, may induce considerable irritability, and thus the amphetamine user, while trying to use barbiturates for sedation in the come-down period, may actually add to the tendency to display violent behavior.

### 4. Tolerance

Amphetamine users seem to develop a tolerance to the euphoric and other "desirable" effects of amphetamine,[43] and to its cardiovascular effects, but not to the "awakeness" or "antisleep" actions of the drug. This is probably because of the undiminished effectiveness of amphetamine in the treatment of narcolepsy,[43] and the state of persistent wakefulness during amphetamine use. Tolerance development may be due in part to the increase in dosage seen during ongoing and progressive use of amphetamine,[21] whereby the user will invariably increase the amount of drug used over a matter of weeks or months, through oral or intravenous injection.[21,30] After the fifth day of continuous amphetamine use, no dose produces the desired effect regardless of its size.[21]

Whether all of this is due to the development of tolerance or to a desire for the intense amphetamine experience, or both, is not clear. Tolerance to the vasoconstrictor actions of amphetamine may be responsible for speed freaks being able to handle 1000 mg of the drug without any untoward physiologic effect. This dosage would be disastrous to the nonuser of amphetamine. No well-documented evidence[14] of cerebrovascular accident caused by intravenous speed[30] exists to date.

It is unclear what amount of speed is required to develop a tolerance in the amphetamine user, or what amount of amphetamine will cause toxicity. More studies are needed in these areas since no systematic studies have been done concerning this aspect of amphetamine use. It is also necessary to determine how long amphetamine tolerance persists after its abstinence. Reports by Bell[29] indicates that tolerance is retained "long after" the last dose of amphetamine has been excreted. One observation showed amphetamine-dependent users who tolerated daily intake of 1700 mg without apparent ill effects. Narcoleptics are able to withstand amphetamine treatment for years with no change in their initial amphetamine dose.

### 5. Compulsive Behavior

An interesting aspect of amphetamine use is its tendency to produce behavior that is repetitive and lasts for a prolonged period. Thus the individual may clean a house again and again, meticulously polish an automobile, or arrange items, taking great care to pay attention to the tiniest of details. On the other hand, however, the individual might take on a destructive characteristic, such as picking the skin to produce extensive ulceration or gritting or gnashing the teeth.

## G. TOXICITY

### 1. Overdose and Mortality (Acute)

When too much of the amphetamine is taken, sometimes called overramping, one or several symptoms may occur; chest pain that lasts minutes or hours, or unconsciousness that lasts minutes or hours, or the user may be awake but unable to talk for hours or even days. More frequently, the user remains unconscious, though the mind is racing. The user is in an ecstatic mood, but unable, or perhaps unwilling, to move. Secobarbital (200 mg) orally or 0.5 gram amytal sodium, slowly I.V., until the desired results occur, can be used to treat acute overdose.[44]

There are very few recorded deaths in which the actual cause was related to an overdose of amphetamines *per se*. The use of the needle can lead to viral hepatitis, tetanus, and infections in the heart and elsewhere, and this may lead to death. In addition, death can be caused by violence because of the paranoid psychoses. Although deaths have occurred in the past, David Smith of the Haight-Ashbury Clinic says that since amphetamine use has increased, there has been a large increase in the number of violent deaths in that district. In those cases where death was related to high doses of amphetamines, there appeared to be a hyperpyrexia (high temperature) shock, acidosis, and death.

There is increasing evidence to suggest that the abuse of drugs intravenously may result in severe vascular abnormalities, thus causing extensive organ damage. This includes brain damage and even death. Most studies have suggested that the CNS stimulants such as methamphetamines may be the most dangerous. The precise role that methamphetamine plays is unclear, since there is usually more than one drug being used and the drug abuser's history is usually unreliable. Furthermore, the drug source, quantity, quality, and diluting agents are unknown. Many times users dissolve drugs in anything from tap water to urine. Foreign matter, including talc used as filler in tablets, is injected and these contaminants can produce small embolization of the lung and lead to pulmonary talc granulomatosis, pulmonary hypertension, and death.[45] Furthermore, in overdoses, various home remedies are used, such as intravenous injections of milk or mayonnaise. It appears that intravenous drug abusers may be subjecting themselves to serious irreversible brain damage. The etiologic basis remains unclear, but methamphetamine is highly suspect. The possibility exists that even the oral use of drugs such as methamphetamine in sensitive individuals may result in vascular abnormalities and brain damage. It is obvious that further investigations are necessary.

### 2. Behavioral Toxicity

Although acute high-dose amphetamine use may induce a toxic hallucinatory state, by far the major behavioral alteration is the chronic amphetamine psychosis that occurs in a state of clear consciousness. Usually the major element of the psychosis is paranoid symptomatology, which includes visual, auditory, and olfactory hallucinations, delusions of persecution, ideas of reference, and body-image changes. Dyskinetic and dystonic reactions have also been described.[45,46] Once the psychosis is manifested, certain symptoms (e.g., delusions) may persist, and the individual has a lower threshold for precipitation of psychosis with subsequent amphetamine use, even after long intervening periods of abstinence.[47–49] Abstinent former abusers have been described as apathetic and psychasthenic.[50]

Abrupt discontinuation of amphetamines taken in high doses may result in severe psychic depression with suicidal tendencies. Although there is no clinical evidence of physical dependence, EEG abnormalities of nocturnal sleep patterns are seen during the withdrawal of a stimulant drug. Drug users refer to the symptoms of withdrawal as a come-down, and many times a second drug is taken to change the discomfort of coming down from the stimulant. Such drugs include heroin and the CNS depressants such as the barbiturates. Although flashback symptoms (that is, a recurrence of a drug's effects at a later date while off the drug) have been commonly reported with the psychotomimetics (LSD, STP, tryptamine, mescaline, morning glory seeds, etc.) and sometimes with marihuana, there have been few reports of flashbacks with amphetamines. This effect would appear, at least at present, to be extremely rare. In addition, there does not seem to be any cross-tolerance between LSD-like drugs and amphetamines.

## 3. Chronic Toxicity

### *a. Abuse Potential*

The properties of individual anorectics have been examined. Griffith and his colleagues[51,52] have extensively tested most of the anorectics for their stimulant, euphoriant, and preference properties in addicts "blind" to the drugs. In general, the results follow clinical impressions in that amphetamine-like compounds have the highest preference with appropriate gradations down to the ring-substituted amphetamine analogs (fenfluramine and chlorphentermine), which apparently do not have any major psychostimulant or sympathomimetic effect. These drugs are perceived as sedatives without euphoriant properties.

Abuse persistence is defined as the abuse pattern's long-term tenacity on the individual. As with narcotics, sedatives, and alcohol, amphetamines demonstrate some capacity for a resolute grip on the individual, even after long periods of abstinence. This stubborn, enduring quality of the stimulant habit does not appear to be as great as that of heroin (or even alcohol) after one or two years. Case histories demonstrate a tendency for the amphetamine habit to "burn out" within a year or so, although some abusers will continue in a sustained pattern for longer. In contrast, the heroin addict[53,54] and alcoholic generally take eight to 16 years for their habit to "burn out" or run its course.

### *b. Pathologic Toxicity in the Chronic Abuser*

Chronic speed users experience weight loss (20 to 30 pounds or more due to periods of total starvation), nonhealing ulcers, abscesses, brittle fingernails (possible secondary causes of malnutrition), and bruxism.[21] Tooth grinding, usually in conjunction with abraded and ulcerative areas of the oral mucosa, can be detected during examination of the drug user. Just as with the heroin addict, frequent encounters with infectious diseases, including hepatitis and endocarditis, are commonly caused by the use of intravenous injections of amphetamine.

High-dose intravenous users suffer from all the problems of dirty needle use (e.g., sepsis and emboli). In addition, the acute overdose hypertensive crisis can precipitate cerebrovascular accidents. On the basis of human and animal studies, Rumbaugh[55] raised the issue of a specific microvascular insult from chronic stimulant intoxication. In animal studies, neuronal chromatolysis, primarily in catecholamine neuron areas[56,57] and a striking permanent depletion (70 percent) of dopamine in the caudate,[58] have been demonstrated following chronic amphetamine intoxication. This evidence of chronic depletion of catecholamine is potentially important for an understanding of (1) the anergia noted in former addicts and (2) the prerequisites of postjunctural supersensitivity. It also raises the nagging question of whether chronic treatment of hyperactive children with moderately high doses (over 1 mg/kg) of amphetamines may have residual effects. Consistent with the chronic behavioral changes noted for humans, there are laboratory data demonstrating that a given stimulant dose induces quantitatively and qualitatively different behaviors than noted with original acute doses. These chronic stimulant intoxication end-stage behaviors include hyperreactive "startle" behaviors, postural abnormalities, and dyskinesias noted in monkeys and cats[59,60] and response augmentation in rats and guinea pigs[61–65]; the increased responsivity persists for several weeks after cessation of chronic treatment. The dyskinesias induced take on considerable relevance, in that Eibergen and Carlson[65] demonstrated that chronic treatment with methadone induces a long-term supersensitivity manifested as amphetamine-induced dyskinesias, at doses that do not have this effect generally. The fact that some methadone maintenance patients abuse amphetamines makes this an important finding. Chronic amphetamine intoxication renders caudate neurons more sensitive to a direct dopamine agonist consistent with the induction of a postsynaptic supersensitivity.[66]

Chronic intraperitoneal administration of amphetamines increases uptake of the last dose into the brain, including a marked increase in striatum and pons.[67] Amphetamines accumulate in tissues during chronic administration. This was further elaborated by Sparber et al.,[68] who reported that chronic amphetamine administration results in 60 percent higher concentrations in adipose tissue than after acute injections. Furthermore moderate stress mobilized the drug stores and led to doubled brain levels of amphetamines in the chronic animals, whereas the acute animals did not show this response. Stress-induced release of mobilizable storage pools may help explain the "conditioned responses" of chronic experimental animals,[60] as well as the sudden panic states (at times with violence) of chronic amphetamine abusers subjected to real and imaginary stress.[69]

## H. CHRONIC ABUSE[12]

### 1. The "Speed Run"

In the late 1970s, there was a sharp increase in the "mainlining" of large amounts of methamphetamine. The so-called "speed freaks" start their "runs" with small amounts of methamphetamine or other stimulants, and then gradually increase their doses. An abuser enjoys the immediate "rush" or "flash" even more than the prolonged feeling of being powerful, hyperalert, and full of energy, and when the "come down" ensues, reinjects. During "speed runs" abusers are disinclined to eat or sleep and they ignore ordinary body care. As much as ten pounds or more may be lost in a week.

Symptoms of the "speed run" include:

1. Overactivity
2. Impulsiveness
3. Defective reasoning
4. Paranoia
5. Delusional thinking
6. Hallucinations
7. Homicidal tendency

The amphetamine psychosis seems to mimic paranoid schizophrenia and, in some individuals, can last beyond the period of amphetamine indulgence. Certain other aspects of amphetamine intoxication are remarkable. Stereotyped behavior is often observed. This may consist of skin picking, bead stringing and unstringing, pacing, or interminable chattering. It is worth noting that all mammalian species will perform stereotyped activities under the influence of amphetamines.

The term "overramping" is used on the street to describe the condition when the amphetamine dosage is raised too rapidly. The "overramped" individual is conscious but unable to move or speak, and has an extremely rapid pulse, elevated temperature, increased blood pressure, and occasionally chest distress. In the tolerant individual, death due to overdosage is infrequent.

Cohen[12] points out:

> Orgasm and ejaculation are delayed or impossible to achieve. As a result, marathon sexual activity is described by some "speed freaks." Others report a complete absence of sexual interest.
>
> After a few days or a week or a "speed" binge, the person becomes so exhausted or so delusional that he or his friends decide that he must "crash." The

withdrawal syndrome to amphetamines consists of a long period of sleep, a marked depression, apathy, a variety of aches and pains, and a ravenous appetite. The depression is so severe that it may initiate another "speed run." Reinjection of amphetamines relieves the distressing symptoms.

The abuse of "speed" (methamphetamine) results in numerous side effects and includes:

1. Necrotizing angiitis
2. Parenchymal liver damage
3. Brain cell injury
4. Malnutrition or cachexia
5. Severe abdominal pain
6. Dyskinesis
7. Hepatitis ("dirty needle syndrome")
8. Paranoid states

In addition, suicide may occur during or after the amphetamine "run." A greater risk exists during the withdrawal phase where the depression is so prolonged and unrelieved that suicide seems to be the only alternative.

### 2. Physical Dependence

In the late '60s and early '70s, a time when the interest in the use (or misuse) of amphetamines increased, supporters of its indiscriminate abuse hailed it as a drug unlike heroin, because no physiological dependence developed. They argued that the fatigue, sleep, and sensation of hunger following withdrawal of the amphetamines were simply physiologic compensations as a result of lack of sleep, starvation, and continuous activity. In the '80s we now have accumulated enough evidence to suggest that the amphetamine hangover is indeed a sign of physical dependence and abstinence.

Although there is a Japanese report suggesting that high-dose amphetamine users may become chronically psychotic, the experience in the United States has usually been that recovery is slow but fairly complete. All of the most severe symptoms disappear within a few days to a week. Some confusion, memory loss, and delusional ideas may remain for six to 12 months. Most commonly, ex-users report slight difficulty in remembering. It is important, then, to recognize that the great majority, if not all, of the severe amphetamine users can recover from even the most profound intellectual disorganization and psychosis by abstaining from six months to a year. Cases of psychosis during amphetamine withdrawal have been reported. These have been described as delirium with confusion, hallucination, delusions of persecution, and disorientation of thoughts. The condition seems to be unusually rare and its relevance to amphetamine use, if any, is obscure.

## I. STIMULANTS AS REINFORCERS: MECHANISMS

Important to a general theory of drug abuse is the concept of stimulants as reinforcers. Since stimulants do not induce severe physiologic dependence and withdrawal, the reinforcing effects are thought to contribute significantly to the stimulants' abuse potential.

A research method to evaluate abuse potential is the self-administration paradigm in animals. Basically this paradigm consists of demonstrating that an animal (e.g., monkey or rat) will work (lever press) for a drug injected through an indwelling intravenous catheter. Certainly any drug that is self-administered by animals, especially monkeys, is highly suspect as to abusable reinforcing properties in humans until proved otherwise.

The reinforcing efficacy of amphetamines and cocaine does appear to be in part mediated by catecholamines, especially dopamine, in that alpha-methyl-tyrosine (αMt) (a known catecholamine neurotransmitter releaser) and pimozide (a dopamine receptor blocker) both increase rates of responding to a given dose in self-administration paradigms.[70-72] Furthermore Antelman and Caggiula[73] have proposed a norepinephrine–dopamine interaction for reinforcing effects, since inhibition of norepinephrine synthesis or lesions of the locus cerulens facilitate lateral hypothalamic self-stimulation.[74,75]

Amphetamines and several of the more potent psychomotor stimulants (including methamphetamine and phenmetrazine) act by selecting and releasing newly synthesized catecholamines, in that αMt, which inhibits tyrosine hydroxylase and thus the synthesis of catecholamines, markedly inhibits the ability of these compounds to induce central stimulant effects.[76-79] Scheel-Kruger[77] and Wallach and Gershon[80] report that unlike amphetamine, methylphenidate, and cocaine, αMt is unable to block the central stimulant effects. Ellinwood[25] discussed the mechanism of action of stimulants. Many stimulants, including d- and l-amphetamine, methamphetamine, methylphenidate, pipradol, and cocaine, have potent catecholamine reuptake blocking actions.[81,82] The stimulant cocaine, like the tricyclics (e.g., desipramine), is similar to amphetamine in its capacity to block reuptake of norepinephrine, but is a weak *in vitro*[83,84] and *in vivo*[85] releaser. The catecholamine reuptake blocking action may potentiate the stimulant effect, but certainly is not the central mechanism underlying the characteristic stimulant behavioral effects.[79] Tricyclic antidepressants are potent norepinephrine reuptake inhibitors[86] and benztropine is a potent dopamine uptake blocker,[87] yet neither induces stereotypy or pronounced locomotor activation in animals. Furthermore they do not induce the characteristic "euphoria," nor are they subject to abuse in humans. Analogously, the monoamine oxidase (MAO) inhibiting actions of amphetamines do not appear independently to contribute to the stimulant effects, since many potent MAO inhibitors do not induce the characteristic stimulant behaviors. Tranylcypromine, an amphetamine analog, has a strong MAO inhibiting capacity as well as some stimulant effects. Most stimulants are not potent MAO inhibitors; like reuptake block, this mechanism may only contribute to the main stimulant effect at higher doses.

With regard to structure–activity relationships, adding methyl groups onto the side chain inhibits MAO degradation, and can even induce MAO inhibition. Halogen substitution on the phenyl ring (e.g., fenfluramine) reduces arousal activation but leaves strong anorectic action through a serotonergic mechanism. Other substitutions induce psychotomimetic activity, reduce arousal and reinforcement effects, or change the stimulant's mode of action in activating catecholamine effects while maintaining reinforcing effects (e.g., methylphenidate and cocaine).

It is quite remarkable that rats and monkeys will not only administer huge amounts of strong stimulants (including cocaine) after only a brief experience with the drug, but will continue to self-administer even though toxic effects have ensued.[88,89]

## J. TREATMENT OF STIMULANT ABUSE[90]

Stimulants, including many amphetamine derivatives, phenmetrazine (Preludin), methylphenidate, cocaine, and others, are more widely abused than generally recognized. In view of their substantial danger of abuse, medically approved stimulants should be prescribed carefully, and only when the benefits exceed the potential dangers implicit in these drugs. When grossly abused, all stimulants produce a similar clinical picture, including some or all of the following signs and syndromes:

1. Insomnia.
2. Anorexia, with possible malnutrition.
3. Hypertension, tachycardia, elevated body temperature.
4. Dilated pupils.
5. Muscular tremor.
6. Possible damage to nasal mucosa (if taken as snuff); extensive needle scars and associated pathology (if taken I.V.).
7. Verbosity—constant "rambling" talk.
8. Impulsivity.
9. Extreme nervousness, suspiciousness, and hostility that may develop into a characteristic stimulant-induced paranoid psychosis. This psychosis is very similar to that of paranoid schizophrenia, but the short-term prognosis is good. With abstinence from the drug, psychotic manifestations usually disappear within a few days, although occasionally they last for several weeks or months. These last should be treated with Haldol.

## 1. Acute Overdose

This condition is rather uncommon with most stimulants and is seen mainly in cocaine abuse. It can include severe hyperthermia, convulsions, cerebrovascular accidents, and possible cardiovascular or respiratory collapse. Treatment must be rapid and appropriate to the symptomatology, including respiratory or cardiac support if indicated, sedation, and aggressive treatment of hyperthermia. Acidification of the urine with ammonium chloride, 12 grams/day P.O. or I.V., significantly enhances amphetamine excretion.

## 2. Chronic Abuse Syndrome

Treatment is primarily psychotherapeutic. In severe psychotic reactions short-term psychiatric hospitalization may be indicated. Minor tranquilizers will control anxiety. Davis, Sekerke, and Janowski[91] recommend haloperidol as possible alleviating psychotic symptomatology. Phenothiazines are not suggested as they retard the excretion of amphetamines.

### *a. Stimulant Withdrawal*

The chronic abuse syndrome usually can be alleviated after a single sleep period (often 24–48 hours long). However, due either to depletion of brain catecholamines or other causes, there might be a withdrawal syndrome that might need additional treatment. This syndrome, which may last weeks or months, is characterized by:

1. Moderate to severe depression, with possible suicidal ideation.
2. Sleep disturbances, lethargy.
3. Postpsychotic suspiciousness or hostility.
4. Mild tremor in extremities; various aches and pains.

### *b. Therapeutic Antidotes*[12]

Certain therapeutic agents are used in the acute as well as chronic treatment of stimulant abuse. Phenothiazines, especially chlorpromazine, are physiologic antidotes. These psychotherapeutic drugs (phenothiazines) should not be used if anticholinergic drugs were taken in addition to amphetamines. Street amphetamines, as Cohen suggests,[12] are unreliable in quality; therefore, certain tranquilizers or barbiturates are safer. For a sedative therapeutic measure, diazepam in initial doses of 10–20 mg intravenously or orally is recommended. The tricyclic antidepressants have been used in the depression associated with amphetamine withdrawal probably due to catecholamine depletion.[92] It is not necessary to reduce the dose of amphetamines gradually because withdrawal symptoms are mild.

### *c. Long-Term Therapy*

Initially treatment should be oriented to restoration of biologic health, including nondependency-producing sedatives at night until a regular sleep cycle is restored; major tranquilizers only if psychosis persists; ample diet, including vitamin supplement; and treatment of associated pathology, such as hepatitis. Antidepressants should be used cautiously during the first week of treatment, as blood levels of stimulant may persist for some time, a situation that creates the possibility of undesirable interaction between the two classes of drugs. They are needed for severe depressive reactions, however. After medical needs are met, there should be referral for long-term care.

The long-term management of the chronic amphetamine abuser is difficult, and relapse is frequent. Abstinence and rehabilitation present complex problems. The user does not readily volunteer for care and in the past community programs offered very little besides enforced abstinence. Many users, following abstinence, will return to drug abuse upon release. The amphetamine should always be withdrawn. However, in severely dependent individuals, the possibility of suicide must be considered. Withdrawal should probably take place in a hospital so the dependent patient can be closely supervised and helped. Since there is a high tendency to relapse, the individual needs to be followed for years with repeated return to clinics and urine examinations, and ongoing psychotherapy. All types of models should be tried, including self-help groups and night clinics.

For example, group therapy has had some success with "speed freaks." According to Cohen[12]: "The chronic amphetamine abuser tends to be a disturbed person who has treated his mood disorder with a highly rewarding euphoriant. His defective life style and inadequate coping mechanisms must be reconstructed if he is to remain drug free."

## K. THERAPEUTIC USES OF STIMULANTS

During the past several years, a variety of new drugs have been introduced as appetite suppressants with little or no CNS stimulation. However, it is now clear that all of these drugs may have CNS stimulating effects (related to the dose) and have abuse potential. It is reasonable, then, to state that any drug with CNS stimulating effects similar to those of amphetamines or related compounds will have abuse potential.[93]

### 1. Miscellaneous Uses

Amphetamine and dextroamphetamine have been replaced as central stimulants for numerous medicinal uses by newer synthetics. Dextroamphetamine has a more intense central action compared to amphetamine, whereas the latter drug is more effective in the peripheral nervous system. Dextroamphetamine has been used clinically in the following conditions: obesity, narcolepsy, hyperkinetic syndrome in children, and Parkinson's disease.

### 2. Hyperactive Behavior

The CNS stimulants such as dextroamphetamine and methylphenidate are widely used to quiet children with hyperactive behavior. The exact reason why stimulant drugs would do this is not known, but is probably related to their stimulation of inhibitory centers in the brain. Although, when used cautiously, these drugs are relatively safe for preadolescent children, there are increasing reports of adverse behavioral reactions with their use. In the literature, three cases of severe behavioral reaction due to methylphenidate have been observed.[94] All three patients had symptoms characteristic of minimal brain dysfunction with hyperactive behavior. In one case, the behavioral reaction was an episode of extreme excitement followed by catatonic withdrawal. In the other two cases, there was drug-induced hallucinosis. The authors state that methylphenidate hydrochloride is often prescribed for children with hyperactive behavior. Some children respond to methylphenidate as they do to dextroamphetamine sulfate with a marked dimunition in their hyperactivity. In some, there is no apparent clinical response. Generally the use of these drugs is no longer indicated beyond puberty in hyperkinetic children, and should be prescribed for adolescents only with the understanding that the drugs may be abused and that excessive stimulation may occur. It is known that paranoid psychotic reactions will occur in adults using large doses of amphetamines and visual, auditory, and tactile hallucinations have been reported in preadolescents receiving the drug. Similar adverse reactions can occur with methylphenidate. The psychotic reactions reported in this study in two children and in one adolescent were severe, dramatic, and very frightening to the families.

There is no doubt that careful use of CNS stimulant drugs such as the amphetamines and methylphenidate is of value in some children with hyperactive behavior. There is also no doubt that serious side reactions can occur. The indiscriminate use of these drugs for children who appear to be behavioral problems in school is a dangerous practice, although increasing numbers of teachers are advocating their use. Adequate statistics are not available, but it is firmly believed that most behavioral problems in school are not attributable to hyperkinetic impulse disorders, but are related to a variety of factors, including problems at home and boredom in school. These problems will not be solved by the use of CNS stimulant drugs, but indicate the need for individual student counseling and for revision of educational curricula. Children should be placed on drugs only after adequate medical work-ups have been performed and indicate that their problems are types that may respond to drug therapy. They should then be followed under medical supervision. The widespread abuse of CNS stimulants, including methylphenidate, by adolescents and adults has created serious medical and social problems. We should be very concerned about the indiscriminate use of these agents in preadolescents as this is indication to our youth that society's difficulties can be solved through chemicals.

A peculiar reaction to the illicit use of methylphenidate (Ritalin) and other drugs has been noticed. This is related to the production of lung abnormalities caused by the I.V. injection of dissolved tablet (oral) forms of certain drugs containing magnesium tricylicate (talc) as filler material. The tablets are dissolved in water and the solution containing drug and talc as a contaminant is injected. The talc produces lesions in the lung, which can lead to chronic fatal changes. Similar lung lesions also have been associated with the abuse of other drugs such as meperidine (Demerol) and "blue velvet," a mixture of paregoric and tripelennamine hydrochloride (Pyroebenzamine) tablets. The talc crystals induce a tumor-like (nodular) reaction in the pulmonary arteries, arterioles, and capillaries. This can lead to vascular scarring, increased blood pressure in the pulmonary arteries, and death.[95,96]

### 3. Anorectics[28]

Do we need anorectics in medicine? The FDA is currently considering the removal of the anorectic indication in the labeling of amphetamine products. However, the cost/benefit ratio for anorectics must take into account the increased mortality and disease morbidity resulting from obesity. The increase in the mortality rates for overweight persons is substantial,[97] and morbidity for hypertension, diabetes, and cerebrovascular and coronary artery disease is much greater.[98-100]

Anorectic treatment does not provide for a sustained weight loss, but neither do other forms of weight control.[101] Preliminary studies indicate that overweight patients who use diet pills typically are people who have experienced difficulty in losing weight with other methods, but there is no evidence of greater drug misuse in this group than in other groups of overweight patients.[102]

The anorectic effects of stimulants, such as amphetamines, are related to at least two neurotransmitter systems. 6-Hydroxydopamine lesions of the ventral noradrenergic bundle to the hypothalamus, which destroys 90 percent of the noradrenergic terminals (but dopamine terminals only slightly), block amphetamine-induced anorexia.[103] Despite the specific noradrenergic findings, evidence is accumulating that bilateral lesions of the dopaminergic nigrostriatal system in the rat induce the same aphagic-adipsic syndrome as reported for the classical lateral hypothalamic lesions.[104-106]

Furthermore, ring substitution on the phenylethylamine nueleus creates pharmacologic characteristics that act on the serotonergic system.[107,108]

According to Ellinwood,[25] the promotion of the selective and discriminate use of anorectics is preferable to a total ban on stimulant substances.

## L. OTHER CNS STIMULANTS

### 1. Cocaine

#### *a. Introduction*

Cocaine is a local anesthetic that has CNS stimulating properties similar to those of the amphetamines. The duration of action, however, is considerably shorter. Cocaine has a high abuse potential and, in high doses, can produce psychotic behavior.

Cocaine's reputation is that of proved clinical efficacy and of abuse as an illicit drug. A historical analysis of the ten recorded centuries of its use reveals a record of coca/cocaine as an emotionally charged subject that has attracted much interest.

Illicit drug use patterns reveal a remarkable upsurge in that for cocaine. Certainly in the 1980s, cocaine has emerged as a subject of intense concern. No longer hidden in the ghetto, it is ubiquitous in middle-class America.

Cocaine is a highly desired drug, and users are often forced to "deal" to support their expensive habit. A survey of 78 recent cocaine abusers admitted to the Haight-Ashbury Free Medical Clinic's Drug Detoxification Project revealed the following demographic breakdown:

Of the 78 cocaine admittees, nine (12 percent) reported secondary abuse of sedative-hypnotics. Cocaine itself was a drug of secondary abuse for 220 (6.1 percent) out of 3363 admittees during 1979–1980. For 87 percent of these 220 individuals, the primary drug of abuse was heroin.

The data also revealed that the cocaine users (when compared with the greater number of primary heroin users) tended to be somewhat younger, and more often single. They also appeared to be of more "privileged" white middle-class backgrounds, were better educated and were employed, and were found to have been significantly younger when they first used drugs. Further, their general drug histories were more extensive.[109]

On a national basis, 4.5 percent of all drug treatment admissions are cocaine related. From 1977 to 1980, cocaine deaths increased from 0 to 56 in Miami (the nation's center for cocaine traffic) and in New York City, from 13 to 79.

Some interesting statistics on cocaine abuse from NIDA[110] reveals that admissions to treatment programs for cocaine abuse increased more than five times from 1975 (2192) to 1980 (11,110), representing the largest admissions increase for any drug or drug type. According to NIDA[110] in a survey of 7000 Americans, experience with cocaine (from 1972 to 1979) doubled among 12- and 17-year-olds and among those over 25. Between the ages of 18 and 25, cocaine use tripled for this period. Fifteen percent of high school seniors surveyed said they had used cocaine.

The amount of cocaine entering the United States increased from 19 metric tons in 1977, to 25 metric tons in 1978, to 31 metric tons in 1979, to 51 metric tons in 1980. In contrast, less than 500 kg per year of cocaine is imported for legitimate medical use.

The smoking of "free base" has become popular and, with this new method of ingestion, aggravated signs of systemic cocaine toxicity are being observed. The "Richard Pryor incident" provided thorough mass media warning against free-base methodology. However, its effect on the problem is currently unknown.

Paola Mantegazza, in 1859, wrote about cocaine: "Borne on the wings of two coca leaves, I flew about in the spaces of 77,438 worlds, one more splendid than another. I prefer a life of ten years with coca to one of a hundred thousand without it."

In 1908, an editorial in *The New York Times* proposed that "It (cocaine) wrecks its victim more swiftly than opium."

### *b. History*[111]

Cocaine is obtained from the leaves of certain trees that are indigenous to Peru and Bolivia. The cocoa leaf was used for many centuries in South America. The Incas apparently used it to appease hunger, impart vigor, and bring joy to the sorrowful. The priests of the Incan empire believed in its divine qualities and employed it on ceremonial occasions, but its use spread rapidly until people from all classes were utilizing cocoa leaves (commonly known as coca) to induce feelings of exhiliration and pleasure. The leaves were commonly used in Peru to relieve fatigue, especially during laborious marches in the mountains. The harmful effects of cocoa became apparent as early as the middle of the 16th century, when attempts were made to stop its use in Chile, Bolivia, and Peru. The cocoa leaves must be mixed with lime to release the drug that is still chewed almost constantly by many of the Indians living in the high Andes. The pure substance, cocaine, was obtained in 1859, and knowledge of it gradually spread throughout the world. It was thought at first to be a cure for alcoholism and morphinism, and was used by the medical profession. Unfortunately many patients developed, in addition to their other habits, a cocaine habit.

One report claims that 90 percent of the adult males and 20 percent of the adult females in the northern Andes are coca chewers. Nine million kilograms of coca leaves are consumed yearly in Peru alone. The plant grows in the foothills but is consumed in the mountains. It is said that mountaineers who come down to the plains to work give up their coca habit.

Scientific study began when cocaine was extracted from coca over 100 years ago. The leaves contain about 1 percent cocaine. Two prominent names have been associated with the earlier work: Sigmund Freud and Sherlock Holmes. The psychic action of synthetic cocaine was first widely advocated by Freud. His publications describing cocaine as a miraculous psychic energizer were publicized widely in Europe and probably were a factor in the subsequent epidemic of cocaine abuse toward the end of the 19th century.

The fictional character Sherlock Holmes took cocaine for many years ("Quick, Watson, the needle"), apparently for his cyclic depressions. It is not known whether or not his creator, Sir Arthur Conan Doyle, shared the cocaine dependence. Eventually both disappeared from the public eye for a three-year period, after which Holmes returned to their readers cured.

It was William Halstead, the pioneer surgeon from Johns Hopkins, who discovered regional anesthesia by blocking peripheral sensory nerves with cocaine. He, too, became a compulsive cocaine user and struggled for a long time to overcome his habit.

During the early part of the 20th century many patent medicines and soft drinks contained small amounts of cocaine. There was a marked increase in the use of cocaine in Europe during World War I, and vigorous preventive measures such as the Harrison Tax Act, were taken by authorities to stop the practice. At present, the Coca-Cola Company extracts the cocaine from the imported leaves and turns it over to the government for medical purposes while using the decocainized leaves as a flavoring agent (see Table 12-2).

### *c. Pharmacology and Street Economics*[109,111–113]

Cocaine is an alkaloid of the deciduous shrub *Erythroxylum coca*, which is extensively cultivated on the eastern slopes of the Andes of Peru and Bolivia; a variety, ipadu, grows in the Amazon basin. A second species, *E. novogranatense*, is cultivated in Colombia; the Trujillo variety is grown along the irrigated desert coast of Peru. The plant grows to ten or more feet in height, but is usually pruned back to four to six feet to facilitate harvesting. The active alkaloid is produced within 18 to 36 months, and continues to be produced for the life span of the plant (almost 40 years). Harvesting is carried out in March, June, and November. The leaves, about one to four inches in length, are plucked from the shrubs and placed in gasoline drums filled with kerosene. The macerated leaves are then subjected to sulfuric acid to make pasta, a crude form of cocaine sulfate. The residual, thick pasta is then ladled into smaller containers and sold to "laboratory agents," who further refine it by portioning the alkaloids into an aqueous acid solution and then removing the nonalkaloid impurities via further solvent extraction. Then the acid solution is neutralized to allow extraction and isolation of the cocaine. One or two further recrystallizations yield cocaine HCl—0.65 to 1.2 percent by weight from the leaves is achieved; 1.0 percent is considered good.[111–113]

Pure "flake" (Merck) wholesale pharmaceutical cocaine retails at from $40.62 to $76.13 per average ounce for "crystal" (Mallinckrodt). In contrast, street cocaine is sold for $100 to $160 per gram; an ounce is sold for $1900 to $2500. As of August 1983, a sealed one-ounce bottle of "Merck" brings $12-15,000 on the illicit market.

According to some investigators,[112,113] cocaine is "cut" with various sugars (mannitol, lactose, glucose, inositol) to increase volume and weight, and by salts of various synthetic local anesthetics for the taste. Other less common adulterants include caffeine, benzocaine, amphetamine, heroin, phencyclidine, and quinine. In 1982 street samples purchased in northern California in the ounce to gram size varied from 30 to 50 percent purity.

In practical terms, one "line" (one by one-eighth inch) of street "coke" weighs between 5 and 20 mg; one "coke spoon" (one sniff/one nostril) contains slightly less. The actual cocaine contained therein depends on the percentage of purity. If the material were 50 percent pure, then "1 gram" snorted or injected over any given time would equal 500 mg of cocaine. Free-basing (smoking of the base in a small

**TABLE 12-2**

**A Medical Chronology of Cocaine**

| | |
|---|---|
| **C. 1500 B.C.** | First anesthetic of the Western World; trephined skulls (with "Inca burr-holes") found in tombs in the Andes. Juice from coca leaves combined with saliva believed to have been used for topical anesthesia. |
| **C. 500 B.C.** | Similar trephined skulls were found in Moche (north coast near Trujillo) and Nazca (near south coast) in Peru. |
| **1580** | Dr. Nicolas Monardes of Spain wrote the first botanical description of the coca plant: "Joyful News out of the new found world, wherein are declared the rare and singular vertues of divers and sundrie herbs, Trees, Oyles, Plants, & Stones. . . ." It is conjectured that Monardes had coca described to him by sailors who had been to the Andes. He stated: "I was desirous to see that herb." |
| **1786** | Lamarck classified the plant as *E. coca.* (The first leaves and plants possibly were brought to Lamarck's laboratory in Europe at that time.) |
| **1836** | Dr. Edward Poeppig of Germany condemned coca chewing, contending that it caused anemia and digestive troubles. |
| **1846–53** | Johann Jacob von Tschudi, Clements Markham, and H. A. Weddell endorsed coca leaf for its power of physical invigoration and its effectiveness in respiratory problems at high altitudes. |
| **1855** | Friedrich Gaedcke of Germany isolated the crystalline "erythroxyline" from coca leaves, a mixture of alkaloids that included cocaine. |
| **1859** | Dr. Paolo Mantegazza said: "Sulle virtu igieniche e medicinali della coca." Italian neurologist who declared coca as a new weapon against disease (toothache, digestive disorders, "neurasthenia"), he had particular influence on Freud. |
| **1859** | K. Scherzer brought active coca leaves to Europe; he gave them to the famous chemist V. Wohler, who passed them on to Albert Niemann. |
| **1860** | Albert Niemann of Göttigen isolated the coca alkaloid "cocaine" and noted its numbing effect on the tongue.<br>William Lossen ascertained the chemical formula of cocaine. |
| **1863** | Angelo Mariani, Corsican chemist, coca botanist, historian, promotional genius, and entrepreneur, introduced "Vin Mariani." He may have come closer to "turning on the world" than any person in history.<br>Testimonials for Vin Mariani and other coca-containing elixirs and specialties were offered by Pope Leo XIII, Sara Bernhardt, Thomas Edison, Ulysses S. Grant, Czar Alexander II, Jules Verne, Henrik |

**TABLE 12-2**

**A Medical Chronology of Cocaine (Continued)**

| | |
|---|---|
| | Ibsen, the Prince of Wales, Emile Zole, Charles Francois Gounod, Jules E. F. Massenet, the Academy of Medicine of France, and a list of over 3000 U.S. physicians, including J. Leonard Corning. |
| **1865** | Dr. Charles Fauvel of Paris endorsed Vin Mariani for ills of the larynx and pharynx (i.e., for numbing the throat). |
| **1868** | Dr. Thomas Moreno y Maiz, Surgeon General of Peru, endorsed cocaine as an invigorating tonic. He also noted cocaine's anesthetic effects on mucous membranes. |
| **1870** | Dr. Charles Gazeau suggested coca leaf for suppression of appetite. |
| **1873** | Alexander Bennett demonstrated the anesthetic properties of cocaine on mucous membranes. |
| **1874–76** | The *British Medical Journal* published editorials praising coca: "A new stimulant and a new narcotic: two forms of novelty in excitement which our modern civilization is likely to esteem." |
| | *Dictionnaire Encyclopedique des Sciences Medicales* published a review of coca/cocaine literature by Bordier, recommending use of coca by armies and in industry. |
| **1879** | Vasili Konstantinovich von Anrep thoroughly studied the pharmacologic properties of cocaine, partly by injecting the skin of his own arm. He suggested the use of cocaine as an anesthetic agent. |
| **1880** | W. H. Bentley wrote in the *Detroit Therapeutic Gazette: "Erythroxylon Coca* is the cure of Opium and Alcohol habits;" "coca (is) the desideratum . . . in health and disease." |
| | Coupart and Bordereau described anesthesia of animals' corneas with cocaine. |
| **1880–84** | Sixteen reports of cures of the opium habit by coca were published in the *Detroit Therapeutic Gazette.* |
| **1882** | *U.S. Pharmacopoeia* listed the fluid extract of coca. |
| **1883** | Theodor Aschenbrandt secretly dosed water of the Bavarian troops. The troops "excelled splendidly" on maneuvers. |
| **1883–85** | "The Great Cocaine Explosion": Cocaine became an enormous fad. Parke-Davis and Merck entered the commercial field; ad campaigns in medical journals touted coca/cocaine as a cure for morphinism and alcoholism. |

**TABLE 12-2**

**A Medical Chronology of Cocaine (Continued)**

| | |
|---|---|
| **1884** | Dr. Sigmund Freud wrote the first of five papers (1884–87), "Uber Coca," enthusiastically extolling the virtues of coca and cocaine.<br><br>On September 15, Dr. Karl Koller, Freud's associate at Vienna General Hospital, presented a three-page paper on the local anesthetic effects of cocaine for ophthalmic surgery. Freud himself states: "Koller can be rightfully considered the discoverer of local anesthesia with cocaine."<br><br>Dr. William Halsted of New York (later of Johns Hopkins University) injected cocaine into nerve trunks, obtaining "nerve blocks," or "conduction" anesthesia. |
| **1885** | Dr. J. Leonard Corning of New York suggested the use of cocaine for spinal anesthesia.<br><br>It was later conjectured that Robert Louis Stevenson wrote the first draft of "Dr. Jekyll and Mr. Hyde" in three days while undergoing treatment for tuberculosis with cocaine. |
| **1885–87** | Dr. Albrecht Erlenmeyer published three monographs denouncing cocaine as "The Third Scourge of Mankind" (after alcohol and morphine). |
| **1886** | *New York Medical Journal:* "No medical technique with such a short history has claimed so many victims as cocaine."<br><br>John Smyth Pemberton invented Coca-Cola and introduced it at his drugstore. |
| **1888** | Asa Griggs Candler purchased Pemberton's rights and introduced Coca-Cola as a "sovereign remedy" and as a "tonic for elderly people who were easily tired." First and most successful of proprietary cocaine-containing "colas"; the soda fountain became part of Americana. |
| **1889** | Magnan and Saury described tactile hallucinations (Magnan's symptom or "cocaine bugs"). |
| **1891** | J. B. Mattison in "Cocaine Poisoning from the Period 1888 to 1891" (*New York Medical Journal*) reported six documented fatalities; by this time, 400 "poisonings" had been reported in the literature. |
| **1892** | Dr. Carl Ludwig Schleich produced infiltration anesthesia by subcutaneous injection of cocaine. |
| **1897** | Dr. George W. Crile of Cleveland used direct infiltration of nerve trunks with cocaine for amputation. |

**TABLE 12-2**

**A Medical Chronology of Cocaine (Continued)**

| | |
|---|---|
| | Dr. Harvey Cushing of Johns Hopkins University performed the first herniorraphy using a similar technique. |
| **1898** | August Bier of Griefswald, Germany, obtained true spinal anesthesia by injecting animals, an assistant, and himself with cocaine. |
| **1898–99** | Drs. Tait and Cagliari of San Francisco and Dr. Rudolph Matas of New Orleans used cocaine for spinal anesthesia in surgical procedures. |
| **1899** | The *Philadelphia Medical Journal* estimated that 30 percent of the "cocainists" in the United States were doctors or dentists. |
| | The American Pharmaceutical Association set up a "Committee on the Acquirement of Drug Habit." Between 1901 and 1903, this committee reported on fear of "negro cocainists." The theme of cocaine-crazed black dope fiends was to persist and play a major role in prohibition campaigns. |
| | Dr. W. Golden Mortimer's *Peru: A History of Coca* was published. A review of coca's history, it also proselytized the varied medical uses for coca/cocaine. The popular and recurring theme of coca as a tonic and restorative, sexual and otherwise, was recounted. The book was dedicated to Mariani. |
| **1902** | Survey by Crothers suggested that only 3 to 8 percent of the cocaine sold in New York, Boston, and other metropolitan areas went into the practice of medicine or dentistry. |
| **1906** | Pure Food and Drug Act required accurate labeling on all proprietary preparations; Coca-Cola went "clean," replacing coca with caffeine. |
| **1908** | August Bier introduced first intravenous anesthesia. |
| **1914** | Harrison ("Narcotics") Tax Act required persons authorized to handle or manufacture drugs to register, pay a fee, and keep a record of all "narcotics" (including cocaine) in their possession. Use of cocaine in proprietary drugs was specifically forbidden; penalties were set for violators. |
| **1922** | Harrison Act amended: penalties increased; cocaine was defined as a "narcotic." (Subsequent drug laws and "acts" have continued this restrictive pattern. Except for strict limited medical use, cocaine has been underground since 1914.) |
| **1923** | Richard Willstatter published his method of synthesis of cocaine, although his experimental work may have taken place as early as |

**TABLE 12-2**

**A Medical Chronology of Cocaine (Continued)**

| | |
|---|---|
| | 1902. Neither Willstatter's original method nor subsequent refinements have thus far proved commercially practicable. |
| **1924** | Emil Mayer documented 26 cocaine deaths in "The Toxic Effects Following the Use of Local Anesthetics" (*Journal of the American Medical Association*). Mayer's committee declaimed "cocaine-mud" and subcutaneous or submucous injection of cocaine. |
| **1930** | Webster's *Legal Medicine and Toxicology* discussed fatal cocaine poisonings from 1900. (Until Finkle and McCloskey's elegant work in 1977, no major toxicologic study of cocaine deaths had been attempted in recent years, although isolated case reports continued to appear.) |
| **1970** | Comprehensive Drug Abuse Prevention and Control Act categorized drugs in "schedules" according to perceived "abuse potential." |

From Gay, G. R. *J. Psychoactive Drugs* 13 (4), 311, 1981. With permission.

pipe) usually involves a single ''hit,'' or dose of less than a ''fifteenth'' (1⁄15 gram, or about 67 mg; a ''tenth'' would be 100 mg).

According to the U.S. Comprehensive Drug Abuse and Drug Act of 1970 (Public Law 91-513), cocaine is legally classified as a ''schedule II'' drug (''high abuse potential with small recognized medical use'') along with opium, opiates (morphine, meperidine, etc.), amphetamines, methaqualone, several barbiturates, methylphenidate, and phenmetrazine. Previously cocaine had been erroneously labeled as a ''narcotic.''

### *d. Chemistry*[109]

Cocaine is the methylbenzoylecgonine, or structurally, 2-beta-carbomethoxy-3-beta-benzoxytropane, with the empirical formula $C_{17}H_{21}NO_4$. Its chemical structure is:

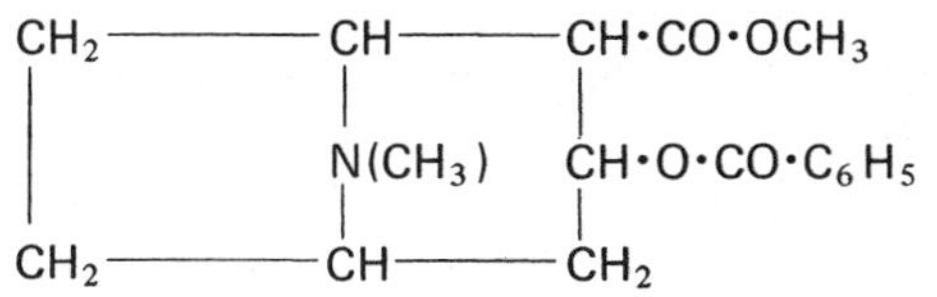

```
CH2 ———————— CH ———————— CH·CO·OCH3
 |            |            |
 |          N(CH3)       CH·O·CO·C6H5
 |            |            |
CH2 ———————— CH ———————— CH2
```

Cocaine is the only naturally occurring local anesthetic known. It is an ester of benzoic acid and the nitrogen-containing base, ecgonine. As a tropane, cocaine is chemically related to the psychoactive alkaloids produced by the Solanaceae family: belladonna or ''deadly nightshade'', henbane, jimson weed or ''thorn apple'' (*Datura stramonium*), and mandrake. Atropine, scopolamine, and hyoscyamine are thus structurally related although they possess very different pharmacologic actions.

In the form of its hydrochloride salt (cocaine HCl), it is a white crystalline powder with a melting point of 195 C (approximately 400 F). One gram of cocaine dissolves in 0.4 ml of water, 3.2 ml of cold ethanol, or 12.5 ml of chloroform; the drug is also soluble in glycerol and acetone, but is insoluble in ether or oils.

Cocaine HCl is prepared by dissolution in hydrochloric acid, forming the water-soluble salt that is commonly sold for medicinal purposes. It is stable at ordinary room temperature and on exposure to sunlight. In its powdered form, however, the salt must be covered, as the moisture in room air will dissolve it. Also, molds decompose it (a process that is enhanced when it is mixed, or ''cut'' with sugars).[114–116]

Pure cocaine (base or free base) is a colorless, odorless, transparent crystalline substance almost totally insoluble in water, but freely soluble in diethyl ether. Further, the melting point of free base (98 C) is much lower than that of its salt.[117] Free base is smoked in cigarettes or, more commonly, in pipes.

### *e. Pharmacokinetics and Metabolism*[109]

Cocaine is absorbed from all sites of application, including mucous membranes such as the nasal and vaginal mucous. Thus cocaine can be absorbed when sniffed, or put into the vagina. When taken orally cocaine is broken down largely in the gastrointestinal tract and is not effective. After absorption, cocaine is metabolized by the liver and may be excreted both as a metabolite and unchanged. Its metabolism is rapid and has a very short duration of action. When used intravenously for psychoactive effects, it must be injected at frequent intervals of less than one hour.

Cocaine undergoes rapid biotransformation in the human body. Plasma pseudocholinesterases and live enzymes produce hydrolysis, and N-demethylation takes place in the liver. The resulting metabolites are benzoylecgonine, ecgonine, ecgonine methyl ester, and several N-demethylated substances, the most important of which is norcocaine (shown to have cocaine-like CNS stimulant activity in animal models). Indeed, cocaine and norcocaine are highly lipophilic, accounting for a rapid crossing of the blood–brain barrier; benzoylecgonine and ecgonine are highly polar and do not significantly cross this barrier. These two latter metabolites, therefore, are found excreted in the urine (in amounts equivalent to one quarter to one half of the original dose of cocaine) within 24 to 36 hours.[117,118]

Depending on urine acidity (greater excretion with lower pH), from 9.5 to 20 percent of cocaine is excreted unchanged in the urine. Cocaine can also be detected in the bile.[117]

Kogan et al.[119] demonstrated that after 100 mg of cocaine was given intravenously, a plasma peak occurred at five minutes, then declined over a five- to six-hour period, with a distributional half-life in the plasma of 20–40 minutes (corresponding to the demonstrated psychologic effects of the drug). Mean plasma biologic half-life was 2.8 hours. In this same study, benzoylecgonine was detected in the urine within five minutes of administration of cocaine, and even after 24 hours could still be detected in the urine.

Cocaine is metabolized quite rapidly *in vitro* by serum pseudocholinesterases (at room temperature, 45 percent of cocaine in plasma may be lost within an hour). Therefore, sophisticated analytical methods for detecting cocaine and its principal metabolite, benzoylecgonine, must be initiated quite promptly on both urine and serum samples for a proper identification. Laboratory methods currently employed include[120–123]:

1. Thin-layer chromatography (TLC). Rapid and cheap, its problem is sensitivity.
2. Enzyme-multiplied immunoassay technique (EMIT). Very rapid for screening of urine for benzoylecgonine, but insensitive to cocaine and not applicable for blood or serum.
3. Gas-liquid chromatography (GLC). Slow and expensive, but quite sensitive.
4. Gas chromatography (GC) and an internal standard. Used for quantitative analysis.

### *f. Pharmacologic and Toxicologic Properties*[120]

(1) *General Actions*: The pharmacology and toxicology of cocaine are very similar to those of the amphetamines. The primary effects are immediate action with a subjective feeling of greater mental agility, greater precision of thought and action, immunity to fatigue, and greater muscular power. These effects are virtually identical to those of amphetamine. Also similar to amphetamine, after one is high on cocaine and then stops the drug, there ensues a profound crash or depression period, the duration of which appears to be related to the length of time that the subject had been intoxicated by cocaine. The chronic use of cocaine can also produce effects similar to those of amphetamine, such as stereotype compulsive behavior; paranoid psychoses with tactile, visual, and auditory hallucinations; and aggressive behavior. To counteract some of these effects,

cocaine users frequently use depressants such as heroin or morphine. In the United Kingdom, cocaine dependence has increased due to the primary use of the drug with heroin. This combination was initiated through a mistaken belief on the part of some doctors and drug-taking individuals that a combination was safer and less potent than either drug alone. This is not true, however, and the combination is even more dangerous and is extremely difficult to treat.

(2) *Acute Effects*: The central stimulant and sympathomimetic effects of cocaine are familiar: euphoria, confidence, energy, increased heart rate and blood pressure, dilated pupils, constriction of peripheral blood vessels, and rise in body temperature and metabolic rate.

A report on the effects of intravenous cocaine in rhesus monkeys at doses of 0.05 to 5 mg/kg indicates increases in respiratory rate and body temperature, and with the highest dose in the heart rate. Increases in pupil size and changes in motor activity and other behavior begin at 0.2 mg/kg. Changes in behavior were more clearly correlated with dose than were physiologic changes, and they occurred at much lower doses; for example, monkeys would press levers for a dose as low as 0.05 mg/kg.[124]

In humans, the most common undesirable effect is a feeling of irritability and lassitude after the euphoria subsides, with a desire for more of the drug. Physicians in attendance at rock music concerts and elsewhere have reported an acute anxiety reaction with symptoms including high blood pressure, racing heart, anxiety, and paranoia.[125] More severe effects, such as tactile and other hallucinations and delusions, are not common but they do occur. Hospitals rarely see cases of cocaine psychosis, but a few have been reported, mainly in habitual cocaine abusers.[126] It is qualitatively similar to amphetamine psychosis but lasts a shorter time, and for that reason, among others, rarely comes to the attention of physicians.

In high doses, cocaine can cause depression of the medullary centers and death from cardiac or, more often, respiratory arrest. Severe physical poisoning and death from the toxic effects are rare. There are no well-documented anaphylactic (allergic) reactions.[127] The reader should review the reports on cocaine-induced death.[118,128,129] These studies reveal that deaths from opiates and cocaine in combination are more common than from cocaine alone.

There is no clear evidence that cocaine induces violent behavior.[112] In fact, animal studies reveal that, like caffeine and nicotine, cocaine increases nonattack behavior produced by a noxious stimulus more than it increases attack behavior; in contrast, dextroamphetamine causes a relative increase in attack responses. Thus cocaine is pharmacologically a nonaggressive agent relative to alcohol, barbiturates, and amphetamines.[130]

(3) *Chronic Effects*: If cocaine is used no more than two or three times a week, it creates no serious problems.[131] Taken daily in significant amounts, it can disrupt eating and sleeping habits, produce minor psychologic disturbances including the inability to concentrate, and can create a serious psychologic dependence.[131,132]

Cocaine does not produce physical dependence in the sense that alcohol or heroin does, but sometimes mild withdrawal symptoms such as anxiety and depression arise. Perceptual disturbances (especially pseudohallucinations) and paranoid thinking occur in chronic users. Sometimes, though rarely, psychoses may appear.[131] A runny or clogged nose is common and can be treated with nasal decongestant sprays. The nose may become inflamed, swollen, or ulcerated; in the older literature, there are reports of perforated septa, but they are rarely found today. Undesirable effects are much more common when intravenous injection is used.

It is noteworthy that, in experiments where unlimited access to intravenous cocaine is provided, animals will kill themselves by voluntary injections.[133] Dependence potential varies with the route of administration. For example, animal experiments continue to show that intravenous cocaine is one of the most powerful, and possibly the most powerful, of drug reinforcers.[134–136]

Usual recreational doses on a chronic basis do not induce tolerance to the euphoric effects of cocaine. Certainly tolerance with high doses has been reported in both humans[28] and animals.[137] However, other studies reveal the phenomena of reverse tolerance.[64] Castellani et al.[138] have demonstrated that reverse tolerance for electrophysiologic responsivity and seizures is absent with cocaine when the intravenous route of administration is used.

According to Grinspoon and Bakalar,[139] most cocaine users have learned ways to take the drug that obviate adverse effects. In addition, cocaine seems to be less dangerous than amphetamines but it presents similar problems.

(4) *Special Actions*:

(a) *The nose.*[109] Nasal mucosa is variably sensitive to street cocaine and its adulterants. This is manifested by symptoms of acute and chronic rhinitis, with sneezing and sniffling. The intense vasoconstrictive properties of cocaine can cause septal necrosis, although this rare condition has been exaggerated. Plastic surgical repair is possible in these cases. Of much greater concern is the profound rebound hyperemia following cocaine sniffing.

A chronic rhinitis with secondary chronic sinusitis is often the result seen in the cocaine sniffer. In general such users are much more prone to upper respiratory infection. Some chronic sniffers are unable to tell when, or even if, they have had a cold. A practice among sniffers is to rinse their nasal passages with tap water or saline. Vitamin E oil or glycerine are favorite balms to prevent drying, cracking and bleeding of the nasal mucosa.

(b) *Cardiovascular system.*[109] Sudden death has occurred following intravenous injection of cocaine.[118] Death in such cases may be due to ventricular fibrillation.

(c) *Sex.* Coca is highly esteemed by the Indians of Peru and Bolivia as an aphrodisiac. Carroll[140] reports that cocaine is said to ensure longevity, with unimpaired sexual powers. After prolonged love making, the cocaine user may enter a medical facility for sexually related problems, including bites, bruises, and scratches on the skin; mucosal tears and bleeding may be apparent.

(d) *The cocaine reaction.*[109] Systemic toxicity to cocaine may be due to an overwhelming adrenergic (or sympathetic) stimulation of the central nervous, cardiovascular, and respiratory systems, as illustrated in Table 12-3 (prepared by Gay[109]).

(5) *Neuropharmacologic Mechanism(s)*[109]: Cocaine interacts with the catecholamine neurotransmitters, norepinephrine and dopamine, and alters the normal interneural communication. It augments the effects of these catecholamines, probably by blocking (or prolonging) reuptake at the synaptic junction, leaving an excess of these neurotransmitters to restimulate receptors.

Cocaine is "sympathomimetic,"[141] and its pharmacologic as well as toxicologic profile seems to be mediated via alteration of neurotransmitter function.

Norepinephrine is found in both the CNS and peripheral nerves. Dopamine is a biosynthetic precursor of norepinephrine and is found in the CNS (specifically the corpus striatum—part of the network governing motor functions—and in that portion of the hypothalamus regulating thirst and hunger). Norepinephrine is the prime neurotransmitter of the ascending reticular activating system (RAS), regulating mechanisms of external attention and arousal, and serving as the pathway to cerebral awareness. It acts as a vital transmitter as well in the hypothalamus, which regulates thirst and hunger, body temperature, sleep, and sexual arousal, and, in general, mediates emotional expression. It also mediates neural activation in the median forebrain bundle of the hypothalamus, which is felt to serve as an individual's "pleasure center."

### *g. Treatment of Acute and Chronic Cocaine Toxicity*

(1) *"Cocaine Reaction"*: The potentially lethal complications of cocaine-induced overdose require immediate resuscitative efforts directed to the support of cardiovascular and respiratory functions.[109] Diazepam (Valium) appears to be useful for the overramped cocaine user. Because of its sedative properties and its action on the central reticular formation, the specific adrenergic reinforcing mechanisms of cocaine are counteracted. Diazepam in oral doses of 15–20 mg every six to eight hours is usually effective. According to Gay,[109] for nighttime medication, a dosage of approximately 20 mg per night should be given initially, decreasing to 10 mg per night over the first week.

(2) *Propranolol Method in Adrenergic Crisis in Chronic Cocaine Toxicity*: A common clinical

## TABLE 12-3

### The Cocaine ("Caine" or Casey Jones") Reaction

| Phase | Central Nervous System | Circulatory System | Respiratory System |
| --- | --- | --- | --- |
| I. Early stimulation | Euphoria; stated feelings of "soaring," well-being<br>Elation, expansive good humor, laughing (this phase may exhibit as an introverted and withdrawn elation)<br>Mydriasis<br>Talkative, garrulous<br>Excited, flighty, emotionally unstable<br>Restlessness; irritable, apprehensive; inability to sit still<br>Stereotyped movements (such as "picking" or "stroking"); bruxism (teeth grinding)<br>Nausea, vomiting, vertigo<br>Sudden headache<br>Cold sweats<br>Tremor (nonintentional)<br>Twitching of small muscles, especially of the face, fingers, and feet<br>Tics, generalized<br>Preconvulsive movements; tonic and clonic "jerks"<br>Phenomena seen in alcoholic toxicity:<br>Possible "pseudohallucinations" e.g., tactile ("snow lights"), auditory, gustatory, olfactory<br>Possible "cocaine psychosis" resembling paranoid schizophrenia<br>Core body temperature rises<br>Verbalization of impending doom: "Something is terrible wrong. I'm going to die." This precedes imminent total collapse and demands immediate intervention. | Pulse varies at first, may immediately slow due to reflex vagal effect; will increase 30–50% above normal with systemic absorption of 25 mg of cocaine (per nares, injected or smoked)<br>Blood pressure usually elevates 15–20% above normal with similar dosages as noted above<br>Skin pallor due to vasoconstriction<br>Premature ventricular contraction(s)<br>Salvos of premature ventricular contractions | Increased respiratory rate and depth<br>Dyspnea |

**TABLE 12-3**

**The Cocaine ("Caine" or Casey Jones") Reaction (Continued)**

| *Phase* | *Central Nervous System* | *Circulatory System* | *Respiratory System* |
|---|---|---|---|
| II. Advanced Stimulation | Unresponsive to voice; decreased responsiveness to all stimuli<br>Deep tendon reflexes greatly increased<br>Generalized hyperflexia<br>Convulsions: tonic and clonic<br>Stratus epilepticus<br>Incontinence<br>Malignant encephalopathy possible | Both pulse and blood pressure continue to increase (CNS); hemorrhage is a rare but deadly complication of increased blood pressure) (high output congestive heart failure possible)<br>Blood pressure falls as ventricular arrhythmias supervene and inefficient cardiac output results<br>Pulse becomes rapid, weak, and irregular<br>Peripheral, then central cyanosis | Gasping, rapid and/or irregular respiration (viz., Cheyne-Stokes)<br>Progressive hypoxia |
| III. Depressive | Flaccid paralysis of muscles<br>Coma<br>Pupils fixed and dilated<br>Loss of reflexes<br>Loss of vital support functions<br>Paralysis of medullary brain center<br>Exitus | Ventricular fibrillation<br>Circulatory failure<br>Ashen-gray cyanosis<br>No palpable pulse<br>Cardiac arrest<br>Paralysis of medullary brain center<br>Exitus | Agonal gasps<br>Respiratory failure<br>Gross pulmonary edema<br>Paralysis of medullary brain center<br>Exitus |

From Gay, R. G., *J. Psychoactive Drugs*, 13 (4), 306, 1981. With permission.

phenomenon is a patient who is three to 14 days into a cocaine "run" or "binge" displaying signs of an adrenergic crisis, including hyperkinetic behavior, tachycardia, hypertension, dyspnea, jerks and tremors, stereotypical movements, distorted perception, and potentially violent delusioned protective behavior. Rappolt et al.[142] propose that such cases of "adrenergic" or "dopaminergic" storm respond quite well to the lytic effects of propranolol.

(3) *Other Treatment Considerations*: The use of phenothiazines, especially chlorpromazine (Thorazine), and the butryophenone haloperidol (Haldol) have specifically been avoided because of their propensity to lower seizure threshold. The tricyclic antidepressants are avoided because of the danger of life-threatening cardiac arrythmias in these already sensitized patients. Anticonvulsants are not effective in preventing cocaine-induced seizures.

Certainly psychologic counseling is indicated, but must be tailored to the patient's needs. The primary problem is that, to determine the exact treatment protocol, the pattern of abuse must be known. In this regard, the following patterns of abuse can be identified: (a) the pure "cokehead"; (b) polydrug users of cocaine; (c) in combination with heroin—the "speedball"; (d) in connection with methadone maintenance.

Finally, Cohen[143] believes that large amounts of cocaine are being smuggled into the United States. The distribution pattern seems to be concentrated in the larger cities, particularly New York, Miami, Los Angeles, and San Francisco. Cohen also suggests that the principal consumers are multiple-drug users, with only small numbers exclusively using cocaine.

## 2. Caffeine

### *a. Introduction*

Caffeine is a CNS stimulant that is used to increase alertness and to reduce fatigue, and is generally ingested in the form of coffee, tea, or cola drink, or taken in pill form such as No-Doz and similar products (See Table 12-4).

### *b. History*

The earliest history of drinks containing caffeine and other closely related chemicals is difficult to determine and abounds in mythical stories. The legend is that coffee was discovered by a holy man in an Arabian convent. Shepherds reported to him that goats that had eaten the berries of the coffee plant jumped and ran about all night, instead of sleeping. The holy man, remembering the long nights of prayer that he had to endure, asked the shepherds to pick the berries so that he could make a beverage from them. The success of his experiment has led to the consumption of over three billion pounds per year in the United States alone.

### *c. Absorption, Metabolism and Excretion*

Caffeine is readily absorbed from the gut, distributed throughout the body, and rapidly taken up by the brain. It is metabolized by the liver, and is excreted both free and as a metabolite by the kidneys. Caffeine is relatively nontoxic, and only three human fatalities have been reported. The primary use of caffeine in the United States is as a CNS stimulant to increase alertness and to reduce fatigue. There is a potential for tolerance that leads to an increasing dosage and a moderate psychologic dependency. Although no specific physical dependency appears to arise, many patients on withdrawal complain of increased insomnia, irritability, cardiac palpitation, tremor, flushing, anorexia, dehydration, diuresis, fever, albuminuria, and abdominal discomfort.[144]

### *d. Pharmacology*

Some 150 to 250 mg of caffeine, or about two cups of coffee, is sufficient to activate the central nervous system. The observation that the cortical neurons are stimulated is shown by the cortex activation and EEG arousal pattern. In the absence of tolerance, there is an increase in the wakeful state, mood elevation, and the length of time it takes to fall asleep. At higher doses, about 500 mg, caffeine stimulates the autonomic centers of the brain, heart rate, and respiration. The cardiovascular system works in opposition to the effect of caffeine upon the autonomic centers. Hypertensive headaches may be reduced by caffeine. This may be due to the effects of vascular muscular dilation and blood vessel constriction caused by the autonomic centers. Although peripheral dilation usually occurs, blood vessel constriction takes place in the brain. Caffeine users have a lower heart rate, higher blood pressure, and a slightly higher basal metabolic rate than nonusers. Nonusers of caffeine experience a significantly reduced heart rate at about 150 to 250 mg of caffeine. A higher blood level of lipids and glucose develops in heavy coffee users and this may cause a higher incidence of angina and myocardial infarction than in moderate coffee users or abstainers. Ironically, this may be helpful in surviving a myocardial infarction.[145]

Even higher doses, about eight cups of coffee, cause an increase in synthesis of microsomal enzymes in the liver. The stimulation of drug metabolism has been shown and it may be true that heavy coffee or tea users also have increased liver microsomal activity.[146]

### *e. Behavioral Actions*

Stating precisely how caffeine affects behavioral performance is difficult since individuals are affected in various ways. One report shows contrasting effects between users and nonusers. Heavy coffee drinkers experienced irritability and sleepiness when given a placebo, but were alert and content[147] with caffeine. Nonusers given 150 to 300 mg of caffeine had upset stomachs, and were jittery and nervous. Caffeine works much like amphetamines, increasing the individual's level of physical performance, mitigating boredom, and increasing attention. There is cortical stimulation, reduced drowsiness, and greater alertness and reactivity, but there may be irritability and excitability, which can disrupt behavior.

Generally 200 to 300 mg of caffeine, or about two cups of coffee, is a sufficient therapeutic dose to offset fatigue, and improve the performance of motor tasks. This may be partly due to caffeine's action on the agent muscle.

### *f. Toxicology*

Many investigators feel that caffeine does little more than restore performance to control levels, or reduce fatigue but there are some reports that caffeine, after a 200- to 300-mg dose, increases the individual's ability to associate words and to process sense information.

### *g. Adverse Reactions*

The beneficial effects of caffeine outweigh its detrimental effects. Caffeine stimulates the CNS and can ward off fatigue or hypertensive headaches. Extremely high doses of caffeine, however, can be toxic and result in convulsions, or even respiratory failure. An oral dose of 10 grams can be fatal and one death from an intravenous injection of 3.2 grams of caffeine has been reported. The CNS stimulation is blocked by CNS depressants.[149]

### *h. Tolerance and Dependency to Caffeine*

A strong tolerance does not develop from caffeine. There is usually less tolerance to the CNS stimulation effect of caffeine than to most of its other effects. The tolerance that develops to caffeine can be eliminated by either increasing the dose or by complete abstinence. Increasing the dose two or four times also eliminates tolerance buildup. Caffeine's effect on the kidneys shows an increase in urine output and in the salivary flow but there is no tolerance development.

Dependence on caffeine is real, and one withdrawal symptom that has been well substantiated is headache, which generally develops in habitual users (five cups or more of coffee per day) after about 18 hours of abstinence. Some reports suggest that nausea and lethargy may precede the actual headache, but the only clear symptom is the headache. It has been produced experimentally by giving caffeine chronically to noncaffeine users and then substituting a placebo, as well as by withholding coffee from habitual users.[150,151]

### 3. Methylphenidate (Ritalin)

#### *a. General Introduction*

Methylphenidate (Ritalin) is a stimulant, but is less abused than either amphetamines or cocaine, and will be discussed only briefly. The substance is widely used in medicine for mild depression, minimal brain dysfunction (MBD) in children, narcolepsy, and sedative-induced lethargy. Ciba-Geigy manufactures the product in 5-, 10-, and 20-mg tablets, and in a multiple-dose vial containing 100 mg. The major problem with its availability is its overprescribed use for minimal brain dysfunction (hyperactivity) and abuse by drug-dependent people. Certainly the controversy over the former problem revolves around the issue of whether overactive children without definite neurologic deficits should be treated with stimulants. In spite of this issue, some schools report that more than 10 percent of the pupils have been diagnosed as MBD and have been given Ritalin or some other stimulant.

#### *b. Abuse Problem*[153,154]

The abuse of Ritalin has increased significantly. It is believed that supplies of the drug have been acquired by forging prescriptions on stolen blanks, robbing drug stores and hospitals, and "ripping off" jobbers and wholesalers by shipment diversion and warehouse theft. Interestingly, Ritalin has never been found to be privately manufactured for the "street" market. Ritalin abuse has been reported by a number of cities across the United States.

The rationale for Ritalin abuse is that it is similar to amphetamines. An initial "rush" is followed by an exuberant feeling of well-being that culminates in a "down."

According to Cohen[155]:

> One special problem for the intravenous user is that Ritalin is manufactured using talcum as a filler and binder. Talc is an insoluble, irritant crystal which can produce abcesses when it is injected under the skin. If it is instilled into a vein, the lung capillaries prevent its further passage. Pulmonary abcesses and fibrosis are occasional results of multiple injections, and lungs have had to be removed for large abcesses. A septic thrombophlebitis adds to the danger of lung infection. A dozen deaths are supposed to have occurred in the Seattle area during 1971 due to the use of intravenous Ritalin. Ritalin has been combined with heroin and methadone to produce a more intense high. There is some anecdotal evidence that it prolongs the action of heroin.

Since Ritalin, Preludin, and the amphetamines have been transferred to Schedule II (requiring a narcotic-type prescription that cannot be renewed), the possibility for illicit use should be reduced, but not eliminated.

**TABLE 12-4**

**Amount of Caffeine in Beverages**

| *Beverage* | *Amount, Oz.* | *Amount of Caffeine (milligrams)* |
|---|---|---|
| *Regular coffee* | *5* | *90–125* |
| *Instant coffee* | *5* | *60–80* |
| *Decaffeinated coffee* | *5* | *30–70 (typical; some are quite low)* |
| *Tea* | *5* | *30–70* |
| *Cocoa* | *5* | *Less than 5 (about 100 mg theobromine)* |
| *Coca-Cola* | *12* | *45* |
| *Pepsi-Cola* | *12* | *30* |
| *Chocolate bar* | *1-ounce bar* | *22* |

From Ray, O. *Drugs, Society and Human Behavior.* St. Louis: C. V. Mosby, 1972. (With permission)

## M. POLITICS OF STIMULANT ABUSE

Most physicians and individuals involved in the dispensing and control of psychoactive drugs agree that stimulants have a substantial potential for abuse. The definition of what constitutes abuse, however, is the subject of marked differences in opinion. The term ''abuse'' has a moral overtone.

The abuse of drugs available only by prescription is more difficult to define than abuse of heroin, where use and abuse are usually considered synonymous. While almost everyone would agree that high-dose intravenous amphetamine use would constitute abuse of these drugs, there is much disagreement on how to label the individual who self-medicates with commonly used therapeutic doses of amphetamines or the individual who obtains drugs by prescription but takes more than the amount prescribed.

Commonly used definitions of abuse of psychoactive drugs reflect either a sociologic or medical perspective. The sociologic perspective indicates that drug abuse constitutes the consumption of a socially unsanctioned drug (the prototype for the most illegal drug being heroin) or the use of a socially sanctioned drug in such a way as to be a detriment to society or the individual. An example would be the overuse of alcohol to the point where an individual's capacity to function as a constructive member of society is grossly impaired. Definitions reflecting the medical perspective of psychoactive drug abuse imply situations wherein nonprescribed use of a particular drug exposes the individual to medical or psychologic harm. Some definitions use elements of both perspectives. Blum et al.,[152] for example, define drug abuse as ''the regular, excessive use of a drug to the extent that it is damaging to a person's social or vocational adjustment or to his health, or is otherwise specifically detrimental to society.''

The World Health Organization's Expert Committee on Drug Dependence defines drug abuse in relation to medical practice as ''persistent or sporadic excessive drug use inconsistent with or unrelated to acceptable medical practice.''

Discussions of amphetamine abuse frequently fail to draw consistent lines of definition within differing subcultures of society. Because of the social–political implications of being labeled a ''drug abuser,'' this label is more likely to be applied to individuals on the fringes of the dominant culture rather than to those within it who may well be demonstrating a similar pattern of drug use. The drug-taking behavior of members of the dominant culture is more likely to be labeled ''misuse'' or ''overuse.'' Ultimately the distinction between abuse, misuse, and overuse of medically prescribed drugs is a complex value judgment.

Wesson et al.[156] suggest that legislation for amphetamines be established that essentially parallels that for alcohol addiction and intoxication. The Uniform Alcoholism and Intoxication Treatment Act (NCCUSL 1971)[157] would be very appropriate for amphetamines. This Act, which also was approved by the American Bar Association as of February 7, 1972, contains reasonable guidelines and safeguards for commitments, voluntary treatment, and decriminalization of alcoholism. Within the Act, treatment is broadly defined to include a wide range of social, medical, rehabilitative, and psychologic services.

Political consciousness concerning alcoholism has developed largely because of our cultural viewpoint that alcohol is not a drug. (see Chapter 11). It is essential to examine the politics, causes, and social issues of all psychoactive agents, including amphetamines and other stimulants, in a uniform way, and to consider the possibility that all are part of the same drug-seeking phenomenology.

Figure 12-1 shows an analysis of the legal and illegal distribution patterns for both depressants (barbiturates) and stimulants (amphetamines).[156]

The patterns are essentially the same for both barbiturates and amphetamines, with this exception: There is evidence of illegal domestic manufacture of methamphetamine, whereas there is no evidence of illegal domestic manufacture of barbiturates at the present time. Points indicated by an (X) in Figure 12-1 are possible sources of diversion. In essence, any time a shipment of bulk quantities of drugs is made from one point to another, there is the possibility that part or all of the shipment will be diverted

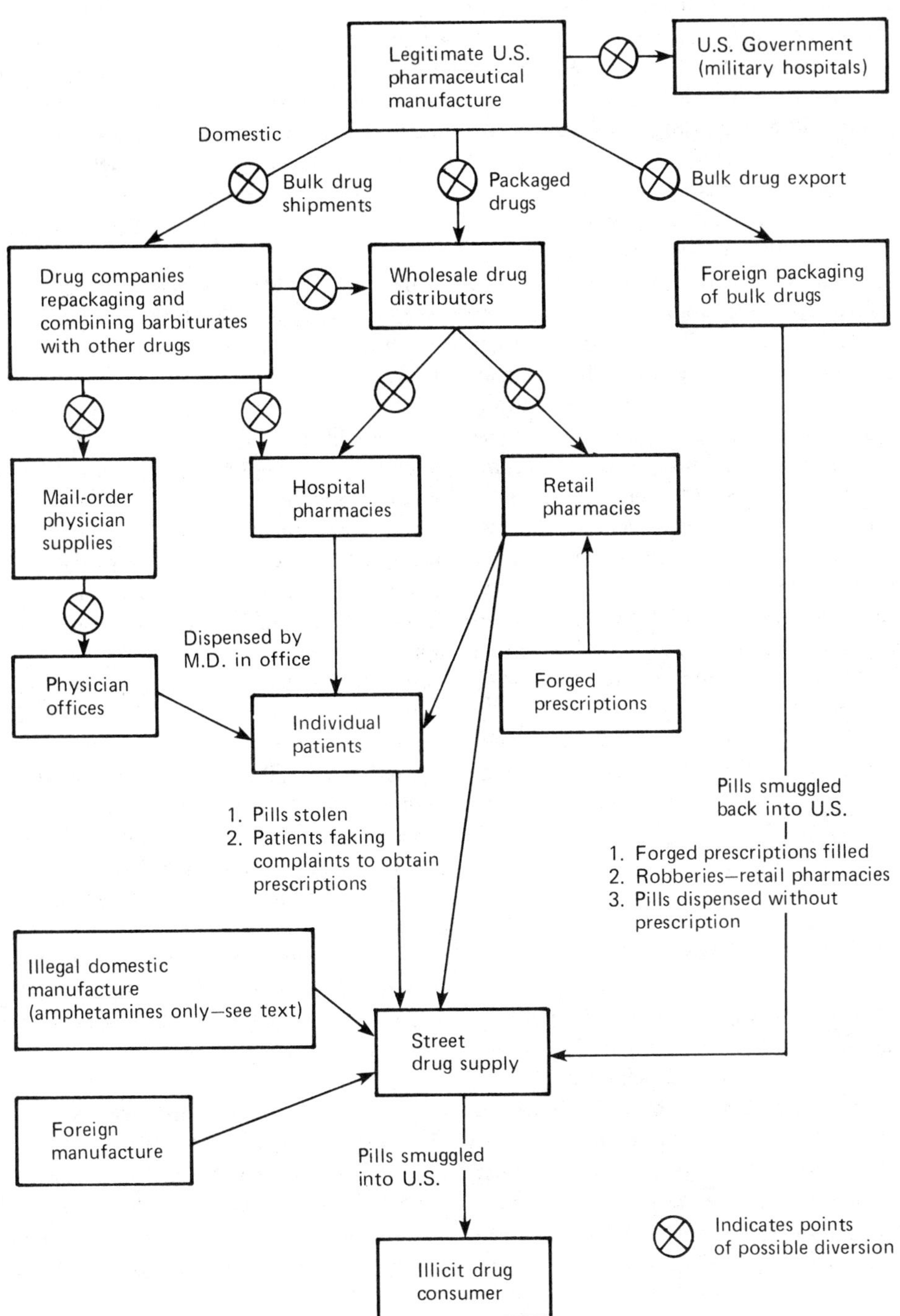


**Figure 12-1. Routes by which amphetamines and barbiturates reach the blackmarket.**

From Wesson, D., et al., *Uppers and Downers*, Englewood Cliffs, NJ: Prentice-Hall, 1973 (with permission).

into the black market. Diversion of bulk shipments accounts for a major portion of the drugs that reach the black market and a well-organized plan is required to effect such massive diversion.

At the bottom of the diagram are examples of small-scale diversion such as forged prescriptions, and burglaries of drugstores, drug warehouses, and physicians' offices. In addition, there are "pseudo-patients" who go from physician to physician obtaining prescriptions or samples of barbiturates and amphetamines.

Some barbiturates and amphetamines are manufactured in other countries and smuggled into the United States. The quantities of drugs that find their way through each particular channel to the black market are impossible to determine at present. There is, however, ample evidence that all of these routes are used to some extent, and an analysis of control measures of one route must take into consideration the possible consequences concerning other routes of diversion and procurement. For example, if the available supplies diverted from domestic legitimate manufacturers are controlled effectively, increasing quantities may reach the black market from other sources.

A suggested alternate distribution of amphetamines and barbiturates is depicted in Figure 12-2.[156]

## N. GENERAL COMMENTS

It is urgent that the pharmaceutical industry assume much more responsibility in its advertising and distribution of psychoactive drugs. Physicians could certainly be more informed concerning the complexities of drug use and, it is hoped, become part of the solution rather than part of the problem. Law enforcement agencies should focus more of their resources on "corporate drug pushers" rather than continually diverting control efforts to highly publicized, but peripheral, areas of America's drug culture.

As for amphetamines, their use in medicine has been steadily decreasing. The current medical indications for these drugs are minimal. However, the manufacture of these compounds should not be completely stopped unless alternative, safer drugs are available for every condition for which amphetamines are now prescribed. Certainly the newer, more expensive synthetic stimulants, such as methylphenidate (Ritalin), do not possess any advantage or additional safety factor over amphetamines.

In general, certain trends have emerged and, as cited by Cohen,[12] include the following:

1. Federal legislation has tightened controls over amphetamine manufacture, transportation, and distribution, but street supplies remain plentiful.
2. A few county medical societies have asked their members to discontinue prescribing amphetamines, except for narcolepsy and hyperkinetic children.
3. Efforts to provide a drug that depresses the appetite regulatory centers without producing central stimulation have been partially successful. We can look forward to a nonstimulating appetite suppresant.
4. The mechanism of action of the amphetamines has been tentatively clarified. They increase the release of catecholamines into the synaptic cleft and retard their reuptake into the neurone. A so-called false transmitter has been isolated from the spinal fluid following amphetamine administration. It is p-hydroxynorephedrine, but its significance remains to be determined.
5. A recent study indicates that children given amphetamines until adolescence for hyperkinesis do not tend to abuse amphetamines when they grow up.

Finally, it is noteworthy that, as predicted from animal experimentation, cocaine would emerge in the 1980s as "the champagne of drugs" for social and sexual occasions. The fact that this highly abused substance can make the unbearable seem bearable is reflected in its black market distribution. Profitability is high. For example, on June 24, 1982, Long Island, (N.Y.) police made the largest drug bust ever by confiscating cocaine worth over $30 million in the "street" market. Stimulants will continue to be abused.

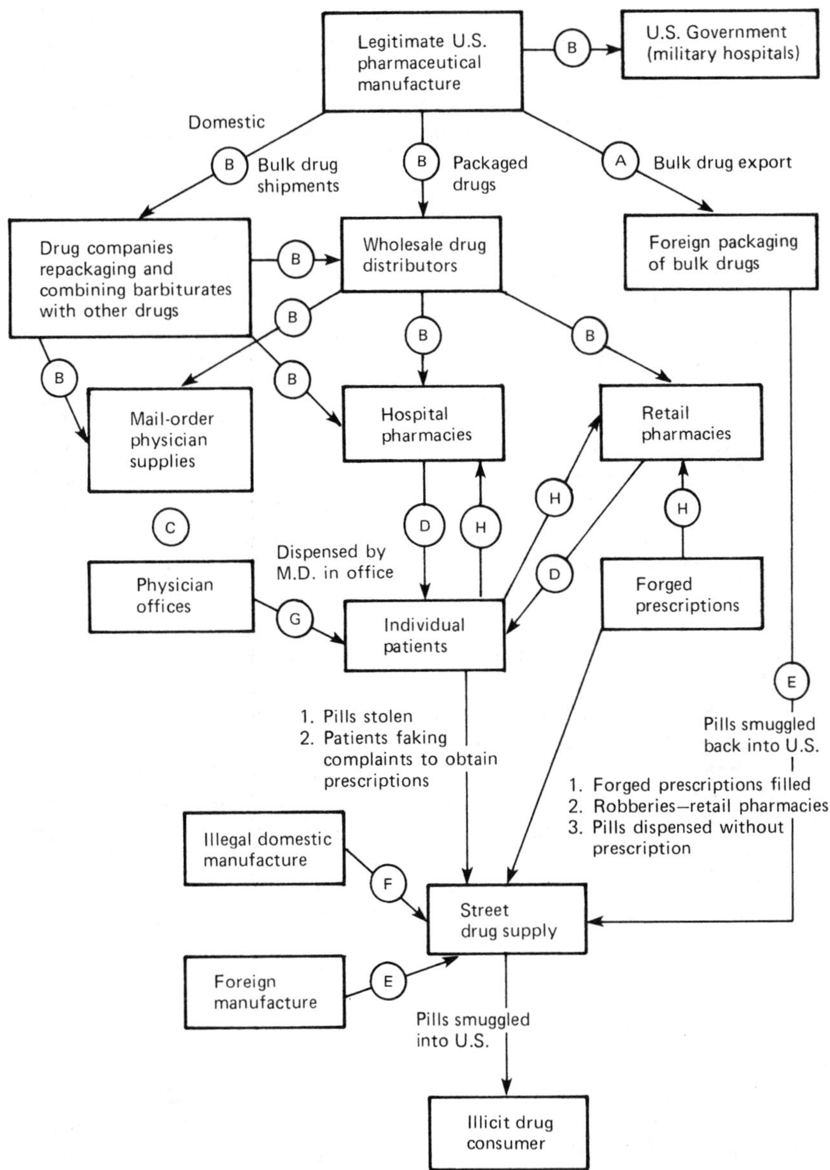


**(A.)** Export quotas made consistent with "medicinal needs" in country being supplied, and assurances that receiving country's government or other appropriate drug-control agency will account for shipments and monitor repackaging and export. **(B.)** Accountability records matched at shipping and receiving points by independent agency audit. **(C.)** This route of delivery is not generally needed for amphetamines and barbiturates. **(D.)** Positive patient identification required for filling of barbiturate or amphetamine prescriptions. **(E.)** Customs inspection and control. **(F.)** Control by local narcotics agencies of BNDD. **(G.)** Education of physician and retraining of prescribing habits to other more effective drugs with lower abuse potential and to sharpen prescribing skills in treatment of anxiety, sleep disorder, obesity, etc., and altering of advertising and "detailing" practices to physicians from drug manufacturers. Physicians would encourage patients to deal with the "symptoms" in a nondrug manner whenever possible. **(H.)** Hand-written BNDD number as well as signature required on prescriptions.

From Wesson, D., et al. ***Uppers and Downers*, Englewood Cliffs, NJ: Prentice-Hall, 1973 (with permission).**

## REFERENCES


1. Ellinwood, E. H., Jr., and Kilbey, M. M. (Editors) *Cocaine and other Stimulants*. New York: Plenum, 1977.
2. Hofmann, F. G. *A Handbook on Drug and Alcohol Abuse: The Biomedical Aspects*. New York: Oxford University Press, 1975.
3. Smith, D. E., and Wesson, D. R. *Uppers and Downers*. Englewood Cliffs, N.J.: Prentice-Hall, 1973.
4. Blum, K., Ehrempreis, S. H., and Briggs, A. H. *Social Pharmacological Perspectives of Uppers (Stimulants)*. Beloit, Wis.: STASH Pamphlet Publications, 1979.
5. Kramer, J. Introduction to amphetamine abuse. *J. Psychedel. Drugs* 2:8, 1969.
6. Caret, J., and Mandel, J. A San Francisco Bay area "speed" scene. *J. Health Soc. Behav.* 9:164, 1968.
7. Smith, R. C. Traffic in amphetamines: Patterns of illegal manufacture and distribution. *J. Psychedel. Drugs*, 2:20, 1969.
8. Hennessee, J., et al. Project Speed Syllabus. Sponsored by the Iowa Regional Medical Program, University of Iowa, Iowa City, 1971.
9. Griffith, J. D. Cited in: Crime in America—Why eight billion amphetamines? Hearings before the Select Committee on Crime, House of Representative, 91st Congress, First Session. Washington, D.C.: U.S. Government Printing Office, 1970, p. 17.
10. Fishburne, P.M., Abelson, H. I., and Casin, I. *National Survey on Drug Abuse: Main Findings: 1979*. Washington, D.C.: NIDA, U.S. Government Printing Office, 1980, p. 83.
11. Kramer, J. C. Amphetamine use and misuse: A medicolegal view. In D. E. Smith and D. R. Wesson, *Uppers and Downers*. Englewood Cliffs, N.J.: Prentice-Hall, 1973, p. 9.
12. Cohen, S. *The Substance Abuse Problems*. New York: Haworth Press, 1981, pp. 146–149.
13. Connell, P. H. *Amphetamine Psychosis* (Maudsley Monographs, no. 5). London: Oxford University Press, 1958.
14. Cox, C., and Smart, R. G. The nature and extent of speed use in North America. *Can. Med. Assoc. J.* 102:724, 1970.
15. Bell, D. S. Comparison of amphetamine psychosis and schizophrenia. *Br. J. Psychiat.* 111:701, 1965.
16. Griffith, J. D., et al. Dextroamphetamine: Evaluation of psychomimetic properties in man. *Arch. Gen. Psychiat.* 26:97, 1972.
17. Goodman, S. J., and Becker, D. P. Intracranial hemorrhage associated with amphetamine abuse. *JAMA* 212:480, 1970.
18. Dimijian, G. C. Contemporary drug abuse. In: A. Goth, ed., *Medical Pharmacology*. 11th ed. St. Louis: C. V. Mosby, 1984.
19. Isbell, H., and White, W. M. Symposium on drug addiction: Clinical characteristics of addictions. *Am. J. Med.* 14:558, 1953.
20. Edison, G. R. Amphetamines: A dangerous illusion. *Ann. Intern. Med.* 74:605, 1971.
21. Kramer, J. C., Fischman, V. S., and Littlefield, D. C. Amphetamine abuse. *JAMA* 201:305, 1967.
22. Ritchie, J. The central nervous system stimulants II: Xanthines. In L. Goodman and A. Gilman, eds., *The Pharmacological Basis of Therapeutics*. Toronto: Macmillan, 1970.
23. Ritchie, J., et al. Cocaine: Procaine and other synthetic local anesthetics. In L. Goodman and A. Gilman, eds., *The Pharmacological Basis of Therapeutics*. Toronto: Macmillan, 1970.
24. Esplin, D., and Zablocke-Esplin, B. Central nervous system stimulants I. In L. Goodman and A. Gilman, eds., *The Pharmacological Basis of Therapeutics*, 4th ed. Toronto: Macmillan, 1970.
25. Ellinwood, E. H. Amphetamines/anoretics. In *Handbook of Drug Abuse*.
26. Innes, I., and Nickerson, M. Drugs acting on postganglionic adrenergic nerve endings and structures innervated by them (sympathomimetic drugs). In L. Goodman and A. Gilman, eds., *The Pharmacological Basis of Therapeutics*. Toronto: Macmillan, 1970.
27. Shulgin, A. Psychotomimetic agents related to the catecholamines. *J. Psychedel. Drugs* 2:63, 1969.
28. Connell, P. H. Clinical manifestations and treatment of amphetamine type of dependence. *JAMA*, 196:718, 1966.
29. Bell, D. S. Addiction to stimulants. *Med. J. Austral.* 1:41, 1967.
30. Non-medical use of drugs, with particular reference to youth. Report of the Special Committee on Drug Misuse, Council on Community Health Care, Canadian Medical Association, *Can. Med. Assoc. J.* 101:804, 1969.
31. Black, J. The "speed" that kills—or worse. *N.Y. Times Magazine*, June 21, 1970, p. 14.
32. Medical Staff Conference. Changing drug patterns in the Haight-Ashbury. *Calif. Med.* 110:151, 1969.
33. Food and Drug Administration. Amphetamines. *Fed. Reg.*, 42(199):55374, Oct. 14, 1977.

34. National Prescription Audit. *Therapeutic Category Report.* Ambler, Pa.: IMS, 1976.
35. Drug Enforcement Administration. DEA laboratory analyses: Schedule II, III and IV Anorectics. (unpublished paper). Washington, D.C.: Office of Compliance and Regulatory Affairs, March 16, 1976.
36. Johnson, L.D., Bachman, J. G., and O'Malley, P. M. *Highlights from: "Drug Use Among American High School Students 1975–1977.* Washington, D.C.: National Institute on Drug Abuse, 1977.
37. National Institute on Drug Abuse. *An Investigation of Selected Rural Drug Abuse Programs.* DHEW Publication no. ADM 77-451. Washington, D.C.: U.S. Government Printing Office, 1977.
38. Thomas, C. E. (Editor) *The Amphetamines. Toxicology and Addiction.* Oriana Josseau Kalant, 1966.
40. Smith, C. B. The role of monoaminoxidase in the intraneuronal metabolism of norepinephrine released by indirectly-acting sympathomimetic amines or by adrenergic nerve stimulation. *J. Pharmacol. Exp. Ther.* 151:207, 1966.
41. Oswald, I. Drugs and sleep. *Pharmacol. Rev.* 20:273, 1968.
42. Toman, J. E. P., and Davis, J. P. The effects of drugs upon the electrical activity of the brain. *Pharmacol. Rev.* I:425, 1949.
43. Kosman, M. E., and Unna, K. R. Effects of chronic administration of the amphetamines and other stimulants on behavior. *Clin. Pharmacol. Ther.* 9:240, 1968.
44. *Journal of Psychedelic Drugs.* "Speed Kills." A review of amphetamine abuse. Vol. II. The Haight-Ashbury Medical Clinic, 1969.
45. Ellinwood, E. H., Jr. Amphetamine and stimulant drugs. In National Commission on Marihuana and Drug Abuse, *Drug Use in America: Problem in Perspective.* Washington, D.C.: U.S. Government Printing Office, 1973, pp. 140–157.
46. Schiorring, E. Changes in individual and social behavior induced by amphetamine and related compounds in monkey and man. In E. H. Ellinwood, Jr., and M. M. Kilbey, eds., *Cocaine and Other Stimulants.* New York: Plenum, 1977, pp. 481–522.
47. Kramer, J. C. Introduction to amphetamine abuse. *J. Psychedel. Drugs* 2:1, 1969.
48. Bell, D. S. The experimental reproduction of amphetamine psychosis. *Arch. Gen. Psychiatry* 29:35, 1973.
49. Utena, H. On relapse-liability, schizophrenia, amphetamine psychosis and animal model. In H. Mitsuda and T. Fukuda, eds., *Biological Mechanisms of Schizophrenia and Schizophrenia-Like Psychoses.* Tokyo: Igaku Shoin, 1974, p. 285.
50. Utena, H. Behavioral aberrations in methamphetamine intoxicated animals and chemical correclates in the brain. *Prog. Brain Res.* 21B:1902, 1966.
51. Griffith, J. D. Structure–activity relationships of several amphetamine drugs in man. In E. H. Ellinwood, Jr., and M. M. Kilbey, eds., *Cocaine and Other Stimulants.* New York: Plenum, 1977, pp. 705–715.
52. Griffith, J. D., Nutt, J. G., and Jasinski, D. R. A comparison of fenfluramine and amphetamine in man. *Clin. Pharmacol. Ther.*, 18:563, 1975.
53. Vaillant, G. E. A twenty year followup of New York narcotic addicts. *Arch. Gen. Psychiatry* 29:237, 1973.
54. Winick, C. Maturing out of narcotic addiction. *Bull. Narcot.* 14, 1962.
55. Rumbaugh, C. L. Small vessel cerebral vascular changes following chronic amphetamine intoxication. In E. H. Ellinwood, Jr., and M. M. Kilbey, eds., *Cocaine and Other Stimulants.* New York: Plenum, 1977, pp. 241–251.
56. Duarte-Escalante, O., and Ellinwood, E. H., Jr. Effects of chronic amphetamine intoxication on adrenergic and cholinergic structures in the central nervous system: Histochemical observations in cats and monkeys. In E. H. Ellinwood, Jr., and S. Cohen, eds., *Current Concepts on Amphetamine Abuse.* Washington, D.C.: U.S. Government Printing Office, 1972, pp. 97–106.
57. Duarte-Escalante, O., and Ellinwood, E. H., Jr. Central nervous system cytopathological changes in cat with chronic methedrine intoxication. *Brain Res.* 21:151, 1970.
58. Seiden, L. S., Fischman, M. W., and Schuster, C. R. Changes in brain catecholamines induced by longterm methamphetamine administration in rhesus monkeys. In E. H. Ellinwood, Jr., and M. M. Kilbey, eds., *Cocaine and Other Stimulants.* New York: Plenum, 1977, pp. 179–185.
59. Ellinwood, E. H., Jr. Effect of chronic methamphetamine intoxication in rhesus monkeys. *Biol. Psychiatry* 3:25, 1971.
60. Ellinwood, E. H., Jr., and Kilbey, M. M. Amphetamine stereotypy: The influence of environmental factors and prepotent behavioral patterns on its topography and development.

*Biol. Psychiatry* 10:3, 1975.

61. Segal, D. A., and Mandell, A. J. Long-term administration of d-amphetamine: Progressive augmentation of motor activity and stereotypy. *Pharmacol. Biochem. Behav.* 2:249, 1974.
62. Klawans, H. L., and Margolin, D. I. Amphetamine-induced dopaminergic hypersensitivity in guinea pigs. *Arch. Gen. Psychiatry* 32:725, 1975.
63. Kilbey, M. M., and Ellinwood, E. H., Jr. Reverse tolerance to stimulant-induced abnormal behavior. *Life Sci.* 20:1063, 1977.
64. Stripling, J. S., and Ellinwood, E. H., Jr. Augmentation of the behavioral and electrophysiologic response to cocaine by chronic administration in the rat. *Exp. Neurol.* 54:546, 1977.
65. Eibergen, R. D., and Carlson, K. R. Dyskinesias elicited by methamphetamine: Susceptibility of form methadome. *Consumer Monkeys Sci.* 190:588, 1975.
66. Groves, P. M., and Rebec, G. V. Changes in neuronal activity in the neostriatum and reticular formation following acute or long-term amphetamine administration. In E. H. Ellinwood, Jr., and M. M. Kilbey, eds., *Cocaine and Other Stimulants*. New York: Plenum, 1977, pp. 269–301.
67. Kuhn, C. M., and Schanberg, S. M. Distribution and metabolism of amphetamine in tolerant animals. In E. H. Ellinwood, Jr., and M. M. Kilbey, eds., *Cocaine and Other Stimulants*. New York: Plenum, 1977, pp. 161–178.
68. Sparber, S. B., Nagasawa, S., and Burklund, K. E. A. A mobilizable pool of d-amphetamine in adipose after daily administration to rats. *Res. Commun. Chem. Pathol. Pharmacol.* 18:423, 1977.
69. Ellinwood, E. H., Jr. Assault and homicide associated with amphetamine abuse. *Am. J. Psychiatry* 127:1170, 1971.
70. Pickens, R. Self-administration of stimulants by rats. *Int. J. Addict.* 3:215, 1968.
71. Yokel, R. A., and Wise, R. A. Increased lever pressing for amphetamine and pimozide in rats: Implication for a dopamine theory of reward. *Science* 187:547, 1975.
72. Schuster, C. R., and Wilson, M. W. The effects of various pharmacological agents on cocaine self-administration by rhesus monkeys. In E. H. Ellinwood, Jr., and S. Cohen, eds., *Current Concepts on Amphetamine Abuse*. Washington, D.C.: U.S. Government Printing Office, 1972, pp. 37–42.
73. Antelman, S. N., and Caggiula, A. R. Norephinephrine dopamine interactions in behavior. *Science* 195:646, 1977.
74. Fuxe, K., et al. Central catecholamine neurons, behavior and neuroleptic drugs: An analysis to understand the involvement of catecholamines in schizophrenia. *J. Psychiatr. Res.* 11:151, 1974.
75. Koob, G. F., Balcom, G. J., and Meyerhoff, J. L. Increase in intracranial self-stimulation in the posterior hypothalamus following unilateral lesions in the locus caeruleus. *Brain Res.* 101:554, 1976.
76. Dominic, J. A., and Moore, K. E. Acute effects of -methyltyrosine on brain catecholamine levels and on spontaneous and amphetamine-stimulant motor activity in mice. *Arch. Intern. Pharmacodyn. Ther.* 178:166, 1969.
77. Scheel-Kruger, J. Comparative studies of various amphetamine analogues demonstrating different interactions with the metabolism of the catecholamines in the brain. *Eur. J. Pharmacol.* 14:47, 1971.
78. Scheel-Kruger, J., et al. Cocaine: Discussion on the role of dopamine in the biochemical mechanism of action. In E. H. Ellinwood, Jr., and M. M. Kilbey, eds., *Cocaine and Other Stimulants*. New York: Plenum, 1977, pp. 373–408.
79. Sayers, A. C., and Handley, S. L. A study of the role of catecholamines in the response to various central stimulants. *Eur. J. Pharmacol.* 23:47, 1973.
80. Wallach, M. B., and Gershon, S. The induction and antagonism of central nervous system stimulant-induced stereotyped behavior in the cat. *Eur. J. Pharmacol.* 18:22, 1972.
81. Ferris, R. M., Tang, F. L. M., and Maxwell, R. A. A comparison of the capacities of isomers of amphetamine deoxypipradol and methylphenidate to inhibit the uptake of tritiated catecholamines into rate cerebral cortex slices synaptosomal preparations of rat cerebral cortex, hypothalamus and striatum into adrenergic nerves of rabbit aorta. *J. Pharmacol. Exp. Ther.* 181:407, 1972.
82. Hendley, E. D., et al. Stereoselectivity of catecholamine uptake by brain synaptosomes: Studies with ephedrine, methylphenidate and phenyl-l-peperidyl carbinol. *J. Pharmacol. Exp. Ther.* 183:103, 1972.
83. Azzaro, A. J., Ziance, R. J., and Rutledge, C. O. The importance of neuronal uptake of amines for amphetamine-induced release of $^3$H-norepinephrine from isolated brain tissue. *J. Pharmacol. Exp. Ther.* 189:110, 1974.

84. Heikkila, R. E., et al. Amphetamine: Evaluation of d- and l-isomers as releasing agents and uptake inhibitors for $^3$H-dopamine and $^3$H-norepinephrine in slices of rat neostriatum and cerebral cortex. *J. Pharmacol. Exp. Ther.* 194:47, 1975.
85. Carr, L. A., and Moore, K. E. Release of norepinephrine and normetanephrine from cat brain by central nervous system stimulants. *Biochem. Pharmacol.* 19:2671, 1970.
86. Koe, B. K. Antidepressant drugs on brain catecholamines and serotonin. In S. Fielding and H. Lal, eds., *Antidepressants.* Mount Kisco, N.Y.: Futura, 1975, pp. 143–180.
87. Coyle, J. T., and Snyder, S. H. Antiparkinsonian drugs: Inhibition of dopamine uptake in the corpus striatum as a possible mechanism of action. *Science* 166:899, 1969.
88. Deneau, G. A., and Yanagita, T., and Seevers, M. H. Psychogenic dependence to a variety of drugs in the monkey. *Psychopharmacologia* 6:183, 1964.
89. Aigner, T., and Balster, R. L. Choice behavior in rhesus monkeys: Cocaine vs food. *Science* 201:534, 1978.
90. Lewis, D. C., and Senay, E. L. Treatment of drug and alcohol abuse. Medical Monograph Series (C. Buckwald, D. Katz, and J. F. Callahan, eds.). Washington, D.C.: NIDA, U.S. Government Printing Office, 1981, pp. 35–36.
91. Davis, J., Sekerke, J., and Janowski, D. Drug interactions involving drugs of abuse. In National Commission of Marijuana and Drug Use, *Drug Use in America: Problems in Perspective*, (second report of the National Commission on Marijuana and Drug Use). Washington, D.C.: U.S. Government Printing Office, 1973.
92. Blum, K. Depressive states induced by drugs of abuse: Clinical evidence, theoretical mechanism(s) and proposed treatment, Part II. *J. Psychedel. Drugs*, 1976.
93. Costa, E., and Garatinni, S. *International Symposium on Amphetamines and Related Compounds.* Raven Press, 1970.
94. Lucas, A. R., and Weiss, M. Methylphenidate hallucinosis. *JAMA* 217, 1971.
95. Hahn, H. H., Schweid, A. E., and Beaty, H. N. Complications of injecting dissolved methylphenidate tablets. *Arch. Intern. Med.* 123:656, 1969.
96. Hopkins, G. B., and Taylor, D. G. Pulmonary talc granulomatosis, a complication of drug abuse. *Am. Rev. Resp. Dis.* 101:101, 1970.
97. Shepard, W. P., et al. *Overweight—Its Prevention and Significance* (Statistical Bulletin). New York: Metropolitan Life Insurance Co., 1960.
98. Kannel, W. B., Brand, N., and Skinner, S. S. Relationship of adiposity to blood pressure and development of hypertension: Framingham study. *Ann. Intern. Med.* 67:48, 1967.
99. Heyden, S., Hames, C. G., and Bartel, A. Weight and weight history in relationship to cerebrovascular and coronary heart disease. *Arch. Intern. Med.* 128:956, 1971.
100. Marks, H. H. Influence of obesity on morbidity and mortality. *Bull. N.Y. Acad. Med.* 36:296, 1960.
101. Leon, G. R. Current direction in the treatment of obesity. *Psychol. Bull.* 83:557, 1976.
102. Angle, H. V., Carroll, J. A., and Ellinwood, E. H., Jr. Psychoactive drug use among psychiatric patients: Problem aspect of anorectic drugs. *Addict Dis.*, in press.
103. Akiskos, J. E., and Hoebel, B. G. Overeating and obesity from damage to a noradrenergic system in the brain. *Science* 182:166, 1973.
104. Marshall, J. F., and Teitelbaum, P. A comparison of the eating in response to hypothermic and vlucoprivic challenges after nigral 6-hydroxydopamine and lateral hypothalamic electrolytic lesions in rats. *Brain Res.* 55:279, 1973.
105. Fibiger, H. C., Zis, A. P., and McGeer, E. G. Feeding and drinking deficits after 6-hydroxydopamine administration in the rat: Similarities to the lateral hypothalamic lesion. *Brain Res.* 55:135, 1973.
106. Carey, R. J., and Goodall, E. B. Attenuation of amphetamine anorexia by unilateral nigral striatal lesions. *Neuropharmacology* 14:827, 1975.
107. Blum, K., Wallace, J. E., and Schwertur, H. A. Intensification of amphetamine-induced excitation by methyserside, a serotonergic receptor blocker. *Experientia* 33:213, 1977.
108. Clineschmidt, B. V. 5, 6-dihydroxytryptamine: Suppression of the anorexigenic action of fenfluramine. *Eur. J. Pharmacol.* 24:405, 1973.
109. Gay, G. R. You've come a long way, baby! Coke time for the new American lady of the eighties. *J. Psychoact. Drugs* 13(4):297, 1981.
110. National Survey on Drug Abuse: Main Findings 1979. NIDA, U.S. Department of Health and Human Services. Washington, D.C.: U.S. Government Printing Office, 1980, p. 24.
111. Blejer-Prieto, H. Cocoa leaf and cocaine addiction—Some historical notes. *Can. Med. Ass. J.* 93:700, 1965.
112. Grinspoon, L., and Bakalar, J. B. *Cocaine: A*

*Drug and Its Social Evolution*. New York: Basic Books, 1976.

113. Lingeman, R. R. *Drugs from A to Z—A Dictionary*. New York: McGraw-Hill, 1969.
114. Foltz, R. L., Fentiman, A. F., Jr., and Foltz, R. B. *GC/MS Assays for Abused Drugs in Body Fluids*. NIDA Research Monograph 32, Washington, D.C.: U.S. Government Printing Office, 1980.
115. Ritchie, J. M., and Greene, N. M. Local anesthetics. In L. S. Goodman, and A. Gilman, eds., *The Pharmacological Basis of Therapeutics*, 6th ed. New York: Macmillan, 1980.
116. Gay, G. R., et al. Cocaine: History, epidemiology, human pharmacology and treatment. A perspective on a new debut for an old girl. *Clin. Toxicol*. 8(2):149.
117. Barash, P. G. Cocaine in clinical medicine. In R. C. Petersen, and R. C. Stillman, eds., *Cocaine: 1977*, NIDA Research Monograph 13. Washington, D.C.: U.S. Government Printing Office, 1977.
118. Finkle, B. S., and McCloskey, K. L. The forensic toxicology of cocaine. In R. C. Petersen and R. C. Stillman, eds., *Cocaine: 1977*, NIDA Research Monograph 13. Washington, D.C.: U.S. Government Printing Office, 1977.
119. Kogan, J. J., et al. Quantitative determination of benzoylecgonine and cocaine in human biofluids by gas–liquid chromatography. *Anal. Chem*. 49(13):1965, 1977.
120. Grinspoon, L., and Bakalar, J. B. Cocaine. In R. I. DuPont, A. Goldstein, and J. O'Donnell, eds., *Handbook on Drug Abuse*. Washington, D.C.: NIDA, U.S. Government Printing Office, 1979, pp. 241–247.
121. Wallace, J. E., et al. Thin-layer chromatographic determination of cocaine and benzoyleugonine in urine. *J. Chromatography* 114:443, 1975.
122. Wallace, J. E., Blum, K., and Singh, J. M. Determination of drugs of abuse in biologic specimens: A review. *Clin. Toxicol*. 7(5):483, 1974.
123. Wallace, J. E., et al. Drug identification: Spectroscopy, colorimetry and flurometry. *J. Pharmaceut. Sci*. 63(2):741, 1974.
124. Wilson, M. C., et al. Acute pharmacological activity of intravenous cocaine in the rhesus monkey. *Psychopharmacol. Commun*. 2:251, 1976.
125. Rappolt, R. T., Gay, G. R., and Inaba, D. S. Propranolol in the treatment of cardiopressor effects of cocaine. *N. Engl. J. Med*. 295:448, 1976.
126. Wesson, D. R., and Smith, D. E. Cocaine: Its use for central nervous system stimulation including recreational and medical uses. In R. C. Petersen and R. C. Stillman, eds., *Cocaine 1977*. Washington, D.C.: U.S. Government Printing Office, 1977.
127. Van Dyke, C., and Byck, R. Cocaine: 1884–1974. In E. H. Ellinwood, Jr., and M. M. Kilbey, eds., *Cocaine and Other Stimulants*. New York: Plenum, 1977.
128. Price, K. R. Fatal cocaine poisoning. *J. Forensic Sci. Soc*. 14:329, 1974.
129. Lundberg, G. D., et al. Cocaine-related death. *J. Forensic Sci*. 22:402, 1977.
130. Hutchinson, R. R., Emley, G. S., and Krasnegor, N. A. The effects of cocaine on the aggressive behavior of mice, pigeons, and squirrel monkeys. In E. H. Ellinwood, Jr., and M. M. Kilbey, eds., *Cocaine and Other Stimulants*. New York: Plenum, 1977.
131. Siegel, R. K. Cocaine: Recreational use and intoxication. In R. C. Petersen and R. C. Stillman, eds., *Cocaine 1977*. Washington, D.C.: U.S. Government Printing Office, 1977.
132. Waldorf, D., et al. *Doing Coke: An Ethnography of Cocaine Users and Sellers*. Washington, D.C.: Drug Abuse Council, 1977.
133. Johanson, C. E., Balister, R. L., and Bonese, K. Self-administration of psychoactive drugs: The effects of unlimited access. *Pharmacol. Biochem. Behav*. 4:45, 1976.
134. Woods, J. Behavioral Effects of cocaine in animals. In R. C. Petersen and R. C. Stillman, eds., *Cocaine 1977*. Washington, D.C.: U.S. Government Printing Office, 1977.
135. Goldberg, S. R., and Kelleher, R. T. Reinforcement of behavior by cocaine injections. In E. H. Ellinwood, Jr., and M. M. Kilbey, eds., *Cocaine and Other Stimulants*. New York: Plenum, 1977.
136. Johanson, C. E., and Schuster, C. R. A choice procedure for drug reinforcers: Cocaine and methylpheridate in the rhesus monkey. *J. Pharmacol. Exp. Ther*. 193:676, 1975.
137. Post, R. M., and Rose, H. Increasing effect of repetitive cocaine administration in the rat. *Nature* 260:731, 1976.
138. Castellani, S. A., Ellinwood, E. H., Jr., and Kilbey, M. M. Tolerance to cocaine-induced convulsions in the cat. *Eur. J. Pharmacol*. 47:57, 1978.
139. Grinspoon, L., and Bakalar, J. B. *Cocaine: A Drug and Its Social Evolution*. New York: Basic Books, 1976.
140. Carroll, E. Coca: The plant and its use. In R.

C. Petersen and R. C. Stillman, eds., *Cocaine: 1977*. NIDA Research Monograph 13. Washington, D.C.: U.S. Government Printing Office, 1977.
141. Drelsbach, R. H. *Handbook of Poisons*. 10th ed. Los Altos, Calif.: Lange, 1980.
142. Rappolt, R. T., Gay, G. R., and Inaba, D. Propranolol: A specific antagonist to cocaine. *Clin. Toxicol.* 10(3):265, 1977.
143. Cohen, S. *The Substance Abuse Problems*. New York: Harworth Press, 1981, pp. 75–80.
144. Reimann, H. A. Caffeinism, a cause of long-continued low-grade fever. *JAMA* 202:131, 1967.
145. Paul, O. Stimulants and coronaries. *Postgrad. Med.* 44:196, 1968.
146. Miltoma, C., et al. Nature of the effect of caffeine on the drug-metabolizing enzymes. *Arch. Biochem. Biophys.* 134:434, 1969.
147. Goldstein, A., Kaiser, S., and Warren, R. Psychotropic effects of caffeine in man. I. Individual differences in sensitivity to caffeine-induced wakefulness. *J. Pharmacol. Exp. Ther.* 149:(1):156, 1965; Psychotropic effects of caffeine in man. II. Alertness, psychomotor coordination, and mood. *J. Pharmacol. Exp. Ther.* 150(1):146, 1965.
148. Weiss, B., and Laites, V. Enhancement of human performance by caffeine and the amphetamines. *Pharmacol. Rev.* 14(1):1–36, 1962.
149. Peters, J. M. Factors affecting caffeine toxicity. *J. Clin. Pharmacol.* 7:131, 1967.
150. Goldstein, A., and Kaizer, S. Psychotropic effects of caffeine in man. III. A questionnaire survey of coffee drinking and its effects in a group of housewives. *Clin. Pharmacol. Ther.* 10(4):477, 1969.
151. Goldstein, A. Wakefulness caused by caffeine. Naunyn-CchiedebergsArch. für Exper. Pathol. Pharmakol. 248:269, 1964.
152. Blum, R., et al. *Drug 1: Society and Drugs*. San Francisco: Jossey-Bass, 1970.
153. Hearings: Subcommittee to Investigate Juvenile Delinquency. Amphetamine Legislation, July 15, 16, 1971, U.S. Government Printing Office, Washington, D.C., 1972.
154. Lucas, A. R., and Weiss, M. Methylphenidate hallucinosis. *JAMA* 212:1079, 1971.
155. Cohen, S. *The Substance Abuse Problems*. New York: Haworth Press, 1981, pp. 151–156.
156. Wesson, D. R., Smith, D. E., and Gay, G. R. The politics of barbiturate and amphetamine abuse. In D. E. Smith, and Wesson, D. R., eds., *Uppers and Downers*. Englewood Cliffs, N.J.: Prentice-Hall, 1973, pp. 97–107.

CHAPTER 13

# Tranquilizing Agents

## A. INTRODUCTION

The practice of psychiatry prior to the 1950s was more reminiscent of the 18th century bedlams than of modern psychiatric facilities. There were insulin rooms, laboratory wards, locks on the doors, beatings for patients, and rampant violence. With the development of drugs such as the antipsychotics, antidepressants, and antianxiety drugs with proven ability to act on mental disorders, the entire concept of the treatment of the psychiatric disorders has undergone a radical change since the second half of the 20th century.

Many substances that act on the central nervous system (CNS) are liable to be abused and are also psychotoxic. Coffee, tobacco, alcohol, LSD, and marihuana are only a few examples of the more often abused and habit-forming natural substances with no specific therapeutic use. On the other hand, substances such as opium and barbiturates have proved therapeutic use as sedatives or hypnotics, but are still liable to be abused. The aim of this chapter is to discuss the drugs used in mental disorders (the psychotropic drugs), with special emphasis on the tranquilizers and the antianxiety drugs.

Usdin, in 1978, classified more than 1500 compounds as psychotropic. The psychotropic drugs may be divided into three broad categories—neuroleptic or antipsychotic, sedative or antianxiety, and mood-elevating or antidepressant agents (see Chapter 14). The tranquilizing agents comprise the first two categories; the antipsychotic drugs are called the "major tranquilizers" (e.g., phenothiazines, thioxanthenes, and butyrophenones) and the antianxiety agents are termed the minor tranquilizers (e.g., the benzodiazepines and meprobamate).

The efficiency of a neuroleptic or antipsychotic drug is based on its specific targeted action in changing the psychotic disorder rather than its sedative or stupifying effect on the patient. All the neuroleptic drugs are effective dopamine receptor blockers and their therapeutic efficacy arises mostly out of this pharmacologic property. There is evidence to indicate that disorders such as schizophrenia are the result of an excessive firing of the dopaminergic neurons in the limbic system. Although most marketed tranquilizers seem to be effective, the major problem associated with their use is the risk of producing neurotoxic effects that mimic neurologic diseases.

The antianxiety drugs such as the benzodiazepines may not be basically different from the sedative-hypnotics, except for their greater popularity and wider abuse. Although their addictive nature is well known, they are less likely to produce tolerance and physical dependence and they are much safer than the sedative-hypnotics when taken in suicidal (large) doses.

The antidepressants or the mood elevators (e.g., the lithium salts) are effective in the treatment of manic disorders. These drugs are not known to produce physical dependence and thus have a low abuse profile.[2] (See Chapter 14.)

## B. HISTORIC DEVELOPMENT

The use of the psychotropic drugs historically has been the result of a quest for change in normal behavior during religious rites or household ceremonies, and also in cases of mental ailments. The story of the development of many psychotic drugs can be ascertained from reviews by Efron and his group of workers,[3] Caldwell,[4] and Schultes.[5] Studies on insanity were initiated by Moreau (hashish intoxication, 1845), Freud (studies on cocaine, 1875), and Sen and Bose[6] (use of *Rauwolfia serpentina* in the treatment of insanity, 1931). Today there is sufficient evidence to show that *Rauwolfia serpentina* alters the pharmacodynamics of the brain peptidyl opiates, which are substances possibly involved in mental disorders. The invention of electroconvulsive therapy in 1937 triggered the treatment of mental depression and schizophrenia (a psychotic group of disorders involving altered ideas of reality, delusions, and hallucinations). The psychic effects of LSD (lysergic acid diethylamide) were first discovered by Hofmann.

The use of lithium in the treatment of manic disorders was first suggested by Cade[7] in 1949. And the first reports on the use of chlorpromazine in psychiatric disorders by Delay and Deniker[8] appeared in 1952, just two years after its synthesis provided the basis for a new era in the treatment of mental disorders. These were soon followed by reports on meprobamate[9] and by Kuhn in 1958 on imipramine[2] to keep up the tempo of the new revolution. The development of the first antianxiety drug chlordiazepoxide (a benzodiazepine) in 1957 by Sternbach,[10] and the discovery of haloperidol (a butyrophenone) resulted in the availability of yet another class of antipsychotic agents. A detailed account of these drugs is presented in Chapter 14.

## C. PATHOGENESIS OF MENTAL ILLNESS

The hypotheses leading to a clear understanding of mental disorders are based on the study of the modes of action of several psychopharmacologic agents that are used either as psychotropic drugs or to mimic the symptoms of mental disorders. One of the hypotheses indicates that the deficiency of biogenic amine transmission in the CNS causes mental depression while an excess of the same causes manic disorders.

The physiologic and pharmacologic modifications of the brain regions, including the cortex, hypothalamus, and limbic system, result in important behavioral changes such as in autonomic functions, consciousness, and arousal. There is evidence that implicates the brain amines,[12] and in particular the catecholamines (dopamine and norepinephrine) in schizophrenia and similar psychiatric disorders. Amphetamine, a drug belonging to the class of catecholamines, produces certain psychotoxic effects that cannot be easily distinguished from certain manifestations of schizophrenia. Further, the phenothiazines and butyrophenones can block the adrenergic or the dopaminergic receptors. Additional evidence indicates that the inhibition of the synthesis of catecholamines by the administration of (alpha) methyltyrosine potentiates the effects of phenothiazines in schizophrenics. Although it is premature to formulate a general hypothesis of the chemical basis of mental illness, there is evidence to implicate some imbalance between dopamine and norepinephrine as part of "the biologic vulnerability in schizophrenia."

The biologic basis of the affective disorders has been reviewed by Schildkraut,[13] Kiev,[14] and Blum et al.[15] The biogenic amines, norepinephrine, dopamine, and serotonin have all been implicated in these disorders. Rational therapy involves the use of MAO (monoamine oxidase) inhibitors, enzyme inhibitors that raise the levels of brain biogenic amines, and tricyclic antidepressants, agents that raise the levels of biogenic amines at postjunctional sites (see Chapter 14).

Although the actual etiology of the psychiatric disorders is not yet fully known, the following major developments undoubtedly can further our understanding of the concept. The discovery of specific binding sites for the benzodiazepines (antianxiety drugs) in the brain by Squires and Braestrup[16] and Mohler and Okada[17] in 1977 resulted in a plausible theory to explain how the benzodiazepines may interact in the CNS. The finding has sparked the idea that anxiety may be a biochemically connected genetic disorder. The second development in the field of brain research was more social and political in nature. In 1979 the U.S. Senate Subcommittee on Health and Scientific Research hearing known as the "Valium hearing" focused on the growing problem of drug abuse. The hearing helped to make the public more aware of the serious, adverse effects of the dependence liability of many of the psychotic agents.

## D. THE ANTIPSYCHOTIC AGENTS

The drugs used in the treatment of psychosis, schizophrenia, and manic illness belong in this category. The different classes of drugs that can be listed are the phenothiazines, dibenzoxazepines, butyrophenones, indolones, and other heterocyclic compounds, and the Rauwolfia alkaloids (e.g., reserpine).

The almost simultaneous introduction of two highly potent drugs, reserpine and chlorpromazine, opened up the vast field of tranquilizers. The alkaloid reserpine was isolated in 1952 from the plant *Rauwolfia serpentina*, the preparations of which had been in wide use in India for centuries. Chlorpromazine was synthesized in France as a consequence of the study of certain antihistamine compounds having the basic structure of phenothiazine (e.g., promethazine). Both reserpine and chlorpromazine were found to be highly effective in their calming effects, even at doses much below the hypnotic levels. Knowledge of the extraordinary efficacy of these drugs in taming wild animals prompted the screening of many other drugs of a tranquilizing nature.

Research on the antihistamine agents resulted in the development of drugs of the basic phenothiazine structure. The typical representative drug chlorpromazine was observed to be closely related to promethazine (Phenergan) in its antipsychotic effects without excessive sedation and physical dependence. Most of the phenothiazine group of drugs are also known to be antiemetics and antipruretics.

### 1. Phenothiazines as Antipsychotic Agents

The antipsychotic drugs are basically comprised of the phenothiazines, thioxanthenes, and butyrophenones; the present discussion will be limited primarily to the phenothiazenes. The advantages and disadvantages of the use of antipsychotic drugs have been discussed by Gardos and Cole.[18] Such use of the antipsychotic drugs has been widespread in recent times.

The phenothiazines, also recognized as the major tranquilizers, include chlorpromazine (Thorazine), thioridazine (Mellaril), trifluoperazine (Trilafon), and promazine (Sparine). The prolonged administration of these drugs in high doses does not induce physical dependence. There is one report[19] of adverse effects when there is an abrupt discontinuation of phenothiazines. The report cites insomnia, anxiety, and gastrointestinal disturbances but there seem to be no gross physiologic disturbances as with amphetamine withdrawal. The issue of whether or not to call this syndrome an "abstinence syndrome" is largely a matter of semantics.

It is observed that moderate tolerance develops to the sedative effects of the phenothiazines. The potent tranquilizing and antiemetic activity of chlorpromazine has led to its widespread use in several other areas of medicine. Many other phenothiazines have been developed, of which at least a dozen are now in clinical use.

#### *a. Chemistry*

The phenothiazines are classified into three groups on the basis of their chemistry and pharmacology. Their structural differences result from substitutions on the nitrogen in the phenothiazine ring. The aliphatic or dimethylaminopropyl compounds include chlorpromazine

(Thorazine), promazine (Sparine), and triflupromazine (Vesprin). The piperidine derivatives are represented by thioridazine (Mellaril) and mesoridazine (Serentil). Among the many piperazine compounds, some of the most widely used are prochlorperazine (Compazine), trifluoperazine (Stelazine), perphenazine (Trilafon), fluphenazine (Prolixin, Permitil), and thiopropazate (Dartal).

Numerous phenothiazine derivatives are in current use. They resemble chlorpromazine in action but differ from it in potency, clinical indications, and toxicity. (See Table 13-1.)

Other clinically useful antipsychotic drugs include the thiozanthene group and the butyrophenones. Aliphatic or dimethylaminopropyl derivatives such as thiothixane (Navane) resemble the phenothiazines in most respects but have greater sedative action and thus are more effective than phenothiazinetype compounds in agitated schizophrenics.

Haloperidol (a butyrophenone known clinically as Haldol) is pharmacologically similar to the phenothiazines except for its antidopaminergic property, which is more potent.

In terms of structure–activity relationships, the piperazine group of compounds may be more useful in depressed or withdrawn schizophrenics. The aliphatic compounds and the piperidyl group resemble each other in more respects. It is noteworthy that the various classes of phenothiazines differ in their abilities to induce specific adverse effects.

The aliphatic group can cause parkinsonism in addition to drowsiness. However, thioridazine (Mellaril) of the piperidyl class is not likely to do so. Extrapyramidal symptoms, as well as dyskinesia, have been clinically observed with the piperazine compounds.

Chlorpromazine, as a prototype phenothiazine, has the following properties: The hydrochloride is a gray-white crystalline powder, with a molecular weight of 355.32. It is 100 percent soluble in water at 26°C (1000 mg/ml). The 5 percent and saturated aqueous solutions, with pH values of 4.9 and 4.6, respectively, are stable for more than 24 hours. The substance is photosensitive.

Chlorpromazine was synthesized in France in 1950 and it is chemically related to the antihistaminic agent, promethazine. Interestingly, the well-known French lytic cocktail, used by Laborit for production of artificial hibernation, consisted of promethazine, meperidine, and chlorpromazine. Profound inhibition of the autonomic nervous system resulted from the administration of this mixture.

### *b. Drug-Induced Responses (Pharmacology)*

Phenothiazine tranquilizers are known for their complex pharmacologic effects. Aside from their potent effects on behavior, these drugs are antiemetics and also act on the autonomic nervous system. In large doses, they produce significant toxic side effects such as parkinsonism. It is believed that chlorpromazine (Thorazine) acts principally at the higher neural centers, particularly in the hypothalamus and reticular substance in the general area of the diencephalon. The drowsiness caused by chlorpromazine may be attributed to the fact that it inhibits the reticular activating system. However, the tranquilizing effect is the result of its activity in the other areas of diencephalon, including the basal ganglia. The antiemetic effect of chlorpromazine is believed to be attributable to its medullary activity in a selective inhibition of the chemoreceptor trigger zone. In high doses, chlorpromazine induces characteristic cataleptic immobility as is observed in experimental animals. The lethal dose is extraordinarily high and, interestingly enough, phenothiazines do not induce coma. Further information on the pharmacologic properties of the antipsychotic drugs can be obtained from the review by Fielding and Lal.[20]

(1) *Acute Toxicity*: No significant toxic effects of phenothiazines are seen when they are administered in low doses. In animals a considerable reduction in operant behavior without change in spinal reflexes is noticed. Responses to different stimuli and exploratory behavior are diminished considerably but not completely. Conditioned avoidance (escape) behavior is selectively inhibited but unconditioned avoidance response is not. The highly reinforcing self-stimulation property and the behavioral activation of the brain are blocked by these drugs.

# TABLE 13-1
# Tranquilizing Agents

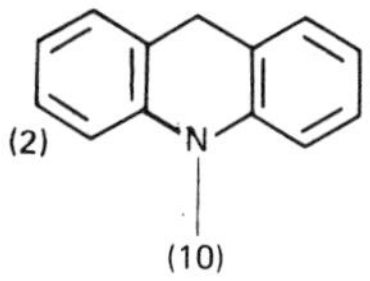

(2) (2)

(10)

penothiazine nucleus

| | Substitution in (2) | Substitution in (10) | Average oral dose (mg) |
|---|---|---|---|
| | | aliphatic | |
| Chlorpromazine (Thorazine) | Cl | $CH_2-CH_2-CH_2-N-(CH_3)_2$ | 25-50 |
| Promazine (Sparine) | — | $CH_2-CH_2-CH_2-N-(CH_3)_2$ | 25-50 |
| Triflupromazine (Vesprin) | $CF_3$ | $CH_2-CH_2-CH_2-N-(CH_3)_2$ | 10-25 |
| Mesoridazine (Serentil) | $SCH_3$ 0 | 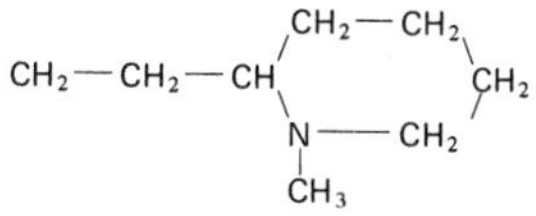 $CH_2-CH_2-CH$ (piperidine ring: $CH_2-CH_2$, $CH_2$, $N-CH_2$, N–$CH_3$) | 50-200 |
| Thioridazine (Mellaril) | $SCH_3$ | 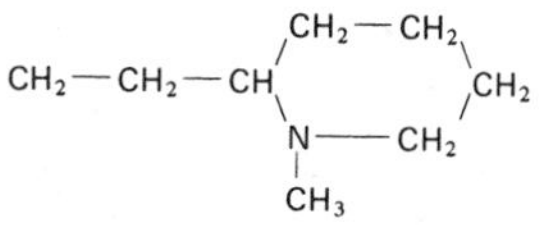 $CH_2-CH_2-CH$ (piperidine ring: $CH_2-CH_2$, $CH_2$, $N-CH_2$, N–$CH_3$) | 25-100 |
| | | piperidine | |
| Prochlorperazine (Compazine) | Cl | 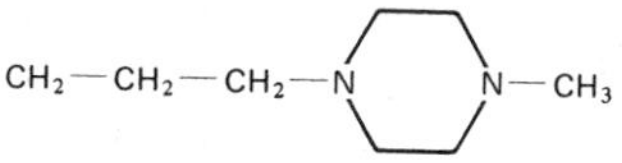 $CH_2-CH_2-CH_2-N$ (piperazine) $N-CH_3$ | 5-10 |
| Trifluoperazine (Stelazine) | $CF_3$ | 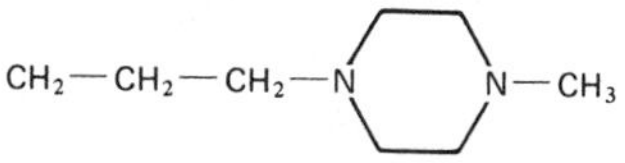 $CH_2-CH_2-CH_2-N$ (piperazine) $N-CH_3$ | 2-10 |
| Perphenazine (Trilafon) | Cl | 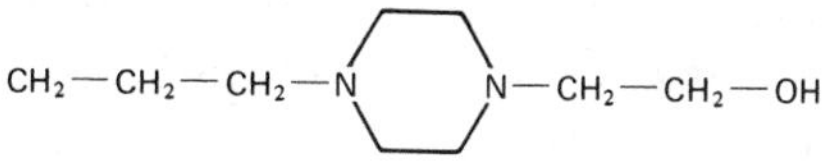 $CH_2-CH_2-CH_2-N$ (piperazine) $N-CH_2-CH_2-OH$ | 4-8 |
| Fluphenazine (Prolixin, Permitil) | $CF_3$ | 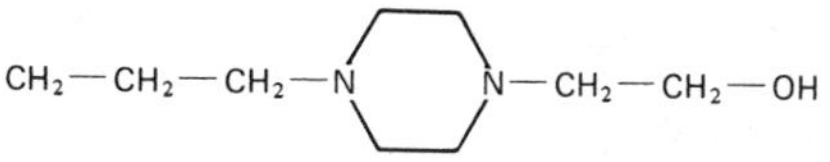 $CH_2-CH_2-CH_2-N$ (piperazine) $N-CH_2-CH_2-OH$ | 0.25-0.5 |
| Thiopropazate (Dartal) | Cl | 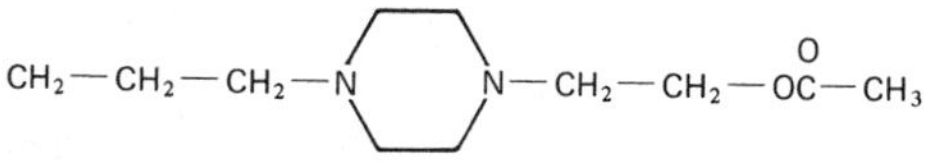 $CH_2-CH_2-CH_2-N$ (piperazine) $N-CH_2-CH_2-OC(=O)-CH_3$ | 10 |
| | | piperazine | |

(Modified from Goth, A. *Medical Pharmacology,* 10th ed. St. Louis: C. V. Mosby Co., 1981. With permission)

### $LD_{50}$ (14-Day) Values of Phenothiazines in Rats

| *Route of Administration* | *$LD_{50}$* (mg/kg) |
|---|---|
| Intraperitoneal | 75 to 100 |
| Subcutaneous | 540 |
| Oral | 492 |
| Intravenous | 25 |

In humans almost all the neuroleptic agents can diminish spontaneous motor activity. Chlorpromazine causes skeletal muscular relaxation in some types of spastic conditions. Since the drug has little effect at spinal levels, its action on motor activity must be mediated at a higher level, possibly on the basal ganglia. On an acute basis, the drug does not block the neuromuscular junction.

2. *Chronic Toxicity*: In chronic doses, in humans, chlorpromazine results in a striking lack of initiative, disinterest in the environment, little display of emotion, and a limited range of effects. Initially drowsiness might become evident. However, subjects are easily aroused, are capable of giving appropriate answers to diverse questions, and their intellectual functions are intact. There is no ataxia, incoordination, or dysarthia. Toxic side effects include aggressive and impulsive behavior, psychotic symptoms or hallucinations, delusions, disorganized thinking, bradykinesia, mild rigidity, tremor, and akathisia (parkinsonism-like). Upon continued administration, many of these side effects gradually disappear, possibly as a result of tolerance to the drug.

When chlorpromazine was given daily to rats and dogs at a dosage of 10 mg/kg orally and to guinea pigs at a dosage of 10 mg/kg subcutaneously, all of the test animals showed a slight depression in growth rate during the latter half of the test period. This effect may have been caused by the decreased food intake brought about by the depressant action of the substance. The guinea pigs showed no significant difference in growth rate from the controls. All of the dogs continued to gain weight throughout the test.

In summary, the most important side effects induced by chronic administration of neuroleptic agents are those on the CNS, cardiovascular system, autonomic nervous system, and endocrine functions.

3. *Dependence and Tolerance*: Phenothiazines and most other antipsychotic drugs do not lead to addiction. However, sleeplessness and muscular discomfort are reported in some cases when the drugs are withdrawn abruptly. Nevertheless, no electroencephalographic (EEG) changes are detected upon withdrawal. Baldessarini and Tarsy[21] demonstrated tolerance and cross-tolerance to the effects of phenothiazines on dopaminergic receptors in the basal ganglia. This tolerance is not observed as often in the limbic region of the forebrain. The development of "disuse supersensitivity" and choreoathetosis is observed in the forebrain regions, upon abrupt withdrawal from chlorpromazine.[22] Yet another problem that often arises due to the quick clinical changes (in high doses) from one drug to another involves changes in the autonomous effects, hypotension, and pyramidal reactions.

4. *Effects on Organ Systems*: The most interesting aspect of the pharmacology of chlorpromazine is its effect on the central nervous system. In intact animals, chlorpromazine causes a decrease in motor activity and loss of aggressive behavior without inducing hypnosis or anesthesia. In decerebrate animals displaying sham rage, chlorpromazine reduces the intensity of the rage.

It is important to understand that chlorpromazine has the unusual ability to block responses to conditioned stimuli in doses that do not alter responses to unconditioned stimuli. In rats trained to climb a pole at the sound of a bell, pretreatment with chlorpromazine in doses of 10 mg/kg blocked this conditioned response to the bell in 85 percent of the test animals. The rats, however, continued to respond normally to the unconditioned stimulus, and electric shock to the feet.

Electroencephalographic records of animals given chlorpromazine resemble those observed in a normal state of drowsiness or sleep, with rapid and normal-appearing arousal in response to stimuli.

Chlorpromazine provides protection against the emetic effect of drugs that have medullary activity. In dogs chlorpromazine decreased the frequency of vomiting 82 to 94 percent when given subcutaneously in doses of 0.5, 1, and 2 mg/kg one hour prior to apomorphine. Oral doses of 2, 3, and 5 mg/kg prior to apomorphine decreased the frequency of vomiting 40 to 100 percent. By comparison, diphenhydramine hydrochloride produced only an 11 percent decrease in vomiting at the maximum tolerated oral dose of 20 mg/kg.

Drugs that cause emesis through an effect on the nodose ganglion, or locally on the gastrointestinal tract, are not antagonized by chlorpromazine.

### *c. Regional Specific Effects on the Nervous System*

Certainly, the antipsychotic drugs have profound effects through the central nervous system. In this section, we explore three important aspects of psychotropic interaction with various specific target brain sites. First, an introduction to the development of chemotherapy of psychology, second, the effects summarized at various brain sites, and finally the mechanism of action (biochemical and pharmacological mechanisms) of antipsychotic drugs.

With the synthesis of chlorpromazine in 1950 (and the beginning of the modern era in our understanding and treatment of psychosis)[8], the recognition that chlorpromazine had central actions, such as the lowering of body temperature, contributed to the initial enthusiasm for the drug as a pre-anesthetic sedative. Furthermore, it was observed that certain agitated psychotic patients respond to cold pack treatment (hypothermia producing) and this provided the impetus to utilize chlorpromazine in the treatment of psychosis. Interestingly, although administration of chlorpromazine to psychotic patients at doses of 75 to 150 mg. per day by injection failed to produce significant hypothermia, there was a significant reduction in psychotic agitation.[8]

It was also soon noticed that chlorpromazine produced antipsychotic effects without concomitant sedation in the patients. However, since chlorpromazine did produce other adverse effects such as the lowering of blood pressure at extrapyramidal effects, other newer and more beneficial drugs were soon developed.

The effects of chlorpromazine on the different regions of the nervous system, with regard to the pharmacologic mechanisms, will now be described.

### 1. EEG and Cortex

Fink reviewed[23] the effect of antipsychotic drugs on EEG patterns. Chlorpromazine, thioxanthenes, thioridazine and haloperidal produce the same kind of effects. To simply enumerate the most important actions they are as follows: 1) slowing down of the EEG patterns; 2) reduction of alpha and theta waves; 3) speeding up the beta, burst and spiking activity; 4) reduction in the variability of the EEG frequencies with an enhancement in the voltage.

In contrast to the above effects, other antipsychotic agents such as promazine and prochlorperazine produce the typical slowing of the EEG pattern, increases alpha but also decreases seizure activity.[23,26] In the cortex, these drugs inhibit the uptake of monoamines but not GABA. Other reviews of the subject include the work of Long,[24] and Shagass and Straumani[25].

### 2. Excitation Threshold (seizure activity)

The basic pharmacological response of chlorpromazine and other antipsychotic drugs (aliphatic phenothiazines) with regard to seizure activity is that there is a lowering of the excitation or convulsive threshold. This effect restricts the use of antipsychotics to now-epileptic patients. Other neuroleptics such as piperazines, phenothiazines (now aliphatic) and thioxanthenes as well as butyrophenones do not affect seizure activity similarly.

### 3. Basal Ganglia, Hypothalamus, Limbic System and Brain Stem

a. *Basal Ganglia*: All the antipsychotic drugs with the exception of reserpine, are thought to relieve psychotic symptoms by interfering with dopaminergic neurons in the basal ganglia. The antipsychotics such as chlorpromazine, other phenothiazines and haloperidol, block the dopamine receptor and increase the production of dopamine in the corpus striatum.''

Evidence is accumulating whereby the major site of action of antipsychotic agents in the caudate nucleus may be the ''dopamine receptor,'' and a dopamine-sensitive adenylate cyclase.[27,28] The effect of the antipsychotic agents on the dopamine-stimulated adenylate cyclase activity should prove useful as an industrial screening method. The findings of Greengard,[30] Snyder et al.,[31] and Baldessarini[32] strongly support the hypothesis that the antipsychotic drugs interfere with the role of dopamine as a synaptic transmitter.

### b. Hypothalamus

Once again due to a dopaminergic mechanism, chlorpromazine and other antipsychotics inhibit the release of growth hormone and stimulate prolactin release[33], decrease secretion of corticotropin regulatory hormone in response to stress[34], and interfere with hypothalamic temperature regulation. Important reviews on the role of neuroleptics on hypothalamic function include Martin et al.,[35] Sachar,[36] and Overall.[37]

### c. Limbic System

A very major action for the antipsychotics in the limbic system is an increase in the dopamine production (turnover) rate.[38] It has been speculated that the center of action for use of these drugs in schizophrenia lies in their ability to alter dopaminergic function. The work by Clement-Cormier and associates,[39] showing that phenothiazines block dopamine-induced stimulation of adenyl cyclase activity in the caudate nucleus, along with other work[40] from her laboratory, helped explain differences between therapeutic efficacy and the inherent inclination of certain anti-psychotic drugs to produce extrapyramidal symptoms. Barchas et al.[41] and Carlsson[42] have reviewed the effects of antipsychotics in the limbic system.

### *d. Brain Stem*

The effects of chlorpromazine on the brain stem is quite complex, even more so than those produced by barbiturates. Briefly, the phenothiazines generally in usual clinical doses do not depress respiration when taken orally but could depress respiration if injected.[43] There might be a centrally mediated fall in blood pressure as a result of chlorpromazine-induced depression of brain stem vasomotor reflexes. Additionally, chlorpromazine may enhance reticular activity by stimulating specific faltering mechanisms that control external stimuli.[44]

4. *Anti-emetic Actions* (Chemoreceptor Trigger Zone)

Since apomorphine is a dopamine agonist, it is not unexpected that chlorpromazine can block apomorphine-induced emesis via a chemoreceptor trigger zone (CTZ) mechanism. Thioridazine is not useful as antiemetic in humans but blocks apomorphine emesis.

5. *Spinal Cord*

The current opinion is that the antipsychotics have no significant action on spinal cord activity.

6. *Peripheral Autonomics*

a. Local Anesthetic Action

Through what has been termed ''membrane-stabilization'' effects, the antipsychotic agents act as local anesthetics but are not used in the clinic for this action.[45]

b. Anti-adrenergic effects

These include postural hypotension with reflex tachycardia, inhibition of ejaculation, and nasal congestion. Intramuscular administration usually results in marked blood pressure effects. Chlorpromazine, due to alpha adrenergic blocking action, cause consistent hypotensive effects in the elderly, whatever the route of administration.

The antipsychotic drugs may be arranged in the following order of decreasing potencies in their adrenergic antagonist activity based on the radio ligand binding assays.[2]

(1) strong drugs:
piperacetazine > droperidol > triflupromazine > chlorpromazine

(2) moderate drugs:
thioridazine > fluphenazine > haloperidol

(3) weak drugs:
trifluoperazine > clozapine > pimozide

### *c. Anticholinergic effects*

Chlorpromazine is a weak peripheral cholinergic blocker which could induce dry mouth, urinary hesitancy, and retention, constipation, reduced sweating, blurred vision and infrequently the precipitation of glaucoma.

### *d. Miscellaneous Actions*

According to Baldessarini,[2] the antihistaminic and antitriptaminergic actions are well documented.

Chlorpromazine exhibits a variety of other antagonistic actions at other receptor sites. The drug has only slight antihistaminic effects. Chlorpromazine blocks the actions of 5-HT quite effectively, both *in vivo* and *in vitro*; however, it remains to be demonstrated whether this antagonism plays any role in the therapeutic efficacy of the phenothiazines. There is little, if any, ganglionic blocking effect.

For further discussion of the autonomic pharmacology of the phenothiazines, Gordon's[46] extensive monograph should be consulted. Various reviews also describe the autonomic side effects of numerous psychotropic drugs.[47–49]

(e) *Effect on Gonads and Pregnant Animals*. Chlorpromazine produced a slight decrease in liver weight and an increase in testes and adrenal weights in treated rats. Male guinea pigs showed a decrease in thymus weight; all other organs and glands were unaffected.

Semimonthly hematologic tests, conducted on all dogs used, revealed no significant variations in the blood pressure. Histopathologic studies on organs removed from sacrificed animals showed no pathologic changes that could be attributed to chlorpromazine. Pregnant rabbits received 5 mg/kg daily by subcutaneous injection until the litters were born. There was no significant difference in size or viability of litters in the treated and control groups.

Female rats were given chlorpromazine from the time of conception by incorporating the drug into their diet. Feedings were regulated so that each animal received about 10 mg/kg daily. There were no deleterious or toxic effects on the pregnant animals or the litters. Second-generation studies did not show adverse effects either.

(f) *Endocrine Effects*. Secondary to its inhibitory effects on the hypothalamus, chlorpromazine decreases or prevents pituitary secretion of ACTH, gonadotropins, and probably other hormones. Other endocrine effects of the neuroleptics are the subject of the works of Schyve et al.,[50] Erle et al.,[51] and Dimond et al.[52]

(g) *Gastrointestinal Effects*. Chlorpromazine decreases gastric secretory volume, but has little effect on acid secretion; it does not block gastric responses to histamine. It is a moderately effective smooth muscle relaxant. No adverse effects on liver function have been observed in animals, but jaundice has developed in some patients on chlorpromazine, possibly as an allergic reaction.

(h) *Effect on Body Temperature*. Body temperature in small animals exposed to cold is lowered further by chlorpromazine, probably as a result of vasodilation (with resulting increased heat loss) and muscular relaxation (with decreased heat production).

(i) *Metabolic Effects*. Basal metabolic rate is decreased in proportion to the fall in body temperature. Chlorpromazine appears to have little effect on gross metabolism, although certain enzyme systems are inhibited.

(j) *Heart Actions*. Chlorpromazine produces peripheral vasodilation and a fall in blood pressure, mainly because of its adrenolytic action. It has little effect on the heart in ordinary doses, except for occasional tachycardia.

(k) *Antishock Effect*. As do adrenergic blocking agents, chlorpromazine gives excellent protection against hemorrhagic and traumatic shock in animals.

(10) *Effect on Activity of Other Drugs*: The depressant effects of barbiturates, anesthetics, and alcohol, and the analgesic effects of various drugs, are increased and prolonged by chlorpromazine. Chlorpromazine does not, however, potentiate the anticonvulsant action of barbiturates.

Additional information on psychotropic drug interactions can be found in Chapter 18.

## 8. Pharmacologic Summary

The profile of the overall antipsychotic drug therapy in humans (taking 25 to 50 mg. chlorpromazine) include numerous effects which can be described as follows.

Cardiac arrhythmias may occur, EEG changes in the form of prolongation of the QT internal and T wave blurring have been noticed, depression of mood and weight gain have been seen, galactorrhoea and amenorrhea are induced in some females; hypothermia occurs in the elderly, there are reports of increased frequency of seizures in epileptic subjects, induced photosensitivity and accumulation of pigment in the skin, cornea and lens, cholestatic jaundice and agranulolytosis occurs infrequently, high doses may cause retinal degeneration (usually seen with thioridazine).

For persons with schizophrenia, chlorpromazine will improve their thought disorders, change their blunted effects, alter their withdrawal and autistic behavior, and relieve their hallucinations, hostility, and resistiveness.[53]

(13) *Biochemical and Pharmacologic Mechanisms of Phenothiazines*: Chlorpromazine exerts important effects on the central nervous system. In addition, it has some adrenergic blocking effects, together with weak antihistaminic, anticholinergic, and antispasmodic actions. It potentiates the hypnotics and blocks the emetic action of apomorphine.

The actions on the CNS are still not well understood although they have been studied extensively through the use of psychologic and neurophysiologic techniques. The drug tends to inhibit conditioned reflexes in animals, decreasing hostility and spontaneous motor activity. It tends to oppose the psychomotor stimulant actions of caffeine and amphetamine, but will not block the convulsant actions of strychnine.

The difference between chlorpromazine and a barbiturate is illustrated in an experiment proposed by Lasagna and McLaun.[54] This experiment is based on the previous observation that the toxicity of amphetamine in mice is markedly influenced by the environment. The $LD_{50}$ of amphetamine for isolated mice was found to be 111 mg/kg when injected intraperitoneally. When three mice were placed in a small cage, a much smaller dose of amphetamine, about 15 mg/kg, produced death. Apparently the anxiety induced by the hyperactive neighbors added to the central stimulant actions of amphetamine.

When either phenobarbital or chlorpromazine was injected in addition to amphetamine, the results in the grouped mice were similar to those obtained with the isolated mice. In other words, the $LD_{50}$ of amphetamine in the grouped mice now went up to about 110 mg/kg, essentially the same as for isolated mice. This may be interpreted as a reduction in the damaging influence of crowded conditions on amphetamine toxicity. There was a great difference, however, between phenobarbital and chlorpromazine in this respect. Phenobarbital had to be raised to anesthetic levels to obtain protection, whereas chlorpromazine prevented the lethal actions of amphetamine even at dose levels that did not produce unconsciousness. This is a remarkable example of a tranquilizing drug reducing the adverse effects of the environment. It should be emphasized that these results cannot be explained on the basis of pharmacologic antagonism to amphetamine, since in single mice neither phenobarbital nor chlorpromazine produced any great increase in the $LD_{50}$ of amphetamine.

It is quite likely that chlorpromazine acts on many different portions of the brain. Its ability to block vomiting induced by apomorphine suggests that it has an effect on the chemoreceptor trigger area.[55] The drug also may interfere with vasomotor reflexes mediated through the hypothalamus.[56]

Among the peripheral actions of chlorpromazine, perhaps the most important is its adrenergic blocking effect. Of less importance is its ability to antagonize to a slight extent the actions of histamine, serotonin, and acetylcholine.

Although the exact mechanism of the antipsychotic effect of chlorpromazine and other phenothiazines is not known, the blocking action of these drugs on central catecholamine receptors is currently being emphasized. This is in line with some current thinking that attributes schizophrenic disorders to a possible overactivity of dopamine, an insufficiency of norepinephrine at appropriate synapses, or an imbalance between the two.[53]

Assuming that the antipsychotic effect of the phenothiazines is related to blockade of central catecholamine receptors, what would be an effect of inhibition of catecholamine synthesis on the efficacy of phenothiazines? This problem was put to a test. The antipsychotic actions of thioridazine and chlorpromazine were markedly potentiated by the tyrosine hydroxylase inhibitor, alpha-methyltyrosine. The dosage of the phenothiazine could be greatly lowered under these conditions. Although this study was performed in only five schizophrenic patients, its implications are far reaching.

The phenothiazines and other antipsychotic drugs interact with central neurohormones other than dopamine. Many neuroleptics enhance the turnover of acetylcholine in the basal ganglion. There is an inverse relationship between antimuscarinic potency of antipsychotic drugs in the brain and extrapyramidal effects. Sulser and Robinson[57] suggested that beta-adrenergic blockade may contribute to central actions of neuroleptic drugs. In addition, other amines (such as serotonin), amino acids (such as GABA), or peptides (substance P, endorphins) that are known to affect dopamine neurons may also be involved in the action of antipsychotics.

### *d. Pharmacokinetics and Metabolism*

Antipsychotic drugs, like chlorpromazine, are well absorbed, mainly from the jejunum. The drugs are metabolized in the liver. When they are taken orally, part of this metabolism is completed as they pass through the portal system on their way to the systemic circulation (first pass metabolism). With chlorpromazine 75 percent of the drug is metabolized like this, whereas with other antipsychotic drugs, it is less. There are approximately 168/metabolites of chlorpromazine which have been detected in the urine. Only two principle metabolites, (one which is not therapeutically active) chlorpromazine sulphoxide and 7-hydroxychlorpromazine, retain therapeutic activity.

Combinations of active and inactive metabolites also occur with other antipsychotic drugs. Chlorpromazine induces liver enzymes that tend to enhance or speed up its own metabolism (barbiturates will do the same thing).

Age is an important determinant of the rate of metabolism and excretion of antipsychotic drugs. Morselli[58] points out that the fetus, the infant, and the elderly have diminished capacity to metabolize and eliminate phenothiazines.

The pharmacokinetics of antipsychotic drugs has been reviewed by Morselli,[58] Hollister,[59] May and Van Patten,[60] and Baldessarini.[61]

There is less information about other antipsychotic drugs. For example, Gottschalk[62] reports that thioridazine has similar pharmacokinetic and metabolic properties to those of chlorpromazine. In general the thioxanthenes are similar to chlorpromazine, except that metabolism to sulfoxides is common and ring-hydroxylated products are uncommon.

Haloperidol and other butyrophenones are metabolized by an N-dealkylation reaction. The resultant fragments can be conjugated with glucuronic acid, and it is believed that all of the metabolites of haloperidol are inactive.[63]

### *e. Therapeutic Uses*

The drug is used for many purposes, but the most common are based on its tranquilizing and antiemetic properties. Agitated psychotic and psychoneurotic patients may be calmed and made more receptive to psychotherapy. The drug is also useful in toxic psychosis. The agitation of alcoholics may be controlled with this medication.

As an antiemetic, chlorpromazine is particularly effective against nausea and vomiting induced by certain drugs and by certain disease states. It is not particularly effective in motion sickness; antihistaminics and scopolamine are distinctly superior.

The drug is effective against vomiting caused by narcotics and anesthetics but not against nausea induced by veratrum alkaloids and digitalis. It has been used successfully as an antiemetic in uremia and hyperemesis gravidarum.

The dose of chlorpromazine is usually 25 mg by mouth, three or four times a day. Similar doses may be given parenterally, but precautions must be taken to avoid orthostatic hypotension.

In psychiatric practice, markedly larger doses of chlorpromazine have been used, even several grams a day. This application of the tranquilizers has done much to decrease the patient load in mental hospitals.

In the past, chlorpromazine had been recommended for treating LSD ''bad'' trips or for treatment of drug withdrawal.[64] However, the use of the drug in the abuse area is limited by recent restraints. In this regard, antipsychotic drugs are not useful in the management of withdrawal from opioids, barbiturates, or alcohol, because of the risk of seizures.

Antipsychotic drugs are helpful in certain rare movement disorders such as Gilles de la Tourette's disease and Huntington's chorea.

### *f. Clinical Adverse Effects*

Chlorpromazine is a potentially dangerous drug and it has caused adverse effects of many different types. These include extrapyramidal symptoms, orthostatic hypotension, dryness of mouth, photosensitivity, cholestatic hepatitis, and blood dyscrasias. By its potentiation of other CNS depressants, it can cause adverse effects in patients who are taking such drugs as barbiturates and alcohol. Because of its atropine-like actions, chlorpromazine is contraindicated in patients with glaucoma or prostatic hypertrophy.

(1) *Hypotention*: Hypotension can be marked, particularly when the drug is given parenterally. The orthostatic nature of the hypotensive response is suggested by the observation that it is particularly likely to occur in ambulatory patients. Marked hypotension has been seen in patients who received general anesthesia following chlorpromazine administration.

(2) *Jaundice*: Jaundice has been observed in approximately 2 percent of the patients taking the drug. Surprisingly, liver function studies have shown that this jaundice resembles the obstructive type rather than the hepatocellular type. Apparently the bile canaliculi become edematous and inflamed in these patients, a condition leading to obstructive jaundice. It is believed that this is a peculiar allergic response to the drug, similar to what has been observed following use of arsphenamine and methyltestosterone. The jaundice usually disappears when the drug is discontinued. It has persisted, however, in some cases, and a few patients have died as a consequence of liver failure. Such an outcome is more likely in the presence of preexisting liver damage.

According to the Smith, Kline and French Laboratories,[66] jaundice due to chlorpromazine of the so-called ''obstructive'' type is without parenchymal damage, and is usually promptly reversible upon the withdrawal of chlorpromazine.

(3) *Drug Hypersensitivity*: Hypersensitivity to chlorpromazine may occur. Dermatitis and light sensitization have been reported. Agranulocytosis fortunately is rare.

(4) *Other Toxic Effects*: The potentiation of the action of hypnotics and anesthetics can lead to toxic complications. Gastrointestinal disturbances may develop. In rare cases, gynecomastia

in males and lactation in females have been reported as complications of chlorpromazine therapy.

(5) *Chlorpromazine and Agranulocytosis*: Agranulocytosis, although rare, has been reported in patients on Thorazine therapy. Some investigators believe that patients who show signs of sensitivity (such as fever or rash) may be more susceptible. Patients receiving chlorpromazine should be monitored frequently and asked to report at once a sudden appearance of sore throat or other signs of infection. If white blood counts and differential smears give an indication of cellular depression, the drug should be discontinued, and antibiotic and other suitable therapy instituted.

It is important to note that there is little possibility of chlorpromazine causing agranulocytosis during short-term therapy. Most reported cases have occurred between the fourth and tenth weeks of therapy. Thus patients on prolonged therapy should be observed closely during that period.

A moderate suppression of total white blood cells is sometimes observed in patients on chlorpromazine therapy. If not accompanied by other symptoms, it is not an indication for discontinuing the drug.

(6) *Potentiation*: Chlorpromazine prolongs and intensifies the action of many CNS depressants such as barbiturates, narcotics, and anesthetics. Although this action is usually desirable, certain initial precautions should be followed.

It is advisable to stop administration of such depressants before initiating chlorpromazine therapy. The depressant agents may be reinstated later, starting with low doses, and increasing them according to the response. Approximately one fourth to one half of the usual dosage of such agents is required when they are given in combination with chlorpromazine.

It is important to remember that chlorpromazine does not potentiate the anticonvulsant action of barbiturates.

7. *Extrapyramidal Effects*

The extrapyramidal effects are generally related to the anti-dopaminergic action of the drugs. The therapeutic effects may also come from their anti-dopaminergic action through a site other than the basal ganglia. Thus, it is very difficult and so far not possible to create active psychotic drugs with no side effects of the extrapyramidal type.

In general there are four kinds of extrapyramidal syndromes associated with the use of antipsychotic drugs: a) acute dystonia b) akathisia c) parkinsonian syndrome, and d) tardive dyskinesia.

(a) *Acute dystonia*

This adverse reaction occurs soon after treatment begins, for the most part in young men. It is seen most with butyrophenones and with the piperazine moiety of the phenothiazine group. The prime observable effects include opisthotonus, grimacing, tongue protrusion, torticollis. This clinical picture is so odd that it could easily be mistaken for hedistic behavior. It can be treated with biperiden lactate 2–5 mg. orally or by slow intravenous injection.

(b) *Akathisia*

This is characterized by uncontrollable physical restlessness with an unpleasant feeling of being unable to keep still. This behavior can easily be mistaken for the general symptoms of agitation in psychotic patients. It occurs in the first two weeks of treatment. It is not controlled by antiparkinsonian agents.

(c) *Parkinsonian syndrome*

This frequent side effect is sometimes difficult to distinguish from idiopathic Parkinsonian. It is characterized by akinesia, a lack of associated movements when walking, rigidity, coarse tremor, stooped posture, and gait. This is a rather late side effect which takes about two or more weeks to appear. Sometimes even with reduced antipsychotic therapy or antiparkinsonian drugs, the effect diminishes. It is not recommended to prescribe antiparkinsonian drugs as a prophylactic measure because there are serious side effects with antiparkinsonian drugs, such as acute organic syndrome and increased risk of tardive dyskinesia.

(d) *tardive dyskinesia*

This syndrome is very serious because recovery is difficult. Observable effects include chewing, sucking movements, grimacing, and choreoathetoid movements. It is very common among young people who have taken high doses of antipsychotic drugs for years. Young women who have brain pathology are the greatest risk. Only 50 percent of patients treated by discontinuation of the antipsychotic drugs recover. Autopsies of patients who died with the syndrome revealed the existence of lesions in the substantia nigra.[65] The cause of the syndrome is uncertain but it could be super-sensitivity to dopamine resulting from prolonged dopaminergic blockade.

The use of minimal effective doses of the antipsychotic drugs during long-term therapy and their prompt discontinuation when clinically indicated seem to be the best preventive practice.

(8) *Special Cautions*:

(a) *Hypotensive Effect of Chlorpromazine*. Postural hypotension and simple tachycardia may be noted in some patients. They may experience momentary fainting spells and some dizziness, usually shortly after the first parenteral dose, and occasionally after a subsequent parenteral dose, but rarely following the first oral dose. In most cases, recovery is spontaneous and all symptoms disappear within one-half to two hours with no subsequent ill effects. Occasionally, however, this hypotensive effect may be more severe, and in a few cases it may produce a shock-like condition.

Because of possible hypotensive effects, the patient should be kept under observation (preferably lying down) for some time after the initial parenteral dose. If hypotension does occur, it ordinarily can be controlled by placing the patient in a slight Trendelenburg position. If it is desirable to administer a vasopressor drug, levarterenol (Levophed) and phenylephrine (Neo-Synephrine) are the most suitable. Other pressor agents, including epinephrine, are not recommended because phenothiazine derivatives may reverse the usual elevating action of these agents and cause a further lowering of blood pressure. When the patient's blood pressure has returned to a normal level, chlorpromazine therapy may be resumed, using smaller doses.

In patients with arteriosclerosis, cardiovascular disease, or similar conditions, chlorpromazine should be used with caution. In such patients any sudden change in blood pressure can lead to serious complications of the cardiovascular system.

(b) *Chlorpromazine and Jaundice*. Of the more than 14 million patients who have been treated with chlorpromazine in the United States, the incidence of jaundice regardless of indication, dosage, or mode of administration has been low. In quantitative terms the occurrence of jaundice appears to be related to duration of therapy.

Incidence figures were developed through the statistical analysis of 165 published articles and 21 unpublished studies reporting on the administration of chlorpromazine to a total of 45,000 patients.[66]

(c) *Lactation*. Moderate enlargement of the breast with lactation may occasionally occur in female patients receiving very large doses of chlorpromazine. This, however, is a transitory condition that disappears on reduction of dosage or temporary withdrawal of the drug.

(d) *Contraindications to Chlorpromazine*. Chlorpromazine is contraindicated in comatose states caused by CNS depressants (alcohol, barbiturates, narcotics, and the like), and also in patients under the influence of large amounts of barbiturates or narcotics.

## 2. Other Antipsychotics

### *a. Antiemetic Actions of Phenothiazine Derivatives*

Although the phenothiazines are ineffective in the prevention of motion sickness they are potent in blocking the effect of drugs on the chemoreceptor trigger zone. Thus the antihistaminic and anticholinergic drugs are most widely used for this purpose. For example, the antihistaminic phenothiazine, promethazine (Phenergan), is useful in motion sickness. Drug-induced nausea, nausea following surgical operations, radiation sickness, and some disease states are effectively prevented by phenothiazines.

A list of phenotiazine antiemetics includes: chlorpromazine (Thorazine), fluphenazine dihydrochloride (Prolixin, Permitil), perphenazine (Trilafon), prochlorperazine (Compazine), thiethylperazine (Torecan), and triflupromazine hydrochloride (Vesprin).

### *b. Antipuritic Action of Phenothiazine Derivatives*

The antihistaminic promethazine hydrochloride is a good example of a phenothiazine derivative having the ability to relieve itching of various skin diseases. The phenothiazine Trimeprazine is commonly used as an antipuritic. Generally these antihistaminic phenothiazines can cause drowsiness and induce the previously mentioned toxic reactions.

### *c. Derivatives of Thioxanthene*

The derivatives of thioxanthene such as chlorprothixene (Taracton) and thiothixene (Wavane) are similar chemically and pharmacologically to the phenothiazine derivatives. The structural difference between the thioxanthene drugs and the phenothiazines is that a carbon is substituted for the nitrogen present in the central ring of the phenothiazine.

Chronic schizophrenics who are apathetic can be effectively treated with thiothixene (Navane). The drug is also effective in psychotic conditions in which agitation and anxiety are prominent symptoms.

The drug is available in capsules containing 1, 2, 5, and 10 mg. It is also available in tablets of 10, 25, 50 and 100 mg and in solutions for injection containing 12.5 mg/ml.

### *d. Butyrophenones*

Since 1956, substituted butyrophenones synthesized in Belgium have been used as antipsychotic agents in psychiatry and anesthesiology.[67]

The structure of haloperidol (Haldol), the prototype of this class of drugs, is as follows:

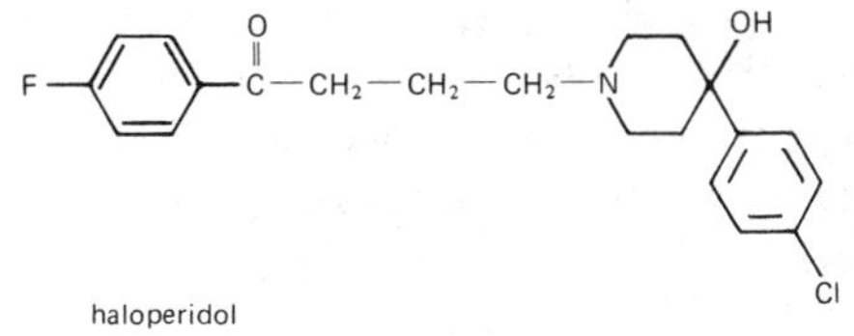

haloperidol

Besides major tranquilizing properties, haloperidol is a potent antiemetic which blocks apomorphine-induced vomiting, probably by actions on the chemoreceptor trigger zone.

Haloperidol, an effective antipsychotic agent like the phenothiazines, induces frequent extrapyramidal reactions. The drug is usually administered to adults in doses of 1 to 2 mg two or three times daily.

Butyrophenones are used in anesthesiology in combination with a potent opiate analgesic. For example, droperidol, in combination with a meperidine-like analgesic (Fentanyl) has been introduced for so-called neuroleptonalgesias under the trade name Innovar.

### 3. Haloperidol: A Butyrophenone Prototype

#### *a. Pharmacologic Actions*

In normal humans, haloperidol is effective both in the treatment of schizophrenia and in the manic phase of manic depressive illness. The presumed mechanism of action of haloperidol and piperazine phenothiazines appears to be similar in that both agents block the effects of dopamine and increase its turnover rate.

#### *b. Brain Effects*

Similar to chlorpromazine, haloperidol induces EEG slowing with an increase in theta waves. The drug also calms and causes sleep in excited patients, an effect less prominent than that of chlorpromazine. Haloperidol lowers convulsive threshold and blocks apomorphine-induced emesis.

#### *c. Autonomic Effects*

Haloperidol possesses little anticholinergic activity but can cause blurring of vision. The drug blocks the activation of alpha receptors by sympathomimetic amines but its autonomic actions are generally less prominent than other antipsychotic drugs such as chlorpromazine.

#### *d. Respiratory and Cardiovascular Actions*

Similar to the phenothiazines, haloperidol potentiates other respiratory depressant drugs. With regard to cardiovascular effects, hypotension occurs with the administration of haloperidol but is less common and severe than that observed with phenothiazines. Tachycardia has been noticed with the use of haloperidol but EEG changes attributable to the drug have not been reported.

#### *e. Effects on Endocrine System*

Haloperidol does not induce weight gain but galactorrhea and other endocrine responses common to the phenothiazines have been observed.

#### *f. Pharmacokinetics and Metabolism*

Peak plasma levels of haloperidol following absorption from the gastrointestinal tract occur within two to six hours and may plateau for as long as 72 hours with persistence of detectable levels for weeks. Approximately 15 percent of a given dose is concentrated in the liver and then excreted in the bile. During the first five days after a single dose, 40 percent is eliminated by the kidneys.

#### *g. Toxicity and Adverse Reactions*

Since haloperidol produces a high incidence of extrapyramidal reactions, especially in younger patients, therapy with this drug should be initiated with caution. Depression as a result of this drug may represent a true side effect or a reversion from a manic state. Side effects from the use of the drug include leukopenia and agranulocytosis. The incidence of jaundice is so low that a casual relationship is hard to establish. It has been suggested that until it is certain that the drug has no teratogenic effect on the fetus,[68] the use of haloperidol in pregnant women should be avoided.

*h. Medical Uses*

Haloperidol is useful in the treatment of psychosis, and for the Gilles de la Tourette syndrome [a neurologic disorder manifested by violent muscular jerks, grimacing, and explosive utterances of foul expletives (corprolalia)].

*i. Alcohol Withdrawal Reactions*

Although there are some reports that recommend haloperidol for the treatment of acute alcohol withdrawal, others[67] indicate the possibility of enhanced convulsions and hyperexcitability following haloperidol therapy, possibly due to the effect of haloperidol on the noradrenergic system.[69] Blum and associates[64] reported enhancement of alcohol withdrawal reactions in mice with haloperidol.

## E. GENERAL SUMMARY ON DRUGS IN THE TREATMENT OF PSYCHOSIS

Cohen[70] points out that it is important to recognize that we have not utilized the neuroleptics to the full extent of their potential. Further, dosage schedules during maintenance are not flexible enough—some patients are overdosed, others are undermedicated. Certainly early identification of side effects remains to be understood, and because the neuroleptics are pharmacologically complex, more skill and thought should be employed in their use.

## F. ANTIANXIETY DRUGS

### 1. Introduction

Substances with useful antianxiety effects are the most frequently prescribed drugs in the United States. For example, the benzodiazepine diazepam (Valium) is the most prescribed drug in the country, with 75 percent of the prescriptions written by nonpsychiatrists. Correct generic terms for this group of agents include antianxiety or anxiolytic; the old term "minor tranquilizers" seems less appropriate. But although the benzodiazepines have unique antianxiety properties, in high doses they share some of the properties of common sedatives.

The diversity of compounds used to treat anxiety greatly complicates attempts to make generalizations about them. Some of the pharmacologic properties are mentioned in Chapter 9, and more extensive reviews on the pharmacology of these drugs, particularly the benzodiazepines, are available.[71,72]

### 2. History[73]

Throughout time, people have sought chemical agents to modify the effects of stress, tension, discomfort, and anxiety. In this regard, some of the agents utilized include ethanol, bromide salts, barbiturates, paraldehyde, and chloral hydrate. By the 1950s great concern about the safety of these drugs led to the development of newer agents such as propanediol carbamates (meprobamate and congeners). This set the scene for the discovery of chlordiazepoxide and other benzodiazepines.

The antianxiety drug market in the United States has resulted in approximately 75 million prescriptions annually at a cost of about $500 million.

### 3. The Benzodiazepines

The following benzodiazepine derivatives are used in the treatment of anxiety: diazepam

(Valium), oxazepam (Seran), flurazepam (Dalmane), chlorazepam (Clonopin), chlorazepate (Tranxene), and chlordiazepoxide (Librium).

The first of the benzodiazepines to be developed was chlordiazepoxide (Librium) in the 1950s. It was found to have excellent muscle relaxant and spinal reflex blocking properties. The successful taming effect on monkeys and wild animals sparked clinical trials in humans. More than 2000 benzodiazepine derivatives have been synthesized so far. Figure 13.1 shows the structures of some select benzodiazepine derivatives used as antianxiety drugs.

### *a. Pharmacology of the Antianxiety Drugs*

The pharmacology of the antianxiety drugs will be discussed here, taking chlordiazepoxide and diazepam as typical representatives of the class.

(1) *General Brain Effects*

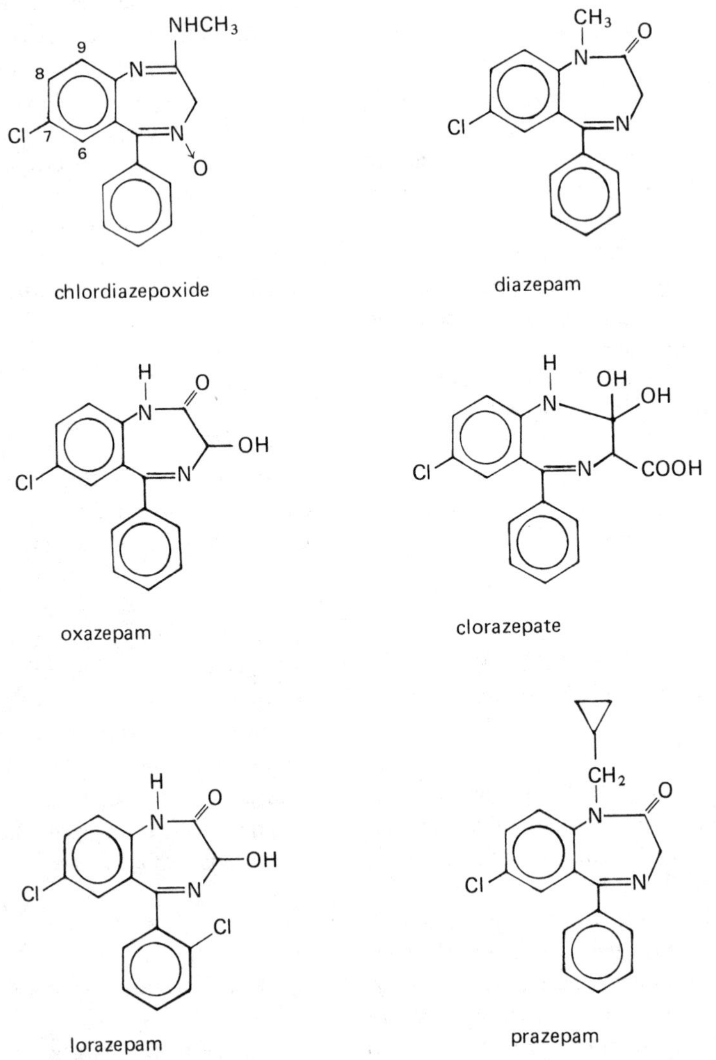

**Figure 13-1**

Generally, benzodiazepines are anxiolytic, sedative, and hypnotic in large doses. They also induce muscle relaxation and are anticonvulsant. Their prime site of action is at the reticular and limbic system, having less effect on the cortex. The above actions seem to be related to their property of potentiating the inhibitory neurotransmitter gamma-aminobutyric acid (GABA), as well as effecting serotonin and dopamine mechanisms.

(2) *Specific Brain Effects*

(a) *Receptorology*—Benzodiazepines interact at specific brain sites or receptors. The evidence accumulated so far shows that benzodiozepine interacts at glycine receptors in the brain: acetylcholine brain receptor, brain, β-adrenergic receptor and certainly the benzodiazepine-GABA receptor complex. The psychophysiological theories of anxiety which point towards potential new directions for research has been detailed by Lader.[74]

(b) *Behavioral pharmacology*. A "conflict test" to assess the anxiolytic effect of drugs was developed by Geller and Seifter,[75] which demonstrate the effectiveness of the benzodiazepines in relieving anxiety. In what is known as the conflict-punishment test, the benzodiazepines markedly reduce the suppressive effects of punishment, while the antipsychotic and the anti-depressant drugs do not show positive effects in these experiments.

(c) *Neurophysiological Actions*. The action of the anxiolytic drugs is somewhat similar to that of the barbiturates. Chlordiazepoxide blocks EEG arousal from stimulation of the brain-stem reticular formation as the barbiturates do. Diazepam and the other benzodiazepine derivatives exhibit their depressant actions on the spinal reflexes partly through the brain-stem reticular system similar to the barbiturates. Chlordiazepoxide depresses the duration of the electric afterdischarge in several regions of the CNS, primarily in the limbic system, septal region, amygdala, hypothalamus, and hippocampus. Many laboratories have reported on the potentiation of the effects of GABA and other inhibitory transmitters in the CNS by the benzodiazepines.[76–78]

(d) *Hypnotic Effects*. The anxiolytic drugs act as hypnotics. Benzodiazepines suppress the deeper phases of sleep, especially stage IV, while increasing the total sleep time. Diazepam is employed in the treatment of "night terrors" that arise out of stage IV sleep.

(e) *Seizure Threshold*. Benzodiazepines increase the seizure threshold and are anticonvulsants. They increase the fast beta activity of the EEG with an increase in amplitude. This effect is also similar to that of the barbiturates.

The antianxiety drugs are widely used in cardiac patients. Generally the cardiovascular effects of benzodiazepines are minimal. It is unlikely that there is significant depression of cardiovascular function when the benzodiazepines are given in usual therapeutic doses by the oral route. However, diazepam in an intravenous dose of 5 to 10 mg., causes a slight decrease in respiration, blood pressure, and left ventricular stroke work. This drug can also increase the heart rate and decrease cardiac output.

(4) *Skeletal Muscle*: Although it is difficult for controlled studies to show an actual advantage in benzodiazepines over either placebos or aspirin, diazepam is widely used as a muscle relaxant.

(5) *Endocrine Function*: Long-term experiments with diazepam in rats revealed no disturbances of endocrine function.

(6) *Lethality*: Oral $LD_{50}$ of diazepam (as an example) is 720 mg./kg. in mice and 1240 mg./kg. in rats. Intraperitoneal administration of 400 mg./kg. to a monkey resulted in death on the sixth day.

(7) *Reproduction Studies*: A series of rat reproduction studies were performed with diazepam, by scientists at Roche Laboratories, in oral doses of 1, 10, 80, and 100 mg./kg. At 100 mg./kg., there was a decrease in the number of pregnancies and survival of offspring Neonatal survival of rats at doses lower than 100 mg./kg. was studied and several of the neonates showed skeletal or other defects. Further studies in rats at doses up to and including 80 mg./kg./day revealed no teratologic effects on the offspring. In humans measurable blood levels of diazepam were obtained in material and cord blood, indicating placental transfer of the drug.

### b. *Pharmacokinetics and Metabolism*

Many of the clinical effects of benzodiazepines can be understood if consideration is given to certain chemical and pharmacokinetic characteristics.

(1) *Chlordiazepoxide*: Chlordiazepoxide is a weak basic substance supplied for clinical use as a water-soluble hydrochloride salt. The drug is unstable, both in solution and when exposed to ultraviolet light. Under these conditions, isomerization to a cyclic 4, 5-oxaziridine occurs. It is noteworthy that this isomer has much less psychopharmacologic activity. Chlordiazepoxide is absorbed relatively slowly following oral administration. In the majority of subjects, peak blood concentrations are reached within four hours of the dose.

In most normal subjects, the half-time is between six and 30 hours. Elderly persons and those with severe hepatic disease probably metabolize the drug more slowly. Demethylation of the 2-methamino side chain yields an initial metabolite, desmethyl chlordiazepoxide, which slowly undergoes oxidative deamination to form a 2-ketone derivative, demoxepam. The psychopharmacologic activity of both metabolites approaches that of chlordiazepoxide. Chlordiazepoxide is, like other benzodiazepines, excreted almost entirely in the urine and in the form of oxidized and glucoronide-conjugated metabolites. Repeated dosage of chlordiazepoxide yields cumulative clinical effects because of its accumulation in the body and its two active metabolites.

(2) *Diazepam*: Diazepam is lipid soluble and water insoluble. Absorption of intramuscular diazepam is slow, incomplete, and erratic. Diazepam, when taken orally, is one of the most rapidly absorbed benzodiazepines, reaching peak concentrations in about an hour in adults, and as quickly as 15 to 30 minutes in children. According to Baldessarini,[2] this property may largely account for the euphoriant or intoxicating effect of large doses of diazepam that contribute to its popularity as a "street drug."

Metabolism of diazepam proceeds slowly, with a half-life of between 20 and 40 hours in most subjects, but as long as 50 hours in others. The major metabolic produce, desmethydiazepam, is formed by removal of the N-1 methyl group. This substance is biologically active and is biotransformed even more slowly than diazepam. Repeated dosage of diazepam leads to accumulation of diazepam and desmethyldiazepam in plasma. In fact, steady-state concentrations are usually reached after five to ten days of therapy. A clinically relevant fact is that the distributive (alpha) half-life of diazepam is about 2.5 hours, whereas the elimination (beta) half-time is initially about 1.5 days, and even longer after prolonged treatment.

(3) *Oxazepam*: Oxazepam is slowly absorbed following oral administration. Biotransformation is facilitated by the 3-hydroxy substitution. The compound is directly conjugated with glucuronide and excreted in the urine. No metabolic intermediates have been identified in human beings. Biotransformation half-times in "normal" individuals range between three and 21 hours. Cumulative effects during chronic therapy are much less important than with chlordiazepoxide or diazepam because of the formation of inactive metabolic products.

(4) *Flurazepam*: Flurazepam is supplied as a water-soluble dihydrochloride salt for oral administration only. It is very rapidly metabolized by degradation and removal of the N-1 side-chain. Its N-1 unsubstituted analog is biologically active and undergoes slow biotransformation with a half-time of between 50 and 100 hours. Thus this metabolite leads to cumulative clinical effects.

(5) *Chlorazepate*: The drug is very rapidly hydrolized to the N-1 demethylated analog of diazepam. Since desmethyldiazepam is slowly biotransformed in humans, long-lasting cumulative effects occur with clorazepate treatment.

Additional information about the pharmacokinetic properties at metabolism of the benzodiazepines is given by Garattini and associates,[73] Greenblatt and Shader,[79] and Hollister.[59]

### c. *Tolerance and Addiction*

Benzodiazepines are prone to be habituated. They exhibit marked withdrawal symptoms similar to those observed with barbiturates and alcohol. Abdominal cramps, vomitings, insomnia, sweating, convulsions, and tremor have been observed following abrupt withdrawal of diazepam. However, according to Allquander,[80] the benzodiazepines must be administered in high doses for long periods for withdrawal symptoms, including seizures, to occur. Particular attention has to be paid to the potential of some individuals to become addicted to the use of benzodiazepines, due to a predisposition to such a dependence. There is growing concern over the tendency of benzodiazepines to cause a high incidence of dependence.[81–85]

### *d. The Abuse of Benzodiazepines*

For the past ten years, diazepam (Valium) has been used in the drug subculture to treat complications of illicit drug use. Psychedelic drug takers generally have a few tablets around in case of a "bummer." A speed freak might keep a "stash" of Valium to ease the "crash" at the end of an amphetamine binge.

Diazepam alone, in doses of 100 to 500 mg, produces an intoxicated high.[84] When compared with its level of medical use, the misuse/abuse of Valium appears to be of the same magnitude as other common sedative drugs.

### *e. Toxicity and Side Effects*

The anxiolytic effects of diazepam start at a blood concentration of about 500 ng/ml (nanograms per milliliter) and the gross CNS intoxication occurs at a concentration of about 900–1000 ng/ml.[58] Chlordiazepoxide causes intoxication at about the same concentrations. The possible side reactions of the antianxiety drugs are nothing but extensions of their pharmacologic actions. All the benzodiazepines (with the exception of oxazepam) increase hostility and irritability in patients and cause disturbing dreams. In older patients reversible confusional states are observed as a result of the use of all kinds of sedatives, including the benzodiazepines.

### *f. Clinical Aspects of Benzodiazepines*

Diazepam (Valium) and chlordiazepoxide (Librium) are important psychoactive products that are offered to approximately one in five adults in the United States.

(1) *Therapeutic Indications*: Diazepam (Valium) is useful in the symptomatic relief of tension and anxiety states resulting from stressful circumstances or somatic complaints that are concomitants of emotional factors. It is of value in psychoneurotic states manifested by tension, anxiety, apprehension, fatigue, depressive symptoms, or agitation.

In acute alcohol withdrawal, diazepam may be useful in the symptomatic relief of acute agitation, tremor, impending or acute delirium tremens, and hallucinosis. It is also utilized as an adjunct in the relief of skeletal muscle spasm caused by reflex to local pathology (such as inflammation of the muscles or joints, or secondary to trauma); spasticity caused by upper motor neuron disorders (such as cerebral palsy and paraplegia); athetosis; and stiff-man syndrome. Oral Valium may be employed adjunctively in convulsive disorders, although it has not proved useful as the sole therapy.

(2) *Adverse Reactions*: Side effects most commonly reported are drowsiness, fatigue, and ataxia; sometimes though infrequently encountered are confusion, constipation, depression, diplopia, dysartria, headache, hypotension, incontinence, jaundice, changes in libido, nausea, changes in salivation, skin rash, slurred speech, tremor, urinary retention, vertigo, and blurred vision. Paradoxic reactions such as acute hyperexcited states, anxiety, hallucinations, increased muscle spasticity, insomnia, rage, sleep disturbances, and stimulation have been reported. If any of these should occur, use of the drug should be discontinued.

Because of isolated reports of neutropenia and jaundice, periodic blood counts and liver function tests are advisable during long-term therapy. Minor changes in EEG patterns, usually low-voltage fast activity, have been observed in patients during and after diazepam (Valium) therapy but are not considered significant.

Among the other toxic reactions seen with chlordiazepoxide are agranulocytosis (rarely) and women failing to ovulate.

(3) *Usage in Pregnancy*: An increased risk of congenital malformations associated with the use of minor tranquilizers (diazepam, meprobamate, and chlordiazepoxide) during the first

trimester of pregnancy has been suggested in several studies. Thus, because such use is rarely a matter of urgency, it almost always should be avoided. The possibility that a woman of child-bearing potential may be pregnant at the time of institution of therapy should be considered. Patients who become pregnant during therapy, or intend to become pregnant, should be advised to ask their physicians about potential dangers of continuing the drug.

(4) *Teratogenic Effects*: Important reviews considering the teratogenic effects of benzodiazepines have been written.[86,87] There may be a slight increase in the risk of midline cleft deformities of the lip or palate.

(5) *Management of Overdosage*: A few deaths have been reported with doses of diazepam or chlordiazepoxide greater than 700 mg. The striking advantage of this group of drugs is the remarkable margin of safety.

Manifestations of diazepam overdosage include somnolence, confusion, coma, and diminished reflexes. Although these effects are rare, respiration, pulse, and blood pressure should be monitored, as in all cases of drug overdosage. General supportive measures should be employed, along with immediate gastric lavage. Intravenous fluids should be administered and an adequate airway maintained. Hypotension may be combated by the use of levarterenol (Levophed) or metaaminol (Aramine). Methylphenidate (Ritalin) or caffeine and sodium benzoate may be given to combat CNS-depressive effects. Dialysis is of limited value. As with the management of intentional overdosage with any drug, it should be recognized that multiple agents may have been ingested.

(6) *Effect of Other Drugs on Benzodiazepines*. Interactions of benzodiazepine with other drugs are usually not significant. However, if diazepam is to be combined with other psychotropic agents or anticonvulsant drugs, careful consideration must be given to the pharmacology of the agents to be employed, particularly in compounds that may potentiate the action of diazepam, such as phenothiazines, narcotics, barbiturates, MAO inhibitors, and other antidepressants. The usual precautions are indicated for severely depressed patients or those in whom there is evidence of latent depression. Recognition of suicidal tendencies is especially important as protective measures may be necessary. The standard precautions in treating patients with impaired renal or hepatic function should be observed.

### g. *Current Biochemical Research on Benzodiazepines*

In 1979, 62.3 million prescriptions for antianxiety drugs were filled (National Prescription Audit, 1979). Because of the sheer volume of traffic in these drugs, their potential for misuse and abuse, and the public health problem created by them, numerous important research reports have appeared in the literature.

Biochemical research on benzodiazepine receptors in the brain and their relation to neurotransmitter mechanisms has rapidly become one of the most active areas of psychopharmacology.

The high-affinity and stereospecific binding sites for benzodiazepines in the brain seem to represent the places where benzodiazepines exert their pharmacologic effects. This concept is based upon the high degree of correlation between the ability of an extensive series of benzodiazepines to displace binding of ($^3$H) diazepam from the high-affinity sites in the brain and their activity in a number of behavioral tests, including conflict muscle relaxant and anticonvulsant tests.[88] One of the most potent benzodiazepines is clorazepam, 5-(0-chloropenyl)-1, 3-dihydro-7-nitro-2H-1, 4-benzodiazepine-2-1. It is also a potent displacer of ($^3$H) diazepam binding to brain specific sites.[89]

Initial investigations of the binding of ($^3$H) diazepam indicated that specific high-affinity binding of ($^3$H) diazepam could be obtained not only to the brain, but also to several peripheral tissues, including kidney.[90]

In addition to the distinction between peripheral and central receptors, some investigators have examined the possibility of multiple central sites based on thermostability studies.[91] The literature reveals that two such sites exist in cerebral cortex and one in cerebellum.

At the receptor level, chronic (several weeks, not months) administration of high doses of benaodiazepines leads to a modest decrease in the apparent number of binding sites in brain.[92,93]

One study disagrees with this finding, however.[94]

In a study combining the electron microscopic autoradiographic localization of benzodiazepine receptors and the immunocytochemical localization of glutamic decarboxylase, it was found that a large fraction of benzodiazepine receptors was associated with GABAergic terminals. On this level benzodiazepine drugs have a profound effect on GABAergic transmission.[78]

As a class, the benzodiazepines are able to maintain their behavior on self-administration but do not appear to be as strong in this regard as other classic drugs of abuse, such as cocaine and pentobarbital. The conclusion is that although there are a number of reports describing human abuse of these drugs, the abuse liability of benzodiazepines is generally considered to be relatively low.[96]

The pharmacokinetic properties of most benzodiazepines (i.e., a long half-life, active metabolites, accumulation in the blood and tissues, and anticonvulsant properties) may help to explain why they are only rarely associated with serious withdrawal phenomena and have a low dependency-producing potential.

The implication of the receptor theory is that human beings must have a built-in calming and anticonvulsive chemical substance that is an endogenous ligand that has not yet been discovered. We can speculate that such ligands are suppressed during benzodiazepine treatment. Consequently the abrupt discontinuation of long-term treatment may not allow for the immediate availability of enough endogenous ligands to replace the benzodiazepines at the receptor sites.

## G. GENERAL COMMENTS ON ANTIANXIETY AGENTS

Dependence is probably less frequent with the current use of benzodiazepines than was the case when barbiturates were the primary sedative-hypnotic drugs, although it still occurs in the context of other types of drug abuse. The withdrawal syndrome produced by most of these drugs is mild and attenuated, and seldom leads to any serious consequences. Most reports of physical dependence on benzodiazepines involve diazepam or chlordiazepoxide, a proportion that reflects the extent of their use. The short-acting derivatives, oxazepam and chlorazepam, produce a similar withdrawal reaction. According to Hollister,[96] benzodiazepine dependence is an avoidable problem.

## REFERENCES


1. Cooper, I.S. (Editor) *Symposium. Cerebellar Stimulation in Man.* New York: Raven Press, 1978.
2. Baldessarini, R. J. Drugs and the treatment of psychiatric disorders. In A. G. Gilman, L. S. Goodman, and A. Gilman, eds., *The Pharmacological Basis of Therapeutics*, 6th ed. New York: Macmillan, 1980, pp. 391–447.
3. Efron, D. H., Holmstedt, B., and Kline, N. S. (Editors) *Ethnopharmacologic Search for Psychoactive Drugs.* Public Health Service Publication no. 67-1645. Washington, D.C.: U.S. Government Printing Office, 1967.
4. Caldwell, A. E. History of psychopharmacology. In W. G. Clar and J. del Guidice, eds., *Principles of Psychopharmacology*, 2nd ed. New York: Academic Press, 1978, pp. 4–40.
5. Schultes, R. E. Ethnopharmacological significance of psychotropic drugs of begetal origin. In W. G. Clark and J. del Guidice, eds., *Principles of Psychopharmacology*, 2nd ed. New York: Academic Press, 1978, pp. 41–70.
6. Sen, G., and Bose, K. L. *Rauwolfia serpentina*, a new Indian drug for insanity and high blood pressure. *Indian Med. World* 2:194, 1931.
7. Cade, J. F. J. Lithium salts in the treatment of psychotic excitement. *Med. J. Aust.* 2:249, 1949.
8. Delay, J., and Deniker, P. Trente-huit cas de psychoses traitees par la cure prolongee et coutinue de 4560 RP. Le Congres des Al. et Neurol. de Langue Fr. In *Compte Rendu du Congres.* Paris: Masson et Cie, 1952.
9. Berger, F. M. The pharmacological properties of 2-methyl-2-N-propyl-1, 3 propanediol dicarbonate (Miltown), a new interncuronal blocking agent. *J. Pharmacol. Exp. Ther.* 112:413, 1954.
10. Sternbach, L. H. Chemistry of 1, 5-benzodiazepines and some aspects of the structure-activity relationship. In S. Garattini, E. Mussini, and L. O. Randall, eds., *The Benzodiazepines.* New York: Raven Press, 1973, pp. 1–20.
11. Jansen, P. A. Butyrophenones and diphenyl bu-

tyrophenones. In M. Gordon, ed., *Psychopharmacological Agents*, vol. 3. New York: Academic Press, 1974, pp. 128–158.

12. Barchas, J. D., et al. The biochemistry of affective disorders and schizophrenia. In W. G. Clark and J. del Guidice, eds., *Principles of Psychopharmacology*, 2nd ed. New York: Academic Press, 1978, pp. 105–132.
13. Schildkraut, J. J. The catecholamine hypothesis of affective disorders: A review of the supporting evidence. *Am. J. Psychiatry* 122:509, 1965.
14. Kiev, A. Depression as a treatable illness, part II. *Drug Ther.* 1975.
15. Blum, K., et al. Possible rationale for differential chemotherapy of depression in humans: A review on the biogenic amine hypothesis, part I. *J. Psychedel. Drugs* 8(3):223, 1976.
16. Squires, R., and Brestrup, C. Benzodiazepine receptors in rat brain. *Nature* 266:732, 1977.
17. Mohler, H., and Okada, T. Benzodiazepine receptor: Demonstration in the central nervous system. *Science* 198:849, 1977.
18. Gardos, G., and Cole, J. O. Maintenance antipsychotic therapy: Is the cure worse than the disease? *Am. J. Psychiatry* 133:32, 1976.
19. Brooks, G. W. Withdrawal from neuroleptic drugs. *Am. J. Psychiatry* 115:931, 1959.
20. Fielding, S., and Lal, H. Behavioral actions of neuroleptics. In L. L. Iversen, S. D. Iversen, and S. H. Snyder, eds., *Handbook of Psychopharmacology*, vol. 10. New York: Plenum Press, 1978, pp. 91–128.
21. Baldessarini, R. J., and Tarsy, D. Tardive dyskinesia. In M. A. Lipton, A. DiMascio, and K. F. Killam, eds., *Psychopharmacology: A Generation of Progress*. New York: Raven Press, 1978, pp. 993–1004.
22. Jacobson, G., Baldessarini, R. J., and Manschreck, T. Tardive and withdrawal dyskinesia associated with haloperidol. *Am. J. Psychiatry* 131:910, 1974.
23. Fink, M. EEG and human psychopharmacology. *Ann. Rev. Pharmacol.* 9:241, 1969.
24. Longo, V. G. Effects of psychotropic drugs on the EEG of animals. In W. G. Clark, and J. del Guidice, eds., *Principles of Psychopharmacology*, 2nd ed. New York: Academic Press, 1978, pp. 247–260.
25. Shagass, C., and Straumanis, J. J. Drugs and human sensory evoked potentials. In M. A. Lipton, A. DiMascio, and K. F. Killem, eds., *Psychopharmacology: A Generation of Progress*. New York: Raven Press, 1978, pp. 699–709.
26. Itil, T. M. Effects of psychotropic drugs on qualitatively and quantitatively analyzed human EEG. In W. G. Clark and J. del. Guidice, eds., *Principles of Psychopharmacology*, 2nd ed. New York: Academic Press, 1978, pp. 261–277.
27. Kalabian, J. W., Petzold, G. L., and Greengard, P. Dopamine-sensitive adenylate cyclase in caudate nucleus of rat brain, and its similarity to the "dopamine receptor." *Proc. Nat. Acad. Sci. U.S.A.* 69:2145, 1972.
28. Garelis, E., and Neff, H. H. Cyclic adenosine monophosphate: Selective increase in caudate nucleus after administration of L-dopa. *Science* 183:532, 1974.
29. Christie, J. E., and Crow, T. J. Turning behaviour as an index of the action of amphetamines and ephedrines on central dopamine-containing neurones. *Br. J. Pharmacol.* 43:658, 1971.
30. Greengard, P. *Cyclic Nucleotides, Phosphorylated Proteins, and Neuronal Functions*. New York: Raven Press, 1978, pp. 25–37.
31. Snyder, S. H., U'Pritchard, D., and Greenberg, D. A. Neurotransmitter receptor finding in the brain. In M. A. Lipton, A. DiMascio, and K. F. Killam, eds., *Psychopharmacology: A Generation of Progress*. New York: Raven Press, 1978, pp. 361–370.
32. Baldessarini, R. J. Schizophrenia. *N. Engl. J. Med.* 297:988, 1977.
33. Martin, J. B. Neural regulations of growth hormone secretion. *N. Engl. J. Med.* 288:1384, 1973.
34. Frohman, L. A. Clinical neuropharmacology of hypothalamic releasing factors. *N. Engl. J. Med.* 286:1391, 1972.
35. Martin, J. B., et al. Neuroendocrine organization of growth hormone regulation. In S. Reichlin, and J. B. Martin, eds., *The Hypothalamus*. Association for Research in Nervous and Mental Disease Publications, vol. 56. New York: Raven Press, 1978, pp. 329–357.
36. Sachar, E. J. Neuroendocrine responses to psychotropic drugs. In M. A. Lipton, A. DiMascio, and K. F. Killam, eds., *Psychopharmacology: A Generation of Progress*. New York: Raven Press, 1978, pp. 499–507.
37. Overall, J. E. Prior psychiatric treatment and the development of breast cancer. *Arch. Gen. Psychiatr.* 35:898, 1978.
38. Anden, N. E. Dopamine turnover in the corpus striatum and the limbic system after treatment with neuroleptic and antiacetylcholine drugs. *J. Pharm. Pharmacol.* 24:905, 1972.
39. Clement-Cormier, Y. C., et al. Dopamine-sensitive adenylate cyclase in mamalian brain: A possible site of action of antipsychotic drugs. *Proc. Natl. Acad. Sci. U.S.A.* 71:1113, 1974.

40. Snyder, S. H., et al. Drugs, neurotransmitters, and schizophrenia. *Science* 184:1243, 1974.
41. Barchas, J. D., et al. The biochemistry of affective disorders and schizophrenia. In W. G. Clark and J. del Guidice, eds., *Principles of Psychopharmacology*, 2nd ed. New York: Academic Press, 1978, pp. 105–132.
42. Carlsson, A. Mechanism of action of neuroleptic drugs. In M. A. Lipton, A. DiMascio, and K. F. Killam, eds., *Psychopharmacology: A Generation of Progress*. New York: Raven Press, 1978, pp. 1057–1070.
43. Dobkin, A. B., Gilber, R. G. B., and Lamoureu, L. Physiological effects of chlorpromazine. *Anaesthesia* 9:157, 1954.
44. Killam, K. F. and Killam, E. K. Drug action on pathways involving the reticular formation. In H. H. Jasper, et al., eds., *Reticular Formation of the Brain*. Boston: Little Brown, 1958, p. 111.
45. Creese, I., Burt, D., and Snyder, S. H. Biochemical actions of neuroleptic drugs: Focus on dopamine receptor. In L. L. Iversen, S. D. Iversen, and S. H. Snyder, eds., *Handbook of Psychopharmacology*, vol. 10. New York: Plenum Press, 1978, pp. 37–89.
46. Gordon, M. *Psychopharmacological Agents*, vol. II. New York: Academic Press, 1976.
47. Sigg, E. B. Autonomic side-effects induced by psychotherapeutic agents. In D. H. Efron, J. O. Cole, J. Levine, and J. R. Wittenborn, eds., *Psychopharmacology: A Review of Progress, 1957-1967*. Public Health Service Publication no. 1836. Washington, D.C.: U.S. Government Printing Office, 1968, p. 581.
48. Klein, D. F., and Davis, J. M. *Diagnosis and Drug Treatment of Psychiatric Disorders*. Baltimore: Williams & Wilkins, 1969.
49. Shader, R. I., and DiMascio, A. *Psychotropic Drug Side Effects: Clinical and Theoretical Perspectives*. Baltimore: Williams & Wilkins, 1970.
50. Schyve, P. M., Smithline, F., and Meltzer, H. Y. Neuroleptic-induced prolactin level elevation and breast cancer: An emerging issue. *Arch. Gen. Psychiatr.* 35:1291, 1978.
51. Erle, G., et al. Effects of chlorpromazine on blood glucose and plasma insulin in man. *Eur. J. Clin. Pharmacol.* 11:15, 1977.
52. Dimond, R. C., et al. Chlorpromazine treatment and growth hormone secretory responses in acromegaly. *J. Clin. Endocrinol. Metab.* 36:1189, 1973.
53. Kety, S. S. Toward hypotheses for a biochemical component in the vulnerability to schizophrenia. *Sem. Psychol.* 4:233, 1972.
54. Lasagna, L., and McLaun, W. Effect of tranquilzing drugs on amphetamine toxicity in aggregated mice. *Science* 125:1241, 1957.
55. Glaviano, V. V., and Wang, S. C. Dual mechanism of the anticuretic action of chlorpromazine. *Fed. Proc.* 13:358, 1954.
56. Dasgupta, S. R., and Weaver, C. Inhibition of hypothalamic medullary and reflex vasomotor responses by chlorpromazine. *Br. J. Pharmacol.* 9:389, 1954.
57. Sulser, F., and Robinson, S. E. Clinical implications of pharmacological differences among antipsychotic drugs. In M. A. Lipton, A. DiMascio, and K. F. Killam, eds., *Psychopharmacology: A Generation of Progress*. New York: Raven Press, 1978, pp. 943–954.
58. Morselli, P. L. Psychotropic drugs. In P. L. Morselli, ed., *Drug Disposition During Development*. New York: Spectrum Publications, 1977, pp. 431–474.
59. Hollister, L. E. *Clinical Pharmacology of Psychotherapeutic Agents*. New York: Churchill-Livingstone, 1978.
60. May, P. R. A., and Van Putten, T. Plasma levels of chlorpromazine in schizophrenia: A critical review of the literature. *Arch. Gen. Psychiatr.* 35:1081, 1978.
61. Baldessarini, R. J. Status of psychotropic drug blood level assays and other biochemical measurements in clinical practice. *Am. J. Psychiatry* 136:1177, 1979.
62. Gottschalk, L. A. Pharmacokinetics of the minor tranquilizers and clinical response. In M. A. Lipton, A. DiMascio, and K. F. Killam, eds., *Psychopharmacology: A Generation of Progress*. New York: Raven Press, 1978, pp. 975–185.
63. Forsman, A., and Ohman, R. On the pharmacokinetics of haloperidol. *Nord. Psykiatr. Tidskr.* 28:441, 1974.
64. Blum, K., et al. Enhancement of alcohol withdrawal reactions in mice by haloperidol. *Clin. Toxicol.* 1975.
65. Chriastiansen, E., Moller, J. E., and Eaurbye, A. Neuropathological investigation of 28 brains from patients with dyskinesia. *Acta Psychiatr. Neurol. Scand.* 46:14, 1970.
66. *An Introduction to Three Phenothiazine Derivatives*. Philadelphia: Smith, Kline, and French Laboratories, undated.
67. Detre, T. P., and Jarecki, H. C. *Modern Psychiatric Treatment*. Philadelphia: Lippincott, 1971.
68. Kopelman, A. E., McCullar, F. W., and Heggeness, L. Limb malformations following maternal use of haloperidol. *JAMA* 231:62, 1975.

69. Iversen, L. L. Inhibition of norepinephrine uptake by drugs. *J. Pharm. Pharmacol.* 17:62, 1965.
70. Cohen, S. *The Substance Abuse Problems*. New York: Haworth Press, 1981, p. 141.
71. Greenblatt, D. J., and Shader, R. I. *Benzodiazepines in Medical Practice*. New York: Raven Press, 1973.
72. Baldessarini, R. J. *Chemotherapy in Psychiatry*. Cambridge, Mass.: Harvard University Press, 1977.
73. Garattini, S., Mussini, E., and Randall, L. O. (Editors) *The Benzodiazepines*. New York: Raven Press, 1973.
74. Lader, M. Current Psychophysical Theories of Anxiety. In M. A. Lipton, A. DiMascio, and K. F. Killam, eds., *Psychopharmacology: A Generation of Progress*. Raven Press, New York, 1978, p. 1375.
75. Geller, I., and Seifter, J. The effects of meprobamate, barbiturates, amphetamine and promazine on experimentally induced conflict in the rat. *Psychopharmacogia* 1:482, 1960.
76. Bloom, F. E. Neural mechanisms of benzodiazepine actions. *Am. J. Psychiatry* 134:669, 1977.
77. Iversen, L. L. Biochemical psychopharmacology of GABA. In M. A. Lipton, A. DiMascio, and K. F. Killam, eds., *Psychopharmacology: A Generation of Progress*. New York: Raven Press, 1978, pp. 25–38.
78. Tallman, J. F., et al. Receptors for the age of anxiety: Pharmacology of the benzodiazepines. *Science* 207:274, 1980.
79. Greenblatt, D. J., and Shader, R. I. Benzodiazepines. *N. Engl. J. Med.* 291(19):1011, 1974.
80. Allquander, C. Dependence on sedative and hypnotic drugs. *Acta Psychiatr. Scand.* 270:1(suppl.), 1978.
81. Bindeglas, P. M. Valium addiction (?) (Questions and Answers). *Drug Ther.* 8:141, 1975.
82. Fink, Knolt, and Beard, Sedative-hypnotic dependence. *Am. Fam. Phys.* 10:115, 1974.
83. Kantman, A., and Brikner, P. Tranquilizer control (letter). *JAMA* 224:1, 1973.
84. Patch, V. D. The dangers of diazepam. A street drug. *N. Engl. J. Med.* 190:807, 1974.
85. Dysken, M. W., and Chan, C. H. Diazepam withdrawal psychosis. A case report. *Am. J. Psychiatry* 134:5, 1977.
86. Safra, J. J., and Oakley, G. P., Jr. Association between cleft lip with or without cleft palate and prenatal exposure to diazepam. *Lancet* 2:478, 1975.
87. Goldberg, H. L., and DiMascio, A. Psychotropic drugs in pregnancy. In M. A. Lipton, A. DiMascio, and K. F. Killam, eds., *Psychopharmacology: A Generation of Progress*. New York: Raven Press, 1978, pp. 1047–1055.
88. Braestrup, C. Brain specific benzodiazepine receptors. *Br. J. Psychiatr.* 133:249, 1978.
89. Braestrup, C., and Squires, R. F. Specific benzodiazepine receptors in rat brain characterized by high affinity (diazepam H-3) binding (affinity binding, anxiolytic activity, brain membrane regional distribution). *Proc. Nat. Acad. Sci.* 74:3805, 1977.
90. Braestrup, C., Albecht, R., and Squires, R. F. High densities of benzodiazepine receptors in human cortical areas. *Nature* 269:702, 1977.
91. Squires, R. F., et al. Some properties of brain specific benzodiazepine receptors—New evidence for multiple receptors. *Pharmacol. Biochem. Behav.* 10(2):825, 1979.
92. Chiu, T. H., and Rosenberg, H. Reduced diazepam binding following chronic benzodiazepine treatment. *Life Sci.* 23:1153, 1978.
93. Rosenberg, H., and Chiu, T. H. Decreased diazepam $H^3$ binding is a specific response to chronic benzodiazepine treatment. *Life Sci.* 24:803, 1979.
94. Mohler, H., Okada, T., and Enna, S. J. Benzodiazepine and neurotransmitter receptor binding in rat brain after chronic administration of diazepam or phenobarbital. *Brain Res.* 156:391, 1978.
95. Tick, M. K., and Davis, W. C. Effect of valproic acid on [$^3$H] diazepam and [$^3$H] dihydropicrotoxinin binding sites at the benzodiazepine-GABA receptor-ionophore complex. *Brain Res.* 223:218, 1981.
96. Hollister, L. E. Dependence on benzodiazepines. In *Benzodiazepines: A Review of Research Results, 1980*. NIDA Research Monograph no. 33, U.S. Department of Health and Human Services. Washington, D.C.: U.S. Government Printing Office, 1981, p. 840.

# Chapter 14

# Antidepressants and Antimania Drugs (Mood Elevators and Stabilizers)

## A. INTRODUCTION

In this chapter, we deal with the drugs that are used in treating two important affective disorders—depression and mania.

The most common mental disorder is "depression," which is a manifestation of worry, sadness, and pessimism. In the United States about four million people annually undergo treatment for mental depression. The drugs used for its treatment are usually the MAO (monoamine oxidase) inhibitors such as phenelzine and the triaydic antidepressants such as the dibenzazepines and dibenzocycloheptadiene derivatives.

The second affective disorder is mania, or hyperactivity of mind. It is a manifestation of uncontrolled thought and speech caused by abnormal changes of mind. The drugs used for the treatment of mania are a combination of the antipsychotic drugs and lithium carbonate.

Depression is broadly classified into two types: exogenous or reactive depression and endogenous or regressive depression. Exogenous depression is caused by external disturbing factors such as the death of a loved one, loss of job, or a major illness. Endogenous depression is not related to any significant external event but is caused by regression, inactivity, and inborn psychotic disorders. Sometimes mania accompanies depression (in which case it is called manic depression).

The more frequent symptoms of depression are anguished facial expressions and soft speech manifested by fear and despondency. Symptoms such as feelings of inferiority, unworthiness, and suicide are less frequent but significant.

According to Hussan,[1] depressive symptoms are mild in some and often self-limited; however, others with more severe problems such as delusions of guilt, hallucinations, and suicidal tendencies require prompt treatment. Depression is often cyclic—nondepressed periods alternating with periods of depression. Therefore, it cannot be assumed that successful control of acute symptoms has "cured" the condition inasmuch as relapses are common.

## B. ANTIDEPRESSANT AND ANTIMANIC DRUGS

Antidepressant drugs have therapeutic benefits in disorders of mood or depressive illness, but they do not have instant mood-stimulatory effects of the kind produced by dextroamphetamine. In this chapter monoamine oxidase inhibitors are considered first, followed by trycyclic antidepressants and then lithium.

The treatment of depression with drugs is a somewhat controversial issue. The MAO inhibitors were introduced as the first antidepressants. Iproniazid was soon replaced by somewhat less toxic MAO inhibitors such as phenelzine (Nardil), isocarboxazid (Marplan), nialamide (Niamid), and tranylcypromine (Parnate).

The tricyclic antidepressant imipramine (Tofranil) was discovered accidentally during clinical testing of antipsychotic drugs. It was followed by related drugs such as amitriptyline (Elavil) and protriptyline (Vivactil) and their demethylated metabolites, such as desipramine (Pertofrane) and nortriptyline (Aventyl).

In addition to these groups of antidepressants, sympathomimetic drugs, such as dextroamphetamine (Dexedrine) and methylphenidate (Ritalin), are still used occasionally in depressed patients.[2]

The mechanism of action of all of these drugs is attributed to the catecholamine hypothesis. The various antidepressants increase the catecholamines in the central nervous system. Thus the MAO inhibitors increase the concentration of catecholamines in the brain, whereas the tricyclic antidepressants interfere with the catecholamine reuptake after its release from nerve endings. Finally, the sympathomimetic amines such as dextroamphetamine release catecholamines and may act directly on central catecholamine receptors.

Blum[3] reviewed the biogenic amine hypothesis and also discussed the relationship between catecholamines and serotonin in the affective disorders. Physicians and staff in drug programs are referred to this article for clarification of this important subject, especially as it relates to drug-induced therapy: postmethadone depression, heroin depression, amphetamine depression, etc.

## C. TYPES OF ANTIDEPRESSANTS

### 1. Monoamine Oxidase Inhibitors

As a class of drugs, the MAOI have the ability to block deamination of naturally occurring monoamines. Although MAOI's have been used in psychiatry, its risk/benefit ratio is still being questioned. There is little argument that these drugs are anxiolytic but they may only be weak antidepressants. In fact, an antidepressant action has not been proved conclusively. Indeed, reported relief from patients may be due simply to their anxiolytic rather than to their antidepressant action.

Among the many disadvantages of the MAOI's are: a) slow action b) hepatoxicity c) over-stimulation d) postural hypotension e) insomnia f) weight gain g) constipation h) paradoxical behavior, and i) inducing severe toxic reactions in combination with other drugs and food-derived amines.[4,5] These interactions are serious enough to not use monoamine oxidase inhibitors as the first drug of choice to treat depression. Thus, MAOI's are used when tricyclic antidepressants give an unsatisfactory result and when electric convulsive shock therapy (ECT) is refused.

#### *a. History:*[6,7]

The antidepressant effect of *Iproniazid (marsilid)*, which was synthesized in 1951 as a chemotherapeutic agent for tuberculosis, was initially observed in tuberculous patients. It was observed that patients receiving this drug became energized and hyperactive.[6] Others found that iproniazid (Isopropyl isoniazid) was capable of inhibiting the enzyme MAO.[7] Following the initial double blind studies by Klein and

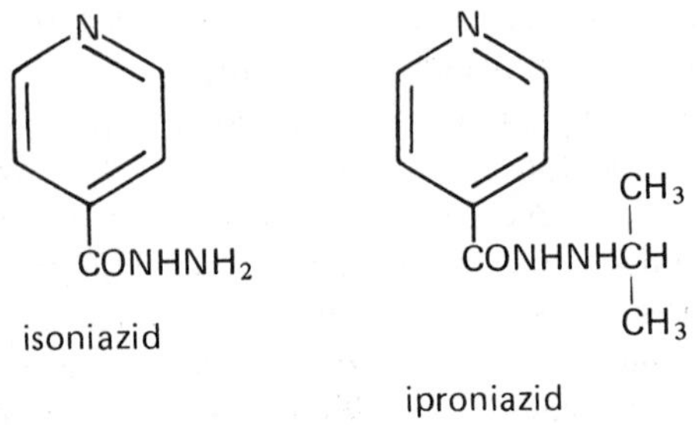

**Figure 14-1.**

associates, which yielded encouraging results, the drug has been employed in psychiatry as a potential mood elevator.[5] Some of the earlier MAOI commercially available—because of severe hepatocellular damage, including ipromiazid—have been withdrawn from the U.S. marketplace. The most feared adverse effect of these drugs was their ability to produce a hypertensive reaction which could result in a cerebrovascular accident.

### *b. Chemistry of MAO Inhibitors*

Biel and associates[8] reviewed the chemistry and structural-activity relationship of a series of MAOI's. The structures of some of the MAO inhibitors now in use in the United States are given in Figure 14–2. In searching for the ideal mood elevator it was first thought that a non-hepatotoxic substitute-like moiety might reside in the amphetamine. As previously mentioned, the hydrazine derivatives were the first to be utilized as MAO inhibitors in the treatment of depression. However, cyclization of the side chain of amphetamine resulted in the non-hydrazine MAO inhibitor tranylcypromine.

### *c. Pharmacology of MAO Inhibitors*

Mono amine oxidase is an enzyme containing the flavin skeleton, located in the mitochondrial membranes. It is distributed throughout the body. In its action it resembles the aldehyde reductases. Its function is the oxidative deamination of compounds such as serotonin, dopamine, and tyramine. Monoamine oxidase supposedly exists in two forms, MAO-A and MAO-B, based on its selective sensitivity to different substrates.

Monamine oxidase is inactivated by MAOI's. The primary role of MAO is to oxidize neurotransmitters such as norepinephrine, 5-hydroxytryptamine (serotonin) and other widely distributed amines taken into the body in foodstuff or drugs. MAOI's also inhibit hydroxylases in the liver which metabolizes other depressant drugs and other antidepressants as well as antiparkinsonian compounds.[9] It is noteworthy that, although inhibition of MAO occurs relatively fast, when MAOI's are withdrawn, it can take two weeks before the enzyme recovers its pre-drug level, so that there is danger of drug interactions which may persist for this time.

The hydrazines—for example, isocarboxazid and phenelzine—bind to MAO in an irreversible fashion, thus delaying not only the antidepressant effect of these drugs, but also their potential reversal effect. On the other hand, the nonhydrazine MAOI's such as tranylcypromine reversibly bind the MAO.

Nonhydrazine derivatives, especially tranylcypromine, cause overstimulation and for this reason they are administered in combination with the phenothiazines. Tranylcypromine was found to cause excessive hypertension in patients following the ingestion of aged cheese.[10] The excessive hypertension is attributed to the

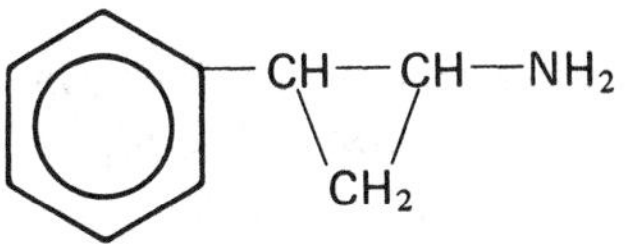

CH—CH—$NH_2$
$CH_2$

tranylcypromine

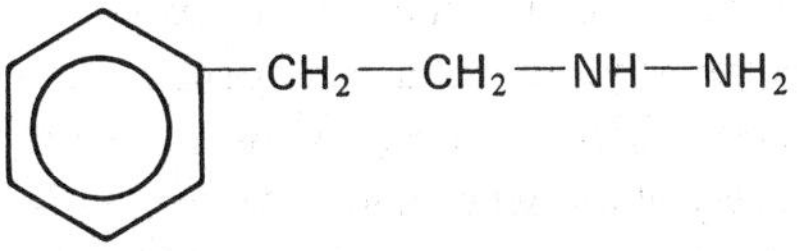

$CH_2$—$CH_2$—NH—$NH_2$

phenelzine

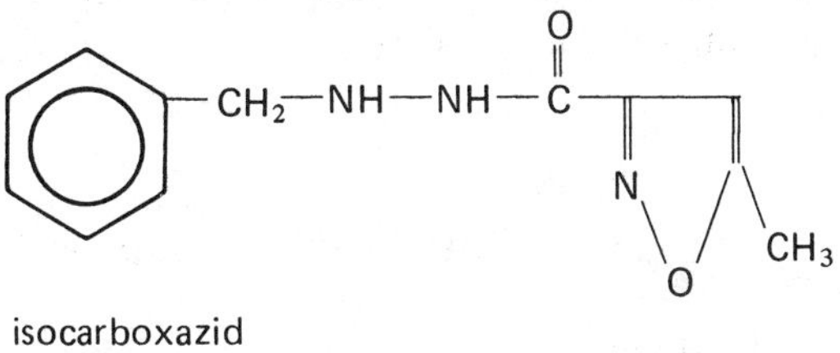

O
$CH_2$—NH—NH—C
N
O
$CH_3$

isocarboxazid

**Figure 14-2.**

accumulation of tyramine and other monoamines that otherwise would be detoxified by MAO. Tranylcypromine has to be administered at an average daily dose of 20 mg for several weeks for the treatment of mood disorders. The exact reason for the delayed action of many MAO inhibitors is yet to be ascertained.

In general, CNS stimulation, euphoria, loss of appetite, and dizziness are the reactions observed during the administration of the MAO inhibitors. Common autonomic nervous system side effects are hypotension, constipation, and dryness of mouth. Other toxic effects are skin rash and hepatic disorders.

The effect of a single dose of tranylcypromine or any MAO inhibitor in experimental animals is not significant by itself. However, a combination of the drug with other psychotic agents exerts marked influence on the behavior and CNS function. Tranylcypromine acts as a stimulant on EEG. Other MAO inhibitors have no significant effects on EEG and sleep.[11] They all lower blood pressure.

### *d. Pharmacodynamics and Metabolism of the MAO Inhibitors*

MAOI's are rapidly absorbed when taken orally and are distributed widely. The MAOI's of the hydrazine type are inactivated by acetylation of their side chain in the liver. According to Vesell[12], the speed of this acetylation varies between individuals determined by the patient's genotype. Support for this pharmacogenetic difference is derived from reports of people who are slow acetylators who show better antidepressant effects even at usual doses. MAOI's are never injected, and human biopsy samples show that these agents produce maximal inhibition of MAO within five to ten days. In addition, tranylcypromine is rapidly metabolized and eliminated in 24 hours.

### *e. Toxicity and Precautions*[1]

Overstimulation of the CNS, hallucinations, and convulsions are some of the toxic effects of the MAO inhibitors when administered in excessive doses. They bring about abnormal changes in blood pressure and hence should not be used in elderly, debilitated, or hypertensive patients. The MAO inhibitors should not be given to patients who suffer from frequent headaches. Prolonged ejaculation time, obstructed urination, and blurred vision are some other adverse reactions of the MAO inhibitors. The reasons for the wide range of the toxic effects are not clear. An important cardiovascular side effect is orthostatic hypotension; if this occurs, the drug must be discontinued immediately. In case of serious hypertensive side effects, 5 mg of phentolamine (Regitine) should be injected intravenously.

(1) *Drug Interactions*: The MAO inhibitors interact with a variety of other enzymes, thereby interacting with many other drugs through a prolongation and intensification of the activity of other drugs. When the activity of monoamine oxidase is inhibited, there is an increase in the amount of norepinephrine stored in adrenergic neurons. This results in an exaggerated activity of a drug that is capable of releasing norepinephrine from its storage sites. The interactions between the indirectly acting sympathomimetic amines (e.g., amphetamine and the MAO inhibitor) presumably occur by this mechanism. Thus when amphetamine is administered simultaneously with an MAO inhibitor, severe hypertensive reactions and cardiac arrhythmia will result. Similar reactions are observed when methyldopa and levodopa are used with an MAO inhibitor.

Although most sympathomimetic amines are to be used only under the constant supervision of a physician, compounds such as phenylephrine, phenyl propanolamine, and ephedrine, which are capable of interacting with the MAO inhibitors, are present in popular over-the-counter nonprescription medications such as cold and allergy remedies and hence are prone to abuse. Patients undergoing treatment with the MAO inhibitors should be restricted from using these medications.

Certain food materials containing considerable amounts of dopa, tyramine, and other amines capable of interacting with MAO inhibitors should be avoided by patients undergoing treatment with the MAO inhibitors.[13,14] Foods such as aged cheese, sour cream, canned figs, and broad beans and beverages such as beer, chianti wine, and coffee should be restricted for these patients.

While amphetamine is unaffected by MAO, tyramine is readily metabolized by it. Thus in the presence of MAO inhibitors large amounts of tyramine accumulate and result in the release of norepinephrine from adrenergic neurons.

Some of the substances that interact with MAO inhibitors are alcohol, barbiturates, and narcotics. The use of these drugs in combination with the MAO inhibitors should be avoided.

Other noteworthy interactions by the MAO inhibitors are enhancement of the activity of the anticholinergic agents and of the antihypertensive agents. The hypoglycemic effect of insulin is also increased by the presence of MAO inhibitors. With phenothiazines, severe extrapyramidal side effects are reported when these compounds are concurrently used with the MAO inhibitors. A more detailed account of the drug interactions of the MAO inhibitors is given in Chapter 19.

Because of the numerous toxic reactions, drug interactions, and side effects, MAO inhibitor therapy should be undertaken only when there is a thorough knowledge of the drug, its indications, and its contraindications. The diet of the patient should be supervised and any problems should be immediately tackled with proper antidotes.

In spite of these toxic reactions and side effects, MAO inhibitors are still recognized for their use in the treatment of depressive disorders and in certain phobic anxiety states.

### *f. Contraindications and Medical Uses*

There are numerous contraindications for MAOI's that include liver disease, congestive heart failure, and their combination with any drug which reacts with MAOI.

Medical use of the MAOI's include treatment of depression and certain anxiety states; sometimes it is prescribed in narcolepsy.

### *g. Products, Preparations, and Dosages*

As previously mentioned, although a number of MAO inhibitors have been on the U.S. market over the years, only three are still indicated for use as antidepressants. Chemically these drugs are either hydrazine derivatives (isocarboxazid/Marplan, phenelzine/Nardil) or nonhydrazine derivatives (tranylcypromine/Parnate).

(1) *Isocarboxazid and Phenelzine*: Hydrazine derivatives have been effective in a number of patients with moderate to severe depression and their recommended dosages as well as the forms in which they are available are noted in Table 14-1.

**TABLE 14-1**

**Monoamine Oxidase Inhibitor Antidepressants**

| *Generic Name* | *Dosage** | *Product* |
|---|---|---|
| Isocarboxazid | Usual initial: 30 mg/day in single or divided doses<br>Usual maintenance: 10–20 mg/day or less; doses above 30 mg/day not recommended | Tablets: 10 mg |
| Phenelzine | Usual initial: 15 mg t.i.d.<br>Usual maintenance: 15 mg/day; doses above 75 mg/day not recommended | Tablets: 15 mg |
| Tranylcypromine | Usual initial: 20 mg/day (10 mg in the morning and 10 mg in the afternoon)<br>Usual maintenance: 10–20 mg/day; adverse effects are more likely with doses over 30 mg/day | Tablets: 10 mg |

*Dosages were obtained from the product literature and apply to the oral use of the drug.
(From Hussan, D. A. The drug therapy of depression, a monograph. In *Therapeutics.* New York: Biomedical Information Corp., 1974, p. 12. With permission.)

(2) *Tranylcypromine*: Tranylcypromine, which is not a hydrazine derivative, is chemically related to amphetamine. It has a more rapid onset of activity than the hydrazine derivatives and is probably the most useful of the MAO inhibitor antidepressants. At one time tranylcypromine was withdrawn from the market because of its toxicity. However, it was again made available, especially for use in patients refractory to other therapeutic approaches. They are hospitalized or kept under close supervision during therapy with this drug.

It is probably because of its close chemical similarity to amphetamine that tranylcypromine is found to have some stimulant activity. At doses above 30 mg daily orthostatic hypotension is a major side effect.

## 2. Tricyclic Antidepressants

### *a. Introduction*[1]

The term "antidepressant" is usually applied to those tricyclic agents and MAO inhibitors that are used in the management of depression. However, other drugs, such as methylphenidate (Ritalin) and the amphetamines, are sometimes included in this category, although their role in the treatment of these disorders is less important. Certain agents that are not "antidepressants" can also be quite useful in treating some depressive disorders. For example, antipsychotic agents such as chlorpromazine (Thorazine) and antianxiety agents such as chlordiazepoxide (Librium) are often useful in the management of "anxious" and "hostile" depressions.

Treating depressed patients with tricyclic compounds or MAO inhibitors often decreases the intensity of symptoms, reduces the danger of suicide, alleviates the patient's discomfort, and promotes social adjustment and occupational rehabilitation. Signs of specific improvements usually include elevation of mood, increased physical activity, increased mental alertness, improved appetite, and improved sleep patterns. But even though a patient's condition is improving, it should be remembered that the risk of suicide is as high in the late stages of the depressive cycle when symptoms are subsiding as it is in the early stages of depression.

The primary indication for antidepressant drug therapy is endogenous depression. Unless there is some factor that would preclude its use, a tricyclic antidepressant is the preferred drug. The tricyclics have been consistently effective in the treatment of this condition and it is estimated that approximately 80 percent of patients benefit from this type of therapy. Although these compounds do not seem to be very effective in the management of reactive depression, some patients with this condition do respond well to drug therapy, particularly if the symptoms are similar to those of endogenous depression. In general, these agents are regarded as more effective and safer to use than MAO inhibitors.

However, in some patients who are refractive to tryclic antidepressants of the imipramine type, administration of L-tryptophan or chlorpromazine (a 5-HT neuronal pump blocker) appears useful.[15]

The basic pharmacology of imipramine and amitriptyline is quite complex. These drugs do not inhibit MAO but they do have anticholinergic, antiserotonin, and antihistaminic actions. In fact, amitriptyline is a potent antihistaminic. The basic mechanism of their antidepressant action may be related to the fact that imipramine can block the uptake of norepinephrine by the brain and other organs.[16]

Imipramine and related drugs have a cocaine-like effect on the uptake and binding of injected norepinephrine *in vivo*. One could speculate that the common denominator between the actions of the MAO inhibitors and imipramine is the presence of elevated free norepinephrine levels in the brain.

Imipramine and amitriptyline are metabolized in the body to N-desmethyl derivatives, which are pharmacologically active. These derivatives have been introduced into therapeutics under the names desipramine hydrochloride (Pertofrane) and nortriptyline hydrochloride (Aventyl). A closely related antidepressant is available as protriptyline hydrochloride (Vivactil).

Desipramine chemically is a tricyclic antidepressant and is pharmacologically related to imipramine. In fact, it is a metabolic product of the latter. The adverse reactions are also similar but may occur less frequently. Some adverse reactions are atropine-like dryness of the mouth, blurred vision, and constipation. In addition, there may be other adverse reactions to both imipramine and desipramine, including ataxia, orthostatic hypotension, parkinsonism-like symptoms, agitation, and anxiety.

The common adverse effects after the use of tricyclic antidepressants are related to autonomic nervous system dysfunction and include dryness of the mouth, constipation, urinary retention in men, and hypotension. Cholestatic jaundice has been reported as a result of the use of these drugs. First-degree atrioventricular block indicates that these drugs can slow atrioventricular conduction.

Currently imipramine (a dibenzazepine derivative), amitriptyline (a dibenzocycloheptadiene derivative), and other closely related compounds are the most widely used drugs for the treatment of depression. Because of their structures, they are often referred to as the tricyclic antidepressants. Their efficacy in alleviating depression has been well established.

The tricyclic antidepressants such as imipramine (Tofranil) and amitriptyline (Elavil) and their desmethyl derivatives are chemically similar to the phenothiazines. Their pharmacologic properties are also similar but empirically they have been found useful as antidepressants.

### *b. Historical Background and Chemistry*

The basic molecular unit of the tricyclic antidepressants is iminodibenzyl, which was first synthesized in 1889.[2] It was not until 1948 that its great pharmacologic importance was recognized, by Hafliger and Schindler, through the synthesis and screening of a vast number of iminodibenzyl derivatives for their therapeutic use as antihistamines, sedatives, and analgesics.

The most important and valuable tricyclic antidepressant drug among the iminodibenzyl derivatives is imipramine, which is successfully employed today for endogenous type of depressions.[7,8]

(It may be noted that the chemical structure of imipramine is analogous to the basic phenothiazine structure in which the sulfur atom is replaced by a $CH_2$-$CH_2$-unit.) Since imipramine is a dibenzazepine compound, attempts were made to synthesize other dibenzazepine derivatives analogous to imipramine. Thus compounds such as desipramine, amitriptyline and doxepin have come in to the market as alternative drugs to imipramine.

The structures of some of the tricyclic antidepressants are depicted in Figure 14-3.

The physicochemical characteristics of promazine (a phenothiazine derivative) and imipramine are strikingly similar except that in promazine the sulfur atom connecting the two benzene rings facilitates conjugation, while in imipramine the $CH_2$–$CH_2$ link prevents the same. Desipramine is a metabolite of imipramine and is believed to be responsible for the antidepressant effects of imipramine in vivo.

In another pair of the tricyclics (amitriptylene and nortriptylene) the nitrogen atom in the central ring of imipramine is replaced by a carbon atom and these are the structural homologs of thioxanthenes without an asymmetric center in their structures. Another pair of active tricyclics are the *cis* and *trans* isomers of doxepin, which are in use as antidepressants.

One of the homologs of chlorpromazine, clopramine, is nothing but the 3-chloro analog of imipramine. It is used as a strong sedative. These examples illustrate the relationship between the chemical structures and the pharmacologic activities of the tricyclic antidepressants. Further information on the topic can be obtained from the reports of Gelder et al.[17]

### *c. Pharmacology*

The basic chemistry of the tricyclic antidepressants dictate the overall pharmacologic profile of the various chemicals in this group. Generally, their antidepressant qualities are a function of the central ring structure. Variations in the side chain alter their potency and sedative properties. A tetracyclic is also commercially available which has four rings attached in its structure. The therapeutic actions are due to their common property of augmenting the functional status of the catecholamines at their respective receptor sites via blocking the reuptake of catecholamines into the presynaptic nerve terminals. Interestingly, most recently two potent antidepressants, inprindole and mianserin, have only a slight effect on receptacle mechanisms which effect both adrenergic and serotonergic neuropathways.

The inhibition of reuptake amine pump occurs much sooner than the onset of therapeutic benefits—approximately two to three weeks.

In normal subjects the acute side effects of imipramine and chlorpromazine appear to be similar.[19,20] Whereas the MAOI's act by euphoric stimulation, the tricyclic antidepressants are known to act by a reduction of the depressive mental state. It has been reported[21,22] that patients treated with imipramine have been observed to have a higher incidence of manic reactions.

Tricyclic antidepressants are known to be sedatives and hence they are occasionally substituted for hypnotics and employed for increasing stage IV sleep. They decrease REM time.[23,24]

In experimental animals the tricyclic antidepressants depress the spontaneous motor activity in a manner similar to the phenothiazines. The typical representative of the class, imipramine, prolongs alcohol narcosis and hexobarbital sleeping time. When administered in experimental animals prior to treatment with reserpine, the tricyclic antidepressants block the reserpine-induced depression, facilitating 5-HT and norepinephrine in the brain. The correlation between this and the blocking effect in human beings is yet to be clarified. Other stimulant-like effects, such as the potentiation of adrenergic agonists, augmentation of some operant-behavior, and self-stimulation of brain, are observed following the administration of imipramine[25] in animals.

(1) *The Biogenic Amine Hypothesis*: The basic generalizations that constitute the biogenic amine hypothesis with reference to the tricyclic

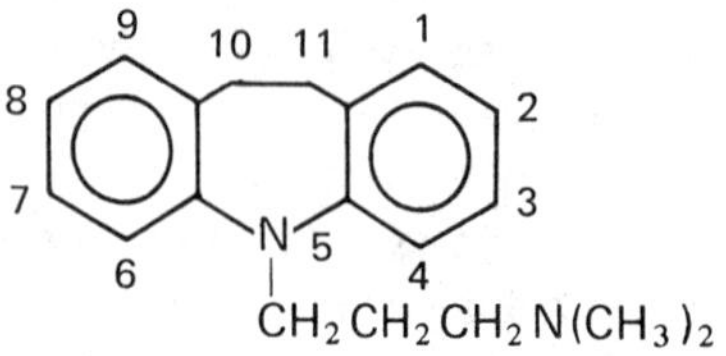

9 10 11 1 8 2 7 3 N 5 6 4

$CH_2CH_2CH_2N(CH_3)_2$

imipramine

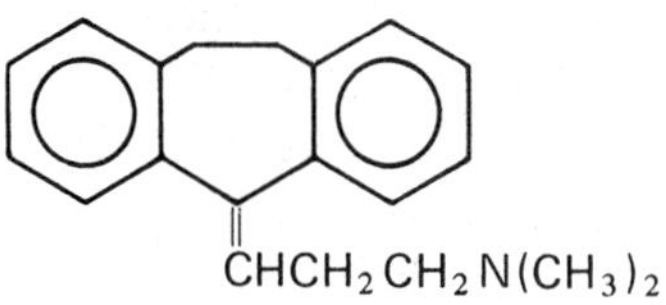

$CHCH_2CH_2N(CH_3)_2$

amitriptyline

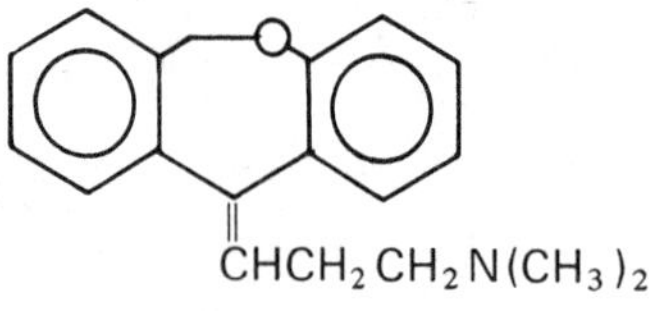

O

$CHCH_2CH_2N(CH_3)_2$

doxepin

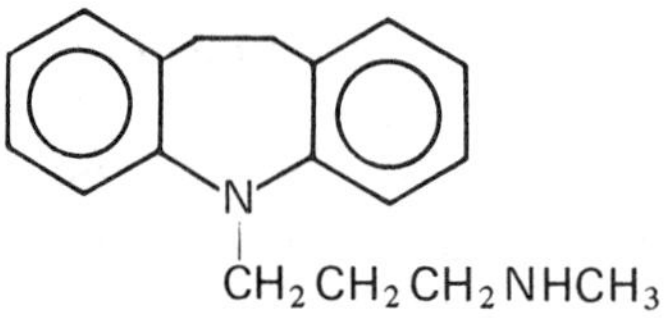

N

$CH_2CH_2CH_2NHCH_3$

desipramine

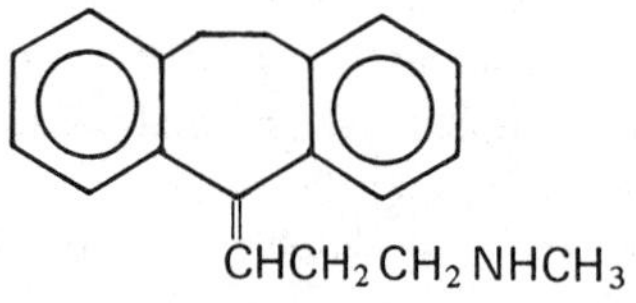

$CHCH_2CH_2NHCH_3$

nortiptyline

$CH_2CH_2CH_2NHCH_3$

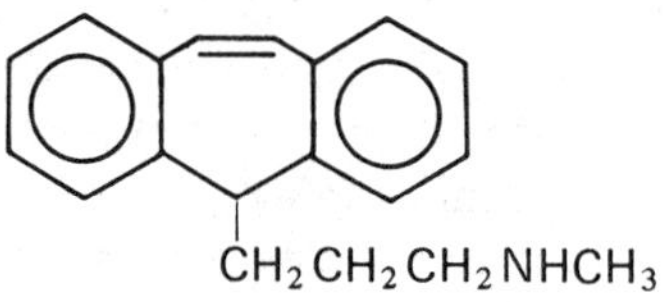

protriptyline

**Figure 14-3.**

antidepressants are as follows: (a) All tricyclic antidepressants block the neuronal uptake of norepinephrine and serotonin. (b) They potentiate the effects of the sympathomimetic amines that act directly on the central nervous system. (c) The tricyclic antidepressants block the effects of the indirectly acting amines such as tyramine to cause the release of norepinephrine. The reviews by Davis,[26] Schildkraut,[27] and Baldessarini[2] may be consulted for further reading on the action of the tricyclic antidepressants on the brain amines.

The tricyclic antidepressants do not seem to have a significant effect on the dopamine receptors. However, they are known to block the uptake of norepinephrine by the adrenergic nerve terminals. The demethylated analogs are more potent in this action.

Two noteworthy drawbacks of the biogenic amine concept are that (a) the validity of the concept in humans is not yet thoroughly established even though many animal models are tested with considerable success, and (b) there is still doubt as to whether the therapeutic actions of the tricyclic antidepressants are exactly linked to the biogenic brain amines, since some of the nonantidepressant compounds such as cocaine and amphetamine also inhibit the transportation of norepinephrine. Moreover, related hypotheses have emphasized the interactions of antidepressants with other CNS amines, particularly serotonin and acetylchroline (ACH).

Since some antidepressants (amintriptyline, imipramine, and especially clomipramine) block the uptake of 5-HT, this CNS neurohumor may be involved in the effects of certain antidepressants.[28] Nevertheless, the physiologic importance of reuptake of 5-HT versus its enzymatic deamination by MAO is uncertain, and many effective antidepressants have little apparent interaction with tryptaminergic neurons.

Janowsky et al.[29] observed that physostigmine, a choline esterase inhibitor, has antimanic effects and might aggravate depressive mood disorders. This observation supports the view that the antimuscarinic action of the tricyclic antidepressants is responsible for their manifold pharmacologic effects. However, the anticholinergic activity of the antidepressants correlates poorly with their main effects,[30] and other strongly antimuscarinic compounds, such as atropine, scopolamine, and many anticholinergic antiparkinsonian agents, are not effective antidepressants. The concept is still under investigation.

The demethylated antidepressants are thought to be much more selective in blocking the uptake of norepinephrine, and accordingly to reduce its turnover and the firing rate of adrenergic neutrons in the locus ceruleus.

In contrast, clomipramine is a rather selective blocker of 5-HT transport and causes a decreased turnover of the amine in the tryptaminergic-containing neurons of the midbrain raphe nuclei. In turn, their firing rate is decreased.

The aminergic pathophysiology of depression is presented here in an attempt to explicate the actions of the antidepressant drugs. A disorder of amine metabolism that exists in a subgroup of depressed patients is as yet not clearly defined.[31-34] It is presumably these patients who respond favorably to the antidepressant drugs. A disorder of amine metabolism may also afflict some patients with mania. Although other neurotransmitter substances may be involved, it is known that all drugs and treatments that modify depression or mania have significant effects on the metabolism of norepinephrine. No more explicit statement can be made at this time but there is considerable hope that eventually a consistent explanation of depression and its treatment will evolve. For a review on the subject see Blum and associates.[35] A summary of this review is presented in Table 14-2.

As shown in Table 14-2, certain depressed patients may have a high serotonergic but low catecholaminergic receptor responsivity (a 5-HT deficit). These patients would be responsive to drugs that elevate functional levels of 5-HT but less responsive, or refractive, to drugs that elevate the functional level of norepinephrine, such as the tricyclic antidepressants. Other patients may have a high catecholaminergic but low sertonergic receptor responsivity (a norepinephrine deficit). They may be responsive to drugs that elevate functional levels of norepinephrine but less responsive, or refractive, to drugs that elevate the functional level of 5-HT, such as L-tryptophan or compounds that specifically block the 5-HT neuronal pump.

(2) *Autonomic, Cardiovascular, and Respiratory Actions*: Unlike the phenothiazines, tri-

cyclic antidepressants have remarkably prominent anticholinergic effects. Side effects include the blurring of vision, urinary retention, and drying of the mouth. Some of these accompany depressive disorders as well. Hence the true effects of the tricyclic antidepressants on the autonomic nervous system should be carefully confirmed. Desipramine has the fewest anticholinergic side effects and amitriptyline causes the maximum effects.[36]

The tricyclic antidepressants lower various cardiovascular reflexes and lower the blood pressure.[37] Patients develop arrhythmia leading to fatality.[38] The property of blocking the brain amine reuptake by these drugs may be considered as the cause of this and other side effects in the cardiovascular system, such as myocardial infarction, orthostatic hypotension, and tachycardia. The T-waves show a sudden flattening in the ECG after administration of the tricyclic antidepressants, particularly imipramine. The tricyclic antidepressants enhance the effects of certain other cardiac depressant agents. The tricyclic antidepressants have no significant effect on respiration in therapeutic doses.

#### *d. Pharmacokinetics and Metabolism*

The tricyclic antidepressant drugs are strong anticholinergic agents and hence affect gastrointestinal activity. Although they are well absorbed by oral ingestion high doses can cause complications such as slowing down the gastric emptying time.

The tricyclics are similar to the phenothiazines in their pharmacokinetic properties. They are highly lipophilic in nature and hence are strongly bound to plasma proteins and other tissue constituents. They are widely distributed over the body.

They are metabolized by N-demethylation, oxidation, and hydroxylation in the aromatic ring. The pharmacologically active metabolic products of imipramine are highly bound to the plasma proteins,[40] sometimes in concentrations higher than the parent drugs themselves.

Patients administered with the same doses of the tricyclic antidepressants often show varying plasma concentrations. This may be attributed to genetic factors.[41] Administration of certain drugs that inhibit the heptaic hydroxylating

**TABLE 14-2**

**A Schematic Rationale for Differential Chemotherapy of Depressions in Humans[35]**

**Depressed Patients**

| *Subgroup N* | *Subgroup S* |
|---|---|
| 1. High catecholaminergic receptor responsivity | 1. High serotonergic receptor responsivity |
| 2. Low serotonergic receptor responsivity | 2. Low catecholaminergic receptor responsivity |
| 3. A norepinephrine (NE) deficit | 3. A serotonin (5 HT) deficit |
| 4. Low levels of NE metabolites (e.g., VMA, MHPG) | 4. Low levels of 5 HT metabolites (e.g., 5 HIAA) |
| 5. Responsive to drugs that elevate functional levels of NE such as tricyclic antidepressants, MAO inhibitors | 5. Responsive to drugs that elevate functional levels of serotonin such as L-tryptophan, drugs that block 5-HT neuronal pump, MAO inhibitors, etc. |
| 6. Refractive to L-tryptophan, etc. | 6. Refractive to tricyclic antidepressants that block NE neuronal pump, etc. |

As shown in Table 14-2, certain depressed patients may have a high serotonergic but low catecholaminergic receptor responsivity (a 5-HT deficit). These patients would be responsive to drugs that elevate functional levels of 5-HT but less responsive, or refractive, to drugs that elevate the functional level of norepinephrine, such as the tricyclic antidepressants. Other patients may have a high catecholaminergic but low serotonergic receptor responsivity (a norepinephrine deficit) and may be responsive to drugs that elevate functional levels of norepinephrine but less responsive, or refractive, to drugs that elevate the functional level of 5-HT, such as L-tryptophan or compounds that specifically block the 5-HT neuronal pump.

(From Blum, K. et al. Possible rationale for differential chemotherapy on depression in humans. A review on the biogenic amione hypothesis. Part I. *J. Psychedelic Drugs* 8(3):223, 1976. With permission.)

agents, simultaneously with the tricyclic antidepressants, cause an increase in the plasma concentrations of the latter drugs.[42,43] The pharmacokinetic properties of the tricyclics can be further understood from the reviews by Morselli[44] and Hollister.[45]

Since the tricyclic antidepressants have a long action, there is the possibility of persistent side reactions. These drugs are given only once a day. Once again, patients differ in their ability to metabolize the tricyclic compounds. However, it has been shown unexpectedly that the excretion of the tricyclic antidepressants is relatively fast, such as 80 percent within the first 24 hours. Imipramine is the fastest to be inactivated and eliminated; protriptyline is the slowest. With nortriptyline, tenfold differences in blood concentrations have been noted in different people all receiving the exact same dose of the drug. Doxepin is demethylated and converted into an active metabolite nordoxepin.[46] Although there are notable exceptions[47,48] most tricyclic antidepressants should be inactivated and excreted within a week after termination of treatment.

### e. Addiction (Tolerance and Dependence)

The tricyclic antidepressants may occasionally develop physical dependence by some patients due to prolonged administration (for years).[49] Patients are known to develop tolerance to the anticholinergic effects during prolonged treatment.

When imipramine is withdrawn abruptly after administration in high doses for sufficiently long periods, a syndrome manifested by severe muscular pain, chill, and coryza will result. In general the liability of the tricyclics for abuse is less compared with the other antidepressant drugs.

In terms of abuse potential, the tricyclic antidepressant drugs are low risk relative to other classic substances of abuse (i.e., cocaine, alcohol, barbiturates).

### f. Toxic Effects and Precautions

The tricyclic antidepressants are known to have significant toxic side reactions, including cerebral and cardiac toxicity as a result of their antimuscarinic activity. The incidence is approximately 5 percent.[50] The antimuscarinic activity is highest in amitriptyline and lowest in protriptylene and desipramine in the following order.

Amitriptyline > imipramine > doxepin = nortriptyline > desipramine = protriptyline[30]

In comparison with the MAO inhibitors, the tricyclic antidepressants show a higher incidence of minor side effects such as drowsiness, agitation, and disorientation but a lower incidence of the relatively more serious side effects such as cardiac failure and brain toxicity. Besides the side effects such as blurred vision, constipation, and urinary retention already mentioned, other anticholinergic side effects include glaucoma, tachycardia, palpitations, and excessive sweating. Precautions should be taken while administering these drugs in older patients as they seem to develop these reactions more easily than others. Caution should be used when treating patients with prostatic hypertrophy, hypertension, and cardiac disorders.

Since most of the tricyclics cause sedation, the least sedating drugs should be selected depending upon the physical and mental alertness of the patient. Doxepin has the maximum sedative effect, followed by amitriptyline.

The tricyclics cause tremors and seizures occasionally. Hence patients with a history of convulsive disorders should be closely monitored while using these drugs.

Cases of hepatotoxicity (e.g., jaundice), hematologic disorders (e.g., thrombocytopenia), allergic reactions (e.g., rash and photosensitization), and psychiatric disorientation (e.g., hallucinations) associated with the use of tricyclics have been reported but are not frequent. Whether or not it is safe to use tricyclics in pregnant women has not yet been clearly established.

Tricyclic antidepressants in doses dangerous enough to be lethal are readily available to patients with mood disorders. Hence acute poisoning or suicide can easily result. A gram of imipramine is usually enough to cause severe toxicity and 2 grams can be fatal.[51,52,54]

Antidepressants are not generally recommended for use in children, but in special cases, such as enuresis, they have been prescribed.

Children are vulnerable to cardiotoxic and seizure-inducing effects of high doses of tricyclic substances and deaths have occurred in children after overdosage of only a few hundred milligrams a day.

### *g. Drug Interactions*

Administration of tricyclic antidepressants concurrently with or shortly after treatment with MAO inhibitors has resulted in severe reactions consisting of signs and symptoms resembling those of atropine toxicity. A dose as low as 25 mg of imipramine, taken three days after the discontinuation of therapeutic doses of tranylcypromine, are capable of producing a severe reaction characterized by convulsions, coma, and hyperpyrexia. Their concurrent use is thus contraindicated. Ten days to two weeks should elapse between discontinuance of MAO inhibitors and initiation of tricyclic antidepressant therapy. If the situation is desperate, electroshock therapy may be employed during the interval.

Other interactions include the potentiation of central depressant drugs, blockade of the antihypertensive effects of guanethidine, and augmentation of the pressor effects of sympathomimetic amines. Interactions with thyroid preparations, methylphenidate, and phenothiazines, all of which may enhance the therapeutic effect of the tricyclic antidepressants, have been reported. Antidepressants are also known to potentiate the effects of alcohol, and probably other sedatives as well.[55]

The tricyclic antidepressants also interfere with the antihypertensive effects of clonidine, but do not interact with the beta-adrenoceptor antagonists.

### *h. Therapeutic Uses*

The use of the tricyclics for the treatment of depression is well established. Other ailments that are treated with antidepressants include *enuresis in childhood* and *severe obsessive compulsive neurosis*.[56]

**TABLE 14-3**

**Tricyclic Antidepressants**

| *Generic Name* | *Dosage** | *Product* |
|---|---|---|
| Imipramine | Hospitalized patients: 100–200 mg/day in divided doses; if needed, can increase to 250–300 mg/day<br>Outpatients: usual maintenance, 50–150 mg/day; doses above 200 mg/day not recommended<br>Parenteral: up to 100 mg/day I.M. in divided doses | Tablets: 10-, 25-, 50-mg ampuls: 25 mg/2 cc |
| Imipramine pamoate | 75–150 mg/day | Capsules: 75, 150 mg |
| Desipramine | Usual: 50 mg t.i.d.; can be increased to 200 mg/day in divided doses | Tablets, capsules: 25, 50 mg |
| Amitriptyline | Hospitalized patients: 100–200 mg/day; if needed, can increase to 300 mg/day<br>Outpatients: usual maintenance, 25 mg two to four times/day; can be increased to 150 mg/day.<br>Parenteral: 20–30 mg I.M. q.i.d. | Tablets: 10, 25, 50 mg<br>Vials: 10 mg/ml (10 ml) |
| Nortriptyline | Usual: 25 mg three to four times/day; doses above 100 mg/day not recommended | Capsules: 10, 25 mg<br>Liquid: 10 mg/5 ml |
| Protriptyline | Usual: 5–10 mg three to four times/day; doses above 60 mg/day not recommended | Tablets: 5, 10 mg |
| Doxepin | Usual: 25–50 mg t.i.d.; doses above 300 mg/day not recommended | Captules: 10, 25, 50, 100 mg |

*Dosages were obtained from the product literature and apply to the oral use of the drug unless otherwise indicated. Lower doses are indicated in adolescent and geriatric patients.

(From Hussan, D. A. The drug therapy of depression, a monograph. In *Therapeutics.* New York: Biomedical Information Corp., 1974, p. 6. With permission.)

### *i. Other Tricyclic Antidepressants*

Table 14-3 represents the generic name, dosage, and products available of other known tricyclic antidepressants. *Doxepin*, which is a relatively new antidepressant, will be the only one discussed in somewhat more detail.

1. *Dibenzoxepines*: Just as the tricyclic antidepressants resulted from modifications of the central ring of the *phenothiazines*, an additional modification has led to a new family of psychotherapeutic agents—the dibenzoxepines. *Doxepin* (*Sinequan*) is claimed to have a mixture of antipsychotic and antidepressant properties. The drug is administered in a daily dosage range of 25 to 300 mg in three divided doses. Its exact position in relation to the *phenothiazines* and the other tricyclic antidepressants is difficult to assess at the present.

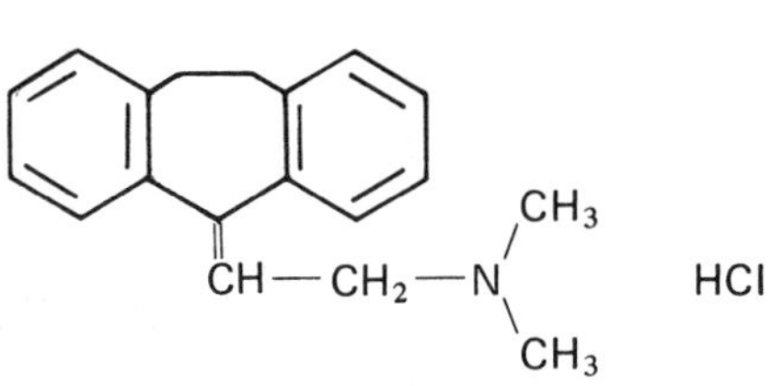

$CH—CH_2—N(CH_3)_2$ · HCl

doxepin hydrochloride

(a) *Doxepin*, (Sinequan, Adapin), the newest tricyclic derivative, possesses in addition to its antidepressant action an antianxiety activity that apparently is more pronounced than that of amitriptyline. It has been suggested that doxepin be used in situations that previously required the use of both an antidepressant and a tranquilizer. If, as more experience is gained, doxepin proves to be as effective as or superior to combinations of other antidepressants with tranquilizers, therapy with doxepin will have two advantages: The dosage of only one agent will have to be adjusted, and side reactions will be less severe because the adverse effects of doxepin are milder than those of the phenothiazines. The use of doxepin as the primary agent in treating anxiety and tension in patients who are not depressed is not recommended as it appears to be less effective than chlordiazepoxide (Librium) or diazepam (Valium) in adequate doses.

Drowsiness is a fairly frequent complication in doxepin therapy but tends to disappear as treatment is continued. It is preferred over other tricyclics for patients taking guanethidine (Ismelin), because doxepin seems less likely to inhibit the activity of this agent when usual doses are employed.

## 3. Lithium Salts

### *a. Introduction*

The inorganic element, lithium, and its salt have been employed in medicine for over a century. Initially, it was used as a cardiac salt substitute. As a treatment for mania, lithium salts were first used by Cade[60] in 1949. However, the work of Schou in Denmark[17] resulted in its acceptable use in the treatment and prevention of affective disorders.[58,59] The rationale for the use of lithium is to prevent the relapse of both mania and depression.

### *b. Chemistry*

Lithium is the lightest of the alkali metals, resembling sodium and potassium in many of the chemical properties of its salt.

### *c. Pharmacology of the Lithium Salts*

Lithium salts do not exhibit any of the common effects that are the prime characteristics of most of the psychotropic agents in normal human subjects such as sedation, depression, and euphoria. Lithium ion inhibits the calcium-dependent release of norepinephrine and dopamine but has no effect on the 5-H tryptamine when administered in milliequivalent concentrations It shows no effect on adenylate cyclase activity but does on the hormonal responses that are mediated by the enzyme. Lithium influences the distribution of the divalent cations but whether or not this is related to its antimanic effects is not yet clear.[59] Pert et al.[61] found that lithium inhibits the effects of receptor blocking agents in the adrenergic receptor systems.

One advantage in using lithium in the treatment of depressive disorders is that it corrects irregular sleep patterns. However, the REM sleep phase is slightly suppressed. Lithium is known to cause ECT changes, sometimes resulting in increased epileptiform discharge. In EEG, high-voltage slow waves with fast beta activity are reported.

### *d. Mechanism of Action of Lithium in Mania*

The mechanism of action of lithium carbonate in manic psychosis is not fully understood. Since there are many similarities in the biologic actions of sodium and lithium, and because sodium is required for catecholamine uptake by the amine pump, current research is focusing on the possible effect of lithium on catecholamine uptake. Lithium appears to accelerate the uptake of norepinephrine by isolated nerve-ending particles (synaptosomes).

### *e. Pharmacokinetics Metabolism*

Since lithium is readily absorbed from the gastrointestinal tract, it diffuses throughout the body fluids and tissues, displaces sodium and potassium, and interferes with magnesium and calcium. Lithium is excreted through the kidney, and it moves in and out of cells more slowly than sodium. Lithium, similar to sodium, is filtered and reabsorbed incompletely by the kidney. One factor which enhances its absorption is that when the proximal tubule absorbs more water, this dehydration effect causes plasma lithium concentrations to rise. When sodium concentration falls, lithium concentration, which is subsequently absorbed, increases.

In elderly patients the rate of excretion is comparatively slow.

In comparison with sodium, lithium is excreted only in very low quantities in feces and sweat (less than 1 and 5 percent respectively) but it is eliminated in higher concentrations through saliva. Lithium shows very feeble effects on carbohydrate metabolism.[62]

### *f. Toxicity and Precautions*

In the initial stages of treatment with lithium, the excretion of sodium, potassium, water,[63] and 17-hydroxy corticosteroids increases but is controlled after two or three days. Lithium treatment with acute doses causes intoxication, the signs of which appear as vomiting, drowsiness, ataxia, diarrhea, and even coma, depending upon the plasma concentrations of the ion.

Cooper and Simpson[64] suggested that a test dose of lithium carbonate could be ingested into a single patient and the plasma levels of it tested after 24 hours to facilitate the determination of the optimal dose requirement of the individual.

Lithium causes allergic reactions such as dermatitis and vasculitis in certain individuals and a reversible increase of blood leukocytes in chronic patients as well as benign and reversible depression of the T-wave of the ECG.[65] Toxic effects of lithium are in general dose dependent and severe reactions result when the serum levels of lithium reach 2.5 mEq/liter. These reactions include mental confusion, dysarthria, seizures, coma, and even death.[66] According to Goldfield and Weinstein,[67] lithium intoxication is observed more commonly in pregnant women using natriuretics and on low-sodium diets. The toxic effects in pregnant women include neonatal goiter, CNS depression, and hypotonia. The newborn is prone to suffer from certain cardiovascular anomalies. Hence lithium treatment is not recommended during pregnancy.

Renal failure is another dangerous side effect of lithium therapy.[69]

### *g. Drug Interactions*

Although thiazide diuretics may correct the nephrogenic (kidney) *diabetes insipidus* induced by lithium, diuretics in general have been known to precipitate lithium toxicity, and should not be given with lithium. Lithium decreases the pressure response to norepinephrine in humans. There have been several reports of serious toxic reactions when lithium is combined with haloperidol.[69] Special caution must be executed when doses of haloperidol above 40 mg./day are combined with lithium concentrations greater than 1 MMOL./liter. A sign of lithium toxicity is nausea. Urinary retension due to the anticholinergic effects of the tricyclic antidepressants can become particularly uncomfortable in the presence of lithium-induced diuresis.

### *h. Therapeutic Uses*

Lithium carbonate is available in capsules (*Eskalith; Lithonate*) and in tablets (*Lithane*), all containing 300 mg of the drug.

Lithium therapy for acute mania or the prevention of recurrences of bipolar manic-depressive illness are the only indications approved in the United States. Davis,[70] in 1976, suggested its use as an alternative to tricyclic antidepressants for severe recurrent unipolar manic-depressive illness as well. Lithium treatment is ideally conducted *only* in patients with normal cardiac and renal function.

## D. GENERAL COMMENTS AND SUMMARY

Hussan[1] has concluded that:

> Drug therapy of depression is the preferred and most convenient form of treating depression and the only mode of treatment that can be used on a scale vast enough to reach the millions of people who are affected by these disorders. Tricyclic antidepressants are the drugs of choice. Because of their toxicity and great potential to interact with other agents, MAO inhibitors should be reserved for patients refactory to tricyclic antidepressants. The chief disadvantage of the antidepressants is their long latency. Therefore, electroconvulsive therapy, which acts faster than antidepressants, is sometimes preferred for the treatment of individuals with suicide tendencies. This type of therapy should also be considered for non-complying patients and for those who do not respond to drug therapy. Electroconvulsive therapy is unacceptable to many patients because of the risks and side effects (memory loss, confusion) associated with its use. The convulsant drug flurothl (Indoklon) has been used in some situations as an alternative to electroconvulsive therapy. The change in prognosis of depression that pharmacotherapy has brought cannot be overemphasized. But pharmacotherapy cannot influence the patient's milieu. Psychologically disturbed patients will need help from as many quarters as possible, including psychotherapy and family counseling.

In conclusion, both clinicians and researchers agree that in the practice of psychiatry today in many patients showing typical symptomatology of affective disorders these are drug induced, particularly those psychoactive agents showing marked abuse potential.[71] Therefore, it is advisable that the medical staffs of drug programs become very familiar with the pharmacology of drugs used in the treatment of psychosis (schizophrenia) and the affective disorders, such as mania and depression.

## REFERENCES

1. Hussan, D. A. *The Drug Therapy of Depression, A Monograph in Therapeutics*. Philadelphia: Smith, Kline, and French Laboratories, 1974.
2. Baldessarini, R. J. Drugs and the treatment of psychiatric disorders. In A. G. Gilman, L. S. Goodman, and A. Gilman, eds., *The Pharmacological Basis of Therapeutics*, 6th ed. New York: Macmillan, 1980, pp. 391–447.
3. Blum, K. Depressive states induced by drugs of abuse: Clinical evidence, theoretical mechanism(s) and proposed treatment, Part II. *Psychedel. Drugs* 8(3):235, 1976.
4. Robinson, D. S., et al. Clinical psychopharmacology of phenelzine: MAO activity and clinical response. In M. A. Lipton, A. DiMascio, and K. F. Killam, eds., *Psychopharmacology: A Generation of Progress*. New York: Raven Press, 1978, pp. 961–973.
5. Bernstein, J. G. *Handbook of Drug Therapy in Psychiatry*. Boston: John Wright-PSG, Inc., 1983.
6. Weil-Malherbe, H. The biochemistry of the functional psychoses. *Adv. Enzymol.* 29:479, 1967.

7. Baldessarini, R. J. *Chemotherapy in Psychiatry*. Cambridge, Mass.: Harvard University Press, 1977.
8. Biel, J. H., Bopp, B., and Mitchell, B. D. Chemistry and structure-activity relationships of psychotropic drugs. In W. G. Clark and J. del Guidice, eds., *Principles of Psychopharmacology*. New York: Academic Press, 1978, pp. 140–168.
9. Costa, E., and Sandler, M. (Editors) *Monoamine Oxidases—New Vistas. Advances in Biochemical Psychopharmacology*, vol. 5. New York: Raven Press, 1972.
10. DiMascio, A., Heninger, G., and Klerman, G. L. Psychopharmacology of imipramine and desipramine: A comparative study of their effects in normal males. *Psychopharmacologia* 5:361, 1964.
11. Wyatt, R. J., Termini, B. A., and Davis, J. M. Biochemical and sleep studies of schizophrenia. *Schizophr. Bull.* 4:10, 1971.
12. Vesell, E. S. Pharmacogenetics. *N. Engl. J. Med.* 287:904, 1972.
13. Marley, E., and Blackwell, B. Interactions of monoamine oxidase inhibitors, amines, and foodstuffs. *Adv. Pharmacol. Chemother.* 8:185, 1970.
14. Ayd, F. J., Jr., and Blackwell, B. (Editors) *Discoveries in Biological Psychiatry*. Philadelphia: Lippincott, 1970.
15. Sulser, F., and Sanders-Bush, E. Effects of drug on amines in the CNS. *Ann. Rev. Pharmacol.* 11:209, 1971.
16. Prien, R. F., Caffey, E. M., Jr., and Klett, C. J. Relationship between serum lithium level and clinical response in acute mania treated with lithium. *Br. J. Psychiat.* 120:409, 1972.
17. Gelder, M., Gath, D., and Mayou, R. *Oxford Textbook of Psychiatry*. Oxford: Oxford Medical Publications, 1983, p. 543.
18. Kaiser, G., and Zirkle, C. L. Antidepressant drugs. In A. Burger, ed., *Medicinal Chemistry*, 2nd ed. New York: Wiley, 1970, pp. 1470–1497.
19. Mandel, M. R., and Klerman, G. L. Clinical use of antidepressants, stimulants, tricyclics and monoamine oxidase inhibitors. In W. G. Clark and J. del Guidice, eds., *Principles of Psychopharmacology*, 2nd ed. New York: Academic Press, 1978, pp. 537–551.
20. Grunthal, E. Untersuchungen uber die besondere psychologische Wirkung des Thymolepticums Tofranil, *Psychiat. Neurol. Wischr.* 136:402, 1958.
21. Lowe, M. C., et al. Preclinical pharmacology of antidepressants. Tricyclics. In W. G. Clark and J. del Guidice, eds., *Principles of Psychopharmacology*, 2nd ed. New York: Academic Press, 1978, pp. 311–323.
22. Lehmann, H. E., Cahn, C. H. and de Veteouil, R. L. The treatment of depressive conditions with imipramine (G22355). *Can. Psychiat. Assoc. J.* 3:155, 1958.
23. Itil, T. M. Effect of psychotropic drugs on qualitatively and quantitatively analyzed human EEG. In W. G. Clark and J. del Guidice, eds., *Principles of Psychopharmacology*, 2nd ed. New York: Academic Press, 1978, pp. 261–277.
24. Longo, V. G. Effects of psychotropic drugs on the EEG of animals. In W. G. Clark and J. del Guidice, eds., *Principles of Psychopharmacology*, 2nd ed. New York: Academic Press, 1978, pp. 247–260.
25. Iversen, L. L., Iversen, S. D., and Snyder, S. H. (Editors) *Handbook of Psychopharmacology*, 14 vols. New York: Plenum Press, 1976–1978.
26. Davis, J. M. The efficacy of the tranquilizing and antidepressant drugs. *Arch. Gen. Psychiat.* 13:552, 1965.
27. Schildkraut, J. J. The catecholamine hypothesis of affective disorders, a review of supporting evidence. *Am. J. Psychiatr.* 122:509, 1965.
28. Praag, H. M. van. Amine hypotheses of affective disorders. In L. L. Iversen, S. D. Iversen, and S. H. Snyder, eds., *Handbook of Psychopharmacology: Biology of Mood and Antianxiety Drugs*, Vol. 13. New York: Plenum Press, 1978, pp. 187–297.
29. Janowsky, D. S., El-Yousef, M. K., and Davis, J. M. Acetylcholine and depression. *Psychosom. Med.* 36:248, 1974.
30. Snyder, S. H., and Yamamura, H. I. A. Antidepressants and the muscarinic acetylcholine receptor. *Arch. Gen. Psychiatry*, 34:236, 1977.
31. U'Prichard, D. C., et al. Tricyclic antidepressants: Therapeutic properties and affinity for alpha-noradrenergic receptor binding sites in the brain. *Science* 199:197, 1978.
32. Crews, F. T., and Smith, C. B. Presynaptic alpha-receptor subsensitivity after long-term antidepressant treatment. *Science* 202:322, 1978.
33. Svessen, T. H., and Usdin, T. Feedback inhibition of brain noradrenaline neurons by tricyclic antidepressants: Alpha-receptor mediation. *Science* 202:1089, 1978.
34. DeMontigny, C., and Aghajanian, G. K. Tricyclic antidepressants: Long-term treatment increases responsivity of rat forebrain neurons to serotonin. *Science* 202:1303, 1978.
35. Blum, K., et al. Possible rationale for differential chemotherapy on depression in humans: A re-

view of the biogenic amine hypothesis. Part I. *J. Psychedel. Drugs* 8(3):223, 1976.

36. Blackwell, B., Stefopoulos, A., and Enders, P. Anticholinergic activity of two trycyclic antidepressants. *Am. J. Psychiatry* 135:722, 1978.
37. Raisfeld, I. H. Cardiovascular complication of antidepressant therapy. Interaction at the adrenergic neuron. *Am. Heart J.* 83:129, 1972.
38. Williams, R. B., and Sherter, C. Cardiac complications of tricyclic antidepressant therapy. *Ann. Intern. Med* 74:395, 1971.
39. Bigger, J. T., Giardina, E. G., and Perel, J. J. Cardiac antiarrhythmic effect of imipramine hydrochloride. *N. Engl. J. Med.* 296:206, 1977.
40. Glassman, A. H., and Perel, J. M. The clinical pharmacology of imipramine. Implications for therapeutics. *Arch. Gen. Psychiat.* 28:649, 1973.
41. Alexanderson, B., and Sjoqvist, F. Individual differences in the pharmacokinetics of monomethylated tricyclic antidepressants: Role of genetic and environmental factors and clinical importance. *Ann. N.Y. Acad. Sci.* 179:739, 1971.
42. Asberg, M., Cronholm, B., Sjoqvist, F., and Tuck, D. Relationship between plasma level and therapeutic effect of nortriptyline. *Br. Med. J.* 3:331, 1971.
43. Glassman, A., et al. Imipramine steady-state studies and plasma binding. In *Proceedings of the Third International Symposium on Phenothiazines and Structurally Related Compounds*. New York: Raven Press, 1974, p. 457.
44. Morselli, P. L. Psychotropic drugs. In P. L. Morselli, ed., *Drug Disposition During Development*. New York: Spectrum Publications, 1977, pp. 431–474.
45. Hollister, L. E. Tricyclic antidepressants (first of two parts). *N. Engl. J. Med.* 299:1106, 1978.
46. Ziegler, V. E., Biggs, J. T., and Wylie, L. T. Doxepin kinetics. *Clin. Pharmacol. Ther.* 23:573, 1978.
47. Spiker, D. G., and Biggs, J. T. Tricyclic antidepressants: Prolonged plasma levels after overdose. *JAMA* 236:1711, 1976.
48. Vohra, J., and Burrows, G. D. Cardiovascular complications of tricyclic antidepressant overdosage. *Drugs* 8:432, 1974.
49. Shatan, C. Withdrawal symptoms after abrupt termination of imipramine. *Can. Psychiat. Assoc. J.* 11:150, 1966.
50. Boston Collaborative Drug Surveillance Program. Adverse reactions to tricyclic-antidepressant drugs. *Lancet* I:529, 1972.
51. Noble, J., and Matthew, H. Acute poisoning by tricyclic antidepressants: Clinical features and management of 100 patients. *Clin. Toxicol.* 2:403, 1969.
52. Crome, P., Dawling, S., and Braithwaite, R. A. Effect of activated charcoal on absorption of nortriptyline. *Lancet* 2:1203, 1977.
53. Granacher, R. P., and Baldessarini, R. J. Physostigmine in the acute anticholinergic syndrome associated with antidepressant and antiparkinson drugs. *Arch. Gen. Psychiatry* 32:375, 1975.
54. Baldessarini, R. J., and Gelenber, A. J. Using physostigmine safely. *Am. J. Psychiatry* 136:1608, 1979.
55. Seppala, T., et al. Effect of tricyclic antidepressants and alcohol on psychomotor skills related to driving. *Clin. Pharmacol. Ther.* 17:515, 1975.
56. Detre, T. P., and Jarecki, G. H. *Modern Psychiatric Treatment*. Philadelphia: Lippincott, 1971.
57. Hardesty, A. S., and Burdock, E. I. Quantitative clinical evaluation in psychopharmacology. In M. A. Lipton, A. DiMascio, and K. F. Killam, eds., *Psychopharmacology: A Generation of Progress*. New York: Raven Press, 1978, pp. 871–878.
58. Johnson, F. N. (Editor) *Lithium Research and Therapy*. New York: Academic Press, 1975.
59. Johnson, F. N., and Johnson, S. *Lithium in Medical Practice*. Baltimore: University Park Press, 1978.
60. Cade, J. F. J. Lithium salts in the treatment of psychotic excitement. *Med. J. Aust.* 2:349, 1949.
61. Pert, A., et al. Long-term treatment with lithium prevents the development of dopamine receptor super-sensitivity. *Science* 201:171, 1978.
62. White, M. G., and Fetner, C. D. Treatment of the syndrome of inappropriate secretion of antidiuretic hormone with lithium carbonate. *N. Engl. J. Med.* 292:390, 1975.
63. Haugaard, E. S., Mickel, R. A., and Haugaard, N. Actions of lithium ions and insulin on glucose utilization, glycogen synthesis and glycogen synthase in the isolated rat diaphragm. *Biochem. Pharmacol.* 23:1675, 1974.
64. Cooper, T. B., and Simpson, G. M. Kinetics of lithium and clinical response. In M. A. Lipton, A. DiMascio, and K. F. Killiam, eds., *Psychopharmacology: A Generation of Progress*. New York: Raven Press, 1978, pp. 923–931.
65. Demers, R. G., and Heninger, G. R. Electrocardiographic T-wave changes during lithium carbonate treatment. *JAMA* 218:381, 1971.
66. Saron, B. M., and Gaind, R. Lithium. *Clin. Toxicol.* 6:257, 1973.

67. Goldfield, M. D., and Weinstein, M. R. Lithium carbonate in obstetrics: Guidelines for clinical use. *Am. J. Obstet. Gynecol.* 116:15, 1973.

68. Jefferson, J. W., and Greist, J. H. Lithium and the kidney. *Sem. Psychiatry* 81, 1979.

69. Tupin, J. P., and Schuller, A. B. Lithium and haloperidol incompatibility reviewed. *Psychiatr. J. Univ. Ottawa* 3:245, 1978.

70. Davis, J. M. Overview, maintenance therapy in psychiatry. II. Affective disorders. *Am. J. Psychiatry* 133:1, 1976.

71. Blum, K. Depressive states induced by drugs of abuse: Clinical evidence, theoretical mechanisms and proposed treatment. Part II. *J. Psychedel. Drugs* 8(3):235, 1976.

## SUGGESTED READING

Bassak, E. L., and Gelenberg, A. J. (Editors) *The Practitioner's Guide to Psychoactive Drugs*. New York: Plenum Press, 1983.

Cooper, J. R., and Bloom, F. *The Biochemical Basis of Neuropharmacology*, 2nd ed. Baltimore: Williams & Wilkins, 1980.

Gairgen, C. E. *Fundamentals of the Pharmacology of the Mind*. Springfield, Ill.: C. C. Thomas, 1981.

Kalinowski, et al. *Biological Treatments in Psychiatry*. New York: Grune & Stratton, 1982.

Klawans, H. L. *Textbook of Clinical Neuropharmacology*. New York: Raven Press, 1981.

Leavitt, F. *Drugs and Behavior*, 2nd ed. New York: Wiley, 1982.

Chapter 15

# Tobacco and Smoking Behavior

## A. INTRODUCTION

Since the dawn of civilization, the interaction of human beings with their environment has provoked a feeling of hostility. Throughout the ages, people had to fight to meet their basic needs for survival—a battle involving the earth, plants, rocks, and the very air. Today we appear to be out of touch with these basic environmental needs. We get close to nature by acquiring pets, plants, and even "pet rocks." Tennant and Day[1] suggest that cigarette advertising supplies our idea of "the good life," that which we have been told we are entitled to; it also suggests a path to instant gratification, one of which we were unaware in infancy and in the process of becoming adult. That path is tobacco.

On the surface, and knowing what we do about it, it seems incongruous that a rational human would absorb, sniff, inhale, or chew tobacco or any of its relatives. The prime question becomes then: What psychosocial advantage can be derived from a substance known to be harmful at best, and lethal at worst?

In the years since the 1964 Advisory Committee's report to the Surgeon General on smoking, awareness of the important effect of this widespread behavior on America's health has triggered significant trends. But William Pollin,[2] director of the National Institute on Drug Abuse, in reviewing the complexity of this medical/social problem suggests that the national effort to cope with it has been defective.

In 1964, a distinct drop in cigarette consumption occurred, and since then it has continued to decrease for adults—from 52 to 39 percent for males and from 32 to 29 percent for females. A 1975 investigation revealed that the number of physicians still smoking had decreased from 30 percent in 1967 to 21 percent; of dentists, from 34 to 23 percent; and of pharmacists, from 35 to 28 percent. In contrast, smoking by girls between the ages of 12 and 18 nearly doubled between 1968 and 1974. The age at which children begin regular smoking is down to 11 to 12 years. This statistic becomes important when we consider that early onset of a drug (smoking) habit is often predictive of stronger substance misuse.

According to the National Survey on Drug Abuse of 1979,[3] more than eight in ten young adults (82.8 percent) and older adults (83.0 percent) and more than half of youths (54.1 percent) had tried cigarettes. Only 14.9 percent of youths, 53.6 percent of young adults, and 59.2 percent of older adults, however, reported having smoked as many as five packs in their lifetimes. Current smoking is reported by less than one half of 18- to 25-year-olds (42.6 percent), about one third of those aged 26 and older (36.9 percent), and about one eighth of the 12 to 17 year olds (12.1 percent). The report also states that current smoking, like current drinking (alcohol), is related to chronologic age, with only 2 percent of the 12- to 13-year-olds reporting current use compared with 9 percent of the 14- to 15-year-olds, 24 percent of the 16- to 17-year-olds, 40 percent of the 18 to 21 age group, and 45 percent of the 22 to 25 year olds. The rate drops off among older adults, with 41 percent of the 26- to 34-year-olds reporting current use and just 26 percent of those aged 35 and older doing so. The report further states that current smokers are more likely than nonsmokers to have used alcohol, marihuana, psychotherapeutic pills, or ''stronger'' drugs (hallucinogens, cocaine, heroin). The largest differences occur among youths and young adults. Among youths, at least one third of current smokers have used stronger drugs (36.8 percent) or psychotherapeutic pills (35.1 percent), while fewer than one out of 20 nonsmokers have ever used these substances. Furthermore eight in ten youths who smoke cigarettes have had marihuana experience (80.9 percent), compared with fewer than one in four nonsmokers (23.9 percent). Ninety-four percent of youths who smoke have used alcohol; only two thirds of nonsmokers have done so (67.0 percent). Usage rates are even higher among young adults who are current smokers—nearly all (98.9 percent), 85.1 percent report using marihuana (nonsmokers, 55.6 percent), almost half (47.3 percent) say they have used stronger drugs (nonsmokers, 22.8 percent), and 43.0 percent report use of psychotherapeutic pills (nonsmokers, 19.6 percent).

Other startling statistics include the fact that the number of people who die prematurely from smoking is estimated at 300,000 annually. For comparison, annual automobile fatalities are estimated at about 55,000, and overdose deaths attributed to barbiturates at about 1400 and to heroin at about 1750. Over 37 million people (one of every six Americans alive in 1979) will die from cigarette smoking years before they would otherwise.

Interestingly Pollin[2] points out that if tobacco-related deaths were elimated, there would be:

- Some 300,000 Americans each year who would not die prematurely.
- One third fewer deaths of males between 35 and 59.
- Eighty-five percent fewer deaths from bronchitis or emphysema.
- One third fewer deaths from arteriosclerosis.
- One third fewer deaths from heart disease.
- Ninety percent fewer deaths from cancer of the trachea and lungs.
- Fifty percent fewer deaths from cancer of the bladder.

In spite of these data, more than 50 million Americans still are smoking.

Smoking is a problem not only in the United States. More than a decade ago, in 1971, a report by Great Britain's Royal College of Physicians on ''Smoking and Health Now'' pointed to cigarette smoking as the greatest preventable cause of illness, disability, and premature death in this century. Tennant[1] notes the mystique of tobacco and its healing powers. And its association with machismo and Marlboro Country may serve to override increasing evidence of potential danger. Tennant believes that the motivation for its use may be derived in part from advertisements portraying ''true, red-blooded Americans'' in youthful abandon, running through the woods, herding cattle, being ''cool,'' ''hip,'' ''together,'' and ''sexy,'' puffing on the ''death-dealing weapon'' of their choice.

In terms of its pharmacognosy, tobacco is a leafy green plant that belongs to the genus *Nicotiana*, of which there are more than 60 species. Only two of these, however, *N. rustica* and *N. tabacum*, possess the attributes that make them desirable for smoking or other human consumption. The *N. rustica* species is grown extensively in eastern Europe and Asia Minor.[4] *Nicotiana tabacum*, a complex hybrid, provides all the common tobaccos consumed in the United States. The different types, such as burley, oriental, and cigar tobaccos, are the result of differences in cultivation and processing as well as of different manifestations of the genetic complexities of the *N. tabacum* species.

Generally the tobacco leaf is harvested green and then subjected to the desired curing and fermentation processes. Subsequently the prepared tobacco is converted into the various tobacco products—cigarettes, cigars, snuff, chewing tobacco, and pipe tobacco. Production of the latter three products involves the addition of aroma and flavoring agents such as sugar, honey, molasses, and licorice to the processed tobacco.

The different tobacco products available are consumed in ways that are as unique as the products themselves. Cigarette smoke is inhaled into the lungs. Pipe and cigar smoke is quite alkaline and generally is not inhaled. The cigar represents a middle ground, however, in that the butt is chewed. Snuff either is sniffed into the nose, placed between the lower lip and the gum, or inserted between the cheek and gum with a moistened toothbrush. Chewing tobacco is macerated slowly and the juice spat out.

Tobacco, regardless of its form of administration, introduces a multitude of potent organic chemicals into the body of the consumer. This results in a very complex situation since the study of even one drug involves the examination of a myriad of many different effects. The drug can be studied relative to its physiologic effects on the various organs and organ systems, its behavioral effects, and its specific biochemical reaction effects, among others. When, as in the case of tobacco, many potent chemicals are introduced, many potential effects are available. Thus a comprehensive statement regarding the etiology of the effects of tobacco smoking must consider the synergistic and antagonistic, as well as individual, effects of its various chemical agents. Obviously a problem of this complexity only can be attacked piecemeal, with that part of more significant sociologic and scientific import receiving priority.

Of all the constituents of tobacco, nicotine has received the widest scientific attention by far. First of all, it is the main component of tobacco that has a broad and immediate pharmacologic action. Also this drug is so strong a poison that only about 60 mg represents a lethal dose for humans. Tobacco smoke contains a minute amount of nicotine and the body rapidly biotransforms (metabolizes) it to a nontoxic state. Otherwise smoking would cause serious, and perhaps fatal, complications. This can be emphasized by the fact that some cigars contain enough nicotine for two lethal doses.[5] Nicotine has no recognized therapeutic value. It is generally credited, however, with producing the pleasant aspects of tobacco consumption. Nicotine was first isolated in 1828 by two French chemists and named for Jean Nicot—the Frenchman credited with introducing tobacco in France.

As with any drug, to exert its effect nicotine must have a route into the body (absorption) and be distributed to the sites of its pharmacologic action. It is then metabolized to products that are less active and/or more readily excreted from the body.

Of late, other chemical constituents of tobacco have generated considerable interest. This is attributable to the recognized carcinogenicity of cigarette tar preparations, and particularly of the polynuclear aromatic hydrocarbons. The Surgeon General's epidemiologic study has concluded that cigarette smoking is a health hazard, with smokers running a statistically high risk of lung cancer and cardiovascular disease. Some studies[6] have shown a positive correlation between pipe smoking and tobacco chewing and the incidence of certain forms of oral cancer. Present efforts are directed at delineating clear mechanisms by which these other tobacco constituents effect carcinogenism.

A close look at tobacco's use and abuse shows that it does fit into the American myth heritage of risk taking and is conjoined with a wide spectrum of destructive health behaviors.

## B. HISTORY

Tobacco, although once considered a drug that was listed in the *Pharmacopeia*, is now seldom considered to fit that definition. In essence, the consumer does not consider the tobacco habit a "drug habit." The indifferent attitude of most tobacco abusers is also reflected at the governmental level, since there is no definitive agency to legislate or control tobacco usage. It is neither imbibed nor ingested, and thus is removed from regulatory agencies that control food and beverage consumption.

The exact origin of tobacco use by humans is not recorded. But it is possible to envision its pleasures being discovered in some accidental manner, perhaps along the lines of the legendary discovery of the taste of cooked pork after the pigs had been roasted when the sty burned down. At any rate, tobacco smoking was a well-developed native custom by the time Columbus arrived in the New World. Tobacco was introduced to Europe in the ensuing years, and by that time the English had made attempts to colonize Virginia.

The highly desirable *N. tabacum* was native to South America. The Spanish arrived there first and quickly established a monopoly on the world's tobacco production, which they retained for over 100 years. This rankled the British, especially in light of the fact that their own initial attempts to establish a tobacco colony in Virginia had failed. In 1612, John Rolfe, the leader of the Virginia colony, obtained some seeds from the *N. tabacum* species and planted them in Virginia. The new species flourished, and within a few years as much Virginia as Spanish tobacco was being sold on the London markets.

The several forms of tobacco use have waxed and waned over the years. A type of cigarette—a thin reed filled with tobacco—was in use by Central American Indians in the early 16th century. However, pipe smoking was the thing to do in Elizabethan England. But by the latter part of the 17th century and continuing through the 18th century, smoking declined in popularity, and snuff "dipping" came into vogue. Probably one impetus for this change was the belief that snuff afforded some protection to its users during the Great Plague of 1665. After the American Revolution, chewing tobacco began to replace snuff, and become particularly popular among cowboys of the early West.

In more recent times, tobacco chewing gradually has given way again to smoking. As with most changes, the conversion from chewing to smoking proceeded slowly and involved a transition state—cigars. The cigar butt is chewable and the cigar smokable. Although cigarettes were among the earliest forms of tobacco use, their popularity has increased only since the middle of the last century. Cigarette smoking gradually overtook cigar smoking, and then far surpassed it in popularity. It remains the most prevalent form of tobacco use.

A discussion of the history of tobacco cannot overlook the extent to which tobacco in various forms was once considered a potent medicine. The 16th, 17th, 18th, and part of the 19th centuries saw the tobacco leaf treated almost as a therapeutic panacea. Tobacco dentifrice was recommended for toothache, tobacco poltices for the pain of childbirth, and snuffing tobacco into the nose for treatment of headache. The slow advance of medical science eventually discredited the supposed attributes of tobacco therapeutics.

Some of the landmarks in the discovery of tobacco are listed in Table 15-1.

During the history of tobacco in this country, there have been three regulatory thrusts: (1) at production, (2) at revenue, and (3) at consumption. In early Virginia, tobacco was used instead of money, and in 1696 it was even put into law that ministers be paid at the rate of 1600 pounds of tobacco annually.[7]

The first proposal for an American federal excise tax on tobacco was written in 1774, and further tax increases were instituted in 1862, 1865, 1866, and 1875. By 1880 the taxes had stabilized and equaled 31 percent of the total federal tax receipts: From 1910 to 1920, in only one decade, they had increased by more than 500 percent, and in the 1920s represented $2.1 billion. Of interest is the fact that, in 1880, only 2 percent of the total federal tobacco revenue was derived from cigarette consumption, the remainder primarily coming from pipe, snuff, and cigar usage. In 1970, a reverse trend occured, with 97 percent of the total tobacco revenue being derived from the sale of cigarettes.[6]

In the first half of 1975, 305 billion cigarettes were smoked in the United States.

Breechen[8] has termed the world of the 19th century and its attitude toward drugs "a dope fiend's paradise." Opiates at one time were prescribed generously for everything from alcoholism to vaginismus, and could be obtained openly and freely through a physician or over the counter. Tennant[1] suggests that the tranquilizing actions of the opiates tended to overshadow the consequences of dependence. The open and widespread usage of tobacco is quite analogous to the early usage of opiates. While the documentation of its deleterious physiologic effects continues to accumulate, its tranquilizing aspects, not to mention economic pressures and advertising, seem to be a subverting influence.

In terms of smoking and the law, as early as 1632, the General Court of Massachussetts Bay enacted a law that forbade smoking in public. This was expanded in 1638 to include public inns and public houses, and was followed by other laws, which subsequently were repealed.[7] Along these lines, laws regulating cigarette advertising on television, signed by President Nixon, and bans in Czechoslovakia, Italy, and England, only temporarily slowed the persistent rise in tobacco consumption. In addition, state-enforced prohibitions have been repealed, and several states have lowered the age restrictions from 18 years to 15 because of enforcement difficulties. Even with the advent of special smoking sections in schools, restaurants, and on airplanes, other factors, such as the widespread use of vending machines, have offset the fight against tobacco's social use.

The net result is that these laws have done little to suppress smoking, and can be but loosely enforced at best.

## C. CHEMICAL COMPOSITION OF TOBACCO[9]

At the onset smoking cigarettes may seem fairly innocent. Advertising encourages cigarette smoking as soothing and relaxing, and to be enjoyed. Subsequent serious health complications are well known, however. Lung cancer, a number one risk in cigarette smoking, is thought to be caused by polonium-210 and nickel present in the smoke of tobacco.[9]

Interestingly, carbon monoxide (CO) may turn out to be a more toxic component in cigarette smoke than nicotine. It is well known that smoking one pack of cigarettes yields about 260 mg. of CO to the user, and this amount can convert 5 to 10 percent of the normal hemoglobin to carboxyhemoglobin. Although it is difficult to pinpoint the exact causes of cigarette smoking, there are other toxic components besides nicotine that may be implicated. Nicotine, the main toxic ingredient, comprises from 0.5 to 8.0 percent. In the future, safer cigarettes should filter out the other 500 or more compounds which have been isolated from the particulate and gaseous phases of tobacco smoke. These include a family of isoprenoid compounds, pyridine and other nitrogenous bases,

**TABLE 15-1**

**Some Landmarks in the Discovery of Tobacco**

| | |
|---|---|
| 1492 | Columbus' sailors observe Indians smoking. |
| 1512 | Juan Ponce de Leon brings tobacco to Portugal. |
| 1556 | Andre Thevet, upon returning from Brazil, introduces tobacco and brings tobacco seeds to France. |
| 1558 | Tobacco is cultivated in Portugal.<br>Francesco Hernandez of Toledo brings tobacco to Spain. |
| 1559 | Damien de Goes gives tobacco plants to Jean Nicot, who describes the "medicinal properties" of the plant. |
| | Francisco Hernandez, private physician to Philip II, returns from Mexico and plants tobacco in Spain. |
| 1565 | Sir John Hawkins brings tobacco seeds to England.<br>Sir Walter Raleigh introduces smoking in England.<br>Konrad Gesner introduces tobacco in Zurich. |
| 1573 | Tobacco is cultivated in England. |
| 1603–1617 | Smoking is introduced in Turkey. |

(From J.L. Van Lancker. Smoking and disease In NIDA Research Monograph no. 17. M.E. J.W. Jarvick et al. eds. Washington, D.C., U.S. Government Printing Office, 1977, p. 231.)

volatile acids, phenolic substances, furfural, and acrolein.

Smoking one cigeratte yields at least 6–8 mg of nicotine (compared with a cigar, which yields from 15 to more than 40 mg nicotine) and about 90 percent of the nicotine is absorbed when inhaled, while only 25–50 percent of nicotine is absorbed when drawn into the mouth and then exhaled. Enough nicotine from even one cigarette is absorbed to warrant immediate consideration of abstinence.

The amount of nicotine found in tobacco depends upon the brand of tobacco, humidity, the nature of the soil, and species, as well as on the habits of the smoker.[10] Unless the tobacco is chewed or snuffed it is the amount of nicotine that appears in the smoke that is critical.[11,12]. The least noxious form of tobacco smoking is the pipe while the most harmful is the cigarette. McNally,[13] in 1932, recognized the importance of temperature and today it is known that high temperatures of burning tobacco might play an important role in the pathogenesis of cancer in pipe smokers.

## D. TOXICOLOGY OF TOBACCO COMPONENTS

### 1. Carbon Monoxide

Carbon monoxide is a colorless, odorless, nonirritant gas. Its toxicity stems from its binding to hemoglobin to form carboxyhemoglobin, which is 2.10 times stronger than the binding of oxygen to hemoglobin to form oxyhemoglobin. Thus repeated exposure to even small amounts of carbon monoxide can dramatically reduce the amount of hemoglobin available for combination with oxygen and cause anoxemia of all tissues. Certainly the heart and the brain, which are heavily dependent on aerobic respiration for function, are the first victims of anoxemia. Goldsmith and Landau[14] in 1968 reported that carbon monoxide binds not only to hemoglobin, but also to many other iron proteins, including the cytochromes, and major electron transporters.

In addition, carbon monoxide interferes with the homeostatic mechanism by which 2, 3-diphosphoglycerate controls the affinity of hemoglobin for oxygen.

Interestingly the deleterious effects of carbon ıonoxide may not be restricted to the smoker. Studies by Chevalier et al.[15] and Russell et al.[16] have shown that inhalation of smoke in an unventilated room for 78 minutes is equivalent to the absorption of the amount of carbon monoxide that would emanate from the smoking of one cigarette.

The greatest concentrations of carbon monoxide in the smoke are obtained during cigar smoking, and the concentration in the lung will be 0.04 percent. The smoking of one cigar is equal to the loss of 250 cc of blood because of the carbon monoxide buildup.[17]

Although such an alteration may be of little significance, it becomes important in persons with severe artherosclerosis or who suffer from other diseases that cause anoxemia.

### 2. Other Compounds

The fermentation of the polysaccharide pectin, found in the tobacco plant, yields methyl alcohol. It is estimated that 40 mg of methyl alcohol is absorbed after one smokes 20 unfiltered cigarettes and 42 mg is absorbed after the smoking of ten cigars.

Other tobacco by-products include ammonia, formaldehyde, phenols, creosote, anthracen, and pyrene and hydrocyanic acids. An increase in thiocyamate in the blood of smokers has been observed, which is excreted through the saliva.[18]

It is noteworthy that fertilizers and insecticides may add arsenic and lead to the tobacco. Half of the arsenic in tobacco enters the smoke, the rest remaining in the ash. The amount of arsenic in the inhaled smoke ranges from 3.3 to 10.5 mg per cubic meter of smoke.[19]

### 3. Nicotine

#### *a. Introduction*

In 1828, nicotine was isolated from tobacco by Posselt and Reinmann.[20] There is no therapeutic indication for its use. The structure of nicotine is shown in Figure 15-1. In terms of structure–activity relationships, both d and l forms are equipotent.

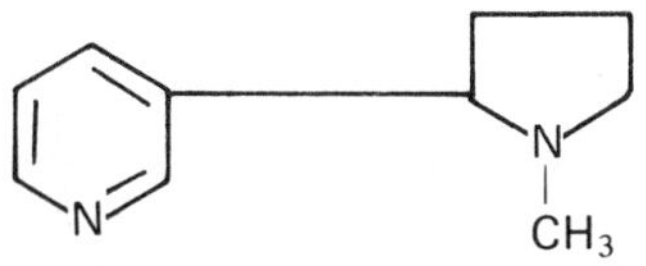

**Figure 15-1. Chemical structure of nicotine: 1-methyl-1-(3-pyridyl)pyrrolidine.**

The naturally occurring liquid alkaloid, 1-methyl-1-(3-pyridyl) pyrrolidine, commonly known as nicotine, is volatile and colorless. An ingredient in tobacco, upon oxidation, it turns brown and smells like burning tobacco. Nicotine is very poisonous; in fact, a cigar contains enough nicotine for two lethal doses. However, through smoking, the nicotine is not delivered in a short enough time to prove fatal to an individual. Death due to nicotine poisoning, like cyanide, is very quick, and the lethal dose in non-tolerant people is about 60 minutes.

### *b. Chemistry*

Nicotine is a beta-pyridyl-alpha-N-methyl pirrolidine. The chemical formula is depicted in Figure 15-1. When it is fresh, nicotine is a colorless oil with an unpleasant odor and is very soluble in water. Upon exposure to air, it becomes brown.

### *c. Pharmacokinetics and Metabolism*

Absorption of the nicotine from tobacco seems to take place via most of the membranes of the body.[21,22] Those of particular interest are in the mouth, nose, and lungs. The absorption of nicotine through the mucosa is very dependent on the form in which the alkaloid is present.

Figure 15-2 shows the alkaline (I) and acid (II) forms of nicotine. If the medium in which it is presented is more alkaline, more of the alkaloid is in form (I) and is thus more soluble in the nonionic lipid of the mucosal cell walls.

Studies of the frequency of inhalation or puffing by cigarette smokers have indicated that there is a tendency to optimize the amount of nicotine delivered to the smoker. These studies can be extended to the other forms of tobacco use. Although nicotine is less readily absorbed by the oral mucosa, cigar smoke is more alkaline than that of the cigarette, and thus presents more of the nicotine in the free base form. As such, it is more soluble in the fat-rich mucosal cell walls, and accordingly is more readily absorbed. In the cases of snuff and chewing tobacco, these forms of tobacco use involve prolonged contact with the mucosa, and thus more chance for nicotine absorbtion.

These statements regarding tobacco use by humans seem to be substantiated by controlled experiments using animals. In experiments with dogs, a greater hypertensive response was elicited when cigarette smoke was directed into the lungs than when the smoke was directed into the upper respiratory passages. Another experiment—using rabbits—showed that inhalation of cigarette smoke caused marked respiratory and cardiovascular effects; these were greatly reduced when the smoke was merely circulated through the animal's mouth. Thus the nicotine available in the smoke streak of a cigarette seems to be absorbed by the lungs and bronchi to a much greater extent than by organs and tissue in the mouth and nose.

Smoking one cigarette causes small increases in heart rate and blood pressure. These effects can be credited to the fact that nicotine causes a release of adrenaline from the adrenal gland and other storage sites. One cigarette contains about 25 mg of nicotine, of which some 10 percent is absorbed by the inhaling smoker. These effects can be approximated by the intravenous injection of 1 mg of nicotine.

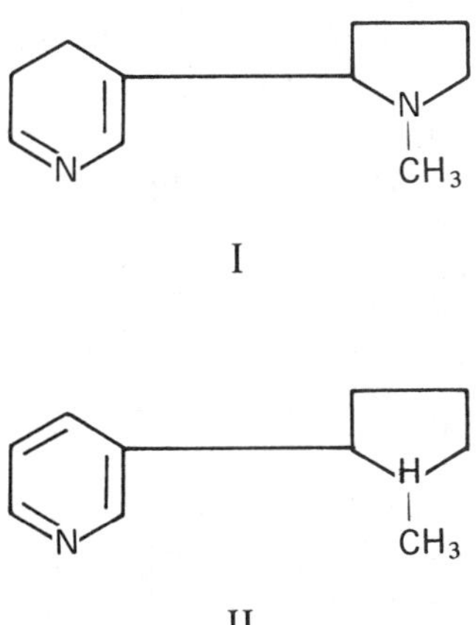


**Figure 15-2. Alkaline and acid forms of nicotine.**

Once nicotine has been absorbed into the bloodstream, it is circulated throughout the systemic blood. It is then available to its various sites of pharmacologic action. At the same time, the drug is passing through the liver, where it is biotransformed (metabolized). Biotransformation of a drug results, generally, in its conversion into chemicals that are less toxic and more water soluble than the precursor. The increase in water solubility renders the compound more soluble in the urine, and thus it is more readily excreted from the body. Nicotine is converted to a number of such metabolites. Some 10 to 20 percent of ingested nicotine is excreted unchanged via the urinary tract.

The liver is the major organ that deactivates nicotine. It is well established that approximately 85 percent of the drug is modified prior to excretion via the kidneys. Since nicotine acts on the hypothalamus to cause a release of the hormone that reduces the loss of body fluids, it tends to slow excretion of itself.

Today the typical filter cigarette still contains between 1 and 20 mg of nicotine. The individual who smokes the cigarette and inhales will absorb 10 percent of that. In this regard, a l-mg intravenous injection of nicotine can induce the physiologic effects of smoking. Ninety percent of inhaled nicotine is usually absorbed.

A significant fraction of inhaled nicotine is metabolized by the lung.[23] The major metabolites of nicotine are cotinine and nicotine-1$^1$-N-oxide, which result from oxidation of the carboal N-oxidation of the pyrrolidine ring. The half-life of nicotine following inhalation or parenteral administration is 30 to 60 minutes. Russell and Feyerbend[24] report that these nicotine metabolites are rapidly eliminated in the kidney. Nicotine is also excreted in the milk of lactating women who smoke. The milk of heavy smokers may contain up to 0.5 mg per liter of nicotine.

### d. Pharmacologic Properties of Nicotine

1. *Overview:* Nicotine is considered to be one of the most toxic of all drugs. Generally the major pharmacologic effects include elevated blood pressure, increased bowel activity, and an antidiuretic action. Nicotine, after prolonged use, produces moderate tolerance and a mild to moderate development of physical dependence.

Nicotine causes a release of noradrenaline from the adrenal glands and other sympathetic sites. This release of the catecholamine noradrenaline increases heart rate, blood pressure, coronary blood flow, and produces vasoconstriction of the skin. Due to the biphasic action of nicotine on ganglionic transmission, sensory receptors (chemical receptors, found in some large arteries) and pain and temperature receptors are first stimulated, then blocked, by nicotine.

Nicotine is known to first stimulate, and then block, central nervous system synapses. Nicotine is a cholinergic agonist via interaction on the cholinergic receptor site, thereby mimicking the actions of acetylcholine. Because nicotine is slowly deactivated, its continued occupation at the receptor site leads to potential paralysis at that site.

In animal studies, nicotine has been shown to alter the electrical discharge of the reticular formation. The drug shifts the EEG to an arousal pattern, thereby acting at the level of the cortex to augment the frequency of the electrical activity.

Low doses of nicotine stimulate oxygen receptors in the carotid artery. The signs associated with acute nicotine poisoning include paralysis of respiratory muscle, convulsions, and tremors.

2. *Effect on organ systems.* The complex and often unpredictable changes that occur in the body after administration of nicotine are due not only to its effects in many neuroeffector and chemosensitive sites, but also to the fact that the alkaloid (nicotine) has both depressant and stimulant phases of actions.[25]

Three fourths of the nicotine in cigarettes is delivered to the peripheral nervous system.

As previously mentioned, nicotine, due to its unusual pharmacology, produces complex and often unpredictable effects. Most of these effects are due to the biphasic nature of nicotine (exhibiting both inhibitory as well as excitatory actions.[25]

The chemosensitive sites are usually affected by approximately 75 percent of the nicotine in cigarettes which is delivered to the peripheral nervous system.

The prime action of nicotine initially is transient stimulation and subsequently persistent depression of all autonomic ganglia. Small amounts of nicotine induce a direct facilitory stimulation of the ganglion cells, whereby high doses produce a very transient stimulation followed by a blockade of transmission. With regard to the adrenal medulla, a biphasic action is observed with nicotine. In response to splanchinic nerve stimulation, large doses prevent catecholamine release, whereas small doses *induce* the release of catecholamines.

Burn et al., in 1959,[26] and later Ferry, in 1963,[27] reported that nicotine also causes the release of catecholamines in a number of isolated organs.

The effects of nicotine on the neuromuscular junction are similar to those on ganglia. In essence, the stimulant phase is obscured by the rapidly developing paralysis.

Nicotine stimulates a number of receptors, such as mechanoreceptors that respond to stretch or pressure of the skin, mesentery, tongue, lung, and stomach; chemoreceptors of the carotid body; thermal receptors of the skin and tongue; and pain receptors.[28]

3. *General Brain Effects*. Nicotine has been proposed as the primary incentive in smoking.[29] It is rapidly extracted by the alveolar capillaries, enters the pulmonary circulation, and is pumped to the aorta, where it stimulates the aortic and carotid chemoreceptors and may produce reflex stimulation of the respiratory and cardiovascular centers in the brain stem. According to Oldendorff,[30] within one circulation time one fourth of the nicotine inhaled passes through the brain capillaries and, since it is highly permeable to the blood–brain barrier, passes quickly into the brain.

Once in the brain, nicotine markedly stimulates nicotinic cholinergic (ACH) synapses and produces tremors, and even convulsions, in both laboratory animals and humans. In terms of mechanism of action, nicotine also releases various biogenic amines, including catecholamines and 5-hydroxytryptamine (serotonin). The excitation of respiration is a particularly prominent action of nicotine, although large doses act directly on the medulla oblongata. Smaller doses, as already mentioned, work indirectly via chemoreceptors.[31] Stimulation of the CNS is followed by depression, and death results from failure of respiration due to both central paralysis and peripheral blockade of muscles or respiration.

Nicotine stimulates the emetic chemoreceptor trigger zone in the medulla and it causes nausea and vomiting in novices. It exerts an antidiuretic action as the result of stimulation of the hypothalamic neurohypophyseal system, with the concomitant release of antidiuretic hormone (ADH).

Studies from a number of laboratories indicate that nicotine can have a facilitating effect upon learning and memory in animals,[32, 33] and possibly in humans.[34] Centrally nicotine may even act as a mild tranquilizer, allowing individuals to make proper choices.[33]

Although nicotine makes up 93 percent of the alkaloid fraction of cigarette smoke, 13 other alkaloids are present that have a variety of pharmacologic effects. Battig[35] has shown a differential effect of nicotine and tobacco smoke alkaloids upon swimming endurance of the rat. Possibly through a central effect, nicotine improved performance whereas total alkaloids impaired it.

4. *Heart and Circulatory Actions*. At 6 to 8 mg. of nicotine there is a considerable effect on the cardiovascular system due to stimulation of sympathetic ganglia and the adrenal medulla as well as release from chromatin tissue and peripheral sympathetic nerve endings. Gebber,[36] in 1969, provided the neurogenic basis for nicotine-induced augmentation of blood pressure in animals. Accordingly, the concomittant release of body catecholamines and their subsequent activation of the chemoreceptors of the aortic and carotid bodies result in vasoconstriction, tachycardia, and elevated blood pressure.

5. *Gastrointestinal tract*. In constrast to the cardiovascular effects of nicotine, the actions of the drug on the gastrointestinal tract are largely the result of parasympathetic stimulation. The combined activation of parasympathetic ganglia and cholinergic nerve endings results in increased tone and motor activity of the bowel. Systemic absorption of nicotine may produce nausea, vomiting, and diarrhea. Inhibition of stomach contractions resulting from hunger is another pharmacologic effect of nicotine. This partially explains the increased hunger and weight gain when one ceases cigarette consumption. One report showed that when over-a-pack-a-day smokers stopped smoking, there was a three-beat-per-minute decrease in heart rate and a 10 percent decrease in oxygen consumption. Slowing of the heart rate de-

creases, to some extent, the energy needs of the body. It seems more probable that the decrease in oxygen consumption resulted from a general decrease in the rate at which food is utilized for energy, so that with the same food intake, more will be shifted into fat-storage depots.[37]

6. *Effects on Exocrine Glands*. Nicotine can directly stimulate muscurinic acetyl-choline receptor sites in the salivary and bronchial glands. Both these glands are initially stimulated, then inhibited, by nicotine. However, it is usually the irritating properties of cigarette smoke rather than nicotine per se which induce reflex salivation.

## E. THEORIES ON THE USE OF TOBACCO

### 1. Pharmacologic and Behavioral Correlates

The possible psychologic basis for the tobacco habit may be a need for oral stimulation. There seems to be a correlation between smoking and other oral habits, such as alcohol and coffee intake, and some studies also suggest that early childhood thumb sucking may lead to the smoking habit. There are also some theories supporting the idea that a smoker who had been breastfed longer smokes less and finds it easier to stop.

Other theories suggest that because smokers maintain an optimal dose in a consistent way—for example, one to two puffs per minute with a volume of 25 ml, which delivers from 1 to 2 mg/kg of nicotine with each puff—a real physiologic basis for smoking may exist.

It appears that in cats 2 mg/kg of nicotine administered intravenously every 30 seconds results in EEG activation in approximately three fourths of the animals tested. Experiments in animals suggest that cortical arousal may act as the reward in humans and that it is this pharmacologic effect of nicotine that is the basis of smoking behavior.

Cortical activation appears to be related to levels of stress and tension. Numerous investigators[33,38–41] have shown that compared with non-smokers, heavy smokers have a higher level of cortical actuation, even in the absence of smoking. Nicotine may induce a brief period of cortical deactivation or tranquilization. In terms of an explanation for chain-smoking behavior, the above mechanism correlates with reports of increased cigarette smoking during periods of tension and stress. In fact, radioactive (traced) nicotine injected into rats lasts only approximately 15–30 minutes in the brain. Chain smokers average about one cigarette per half an hour.

On the negative side, however, the smoker may have tremors, shortness of breath, nose and throat irritations, increased incidence of coronary disease, a predisposition to tumors and lung cancer, and a shortened life span. On the other hand, incentives for continued smoking include relief of constipation, anorexia, hand–mouth activity, alteration of taste and olfaction, stimulation, tranquilization, and pacification. Tennant[1] points out that one has only to watch television to be frequently reminded that constipation is unhealthy and obesity undesirable, and that tranquility is a commodity much to be sought after.

### 2. Smoke as a Reinforcer

Much of the evidence for the role of nicotine as the primary reinforcer in cigarette smoke is circumstantial. Smokers clearly prefer cigarettes with nicotine to those without,[42] but they will smoke nicotine-free cigarettes, although grudgingly. In Figure 15-3, it can be seen that in 1973 the most popular cigarettes had a nicotine content between 1.25 and 1.49 mg per cigarette, and in the 1980s this has not significantly changed.

Interestingly cigarettes with a nicotine content of less than 0.3 mg per cigarette do not do well on the market. Jarvik[43] believes that tobacco-free cigarettes are doomed to oblivion unless they are made of marihuana. Lettuce cigarettes had a brief vogue in the United States, but the two companies that produced the two brands available went bankrupt. It is the rare smoker who continues to smoke cigarettes that lack nicotine when high-nicotine cigarettes are available. Thus nicotine appears to be a reinforcer.

Studies in humans to determine reinforcing properties of nicotine include direct positive responses[44–47] and suppression of smoking,[47] but these studies have not been entirely convincing.

### 3. Social Incentives

The tobacco industry has capitalized on the subtle interaction of socially encouraged behaviors, appearance, and image. Glasser[48] has developed the idea that identity ads promote an individuality that stresses social and sexual desirability. Cigarette advertising promulgates the image of the individual who is youthful, self-satisfied, attractive, "tough," and enjoying the "good life." Shafe[7] suggests that cigarette ads are not designed to persuade a smoker of one brand to smoke another, but rather to reinforce the quest for a successful self-image and to entice the nonsmoker into becoming a smoker. It is noteworthy that in the year (1972) in which the ban on television ads was enacted, the cigarette advertising industry was doing a $220 billion business. The outdoor or billboard advertising business is capitalizing on cigarette advertising today.

## F. ACUTE TOBACCO AND NICOTINE POISONING

The acutely fatal dose of nicotine for an adult is probably about 60 mg of the base. Smoking tobacco usually contains 1 to 2 percent nicotine. When smoked, cigarettes currently manufactured in the United States usually deliver 0.25 to 2.5 mg of nicotine (see Figure 15-3).

The symptomatology of acute nicotine or tobacco poisoning is quite variable. Generally nicotine-poisoned individuals exhibit nausea,

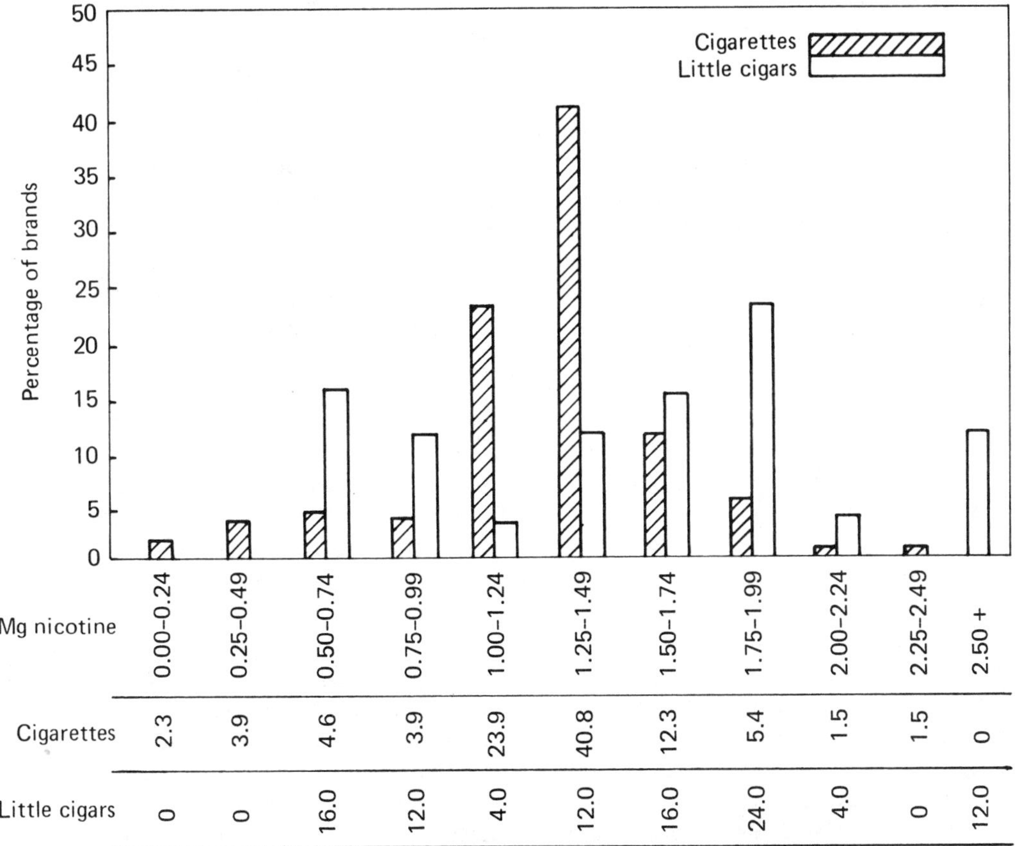


| Mg nicotine | 0.00–0.24 | 0.25–0.49 | 0.50–0.74 | 0.75–0.99 | 1.00–1.24 | 1.25–1.49 | 1.50–1.74 | 1.75–1.99 | 2.00–2.24 | 2.25–2.49 | 2.50 + |
|---|---|---|---|---|---|---|---|---|---|---|---|
| Cigarettes | 2.3 | 3.9 | 4.6 | 3.9 | 23.9 | 40.8 | 12.3 | 5.4 | 1.5 | 1.5 | 0 |
| Little cigars | 0 | 0 | 16.0 | 12.0 | 4.0 | 12.0 | 16.0 | 24.0 | 4.0 | 0 | 12.0 |

**Figure 15-3. Percent distribution of 130 brands of cigarettes and 25 brands of little cigars by nicotine content. [From Jarvik, M.E. Biological factors underlying the smoking habit. In M.E. Jarvik et al., eds., *Research on Smoking Behavior* (NIDA Research Monograph no 17). Washington, D.C.: NIDA, 1977, p. 131.]**

vomiting, dizziness, and general weakness. These conditions, to some extent, are all too familiar to the novice smoker attempting to enjoy that first strong cigar. Severe nicotine poisoning can quickly result in convulsions, unconsciousness, and possibly death. In fact, it appears that in some instances coma and death occur before all the symptoms of nicotine poisoning manifest themselves. This may in some measure account for the observed variety in symptom patterns.

Documentation of the past medical therapeutic usage of tobacco is replete with cases of nicotine overdose. Infusion of a tobacco decoction into the rectum sometimes resulted in fatal nicotine poisoning due to rapid absorption of nicotine by the rectal tissue. Application of hot tobacco leaves to the skin sometimes gave the same result, but often over a longer period of time owing to the slower absorption of nicotine through the skin. Cases of serious nicotine poisoning have been recorded wherein users of nicotine sulfate insecticide sprays inadvertently allowed their skin to come into contact with the solution.

Small children who play with old smoking pipes provide another source of sometimes fatal dosages of nicotine. The child who uses his or her father's pipe to blow soap bubbles is courting death with an intensity that is not generally appreciated.

## G. CHRONIC TOXICITY OF TOBACCO AND NICOTINE

### 1. Overview

Not only does cigarette smoking cause cancer of the lungs,[4] it also causes cancer of the oral cavity, larynx, esophagus, and the mucosal epitheliomas. Heavy cigarette smoking takes its toll, with male smokers versus nonsmokers dying from lung cancer in a ratio of 11 to 1, in America. Women also suffer from cigarette smoking health complications. Reproductive disorders include preeclampsia, fewer pregnancies, more natural abortions, and a higher incidence of neonatal mortality, as well as low-birth-weight infants.[22] Many of the health problems associated with cigarette smoking are also found in nonsmokers; however, the risks for the smokers are obviously higher. Smokers, for example, have higher incidences of respiratory, pulmonary, cardiovascular, ulcer, and even vision problems. The respiratory syndrome is characterized by dyspnea, wheezing, pharyngeal constriction, pain in the chest, and frequent upper respiratory infections, often mistaken for asthma, which disappears after smoking is eliminated. It is thought that the respiratory syndrome is caused by a depression of the ciliary defense mechanism of the respiratory tract. Ventilatory efficiency may also be impaired. Chronic obstructive pulmonary disease was observed in smokers, and pulmonary damage occurred in high school students who had smoked for at least one to five years.[49]

Another considerable health risk from cigarette smoking involves the cardiovascular system. More and more smokers are dying from coronary disease. Levine[50] found evidence of increased thrombus formation due to tobacco smoke, which also contributed to coronary heart disease. Additionally, cerebrovascular disorders are frequent, causing premature systoles, paroxysmal attacks of atrial tachycardia, or a decrease in amplitude or an inversion of the T-wave. More than 90 percent of patients with thromboangitis obliterans are smokers. Observations also show that smoking causes peripheral vasoconstriction, especially in the skin, and is implicated, although not definitively, in Buerger's disease.[4]

Psychologic factors and high levels of gastric acid cause the development of peptic ulcers. Although an increase in gastric acid does not occur from cigarette smoking, there is a decrease in bicarbonate in the small intestine, apparently due to nicotine, and this may contribute to the formation of peptic ulcers as a result of cigarette smoking.[51, 52] A gradual or sudden decrease in visual acuity, mostly in the central field and especially for colored objects, may eventually lead to optic nerve atrophy and permanent injury to vision. Fortunately, tobacco amblyopia is not a frequent occurrence.

Tolerance development and toxicity of nicotine, and other chemicals in tobacco are extremely dangerous effects that cannot be overemphasized. A person's life is shortened by 14 minutes for every cigarette smoked; moreover, in the United States alone, it is estimated that 360,000 persons die each year from tobacco use.[41] The high incidence of a variety of medical problems from tobacco smoking is well correlated in *Smoking and Health* and *The Health Consequences of Smoking,* which are detailed and described in authoritative reports by the Surgeon General of the U.S. Public Health Service. Yet a large population still abuses cigarette smoking, which could alternatively be the nation's most preventable cause of death.[53, 54]

## 2. Tolerance and Dependence Liability

Russell,[55] in discussing tobacco smoking as a form of drug dependence, suggested that the modern cigarette is a highly efficient device for self-administering the drug nicotine. Unknown to most, by inhaling, the smoker can get nicotine to the brain more rapidly than the heroin-dependent person can get a "buzz" by shooting heroin into a vein. For example, it takes only seven seconds for nicotine in the lungs to reach the brain compared with the 14 seconds it takes for blood to flow from arm to brain. Additionally the smoker gets a "shot" of nicotine after each inhaled puff. It has been estimated that at ten puffs per cigarette, the pack-a-day smoker gets more than 70,000 nicotine shots to the brain in a year.

When adolescents take up smoking, a variety of psychosocial reasons—including to look "tough" or "grown up" or because "most of their friends smoke"—seem to outweigh the unpleasant effects of nicotine. Tolerance soon develops to the unpleasant side effects and, as this threshold is passed, increasing amounts of nicotine are inhaled so that the smoker progresses to a stage of dependence. In 1967, McKennell and Thomas[56] described the startling statistic that of those teenagers who smoke more than one or two cigarettes occasionally, only 15 percent will avoid escalating to dependent smoking.

As with other addictive psychoactive substances, such as alcohol and heroin, the notion of "once a smoker, always a smoker" is only a slight exaggeration. Only 25 percent of smokers succeed in giving up the habit for good before reaching the age of 60. Only a small minority—2 percent according to one study—for whom smoking is a take-it-or-leave-it affair, and who limit themselves to intermittent or occasional smoking, once or twice a week or less, exists.

An important factor in the degree of "abstinence symptoms" from nicotine withdrawal may be the genetic makeup of the individual. Researchers have been investigating the pharmacogenetics of cigarette smoking and nicotine. According to Dr. Allan Collins, principal investigator on a research project funded by the National Council for Tobacco Research, mouse strains differ in their behavior and physiologic responses to nicotine.[57] Interpretation of these results is that genetic factors infludence both acute and chronic effects of nicotine.

The dependence liability of tobacco smoking clearly is strong, and few other forms of drug taking are as addictive as the puff-by-puff shots of nicotine obtained by smoking cigarettes. Tobacco addiction is so easily acquired relative to alcohol, and possibly even heroin, that cigarette smoking is a drug-addiction problem.

There are a variety of reasons why cigarette smoking is so addictive. These include: (1) rapid and numerous pharmacologic reinforcements afforded by the puff-by-puff nicotine bolus of intake from inhaled cigarette smoking; (2) rapid clearance and metabolism of nicotine in the brain; (3) the sharp "letdown" from those effects that depend on a direct action; (4) the fact that cigarette smoking not only does not impair performance, but actually enhances socialization; and (5) its social acceptability. Although the social climate has changed, cigarette smoking is still, in most social circles, far more acceptable than the use of other drugs, with the exception perhaps of tea and coffee, sleeping pills (taken at night but not by day), and tranquilizers that are medically prescribed. Among other reasons is that, in modern societies. cigarettes are one of the most readily available of all commodities. This availability is linked to low cost—two packs a day are cheaper than a bottle of gin. Also, cigarette smoking combines a pharmacologic effect with a sensorimotor ritual that includes the mouth as a locus of pleasurable self-indulgence.

In view of the changing attitudes toward cigarette smoking, new motivations for wanting to quit smoking have become evident. One is the smoker's feeling of being an unwelcome nuisance. Another reason for wanting to quit is that many people want to avoid the increasingly poor image of the smoker in modern society.

## 3. Chronic Effects of Smoking and Disease

### *a. Cardiovascular System*[58]

Nicotine has a triple effect on the cardiovascular system. It causes a hemodynamic response of the heart, it leads to increased circulation of free fatty acids, and it causes an increase in platelet stickiness and aggregation.[57] Coronary heart disease is the major cause of death among both males and females in the U.S. population. The 1979 Surgeon General's report clearly demonstrated the close association of cigarette smoking and increased coronary heart disease among males. Furthermore a report of the Surgeon General in 1980 reveals that coronary heart disease, including acute myocardial infarction and chronic ischemic heart disease, occurs more frequently in women who smoke. In general, cigarette smoking increases the risk by a factor of about two; in younger women, cigarette smoking may increase the risk severalfold. The use of oral contraceptives by women who smoke cigarettes increases the risk of a myocardial infarction by a factor of approximately ten.

Men and women who smoke low-''tar'' and -nicotine cigarettes experience less risk for coronary heart disease than individuals who smoke high-tar and -nicotine cigarettes, but their risk is still considerably greater than that of nonsmokers.

It is known that increased levels of high-density lipoprotein (HDL) are correlated with a reduced risk for an acute myocardial infarction whereas cigarette smokers have decreased levels of HDL.

Increased incidence and severity of atherosclerosis among smokers are observed at autopsies. Nicotine induces necrosis in the arterial walls, and when it is associated with cholesterol in the diet, endothelial fibrosis takes place. Smoking cessation improves the prognosis of the disorder and has a favorable impact on vascular patency following reconstructive surgery.

Cigarette smokers experience an increased risk for subarachnoid hemorrhage. In females, the use of both cigarettes and oral contraceptives appears synergistically to increase the risk of subarachnoid hemorrhage.

Kjeldsen and Mozes [59] report that Buerger's disease (obstructive vasculitis of the arteries and veins of the lower extremities) is aggravated by smoking.

Cigarette smokers may be more likely to develop severe or malignant hypertension than nonsmokers.

A schematic representation of the pathogenesis of heart disease in smokers is presented in Figure 15-4.

Finally, in Great Britain—as an example of the universality of the problem—52,000 people die from smoking every year, with half of these deaths caused by cardiovascular disease.[60] It is possible that a 20 percent reduction in cigarette consumption by heavy smokers could reduce the number of deaths annually from cardiovascular disease by 8000.

### *b. Respiratory System*

Three types of diseases are classified under the term ''chronic obstructive lung disease'' (COLD): chronic bronchitis, pulmonary emphysema, and reversible obstructive lung disease, or bronchial asthma.

A majority of patients suffering from COLD are cigarette smokers.[61] Women's total risk of COLD appears to be somewhat lower than men's, which may be the result of differences in prior smoking habits.

Ventilatory functions have been shown to be decreased in smokers as compared with nonsmokers.[62] The prevalence of chronic bronchitis varies directly with cigarette smoking, increasing with the number of cigarettes smoked per day.

Kilburn and McKenzie,[63] in an attempt to elucidate the pathogenesis of chronic bronchitis, were unable to determine its exact mechanism.

Smokers and nonsmokers are found in equal numbers in patients with panlobular emphysema, but 98 percent of patients with centrolobular emphysema are smokers.[64] Auerbach et al.[65] have shown that the presence of emphysema at autopsy exhibits a dose–response relationship (one-pack-a-day) with cigarette smoking during life.

There is a close relationship between cigarette smoking and chronic cough or chronic sputum production in both males and females, which increases with total pack-years smoked. Current smokers show poorer pulmonary function on spirometric testing than do ex-smokers or nonsmokers, a relationship that is dose-related to the number of cigarettes smoked.

A schematic representation of the pathogenesis of chronic obstructive pulmonary disease is presented in Figure 15-5.

### *c. Cancer*

The first public awareness of the carcinogenic properties of tobacco resulted from a warning by John Hill, a physician who wrote a note entitled, "Caution Against the Immoderate Use of Snuff," in which cancer of the nostrils was attributed to the use of snuff.[54]

The use of tobacco in any form may cause cancer of the lip, tongue, tonsils, larynx, lung, stomach, intestine, pancreas, and bladder.[66–69]

In almost all countries where the incidence of cancer of the lung has been studied, the number of cigarettes smoked is seen to have risen

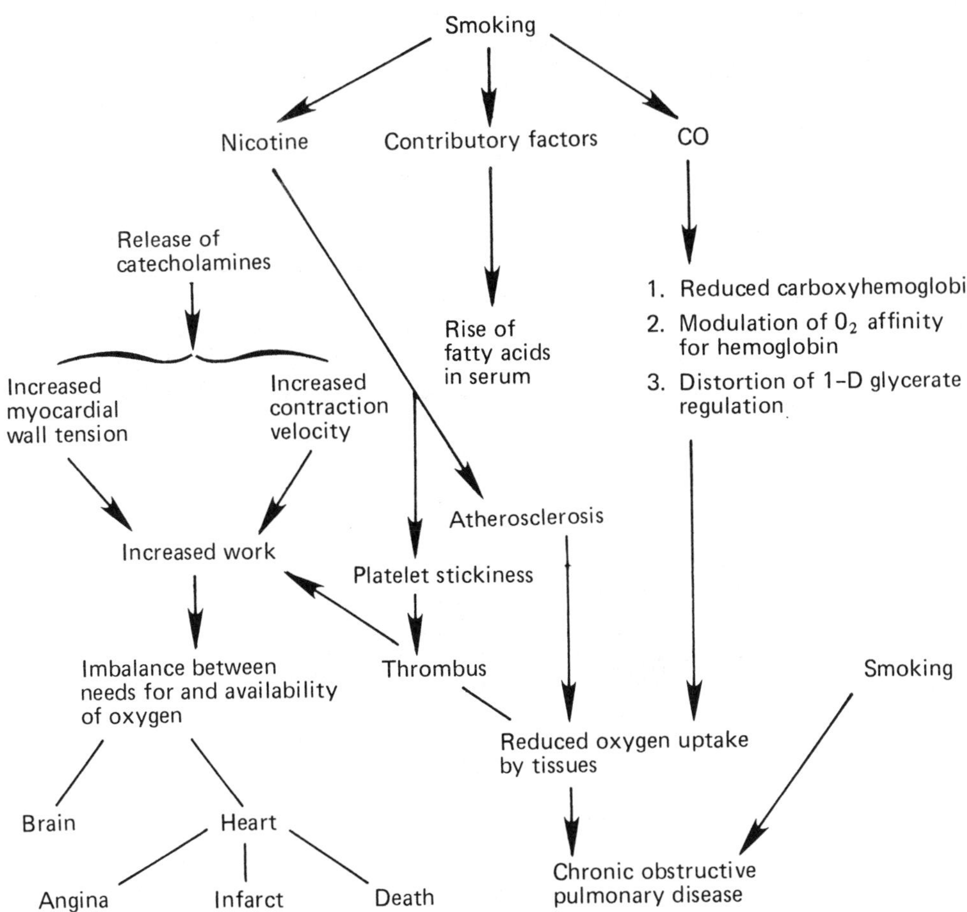


**Figure 15-4. Pathogenesis of heart disease in smokers. [From Van Lancker, J.L. Smoking and disease. In M.E. Jarvik et al., eds., *Research on Smoking Behavior* (NIDA Research Monograph no. 17). Washington, D.C.: NIDA, 1977, p. 252.]**

with the incidence of the cancer.[70] Tennant[71] reported the synergistic effects of smoking tobacco and of smoking hashish on the development of precancerous cells on lung tissue.

A similar combined effect of alcohol and smoking has been observed for cancer of the larynx. The risk of developing cancer of the larynx is ten times greater among tobacco smokers who are also heavy drinkers.

The exact mechanisms by which tobacco or its components cause cancer are unknown. It is believed that chemical carcinogens initiate the alteration of gene expression that is characteristic of cancer by modifying DNA molecules. Some carcinogens, the alkylating agents, for example, enter the cell and bind directly to DNA, but most substances that act as carcinogens are metabolically converted before binding to DNA. Definite identification of the chemical promoters in cigarette smoke is inconclusive. However, volatile phenols, aldehydes, and acids are likely candidates.

An association between cigarette smoking and cancer of the bladder seems to exist, and β-napthylamine, an extablished carcinogen in human bladder cancer, is found in tobacco smoke as a result of pyrolysis of certain α-amino acids.[72]

There are alarming statistics concerning the interrelationship between tobacco utilization and cancer. Cigarette smoking accounts for 18 percent of all cancers newly diagnosed and 25 percent of all cancer deaths in women. The rise in lung cancer death rates is currently much steeper in women than in men. It is projected that age-adjusted lung cancer deaths will surpass those from breast cancer in the early 1980s.

Women cigarette smokers have been reported to have between 2.5 and five times greater likelihood of developing lung cancer than nonsmoking women. The rapid increase in lung cancer rates in women is similar to, but steeper than, the rise that was seen in men approximately 25 years earlier. This probably reflects the fact that women first began to smoke in large numbers 25 to 30 years after the increase in cigarette smoking among men. Thus neither men nor women are protected from lung cancer caused by cigarette smoking. Cigarette smoking has been causally related to all four of the major histologic types of lung cancer in both men and women, including epidermoid, small cell, large cell, and adenocarcino.

The use of filter cigarettes and cigarettes with low levels of tar and nicotine is correlated with a lower risk of cancer of the lung and larynx as compared with the use of high-tar and -nicotine or unfiltered cigarettes. The risk posed by smok-

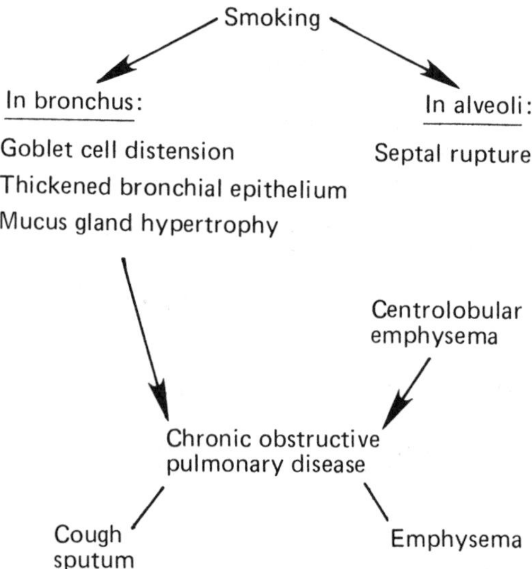


**Figure 15-5. Pathogenesis of COPD in smokers. (From Van Lancker, J.L. Smoking and disease. In M.E. Jarvik et al., eds., *Research on Smoking Behavior* NIDA Research Monograph no. 17). Washington, D.C.: NIDA, 1977, p. 255.]**

ing low-tar cigarettes is clearly greater than that among individuals who have never smoked. Finally, after cessation of smoking, the risk of developing lung and laryngeal cancer has been shown to drop slowly, equaling that of nonsmokers after ten to 15 years.

The pathogenesis of lung cancer as caused by cigarette smoke is shown in Figure 15-6.

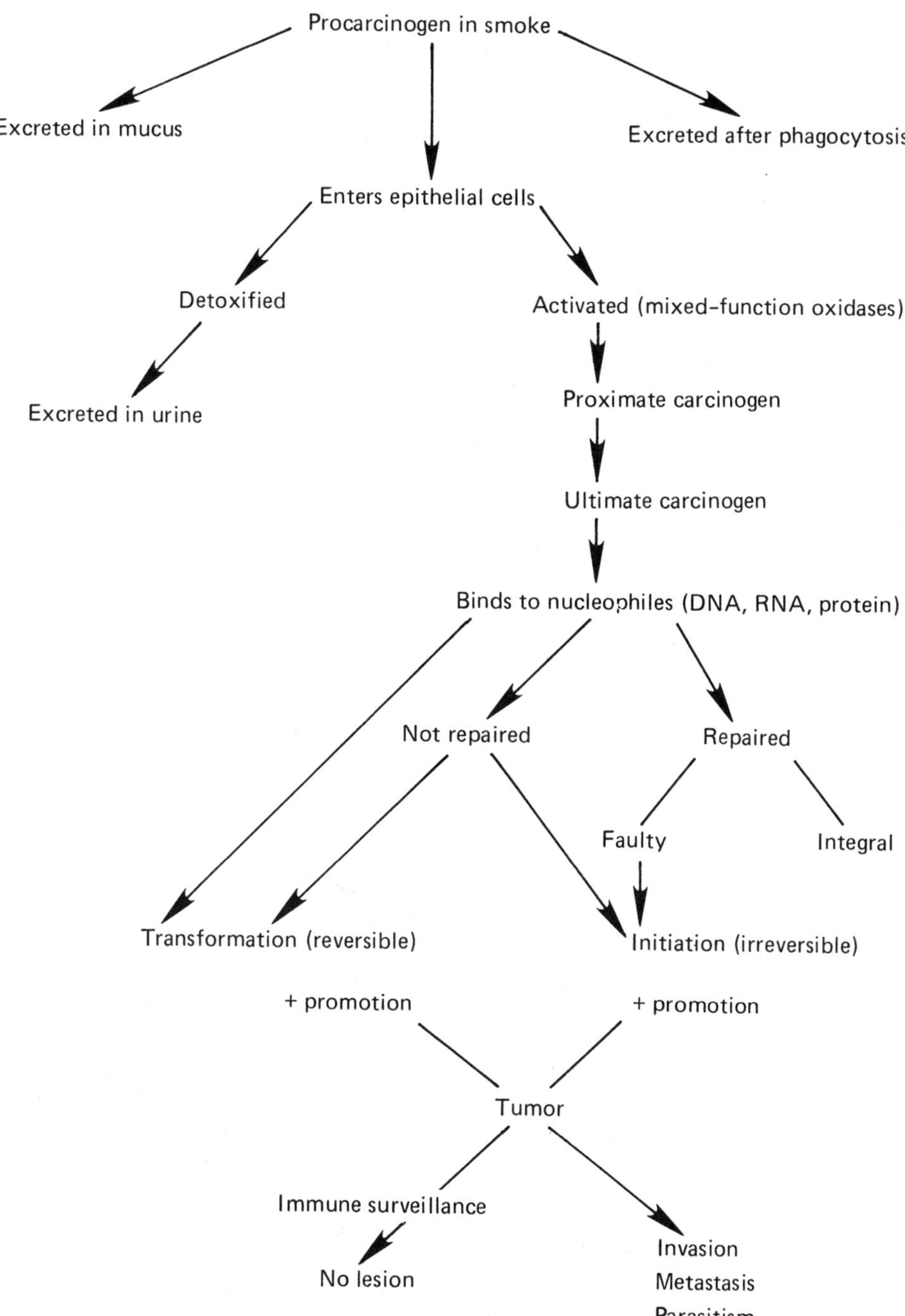


**Figure 15-6. Pathogenesis of lung cancer. [From Van Lancker, J.L. Smoking and disease. In M.E. Jarvik et al., eds., *Research on Smoking Behavior* (NIDA Research Monograph no. 17). Washington, D.C.: NIDA, 1977, p. 262.]**

#### d. Child Development

Infants born to women who smoke during pregnancy are from 70 to 250 grams lighter than children born to comparable nonsmoking women. Maternal smoking during pregnancy may adversely affect the child's long-term growth, intellectual development, and behavioral characteristics. Furthermore maternal smoking during pregnancy exerts a direct growth-retarding effect on the fetus; this effect does not appear to be mediated by reduced maternal appetite, eating, or weight gain.

The mortality in babies of smokers is significantly higher than in babies of nonsmokers for both still births and neonatal deaths. For reasons unknown, mothers who smoke have a reduced incidence of preeclamptic toxemia as compared with nonsmoking mothers.

Increasing levels of maternal smoking result in a highly significant increase in the risk of abruptive placentae, placenta revia, bleeding early or late in pregnancy, premature and prolonged rupture of membranes, and preterm delivery—all of which carry high risks of perinatal loss. Up to 14 percent of all preterm deliveries in the United States may be attributable to maternal smoking.

An infant's risk of developing the "sudden infant death syndrome" is increased by maternal smoking during pregnancy. In addition, studies in women and men suggest that cigarette smoking might impair fertility.

Although there is no evidence that the cigarette smoke is teratogenic *in vivo, in vitro* tests have shown that cigarette smoke contains mutagenic factors for the galmorella microsonal system.[73]

Additional information on the effects of smoking on peptic ulcers, psychosocial aspects, and interactions with drugs, foods, and diagnostic tests can be obtained from a 1980 report of the Surgeon General.[58]

### 4. Mortality and Morbidity[58]

#### a. Mortality

Mortality ratios are generally proportional to the duration of cigarette smoking; the longer an individual smokes, the greater the excess risk of dying. Mortality ratios tend to be higher for those individuals who begin smoking at a young age as compared with those who begin smoking later. Mortality ratios also are higher for those who inhale smoke than for those who do not inhale. Certainly mortality ratios for men and women increase with the tar and nicotine content of the cigarette. Women demonstrate the same dose–response relationships with cigarette smoking as do men.

#### b. Morbidity

The 1979 report of the Surgeon General summarized the information on smoking and morbidity as follows:

1. Current cigarette smokers report more acute and chronic conditions including chronic bronchitis and/or emphysema, chronic sinusitis, peptic ulcer disease, and arteriosclerotic heart disease than nonsmokers.
2. There is a dose–response relationship between the number of cigarettes smoked per day and the frequency of reporting for most of the chronic conditions.
3. The age-adjusted incidence of acute conditions (e.g., influenza) for smokers is 20 percent higher than for nonsmokers.
4. Smokers lose more days of work than nonsmokers.

## H. TRENDS IN SMOKING BEHAVIOR

*Nicotiana tabacum* was introduced by the American Indian into Europe in 1598. Thus the habit pattern that Europeans adopted is 400 years old. Less than 60 years later, tobacco had become a staple agricultural commodity in Virginia and its principal currency.

Cigarette consumption has shown a steady increase throughout the world since 1880. While a decline in cigarettes sold was demonstrated in 1964, it has been suggested that this may have been correlated with the issuance of the report of the Surgeon General that same year, which clearly elucidated that smoking was associated with lung cancer, emphysema, bronchitis, and coronary heart disease.

Historic data on tobacco products in the United States are available through the records of the U.S. Department of Agriculture, which provide estimates of per capita consumption of such products.

Inspection of the data reveals the relative stability of consumption of all tobacco products combined as compared with some of the individual products, even though the overall consumption was actually 2.2 times as great in 1954 as in 1880. Between the years 1880 and 1954, there was a tremendous shift to cigarette use from other forms of tobacco.

In 1969, a decline in cigarette consumption occurred that may have been due to increased sales taxes as well as to the federal government's stand against smoking and the social movement in support of that stand. Shafter[54] reports that the overall trend from 1963 through 1970 reflects an increase of 17.7 billion in total cigarette sales. In 1972, 45.9 percent of the male population 17 years old and older and 30.5 percent of the females in the same age group were smokers.

Data from the Economic Research Service[75] indicate that the total output of cigarettes showed a 2 percent increase, and, in a ten-month period in 1972, as compared with the same period in 1971, smokers consumed 4 percent more cigarettes.

Other changes in trends have been seen with respect to the age and the sex of those smoking. Not only are there more young smokers, but there appear to be increasing numbers of young girls smoking—a practice once thought to be the juvenile male's perogative. Indeed more women have acquired this so-called masculine habit.

From 1965 to 1978, the proportion of adult men cigarette smokers declined from 51 to 37 percent. Estimates of adult men's smoking prevalence for 1979 is 36.9 percent whereas for women it is 28.2 percent. The overall smoking prevalence of 32.3 percent for both sexes in 1979 represents the lowest recorded value in at least 45 years. The proportion of adult smokers attempting to quit smoking declined from 1970 to 1975, but increased in 1978–1979. The proportion of adult smokers using lower tar and nicotine brands has increased substantially. In 1979, 39 percent of adult women smokers and 28 percent of adult men smokers reported primary brands with FTC tar delivery of less than 15.0 mg; surveys of adolescent smoking habits reveal that by ages 17 to 19, smoking prevalence among women exceeds that of men.

It has been suggested by Moersch[76] that women, from a biologic standpoint, show a greater tendency for masochism than do men, which may account for their purported difficulty with smoking cessation. Should evidence appear to support this thinking, it should be readily apparent that the cigarette industry would aim for this target population. In fact, billboard advertising increased markedly following the television ban, with an emphasis on attracting the female population.[77] Physicians now make up the only social group that has stopped smoking in large numbers. Since 1965, approximately two thirds of physicians who smoked have stopped smoking, presumably because they are more aware of its health consequences.

## I. PREVENTIVE AND TREATMENT APPROACHES

With the publication in 1950 of four individual studies linking smoking to lung cancer, cigarette smoking joined the company of other forms of gratification behavior whose abuse leads to serious problems. In its company are the well-known problems posed by sexual behavior, drug use, eating habits, alcohol use, physical risk-taking such as fast driving and hazardous sports, and violence.

In general, one may define this class of behavior as comprising normal, socially acceptable ways of increasing the enjoyment of life, or providing mechanisms for coping with life's problems. They can be useful, even necessary, concomitants of life. They share the characteristic that, when they are carried beyond a certain point or occur at inappropriate times (that is, when they are "abused"), they create problems—either health problems or social problems—for the individual, the individual's associates, and society at large. Yet each of these forms of gratification behavior has its own distinguishing features. For example, eating is a necessary form of behavior to maintain life;

but when it is overgratified, it can lead to obesity, thus creating both social and health problems for the individual.

What distinguishes cigarette smoking from the others is that, after it gained a strong hold on the American population over a period of some 40 years, research reports began to show that what once was considered abusive use (say three or more packs a day) was a serious overestimate. Abuse of cigarettes must now be defined at a much lower level; in fact, we have not been able to identify any threshold, even below a half pack a day, at which serious risks are not encountered.

Because of the hold cigarette smoking has on the adult population (about one half of male adults and one third of female adults are cigarette smokers), and because of the substantial vested interest in the continued use of cigarettes represented by a $1 billion agricultural product, a $9 billion manufacturing industry, and a $300 million advertising investment each year, the forces operating against control are strong. As a consequence, the only practical methods available to bring the situation under control are not those that impose change, but rather those that encourage change by promoting the reduction of smoking and by discouraging the taking up of this practice and its continuation.

## 1. Prevention

Cohen[78] points out that more than 4000 cigarettes are consumed per capita each year in the United States. Furthermore the smoking habit is generally acquired during early adolescence, often on the basis of peer mimicking. We are only too aware of the many gaps in knowledge and the misconceptions that exist in the general population of smokers about the nature and magnitude of the biologic effects of cigarette smoking. It has been shown that not only must one realize that a threat exists, but one must acknowledge its importance, see it as personally relevant, feel capable of stopping, and recognize the value thus to be derived. Interpersonal influences, mass communications, and scientists and physicians and other key groups all can play an important part in the prevention of smoking.

There appears to be a concensus of opinion throughout the literature that (1) education seems to be the most effective approach, (2) innovative educational techniques are needed, and (3) the educational battle against nicotine ''addiction'' should be waged at an early age. Previous studies of the outcomes of drug education would seem to support this stand.[79, 80]

## 2. Secondary Prevention

Manufactured materials that could be substituted for tobacco or mixed with tobacco have been the subject of research for at least two decades. Artificial tobacco substitutes (ATS) may offer one alternative mode of secondary prevention that might reduce the toxicity of tobacco and the degree of dependence.

It is noteworthy that as many as a fourth of former smokers were able to give up the practice through their own devices or with the aid of the numerous antismoking programs. Among the 54 million people in the United States who still smoke, college graduates use filter cigarettes more often than do grammar or high school graduates.[81]

As Cohen[78] suggests, ''Since millions cannot or will not desist from smoking, the development of a less harmful—but not to be understood as safe—cigarette is justified.'' This is done by selective breeding of the plant to produce low-tar, low-nicotine leaves, and the interposition of suitable filters and aerators. Less than 9 mg of tar, 0.6 mg of nicotine, and low levels of the other known hazardous substances should be achieved.

Over-the-counter devices can be found in almost any drugstore. One is a cigarette holder, and includes a programmed approach to decreasing not the amount smoked, but rather the amount inhaled, and the purchaser is promised self-detoxication. Also a chewing gum is on the market that contains lobeline sulfate, and is purported to reduce nicotine craving. Lobeline is a substituted piperidine compound, and has a psychologic effect comparable to that of nicotine but is less potent.

Even with decreased amounts of the toxic

agents, a smoker may counteract any benefits of the less harmful cigarette by inhaling deeply, smoking more units, or smoking each cigarette more completely.

### 3. Tertiary Prevention (Treatment)

There are numerous treatment modalities, including individual and group counseling, hypnosis, acupuncture, and learning theory approaches such as conditioned avoidance techniques. In general, short-term success rates are excellent, but when the clients are followed for one year, the abstainers are found to average about 25 percent.

Periodic reinforcement and contacts over a follow-up period seem to improve the number of favorable outcomes. It has also been found that over the long term, males, older people, light smokers, those with support from spouses, the emotionally stable, and those who feel that stopping will help them personally show the highest success rates.[82]

A number of adversive techniques, such as electric shock, unpleasant odors, warm stale smoke, and imagined noxious experiences, are in vogue. Sensory deprivation has been tried with excellent initial results, but the long-term outcome is not so favorable.

Chemical approaches include lobeline chewing gum, and smoking deterrents such as silver nitrate or potassium permagannate mouth washes.

Among nonchemical approaches used to stop smoking are contingency contracting, relaxation exercises, acupuncture, hypnosis, and even biofeedback. Many of these measures are reviewed by Schwartz.[83]

For most individuals, abrupt discontinuance of smoking is preferable to gradually cutting down to zero cigarettes. The withdrawal symptoms from smoking tobacco are unpleasant and uncomfortable, but they are not life-threatening, and they can be ameliorated by symptomatic management. Like heroin addiction, treatment of the smoker should persist for months, if not years, after abstinence has been achieved.

Certainly cigarette smoking imposes a tremendous economic burden on the economy and a treatment challenge to the United States and other countries. But currently there is no single preferred treatment approach to eliminate smoking that is universally acclaimed. Sadly only a slight dent in the control of a multibillion dollar cigarette addiction has been achieved.

## J. SOCIAL COSTS AND IMPLICATIONS

Cigarette smoking brings about not only changes in the system of the individual, but also in the social system with which that individual interacts. Although the general public is aware of the many health consequences of smoking, few persons are cognizant of the fact that cancers of the larynx, lip, mouth, esophagus, and bladder are found almost solely in cigarette smokers. Other smoking consequences include premature aging and skin wrinkles,[84] erythocytosis,[85] osteoporosis,[86] dental problems,[87] hypertension and stroke,[1] emphysema,[88] noninfluenzal respiratory disease,[86] pneumonia, coronary heart disease,[87] increased perception of pain,[1] high absenteeism rate[89] with cigarette smoking and a lower rate with pipe or cigar smoking, weight change,[90] and high accident–violation proneness.[91]

The present focus on the prenatal effects of smoking reveals that mothers who smoke during pregnancy have a greater risk of giving birth prematurely, and hence of death to the newborn, and that neonates of mothers who smoke weigh less at birth.[6]

The associated costs of smoking, borne by the tax-paying public, stagger the imagination. The number of forest fires that have been set by smokers is unknown, let alone of fires in homes, restaurants, and apartment houses, with the resultant loss of lives. The damage to public property by burns and defacing by smoke coincidental with smoking is costly to the public. Shuman[54] reported in 1965 that 47 percent of deaths from all causes were related to tobacco use. Projections of these figures into the 1980s further exemplify the magnitude and impact this problem has on health care delivery and the public pocketbook throughout the world.[54]

## K. COMMENTARY AND SUMMARY

A quick view of the world in the 1980s reveals a multitude of problems, including economic strife, unemployment, crime, violence, juvenile deliquency, hunger, poverty, inflation, war, and drug and alcohol abuse.

Today drugs of all types are being abused in heretofore unknown proportions, and tobacco—specifically in cigarettes—is only one in that vast array. Cohen[78] suggests that we will become a nation of preponderantly female filtertip cigarette smokers, if present trends continue. Young women are smoking more than ever; and females stop their "addiction" to tobacco to a lesser degree than do males. Insight into this differential phenomenon is derived from an interview with R.G. Hernandez, a director of education for an early child development program, who supervises more than 200 employees, both male and females. A smoker herself, she believes:

> A prime reason for increased smoking by the female population in the United States may be due to a variety of reasons, such as (1) working in a predominantly male chauvinistic business world: (2) competing with males for "high paying" jobs; and (3) maintaining traditional female roles such as parenting, and being a wife and a housekeeper. Taking all these things into account, the young or older female is placed in a more stressful situation than counterpart males in a similar environment.

Interestingly tobacco usage is another example of the point that the facts are not much of a deterrent to practices that have become habitual. Cohen[78] points out that "knowledge does not make people free, it merely makes them guilty about doing something harmful to themselves."

That most smokers want to stop but are unable to do so reflects upon the problems of all addicted people. In this regard, we must be reminded that the degree of dependence on drugs, including tobacco, may be due to the genetic milieu of the subject. Thus some individuals are able to withdraw from tobacco without significant symptoms whereas others have great difficulty with their tobacco detoxification efforts.

Cigarettes are cheap, legal, and readily available. They support multibillion dollar industries, which pay the wages of the many workers associated with them, and are a substantial and continuing source of revenue for federal, state, and local governments.

There are no certain answers or ideal solutions to the smoking habit dilemma. Perhaps insurance companies might be further encouraged to continue their programs whereby lower premiums are paid by nonsmokers. Additionally the use of a tax (nine cents per pack) added to the price of cigarettes could provide funds for basic research and to help defray the rising health care costs incurred by smokers.

Judy Newman[92] describes a modern view of women regarding tobacco use: "Smoking seems to be losing its 'chic' appeal. Attitudes toward smoking have changed in the last five to 10 years. Today's smokers do more than worry about their health—they have to think about their image. For more and more people, smoking is not just a hazard, but an embarassment."

In the past, we have made great strides in reducing tobacco use in the United States. However, even greater efforts, in terms of prevention methods especially targeted at the very young, are a requisite for success in generations to come.

## REFERENCES

1. Tennant, F. S., and Day, C. M. Tobacco and Smoking Behavior. In: Blum, K., and A. M. Briggs, eds. *Social Pharmacology* (in preparation)
2. Pollin, W. Foreword. M.E. Jarvik et al., eds. *Research on Smoking Behavior.* (NIDA Research Monograph 17) Washington, D.C.: NIDA, 1977, p. v.
3. Abelson, H.I., Fishburne, P.M., and Cisin, I. *National Survey on Drug Abuse: 1977; A Nationwide Study—Youth, Young Adults, and Older People.* Vol. I. *Mainfindings.* Rockville, Md.: National Institute on Drug Abuse, 1977, p. 89.
4. *The Health Consequences of Smoking.* Public Health Service Publication no. 1696. Washington, D.C.: U.S. Government Printing Office, 1967.
5. Ray, O.S. *Drugs, Society and Human Behavior.* St. Louis: C.V. Mosby, 1972, p. 95.
6. Padgett, E.C. Oral epidermoid carcinoma: general considerations and etiologic factors. *Int. J. Orthod. Oral Surg.* 22:283, 1936.

7. *Marihuana: A Signal of Misunderstanding: The Technical Papers of the First Report of the National Commission on Marihuana and Drug Abuse*. Washington, D.C.: National Commission on Marihuana and Drug Abuse, 1972.
8. Breechen, E.M. *Licit and Illicit Drugs; The Consumers Union Report on Narcotics, Stimulants, Depressants, Inhalants, Hallucinogens, and Marijuana, Including Caffeine, Nicotine, and Alcohol*. Boston: Little Brown, 1972.
9. Volle, R.L., and Koelle, G.B. Ganglionic stimulating and blocking agents. In L. S. Goodman and A. Gilman, eds., *The Pharmacological Basis of Therapeutics*, 5th ed. New York: Macmillan, 1975, P. 565.
10. Bogen, E. Composition of cigarettes and cigarette smoke. *JAMA* 93:1110, 1929.
11. Bailey, E.M. The thirty-second report on food products and the twentieth report on drug products. *Conn. State Agric. Exp. Stn. Bull.* 295:300, 1928.
12. Lehmann, G., and Michaelis, H.F. Tabakgenuss und Adrenalinspiegal. *Arch. F. Exper. Path. U. Pharmakol.* 202:627, 1943.
13. McNally, W.D. Tar in cigarette smoke and its possible effects. *Am. J. Cancer* 16:1502, 1932.
14. Goldsmith, J.R., and Landau, S.A. Carbon monoxide and human health. *Science* 162:1352, 1968.
15. Chevalier, R.B., Krumholz, R.A., and Ross, J.C. Reaction of nonsmokers to carbon monoxide inhalation. Cardiopulmonary responses at rest and during exercise. *JAMA* 198:1061, 1966.
16. Russell, C.S., Taylor, R., and Law, C.E. Smoking in pregnancy, maternal blood pressure, pregnancy outcome, baby weight and growth, and other related factors. A prospective study. *Br. J. Prev. Soc. Med.* 22:119, 1968.
17. Jongbloed, J. Uber den Kohlenoxydgehalt der Alveolarluft beim Tabakrauchen. *Arch. Int. Pharmacodyn. Therap.* 63:346, 1939.
18. Trasoff, A., Blumstein, G., and Marks, M. Immunologic aspect of tobacco in thromboangiitis obliterans and coronary artery disease. *J. Allergy* 7:250, 1936.
19. Thomas, M.D., and Collier, T.R. Concentration of arsenic in tobacco smoke determined by rapid titrimetric methods. *J. Ind. Hyg. Toxicol.* 27:201, 1945.
20. Apperson, G.L. *The Social History of Smoking*. London, 1914.
21. Konturek, S.J., et al. Effects of nicotine on gastrointestinal secretions. *Gastroenterology* 60:1098, 1971.
22. Butler, N.R., Goldstein, H., and Ross, E.M. Cigarette smoking in pregnancy: Its influence on birth weight and perinatal mortality. *Br. Med. J.* 2:127, 1972.
23. Turner, D.M., et al. Metabolism of nicotine by the isolated perfused dog lung. *Xenobiotica* 75:539, 1975.
24. Russell, M.A., and Feyerbend, C. Cigarette smoking: A dependence on high-nicotine level boli. *Drug Metab. Rev.* 8:29, 1978.
25. Taylor, P. Ganglionic stimulation and blocking agents. In A.G. Goodman, L.S. Goodman, and A. Gilman, eds. *The Pharmacological Basis of Therapeutics*. New York: Macmillan, 1980, p. 211.
26. Burn, J.H., et al. Peripheral effects of nicotine and actylcholine resembling those of sympathetic stimulation. *J. Physiol.* 148:332, 1959.
27. Ferry, C.B. The sympathomimetic effect of acetylcholine on the spleen of the cat. *J. Physiol.* 167:487, 1963.
28. Douglas, W.W., and Gray, J.A.B. The excitant action of acetylcholine and other substances on cutaneous sensory pathways and its prevention by hexamethonium and d-tubocurarine. *J. Physiol.* 119:118, 1953.
29. Jarvik, M.E. Further observations on nicotine as the reinforcing agent in smoking. In W.L. Dunn, Jr., ed., *Smoking Behavior: Motives and Incentives*. Washington, D.C.: Winston, 1973, p. 33.
30. Oldendorf, W.H. Distribution of drugs to the brain. In M.E. Jarvik, ed., *Psychopharmacology in the Practice of Medicine*. New York: Appleton-Century-Crofts, 1977, p. 167.
31. Heymans, C., Bouckaert, J.J., and Dautrebande, L. Sinus carotidien et reflexes respiratoires; sensibilité des sinus carotidiens aux substances chimiques. Action stimulante respiratoire reflexe du sulfure de sodium, du cyanure du potassium, de la nicotine et de la lobeline. *Arch. Int. Pharmacodyn. Therap.* 40:54, 1931.
32. McGaugh, J.L. Drug facilitation of learning and memory. *Ann. Rev. Pharmacol.* 13:229, 1973.
33. Geller, I., Hartmann, R., and Blum, K. Effects of nicotine, nicotine monomethidide, lobeline, chlordiazepoxide, meprobamate, and caffein on a discrimination task in laboratory rats. *Psychopharmacologia* 20:355, 1971.
34. Andersson, K., and Hockey, G.R. Effects of cigarette smoking on incidental memory. *Psychopharmacology* 52:223, 1977.
35. Battig, K. Differential effects of nicotine and tobacco smoke alkaloids on swimming endurance in the rat. *Psychopharmacologia* 18:300, 1970.
36. Gebber, G.L. Neurogenic basis for the rise in blood pressure evoked by nicotine in the cat. *J.*

*Pharmacol. Exp. Ther.* 166:255, 1969.
37. Glauser, S.C., et al. Metabolic changes associated with the cessation of cigarette smoking. *Arch. Environ. Health* 20:377, 1970.
38. Armitage, A.K., Hall, G.H., and Morrison, C.F. Pharmacological basis for the tobacco smoking habit. *Nature* 217:331, 1968.
39. Hall, G.H. Effects of nicotine and tobacco smoke on the electrical activity of the cerebral cortex and olfactory bulb. *Br. J. Pharmacol.* 38:271, 1970.
40. Brown, B.B. Some characteristic EEG differences between heavy smoker and non-smoker subjects. *Neuropsychologia* 6:381, 1968.
41. Vogt, T.M. Smoking behavioral factors as predictors of risk. In M.E. Jarvik et al., eds., *Research on Smoking Behavior* (NIDA Research Monograph no. 17). Washington, D.C.: NIDA, 1977, p. 98.
42. Goldfarb, T.L., Jarvik, M.E., and Glick, S.D. Cigarette nicotine content as a determinant of human smoking behavior. *Psychopharmacologia* 17:89, 1970.
43. Jarvik, M.E. Biological factors underlying the smoking habit. In M.E. Jarvik et al., eds., *Research on Smoking Behavior.* (NIDA Research Monograph no 17). Washington, D.C.: NIDA, 1977, p. 122.
44. Johnston, L.M. Tobacco smoking and nicotine. *Lancet* 2:742, 1942.
45. Jarvik, M.E., Glick, S.D., and Nakamura, R.K. Inhibition of cigarette smoking by orally-administered nicotine. *Clin. Pharmacol. Ther.* 11:574, 1970.
46. Lucchesi, B.R., Schuster, C.R., and Emley, G.S. The role of nicotine as a determinant of cigarette smoking frequency in man with observations of certain cardiovascular effects associated with the tobacco alkaloid. *Clin. Pharmacol. Ther.* 8:789, 1967.
47. Kumar, R., et al. Is nicotine important tobacco smoking? *Clin. Pharmacol. Ther.* 21:520, 1977.
48. Glasser, W. *The Identity Society*. New York: Harper & Row, 1972.
49. Seely, J.E., Zuskin, E., and Bouhuys, A. Cigarette smoking: Objective evidence for lung damage in teen-agers. *Science* 172:741, 1971.
50. Levine, P.H. An acute effect of cigarette smoking on platelet function. A possible link between smoking and arterial thrombosis. *Circulation* 48:619, 1973.
51. Doll, R., Jones, F.A., and Pygott, F. Effect of smoking on the production and maintenance of gastric and duodenal ulcers. *Lancet* 1:657, 1958.
52. *Smoking and Health: A Report of the Surgeon General*. Washington, D.C.: Department of Health, Education & Welfare, 1979 (DHEW Pub. no. PHS 79-50066), p. 1251.
53. Jaffee, J. Tobacco addiction: A review. *Science* 185:1039, 1974.
54. Ochsner, A. The health menace of tobacco. *Am. Sci.* 59:246, 1971.
55. Russell, M.A.H. Tobacco smoking and nicotine dependence. In R.J. Gibbins et al., eds., *Research Advances in Alcohol and Drug Problems*. Vol. 3. New York: Wiley, 1976, p. 1.
56. McKennell, A.C., and Thomas, R.K. *Adults' and Adolescents' Smoking Habits and Attitudes*. London: HMSO, 1967.
57. Hatchell, P.C., and Collins, A. C. Influence of genotype and sex on behavioral sensitivity to nicotine in mice. *Psychopharmacology (Berlin)* 71:45, 1980.
58. Van Lancker, J. Smoking and disease. In M.E. Jarvik et al., eds., *Research on Smoking Behavior* (NIDA Research Monograph 17). Washington, D.C.: NIDA, 1977, p. 230.
59. Kjeldsen, K., and Mozes, M. Buerger's disease in Israel. Investigations of carboxyhemoglobin and serum sholesterol levels after smoking. *Acta Chir. Scand.* 135:495, 1969.
60. Ball, K., and Turner, R. Smoking and the heart. The basis for action. *Lancet* 2:822, 1974.
61. Crowdy, J.P. and Snowden, R.R. Cigarette smoking and respiratory ill-health in the British army. *Lancet* 1:1232, 1975.
62. James, R.H. Prior smoking as a determinant of the distribution of pulmonary ventilation. *Am. Rev. Respir. Dis.* 101:105, 1970.
63. Kilburn, K.H., and McKenzie, W. Leukocyte recruitment to airways by cigarette smoke and particle phase in contrast to cytotoxicity of vapor. *Science* 189:634, 1975.
64. Anderson, D.O., Ferris, B.G., Jr., and Zickmantel, R. The Chilliwack Respiratory Survey, 1963. IV. The effect of tobacco smoking on the prevalence of respiratory disease. *Can. Med. Assoc. J.* 92:1066, 1965.
65. Auerbach, O., et al. Relation of smoking and age to emphysema. Whole-lung section study. *N. Engl. J. Med.* 186:286:853, 1972.
66. Levin, M.L., Goldstein, H., and Gerhardt, P.R. Cancer and tobacco smoking; Preliminary report. *JAMA* 143:336, 1950.
67. Hammond. E.C. Tobacco. In J.F. Fraumeni, Jr., ed., *Persons at High Risk of Cancer: An Approach to Cancer Etiology and Control; Proceedings of a Conference, Key Biscayne, Florida, December 10-12, 1974*. New York: Academic Press, 1975, p. 131.
68. Rothman, K.J. Alcohol. In J.F. Fraumeni, Jr., ed., *Persons at High Risk of Cancer. An Ap-*

*proach to Cancer Etiology and Control; Proceedings of a Conference, Key Biscayne, Florida, December 10–12, 1974*. New York: Academic Press, 1975, p. 139.

69. Wynder, E.L., et al. Interdisciplinary and experimental approaches: Metabolic epidemiology. In J.F. Fraumeni, Jr., ed., *Persons at High Risk of Cancer. An Approach to Cancer Etiology and Control; Proceedings of a Conference, Key Biscayne, Florida, December 10–12, 1974*. New York: Academic Press, 1975, p. 485.
70. Drogendijk, A.C. Smoking and lung cancer. *Triangle* 7:166, 1966.
71. Tennant, F.S., Jr. Histopathologic and clinical abnormalities of the respiratory system in chronic hashish smokers. *Subst. Alcohol Action/Misuse* 1:93, 1980.
72. Miller, R.L., and Stedman, R.L. Essential absence of betanaphthylamine in cigarette smoke condensate. *Tobacco* 165:31, 1967.
73. Kier, L.D., Yamasaki, E., and Ames, B.N. Detection of mutagenic activity in cigarette smoke condensates. *Proc. Natl. Acad. Sci. U.S.A.* 71:4159, 1974.
74. Milmore, B.K., and Conover, A.B. Tobacco consumption in the United States, 1880–1955. *Agric. Econ. Res.*, 8:9, 1956.
75. *Tobacco Situation*. Economic Research Service, U.S. Department of Agriculture, TS-140, June 1972.
76. Moersch, H.J., et al. Counsel for patient who smokes. *Dis. Chest* 54:211, 1968.
77. Schwartz, J.L. The Second World Conference on Smoking and Health: A conference report. *Calif. Health* 19:7, 1972.
78. On the smoking of cigarettes. In S. Cohen, ed., *The Substance Abuse Problems*. New York: Haworth Press, 1981, p. 156.
79. Tennant, F.S., Weaver, S.C., and Lewis, C.E. Outcomes of drug education: Four case studies. *Pediatrics* 52:246, 1973.
80. Gossett, J.T., Lewis, J.M., and Phillips, V.A. Extent and prevalence of illicit drug use as reported by 56,745 students. *JAMA* 216:1464, 1971.
81. Wynder, E.L., and Hoffmann, D. Tobacco and health: A societal challenge. *N. Engl. J. Med.* 300:894, 1979.
82. West, D.W. Correlates of smoking withdrawal in a clinic population: Results of a five-year follow-up Chicago, Il., Presented at the Annual Meeting of American Public Health Associations, Nov. 17, 1975.
83. Schwartz, J.L. Smoking cures: Ways to kick an unhealthy habit. In M.E. Jarvik et al., eds., *Research on Smoking Behavior* (NIDA Research Monograph no. 17). Washington, D.C.: NIDA, 1977, p. 308.
84. Daniell, H.W. Smokers' wrinkles. *Ann. Intern. Med.* 75:873, 1971.
85. Sagone, A.L. Jr., and Balcerzak, S.P. Smoking as a cause of erythrocytosis. *Ann. Intern. Med.* 82:512, 1975.
86. Daniell, H.W. Osteoporosis of the slender smoker. Vertebral compression fractures and loss of metacarpal cortex in relation to postmenopausal cigarette smoking and lack of obesity. *Arch. Intern. Med.* 136:298, 1976.
87. Friedman, G.D., Siegelaub, A.B., and Seltzer, C.C. Cigarettes, alcohol, coffee and peptic ulcer. *N. Engl. J. Med.* 290:469, 1974.
88. Spain, D.M., Siegal, H., and Bradess, V.A. Emphysema in apparently healthy adults. Smoking, age, and sex. *JAMA* 224:322, 1973.
89. Finklea, J.F., et al. Cigarette smoking and acute non-influenzal respiratory disease in military cadets. *Am. J. Epidemiol.* 93:457, 1971.
90. Holcomb, H.S., 3d., and Meigg, J.W. Medical absenteeism among cigarette, and cigar and pipe smokers. *Arch. Environ. Health* 25:295, 1972.
91. Garvey, A.J., Bosse, R., and Seltzer, C.C. Smoking, weight change, and age: A longitudinal analysis. *Arch. Environ. Health* 28:327, 1974.
92. Newmark, J.J. Smoking loses ''chic'' appeal. *San Antonio Light,* June 12, 1983.

Chapter 16

# Over-the-Counter (OTC) Drugs

## A. INTRODUCTION

After reviewing the literature on the over-the-counter (OTC) drug market,[1-4] it becomes apparent that the United States has produced an unlimited resource of degreeless pseudo-self-medicating frustrated doctors. With the availability and sophistication of American health care one might assume that persons who are ill invariably seek the attention of a physician. This is far from true and is made evident by the fact that the fields of herbal medicine and folk healing are growing yearly.[5]

The media have spent millions to teach us that we can relieve all aches, pains, fevers, and colds with the use of drugs or chemicals.

''Better living through chemistry'' has echoed across this nation with great fervor. The result is a chemophillic society. Many Americans can be characterized as coffee-saturated, pill-popping, boozers who are smoking a path to the stars. Americans pour an estimated $5 billion a year into the OTC drug industry.

Many of the cough and cold medications, antacids, laxatives, motion sickness drugs, and arthritis and pain drugs are as strong as prescription drugs. However, other OTC products have little more effect than a placebo. Some contain ingredients that have not been proven to be safe or effective according to reports of the U.S. Food and Drug Administration (FDA). Consumers should be made aware of these ineffective, possibly harmful drugs so that they will be able to make intelligent choices at the pharmacy. A major problem in self-medication practice is that people are ill informed and rarely consult a physician or even a pharmacist about the medications they purchase.

According to many experts,[5-7] the advertisements that provide so many consumers with most of their purchasing information are at best misleading. And a lot of claims made by manufacturers are completely unfounded. It is a fact that the U.S. Government does not provide the consumer protection for OTC drugs that it does for prescription medications. The result is that many drugs sold over the counter do not contain proper restrictions or warnings concerning their use. In 1955, the Consumer's Union published the first edition of its book *The Medicine Show*,[2] subtitled ''Some Plain Truths About Popular Remedies,'' which explored the issue of popular prices versus product composition.

The widespread belief of the public is that ''medicines, or OTC'' can magically solve problems of minor illnesses. This is perpetuated by some manufacturers who refuse to disclose the contents of their drugs on the basis that they are "trade secrets."[8] With regard to this, the American Pharmaceutical Association in 1968 officially went on record as follows:

> Public drug abuse may be enhanced when people are ignorant of the exact list of active ingredients in the abused drug. Imperatively, "pharmacists should recommend only those products on which information on the quantitative amount of all active ingredients is available, such as in the *Handbook of Non-Prescriptive Drugs*, or on the label. A general belief that people are inclined to use OTC drugs as directed on the label is shown by the Food and Drug Administration's attitude that "people are capable of treating some of their illnesses. . . . Mature persons are familiar with the signs and symptoms of the common minor, everyday ailments which can be self-treated successfully."

To reinforce the safe use of OTC drugs by the general public, adequate information on their active ingredients, as well as implicit instructions for their use and any warnings or limitations, are clearly stated on the labels of OTC drug packages. "Discontinue use if pain persists and consult physician," is universally known. A list of the common or generic names and quantities of all active ingredients and alcohol content is also available. Prescription drugs do not require a list of their active ingredients; however, this inconsistency may be corrected with legislative action. Some 750 people in every 1000 are said to experience common everyday ailments. Most bypass medical advice and rely on self-treatment or on OTC drugs. Approximately one third seek professional advice. The National Center for Health Statistics reports that one out of every five individuals under the age of 17 has a chronic medical condition. Adults, for example, have only two colds per year, while children have four.

Consumer rights groups have taken on the responsibility of encouraging the government to examine and to ban from sale those medications with minimal or no proven effectiveness. In 1979, one of Ralph Nader's consumer organizations, the Health Research Group, filed a lawsuit against the FDA challenging its decision to permit the sale of such products.

## 1. OTC Government Regulation

The governmental agency primarily responsible for the control of all drugs is the FDA. In 1972, the FDA began a detailed examination of ingredients used in OTC medications. Seventeen Advisory Panels on OTC drugs were established to investigate the safety and effectiveness of various nonprescription drugs. As of 1982, although the FDA has commented on some medications, much of its work is still in progress and decisions concerning the possible suspension of many products have not yet been reached. Consequently, drugs without proven effectiveness or safety are still permitted to be sold. Because it may take years before final verdicts are reached, consumer groups are compensating by forcing significant changes in the way drugs are advertised. For example, manufacturers no longer advertise that the "antibacterials" in throat lozenges destroy the bacteria that cause sore throats and advertisements for hemorrhoid suppositories no longer claim to cure hemorrhoids; they advertise temporary relief of symptoms.

According to Wigden,[4] both the government and consumer groups can play effective roles in protecting the consumer. The approach would include the following basic requirements prior to the marketing of a particular drug:

1. Medications should be proven to be safe and effective for the purpose for which they are sold.
2. Advertising claims should not exaggerate the anticipated benefit of taking the medication.
3. The purpose of each ingredient should be identified.
4. Effective dosages according to age or weight should be noted.
5. Significant drug interactions with both prescription and nonprescription medications should be listed.
6. Precautions for use of the product by consumers with preexisting medical conditions such as heart disease, diabetes, and glaucoma should be stressed.

Wigden[4] further suggests that a consumer group organize a panel of unbiased experts to "pool their collective experience and opinions to provide consumers with appropriate guidelines for self-treatment and recommendations for OTC drugs."

## 2. OTC and Mass Media

With over 200 new cough and cold products introduced in the 1959 to 1965 period alone, the cough and cold remedy market is big business—to the tune of a half billion dollars or more per year.

Television advertising costs are well over $50 million a year for headache remedies; about $120 million is spent to advertise 48 headache, tension, and drowsiness remedies. It is not the amount of advertising that is of major interest here, but the quality—the focus of the commercials. The two issues involved are misrepresentation and the underlying general attitude and orientation of the ads and commercials.

In 1961, the Federal Trade Commission (FTC) questioned whether Bufferin, Excedrin, Bayer Aspirin, and Anacin could all really be "faster" or "more effective." There is an overabundance of medicinal remedies for ailments such as common cough, cold, and headache, with more than 200 such remedies in the form of pills, liquids, and powders available. It is doubtful that all of them can actually provide the effective relief they proclaim. Of all the toothpaste products produced between 1938 and 1962, only stannous fluoride products were considered effective as an aid in reducing dental caries. Undoubtedly it is the large number of different brands of OTC drugs that breeds competitive and misleading advertisement. Aspirin products, including Bufferin, Excedrin, Bayer Aspirin, and Anacin, are frequently presented as providing "prompt and more effective relief." Concrete evidence of this is dubious since even a placebo drug can be characterized as "faster and more effective." The legislation of strictly controlled common advertising and agreements reached between the FDA and the FTC have helped somewhat.

There is a prevalence of TV commercials that suggest easy solutions to problems of everyday living. Hard-sell ads are aggressive and competitive when pushing their brands as best. This may be confusing to the gullible person who is easily influenced by nonspecific (placebo) effects and symptomatic relief. The underlying offer in advertising is to provide universal and instantaneous solutions to ailments. Pills promise to turn rain to shine, gloom to joy, and depression to euphoria, and to solve problems and dispel doubts. The lax attitude toward commercial advertisements of OTC drugs, in 1970, prompted New York City's mayor John Lindsay to state[8]:

> In a sense, the impulses driving our children to this (drug addiction) are beyond our effective control. How can any institution, for example, compare with the force of television on the mind of a child? We are told that the average family watches television 5½ hours a day. Thus if a city child begins serious watching when he is 2, then by the time he comes into your schools, he has seen some 8000 hours of TV. And what has he been taught? He has been taught to relax minor tensions with a pill; to take off weight with a pill; to win status and sophistication with a cigarette; to wake up, slow down, be happy, relieve tension with some pills—that is, with drugs.

Educating the general population may help curtail the greediness in false and misleading advertising. Drug misuse, illegal drug use, and OTC commercials will be resolved in Congress and in the courts as much as in experiments and surveys. The OTC ads and commercials will also change as the FDA continues to implement the research of the National Academy of Science/National Research Council (NAS/NRC) drug efficacy panels. Legal steps are underway to help remove the ineffective products from the market. Other efforts to stop false and misleading TV ads of OTC drugs such as "stimulants, calmatives, or sleeping aids" are shown by guidelines issued by the National Association of Broadcasting Code Authority in 1970. According to these guidelines, drug advertising must not be sensational in format, nor must it exhibit a casual attitude toward drug use, be addressed to the young in particular, suggest pleasurable effects or instantaneous relief, or invite chronic use of the drug. Although it is difficult to ascertain whether OTC drugs actually contribute to drug abuse, a study of the relationship between illegal drug use and OTC commercials is certainly a worthwhile endeavor.

## B. HISTORY

In ancient civilizations few people knew the compositions of the nostrums sold by self-appointed healers. But even if they had known what went into these "medicines," they would have had very little fundamental knowledge of the pharmacologic actions of the active ingredients.

As the knowledge of medicine and pharmacy advanced, the "secret remedy" grew in popularity. But the introduction of "patent medicines" did not promote disclosure of contents; in fact, patent medicine makers were even more reticent about their formulas than were their predecessors. The compositions of patent medicines varies and pharmacists tried in vain to learn more about the products they were making available to the self-medicating public.

One of the first actions of the American Pharmaceutical Association when it was founded in 1852 was to form a committee to formulate an effective statement of the dangers of unlabeled drugs. The following is a classic example from the compilation of recipes written by pharmacist A. Emil Hiss and published as *A Thesaurus of Proprietary Preparations*.[1] According to Hiss:

> Proprietary preparations, like other medicines, are good or bad according to their respective intrinsic merits as medicinal agents. The reproach of proprietary pharmaceuticals as a class consists primarily in the atmosphere of secrecy and mystery with which many manufacturers attempt to surround their preparations. An open proprietary medicine with a clear descriptive name is entitled to full consideration without prejudice, but a secret compound with a meaningless title is presumptively a fraud. Why conceal the composition of a remedy unless it be to impose upon the physician's credulity, and to maintain a monopoly not based on the excellence of the product? Why a "secret" if not to permit extravagant or fraudulent claims as to therapeutic merit?

## C. PHARMACOLOGY OF OTC PRODUCTS

In one study,[14] OTC drugs were implicated in 32 of 177 (18.1 percent) hospital admissions. The New York Pharmaceutical Society demonstrated that of 10,000 people studied 85 percent either did not follow the advice written on the container or did not comprehend its significance. Because of the multinature of OTC products, it is difficult to understand their pharmacology. In this chapter, many of the products listed are of dubious value. In addition, the listing is selective and for the most part obtained from limited sources.[5,15] Unlike in other sections of this book, pharmacology is discussed only superficially.

Among the OTC products described that have potential for abuse are pain medications, sleeping pills, stimulants and tranquilizers, weight-loss drugs, cough medications, nausea/ vomiting/ motion sickness drugs, and cold and sinus medications. The other OTC drugs presented are not abused.

### 1. Pain and Fever Medications

Normally our consciousness allows us to experience pain at different levels—as mild pain or a sharp pain, for example. This unpleasant feeling may be avoided by either of two classes of drugs that were synthetically produced for the purpose of reducing pain or the awareness of it. These drugs include anesthetics (meaning "without sensibility") and analgesics (meaning "without pain"). Drugs that reduce awareness and block consciousness completely include barbiturates and the volatile anesthetics such as ether; analgesics reduce pain while causing insensibility.

Only four types of pain-relieving ingredients are found in OTC analgesics. The two basic ingredients are aspirin and acetaminophen (Tylenol). The third ingredient, phenacetin, is mostly converted in the body into acetaminophen for its effect. The fourth ingredient, salicylamide, is chemically related to, and less effective than, aspirin and acetaminophen.

The experience of pain is brought on by different kinds of nerve transmission and the type of pain experienced will depend on its place of origin. Pain may be visceral or somatic. Narcotics effectively reduce pain of the former type, which originates from the nonskeletal portions of the body, such as intestinal cramps. Salicylates (aspirin) are effective in reducing pain of the somatic type, which arises from muscle or bone—such as sprains, headaches, and arthritis. Depending on the type of neuron that transmits the pain, a person will experience either a bright, sharp pain; a dull, aching pain; or a burning pain. Large, fast neurons activate the individual and increase sharp pain, and small, slow neurons depress the person and cause anxiety. Neurons intermediate in size and speed are responsible for a burning pain.

The intensity of one's perception of pain may be attributable in part to the level of activity of the brain endorphinergic system (see Chapter 8). It also may be influenced by nonspecific factors. The experience of pain is increased with fatigue, anxiety, fear, boredom, and anticipation of more pain.

When pain was experimentally induced in a laboratory, it was found that redheaded people report pain at lower stimulus intensities than blondes, who in turn are more sensitive than brunettes. When personality tests were used to select introverts and extroverts, introverts were generally found to have lower pain thresholds. It is certain, at least from experiences in combat zones during war, that a high level of arousal and/or intense concentration on a task crucial for survival can completely block the experience of pain. During combat, severe wounds would be incurred, but it was only after the attack ended that the victims would become aware of these wounds. The molecular explanation for this may be related to brain activity of endogenous peptidyl opiates.

In terms of a placebo effect, consensus of the literature indicates that about 35 percent of patients studied had their pain "satisfactorily relieved" by placebos. The psychologic force of the placebo effect is a predominant factor, as evidenced by reports stating that although 35 percent of patients did receive satisfactory relief from pain, 75 percent experienced relief only after receiving morphine. But even in stressful situations, placebos are effective in reducing pain. The conclusion is that placebos are more effective in real-life or pathologic situations than with experimental pain. However, the internal analgesics have been shown repeatedly to be more effective at therapeutic doses than placebos for certain kinds of pain.

Americans use about 45 billion tablets of aspirin each year. That averages out to about 200 tablets for each man, woman, and child. In 1977, aspirin accounted for over $539 million in retail sales. According to the statistics of *Product Marketing*, sales of acetaminophen (Tylenol and other brands) amounted to almost $157 million. Effervescent compounds added about $11 million more in sales.

It is evident that analgesics are self-administered in a variety of circumstances. Indications include headache, arthritis, fever, and muscle ache, and for "not feeling well."

The potential dangers associated with the use of headache aids are not appreciated by the majority of persons who use these products for self-medication. In hypersensitive people, headache aids may produce gastrointestinal disturbances and toxicity. Untoward side effects produced by these compounds are:

| | |
|---|---|
| Salicylates: | gastric bleeding |
| Aminopyrine: | agranulocytosis |
| Phenacetin: | kidney damage |

A summary of common brands, usual adult dosage, strength for pain relief, ability to reduce fever, ability to relieve inflammation of arthritis, advantages, side effects, and disadvantages is presented in Table 16-1.

### *a. Aspirin and Acetaminophen*

Aspirin is an excellent pain reliever and fever reducer. It also reduces inflammation. These advantages are accompanied by several common side effects. About 5 percent of the population using this drug may experience stomach upset and heartburn. Aspirin causes gastrointestinal bleeding, which for the most part goes unnoticed.

## TABLE 16-1
## Adult Pain and Fever Medications

| *Category* | *Common Brands* | *Usual Adult Dosage* | *Strength for Pain Relief* | *Ability to Reduce Fever* | *Ability to Relieve Inflammation of Arthritis* | *Advantages* | *Side Effects and Disadvantages* |
|---|---|---|---|---|---|---|---|
| Aspirin tablets | Bayer<br>Squibb St. Joseph | 2 tablets every 4 hours | Excellent for relief of mild to moderate pain. | Excellent | Good | Usually least expensive | Upset stomach and heartburn in small number of persons. Tends to cause bleeding, expecially of gastrointestinal tract. Not recommended for persons with ulcers. |
| Buffered aspirin tablets | Arthritis Pain Formula<br>Ascriptin<br>Bufferin | 2 tablets every 4 hours | Excellent for relief of mild to moderate pain. | Excellent | Good | Less tendency to upset gastrointestinal tract than plain aspirin. | Same side effects as aspirin. |
| Acetaminophen tablets or liquid | Tempra<br>Tylenol | 2 tablets every 4 hours. For liquid, see directions on package. | Excellent for relief of mild to moderate pain. | Excellent | None | No stomach upset or heartburn. No gastrointestinal bleeding. Liquid form available. | Overdosage can cause liver damage. |
| Effervescent tablets and powder | Alka-Seltzer<br>Bromo Seltzer<br>Fizrin Powder | See directions on package. | Excellent for relief of mild to moderate pain. | Excellent | Good | Causes least gastro intestinal bleeding of products that contain aspirin. Less tendency than plain aspirin to upset stomach and cause heartburn. | Same side effects as aspirin. High sodium (salt) content. |

(Adapted from Wigden, H. N. *A Guide to Over-the-Counter drugs.* New York: Delta, 1979, p. 32.)

Aspirin has many qualities of which the public is not generally aware. Allergic reactions to aspirin can occur. Allergy to aspirin may be found in as many as 5 percent of asthmatics. It also causes adverse side effects when taken with other medications (see Chapter 18). In combination with alcohol aspirin is likely to result in gastrointestinal bleeding, and thus is not recommended for a hangover. When taken with diabetic medications such as insulin, chlorpropamide (Diabinease), tolazamide (Tolynase), or colbutamide (Orinase) aspirin induces enhanced hypoglycemia. Aspirin also increases the action of anticoagulants such as warfarin (Coumadin); cancer patients who are treated with methotrexate should be advised that aspirin increases its toxicity.

Powdered aspirin, dissolved in water, is quickly absorbed from the gastrointestinal tract and results in less gastrointestinal bleeding. However, since the powdered form contains large amounts of sodium it is contraindicated for people with high blood pressure or those on a low-salt diet. Aspirin is not sold in liquid form; however, liquid forms of acetaminophen, such as Extra Strength Tylenol Liquid, are available for adults. Other forms of aspirin and acetaminophen include suppositories and time-release capsules.

Although acetaminophen does not reduce inflammation, it is an excellent pain reliever without producing gastrointestinal upset.

### *b. Combinations of Ingredients*

Advertisements would have us believe that a combination of ingredients induces more pain relief than aspirin or acetaminophen alone. Several brands combine all four pain-relieving ingredients (aspirin, acetaminophen, salicylamide, and phenacetin) in varied proportions. But according to Widgen,[4] consensus of the literature reveals that no combination of ingredients is any more effective than a single ingredient.

Another ingredient in many of the combination pain relievers is the stimulant caffeine. According to the FDA,[7] "There is weak evidence that the combination of caffeine and aspirin is more effective than aspirin alone." Supportive clinical evidence for the FDA statement includes the finding by Moertel et al.[16] that caffeine plus aspirin worked no better to relieve pain than aspirin alone. Caffeine has no proven analgesic effect and there is no valid evidence that it potentiates the effect of analgesics nor is there any rationale to include caffeine in analgesic OTC remedies.[17,18] Consumer products that contain or contained caffeine include Anacin, Empirin Compound, Vanquish Caplet, Excedrin, and Cope.

Phenacetin, another pain reliever included in combination remedies, may cause episodic anemia in certain individuals (American blacks) and kidney disease.

### *c. Children's Pain and Fever Remedies*

Children's pain and fever medications consist of either aspirin or acetaminophen, the same medications contained in adult products but in doses designed specifically for children according to age or size. Unlike adult medications, children's products are usually pure and consist of a single ingredient. See Table 16-2.

## 2. Sleeping Pills

Insomnia affects millions of people and in a variety of ways, from minor fatigue the next day to substantial interference with one's job, social life, and state of mind. Sleep disturbances may be caused by serious physical diseases, such as peptic ulcer, congestive heart disorders, epilepsy, asthma, abnormalities of the thyroid gland, and emotional problems. Anxiety or stress and depression account for the majority of sleep problems. Increasing age or senescence is usually associated with changes in sleep cycles and often mistakenly blamed for "insomnia." The amount of total sleep required by elderly people is significantly less than that required by younger persons.

Americans spend over $30 million annually on antihistamines sold as sleep remedies. The prime reason for the use of antihistamines in this regard is their well-known side effect of

**TABLE 16-2**
**Children's Pain and Fever Medications**

| *Category* | *Common Brands* | *Form of Medication* | *Usual Dosage* | *Ability to Reduce Fever* | *Strength for Pain Reflief* | *Advantages* | *Side Effects & Disadvantages* |
|---|---|---|---|---|---|---|---|
| Aspirin | Bayer Children's Aspirin St. Joseph Aspirin for Children | Chewable tablets | Varies with age. For details see previous categories. | Excellent | Excellent for relief of mild to moderate pain. | | Not available in liquid form. May contribute to upset stomach. |
| Acetaminophen | Tempra Drops or Syrup Tylenol (Chewable Tablet, Drops, or Liquid) St. Joseph Fever Reducer for Children | Chewable tablets or liquid | Varies with age. For details see previous categories. | Excellent | Excellent for relief of mild to moderate pain. | Available in liquid form. Does not upset stomach. | Overdose can cause liver damage. |

(Adapted from Wigden, H. N. *A Guide to Over-the-Counter Drugs.* New York: Dell, 1979 p. 43.)

drowiness. A summary of available OTC sleep remedies is given in Table 16-3.

Table 16-3 reveals that other ingredients contained in OTC sleep aids are salicylamide, salicylates such as aspirin, and acetaminophen. One of the side effects of salicylamide is mild drowsiness but in OTC products the amount is not enough to produce sedation in most people. The rationale for inclusion of these analgesics is that alleviation of minor pain will help one sleep.

The extent of abuse of such products as Nervine, Compoz, Sominex, Nytol, and Quiet World is not known, but is assumed to be significant in the adult population. Most people do not realize the abuse potential of these products.

## 3. Stimulants

Caffeine is the prime stimulant found in many OTC products. Like all drugs, caffeine has unpleasant side effects—including inability to fall asleep, nervousness, and irritability. Since coffee and tea contain caffeine, millions of Americans consume these beverages each day either to get started or to keep awake. Some people are under the misconception that caffeine is an antidote for the depressant effects of alcohol, a belief that appears to be unfounded. Substantial sales of decaffeinated coffee indicate that many individuals are experiencing side effects from caffeine. However, the decaffeinated product may be dangerous as well.[19]

Most OTC stimulant medications contain 100 to 250 mg of caffeine in each tablet or capsule. Table 16-4 summarizes available OTC stimulants.

Stimulants, whether coffee, tea, or medication, are of questionable value. Both coffee and OTC stimulants are abused primarily by the adult community.

## 4. Antiobesity Drugs

Obesity is one of the most common problems affecting the health of Americans. It is estimated that approximately one third of all Americans are overweight. Obesity has been associated

**TABLE 16-3**
**Sleeping Pills**

| *Category* | *Common Brands* | *Usual Adult Dosage* | *Advantages* | *Side Effects and Disadvantages* |
|---|---|---|---|---|
| Sleeping pills that contain only an antihistamine | Nervine | Depends on brand chosen. | May make you drowsy. | Probably ineffective. |
| Sleeping pills that also contain scopolamine | Compoz Quiet World Sominex | Depends on brand chosen. | May make you drowsy. | Probably ineffective. Interferes with normal sleep cycles. May contribute to increased eye pressure (glaucoma) and difficulty in urination. |
| Sleeping pills that also contain pain and fever reducers | Nytol Quiet World Sominez | Depends on brand chosen. | May make you drowsy. | Probably ineffective. Contains unnecessary medication. |

(Adapted from Wigden, H. N. *A Guide to Over-the-Counter Drugs.* New York: Dell, 1979, p. 124.)

with several serious medical problems, including diabetes mellitus, hypertension, and cardiovascular disease. One approach to the problem is depression of the appetite. It is believed that hunger is related to the utilization of glucose by cells in hypothalamic centers. This has been termed "glucostatic hypothesis of appetite regulation." Another approach takes into consideration the fact that an empty stomach will stimulate the appetite because it will induce hunger contractions, whereas a distended stomach will depress the appetite because it will not induce hunger contractions. Underlying mechanisms of obesity include peptidyl opiates, such as B-endorphin,[20] and other peptides, such as $CPK_8$ (cholecystotkinin).[20,21]

Although no single plan has been universally successful, numerous schemes that have been devised to induce weight loss. These include fad diets, starvation diets, stimulant medications, and organizations such as Weight Watchers and Take Off Pounds Sensibly (TOPS). All these plans are based on a low calorie intake.

The dangers of fad diets, starvation diets, and protein hemolysate diets have been documented.[4] For example, protein hemolysate diets have been associated with sudden death in young, otherwise healthy, persons. The OTC preparations used in weight control include preparations that fall into six rather diverse groups:

1. Those that increase in the gastrointestinal tract—hydrophilic colloids (phony foods).
2. The so-called "dietaries" or low-calorie foods—canned foods containing not more than 900 calories.
3. Those that contain benzocaine—hydrophilic colloids plus benzocaine.
4. Those that contain glucose, supposedly for the purpose of stimulating the satiety center (Dex-a-diet).
5. Preparations containing phenylpropanolamine (Hungrex, Slender-x, and Diet Trim).
6. The artificial sweeteners—saccharin and sucaryl.

The OTC weight-loss drugs are presented in Table 16-5.

As previously mentioned (see Chapter 12), amphetamines exert their effect on the appetite centers in the brain. Since amphetamines induce CNS stimulation and tolerance develops, long-term use of these drugs is not desirable.

An OTC drug pharmacologically related to amphetamine is phenylpropanolamine, which is a decongestant found in many OTC cold and allergy medications. The amount of this ingredient contained in cold medications can be as great as that in so-called OTC appetite suppressants, and it is probably ineffective as an appetite suppressant in the dosage provided (25 mg).[17] Side effects of this drug include hyperglycemia, hypertension, palpitations, rapid heart beat (tachycardia), insomnia, headache, nausea, and nervousness. Over-the-counter phenylpropanolamine-containing remedies are not recommended for persons with diabetes mellitus, heart disease, hypertension, or thyroid or goiter disease.

**TABLE 16-4**
**Stimulants**

| *Category* | *Common Brands* | *Usual Adult Dosage* | *Advantages* | *Side Effects and Disadvantages* |
|---|---|---|---|---|
| Coffee | Any brand that contains caffeine. | Dosage varies with desired effect. | May help keep you awake. | No substitute for adequate sleep. Nervousness and irritability. |
| Over-the-counter products with caffeine | Nodoz<br>Vivarin | Dosage varies with desired effect. | May help keep you awake. More convenient than making coffee or tea. | No substitute for adequate sleep. Nervousness and irritability. |

Adapted from: Wigden, H. N. "Guide to Over-the-Counter Drugs." Dell Publishing Company, New York, 1979, p. 139.

## 5. Antitussives (Cough Medications)

In the United States, more than $400 million is spent yearly for antitussive medications. Over-the-counter medications are divided into two categories—cough suppressants and expectorants. Narcotics or narcotic-like drugs are cough suppressants that are designed to stop a cough; expectorants eliminate secretions from the lungs.

Manufacturers of most cough remedies include other ingredients, such as antihistamines and analgesics. A common additive to many liquid cough medications is alcohol. Certainly alcohol does not treat coughs, but it may help relieve the uncomfortable "tickle" sensations in the throat. Sugar is another ingredient found in cough medication but the amount is not clinically significant except in cases of uncontrolled diabetes.

Table 16-6 includes information on available OTC cough medications.

Cough-suppressant drugs contain either codeine or dextromethorphan. Common side effects of codeine include constipation, stomach upset, and drowsiness. The drowsiness produced by codeine or dextromethorphan is enhanced by the addition of alcohol and antihistamines.

Compounds such as codeine and dextromethorphan act on the CNS to raise the threshold of the cough center and in this manner the frequency and intensity of the hyperactive cough are reduced. Glyceryl guiacolate, ipecac, and ammonium chloride relieve coughs because of their expectorant effect.

The preparations containing codeine or dextromethorphan should not be used for prolonged periods of time because of their dependence potential. Ipecac should be used with caution in children. Because of the acid-forming properties of ammonium chloride, it has the tendency to produce acidosis and thus should not be used for a great length of time.

Accidental overdosage can cause respiratory depression, especially in chronic pulmonary disease. Ingestion of large amounts of this type of medication may result in disturbances of the level of consciousness. Their abuse potential is great because of the high opiate content and at times they replace street heroin.

## 6. Nausea/Vomiting/Motion Sickness Drugs

According to *Product Marketing*, in 1977 over $21 million worth of motion sickness med-

**TABLE 16-5**

**Weight-Loss Drugs**

| *Category* | *Common Brands* | *Advantages* | *Side Effects and Disadvantages* |
|---|---|---|---|
| Appetite-suppressant drugs | Prolamine | Possibly helpful in weight loss when combined with a weight-reduction diet. | Works best on a short-term basis. Side effects include nervousness, insomnia, headache, restlessness, and a rise in blood sugar. |
| Artificial sweetners<br>Low-calorie candy<br>Low-calorie foods | Ayds<br>Metrecal<br>Slender<br>Sucaryl<br>Weight Watcher Foods | Low-calorie sweeteners, candy, and foods are substitutes for similar products that contain considerably more calories. If these products actually substitute for your higher calorie habits, your total calorie intake will be reduced. This strategy is called dieting. | Saccharin (found in many low-calorie foods) has recently come under scrutiny by the FDA as a possible carcinogen. |

ications were sold. Nausea, vomiting, and dizziness are typical symptoms of motion sickness, and can be reduced by medication taken prior to travel. Major side effects of these OTC motion sickness products are drowsiness, exacerbation of glaucoma, and urinary retention.

The advantages and disadvantages of medications such as dimenhydrinate (Dramamine) and cyclizine (Marezine) are summarized in Table 16-7.

Interestingly, when nausea and vomiting are attributed to indigestion, flu, or gastroenteritis, they are not usually treated with motion sickness drugs.

## 7. Cold and Sinus Medications

### *a. Common Cold*

The common cold is a syndrome characterized by a catarrhal inflammation of the upper respiratory tract, namely, the nose, pharynx, accessory nasal sinuses, and the larynx.[22] Symptoms include running nose, stuffiness, scratchy throat, and cough. There is usually little or no fever. The common cold is the most frequent acute illness and accounts for more time away from work and school than any other cause.[23] Approximately 250 million days are lost each

**TABLE 16-6**

**Cough Medications**

| *Category* | *Common Brands* | *Usual Adult Dosage* | *Advantages* | *Side Effects and Disadvantages* |
|---|---|---|---|---|
| Cough suppressants | Pertussin<br>Robitussin DM<br>Silence is Golden<br>Symptom1 | Depends on patient age and brand chosen. | Strongest medication for stopping coughs. | Produces drowsiness. |
| Cough expectorants | Robitussin | Depends on patient age and brand chosen. | Supposedly helps loosen mucus and secretions. | Not very effective. |
| Throat lozenges that contain a cough suppressant | Hold<br>Robitussin DM Cough Calmers<br>Vicks Cough Silencers<br>Vicks Formula 44 Cough Disks | Depends on patient age and brand chosen. | Convenient form of medication. | Produces drowsiness. Some brands provide inadequate amounts of cough suppressant for an adult. |
| Cough drops | Ludens<br>Smith Bros.<br>Vicks Cough Drops | May be used as often as needed. | Convenient form of medication. Excellent means to relieve "tickle" in the throat. | No better than hard candy or honey, and may be more expensive. |

(Adapted from Wigden, H. N. *A Guide to Over-the-Counter Drugs.* New York: Dell, 1979, pp. 96–97.

**TABLE 16-7**

**Motion Sickness Medications**

| *Category* | *Common Brands* | *Form* | *Advantages* | *Side Effects and Disadvantages* |
|---|---|---|---|---|
| Motion sickness drugs | Dramamine<br>Marazine | Tablet<br>Liquid | Good for motion sickness. | Drowsiness. |

(Adapted from Wigden, H. N. *A Guide to Over-the-Counter Drugs.* New York: Dell, 1979, p. 184.)

year by workers in the United States because of the common cold.

Although it is known that the common cold is caused by a strain of viruses called the rhinoviruses, a cure has not been found. Viruses that cause influenza, measles, and pneumonia are quite distinct from those that cause colds. It is extremely difficult to identify the elusive virus of the cold because of the enormous variety of viruses; more than 100 types have been identified. Rhinoviruses readily change their immunologic reactivity, thus adding to the problem. Experts have successfully developed vaccines against poliomyelitis and measles, and perhaps the next vaccine will overcome the nuisance of the cold.

Statistically more than 250 million acute cold-like illnesses occur each year in the United States and outnumber other ailments 25 to 1.[10] The lack of protective antibodies against a virus is a risk with serious consequences. A viral infection such as influenza is more than just a bad cold. Influenza outbreaks have been recorded as early as the year 1173. Twenty million deaths resulted from influenza in the post-World War I epidemic in 1918–1919. In 1957–1958, the Asian flu was responsible for the deaths of 78,000 persons in the United States.

The experimental animal of choice for studying colds had to be humans. In numerous investigations with human volunteers, three types of findings seem to emerge: (1) Only about one half of those directly exposed to a cold virus develop cold symptoms. (2) Those individuals carrying antibodies to the cold virus may have minor symptoms that last for a brief period (12 to 24 hours) and then disappear.[24] (3) The incidence of colds increases during the winter months, and there may be an early peak in November and then another in February. The incidence curves are similarly shaped for southern and northern United States. According to Tyrrell,[25] the actual temperatures and climates of different areas do not control the frequency of colds, but a change of climate to a cooler, and possibly damper type, might increase their incidence.[17]

The use of cold remedies dates back to World War II. At that time, antihistamines were touted as preventing and curing the common cold, not just as suppressing its symptoms. Before the FDA could step in, most Americans were ascribing to the belief that the antihistaminic drugs were "cold cures." Today antihistamines are just one of many drugs in cold capsules. The most frequently used are the pheniramines, which include brompheniramine and chlorpheniramine. In 1977, according to statistics in *Product Marketing*, Americans spent almost $243 million for cold tablets, capsules, and sinus products. About $100 million was spent just for nasal drops and sprays.

Cold and sinus medications are basically decongestants, and are available in either oral (by mouth) or topical preparations. Both oral and topical medications have advantages and disadvantages, and many find a combination of an oral and topical decongestant the best therapy for a cold. The effectiveness of any decongestant will vary with the individual and the severity of the illness.

Tables 16-8 and 16-9 summarize clinical pharmacologic actions of oral decongestants and topical decongestants respectively.

Oral decongestants, when used in recommended dosages, are usually quite safe, but there are side effects as listed in Table 16-8. These include nervousness, insomnia, headache, rapid heart beat, palpitations, hypertension, and hyperglycemia. These products are contraindicated in patients with overactive endocrin glands, ischemic heart disease or angina, hypertension, or uncontrolled diabetes mellitus.

Oral decongestants interact with digitalis and antidepressants. Combination products usually contain antihistamines.

Topical decongestants are useful in reducing the congestion of colds quickly. However, overuse may result in rebound congestion, that is, the spray itself causes increased nasal congestion.

## 8. Allergy Medications (Allergic Rhinitis)

Allergic rhinitis, commonly referred to as allergy, is primarily caused by ragweed or pollen and is seasonal. People with this problem experience a worsening of symptoms in the spring and late summer. The symptoms include runny nose, sniffles, red and watery eyes, and nasal and sinus congestion. People of all ages are bothered by allergy problems caused by drugs, animals, dust, food, and plants.

According to the July 1978 issue of *Product Marketing*, Americans spent over $43 million on allergy and hay-fever products in 1977. For the most part, OTC allergy medications are formulated to treat the allergic symptoms of hay fever. Treatments of hay fever other than self-medication include moving to another part of the country, using electrostatic air cleaners, or restricting dust, feathers, and pets.

Antihistamines are the drug of choice for treating allergic rhinitis because of their ability to antagonize, to varying degrees, many of the actions of histamine. Histamine is released in a number of conditions, such as rash, seasonal hay fever, and drug reactions. The degree of sedation produced by antihistamines may affect activities such as driving, operating a machine, or climbing stairs or ladders. Gastrointestinal upset—including loss of appetite, nausea, vomiting, constipation, or diarrhea—is frequently observed.

Allergy medications, and their dosage, advantages, and disadvantages, are presented in Table 16-10.

According to Ray,[24] the important observation is that the misuse of cough, cold, and allergy remedies to produce alterations in

**TABLE 16-8**
**Oral Decongestants**

| *Category* | *Common Brands* | *Usual Adult Dosage* | *Advantages* | *Side Effects and Disadvantages* |
|---|---|---|---|---|
| Pure decongestant (pseudoephedrine) | Novafed<br>Sudafed | 2 tablets or 2 teaspoonfuls 4 times a day. | Excellent decongestant—the same medication physicians often prescribe. Does not contain unnecessary ingredients. | Side effects are uncommon at recommended dosages. Palpitations, nervousness, rise in blood pressure. |
| Combination decongestant and antihistamine | A.R.M.<br>Chlor-Trimeton Decongestant Tablets | Dosage varies with produce. See package directions. | No advantage over a pure decongestant for treating a cold. | The antihistamine produces drowsiness. |
| Combination decongestant and antihistamine in time-release capsules | Allerest<br>Contact<br>Dristan Capsules | 1 capsule in the morning and 1 capsule in the evening. | Very convenient form of medication—only requires taking a capsule twice a day. | Dosage of medication may be inadequate to treat some adults for a full 12 hour. |
| Combination medications that also contain pain and fever reducers | Alka-Seltzer Plus<br>Comtrex<br>Coricidin<br>Sinutab | Dosage varies with product. See package directions. | Supposedly, these medications are convenient since they provide ingredients to treat fever and muscle-aches. However, the dosage of aspirin may be inadequate for an adult. | Contains unnecessary medication since most colds produce fever or muscleaches for only a brief period of time during the illness. |

(Adapted from Wigden, H. N. *A Guide to Over-the-Counter Drugs.* New York: Dell, 1979, p. 63–64.)

consciousness is not uncommon. In fact, high doses of sympathomimetic or anticholinergic drugs produce hallucinations. Dextromethorphan in high doses can result in sensations that some may interpret as positive feelings. These OTC compounds often have a relatively high alcohol content and, even without the addition of other psychoactive agents, can cause a high. Furthermore, the antihistamines produce drowsiness, which, for some individuals, induces a feeling of well-being similar to a barbiturate high.

## D. NONABUSABLE CATEGORY

In the previous category of OTC products the designation of abusable refers to the ''psychotherapeutic'' and/or mental properties of the compounds described. However, there are numerous ways to group OTC compounds. Although vitamins and laxatives are not overused because of their ''psychic'' actions, they are misused and/or abused.

Over $200 million was spent in 1967 on vitamins, and since that time vitamin consumption has steadily increased in popularity. Vitamins are not drugs in a strict sense of the term but they do exhibit independent pharmacologic reaction and are considered toxic if taken in excessive amounts and for prolonged lengths of time. Although vitamins are organic chemicals that are not manufactured by the body, they are as essential as enzymes in the body.

Some people use laxatives compulsively as a part of their normal bowel function. Over $200 million is spent for more than 700 OTC laxatives each year. The abuse of laxatives over a long period of time impairs the capability of the body to maintain regularity. ''It is now more generally realized that moderate constipation consti-

**TABLE 16-9**

**Topical Decongestants**

| Category | Common Brands | Usual Adult Dosage | Advantages | Side Effects and Disadvantages |
|---|---|---|---|---|
| Long-acting decongestants | Afrin<br>Dristan Longacting<br>Duration | 2 sprays into each nostril twice a day | Long-acting relief. No drowsiness. | Only desinged to be used for a few days. Overuse can lead to increased congestion (rebound congestion). |
| Short-acting decongestants | Alconefrin<br>Neo-Synephrine | 2 drops or 2 sprays into each nostril 3 or 4 times a day | No advantage over long-acting nasal sprays. No drowsiness. | Only designed to be used for a few days. Overuse can lead to increased congestion (rebound congestion). |
| Aromatics (inhalers) | Dristan Inhaler<br>Vicks Inhaler* | Inhale twice into each nostril 3 or 4 times a day. | No advantage over long-acting nasal sprays. No drowsiness. | Only designed to be used for a few days. Overuse can lead to increased congestion (rebound congestion). |

*Popular recreational days of abuse in the 1960s and 1970s.
(Adapted from Wigden, H. N. *A Guide to Over-the-Counter Drugs.* New York: Dell, 1979, p. p. 65.)

tutes a far smaller menace to health than over-enthusiastic efforts to treat it . . . the abuse of laxatives by the public is still common. . . "[27]

Because the focus of this work is abusable drugs, the nonabusable OTC products will be discussed only briefly. A more detailed account can be obtained from other sources.[4,15,28]

Products to be reviewed include sore throat medications, antacids, laxatives, diarrhea medications, hemorrhoid medications, menstrual products, acne medications, antiseptics, antibiotic ointments, ophthalmic aids and mouth wash products, and medicinal herbs.

## 1. Sore Throat Medications

Over-the-counter treatment of the sore throat usually includes aspirin and lozenges. It must be emphasized that these are designed to provide

**TABLE 16-10**
**Allergy Medications**

| *Category* | *Common Brands* | *Usual Adult Dosage* | *Advantages* | *Side Effects and Disadvantages* |
|---|---|---|---|---|
| Pure antihistamine | Chlor-Trimeton Tablets or Syrup | 1 tablet or teaspoonful every 4–6 hours. | Drug of choice for hayfever (allergic rhinitis) | Commonly produces drowsiness. |
| Combination antihistamine and decongestant | A.R.M.<br>Chlor-Trimeton Decongestant Tablets<br>Novahistine Elixir<br>TGriaminic Syrup | Dosage varies with product. See directions on package. | May be more effective in some persons than a pure antihistamine. | Commonly produces drowsiness. |
| Combination antihistamine and Decongestant in time-release capsules | Allerest Time Capsule<br>Contact<br>Dristan Capsules | 1 capsule in the morning and 1 capsule in the evening. | Convenient dosage schedule—only requires taking 2 capsules a day. | Commonly produces drowsiness. Amount of medication may be inadequate for a full 12 hours. |

(Adapted from Wigden, H. N. *A Guide to Over-the-Counter Drugs.* New York: Dell, 1979, p. 77.)

**TABLE 16-11**
**Sore Throat Medications**

| *Category* | *Common Brands* | *Usual Adult Dosage* | *Advantages* | *Side Effects and Disadvantages* |
|---|---|---|---|---|
| Throat lozenges that contain anesthetic | Cepastat<br>Chloraspetic<br>Chloraseptic<br>Spec-T | Variable. See package insert. | Some benefit in relieving sore throat discomfort. | Provide temporary relief only. Allergic reactions are possible though uncommon. |
| Throat lozenges that contain "antibacterials" | Cepacol<br>Coltrex Troches<br>Sucrets | Varible. See package insert. | Some benefit in relieving sore throat discomfort. | "Antibacterials" do not do what they were designed to do, that is, they do not kill bacteria or viruses that cause sore throats. |

(Adapted from Wigden, H. N. *A Guide to Over-the-Counter Drugs.* New York: Dell, 1979, p. 108.)

relief of the pain associated with viral pharyngitis, strep throat, flu, and infectious mononucleosis. Table 16-11 summarizes sore throat medications.

## 2. Antacids

Antacid products exert their action by general neutralization of the hydrochloric acid present in the gastric fluids as the result of overeating. Some antacids release gas (carbon dioxide) from the stomach, and thus relieve the discomfort. Self-medication for a prolonged period of time with antacids may cause various problems: calcium carbonate—constipation, urinary calculi; sodium bicarbonate—acid rebound and alkalosis; aluminum hydroxide—constipation; magnesium hydroxide—cathartic effect, and neuromuscular, neurologic and cardiovascular impairment.

Antacids are designed to neutralize stomach acid and not as an aid to the digestion of food. They are primarily used in the treatment of ulcers and heartburn. Consumers also use these products for self-medication for a variety of ailments: 51 percent for upset stomach and nausea[4,15]; 29 percent for heartburn; 17 percent for sour stomach; 9 percent for indigestion. Ulcer-related problems motivate only 12 percent. These figures exceed 100 percent since many people use antacids for more than a single symptom.

American consumers of antacids spend over $450 million or more each year according to the July 1978 issue of *Product Marketing*. As summarized briefly in Table 16-12, antacids are sold without prescriptions, and the consumer has over 100 sizes and brands of antacids from which to choose. It has been estimated that the average adult uses these products more than seven times each month.

**TABLE 16-12**
**Antacids**

| *Category* | *Brands* | *Usual Adult Dosage* | *Form of Medication* | *Advantages* | *Side Effects and Disadvantages* |
|---|---|---|---|---|---|
| Aluminum and magnesium antacids | DiGel<br>Gelusil<br>Maalox<br>Mylanta | Variable. See package directions. | Chewable tablets or liquid. | Excellent ability to neutralize acid. | Aluminum products can cause constipation. Magnesium products can cause diarrhea. |
| Calcium carbonate antacids | Pepto-Bismol liquid | See package directions. | Liquid | None | Contains no antacid. |
| | Alka-2*<br>Pepto-Bismol Tablets<br>Tums | See package directions. | Chewable Tablets or Liquid. | Excellent ability to neutralize acid. | May actually increase acid production by the stomach. |
| Antacids that contain aspirin | Alka-Seltzer (original) | See package directions. | Effervescent Tablets or Powder. | Excelelnt ability to neutralize acid. | Aspirin may cause increased stomach upset and bleeding, especially when associated with alcohol ingestion. |

*A substance used to neutralize acod.
(Adapted from Wigden, H. N. *A Guide to Over-the-Counter Drugs.* New York: Dell, 1979, p. 197–198.)

## 3. Laxatives

More than $273 million was spent by the American public in 1978 on laxative products. Laxatives are one of the most abused drugs on the OTC market.

Most people think that transitory constipation should be treated promptly. Drugs that promote defecation are used because constipation is a functional impairment in the normal capacity of the colon to produce properly formed stools at regular intervals. Stimulant laxatives (cascara sagrada, rhubarb), synthetic (phenophthalein, danthrom, oxyphenisatin, biscodyl), saline (magnesium sulfate, tartrate, phosphate, citrate ions), bulk forming (derived from agar), emolient (mineral oil), and enemas are in widespread use.

The stimulant laxatives increase the propulsive peristaltic activity of the intestine by local irritation of the mucosa. The site of action varies from activity limited to the small intestine (castor oil) or colon (anthracene derivatives). The intensity of the action is proportional to the dosage, but individually effective doses of all such compounds vary as much as eightfold. Prolonged use of laxatives leads to habituation. Laxatives should not be used in the treatment of constipation associated with intestinal pathology. Hernia, cardiovascular disease, and hypertension patients should not force defecation. The advantages and disadvantages are pointed out in Table 16-13.

**TABLE 16-13**
**Laxatives**

| *Category* | *Common Brands* | *Form of Medication* | *Approximate Time for Effect* | *Advantages* | *Side Effects and Disadvantages* |
|---|---|---|---|---|---|
| Bulk formers and stool softeners | Colace<br>Maltsupex<br>Metamucil<br>Serutan | Capsule<br>Liquid<br>Powder<br>Tablets | 12 to 72 hours | Mild, safe, and usually effective. | Slow onset of action. |
| Saline (salt) cathartics | Fleet's Phospha-Soda<br>Phillips Milk of Magnesia<br>Sal Hepatica | Liquid<br>Tablets<br>Granules | ½ to 3 hours | Fast acting and effective. | Fleet's Phospha-Soda and Sal Hepatica not recommended for persons on low-salt diets. Not recommended for persons with kidney diseases. Repeated use may result in loss of the body's fluids. |
| Enemas | Fleet's<br>Tucks | Enema | ½ hour | Safe and effective for occasional use. | Chronic use may result in inability to move the bowels without an enema. |
| Stimulants | Carter's Little Pills<br>Dulcolax<br>Ex-Lax<br>Feen-A-Mint<br>Fletcher's Castoria<br>Senekot | Liquid<br>Capsule<br>Suppository<br>Tablet<br>Powder | 1 to 10 hours (suppositories work the fastest). | Effective | May cause abdominal cramps. |

(Adapted from Wigden, H. N. *A Guide to Over-the-Counter Drugs.* New York: Dell, 1979, p. 161–162).

## 4. Diarrhea Remedies

Diarrhea affects most individuals at one time or another, and is perhaps treated as a symptom of an undiagnosed and presumed minor and transient gastrointestinal disorder. The drugs commonly used are adsorbants and astringents. The principal gastrointestinal adsorbants used are kaolin, attapulgite, aluminum hydroxide, magnesium trisilicate, bismuth, subsalts, pectin, and activated charcoal. Sometimes absorbants are combined with resin. These compounds exert their antidiarrheal action by absorbing digestive enzymes, toxins, bacteria, and other noxious material. The adsorption is not a specific action.

Wigden[4] points out that in 1977 American's spent almost $109 million on OTC medications for diarrhea. But the only proven products for the control of diarrhea are not available over the counter in most parts of the United States. These drugs are opiates, and only a few states permit the nonprescription sale of opium and paregoric. All opiate medications sold OTC are required by law to be combined with other ingredients to decrease their drug-abuse potential. The effective adult dosage (decreased for children) for opium is 15–20 mg four times a day. One teaspoonful of paregoric has an approximately equal effect to that of 20 mg of opium.

Table 16-14 includes additional information concerning the effects of diarrhea medications.

## 5. Hemorrhoid Medications

Hemorrhoids are "piles" or a dilated vein that can be palpated around the rectum. The familiar symptoms of pain, inflammation, swelling, and bleeding occur as these veins degenerate. The etiology of hemorrhoids is still unknown. Many experts implicate chronic constipation, straining during bowel movements, excessive use of enemas, pregnancy, diet, liver obstructions, and cathartic laxatives, among other factors. Only surgery can actually eliminate the problem of hemorrhoids. Approximately 100 products are sold throughout the United States and no less than $55 million is spent annually on antihemorrhoid medications. Most hemorrhoidal products contain an anesthetic for the relief of pain. Astringents are also included in the majority of hemorrhoidal medications.

In addition, nearly three quarters of all he-

**TABLE 16-14**

**Diarrhea Medications**

| *Category* | *Common Brands* | *Form of Medication* | *Usual Adult Dosage* | *Advantages* | *Side Effects and Disadvantages* |
|---|---|---|---|---|---|
| Medications that contain opiates | Donnagel-PG | Liquid | Varies with age. | Effective in treatment of diarrhea. | Most states do not allow sale of opiates without a prescription. Chronic use of opiates can be habit forming. Opiate overdosage can cause sedation and even respiratory depression. |
| Medications without opiates | Donnagel<br>Kaolin Pectin Suspension<br>Kaopectate | Liquid | Varies with age. | Something to do while you are waiting for the diarrhea to stop. | No proven efficacy in treating diarrhea. |

(Adapted from Wigden, H. N. *A Guide to Over-the-Counter Drugs.* New York: Dell, 1979, p. 169.)

morrhoidal compounds contain an antiseptic designed to prevent the growth of bacteria. The value of sterilization in the treatment of hemorrhoidal symptoms is questionable.

A brief review of selected hemorrhoid medications is presented in Table 16-15.

## 6. Menstrual Products

Behavioral changes during menstruation occur as the result of hormonal changes. It has been noted that more crimes have been committed in Paris by females, and that 52 percent of all female crimes of violence occur during the seven days prior to menses. The correllation is not absolute.

A prime taboo was shattered when television commercials began to tout the virtues of products designed to relieve ''her'' special problems, including those containing caffeine, ephedrine, and vitamin C, as well as anticholinergics and antihistamines. Some products even contain herbs, alcohol, nasal decongestants, and bronchodilators. Great caution should be exercised when utilizing products that include large doses of caffeine. Sustained use over several days can lead to ''caffeine withdrawal headache'' when medication is discontinued. Modell[26] states that ''a well-controlled study is still needed to establish diuresis as useful therapy for premenstrual tension.'' Also to be considered is the use of diuretics in dysmenorrhea.

Basically the only benefit of menstrual products is the pain relief provided by the aspirin or acetaminophen involved. Millions of dollars are spent on such products; in 1977, according to the July 1978 issue of *Product Marketing*, Americans purchased over $17 million worth of ''menstrual pain relievers.'' (See Table 16-16.)

All things considered, it might be wiser for women to bear some natural discomfort once a month than to use OTC preparations that are of dubious value.

## 7. Antiseptics and Antibiotic Ointment

Antiseptics inhibit the growth of bacteria; they are useful, together with antibiotic ointments, for preventing infections from cuts and abrasions. Antibiotic ointments, or first-aid creams, protect the skin against bacterial contamination during the healing process.

There is a tendency to overuse ointments and antiseptics; most abrasions and minor lacerations heal very well without them. According to *Product Marketing*, in 1977 alone, Ameri-

**TABLE 16-15**
**Hemorrhoid Medications**

| *Category* | *Common Brands* | *Form* | *Advantages* | *Side Effects and Disadvantages* |
|---|---|---|---|---|
| Anesthetics and/or astringents | Americaine<br>Anusol<br>Nupercainal<br>Tucks<br>Wyanoids | Suppository ointment<br>Cream<br>Medicated pad | Anesthetics reduce pain on mucous membranes. Astringents reduce edema and inflammation. | Allergies to anesthetics can develop. |
| Lubricants | Hemorr-Aid<br>Vaseline | Ointment | Soothing effect on irritated skin. | |
| Miscellaneous | Preparation H | Suppository ointment | | Contains ingredients of questionable value in the treatment of hemorrhoids. |

(Adapted from Wigden, H. N. *A Guide to Over-the-Counter Drugs.* New York: Dell, 1979, p. 178.)

cans spent almost $84 million on medications for cuts and abrasions.

A summary of effects of antiseptics is given in Table 16-17; Table 16-18 reviews antibiotic ointments.

## 8. Acne Medications

Over $103 million was spent in 1977 on acne preparations, according to *Product Marketing*. Wigden[4] points out that at least one half of all

### TABLE 16-16
### Menstrual Products

| *Category* | *Common Brands* | *Usual Adult Dosage* | *Advantages* | *Side Effects and Disadvantages* |
|---|---|---|---|---|
| Aspirin or acetaminophen | Bayer<br>St. Joseph<br>Tylenol | 2 tablets every 4 hours | Excellent for relief of mild to moderate pain. | Aspirin can upset the stomach, and should not be taken by persons with bleeding problems or ulcers. |
| All over-the-counter menstrual products | Midol<br>Pamprin | Dosage varies with brand. | None | Contain a host of ingredients of dubious value in the treatment of menstrual cramps. |

(Adapted from Wigden, H. N. *A Guide to Over-the-Counter Drugs.* New York: Dell, 1979, p. 133.)

### TABLE 16-17
### Antiseptics

| *Category* | *Common Brands* | *Effectiveness* | *Advantages* | *Side Effects and Disadvantages* |
|---|---|---|---|---|
| Antiseptics used in hospitals | Betadine<br>Hibiclens<br>Iodine | Excellent | Widely accepted by hospitals and physicians as effective for killing bacteria on the skin. | Betadine may cause skin irritation. |
| Rubbing alcohol | Any brand | Good | Inexpensive | Causes burning or stinging sensation. |
| Hydrogen peroxide | Any brand | Fair | Foaming action helps remove dirt from wounds. | Causes burning or stinging sensation. |
| Mercurochrome | Mercurochrome | Fair | None | Low-strength antiseptic. |
| First aid sprays | Bactine | Fair | Convenient to use. | Sprays are not as effective as scrubbing a wound with an antiseptic. |

(Adapted from Wigden, H. N. *A Guide to Over-the-Counter Drugs.* New York: Dell, 1979, p. 150.)

adolescents and teenagers experience difficulty with acne, but few seek medical advice. Most self-medicate with a variety of OTC products.

Acne is a chronic skin condition that results from overactivity of sebaceous glands under the surface of the skin. It can be treated with OTC medications as indicated in Table 16-19.

## 9. Ophthalmic Products

There are several reasons for using eye drops or eye decongestants. They include esthetic or cosmetic purposes, to clear red eyes and to give a fresh appearance, and for medicinal purposes, such as in eye infections. Eye decongestants are absorbed through the cornea but not the sclera, though the cornea is still relatively resistant to topically applied medications. Fortunately, eye infections from airborne pathogens are curtailed by tearing, which acts to lubricate, hydrate, and remove debris from the ocular surface.

Excessive use of eye decongestants can be hazardous and rebound congestion has been reported. Most OTC ophthalmic preparations include ephedrine, phenylephrine, nephazoline, and tetrahydrazoline. Nephazoline and tetrahydrozoline are harmful if ingested by children. The OTC products containing methylcellulose can be discomforting if used excessively.

**TABLE 16-18**
**Antibiotic Ointments**

| *Category* | *Common Brands* | *Advantages* | *Side Effects and Disadvantages* |
|---|---|---|---|
| Ointments without neomycin | Baciguent<br>Bacitracin<br>Betadine<br>Polysporin | Excellent antibiotic ointments | |
| Ointments with neomycin | Mycitracin<br>Neo-Polycin<br>Neosporin<br>Triple Antibiotic ointment | Excellent antibiotic ointments. | The neomycin in these products may cause allergic reactions in some people. |

(Adapted from Wigden, H. N. *A Guide to Over-the-Counter Drugs.* New York: Dell, 1979, p. 151.)

**TABLE 16-19**
**Acne Medications**

| *Category* | *Common Brands* | *Advantages* | *Side Effects and Disadvantages* |
|---|---|---|---|
| Products with benzoxl peroxide | Benoxyl Lotion<br>Foster Acne Gel<br>Oxy-5<br>Oxy-10 | Strong, effective over-the-counter medications. | Most irritating of all the over-the-counter acne medications. |
| Combinations of sulfur, resorcinol, and salicylic acid | Clearasil<br>Epi-Clear<br>Fostril<br>Pernox Lotion<br>Stri-Dex<br>pHisoAc<br>Fostex Cream | Moderately strong medications. Less irritating than benzoly peroxide. | Most irritating of all the over-the-counter acne medications. |
| Skin cleansers | Bep-Clear Scrub<br>Pernox Cleanser | | Not as potent as benzoyl peroxide. |

(Adapted from Wigden, H. N. *A Guide to Over-the-Counter Drugs.* New York: Dell, 1979, p. 209.)

### 10. Mouth Wash Products

Halitosis became a household word through commercial advertising. It is an alleged causative factor in social, sexual, and positional insecurity. Halitosis is strongest in the morning because of the stagnated food stuffs and bacteria that have remained in the mouth overnight. Since bacteria are involved, the antibacterial agents (hexachlorophene, quaternary ammonium compounds, tyrothricin) and hydrogen peroxide have been recommended. These compounds, if absorbed, eventually can result in harmful effects, such as decalcification of tooth substances. Hydrogen peroxide can lead to the production of black, hairy tongue and decalcification of tooth substances.

## E. HERBAL MEDICINES

Throughout the ages, humans have seriously explored natural materials (drugs, plants) to heal illnesses, both central and peripheral in nature. The renewed interest in traditional medicine with recognition by the World Health Organization (WHO) of the need to integrate traditional healing practices with modern scientific methodology is but one example of the growing popularity of folk medicine and herbal healing. A state-of-the-art review by Meyer and associates[28] is recommended for readers who are seriously interested in this subject.

Today a large assortment of medicinal herbs is available to the general public. However, not all of these herbs are harmless, and some must be considered potentially dangerous.

Many of the herbs used for self-medication are also important to the pharmaceutical industry. Herbs are employed as flavoring agents, and extracted chemical ingredients are active constituents of modern medicinal products. Species of the following genera remain useful to the drug industry: Althera, Carica, Cassia, Cinchona, Cinnamomum, Citrus, Cola, Commiphora, Datura, Dioscorca, Ephedra, Eucalyptus, Gaultheria, Glycyrrhiza, Hydrastis, Plantago, Prunns, Rhamnus, and Ulmus.[29]

A number of herbs that are readily available have been reported to cause intoxication in both humans and animals. Also, self-medication with herbs may cause adverse reactions in an individual who is taking prescription or other nonprescription medicines as well.

One side effect of handling plants or plant parts is dermatitis. According to Sullivan[30] and others,[31-33] the following genera have been involved in producing dermatitis in humans: Achillea, Artemisia, Berberis, Capsicum, Citrus, Euphorbia, Gaillardia, Geranium, Juglans, Humulus, Lavrea, Rhus, Rudbeckia, Ruta, and Xanthium.

Other toxic reactions induced by herbs taken internally include severe nausea, vomiting, and diarrhea. Species of the following genera have been reported to cause a poisonous response in humans: Asclepias, Cassia, Caulophyllum, Clenatis, Datura, Helenium, Ilex, Iris, Lobelia, Lycium, Physalis, Phytolacca, Prunus, Rhamnus, Rumex, Senecio, Solanum, and Tanacetum.[31-33]

In addition to the adverse reactions noted, ''herbal highs'' from natural or legal drugs have been reported. A number of these highs were serious enough to require medical attention.[34] Hallucinations are produced by catnip, juniper, kava-kava, nutmeg, and jimson weed. Mild stimulant action may be obtained from cinnamon, damiana, kola nut, mate, Mormon tea, and the passion flower. Mild tranquilizer effects have been observed with valerian, kava-kava, and wormwood. Euphoria may be obtained from both lobelia and prickly poppy. Peppermint, spearmint, and many of the other common species may also contain psychoactive substances.[35]

Among other herbs that are normally available for culinary or medicinal use are: fennel, garlic, mace, mustard, allspice, basil, bay, cayenne, chili, cream of tartar, cumin, curry, oregano, paprika, parsley, black and white pepper, thyme, tumeric, and vanilla.

According to Sullivan,[30] ''During the past few years there has been a very definite renewal of interest in natural foods and vitamins.'' This is evidenced by the establishment of a large number of natural food stores across the United States. Sullivan[30] is convinced that there is a parallel interest in the use of herbs for the treatment of human maladies.

For a more complete listing and purported uses of herbal medicines, refer to the works of

Burlage,[36] Krochmal and Krochmal,[37] Martinez,[38] and Youngken.[39]

## F. GENERAL COMMENTS[24]

The world of OTC drugs is vast. Perhaps it is more in this drug area than in any other that the consumer, manufacturer, advertiser, and government need increased interaction. The people who use OTC compounds are not sophisticated in drug use and must be guided carefully into the land of safe, symptomatic self-treatment. This will require restraints on advertising as well as on the proliferation of new and safer medications. However, governmental controls on herbs and plants have been seriously questioned. Weil,[40] in discussing the pros and cons of botanical versus chemical drugs, clearly stated that:

> It is not the business of government to deny us access to plants, especially plants that have healing properties. Let them put warnings on things if they wish. Let them print in red letters all over packages of (for example) sassafras tea, "We think this dangerous for you; the purified active principle causes cancer in our rats" . . . that is not the same as not letting people buy it.

Weil[40] additionally points out that using medicinal plants to treat our maladies is a right that must not be interfered with by government. He suggests that to protect this right, people must inform themselves about such matters and be willing to exercise more responsibility in the maintenance of health and the management of illness.

With the expanding demands for better medical care and an ever-greater patient–physician ratio, it appears likely that self-medication will increase along with the potency of the drugs available and in use. It seems essential that some action be taken to plan for the systematic education of the public in the analysis of symptoms and the selection of safe but effective drugs to deal with them.

Have you ever taken a drug without a prescription? The answer to that question for most of us would be "yes." Then another question would be raised, "Why?" Most people believe that self-medication, or taking drugs without prescription, is an integral part of health care. People choose to medicate themselves because self-medication is easy, inexpensive, and convenient. However, the self-medicating public must be made to recognize the approximate boundaries of their therapeutic competence and the dangers inherent in attempting to exceed those limits. When these limits are exceeded the results can be toxic effects or interference with medical diagnosis.

We take nonprescription or OTC drugs because we believe that they will help relieve illnesses. Small bodily discomforts such as headache, indigestion, stomach pain, constipation, or a general ill feeling can be tolerated. But we have learned to expect alleviation and we take drugs to get it. We have had little exposure to the concept that the body has strong defense mechanisms and, to some extent, can take care of minor ailments if given time.

The executive director of the American Pharmaceutical Association has written[6]:

> Self-medication is being practiced today with a degree of sophistication that belongs to the dark ages. It is national policy for us to practice every possible precaution to protect the patient in the case of drugs which require prescription orders. Nevertheless, some drugs are available for self-medication that may not be as potent as legend drugs when compared on paper, but there is abundant evidence their pharmacological action in vivo clearly indicates that they deserve to be labeled "Explosive—handle with care."

## REFERENCES

1. Hiss, A. E. *A Thesaurus of Proprietary Preparations in Pharmaceutical Specialties.* Chicago: G. R. Englehard, 1898.
2. Consumer Reports. *The Medicine Show; Some Plain Truths About Popular Remedies for Common Ailments.* Mount Vernon, N.Y.: Consumers Union, 197
3. *Handbook of Non-Prescription Drugs*, 5th ed. Washington, D.C.: American Pharmaceutical Association, 1977.
4. Wigden, H. N. *Wigden's Guide to Over-the-Counter Drugs: A Critical Comparison of the*

*Effectiveness, Cost, and Safety of the Most Popular and Widely Advertised Brands.* Los Angeles: Tarcher, 1979.
5. Meyer, G. C., Blum, K., and Cull, J. G. (Editors) *Folk Medicine and Herbal Healing.* Springfield, Ill.: Thomas, 1981.
6. Griffenhagen, G. B. *Handbook of Non-Prescription Drugs.* Washington, D.C.: American Pharmaceutical Association, 1969.
7. U.S. Food and Drug Administration. Summary minutes on OTC Panel on Internal Analygesics, Including Antirheumatic Drugs. 18th Meeting, Dec. 9–10, 1974.
8. U.S. Food and Drug Administration. *The Use and Misuse of Drugs.* Publication no. 46, U.S. Department of Health, Education and Welfare. Washington, D.C.: U.S. Government Printing Office, 1968.
9. Grollman, A. Efficacy and therapeutic utility of . . . home remedies. *J. Am. Pharm. Assoc.* 5:586, 1965.
10. Cold remedies around the world. *Am. Assoc. Ind. Nurses J.* 13:29, 1965.
11. Verhulst, H. L., and Crotty, J. J. Survey of products most frequently named in ingestion accidents in 1965. *J. Clin. Pharmacol.* 7:10, 1967.
12. Smith, L. H., Jr. The clinical pharmacology of salicylates. *Calif. Med.* 110(5):410, 1969.
13. Goodman, L. S., and Gilman, A. *The Pharmacological Basis of Therapeutics*, 6th ed. New York: Macmillan, 1980.
14. Caranasos, G. J., Stewart, R. B., and Cluff, L. E. Drug-induced illness leading to hospitalization. *JAMA* 228:713, 1974.
15. Graedon, J. *The Peoples' Pharmacy.* New York: Avon, 1976.
16. Moertel, C. G., et al. Relief of pain by oral medications. *JAMA* 229:55, 1975.
17. *AMA Drug Evaluations.* 3d ed. Littleton, Mass.: Publishing Sciences Group, 1977.
18. Greden, J. F. Anxiety or caffeinism: A diagnostic dilemma. *Am. J. Psychiatry* 131:1089, 1974.
20. Blum, K., et al. Psychogenetics of drug seeking behavior. *Subst. Alcohol Actions/Misuse.* 1(3):255, 1980.
21. Gibbs, J., Young, R. C., and Smith, G. P. Cholecystokinin decreases food intake in rats. *J. Comp. Psychol.* 84:488, 1973.
22. Regnier, E. The administration of large doses of ascorbic acid in the prevention and treatment of the common cold. *Rev. Allergy* 22:835, 1968.
23. Douglas, R. G. Pathogenesis of rhinovirus common colds in human volunteers. *Ann. Otol.* 79:563, 1970.
24. Ray, O. S. *Drugs, Society, and Human Behavior.* St. Louis: C. V. Mosby, 1972.
25. Tyrrell, D. A., Jr. *Common Colds and Related Diseases.* Baltimore: Williams & Wilkins, p. 30.
26. Modell, W. (Editor) *Drugs of Choice, 1970–1971.* St. Louis: C. V. Mosby, 1970, p. 101.
27. Dunlop, D. Abuse of drugs by the public and by doctors. *Br. Med. Bul.* 26:131, 1970.
28. Press, I. Urban folk medicine: A functional overview. *Am. Anthropol.* 80:71, 1978.
29. Tyler, V. E., Jr., Brady, L. R., and Robbers, J. E. *Pharmacognosy.*, 7th ed. Philadelphia: Lea & Febiger, 1976.
30. Sullivan, G. Herbs available to the public. In G. G. Meyer, K. Blum, and J. G. Cull, eds. *Folk Medicine and Herbal Healing.* Springfield, Ill.: C. C. Thomas, 1981, p. 179.
31. Ellis, M. D., ed. *Dangerous Plants, Snakes, Arthropods and Marine Life of Texas.* Washington, D.C.: U.S. Department of Health, Education and Welfare, Public Health Service, 1975.
32. Lampe, K. F. and Fagerström, R. *Plant Toxicity and Dermitis; A Manual for Physicians.* Baltimore: Williams & Wilkins, 1968.
33. Kingsbury, J. M. *Poisonous Plants of the United States and Canada*, 2d ed. Englewood Cliffs, N.J.: Prentice-Hall, 1964.
34. Siegel, R. K. Herbal intoxication. Psychoactive effects from herbal cigarettes, tea, and capsules. *JAMA* 236:473, 1976.
35. Schultes, R. E. *Hallucinogenic Drugs.* New York: Golden Press, 1976.
36. Burlage, H. M. *Index of Plants of Texas with Reputed Medicinal and Poisonous Properties.* Austin, Tx., 1968.
37. Krochmal, A., and Krochmal, C. A. *A Guide to the Medicinal Plants of the United States.* New York: Quadrangle, 1973.
38. Martinez, M. *Las Plantas Medicinales de Mexico.* Mexico: Ediciones Botas, 1956.
39. Youngken, H. W. *A Textbook of Pharmacology*, 6th ed. Philadelphia: Blakiston, 1948.
40. Weil, A. T. Botanical vs. chemical drugs: pros and cons. In G. G. Meyer, K. Blum, and J. G. Cull, eds. *Fok Medicine and Herbal Healing.* Springfield, Ill.: C. C. Thomas, 1981, p. 287.

## SUGGESTED READINGS

Beecher, H. K. Placebo effects of situations, attitudes and drugs: A quantitative study of suggestibility. In K. Rickels, ed. *Non-specific Factors in Drug Therapy.* Springfield, Ill.: C. C. Thomas, 1968.

Boyd, E. M. Analgesic abuse: maximal tolerated daily doses of acetylsalicylic acid. *Can. Med. Assoc. J* 99:790, 1968.

Burn, G. P. A device for measuring the threshold of pain in man. *Br. J. Pharmacol.* 34:251, 1968.

Craig, J. O., Ferguson, I. C., and Syme, J. Infants, toddlers, and aspirin. *Br. Med. J.* 1:757, 1966.

Crotty, J. J. The epidemiology of salicylate poisoning. *Clin. Toxicol.* 1(4):381, 1968.

Dunlop, D. Abuse of drugs by the public and doctors. *Br. Med. Bull.* 26(3):236, 1970.

Ferreira, S. H., Moncada, S., and Vane, J. R. Indomethacin and aspirin abolish prostaglandin release from the spleen. *Nature New Biol.* 231:237, 1971.

Fosdick, W. M., and Shepart, W. L. Enteric-coated microspherules. A clinical appraisal of two forms of aspirin. J. Clin. Pharmacol. 9:126, 1969.

Goddard. Tax drugs to fight abuse. *Am. Drug.* 34, 1970.

Grotto, M., Dikstein, S., and Sulman, F. G. Additive and augmentative synergism between analgesic drugs. *Arch. Int. Pharmacodyn. Ther.* 155(2):365, 1965.

Griffenhagen, G. B. and Hawkins, L. L. (Editors) *Handbook of Non-Prescription Drugs.* Washington, D.C.: American Pharmaceutical Assoc., 1971.

Hasebroock, Mrs. W. H. Home remedies in household management. *Ann. N.Y. Acad. Sci.* 120(2):996, 1965.

Haslam, D. R. Individual differences in pain threshold and level of arousal. *Br. J. Psychol.* 58(1):139, 1967.

Herman, E., and Stenebring, W. (Editors) Second Conference on Antiviral Substances. *Ann. N.Y. Acad. Sci.* (in press).

Keefer, C. S. Summary and conclusions. *Ann. N.Y. Acad. Sci.* 120(2):1005, 1965.

Levy, G. Aspirin, absorption rate and analgesic effect. *Anesth. Analg.* 44:837, 1965.

Meyer, G. G., Blum, K., and Cull, J. G. (Editors) *Folk Medicine and Herbal Healing.* Springfield, Ill.: C. C. Thomas, 1981, p. 000.

Parkhouse, J., et al. The clinical dose response to aspirin. *Br. J. Anaesth.* 40:433, 1968.

Prescott, L. F. Analgesics. *Practitioner* 200:84, 1968.

Purnell, J., and Burry, A. F. Analgesic consumption in a country town. *Med. J. Aust.* 2:389, 1967.

Report of the Commission on Drug Safety, 1964, Subcommittee on Responsibilities of the Public on Drug Safety. Federation of American Societies for Experimental Biology, Washington, D.C., pp. 176, 179.

Salicylates. *Chem. Eng. News* 46:50, 1968.

Should aspirin be put on RX-only status? *Am. Drug.* 161(6):40, 1970.

Smith, G. M., and Beecher, H. K. Experimental production of pain in man: ensitivity of a new method to 600 mg. of aspirin. *Clin. Pharmacol. Ther.* 10(2):213, 1969.

Smith, J. B., and Willis, A. L. Aspirin selectively inhibits prostaglandin production in human platelets. *Nature (New Biol.)* 231:235, 1971.

Stephens, F. O., et al. The effect of food on aspirin induced gastro-intestinal blood loss. *Digestion* 1:267, 1968.

Stevenson, J. M. Aspirin. *J. Indiana State Med. Assoc.* 61:1462, 1968.

Tyrrell, D. A. Hunting common cold viruses by some new methods. *J. Infect. Dis.* 121(5):561, 1970.

Vaccines up the nose. *Br. Med. J.* 1:63, 1970.

Vane, J. R. Inhibition of prostaglandin synthesis as a mechanism of action for aspirin-like drugs. *Nature (New Biol.)* 231:232, 1971.

Wiseman, E. H., and Federici, N. J. Development of a sustained-release aspirin tablet. *J. Pharm. Sci.* 57:1535, 1968.

Wolff, B. B., et al. Response of experimental pain to analgesic drugs. III. Codeine, aspirin, secobarbital and placebo. *Clin. Pharmacol. Ther.* 10:217, 1969.

Woodbury, D. M. Analgesic-antipyretics, anti-inflammatory agents, and inhibitors of uric acid synthesis. In L. Goodman and A. Gilman, eds., *The Pharmacological Basis for Therapeutics*, 4th ed. New York: Mcmillan, 1970, p. 321.

CHAPTER 17

# Marihuana: Heaven or Hell

## A. INTRODUCTION[1]

Indian hemp, or *Cannabis sativa*, is a tall, annual, weedy herb that can be grown in any region with hot summers. There are both male and female plants; in the past the male was used in the making of fibers. The female plant produces the most active pharmacologic ingredients. Although recent studies show that the leaves of both the male and female plants furnish active products, it is the female that has a higher concentration of those products in the flowering tops. Marihuana consists of the dried and crumbled stems, leaves, and seed pods of the female plant. In the United States the materials are usually mixed with tobacco and smoked. In India the uncultivated hemp plant is smoked as marihuana and also used as a drink called "bhang." In other parts of the world, a special cultivated hemp plant known as "ganja" contains an unusually large quantity of active materials. Ganja may be smoked, or brewed and drunk as tea. It can also be made into candy. The pure unadulterated resin from the top of the finest female plants of Indian hemp is known as hashish or charas, and contains a very high concentration of active ingredients. When the female plant is ripe and the temperature is elevated, the flower clusters and the top of the plant are covered by a sticky, golden-yellow resin that has an odor rather like that of mint. This resin, closely allied to the substance hops, is so precious that great pains are taken to harvest it. In the past the resin was obtained by naked men who were driven through the steaming rows of hemp, thrashing their arms about them so that it would stick to them. This was then scraped off. Later the runners were made to catch the resin in large leather aprons. More esthetic methods are now used. The active ingredients are extracted and synthesized and constitute a series of derivatives of tetrahydrocannabinol (THC). The most active one is delta-9-tetrahydrocannabinol ($\Delta^9$-THC). Of course, the potency of a product will depend upon the content of active ingredients. This, in turn, is dependent upon whether the plants are cultivated, and whether the material is pure resin or is derived from other parts of the plant. Prior to 1979 the marihuana used in the United States, which was obtained from uncultivated plants and various parts of the plant, contained few active ingredients.

The potency of "street" marihuana has increased markedly in recent years. Confiscated materials in 1975 rarely exceeded 1 percent $\Delta^9$-

THC content. By 1979 samples with as high as 5 percent THC content were common. ''Hash oil,'' a marihuana extract unavailable a decade ago, has been found to have a THC content as high as 28 percent. More typical samples analyzed by University of Mississippi chemists ranged from 15 to 20 percent THC.

In 1972 a national survey indicated that some 24 million Americans had tried marihuana at least once, and that at least 8.3 million were regular users.[2] Marihuana use now begins at a much earlier age than a decade ago and is more likely to be frequent rather than experimental. The most significant increases are in the 12- to 17-year-old group. Among high school seniors, for example, daily use nearly doubled from the class of 1975 to those of 1978 and 1979 (from 8.5 percent to 10.7 and 10.3 percent for each of these classes). Moreover, the percentage of each of these senior classes that began to use in the ninth grade or earlier has also nearly doubled (from 16.9 percent of the class of 1975 to 30.4 percent of the 1979 class). About one in ten of the 1979 senior class reported daily use.[3]

In 1980 a national survey discovered that only 5 percent of the peak-using 18- to 25-year-old group saw the drug as having ''no bad effects.'' Perceived adverse consequences include performance and health impairment, possible psychologic effects, and the increased likelihood of using stronger drugs. Nearly three quarters (72.2 percent) of young adults believed that being high causes impaired driving performance.

According to Snyder,[4] there was a time in the United States when extracts of cannabis were almost as commonly used for medicinal purposes as aspirin is today. Cannabis was a proprietary medication that could be purchased without a prescription in any drug store. It was also prescribed by physicians for the treatment of a broad variety of medical conditions, from migraines and excessive menstrual bleeding to ulcers, epilepsy, and tooth decay.

Though cannabis was medically advocated in the past, it is now discouraged. The primary reason for discontinuation was the huge variation in the potency of different batches due to variations in the THC content of different plants. Further, the low solubility and delayed action of cannabis resulted in the increased use of morphine, barbiturates, and aspirin in preference to it. Finally, the Marihuana Stamp Act of 1937 put an end to its legal use.

With the isolation and synthesis of delta-1-tetrahydrocannabinol in 1964, new frontiers in the research on the pharmacology of the cannabis derivatives were sighted. The effects of the various derivations of THC with known doses and the structure–activity relationships of its different analogs could be predicted and tested in human subjects.[5] One of the THC analogs is found to lower the blood pressure without too much effect on the mind. Sim and coworkers suggested that this might be a good drug for the hypertensive patient.[5] Many U.S. drug companies are currently attempting to synthesize new analogs of THC with the aim of developing some clinically useful preparations. The trend seems to continue in spite of the official branding of cannabis as a ''dangerous drug.''

## B. HISTORY[2,6,7]

### 1. Overview

The history of cannabis products and their use has been long, colorful, and varied. ''To the agriculturist, cannabis is a fiber crop; to the physician, it is an enigma; to the user, a euphoriant; to the police, a menace; to the trafficker, a source of profitable danger; to the convict or parolee and his family, a source of sorrow.'' The fact is that cannabis has been held simultaneously in high and low esteem at various times throughout recorded history.

The volume of information available on the medical application of cannabis is considerable. Occasionally certain references have been condensed or deleted, but this should not detract from the completeness of the report.

This historic survey of the medical uses of marihuana begins by presenting a broad overview of its use, including brief notes on current and projected research, and then considers specific historical settings and circumstances in ancient China, Egypt, India, Greece, Africa, and the Western World.

*Cannabis sativa* has been used therapeutically from the earliest records, nearly 5000 years ago, to the present day,[31] and its products have been widely noted for their effects, both physiologic and psychologic. Although the Chinese and Indian cultures were aware of the properties of this drug from very early times, this information did not become generally known in the Near and Middle East until after the fifth century A.D., when travelers, traders, and adventurers began to carry news of the drug westward to Persia and Arabia.

Historians claim that cannabis was first employed in these countries as an antiseptic and analgesic. Other medical uses were later developed and spread throughout the Middle East, Africa, and Eastern Europe.

Several years after the return of Napoleon's army from Egypt, cannabis became widely accepted by Western medical practitioners. It had previously been limited to purposes such as the treatment of burns. The scientific members of Napoleon's forces were interested in the drug's pain-relieving and sedative effects. It was used during and, to a greater extent, following his rule in France, especially after 1840 when the work of such physicians as O'Shaughnessy, Aubert-Roche, and Moreau de Tours drew wide attention to this drug. With the rise of the literary movement of the 1840–1860 period in France (Gautier, Baudelaire, Dumas, etc.), cannabis became somewhat popular as an intoxicant of the intellectual classes.

In the United States medical interest in cannabis use was evidenced in 1860 when the Committee on Cannabis Indica of the Ohio State Medical Society reported on its therapeutic applications.[8] Walton states that between 1840 and 1890 more than 100 articles were published that recommended cannabis for some disorder. In India concern about cannabis as an intoxicant led the government to establish the India Hemp Commission of 1893–1894 to examine the question of its use in that country.

In the latter half of the 19th century use of medications superior to cannabis in their effects and more easily controlled as to dose was growing. Consequently cannabis began to lose the support of the medical profession.

In the years between 1856 and 1937, the perception of cannabis changed from that of being medically acceptable to being socially disreputable. Strong public reaction coupled with a campaign in the public press led to a federal antimarihuana law in 1937. (The drug was illegal in many states before that year.) The issue of medical use remained active, however, and Dr. William C. Woodward, Legislative Counsel to the American Medical Association, and an opponent of cannabis use and the only physician to be a witness at the Taxation of Marihuana hearings, stated: "There are exceptions in treatment in which cannabis cannot apparently be successfully substituted for. The work of Pascal seems to show that Indian Hemp has remarkable properties in revealing the subconscious; hence, it can be used for psychological, psychoanalytic and psychotherapeutic research."[9]

Although cannabis drugs are generally regarded as obsolete and rarely employed in "western" medicine today, cannabis is "still used extensively in the Ayruvedic, Unani and Tibbi systems of medicine of the Indian-Pakistani subcontinent."[10] The *Pharmacopoeias* of India mention cannabis use in the recent past. Two preparations of cannabis, a liquid extract and a tincture, are listed in the 1954 and 1966 editions of these *Pharmacopoeias*, which contain descriptions of cannabis and its extract and how it is made.[11]

A more recent source makes reference to the fact that "in contemporary India and Pakistan, there continues to be widespread indigenous medical, 'quasi-medical,' and illicit use of both opium and cannabis."[11] Bouquet notes that hemp resin is occasionally used in the native medicines of the countries where it is collected. He points especially to India where "the medical systems . . . make much use of cannabis as a sedative, hypnotic, analgesic, anti-spasmodic and anti-hemorrhoidal."[12]

Hollister[13] lists a few difficulties with the therapeutic use of cannabis:

(1) The onset of the action of oral doses of THC is often rather slow, contrary to that of conventional sedative-hypnotics.

(2) Doses high enough to produce a marked hypnotic effect are almost always accompanied by some degree of psychotomimetic-like perceptual disorders, which many patients might find disagreeable.

(3) The fine titration of dose required to provide sedative effects is likely to be difficult.

(4) The drug does not have novel effects compared with other sedative-hypnotics.

Despite the many statements discounting cannabis' therapeutic usefulness, some authorities maintain that its medical value might be reborn through further research and/or use. David Solomon, in his foreword to *The Marihuana Papers*,[14] argues that:

> Marihuana should be accorded the medical status it once had in this country as a legitimate prescription item. After 1937, with the passage of the Marihuana Tax Act and subsequent federal and state legislation, it became virtually impossible for physicians to obtain or prescribe marihuana preparations for their patients. Thus, the medical profession was denied access to a versatile pharmaceutical tool with a history of therapeutic utility going back thousands of years.

Mikuriya[7] lists many possible therapeutic uses of THC and similar products in his paper "Marihuana in Medicine: Past, Present and Future." He includes: "analgesic-hypnotic, appetite stimulant, antiepileptic, antispasmodic, prophylactic and treatment of the neuralgias, including migraine and tic douloureaux, antidepressant-tranquillizer, antiasthamatic, oxytocic, antitussive, topical anesthetic, withdrawal agent for opiate and alcohol addiction, child birth analgesic, and antibiotic."

### *a. China*

The oldest known therapeutic description of cannabis was by the Emperor Shen-Nung in the 28th century B.C. in China, where the plant had long been grown for fiber. He prescribed cannabis for beri-beri, constipation, "female weakness," gout, malaria, rheumatism and absentmindedness.[15,16]

### *b. Egypt*

In Egypt, in the 20th century B.C., cannabis was used to treat sore eyes. Additional medical usage was not reported until much later.

### *c. India*

Prior to the tenth century B.C., *bhang*, a cannabis preparation, was used as an anesthetic and antiphlegmatic in India. In the second century a Chinese physician, Hoa-Tho, prescribed it as an analgesic in surgical procedures.[7]

From the tenth century B.C. up to 1945 (and even to the present time), cannabis has been used in India to treat a wide variety of human maladies. The drug is highly regarded by some medical practitioners in that country. The religious use of cannabis in India is thought to have preceded its medical use in that country.[17,18] This use of cannabis is to help "the user to free his mind from worldly distractions and to concentrate on the Supreme Being."[19]

Cannabis is used in Hindu and Sikh temples and at Mohammedan shrines. Besides being utilized as an aid to meditation, it is also employed by the religious mendicants to overcome hunger and thirst. In Nepal it is distributed on certain feast days at the temples of all Shiva followers.[17] The Hindus spoke of the drug as the "heavenly guide" and "the soother of grief." Considered holy, it was described as a sacred grass during the Vedic period.[20]

## 2. History of Medical Use

Despite the fact that marihuana was declared illegal in the United States in 1937, research has continued on the possible medical uses of cannabis and its chemical derivatives. One of the most interesting findings[21] concerns the effect of cannabis in reducing intraocular pressure. It was found that as the dose of marihuana is increased, the pressure within the eye decreases by up to 30 percent. This was seen to occur in normal persons as well as in those with glaucoma, a disease of the eye in which increased intraocular pressure may cause blindness. However, much more research is necessary in connection with this clinical finding.

During the past 20 years in western medicine, marihuana has been assigned antibiotic activity; as a result, several studies relating to this possibility have been undertaken. Murphy,[22] in reporting investigations in Eastern Europe, stated that "it is alleged to be active against gram positive organisms at 1/100,000 dilution, but to be largely inactivated by plasma, so that prospects for its use appear to be confined to E.N.T. [ear, nose, and throat] and skin infections."

Kabelikovi[23] and his co-workers carried out tests on rats, which were similar to tests carried out with penicillin *in vitro*. The alcohol extract of cannabis was bacterially effective against many gram-positive and one gram-negative microorganism. It was also found that a paste form applied externally was successful. According to Kabelikovi, "from a study of 2000 herbs by Czechoslovakian scientists it was found that *Cannabis indica* (the Indian Hemp) was the most promising in the realm of antibiotics."

In a 1959 publication of *Pharmacie*, Krejci[24] stated: "From the flowering tops and leaves of hemp, *Cannabis sativa var indica* bred in Middle Europe, were extracted a phenol and an acid fraction. From the acid fraction, two acids were obtained, of which one preserved its antibiotic properties."

This section on the antibiotic uses of cannabis concludes with a summary of several reports from various countries. In *Pharmacopee Arabe*[25]: "The ground-up seeds are mixed with bread for people with tuberculosis." In Czechoslovakia[26]: "A preparation from seed pulp was . . . introduced by Sirek to act as a roborant diet in treatment of tuberculosis." In Southern Rhodesia the plant is used as an African remedy for malaria, anthrax, sepsis, black water fever, dysentary, blood poisoning, tropical quinine-malarial haemoglobinuria, and as a wart medicine.[27] In Argentina[26]:

> Cannabis is considered a real panacea for tetanus, colic, gastralgia, swelling of the liver, gonorrhea, sterility, impotency, abortion, tuberculosis of the lungs and asthma . . . even the root-bark has been collected in spring, and employed as a febrifuge, tonic, for treatment of dysentery and gastralgia, either pulverized or in form of decoctions. The root, when ground and applied to burns, is said to relieve pain. Oil from the seeds has been frequently used even in treatment of cancer.

In 1949 David and Ramsey reported a study of the effect of THC on epileptic children. The demonstration of anticonvulsant activity of the tetrahydrocannabinol (THC) congeners by laboratory tests[28] prompted clinical trial in five institutionalized epileptic children[29] and could not obtain consistent results.

Dr. Vansim of Edgewood Arsenal has written in *Psychotomimetic Drugs* that the synthetic preparations of cannabis are of interest. There are three areas of medicine in which they may be of definite use.[30] One concerns the use of a cannabis analog that Dr. Walter S. Loewe reported as very effective in preventing grand mal seizures if given in small doses.

The second use refers to cannabis as an antidepressant. Walton,[31] Adams,[32] and Stockings[33] point to the possible use of cannabis and cannabis analogs in relieving dysphoria in depressed patients. Other authors[34] had less success but recommended further research in this field. A report from London in 1968 suggests that cannabis treats the symptoms and not the cause by focusing users' attention on any anxieties and pains without helping the user to resolve them.[35]

The third use is described by Douthwaite, who used hashish in 1947 "for reducing an anxiety and tension in patients with duodenal ulcers." And a report in a 1965 issue of *Medical News*, "Cardiac Glycocides"[36] suggests cannabis as a treatment for a specific form of malignancy.

Cannabis is recognized as an appetite stimulant, which suggests that it might be useful in the treatment of the pathologic loss of appetite known as anorexia nervosa.[37] Similar symptoms exist in terminal cancer patients who, when treated with cannabis over a short period of time, have demonstrated stimulation of appetite, euphoria, an increased sense of well-being, mild analgesia, and an indifference to pain that reduced the need for opiates.[38]

Cannabis has been proposed as an adjunct in the treatment of alcoholics and drug addicts. Adams[32] and Mikuriya[39] have noted that the substitution of smoked cannabis for alcohol may have rehabilitative value for certain alcoholics. It also has been concluded that "pyrahexyl (a synthetic cannabis-like drug) and related compounds are beneficial in the treatment of withdrawal symptoms from the use of opiates to a less marked, but still significant degree.''[40] Blum and associates[41] reported that low doses of THC (0.5 to 2 mg/kg) inhibited ethanol-induced withdrawal reactions in mice, but cautioned that higher doses (up to 3 mg/kg) actually intensified ethanol-induced withdrawal reactions.

In his study of the medical applications of cannabis for Mayor LaGuardia's Committee on Marihuana in New York City, Dr. Samuel Allentuck reported ''favorable results in treating withdrawal of opiate addicts with tetrahydrocannabinol (THC), a powerful purified product of the hemp plants.''[7] Similar results were reported by others.[42]

Roger Adams' detailed studies, as reported by Dr. C. K. Himmelsbach in his 1944 article ''Treatment of the Morphine Abstinence Syndrome with a Synthetic Cannabis-Like Compound,''[43] indicated that ''withdrawal manifestations were considered to be mild.'' He went on to say that: ''The reported therapeutic value of marihuana was attributed to improved appetite, greater sleep, euphoria, and a reduction of the intensity or elimination of abstinence phenomena.'' Himmelsbach, however, was not as successful when he studied the effect of a ''pyrahexyl'' compound on the morphine abstinence syndrome.

Mayor LaGuardia's committee reported two possible therapeutic applications of marihuana: (1) euphoria—possibly active in the treatment of mental depression; and (2) alleviation of withdrawal symptoms in drug addicts.[44]

Some reports indicate that cannabis helps to relieve labor pains, and is used for this purpose among native tribes in South Africa and Southern Rhodesia. ''The Suto tribe fumigates the parturient woman to relieve pain''; the Sotho women of Basutoland ''are reported as smoking cannabis to stupefy themselves during childbirth,'' and have also been known to ''administer the ground-up achene with bread or mealiepap to a child during weaning.''[45]

The use of cannabis in the treatment of leprosy was described in a 1939 dictionary of Malayan medicine: ''Seeds of Hydnocarpus anthelmintica . . . form the basis of the Tai Foong Chee treatment of leprosy. After crushing and sieving, they are mixed with *Cannabis indica* in the proportion of two parts of the seeds to one of Indian hemp.''[25] Likewise, Watt and Breyer-Brandwijk quote Pappe, ''The early colonist employed a decoction in the treatment of chronic cutaneous eruptions possibly in leprosy . . .''[25]

Kabelik, Krejci, and Santavy have reported favorable results ''in stomatitis aphtosa, gingivitis, and in paradentoses with a mouthwash of the following composition: Tinct. Cannabis 20.0, Tinct. Chamomillae, Tinct. jemmarum populi (or another name for example, Tinct. Gallarum) āā 10.0 to be applied in the form of sprays or linaments to the inside of the mouth.''[26]

Dr. R. N. Chopra[46] reports that hemp drugs are popular as household remedies in the amelioration of such ailments as ''poor appetite, indigestion, malarious tracts, gonorrhoea, dysuria, dysmenorrhoea, asthma, infections of eyes, conjunctivitis, swollen joints, orchitis, and other acute inflammatory conditions.''

Tuberculosis, anthrax, tetanus, and menstrual cramps are among the miscellaneous medical uses of cannabis reported. Reports from Mexico indicate the smoking of marihuana ''to relax and to endure heat and fatigue.''[7]

Murphy[22] refers to an article by Lang, ''Treatment of Acute Appendicitis with a Mixture of Ma Jen,'' which says ''the drug has apparently been used in China for the treatment of appendicitis.'' The Xosa tribe of South Africa ''employs it for treatment of inflammation of the feet,''[26] and the Mfengu and Hottentot use the plant as a snake-bite remedy.[45]

Other therapeutic uses attributed to marihuana are for the treatment of migraine headaches, as an analgesic, and as a hypnotic. Hollister[13] states that ''other uses which have been proposed for marihuana include the treatment of epilepsy, as prophylaxis for attacks of migraine or facial neuralgia, or as a sexual stimulant.''

Practically every human complaint has been treated with Indian hemp. Although some of the uses mentioned from various cultures seem outlandish, certain of the ancient uses coincide with the results of careful studies undertaken in modern research institutes.

## 3. History of Intoxicant Use

The preceding history of the medical use of marihuana has provided an outline of how it has been alleged to cure diseases and to relieve pain. This section discusses the nonmedical use of cannabis. The survey includes a discussion of marihuana use in India and elsewhere in Asia, in Africa, in Europe, and in the United States. It concludes with an analysis of its use as an intoxicant in contemporary times—a difficult assessment in view of its importance to many people throughout the world as a folk medicine or a ceremonial adjunct.[47] Aside from caffeine and nicotine, cannabis as an intoxicant is second in worldwide popularity only to alcohol.

### *a. India*

Marihuana was probably first used as an intoxicant in India around 1000 B.C., and soon became an integral part of Hindu culture.[18,48] On the other hand, in China the marihuana plant was used for centuries to make cloth and certain medicines, but it was not recorded as an intoxicant.

Marihuana was also used as an intoxicant in other parts of the world prior to 500 A.D. but this usage is not as well documented as that of opium. The drug "nepenthe" in Homer's *Odyssey* is believed by a number of scholars to have been a brew in which the most active ingredient was hemp. Galen wrote in the second century that it was customary to promote hilarity and happiness at banquets by giving the guests hemp.[49]

Cannabis is used in three different preparations in India.[18] The first is called *bhang*, comparable in potency to marihuana in the United States. It is made from the leaves and stems of uncultivated plants and blended into a pleasant-tasting liquid concoction. The second is *ganja*, which is more potent than bhang. It is made from the tops of cultivated plants. The third and most potent preparation, *charas*, is similar to hashish or "hash" and is obtained by scraping the resin from the leaves of the cultivated plants. Hard blocks pressed from this material are converted for smoking.

High-caste Hindus are not permitted to use alcohol, but they are allowed bhang at religious ceremonies, and also employ it as an intoxicant at marriage ceremonies and family festivals. Bhang is used by laborers in India in much the same way as beer is used in the United States.[19]

The lower classes of India either take a few pulls at a ganja pipe or sip a glass of bhang at the end of the day to relieve fatigue,[47] to obtain a sense of well-being, to stimulate appetite, and to enable them to bear more cheerfully the "strain and monotony of . . . daily routines."[48] This is quite the reverse of the situation in the United States, where marihuana users consider themselves an exclusive and advanced "in group."[25]

### *b. Asia and the Middle East*

From India cannabis spread to other parts of Asia, to the Middle East, and then to Africa and South America, although some believe it may have originated independently in the latter two continents.[20] Cultural values may have played a part in determining its use. Opium and cannabis were equally available in pre-Communist China, but the latter was not popular as an intoxicant.[19] The Chinese spoke of the plant as the "liberator of sin," whereas in India it was called the "giver of life." One author proposed that temperament may have played a role in this determination, suggesting that perhaps the placid, practical Chinese did not appreciate the euphoria produced by cannabis.[19]

Additional evidence of mid-Asian use comes from interpretations of cuneiform tablets that describe use in Persia circa 700–600 B.C. and during Ashurbanipal's Assyrian reign, 669–626 B.C.[49] The drug's popularity as an intoxicant spread to the Middle East and had thoroughly permeated Islamic culture within a few centuries.[48] Because alcohol was prohibited to the followers of Mohammed, cannabis was accepted as a substitute.

### *c. Africa*

Use of cannabis in most parts of Africa developed slowly, most of it during the past 100 years. A report from Africa in 1891,[50] concerned a tribe that used hemp as an intoxicant as part of religious rites and in preparing for battle. A similar use is described in the Congo; in 1964 Simba warriors were said to use a cannabis—alcohol mixture in preparation for battle, both to excite themselves to fight and to guarantee immunity from harm. In Morocco marihuana, called *kif*, has been used as an intoxicant by adult males for centuries, a custom that continues today even though the drug is illegal.[51]

Although moderate use appears to be tolerated in India, North Africa, and the Middle East, excessive use is generally viewed as indicative of serious personality problems.[48]

### d. Europe

One of the more suggestive parallels between 19th century France and the United States today is the fact that the French interest in cannabis was aroused by soldiers and scientists of Napoleon's army returning from Egypt, a source of the drug. A similar interest was seen in the United States after the Korean conflict and it has intensified since Vietnam.[48]

During the 19th century, European interest in cannabis was abetted by two scientific reports, the first by W. B. O'Shaughnessy in 1839, and the second by Queen Victoria's physician, Russell Reynolds. Both recommended its medical use for a variety of ailments and as a mild euphoriant.[47] Cannabis received laudatory testimonials from the contemporary medical profession and was readily available without prescription.[18]

Interest in cannabis was further kindled by popular writers who used and spoke of hashish enthusiastically, including Charles Baudelaire, Arthur Rimbaud, and Pierre Gautier. Gautier and Baudelaire, in fact, were members of the *Club des Hachischins*, in which a number of writers and intellectuals gathered to experiment with hashish.[48]

Although the public delighted in reading about the French writers' drug experiences, most people did not wish to engage in the same kind of activity; to them the experiences were frightening and repugnant. "As a result, the smoking of hashish remained the sub-rosa province of a few European artists until the recent trans-Atlantic phenomenon of the American drug culture."[48]

### e. United States

The events surrounding the introduction of cannabis use to the New World are not at all clear. Some historians say the Spaniards brought the plant with them in the 16th century; others say marihuana smoking came in with the slave trade or with the Asian Indian migration of the late 18th century.

The hemp plant was cultivated in the United States for centuries, apparently without general knowledge of its intoxicating properties.[47] Cannabis was a popular medicine in the United States in the 19th century. Widely prescribed by physicians, it was also easily available without a prescription.[18] The pioneers utilized hemp to cover their wagons. A major crop in Kentucky and Virginia, as well as Wisconsin and Indiana, it was one of the South's more important agricultural products, after cotton. It is still used to make rope, twine, and textiles, and the seed is used as bird food.[48]

Marihuana use as an intoxicant in the United States began slowly in the early part of this century. Puerto Rican soldiers, and then Americans who were stationed in the Panama Canal Zone, are reported to have been using it by 1916. American soldiers fighting Pancho Villa around 1916 also learned to use it. This follows the first reported use in Mexico in the 1880s. Intoxicant use in the United States is also traced to the large influx of Mexican laborers in the 1910s and 1920s.[49]

Cannabis has been rejected by some groups on ascetic grounds. Such puritanical societies as the Wahabil of Arabis and the Senussis of Libya tolerated no smoking of any kind (or the use of coffee). In North Africa, social rank dictated use: The aristocratic Moors scorned both hemp and tobacco smoking, preferring instead, as compatible with high status, opium eating, while Nigerians supported the use of marihuana until Americans indiscriminately exploited it.[52]

In the United States, the decade of the 1960s saw a spectacular and unprecedented spread of marihuana use, chiefly among the youth. In the 1980s we are experiencing its use in all age groups and social classes—a phenomenon that has provoked marked public reaction and the need for more information concerning the effects of the drug.

### *f. Summary*

The extent and nature of cannabis use in the United States are summarized in the National Survey on Drug Abuse 1979. Large-scale marihuana use by Americans is recent[53] and as our experience with tobacco and alcohol demonstrates, it frequently requires many years of use by large numbers of people for long-range effects of a drug to appear. While there are cultures in which cannabis use has been traditional for many years, the drug usually has been used differently than in modern social use, and traditional users rarely include women or the very young. Perhaps the most disquieting development in our society has been the rapid increase in younger users, under the age of 18. Use is beginning earlier and earlier, and is often on a daily basis. Even those who regard occasional use by well-integrated, healthy adults as unlikely to pose serious public health problems agree that use, especially frequent, by children and adolescents can be seriously disruptive.

Despite our increasing awareness, much remains to be learned about the effects of chronic use. Unfortunately our limited knowledge is often interpreted as indicating that marihuana is "safe." There are many areas in which we simply do not know the parameters of risk. We do know that acute use poses hazards in driving and other complex behavior and definitely interferes with memory and intellectual functioning. As use comes to involve both younger and older persons, it becomes increasingly important that we be able to specify the kinds of danger and degree of public health risk posed by cannabis, both now and for the future. It is hoped that this summary of our present knowledge will represent another step toward achieving a better understanding of marihuana's public health implications.

In terms of use, there are indications that the increase has been greatest among young people (under 18). For example, the most notable changes in the 1977 National Survey from its predecessor in 1976 were a 25 percent increase in the total of those between ages 12 and 17 who had ever used marijuana and a nearly 30 percent increase in the number of that age group who were currently using marihuana (i.e., who had used it in the month preceding the survey). Current use in the over-18 population did not increase significantly. Nearly three out of ten (28.2 percent) of 12- to 17-year-olds in 1977 reported having tried marihuana at some point in their lives; nearly one in six (16.1 percent) were current users.[54]

Two thirds of young adults (68.2 percent), three in ten youths (30.9 percent), and one fifth of older adults (19.6 percent) reported having used marihuana. The relationship between marihuana use and chronologic age is marked. Experience increases fourfold between respondents age 12–13 (8 percent) and 14–15 (32 percent), and a majority (51 percent) of youths aged 16–17 report marihuana experience. Young adults aged 18–21 and 22–25 have the highest experience rates of all age subgroups (69 percent and 68 percent respectively). Usage declines among older adults, although almost one half (48 percent) of those aged 26–34 reported using marihuana. Only 10 percent of those aged 35 and older had done so.

Usage is higher among males than females in all three age cohorts: three fourths of young adult males, compared with 61 percent of females in the same age group, reported marihuana use, as did one fourth (26 percent) of older adult males, compared with 14 percent of females. Among youths the gap is much narrower, but still significant—34 percent of males and 28 percent of females.

From 1977 to 1979 there was a significant increase in the lifetime prevalence rates for both young adults (59.9 percent in 1977 to 68.2 percent in 1979) and older adults (15.3 percent in in 1977 to 19.6 percent in 1979). Moreover, within these two major cohorts, three of the four age subgroups (18–21 years, 22–25 years, and 35 or older) showed a significant increase in use.

Youth experience overall did not change significantly between the 1977 and 1979 studies. However, usage among 12–17-year-old residents of nonmetropolitan areas increased 9 percentage points between 1977 and 1979.

Among young adults, the following subgroups registered significant increases: males, females, whites, those who did not graduate from high school, those who had attended college, residents of the north central and southern states, and those from large metropolitan and nonmetropolitan areas. Three of these increases among young adults are particularly striking: whites (61 percent in 1977, 69 percent in 1979); those who were not high school graduates (52 percent in 1977, 67 percent in 1979); and residents of nonmetropolitan areas (48 percent in 1977, 61 percent in 1979).

In rural areas (a subcategory of nonmetropolitan), 60 percent of young adults had had marihuana experience. A significantly greater percentage of those residing in areas of population size 2500 to 24,999 reported such experience (68 percent) than those in areas of 2499 or less (54 percent).

Among older adults significant increases were shown by males, females, whites, college graduates, residents of the southern states, and residents of nonmetropolitan areas. The most striking of these was the increase registered by those in the South: 9 percent in 1977 to 18 percent in 1979.

If one takes the percentages of cannabis users noted in the 1977 survey and extrapolates to the general population, 43 million Americans had tried marihuana as of the spring of 1977, and in 1977 about 16 million were using the drug. A disturbing trend continues to be the tendency toward initial marihuana use at younger ages. For example, 16.9 percent of the class of 1975 had used the drug prior to the tenth grade, but the corresponding percentages in the 1976, 1977, and 1978 classes were 22.3, 25.2, and 28.2 percent. In a senior high school class studied, the 1979 group, 30.4 percent, had used prior to the tenth grade. Thus the percentage of seniors who first used in the ninth grade or earlier has nearly doubled over the past five years.[55,56]

Although overall the use of alcohol and tobacco continues to exceed that of marihuana, *daily* use of marihuana among the class of 1978 (10.7 percent) was nearly double that for alcohol (5.7 percent daily use) and was exceeded only by daily cigarette smoking (27.5 percent). Twice as many males as females were daily marihuana users. However, at lower levels of marihuana use, the sexes do not differ markedly in the percentages using.[55,56]

For the first time the NIDA 1979 Survey included questions about perceived hazards of marihuana use. It is noteworthy that only 5 percent of the peak-using 18- to 25-year-old group saw the drug as having "no bad effects." Perceived adverse consequences include performance and health impairment, possible psychologic effects, and the increased likelihood of using stronger drugs. Nearly three quarters (72.2 percent) of young adults believed that being high causes impaired driving performance.

## C. PHARMACOGNOSY

Marihuana is a preparation derived from the hemp plant, *C. sativa*. The plant is an annual that either is cultivated or grows freely as a weed around the world, including most of the United States. When cultivated in temporate climates, plantings are made in May to June. The seeds germinate in less than a week in moist soil. After thinning, the plants grow as rapidly as 2 feet a week during the peak growing season. They can reach a height of up to 18 feet at maturity, approximately three to five months after planting. Growth is greatly inhibited by inadequate light, water, or soil nutrients.

Marihuana is produced by cutting the stem beneath the lowest branches, air drying, and then stripping away the seeds, bracts, flowers, leaves, and small stems. When stems and seeds are variably removed using a mesh screen, manicured marihuana results. Hashish is produced by scraping the thick resinous material secreted by the flowers.[57]

Many morphologic variations in branching and leaf structure are observed among plants produced by different seed types. The characteristic leaf is palmately compound and contains an odd number of coarsely serrated leaflets. Plants of a given seed type generally grow at similar rates and resemble each other. Thus, botanists believe, *C. sativa* represents a single species that has not stabilized and has many variations.[57]

*Cannabis sativa* is a dioecious species with separate male and female plants, both producing flowers. Some monoecious variants are reported. Pollination appears to be accomplished by air currents. Bees are attracted by male flowers but not by female flowers. Sex cannot be established until flowering begins and the structures of the male and female flowers are distinct. Male plants begin shedding leaves shortly after flowering, then shed their pollen and die. Female plants lose their older leaves as the seed matures. After shedding their seed, they die. Contrary to popular belief, there is no significant difference in drug content between male and female plants at equivalent states of maturity.[58, 59]

The drug content of the plant parts is variable. Generally it decreases in the following order: bracts, flowers, leaves. Practically no cannabinoids are found in the stems, roots, or seeds. Fluctuations in pharmacologic activity of a sample of marihuana depend on the mixture of these plant parts, which is determined by the manicuring process.[58]

Different variants of the plant contain different amounts of psychoactive drug. Variants of *C. sativa* cover a spectrum of drug contents. Generally they can be classified as either drug or fiber genotype. The drug type is high in THC and low in cannabidiol and the fiber type is the converse. The type is determined genetically and transmitted by the seed. Thus seeds from different geographic areas produce plants with a wide range of drug content. For example, under similar conditions, plants grown from seeds from Mexico may contain 15 times more psy-

**Figure 17-1. Natural cannabinoids**

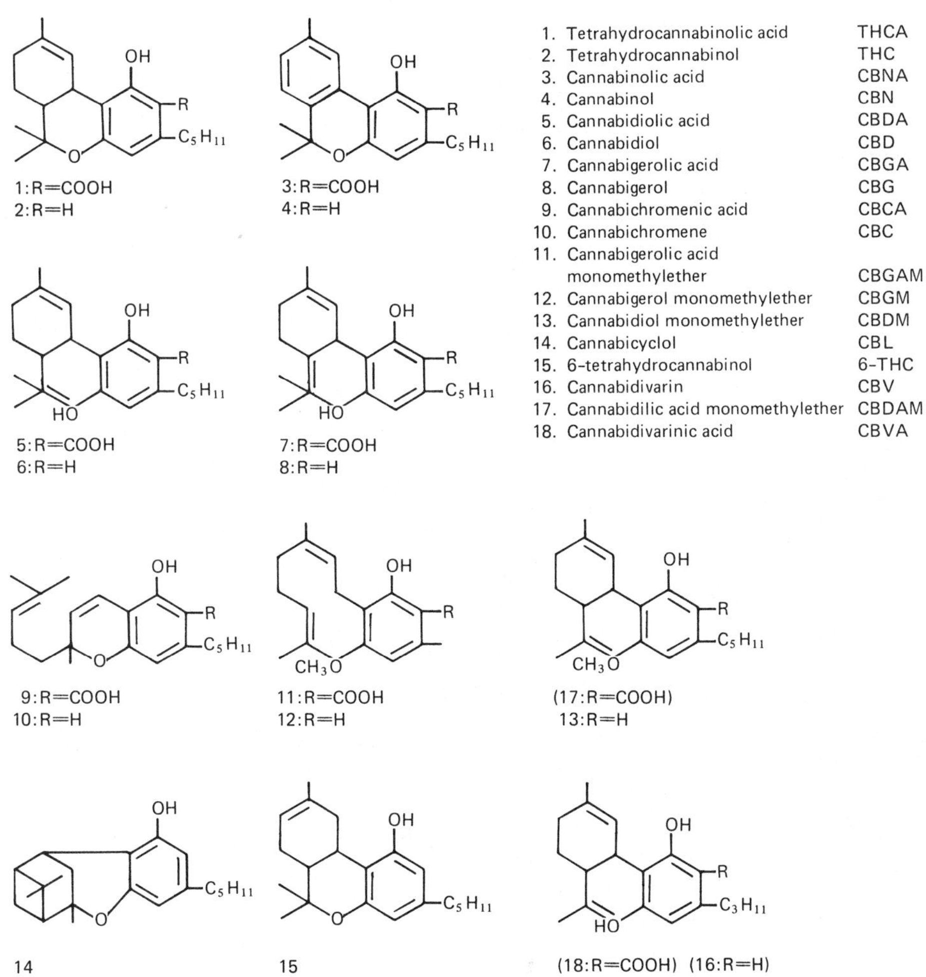

choactive drug than those grown from seeds from Iowa. Of course, individual plants of the same variant also often contain greatly different drug content.[58]

Environmental factors are not as important as heredity in determining type, but they do influence the drug content to some degree. And these factors, including type of soil, water, growing space, temperature, and light, play an important role in determining the size and vitality of the plants.[57,59,60]

This notorious variability of cannabis preparations has hindered detailed and reproducible biologic work. Consequently much effort has been expended to provide a firm chemical basis for furnishing pure and well-defined substances for research.

The major naturally occurring active component of cannabis, 1-$\Delta^9$-trans tetrahydrocannabinol, was not isolated in a pure form or its structure elucidated until 1964.[61-63] In addition, the $\Delta^8$-isomer, which is usually present in small quantities in the natural product, representing less than 10 percent of the combined THC content, has a similar spectrum of activity.[64] These two chemicals, available by industrial synthesis[65,66] or by extraction from the natural plant, apparently can fully reproduce the effects of the crude drug in animals and humans. More than 20 natural cannabinoids have been identified in the plant (Figure 1).[57,67,68]

All but $\Delta^8$- and $\Delta^9$-THC are inactive psychopharmacologically and do not seem to exert potentiating or other effects. However new compounds, cannabinoids and noncannabinoids, are being isolated from the plant and require further investigation. Several studies seem to indicate that some material present in natural marihuana may act synergistically with THC and potentiate its psychologic effect.[69] Paton and Pertwee[70] suggest that cannabidiol may play this role.

The chemical nomenclature of tetrahydrocannabinols is in a state of confusion due to the existence of two numbering systems. The dibenzopyran, or formal, system treats the compound as substituted dibenzopyrans ($\Delta^9$-THC) while the monoterpenoid system considers them as substituted terpenes ($\Delta^1$-THC). The formal system will be used hereafter (Figure 2).

Many of the natural cannabinoids are present in the plant as acids. These acids are believed to be psychopharmacologically inactive. However, they are converted rapidly when heated, and slowly when stored into their respective active neutral components (Figure 3).[71] This conversion (decarboxylation) apparently does not occur when the acids are absorbed after oral consumption.[67]

The proposed biogenesis (Figure 4) of $\Delta^9$-THC appears to proceed through cannabidiol (CBD). Cannabis variates of the fiber type apparently do not perform this conversion. Thus, cannabidiol is the cannabinoid present in the largest percentage on the nondrug variety.[60] Marihuana seems to lose its potency over time because of the conversion of THC to cannabinol (CBN)[67]; this also apparently occurs more

**Figure 17-2. Chemical nomenclature.**

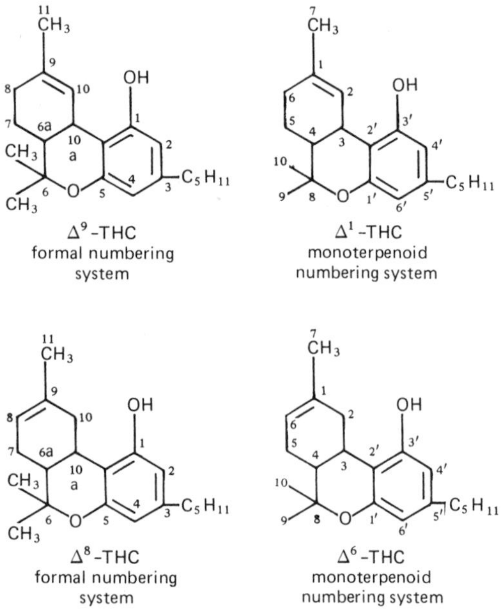

**Figure 17-3. Decarboxylation of THC acid.**

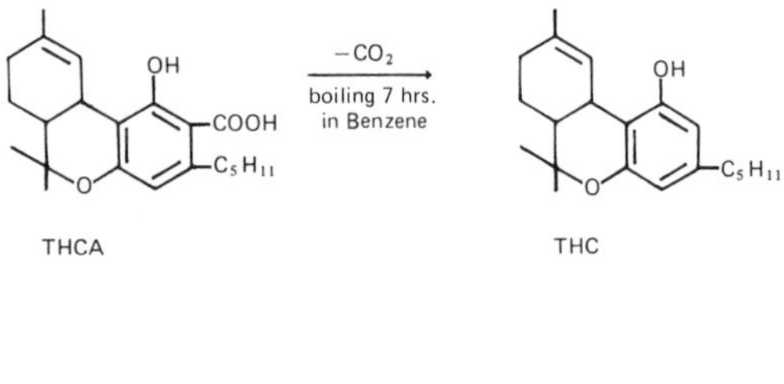

**Figure 17-4. Biogenesis of marihuana components.**

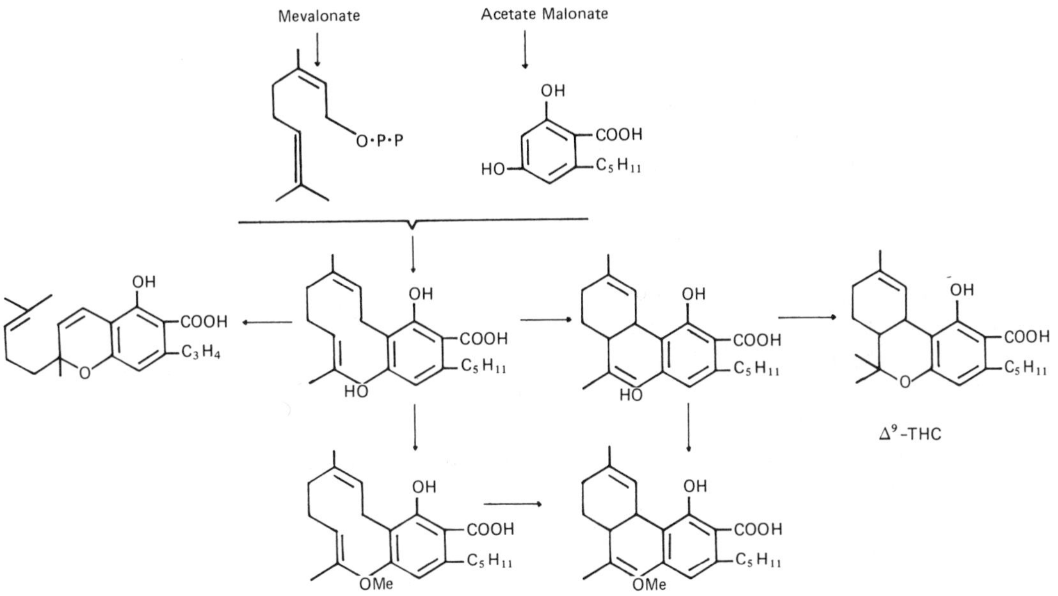

quickly for hashish, implying the presence of a stabilizing substance in the whole plant (Figure 5).

Recently the n-propyl homolog of $\Delta^9$-THC was isolated from crude marihuana. It has about 20 percent of the activity of $\Delta^9$-THC in mice and probably makes only a small contribution to the total marihuana effect.[72] Merkus[73] and Vree[74] recently identified propyl and methyl cannabinol homologs in hashish in extremely small quantities.

In addition, numerous other noncannabinoids have been identified in the natural material. Most of these have little or no psychoactivity.[75,76] Waxes, starches, oils, terpenes, and simple nitrogenous compounds, including muscarine, choline, and trigonelline, as well as volatile low-molecular-weight piperdines, also have been isolated.

**Figure 17-5. Decomposition of THC.**

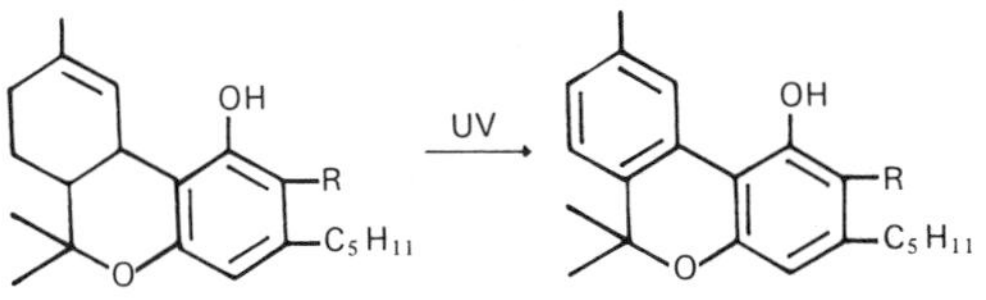

Four more complex nitrogen-containing compounds of the generally accepted alkaloid type have been reported in marihuana leaves in minute concentrations (average 0.002 percent). These produced decreased activity but no acute toxicity in mice.[77] Another laboratory has isolated two steroids and triterpenes from marihuana as well as tyramine amide derivatives from the roots.[57]

Analysis of the smoke obtained from marihuana has been investigated. As in the case of any combustible plant, a gas and a particulate phase are produced. Both phases are delivered to the lung. The gas as well as the particulate phase consist of compounds present in approximately the same percentages as in other burned cellulose-containing materials, except for the cannabinoid fraction. This includes carbon dioxide, carbon monoxide, and hydrogen cyanide gases.[78]

The remaining smoke condensate consists of a complex mixture of relatively nonvolatile compounds. Included in this mixture are the cannabinoids (16 percent), carbohydrates and alcohols (8 percent), fatty and aromatic acids (11 percent), polybasic acids (7 percent), aliphatic amines (1 percent), aromatic phenols (27 percent), aliphatic phenols (6 percent), tannin (6 percent), and unidentified compounds (18 percent).[78]

One group of investigators[79] compared the tar collected from combustion of marihuana cigarettes with the tar from tobacco cigarettes. They reported that the total tar yield from marihuana was slightly less than half that produced by an equal weight of tobacco. The tars contain similar constituents, judging by typical changes produced on the skin of mice.

In addition, there are a multitude of synthetic compounds that are related to the naturally occurring $\Delta^9$-THC derivatives and are much more potent (Figure 6). A large number of homologs have been prepared, all with similar activity, but varying widely in their potency.

In general, the activity of these compounds increases dramatically over that of $\Delta^9$-THC by lengthening the 3 alkyl side chain to 6 and 7 carbons, with additional branching in the alpha and beta positions. The dimethylheptyl analog (EA1476 or DMHP) is the most active, having 50 times the activity of $\Delta^9$-THC. The 1-methyloctyl substitution (MOP, EA1465) is the next most potent compound. The 1,2-dimethylortyl substitution resulted in a 25-fold decreased activity from DMHP.[80,81]

Numerous variations of the basic structures in the cyclohexene moiety of the molecule, as well as the replacement of both methyl groups by hydrogen, resulted in partial, and even complete, loss of activity.[80,81]

Mechoulam[82] has summarized the investigations related to the structure activity relationships of the cannabinoids as follows:

(1) The pyran ring with a hydroxyl group at 1 position and an alkyl group at the 3 position is an essential requirement for psychotomimetic activity, e.g., cannabidiol is inactive.

(2) The aromatic hydroxyl group has to be free or esterified for activity.

(3) The presence of a carboxyl, acetyl or carbomethyoxyl group in position 2 or 4 renders the compound inactive. Substitution with an alkyl group at position 2 retains activity.

(4) Dextrorotary (+) delta-9-THC is inactive whereas its optical isomer levoratary (−) delta-9-THC is active.

(5) Maximal activity is seen if the double bond is in the delta-9 or delta-8 position. The delta-6a, 10a-THC is relatively inactive.

(6) The activity of the delta-6a, 10a-THC can be increased by replacement of the pentyl side chain with a hexyl side chain to form synhexyl which is an active compound. Branching of the side chain may lead to considerable increase in potency. The substitution of a dimethylheptyl side chain for the pentyl side chain in the delta-6a, 10a, analogue of THC to form DMHP or EA1476 results in a marked increase in pharmacologic activity.

(7) Substituents at the 9 and 10 position have to be in the plane of the ring (that is, equatorial) in order that high activity be retained.

**Figure 17-6. Several synthetic cannabinoids.**

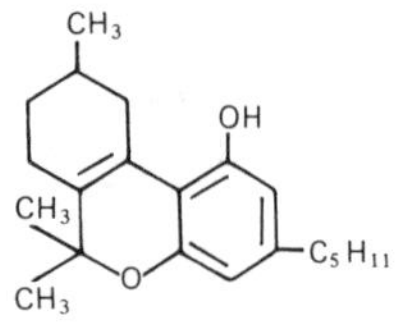

$\Delta^{6a,10a}$–THC or $\Delta^3$–THC

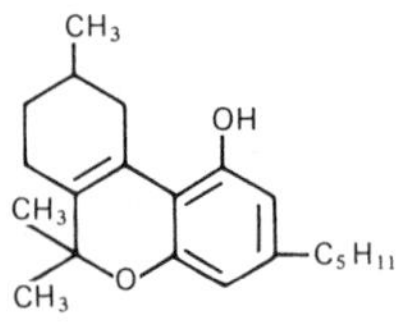

Synhexyl

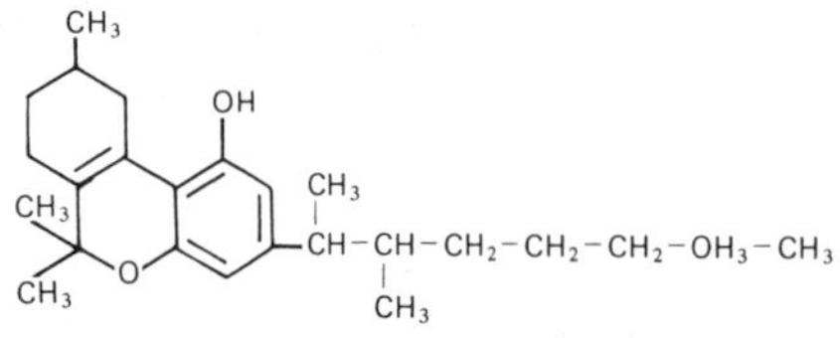

DMHP

## D. CHEMISTRY

### 1. Overview

Although the chemistry and metabolism of marihuana (i.e., the ways in which the drug is broken down and chemically transformed in the body) are technical topics not easily translated into everyday language, they are important. For example, contrary to popular belief, the plant material is quite complex, containing at least 421 individual compounds. Sixty-one of the chemicals that have been identified in the plant—the cannabinoids—are specific to cannabis. Ten are now routinely quantified in identifying cannabis samples. When smoked, some of the chemicals contained are further transformed by burning (pyrolysis) into still other compounds.

Plant material differs widely in the amount of the principal psychoactive ingredient—delta-9-tetrahydrocannabinol (THC, for short)—contained, as well as in the proportions of other chemicals. Although the effects of cannabinoids other than $\Delta^9$-THC have been studied, much remains to be learned about their effects, both alone and in interaction with one another. While for many practical purposes the percentage of $\Delta^9$-THC is a useful guide to the psychoactivity of a drug sample, other chemical ingredients ultimately may prove to be important in modifying THC's effects because of their own impact on the body. A good deal of valuable basic research has been done on THC, but it should be emphasized that it is only one ingredient in the natural material. Thus some of the research on THC may be partially relevant only to the effects of the plant material itself. In addition, the ratios of the different cannabinoids found in cannabis change in response to the passage of time and storage conditions. Plants that have been specifically cultivated for their psychoactivity contain much more $\Delta^9$-THC than do those grown for fiber. Most of the cannabis growing wild in the United States derives from plants that originally were cultivated for their fiber rather than their drug content, so that they could be used in making rope and other nondrug products. Thus the THC content of this cannabis rarely exceeds 1 percent THC.

Although there has been no representative random sampling of illicit marihuana that can provide an accurate indication of changes over time, there is evidence that material now sold is significantly higher in THC content than a few years ago. Chemists at the University of Mississippi who have been analyzing confiscated samples of cannabis for several years have found increases of the order of ten times in potency since 1974. Mexican "brick" (i.e., compressed kilogram quantities of marihuana) samples studied in 1974 averaged about a fifth of 1 percent $\Delta^9$-THC. Mexican samples analyzed in 1979 averaged nearly 2 percent. Other cannabis samples, probably of Colombian origin, that were analyzed in 1979 averaged over 4 percent THC content. Hash oil, a concentrated liquid marihuana extract not available on the street until a few years ago, has been found to have THC levels ranging from nearly 11 percent to 28 percent. Such stronger materials are more likely to lead to higher levels of intoxication and possibly to adverse consequences.

As knowledge of cannabis chemistry and metabolism has increased and the role of various metabolites becomes more important, there has been a corresponding need to synthesize supplies of these substances. Research availability of these materials enables us to tease out their effects from those of other constituents. Several improved methods for synthesizing metabolites have been developed, and these have accelerated work on the detection of marihuana in body fluids, and have enabled the study of the drug's metabolism. By radioactively labeling the substances involved, it is possible to trace their passage through the body.

The chemistry of marihuana smoke has commanded considerable attention in recent years. Some 150 compounds have been identified in the smoke itself. One of them, benzopyrene, known to be carcinogenic, is 70 percent more abundant in marihuana smoke than in tobacco smoke. There is also evidence that more "tar" is found in marihuana cigarettes than in high-tar tobacco cigarettes.

The metabolism of marihuana is only partially understood. Over 35 metabolites of $\Delta^9$-THC have been identified thus far, along with several dozen metabolites of other marihuana constituents. The ability to identify and trace the pathways of these chemicals in the body provides vital information concerning how they are stored and eventually eliminated. Such information is useful in helping determine the possible sites of action for long-term effects of marihuana.

Detection and quantification of cannabinoids and their metabolites in body fluids continue to be important problems. Sophisticated laboratory techniques are available for the precise measurement of cannabinoid levels in blood and other biologic samples. More routine and simpler techniques have also been developed, and are undergoing field testing. When this is completed and the techniques become generally available, they will be useful for such purposes as the routine laboratory detection of marihuana-intoxicated automobile drivers and the screening of individuals in treatment programs for current marihuana use. The earlier, more elaborate, techniques have been important in research as well as in furnishing the necessary standards by which the results of more rapid and convenient techniques can be evaluated.

A good beginning has been made toward understanding marihuana chemistry and metabolism. Researchers have been able to demonstrate that marihuana constituents cross the placental barrier, and so can affect fetal development. The presence of cannabinoids in mother's milk raises the question of possible impact on the infant of the marihuana-using mother. Greater understanding of the chemistry of marihuana has also pointed up the possibility (compare "Therapeutic Aspects") that one or more of the synthesized components of cannabis in its original or chemically modified form may have therapeutic usefulness. Finally, our increased awareness of marihuana's chemical complexity and the ways in which components other than $\Delta^9$-THC modify the drug's effects may shed light on the common street belief that different types of marihuana have different effects not wholly related to their THC content.

## 2. Chemical Identification and Synthesis

### *a. Drug Sources*

The investigation of *C. sativa L.* continued to yield new components. For instance, the biogenic precursor of delta-9-tetrahydrocannabinol—the 2-tetrahydrocannabinolic acid (THCA)—has been isolated in quantity from Mexican cannabis,[83] as has the isomeric 4-acid from an Indian variant[84] and the propyl isomer—delta-9-tetrahydrocannabivarolic acid.[85] Some of the minor, lower molecular weight components of cannabis resin also have been separated and partially characterized by gas chromatography (GC) and mass spectroscopy (MS).[86]

The monomethyl ether of cannabidiol (CBD) has been isolated[87] and the presence of methyl ether of cannabinol (CBN) has been demonstrated.[88] The isolation of additional noncannabinoid components continues in an effort to further elucidate their role in the biologic effects of cannabis. In addition to some phytosterols,[89] several of the high molecular weight hydrocarbons have been isolated.[84]

According to both technical and popular (counterculture) sources, a form of liquid hashish has appeared on the drug market. Sources indicate that it may vary in potency from 22 to 70 percent THC.[90–92] Little investigation of this new material has been done as yet.

Quantities of cannabinoids have been made available to investigators by the National Institute on Drug Abuse. Without this service, most preclinical and human research on the effects of marihuana could not be undertaken. New syntheses of $\Delta^9$-THC have appeared[93] and, perhaps more important, syntheses of the principal hydroxylated metabolites have been achieved.[93–97] The major metabolite present in humans and animals, 11-delta-9-tetrahydrocannabinol-9-carboxylic acid, and the corresponding $\Delta^8$-acid have been synthesized.[98,99]

New radiolabeled cannabinoids have been prepared for essential distribution and metabolism studies. Labeled $\Delta^8$- and $\Delta^9$-THCs, with very high specific activity, were prepared by the incorporation of tritium into the pentyl side chain.[99,100] A new carbon-14 labeled $\Delta^9$-THC was synthesized by a more convenient route than used previously.[99] To make other derivatives available, efforts continue in chemical research.

The chemistry of marihuana can best be understood by breaking all known constituents of the cannabis plant down into classes of chemicals. There are 421 known constituents of cannabis. (Table 17-1).

Not only is the chemistry of marihuana complex because of the large number of chemical constituents, but it is compounded by three distinctly different cannabis chemovariants; each produces a distinctly different marihuana. The three types are fiber, intermediate, and drug. Cannabidiol is the major cannabinoid found in fiber type; the percent by dry weight of cannabidiol is equal to or greater than $\Delta^9$-THC in intermediate cannabis; and $\Delta^9$-THC is the major cannabinoid in the drug type with CBD being absent or present in trace amounts. Cannabichromene is always present in drug types. Ratios of cannabinoids vary hourly, daily, and so on, and thus there are dynamic changes over time.[101]

To understand cannabis chemistry, it is best to look at analyses of several samples of crude drugs from cannabis available on the street, from NIDA and from the United Nations (Table 17-2).

The preparations listed in Table 17-2, with the exception of hashish, are dry forms of cannabis commonly called marihuana and illustrate

## TABLE 17-1

## Chemical Constituents of *Cannabis* Preparations

1. Cannabinoids: *61 known*
   a. Cannabigerol (CBG) type: 6 known
   b. Cannabichromene (CVC) type: 4 known
   c. Cannabidiol (CBD) type: 7 known
   d. Δ⁹-Tetrahydrocannabinol (Δ⁹-THC) type: 9 known
   e. Δ⁸-Tetrahydrocannabinol (Δ⁸-THC) type: 2 known
   f. Cannabicyclol (CBL) type: 3 known
   g. Cannabielsoin (CBE) type: 3 known
   h. Cannabinol (CBN) type: 6 known
   i. Cannabinodiol (CBND) type: 2 known
   j. Cannabitriol (CBT) type: 6 known
   k. Miscellaneous types: 9 knwon
   l. Other cannabinoids: 4 known
2. Nitrogenous compounds: 20 known
   a. Quaternary bases: 5 known
   b. Amides: 1 known
   c. Amines: 12 known
   d. Spermidine alkaloids: 2 known
3. Amino acids: 18 known
4. Proteins, glycoproteins, and enzymes: *9 known*
5. Sugars and related compounds: *34 known*
   a. Monosaccharides: 13 knwon
   b. Disaccharides: 2 known
   c. Polysaccharides: 5 known
   d. Cyclitols: 12 known
   e. Amino sugars: 2 known
6. Hydrocarbons: *50 knwon*
7. Simple alcohols: *7 known*
8. Simple aldehydes: *12 known*
9. Simple ketones: *13 known*
10. Simple acids: *20 known*
11. Fatty acids: *12 known*
12. Simple esters and lactones: *13 known*
13. Steroids: *11 known*
14. Terpenes: *103 known*
    a. Monoterpenes: 58 known
    b. Sesquiterpenes: 38 known
    c. Diterpenes: 1 known
    d. Triterpenes: 2 known
    e. Miscellaneous compounds of terpenoid origin: 4 known
15. Noncannabinoid phenols: *16 known*
16. Flavanoid glycosides: *19 known*
17. Vitamins: *1 known*
18. Pigments: *2 known*

(From Turner, C. E., Elschly, M. A. and Boeren, E. G. A review of the chemical constituents of *Cannabis sativa L. Lloydia* 43(2), 1980.)

## TABLE 17-2

## Cannabinoid Analyses

| *Cannabis* Prep | CBDV[1] | Δ⁹-THCV | CBL | CBD | CBC | Δ⁸-THC | Δ⁹-THC | CBN |
|---|---|---|---|---|---|---|---|---|
| Sinsemilla[2] (fiber) | 0.07 | 0.02 | 0.03 | 4.68 | 0.47 | 0.09 | 0.21 | 0.06 |
| Sinsemilla (inter.) | t[3] | 0.08 | 0.01 | 3.69 | 0.61 | 0.07 | 3.58 | 0.21 |
| Sinsemilla (drug) | — | 0.15 | 0.02 | 0.02 | 0.20 | — | 6.28 | 0.22 |
| Hashish (UN stand.) | 0.03 | 0.03 | 0.03 | 2.89 | 0.38 | 0.22 | 2.22 | 2.50 |
| NIDA[5] (Cig 1) | 0.01 | t | t | t | 0.12 | 0.09 | 0.84 | 0.30 |
| (Cig 2) | — | 0.02 | 0.02 | 0.02 | 0.18 | 0.15 | 1.86 | 0.13 |

[1]CBDV = cannabidivarin: Δ⁹-THCV = (—)-Δ⁹-*trans*-tetrahydrocannabivarin; CBL = cannabicyclol; CBD = cannabidiol; CBC = cannabichromene; Δ⁸-THC = (—)-Δ⁸-*trans*-tetrahydrocannabinol; Δ⁹-THC = (—)-Δ⁹-*trans*-tetrahydrocannabinol and CBN = cannabinol. Cannabigerol (CBG) and cannabigerol monomethylether (CBGM) were excluded but are routinely included in all analyses.

[2]Sinsemilla—a crude drug from the flowering tops of female cannabis plants that have not been pollinated: "Seedless marijuana." Same as *dagga* from the Republic of South Africa. These samples were grown in California.

[3]*t* = trace (less than 0.009%).

[4]Absent.

[5]Standard NIDA Mexican marijhuana cigarette from cannabis grown in Mississippi.

(From Turner, E. L. Chemistry and metabolism. In R. C. Peterson (ed.), *Marihuana: Research Findings: 1980.* (Research Monograph No. 31, NIDA,) Washington, D.C.: U.S. Government Printing Office p. 85.)

the fact that the chemistry of marihuana is not just the chemistry of $\Delta^9$-THC, but at a minimum a combination of cannabinoids. For example, observe the cannabinoid ratios in the three types of *Sinsemilla* listed. Moreover, $\Delta^9$-THC is not the only psychomimetically active compound: $\Delta^8$-THC, $\Delta^9$-THCV, and CBN are active.[102,103] Since the early 1970s, kinetic interactions have been reported to occur among cannabinoids.[104–106] Therefore, the role of other cannabinoids in the pharmacology of marihuana is yet to be determined.

A new subclass of cannabinoids called cannabitriols was discovered, and Chan, Magnus, and Watson[107] provided the first of these compounds: (−)-cannabitriol. Elsholy, El-Feraly, and Turner[108]; Elsohly et al.[109]; and Boeren, Elsohly, and Turner[110] quickly confirmed this work and found four additional cannabitriols. Boeren and colleagues[110] determined the stereochemistry of one compound, cannabiripsol, as well as the presence of other "cannabitriols." These compounds may be of pharmacologic significance because they decompose to CBN and are produced when $\Delta^9$-THC decomposes to CBN.[111,112]

For many years it was believed that alkaloids were responsible for the biologic activity in cannabis preparations.[113,114] Until recently no alkaloids of significance were found in marihuana. Turner and colleagues[112] reported the structure of hordenine and Lotter et al. reported the finding of a spermidine class alkaloid, cannabisativine. In 1978 Elsohly et al.[109] found anhydrocannabisativine. These three alkaloids are present in marihuana produced from many variants of cannabis.[115] Pharmacologic studies on cannabisativine and anhydrocannabisativine have not been carried out. These compounds are unique and believed to be indigenous to cannabis.

Discovery of a new class of spiro-compounds in marihuana[116–121] may solve some of the inconsistencies reported in hormonal research with marihuana as compounds of the spiro type have exhibited estrogenic properties.[122] Moreover, these compounds may be more abundant in marihuana than previously thought.[123]

Burstein et al.[124] reported that eugenol and p-vinylphenol may contribute to the overall activity of marihuana. Both of these compounds are noncannabinoid phenols, as are the spiro-compounds. These compounds are excluded from research programs using only synthetic cannabinoids.

The contribution of X-ray crystallography to research in the field of marihuana chemistry has been demonstrated by Ottersen et al.,[125] Jones et al.,[126] and El-Feraly et al.[123] Structural data obtained by X-ray methods will allow more thorough studies of the possible structural correlations with other classes of drugs. These correlations are presently being investigated with anticonvulsant drugs.[126]

### *b. Progress on Synthetics*

Synthetic production of new analogs of naturally occurring cannabinoids continues at a rapid pace. Handrick et al.[127] synthesized the *cis* isomers of cannabidiols and Uliss et al.[128] reported a procedure to convert *cis* cannabinoid isomers to *trans*. The synthesis of novel cannabinoids,[129] along with other synthetic procedures reported,[130] provides new approaches to the synthesis of metabolites and some elusive cannabinoids.[111]

Microbiologic oxidation of the pentyl side chain to provide a series of metabolites was a significant accomplishment. Refinements of this method,[131] combined with synthetic programs, as described by Pitt et al.[132] and Ohlsson et al.,[133] afford a route to side-chain metabolites.

Another significant development was the synthesis of a C-glucuronide of $\Delta^8$-THC. C-glucuronides may be very significant in determining the nature of water-soluble conjugates.[134] These conjugates have been of particular interest since Harvey, Martin, and Paton[135] reported the identification of 0-glucuronides of seven cannabinoids.

With the synthesis of CBC by Elsohly, Boeren, and Turner,[136] it is now possible to study CBC and its influence on the pharmacology of other cannabinoids. Cannabichromene is one of the four major naturally occurring cannabinoids. Pharmacologic studies were previously restricted because of an insufficient supply. Further work on the separation and quantification of CBC and CBD[137] was carried out and again confirmed that CBC is a major cannabinoid.[111] The report by Coutts and Jones[111] also has important forensic significance because all extracts of suspected cannabis preparations found to be positive using (1) microscopic examination of the material, (2) modified Duquenois-Levine color reaction, and (3) a thin-layer chromatographic examination of the extracts were confirmed in blind experiments using GC-mass spectral data.[138]

### c. *Chemistry of Marihuana Smoke*

Marihuana chemistry is the chemistry of smoke from natural marihuana or special products prepared by coating placebo marihuana with individual synthetic cannabinoids. Research programs may use both products whereas users consume the natural material. In this connection, Mikes and Waser[139] suggested that the cannabinoid composition of marihuana smoke may differ from the leaf analysis. Reports on the amount of $\Delta^9$-THC available in marihuana smoke have been inconsistent[140,141]; however, smoking conditions normally employed by the marihuana user may provide up to 62 percent of the original $\Delta^9$-THC in the smoke.[142] Also, more tar will be produced from a marihuana cigarette than from a tobacco cigarette deliberately chosen to produce high tar levels. Many variables affect the amount of drug (cannabinoids) available to the user via smoking.[142] Lee, Novotny, and Bartle[143] identified 150 compounds in marihuana smoke by using a capillary GC column. Further work on the acidic fraction of marihuana smoke was done by Maskarinec, Alexander, and Novotny.[144] Novotny and coworkers[145] concluded that benzopyrene, a known carcinogen found in tobacco smoke, was 70 percent more abundant in marihuana smoke. Pyrolysis of cannabinoids or nonpolar higher terpenes abundant in marihuana[101] was thought to be the source of the elevated amounts of polynuclear aromatic hydrocarbons found in marihuana smoke. Hofmann et al.[146] provided a detailed comparison between marihuana and tobacco smoke.

Some of the products formed in the pyrolysis of pure CBD have been isolated and characterized.[147–149] The pyrolysis of pure CBD produced many new cannabinoid-like compounds. Rosenkrantz and Hayden[150] found marked changes in animal testicular tissue during acute and subacute inhalation of Turkish marihuana, CBC, and CBD. These findings are indicative of variations in smoke content. Moreover, in a one-year study Fleishman, Baker, and Rosenkrantz[151] found focal granulomatous inflammation and cholesterol-like clefs in rats exposed to marihuana smoke. These two studies illustrate the variable results obtained when smoke from different types of marihuana and synthetic cannabinoids is delivered to research subjects. A striking finding by Rosenkrants and Hayden[150] was that Turkish marihuana smoke was more lethal than placebo impregnated with 10 percent CBC or CBD, which was more lethal than 9 percent $\Delta^9$-THC or placebo. Using standard Mexican marihuana, Zwillich et al.[152] found that marihuana had stimulatory effects on metabolic rate, ventilation, and the ventilatory response to $CO_2$.

The composition of cannabinoids in the marihuana are known but we do not have as yet an adequate understanding of the chemical composition of marihuana smoke and interactions of the cannabinoids within smoke.

## 3. Analytical Techniques: Detection

The development of improved methods for the detection and estimation of cannabinoids, particularly in body tissues and fluids, remains a fundamental goal for all types of marihuana research.

Gas chromatography (GC) continues to be the most often employed technique for identifying and analyzing cannabis constituents, as the large number of studies employing this analytical method demonstrate.[153–160] Using accepted chromatographic conditions it has been shown that the peak representing CBD also contains cannabichromene (CBC). In other experiments using Mexican cannabis, as much as 90 percent of what had been labeled as CBD in the past was found to be CBC. The presence of CBC will require a reevaluation of the current use of

THC and CBD ratios to classify different varieties of cannabis. Additionally, studies indicate that the GC peak corresponding to $\Delta^9$-THC is often contaminated with cannabielsoin, the decarboxylation product of cannabielsoic acid, which is a cyclization product of cannabidiolic acid.[161,162] Identification techniques permit proper research on cannabis alone and in combination with other drugs.[163–172]

Thin-layer chromatography (TLC) studies have appeared.[173–178] Among these, the most significant have used dansylate derivatives to determine THC up to 14 hours after marihuana or hashish has been smoked.[175,176]

A radioimmunoassay that may be applied directly to urine has been developed for $\Delta^9$-THC and its 11-hydroxy metabolite.[179] Unfortunately, for this technique to be used with plasma, an extraction step is required because of the extensive protein binding of the labeled THC. The first reported estimation of THC in human blood levels with a time lapse after smoking marihuana was based on the use of radiolabeled $\Delta^9$-THC.[180] Peak plasma levels of 25–50 ng/ml were indicated. A more definitive study using a gas chromatography/mass fragmentography method was reported.[100] Extracts of plasma required prior purification by Sephadex chromatography. With this procedure as little as 1 ng/ml of THC in blood can be accurately determined. It was found that a peak of 19–26 ng/ml was reached ten minutes after smoking a cigarette containing 10 mg of $\Delta^9$-THC. This level rapidly fell to 5 ng/ml within two hours.

The TLC method has the disadvantage that it requires a specially designed mass spectrometer. Reports of work using a simpler method based on derivatization and electron-capture detection following gas chromatography have appeared.[155,181] With this method as little as 10 ng/ml can be measured.[181] A clean-up procedure utilizing high-pressure liquid chromatography has also been developed. A preliminary pharmacokinetic study of the disposition of a 0.1-mg/kg (intravenous) dose of $\Delta^9$-THC in dogs indicated that there is an initial rapid distribution and metabolism phase (half-life, 7.5 minutes) followed by a slow loss from the blood (apparent half-life, eight hours). This agrees with reported earlier tracer studies in humans.[86]

Further improvements in the area of detection methods would allow for a more detailed understanding of the correlation among the routes of administration, metabolism, and behavioral effects and the serious reader should refer to recent reviews.[182–184]

In summary, determination of cannabinoids and metabolites in biologic fluid can be accomplished by the following principal methods: (1) gas chromatography/mass spectrometry; (2) thin-layer chromatography; (3) high-pressure liquid chromatography; (4) radioimmunoassay (RIA); and (5) gas chromatography. However, the first method, gas chromatography/mass spectrometry, provides the most specific and sensitive assays for cannabinoids in biologic fluids.[185] Both chemical and electron-impact ionization methods are used. Fentiman, Foltz, and Foltz[186] have provided a manual and Rosenthal et al.[187] have compared the methods for quantitating $\Delta^9$-THC in biologic media. Foltz[188] also discusses the use of gas-chromatography chemical ionization in the quantitative analysis of $\Delta^9$-THC. Pirl, Papa, and Spikes[189] have used this method to detect $\Delta^9$-THC in postmorten blood samples.

Both thin-layer and high-pressure liquid chromatography have been used to detect and separate cannabinoids and metabolites, and Kanter, Hollister, and Loeffler[190] have developed a way to quantitate $\Delta^9$-THC by combining these techniques.[191] Maximum sensitivity at 217 mm is about 30 times greater than at 280 mm.

Radioimmunoassay, in general, lacks the specificity and precision of other methods, but it does offer certain advantages as a result of cross-activity between $\Delta^9$-THC and its metabolites and other cannabinoids. A report by Gross and Soares[179] illustrated an RIA method for determining $\Delta^9$-THC in plasma that gave levels corresponding to intoxication. A homogeneous enzyme immunoassay (EMIT) for cannabinoids in urine has been used,[192] and may prove useful in rapid screening programs.

Progress has been slow in the quantitation of pure $\Delta^9$-THC and its metabolites in biologic systems. Moreover, no practical method has been developed as a forensic tool for determining levels of intoxication based on detectable cannabinoids and metabolites when marihuana is used.

## E. PHARMACOKINETICS AND METABOLISM[193-195]

### 1. Overview

Marihuana and hashish can be smoked and are well absorbed through the lungs. The effects are noticeable in one to five minutes, reach a peak within 30 to 60 minutes, and usually dissipate after three or four hours. Both marihuana and hashish can be cooked in foods, usually brownies or cookies, and ingested. In addition, a tealike preparation can be prepared by boiling the small leaves and stems. When marihuana preparations are taken orally, the effects are diminished, but prolonged. Their onset may occur 30–60 minutes after ingestion and last anywhere from five to eight hours or longer, depending on the dose. Rarely do the effects last longer than 12 to 14 hours. Because of the rapid onset of the effects of smoked marihuana, smokers are usually able to regulate dosages and stop when they have reached desired highs. Overdosage is more common after oral administration, when the onset of the effects is delayed.

The smoking of marihuana is an acquired art. The novice must learn the proper way to smoke and what to expect. One must inhale deeply, hold one's breath, and learn to distinguish the early signs of intoxication. First attempts are said to be seldom pleasing, and many people have to smoke numerous "weeds" before having a pleasurable experience. This obviously depends upon the setting and the potency of the product. Studies of the metabolism of the active ingredient $\Delta^9$-THC suggest that one or more metabolic products may also be active.[194,195] The amount of enzyme that produces this change could depend on, and be stimulated by, the presence of $\Delta^9$-THC. This could explain why several exposures are necessary before marked effects are seen. The effects may come on rather rapidly and may last for several hours. There is marked individual susceptibility and striking variations in effect. The solitary smoker usually becomes quieter, and occasionally depressed, whereas the participant in a group may become more outgoing, talkative, and contented. In a group the cigarette is usually passed around and smoked down to the last little scrap. Apparently little tolerance develops initially, and many smokers use less as they learn to obtain the desired results.

Although the effects of marihuana last only for several hours, it can be shown that the products in marihuana (THC and its metabolites), which are only soluble in fat, are stored in body tissues, including the brain, for weeks and months. It is also evident that these products are excreted in the urine for periods as long as two weeks.

### 2. Metabolism

#### *a. Historical Overview*

The development of $\Delta^8$- and $\Delta^9$-cannabinol, cannabidiol, and THC has led to a number of *in vivo* studies on these compounds in experimental animals. A comprehensive review of such research is beyond the scope of this book, and the interested reader is advised to look into several excellent reviews[69,196] for information on the absorption, disposition, excretion, and metabolism of the cannabis derivatives.

From animal and in vitro studies it appears that the liver rapidly changes $\Delta^9$- and $\Delta^8$-THC in a similar manner by hydroxylation to 11-OH THC. This compound appears to be pharmacologically as potent as, or possibly more potent than, the parent compound. The metabolite appears to be rapidly hydroxylated to 8-11 dihydroxy $\Delta^8$-THC (7-11 dihydroxy $\Delta^8$-THC), which is inactive. The 8-OH $\Delta^9$-THC appears to be a minor active metabolite.[197-203] These metabolites are excreted primarily into the bile and then into the feces. Some evidence exists for an enterohepatic circulation returning the drug to the blood.[204,205]

Another metabolic pathway appears to be present that results in a series of acidic metabolites excreted primarily in the urine.[206] Recently Burstein and Rosenfeld[207] isolated and identified a major rabbit urinary metabolite, 11-carboxy-2′-hydroxy-$\Delta^9$-THC. They postulate that other acidic metabolites might be esters or amides of this compound (Figure 17-7).

Nakazawa and Costa[208] demonstrated that Δ⁹-THC was metabolized by lung microsomes forming two unidentified products not found in liver homogenates. Lemberger[209] and Galanter[210] have performed metabolic studies in people using intravenous, oral, and smoked Δ⁹-THC. These studies indicate that the THC disappears from the plasma in two phases. The initial rapid phase has two components and represents metabolism by the liver and redistribution from the blood to the tissues. The slower, second phase represents tissue retention and slow release and subsequent metabolism.

The plasma half-life of THC has been seen to be significantly shorter in daily users than in nonusers at both the first component of phase one (10 minutes versus 13 minutes) and phase two (27 hours versus 56 hours). Tissue distri-

**Figure 17-7. Metabolism of THC.**

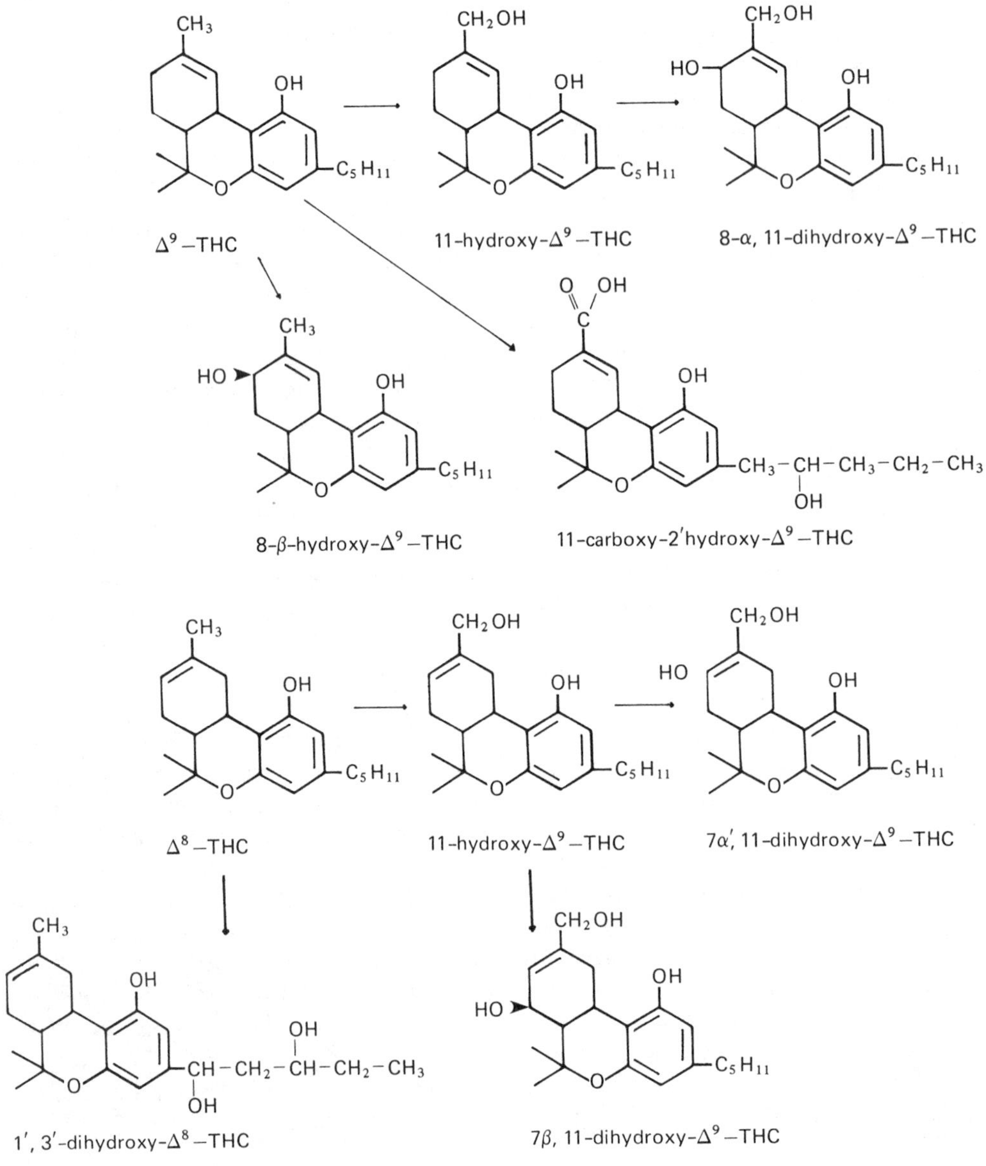

Δ⁹–THC

11-hydroxy-Δ⁹–THC

8-α, 11-dihydroxy-Δ⁹–THC

8-β-hydroxy-Δ⁹–THC

11-carboxy-2′hydroxy-Δ⁹–THC

Δ⁸–THC

11-hydroxy-Δ⁹–THC

7α′, 11-dihydroxy-Δ⁹–THC

1′, 3′-dihydroxy-Δ⁸–THC

7β, 11-dihydroxy-Δ⁹–THC

bution was similar in daily and nonusers (half-life, two hours). Therefore, immediate metabolism of THC and subsequent metabolism is more rapid for daily users than for nonusers, implying specific enzyme induction. THC persists in the plasma for a considerable period of time, at least three days, with a half-life of 57 hours for nonusers and 28 hours for daily users.

The presence of 11-hydroxy THC and more polar metabolites in the plasma of both users and nonusers within ten minutes indicates that the metabolite probably accounts for the pharmacologic activity of marihuana, not THC.

Further metabolism of the 11-hydroxy THC to more polar inactive 8-11 dihydroxy $\Delta^9$-THC metabolite occurs more rapidly in users than nonusers. During the first few hours after injection, unchanged THC, its polar metabolites and nonpolar metabolites in the plasma, decline rapidly, and then level off as they are distributed to the tissues. THC persists in the plasma for at least three days, and both users and nonusers excrete metabolites in the urine and feces for more than a week.

According to Lemberger and associates,[209] $\Delta^9$-THC is extensively metabolized to more polar compounds that are excreted in the urine and feces. Urinary excretion and biliary excretion (reflected a day later in the feces) was found to be greatest during the initial 24 hours, then gradually tapering off. All THC is metabolized since no unchanged THC was excreted in the feces or urine. No difference in total cumulative excretion was observed, but a significantly larger percentage of the metabolites was excreted in the urine of users than in nonusers. About 40–45 percent of the metabolites were collected in the feces in both groups in one week. Urinary excretion in this period accounted for 30 percent in daily users and 22 percent in nonusers.[209]

Perez-Reyes[211] found a similar pattern of excretion of metabolites after oral administration. Urine contained no $\Delta^9$-THC, only a small quantity (3 percent) of 11-hydroxy THC, and 90 percent more polar acidic compounds, as yet unidentified. Preliminary studies by Burstein and Rosenfeld[207] suggest that these human acidic urinary metabolites are identical to the 11-carboxy-2′ hydroxy THC found in rabbits.

In humans, Lemberger[212] found that 11-OH THC and 8-11-OH THC were primarily excreted in the feces. Twenty-two percent of the metabolites in the feces were unchanged 11-hydroxy THC, and slightly less were 8-11-dihydroxy THC. The remainder were unidentified more polar compounds, perhaps conjugates of these metabolites.

All user subjects,[209] but no nonusers, noted a high after intravenous injection of the 0.5-mg dose of $\Delta^9$-THC (5–7 μg/kg). Highs have been noted by Kiplinger[213] with smoking THC which delivers the user a dose of 6.25 μg/kg. The high for some lasted up to 90 minutes. Thus the plasma levels of $\Delta^9$-THC and its metabolites noted after intravenous injection suggest that psychopharmacologic effects are seen in the first component of the rapid phase and are terminated by redistribution and metabolism after the initial phase. The 11-hydroxy $\Delta^9$-THC would be present at this early phase and is probably responsible for the activity of $\Delta^9$-THC in marihuana.

Further evidence that the 11-OH $\Delta^9$-THC is responsible for marihuana's effect was seen in oral and inhalation studies. By the oral route, blood levels of unchanged THC were relatively low compared with the radioactivity levels of the metabolic products at the time of peak subjective effect. While the blood level of unchanged THC at the peak oral effect was identical to that after intravenous injection of the 0.5-mg dose, the psychologic effect was much more pronounced after oral administration of the larger, 20-mg dose of THC. Again after inhalation, the plasma levels of the metabolites correlate temporally with the subjective effects but the plasma levels of unchanged $\Delta^9$-THC do not.[209,210]

To elucidate further the metabolism of the cannabinoids,[214] a series of studies showed that very little of the 11-hydroxy metabolite of $\Delta^9$-THC is seen in the blood after its administration. Rather the principal blood metabolites are the oxidation product—the 9-carboxylic acid—and a variety of side-chain hydroxylated acids.[99,215] These are also the major metabolites found in urine. Several other preclinical studies of metabolism have involved the identification of metabolites and their distribution[214,215–222] after various routes of administration and the part of the enterohepatic system in their excretion.

Studies to ascertain the role played by the metabolites of $\Delta^9$-THC in contributing to its pharmacologic effects were carried out by measuring various animal brain levels.[223–225] Results obtained support the earlier belief that Δ9-THC and its hydroxylated metabolites are all active to varying degrees and collectively account for the observed effects. Study of the individual hydroxylated metabolites continues.

### b. Recent Metabolism Developments[117]

Progress has been made in understanding mechanisms for distribution, storage, and disposition of cannabinoids and their metabolites. This progress is the key to illuminating the short- and long-term effects of marihuana and individual cann binoids on the body.

Initial metabolism of cannabinoids in marihuana smoke takes place in the lungs, whereas initial cannabinoid metabolism of orally consumed marihu na takes place in the liver. Since different enzymes are involved, different initial metabolites are produced. Major lung metabolites are usually side-chain hydroxylated metabolites whereas major liver metabolites are usually hydroxylated derivatives of the cyclohexene ring system. There are over 35 known metabolites of Δ9-THC, 22 metabolites of CBD, and 22 metabolites of CBN. Considerable species variation exists.[226–228] These metabolites were formed by *in vivo* and *in vitro* metabolism and were found in feces, plasma, urine, and homogenized tissues and organs.

We now know several of the biotransformation pathways for Δ9-THC. These include allylic and aliphatic hydroxylations; oxidation of methyl groups to acids, aldehydes, and ketones; conjugations with fatty acids or 8-glucuronic acid; epoxidation of double bonds; and reduction of the terpene double bond.

Some of these metabolites are "psychoactive," but most are not. This does not mean that these "cannabinoids" are not active biologically. Findings on the nonspecific membrane-binding properties of Δ9-THC,[167] the interaction of cannabinoids with model membranes,[171] and the complex pharmacokinetics of distribution, storage, and disposition of cannabinoids and metabolites, strongly suggest biologic activity.

Data show that cannabinoids and their metabolites are distributed throughout the body. Recent experiments by Schou et al.[229] using radiolabeled Δ9-THC in rats have demonstrated that 11-hydroxy-Δ9-THC penetrates the blood–brain barrier more readily than Δ9-THC. Possibly the affinity of 11-hydroxy-Δ9-THC for plasma albumin accounts for this. Delta-9-THC is bound to lipoprotein.

Progress in finding and isolating new metabolites[226–228] has been significant. These advances provide much information on how metabolites are stored in and disposed of by the body. Synthesis of these individual metabolites and subsequent toxicologic testing can be of great help in accurately defining the long-term effects of marihuana.

Our knowledge of how pure Δ9-THC and its metabolites, as well as the crude drug marihuana, affect certain systems of the body is growing. It is clear that the cannabinoids affect brain amine levels,[230] platelet monoamine oxicase activity,[170] and ultrastructural changes in neurons.[231] The cannabinoids interact with ethanol,[163,168,169] cross the blood–brain barrier,[229] and are transferred from the milk of lactating animals to nursing pups.[164] These diverse examples illustrate the complex ways in which pure Δ9-THC and marihuana affect body chemistry and metabolism. Future chemical and metabolic research on marihuana will continue to focus on a "standard" supply of the crude drug marihuana and studies of synthetic metabolites.

The broad spectrum of biologic activity found in marihuana and its components may provide chemical leads for developing therapeutic drugs. However, the lack of current knowledge of the chemistry of marihuana precludes this use.

Other studies with regard to the chemistry and metabolism of cannabis provide more detailed information.[232–243]

## F. PHARMACOLOGY[1,6]

### 1. Classification

The precise pharmacologic classification of marihuana is difficult to determine. The most recent information suggests that many of its properties are similar to that of the sedative-hypnotic group of drugs.[225] In low doses its effects are similar to those of alcohol but Isbell's studies on the active ingredient Δ⁹-THC isolated from hashish suggest that the drug also is hallucinogenic in high doses.[244] The chemistry and pharmacology of marihuana are distinct from other drugs, such as the opiates, alcohol, barbiturates, amphetamines, and hallucinogens, and should be classified separately.

## 2. General Pharmacologic Aspects

Before we consider the specific pharmacologic actions of either natural marihuana or THC, we need to discuss other general pharmacologic aspects (i.e., dose–response relationships, dose–time relationships, route of administration, set and setting, etc.).

### *a. Dose–Response Relationship*

A major advance has been a quantification of dose for THC in relation to clinically observable phenomena. This has been extensively studied over a wide dosage range for marihuana[245–253] and Δ⁹-tetrahydrocannabinol.[254–257]

Investigations by Isbell,[258] Kiplinger,[213] and Renault[259] have clearly demonstrated that when reliable quantities of smoked marihuana or THC are delivered to the subject, a reproducible linear dose-dependent effect occurs on indexes of physiologic, psychomotor, and mental performance, as well as on mood and subjective experiences, over a dose range of 12.50–200 μg of Δ⁹-THC per kilogram of body weight.

For a 154-pound man this is comparable to consuming 0.88–17.5 mg of Δ⁹-THC or 88–1750 mg of marihuana containing 1 percent Δ⁹-THC. It is generally assumed that good-quality marihuana available in the United States contains 1 percent Δ⁹-THC and that an average marihuana cigarette consists of 500 mg of marihuana, and thus 5 mg of Δ⁹-THC.[260]

As with most drugs, the larger the dose taken, the greater is the psychopharmacologic effect. Isbell[258] noted that clinical syndromes vary from a mild euphoric feeling of relaxation at low doses (25 μg/kg) to an intensive hallucinogenic-like experience at high doses (250 μg/kg).

### *b. Dose–Time Relationship*

Similar time–action curves have been demonstrated for smoked Δ⁹-THC and equivalent quantities of smoked marihuana.[213,256,258,259] In these studies, symptoms began almost immediately after smoking (two to three minutes). At lower doses the peak effect is seen at 10 to 20 minutes and the duration of effect is 90 minutes to two hours. At higher doses symptoms persist for three to four hours.

The larger the dose taken, the longer is the action. The subjective symptoms experienced by the subject appear to parallel in time the subjective effects and some physiologic indexes such as pulse rate.[210,213,256–259] Others, such as reddening of the eyes, have a delayed peak response and longer duration.[213]

### *c. Route of Administration*

A second factor that influences the effect experienced by the user is the manner in which the substance is consumed. That is, whether it is smoked, swallowed, or injected.

Isbell[258] demonstrated that smoked material is 2½ to three times as effective as orally consumed marihuana in the form of a 95 percent ethanolic solution in producing equivalent physiologic and subjective effects. In addition, the oral time–action curve is extended, with the onset of symptoms being one-half to one hour after administration. A peak effect is reached in two to three hours and the effect persists for three to five hours at low doses and six to eight hours at larger doses.[211,256,258,259] In general, the effects produced by ingested THC or ingested marihuana extract are comparable to those produced by nearly one third the amount of smoked and inhaled THC or marihuana.[260]

Recent work has been reported that clarifies these findings. Utilizing radioactive labeled THC, Lemberger[257] studied absorption into the blood by three routes of administration: smoking, ingesting in 95 percent ethanolic solution in cherry syrup, and intravenous injection. The first appearance of the drug in the blood was immediate by intravenous administration, almost immediate by inhalation, and delayed for 15 to 30 minutes when ingested.

Perez-Reyes and Lipton,[211] using a labeled $\Delta^9$-THC, demonstrated that the rate of absorption by the gastrointestinal tract and the duration of action are greatly influenced by the vehicle used to ingest the drug. Speed and completeness of absorption varied when the THC was dissolved in 100 percent ethanol or sesame oil or emulsified with a bile salt (sodium glycocholate), and administered to a subject who had fasted 12 hours. With the bile-salt vehicle, the physiologic and subjective effects were noted between 15 to 30 minutes after ingestion and lasted two to three hours. In contrast, the effects with ethanol or sesame oil appeared after one hour and lasted four to six hours. Hollister and Gillespie[261] hypothesize that this delayed gastrointestinal absorption of THC might be accounted for by the nonpolar vehicle required to dissolve THC or marihuana.

Furthermore, Perez-Reyes and Lipton[211] found that the peak levels and duration of radioactivity in the plasma paralleled the physiologic and subjective effects, although the plasma levels remained high longer than the effect. Subjects receiving the drug emulsified in sodium glycocholate or dissolved in sesame oil had three times higher plasma levels of radioactivity, with much less excreted in the feces, than those receiving the drug dissolved in ethanol.

These results indicate that the THC is poorly absorbed from the gastrointestinal tract when given in an alcoholic solution. The sesame oil solution and the glycocholic acid preparation allow more complete absorption and the latter preparation is much faster. It is of interest that the degree of subjective high after ingestion of 37 mg of $\Delta^9$-THC also parallels the plasma radioactivity.

Thus the subjects reported their experience as intense and unpleasant with both the bile salt and the sesame oil, and as moderate and entirely pleasant with ethanol.[211] This correlates well with the earlier findings of Hollister.[256]

### *d. Quantification of Dose Delivered*

The problem in quantifying the THC dose delivered by different routes of administration has been clarified by several studies using radioactive compounds. However, until a method for determining the THC blood concentration is developed, only estimates of amount delivered are possible.

Radioautographic studies clearly demonstrate that intravenous injection gives the most complete and consistent delivery.[212,262–265] These investigators have demonstrated that THC is poorly absorbed from the injection site after intraperitoneal or subcutaneous injection.

As discussed earlier, the completeness of absorption after oral administration of THC appears to depend upon the vehicle. Judged by radioactivity levels, almost complete absorption of the THC occurs with an oil or bile-acid vehicle, but absorption is incomplete with an alcohol vehicle.[211]

Animal studies performed for NIMH indicated that the oral dose necessary to produce comparable gross behavioral changes in laboratory animals is about three times higher than the intravenous dose.[266] Ferraro[267] demonstrated the comparability of effective oral doses of THC in chimpanzees and humans. Furthermore, preliminary work performed in the laboratories of McIsaac,[262] Harris,[268] and Mechoulam[82] appear to indicate that the intravenously administered dose of $\Delta^9$-THC necessary to produce detectable behavioral changes in monkeys (20 to 50 μg/kg) on conditioned learning tasks is comparable to that in humans.[213,269]

When ingested orally, the dose of THC absorbed from natural marihuana extracts is uncertain. It is present as an acid in variable quantities in natural marihuana, but the acid has not been proved to be active. Claussen and Korte[270] reported that the THC carboxylic acid is converted to free THC during the smoking process. Whether these acids are active themselves, are absorbed from the gastrointestinal tract or converted there into THC, or are decarboxylated in the body is not known.

Because inhalation is the most widely used route of administration, several laboratories have investigated the effect of combustion and smoking on marihuana. Techniques and conditions varied between laboratories, however, and so precise quantification of the delivery to the smoker's lungs is uncertain.

It has been calculated that about 50 percent of the THC contained in a marihuana cigarette would be delivered to the smoker's lungs for absorption if the entire cigarette were smoked in ten minutes and each inhalation were retained for 30 seconds with no side-stream loss. Truitt[140] and others[271] found that 50 percent of THC was pyrolyzed and that 6 percent was lost in the side stream, while noting that almost 21 percent of the THC remained in the butt when three fourths of the cigarette was consumed.

In a study by Agurell and Leander[206] using actual smoking subjects, in which only the mainstream smoke was collected, it was found that 14–29 percent of the THC was transferred in the mainstream smoke for a cigarette and 45 percent for a pipe. They stated that these amounts would be comparable however, if no cigarette butt were left.

Agurell and Leander[206] also found that the amount transferred was not affected by depth of inhalation, but that smokers who inhaled deeply retained 80 percent of the transferred THC while those who used superficial inhalation tended to exhale more than 20 percent of the transferred THC. Mikes and Waser[139] found about 22 percent in the mainstream smoke.

### *e. Effect of Pyrolysis on the Cannabinoids*

Several investigators have studied the effect of pyrolysis on the cannabinoids. Most have concluded that only negligible changes occur in the original cannabinoid fractions of marihuana, except for decarboxylation of the acids to the cannabinoids. No evidence was found for isomerization of $\Delta^9$-THC or $\Delta^8$-THC, nor for the formation of any new pyrolysis products.[141,206,270-272] Mikes and Waser[139] suggested that a small percentage of cannabidiol was converted to $\Delta^9$-THC, but this observation was not confirmed by the other groups.

Miras and Coutselinis[204] noted that less THC was destroyed during smoking when $\Delta^9$-THC was the only cannabinoid present than with a resin or a mixture of cannabinoids. This was believed to be at least partially accounted for by the distribution of THC in the cigarette. More destruction occurred when the THC was evenly distributed in the cigarette than when it was in a well-defined lump.

### *f. Set and Setting*

A most important variable encountered when evaluating the effect of marihuana is the interaction of the drug with the nondrug factors, such as set and setting. Set refers to the drug taker's biologic make-up, including personality, past drug experiences, personal expectations of drug effect, and mood at the time of the drug experience. Setting refers to the external surroundings and social context in which the individual takes the drug. Set and setting exert their greatest effect with psychoactive drugs, such as marihuana, with subtle subjective mental effect and minimal physiologic effect. They have a variable but often marked influence on the potential drug effects.[255,273]

The results of a series of experiments by Jones[274] suggest that the subjective state produced by "a socially relevant dose of smoked marihuana, . . . 9 mg THC" is determined more by set and setting than by the THC content of the marihuana. In one experiment, greater variety and more intense pleasurable symptoms occurred in a four-person group allowing unstructured interpersonal interaction than in unstructured solitary test situations. Contrasting behavioral patterns were observed by the investigator and reported subjectively by the individuals. Subjects tested individually demonstrated a relaxed, slightly drowsy, undramatic state as they read, listened to the radio, or sat doing nothing. In the group setting there was elation, euphoria, uncontrolled laughter, a marked lack of sedation, and energetic conversation.[274]

This strongly emphasizes the importance of setting in the marihuana experience and makes clear the reason why marihuana is usually used with other people. However, most investigators studying its effects evaluate their subjects alone in well-controlled, sterile, scientific laboratories.

The importance of the placebo effect (the subject experiences a drug effect from an inert material) to the "social high" obtained from marihuana was studied in another experiment.[252,274] Misjudgments of the pharmacologic potency of both the smoked placebo (marihuana without THC) and active marihuana were commonly made by the subjects, although physiologic and performance indexes routinely matched the distinction correctly. The smoking of a material that smells and tastes like marihuana by individuals with marihuana experience appeared to produce a mental state that is interpreted as being high, if combined with the expectation of becoming high.

The importance of learning to get high was demonstrated when individuals who smoked marihuana less than twice a month were compared with those who used marihuana at least seven times a week. Although both groups rated the active marihuana equally potent, the frequent users rated the placebo as equal to the active drug, while the infrequent users experienced significantly less high from the placebo.

The infrequent users' experiences appear mainly to reflect pharmacologic factors with moderate set–setting influence. However, the frequent users' response to the placebo appears to reflect learned set–setting influence and minimal pharmacologic factors.[274]

Smith and Mehl[275] call learning to get high "reverse tolerance." During the early exposures to marihuana, the individual learns to appreciate the subtle drug effects, and consequently less drug may be required to experience the desired high in the early stages of marihuana use.

Further evidence of this is seen when the familiar smoking route and smell and taste cues are made ineffective by giving the active and inactive material by the oral route.[252] Both groups of users can significantly distinguish the intoxication produced by 25 mg of active material. But the frequent user rates this high significantly poorer than the smoking high while the infrequent user rates them correctly.

## 3. Specific Pharmacology[l]

### a. Central Nervous System

The primary use of the drug in the United States depends on a variety of factors, including curiosity, group conformity, sedation, and intoxication, and for certain therapeutic reasons. Many smoke marihuana for relaxation, as others might use alcohol. In younger people one of the predominant motivations is to get high—the alcohol equivalent of being drunk. The experienced user usually indicates a feeling of inner joy that is described as being high. When alone, the user may be quiet and drowsy, but in company, talkative and hilarious. Awareness, touch, and perception are considerably altered, particularly as they relate to time and space. These effects may last several hours.

Acute effects associated with marihuana are dose related; but the degree depends upon the amount of active ingredients or active principles, presumably derivatives of THC. With adequate dosage and practice, the drug produces a state of intoxication that is characterized by euphoria, time and space distortion, and motor impairment.

Studies indicate that the acute effects of a marihuana high include temporal disintegration and depersonalization.[276,277] Temporal disintegration means that the individual has difficulty in retaining, coordinating, and serially indexing those memories, perceptions, and expectations that are relevant to a pursued goal. Subjectively temporal disintegration is experienced as a confusion of past, present, and future. Depersonalization is the experience of the self as strange and unreal. The two processes are interrelated and are euphorogenic in that the subject feels less concern about future consequences. Impaired immediate memory may account in part for temporal disintegration.

A review of marihuana's acute effects on intellectual functioning indicates that marihuana intoxication interferes with immediate memory and a wide range of intellectual tasks in a manner that might be expected to impair classroom learning among student users. Additionally there is also good evidence that marihuana interferes with driving skills.[278]

### b. Acute Effects of Marihuana

(1) *Memory and Intellectual Functioning*: Although much recent interest has been focused on the possible long-term, chronic effects of marihuana, it is important to recognize that some of the drug's acute effects on intellectual and psychomotor performance have practical significance. This includes the likelihood of impaired learning ability when marihuana is used

by students during the school day, as well as adverse effects on driving and other complex psychomotor performance. Marihuana appears to interfere with the transfer of material from immediate to longer term memory storage.[279]

When marihuana is smoked, the ability to recall material learned while "high" is typically impaired. This impairment occurs with a wide variety of verbal, as well as graphic, material. It is especially true when the task involves recalling the learned material rather than simply its recognition. Dozens of experimental studies have been conducted and they are generally consistent. Marihuana's acute effects on memory and cognition vary with the task and amounts used, but they are almost invariably detrimental.

Although there have been no studies directly assessing the impact of marihuana intoxication on classroom learning, the similarities to laboratory experiments make it virtually certain that the drug does interfere. Since there is now evidence that substantial numbers of high school students are using marihuana during the course of the school day, it is likely that its use is having a detrimental effect on their functioning in the classroom. (2) *Acute Marihuana Intoxication and Complex Psychomotor Performance in Driving and Flying*: There is strong evidence that marihuana use at typical social levels impairs driving ability and related skills. Relevant studies include laboratory assessment of driving-related skills,[280] driver-simulator studies,[281] test-course performance,[282] actual street-driver performance,[283] and, as previously reported, a study conducted for the National Highway Traffic Safety Administration of drivers involved in fatal accidents.[284] As use becomes increasingly common and socially acceptable, and as the risk of arrest for simple possession decreases, more users are likely to risk driving while high. In limited surveys, from 60 percent to 80 percent of marihuana users questioned indicated that they sometimes drive while high.

Marihuana use in combination with alcohol is also quite common and this risk may well be greater than that posed by either substance alone. A study of drivers involved in fatal accidents in the greater Boston area was conducted by the Boston University Accident Investigation Team. It found that marihuana smokers were overrepresented in fatal highway accidents as compared with a control group of nonusers of similar age and sex.[284]

Another study, conducted by the California State Department of Justice, found that of nearly 1800 blood samples taken from drivers arrested for driving while intoxicated, 16 percent were positive for marihuana. Where no alcohol was present in the blood sample (about 10 percent of the samples), the incidence of marihuana detected rose to 24 percent.[285] And while there have been no recent studies, previous research findings indicate that experienced pilots undergo marked deterioration in performance under flight simulator test conditions while high.

A continuing danger common to both driving and flying is that some of the perceptual and other performance decrements resulting from marihuana use may persist for some time (possibly several hours) beyond the period of subjective intoxication. Under such circumstances, the individual may attempt to fly or drive without realizing that his or her ability to do so is still impaired although the high has passed.

### c. *Effects of Chronic Use on Intellectual Functioning*

The question of whether or not enduring effects on memory and other aspects of intellectual functioning occur as a result of chronic use is a difficult one to answer. While three carefully controlled studies of heavy users in Jamaica, Greece, and Costa Rica failed to find evidence of this, several caveats should be mentioned. The numbers studied were small, the testing procedures with the populations studied may have been insensitive to drug-induced decrements, if any, and even the mode of drug use may have differed from American use. Overall the majority of studies have suggested that impairment does occur. Unfortunately the studies in this area have been of dubious quality and so, the issue remains to be clarified, especially with reference to U.S. users.

A retrospective study of an Egyptian prison population of cannabis users compared 850 chronic users with 839 nonusers, utilizing a variety of testing methods for psychologic functioning. Users were reported to be slower in their psychomotor performances and to show impaired visual coordination and memory for designs. These performance deficiencies were found to be more common in younger, better educated users from urban backgrounds than in older, illiterate users from rural areas.[286,287] This study has been sharply criticized for alleged sampling and psychometric deficiencies, and equally sharply defended by its author.[288,289]

A study of chronic cannabis users in northern India has been published that was based primarily on a comparison of 11 male users (out of a larger sample of 23, in turn chosen from 139 longer term cannabis users) with 11 male non-users who were matched in terms of age, occupation, and marital status. Users all had used cannabis equivalent to about 50 mg THC per day (about the equivalent of five to ten "joints" of typical 1 to 2 percent THC content marihuana) for five years or more. They were given physical examinations, including various laboratory tests of blood and urine, chest X-rays, electrocardiograms (EKG), and electroencephalograms (EEG). Subjects were also given a range of psychologic tests of intelligence, memory, and other intellectual functions.

The physical examinations, including all but one of the laboratory tests (for uric acid blood levels, which were found to be somewhat elevated in users), were normal for both users and controls. In the psychologic tests, however, users did significantly less well than nonusers on two measures of intelligence (9 to 11 I.Q. points lower for users), a measure of memory, a task requiring reproduction from memory of geometric figures, a test of combined cognitive psychomotor speed, and a test of time perception.[290]

American studies comparing college student users with nonusers have found little in the way of evidence of intellectual performance decrement associated with cannabis use, at least as such performance is measured by college grades.

(1) *Cardiovascular Effects*: Although cardiovascular effects of marihuana have been investigated extensively, such research in humans has been largely restricted to healthy young male volunteers in whom the effects appear to be limited in duration and generally benign. One such study examined the short-range effects of smoking one to three marihuana cigarettes on 21 male experienced smokers participating in a 94-day in-hospital study of heavy marihuana smoking. They found, as have others, a significant increase in heart rate after smoking, although not as clearly dose related as in previous findings. They attribute the lack of a clear dose relation to tolerance that developed for the cardiovascular effects of the drug as a result of chronic use. The changes they found in heart functioning were secondary to temporarily increased heart rate and appeared to be free of adverse consequences.[291] There is evidence that in patients with already impaired heart function, use of marihuana may precipitate chest pain (angina pectoris) more rapidly and following less effort than with tobacco cigarettes.[292] This response to marihuana by heart disease patients may prove of considerable practical significance if use expands to include older populations or if young adult users continue their habit as they progress through middle life. Despite the limited evidence to date, a warning to patients with impaired cardiac function not to use marihuana continues to be justified.

(2) *Eyes*: Reddening of the eyes is a common effect, which cannot be attributed to irritation by the smoke as it is also seen with the ingestion of marihuana or its pure active ingredients. Although discussed in the literature, pupillary dilation does not appear to accompany either the smoking of marihuana or the administration of its active products. In fact, there is probably a slight but consistent pupillary constriction.

Preliminary evidence would suggest that marihuana may decrease intraocular pressure and thus may be of some use in glaucoma[293] (a disease characterized by increased pressure in the eye).

It has been shown that marihuana causes a marked increase (several hours) in the time it takes to recover from glare. This may indicate a significant hazard in night driving.

(3) *Pulmonary Effects*: Because marihuana typically is smoked, its possible adverse effects on the lung and pulmonary function have long been a matter of concern in America. It is noteworthy that one of the early attempts to assess the health and social implications of cannabis use, the *Report of the Indian Hemp Drugs Commission of 1893-94*, includes observations about its pulmonary effects that are surprisingly sim-

ilar to contemporary views. For example, this report mentions a possible value in the treatment of asthma because of the drug's "pulmonary sedative" qualities. However, it goes on to say that "long continued smoking . . . doubtless results in the deposition of finely divided carbonaceous matter in the lung tissues, and the presence of other irritating substances in the smoke ultimately causes local irritation of the bronchial mucous membrane, leading to increased secretion, and resulting in the condition which is described as chronic bronchitis in ganja smokers." (*Ganja* is the Indian term for a type of smoked cannabis preparation intermediate in potency between marihuana and hashish.)

The report makes still another observation descriptive of present-day marihuana use: "In ganja smoking . . . the inspiratory act is far greater and more prolonged, a larger volume of smoke entering the lungs than in cigarette smoking."[294] Such deep inhalation of marihuana may well offset the typically smaller amounts smoked compared with cigarette smoking. One indication of this is found in a study comparing marihuana and cigarette smokers, which found that smoking less than one "joint" per day decreases vital capacity—the amount of air the lungs can expel following a deep breath—as much as smoking 16 cigarettes per day.[295] Although the ratio needs to be confirmed by more extensive research, it suggests that the mode of marihuana inhalation and the way in which it is consumed may result in disproportionately adverse pulmonary effects. Part of this difference may be accounted for by the fact that present-day cigarettes are filtered and have significantly lower levels of "tar" than was true in the past. Marihuana "joints" are unfiltered and virtually entirely consumed. Moreover, depending on their ready availability the number of "joints" consumed may approach that of tobacco cigarettes (as high as ten per day).[296]

Thus far there is no direct evidence that smoking marihuana is correlated with lung cancer. The American experience has been too brief for this to be determined. Nevertheless there is good reason for concern about the possibility of pulmonary cancer resulting from extended use over several decades. Like tobacco smoke residuals—so-called "tar"—the application of cannabis residuals to the skin of experimental animals has resulted in the production of tumors.[297] Analysis of marihuana smoke has also shown that it contains larger amounts of cancer-producing hydrocarbons. For example, benzypyrene, a known cancer-producing chemical found in tobacco smoke, has been reported to be 70 percent more abundant in marihuana smoke.[298]

Cilia that assist in moving inhaled dust and other small foreign particles from the lungs are adversely affected by marihuana smoke. Following exposure to the smoke, antibacterial defense systems in the lung are found to be less effective against *staphylococcus aureus*, a bacterium causing a serious form of pneumonia.[299]

While similar effects have not yet been demonstrated in humans, it would be surprising if they did not occur. It is expected that the greater the amount used and the frequency of use, the greater is the likelihood of adverse pulmonary (and other) consequences.

Serious effects on the lungs have been discovered in rats exposed to marihuana smoke in quantities producing blood cannabinoid levels similar to those of human daily users. The animals were made to inhale smoke in a specially constructed apparatus at daily intervals for periods corresponding to an eighth to one half of their normal life span. Extensive lung inflammation and degenerative changes were seen that were similar to but more severe than those induced by exposure to tobacco smoke. The authors conclude that in addition to the irritating effects of smoke, the cannabinoids, chemicals specific to marihuana, "may have a direct undesirable effect on pulmonary function."[300]

Several clinical studies of human users have reported such symptoms as laryngitis, cough, hoarseness, bronchitis, and cellular change in chronic marihuana and hashish smokers that resemble the symptoms of heavy tobacco smokers.[301–303] In a study of American soldiers stationed in Europe, these symptoms were serious enough for the chronic hashish users to seek medical treatment.[303,304] While studies of chronic cannabis users in Jamaica, Greece, and Costa Rica did not find evidence of lung pathology, this may have been because traditional users in those countries do not inhale cannabis smoke as deeply and retain it in their lungs as long as American users do.

From the total body of clinical and experimental evidence accumulated to date, it appears likely that daily use of marihuana leads to lung damage similar to that resulting from heavy cigarette smoking. Since marihuana users often smoke both tobacco and marihuana, the effects of the combination require more study.

## 4. Reproductive Effects of Marihuana

Effects on reproduction have been attributed to marihuana as far back as the earliest cannabis commission's scientific report, that of the Indian Hemp Drugs Commission of 1894. While commenting on a sexual ''stimulant'' effect similar to that of alcohol, the report also describes cannabis as ''used by ascetics in this country [India] with the ostensible object of destroying sexu appetite.''

### *a. Males*

With respect to human males, some investigators have found a decrease in levels of serum testosterone correlated with heavy marihuana use, although others have not. One explanation for this apparent discrepancy in experimental findings is that after smoking marihuana the temporarily depressed levels of testosterone may rapidly return to usual levels. Depending on the time schedule in which sampling is done, the effect may be missed. Even when testosterone decreases have been found, the levels have been within normal limits. Whether more persistent chronic use of marihuana might result in permanently depressed levels of serum testosterone is not known.

Two studies of the semen of male chronic users have found abnormalities in sperm count and motility and in the structural characteristics of the sperm examined.[306,307] In one of these, the semen of 16 healthy young males smoking marihuana under controlled conditions was studied.[306] The levels of use while high—eight to 20 joints per day—were comparable to those of other very heavy users in the general population. Decreases in sperm count and motility were found, together with evidence of structural abnormality in the user's sperm. A second study of chronic hashish users also found structural abnormalities in sperm that were associated with heavy use.[307] While the clinical implications of these animal and human findings are by no means certain, decreased fertility might well result, especially in those of already marginal fertility. In the more controlled laboratory study there was an apparent gradual return to normal functioning when marihuana use was discontinued.[306] Scrutiny of the available literature reveals that there have been no published reports of abnormal offspring that have been related to marihuana use by fathers. Whether or not alterations in reproductive function might have greater significance for the developing child or adolescent is not known, although this is a concern since the younger user is probably more vulnerable.

### *b. Females*

With regard to marihuana's effects on the female reproductive system, there is some recent animal experimentation with doses comparable to those in actual societal use that suggests possible adverse consequences. One study, using THC at levels the authors describe as ''equivalent to moderately heavy marihuana usage in the United States,'' found that the rate of ''reproductive loss'' in THC-treated female rhesus monkeys was about four times greater than that in drugfree controls. The majority of these losses represented deaths, abortions, or resorptions of the fetus. No clear pattern of fetal abnormality was evident. The authors conclude that their experimental results ''raise the possibility that exposure of the human female to marihuana in amounts in relatively common use may be associated with an increased risk of reproductive loss.''[308]

A study of female ''street users''—women using marihuana on their own and of unknown potency—has also raised questions about the possible reproductive effects of cannabis on women. In this research 26 women in their 20s who used marihuana three times a week or more for six months or more were compared with a nonusing group of women of similar age. The experimental group had a significantly higher frequency of abnormal menstrual cycles in which they failed to ovulate (i.e., produce a ripened egg) or showed possible evidence of a shortened period of potential fertility—shortened luteal phase of the menstrual cycle. Lowered levels of prolactin—a hormone important after childbirth in producing adequate mother's milk—were also found, suggesting that nursing might be impaired in marihuana-using women. While such findings are of considerable interest, they must be regarded as preliminary. The drug-using women also used larger amounts of alcohol than did the controls, which may have contributed to the result, and there may have been other differences in life-style that contributed to the experimental outcome. Nevertheless both animal and human data raise the distinct possibility that fertility may be impaired in heavy marihuana users. Studies done in countries of more traditional cannabis use are of little value in clarifying this question since male use overwhelmingly predominates among traditional users.

Experiments with radioactively labeled THC (enabling its progress through the body to be traced) clearly indicate that the drug appears in the milk of nursing monkey mothers and in their offspring.[164] There is also good evidence that THC and other cannabinoids pass through the placental barrier, reaching the fetus during uterine development where they tend to concentrate in the fetus' fatty tissue (including the brain).[172] While pre- and postnatal changes related to maternal use have usually been found only with larger doses in animals and have not been reported in humans, there is a distinct possibility that marihuana use during pregnancy might result in abnormal fetal development.

While much remains to be learned about the possible effects of marihuana on reproduction, several points are reasonably clear. Marihuana at higher doses has a range of effects relevant to reproduction in animals. These appear to result from a variety of mechanisms, including the drug's effects on adrenal function and hormone production in testes and ovaries. More recently, at dose levels that might be encountered in the heavy, regular user, possible adverse consequences for fertility in both males and females have been identified. Such effects may be of greater importance for the marginally fertile or the developing adolescent than for the mature, healthy adult. Finally, given the many unknowns concerning possible effects on the human fetus, use of marihuana during pregnancy should be strongly discouraged. For a recent review on the subject, the serious reader should refer to the work of Dalterio and others.[309]

## 5. Marihuana and the Immune Response

Because of the importance of the body's natural defenses against illness, principally the immune response, several animal studies have produced data to show possible trends of immunogenicity. One study showed that rats could be immunized with a protein conjugate of THC against the effects of THC as exhibited in a spontaneous motor activity test.[310] This is presumably caused by the binding of $\Delta^9$-THC to anti-THC antibodies, thus preventing the $\Delta^9$-THC from reaching drug-receptor sites. Another paper presents "evidence for the possible immunogenicity of $\Delta^9$-THC in rodents."[311] The percentage of blast transformation in cultured mice spleen cells observed after 3-H thymidine incorporation was increased by THC, which acts as other antigen substances. Nahas and colleagues hypothesize that "THC might constitute a hapten in vivo which could trigger an immune response, as indicated by blast transformation"[310] and may have implications for human health. Other work[312] indicates that leukocytes from chronic marihuana users have a reduced responsiveness to stimulation by phytohemagglutinin as measured by thymidine uptake in cultured cells. This observation prompted studies on the rejection of skin grafts in mice.[313] Delta-9-THC significantly prolonged the interval before grafts were rejected, suggesting potential usefulness in transplants. This group also reported significant inhibition of solid tumor growth in mice by $\Delta^8$- and $\Delta^9$-THC.[314] It appears that the cannabinoids may interfere with the incorporation of nucleic acids into DNA and that these solid tumor cells are more sensitive than cells from other tissues.

There have been contradictory reports of impairment of this response in humans.[315–319] The animal data, using generally higher doses, have consistently indicated a definite suppression of the test animals' immune responses.[320,321] In humans, even when there have been indications of a diminished response, it has not been found in all users and the clinical implications are unclear. As yet, no epidemiologic research has been undertaken to determine whether marihuana smokers suffer from infections and other diseases to a greater extent than those of similar life-style who do not use the drug. For the present, this important question must be regarded as unresolved.

## 6. Chromosome Abnormalities

There is no new evidence in this area. While there were early reports of increases in chromosomal breaks and abnormalities in human cell cultures, more recent results have been inconclusive. The three positive studies in humans that have been reported have decided limitations.[322,323] All were retrospective—that is, studies of those already using marihuana who were compared with nonusers. Such variables as differences in life-style, exposure to viral infections, and possible use of other drugs, all known to affect chromosome integrity, could not be reliably assessed. In two of the studies, the aberrations observed were found only in a minority of the users.

Three other studies done prospectively (i.e., before and after use) have been reported.[324–326] All were negative, but the results could have been influenced by the fact that all the subjects had at least some prior experience with marihuana. It is possible that the baseline levels of chromosome deficits may have been elevated by earlier casual marihuana use, thus masking a drug-related effect.

A team investigating the effect of marihuana smoke on human lung cells in laboratory culture has found an increase in the number of cells containing an abnormal number of chromosomes.[327] Another investigator who previously reported a high proportion of cells in marihuana smokers with reduced numbers of chromosomes more recently reported that the addition of $\Delta^9$-THC (the principal psychoactive ingredient of marihuana) to human white blood cell cultures also resulted in an increased frequency of cells with abnormally low chromosome numbers.[328] The implications of these findings continue to be uncertain.

## 7. Alterations in Cell Metabolism

The implications of laboratory findings on the inhibition of DNA, RNA, and protein synthesis (all of which are basically related to cellular reproduction and metabolism) are still unknown. Adding $\Delta^9$-THC to various types of human and animal cell cultures has been found to inhibit DNA, RNA, and protein synthesis. No effect on DNA repair synthesis was found although the uptake of the chemical precursors within the cells was reduced by half.[329]

The possibility that cannabis, or one or more of its chemical ingredients, differentially affects the cell metabolism and reproduction of cancer cells in animals was raised by earlier research. One aspect of the mechanism by which this may occur is an inhibition of DNA metabolism in abnormal cells but not in normal cells.

If this preferential inhibition of DNA synthesis in animal tumors also occurs in humans, marihuana might prove of value as an anticancer drug. It should once again be stressed, however, that at this time there is no evidence that cannabis or any of its synthesized or naturally occurring constituents is of value in inhibiting human cancer growth. If animal findings of a depressed cell immunity response that is also related to cell metabolism are substantiated in humans, cannabis, its synthesized components, or chemically related drugs might prove useful in preventing organ rejection in human organ transplant surgery.

## 8. Miscellaneous Pharmacologic Effects

The previously reported anticonvulsive effects of cannabinoids have been confirmed in different laboratories. Cannabinoids were found to be potent anticonvulsive agents in a variety of test procedures (e.g., against audiogenic seizures in rats[330–332] or seizures elicited by electrical stimulation, "kindling" of the limbic cortex and the amygdala,[333,334] as well as against maximal electroshock (MES) or pentylenetetrazol (PTZ)-induced seizures.[335] Although anticonvulsant potencies do not differ significantly, $\Delta^8$-THC is three times more neurotoxic than $\Delta^9$-THC, and both are without effect on minimal seizures and lethality induced by PTZ. However, tolerance is developed after repeated administration and the antiepileptic property of cannabinoids disappears rapidly.[334] The low protective indexes (ratio between neurotoxic and effective dose) that have been found[335] suggest that $\Delta^9$- and $\Delta^8$-THC have poor therapeutic potential as antiepileptic drugs. The anticonvulsive effects of other components of marihuana were highlighted when Izquierdo found that cannabidiol (CBD), like diphenylhydantoin, can produce decreases in hippocampal seizure discharges.[336] Cannabidiol has little psychoactive activity in laboratory animals or humans and may represent a separation effect.

The EEG effects of cannabinoids are highly variable and are related to species, dose, and duration of treatment. As researchers study the other marihuana cannabinoids, new central effects are being discovered. A power spectrum study of EEG changes in rabbits after I.V. infusion of 0.1–2.0 mg/kg $\Delta^9$-THC confirmed previous results, which showed an increase in amplitude of low-frequency components in the delta band and the appearance of either single or multiple spikes mainly in the motor and limbic cortices. These changes in EEG after administration of $\Delta^9$-THC are accompanied by autonomic effects (i.e., rapid fall in blood pressure and bradycardia) that are not seen with other hallucinogenic agents such as LSD-25, mescaline, and DOM. These compounds also evoke EEG desynchronization rather than synchronization, which is mostly localized in the lower brain stem. With $\Delta^9$-THC, the EEG synchronization is generalized, with slowing more prominent in the cortical areas but also seen in subcortical areas. In the same species and at about the same dose levels, $\Delta^9$-THC failed to block the cortical desynchronization (arousal) produced by physostigmine, thus showing that central cholinergic sensitive neurons associated with EEG activation systems are not blocked by THC.[338] In monkeys implanted with deep cortical electrodes, exposure to marihuana smoke induced distinct recording changes in the septal region, occasionally accompanied by changes in recordings from the cerebellum, thalamus, hippocampus, and orbital and temporal cortices.[339] Curiously $\Delta^8$-THC, when administered to cats I.P. or I.V., failed to produce any striking EEG and behavioral effects.[340]

Effects of $\Delta^9$-THC on the sleep–wakefulness cycles of rabbits,[341] cats,[342] and humans[343] have also been reported, with a decrease in REM sleep after acute administration.

Continuing the studies of the effects of $\Delta^9$-THC on the polysensory cortex, Boyd[344] compared the effects of a number of psychoactive drugs such as LSD, mescaline, and phencyclidine on an evoked response sensitive to the effect of $\Delta^9$-THC. This group found that mescaline had effects very similar to those of $\Delta^9$-THC, thus increasing both early and late evoked responses and resembling those of stimulant drugs. These effects may be related to the changes in sensory perception produced by these compounds. A direct cortical site of action for changes in sensory perception was also emphasized by others.[345] Delta-9-THC has been shown to exert a differential effect on lateral geniculate neurons in the rat, outlining the effect of this compound on the visual system.[346] Units that fire when the eye is illuminated are inhibited by the compound, whereas those that discharge in the dark but are inhibited by light either remain unchanged or increase their rate of firing.

Acute administration of pharmacologically active cannabinoids $\Delta^9$-THC, $\Delta^8$-THC, and 11-OH-$\Delta^9$-THC also caused a highly significant but reversible reduction in nuclear membrane —attached ribosomes of infant rat brain cortical cells.[339] Studies on the tolerance to EEG changes have reported inconsistent results after long-term administration.[347,348]

The mechanism of action in THC and its metabolites was further defined in *in vitro* experiments. Delta-9-THC and/or its metabolite, 11-OH-$\Delta^9$-THC, were found to have an inhibitory effect on nerve conduction.[349–351] *In vitro*, they potentiate both the acetylcholine and adrenaline-induced contractions of isolated muscles.[352] Changes in RNA and acetylcholine activity reported earlier in chronic experiments were found to be reversible after cessation of treatment.[353]

The effect of $\Delta^9$-THC on the peripheral sympathetic nervous system was confirmed when it was reported that 20 mg/kg Δ$^9$-THC injected subcutaneously for seven days into rats produced a significant decrease in serum dopamine β-hydroxylase activity.[354] This was also seen with ethanol. These results are critically influenced by environmental setting. In naive animals, Δ$^9$-THC appears to have a sympatholytic effect, whereas in animals subjected to immobilization stress it potentiates the sympathetic response.[354,355] Serotonin (5-HT) seems to be involved in the development of cannabis-elicited aggressive behavior after chronic treatment.[356] After chronic treatment with cannabis extract, the 5-HT brain levels remained unchanged in nonaggressive rats but were significantly decreased in aggressive animals. Continuing his experiments with inhibition of the biosynthesis of prostaglandins by cannabinoids, Burstein[357] has shown that not only Δ$^9$-THC but also other major cannabinoids such as cannabinol and cannabidiol and the precursor olivetol possess the same inhibitory properties. This indicates that the inhibitory power of the cannabinoids resides in the aromatic portion of the molecule.

The neuroendocrine effects of cannabinoids are still unclear and seem to vary with route and duration of administration. Most of the newer studies of the effects of marihuana on neuroendocrine regulation have examined the effects of the drug on the hypothalamic–pituitary axis. These studies have resulted in part because of the observed effects of marihuana on the peripheral endocrine organs that are regulated by the hypothalamic–pituitary axis. For example, the reproductive consequences of prolonged marihuana use include both (1) alterations in reproductive hormones[358] and (2) effects on spermatogenesis[359] or ovulation.[360] Since both of these reproductive processes are controlled by the hormones from the anterior pituitary gland, and since marihuana is a neuroactive drug, it seemed reasonable to assume that the hypothalamic–pituitary axis was the site of action for the reproductive effects of marihuana.

In terms of neuroendocrine effects of marihuana, there is evidence of effects of this cannabis on the hypothalamic–pituitary function[361] in levels of LH and FSH in ovariectomized monkeys[362]; on synthetic gonadotropin-releasing factor[362]; on suppression of ovulation in rats[363] and in rabbits[364]; on prolactin secretion[365–367]; on thrytropin (TSH) secretion[368]; on corticotropin (ACTH) secretion[369–371]; and on hypothalamic neurotransmitters.[372–375]

In several studies, the site of action of the effects of marihuana and THC on hypothalamic–pituitary function has been shown to be at the level of the hypothalamus. In general, it has been shown that the pituitary responds to exogenous releasing factors in the presence of the drugs. This inhibitory effect on hypothalamic–pituitary function is not unique to cannabis derivatives but is a property shared by several CNS depressant drugs, including narcotics, some tranquilizers, and some sedatives. Certain of the cannabis effects, however, are unique, especially the inhibition of prolactin secretion. Virtually every other drug that inhibits LH and FSH levels (including narcotics and sex steroids) stimulates prolactin release. THC inhibits LH, FSH, and prolactin. The hypothalamic–pituitary activity of the cannabis derivatives also appears to be somewhat associated with the psychoactivity or neuroactivity of the compounds. This may not be true among the other CNS depressant drugs. It appears certain that the hypothalamic–pituitary effects of marihuana are somehow related to the effects of the drug on hypothalamic neurotransmitters.

Because of the primary role of biogenic amines, especially dopamine and norepinephrine, in the regulation of hypothalamic releasing factors, it has been postulated that the effects of THC on these transmitters may be important. Several studies have shown that THC can alter levels of biogenic amines in the CNS.[376–378] The effect on these transmitters appears to be mediated by an effect of THC on the reuptake of dopamine, norepinephrine, and serotonin into nerve endings in the brain.[379] This effect of THC apparently results in an increase in serotonin levels in certain areas of the brain[380] and a decreased content of catecholamines in parts of the brain. It is not clear, however, whether THC acts directly on transmitter levels, or even on transmitter uptake, or whether its effects are mediated by secondary effects on neuronal activity. THC has also been shown to alter cholinergic activity in certain brain areas. Studies on the turnover rate of acetylcholine in the rat hippocampus indicate that THC (but not the nonpsychoactive cannabidiol) decreases cholinergic activity.[381] This effect of THC appears to be secondary to an increase in the activity of GABA (gamma-aminobutyric acid), another important central transmitter. The effect of THC on central cholinergic pathways is probably significant in the psychoactive effects of THC. Its role in the disruption of hypothalamic–pituitary function is not known.

Some neuropharmacologic studies have examined the part of hypothalamic neurotransmitters in the neuroendocrine effects of THC. Marks[382] studied the involvement of a hypothalamic cholinergic mechanism by using oxotremorine, a cholinergic muscarinic agonist, in combination with THC. He concluded that the effect of THC on LH levels was not related to its effect on the cholinergic system.

Investigations into the effects of THC on certain metabolic processes and subcellular structures in the rat brain[383] showed that THC, but not the nonpsychoactive cannabinoids, decreases protein and nucleic acid synthesis in the infant rat brain. Studies of the subcellular distribution of the THC indicate that these metabolic effects may be related to the preferential binding of THC to mitochondrial and microsomal fractions in brain cells.

Certain cell membrane processes have been reported to respond specifically to psychoactive cannabinoids.[384] The plasma membrane-bound enzyme, LPC-acyltransferase, which is thought to be responsible for regulating the proportion of saturated fatty acids in the plasma membrane, is inhibited by the psychoactive cannabinoids only. The inhibition of this enzyme in synaptosomes from mouse brain may be responsible for the effects of marihuana on neurotransmitter uptake mechanisms.

Morphologic changes in the ultrastructure of the synaptic cleft region in rhesus monkey brain has also been reported in response to marihuana exposure or THC treatment.[385] These changes consisted of (1) appearance of opaque granular material in the synaptic cleft region, (2) widening of the synaptic cleft, and (3) synaptic vesicle clumping. These ultrastructural changes were consistent with lasting EEG changes produced in the monkey by marihuana or THC. They were observed in various areas of the brain, with the most profound effects seen in the septal region, the hippocampus, and the amygdala.[386] The impact of morphologic changes in the neural effects of THC or marihuana remains to be shown.

Although cardiovascular effects of cannabinoids have previously been discussed, certain animal studies are mentioned here to complete the discussion. Delta-9-THC has been shown to reduce the blood pressure of hypertensive rats. However, tolerance to this effect developed rapidly.[387,388] The hypotensive activity of $\Delta^9$-THC in anesthetized cats and dogs may partially be caused by an attenuation of cardiac output.[389,390] This may be mediated by direct and reflexogenic action on the cardiovascular centers in the brain.[391] Apparently the hypotensive effect of $\Delta^9$-THC may be prevented by hypoxia, but its bradycardic effect is profound and independent of alterations in blood gas parameters.[392] Interactive effects with barbiturates and various sedative hypnotic drugs,[393-395] amphetamines,[396] anesthetic agents,[397] and chloramphenicol[398] have been reported, usually after acute administration. In one study attenuation of effects was seen after subchronic THC treatment.[399] This was probably due to the development of tolerance.

In relation to the differential activities of $\Delta^9$-THC, cannabis extract, and LSD, it was reported that cannabinoids—in contrast to LSD—increase the liver tyrosine–alpha-keto gluterate transaminase (TKT) and tryptophan pyrrolase (TPO) activities.[400]

## 9. Behavioral Pharmacologic Actions

### *Psychologic Effects*

In the past the literature was filled with confusing reports concerned with the animal effects of marihuana on various behavioral pharmacological parameters. The main confusion arose from the indiscriminate interchange of the term marihuana with its prime active ingredient, THC. As basic research expanded from animals to humans, this problem declined. There are available numerous methods to evaluate the effects of THC on the brain and spinal cord.[401]

The discrepancies in attempting to unravel the actual behavioral pharmacological profile of even THC include design of the experiment, variation in THC doses, and route of administration. Other critical factors include previous drug experience, motivations, and the psychological state of the intended subject.[402]

It has now become clear that the atmosphere or setting of a particular drug experiment, especially with THC or marihuana, must be standardized. Galenter and co-workers,[180] reported that people experiencing THC in an "austere" atmosphere compared to a "congenial" atmosphere had greater untoward effects in the former.

The notion that approximately 50 percent of THC in a marihuana cigarette will be absorbed when smoked does not take into account the wide psychogenetic variability of individual smokers. In one carefully controlled study, peak plasma levels of THC following the smoking of known equipotent amounts of marihuana were 69, 37, and 21 mg./ml., which represents 41, 20 and 15 percent actually absorbed by these subjects.[403]

We will now consider some of the common as well as the less common psychologic effects of THC.[4,6,13,402–404]

(1) *Effects on Mentation and Psychomotor Performance*: Characteristic intoxication with psychoactive materials affects psychomotor and mental functions. It is apparent from the subjective assertions of users, and from experimental studies, that marihuana is no exception.[44,210,213,246,247,249-251,271,405-408]

Psychomotor tasks that have been tested include tapping speed, handwriting and freehand drawing, simple and complex reaction time, pursuit rotor and tracking, and continuous performance. Cognitive functions frequently tested are simple arithmetic problems, serial addition or subtraction, fine judgment tasks, digit–symbol substitution, digit-code memory, reading comprehension, speech or verbal output, forward and backward digit spans, goal-directed complex serial subtractions and additions to reach a set end sum, and short-term or immediate memory.

Kiplinger et al.[213] have clearly demonstrated that the degree of impairment is dose related and varies during the period of intoxication, exerting its maximal effect at the peak level of intoxication.

Naive subjects commonly demonstrate greater decrement in performance than experienced users but report less subjective effect.[248] Experienced users appear to compensate better for the effect of the drug, especially in ordinary performance at lower doses.[249-252-277,406,409] Performance of simple or familiar tasks (i.e., simple reaction time) during intoxication is minimally effected. However, on unfamiliar or complex tasks (i.e., complex reaction time), performance decrements occur.[404,406]

Performance decrements are further enhanced when verbal tasks are performed during delayed auditory feedback.[213] Also, marked individual differences in performance are noted between similar subjects.[213,250,271] A cyclical waxing and waning of the intensity of the intoxication and concomitant performance occurs periodically.[246,251] Finally, when subjects concentrate on the task being performed at "normal social high," objective evidence of intoxication is not apparent and the individual may perform better than when drugfree.[245,408]

These observations raise practical doubts regarding an intoxicated individual's ability to function at jobs requiring memory, concentration, and organized thinking.

(2) *The Intoxicated Mental State*: Several investigators have suggested that short-term memory is the mental function most significantly affected by marihuana and contributes to the subtle alterations of mental functioning noted. General impairment of recent or short-term memory is demonstrated,[410,411] and mental tasks requiring immediate information acquisition[412] and/or retrieval[248] are affected.

Abel[413] showed that marihuana blocks the acquisition process involved in the storage of new information but does not interfere with the retrieval of already stored information. Decrements are produced in decisions requiring recent memory or sustained alertness,[251] conversation,[248] calculations, or reading that require retention, coordination, and indexing of sequential information termed temporal disintegration.[246]

Melges[246] theorizes that episodic impairment of immediate memory produces voids that are filled with perceptions and thoughts extraneous to the organized mental processes. He suggests that this leads to temporal disintegration, producing a fragmented and disorganized temporal experience in which past and future time frames are blurred and the present is experienced as prolonged or boundless. Thus depersonalization occurs as the individual experiences himself temporally being placed in a strange and unreal world during marihuana intoxication.

(3) *Unpleasant Reactions*: The substantial cognitive and psychomotor effects are likely to be responsible for many of the acute adverse reactions to marihuana. One of the most common is a heavy, drugged state in which the individual feels mentally and physically sluggish so that every motion and thought seems to require extreme effort.[278] This most frequently occurs after oral ingestion of large doses of drugs or in inexperienced smokers who have not learned to self-titrate their doses to achieve desired highs.

Depression, anxiety, fatigue, short-term memory loss, dizziness, nausea, incoordination, palpitations, and generalized discomfort are common complaints. ''Novice anxiety reactions'' or panic reactions account for a majority of acute toxic reactions to marihuana.[278,414–424]

When dosage, set, and setting are optimal, the distortion of self (depersonalization) and temporal disintegration (timelessness of the present moment) is recognized by the individual as drug-induced and fairly pleasant. But if dose, set, and setting are not optimal, the experience may cause the intoxicated individual to fear that loss of identity and self-control. Acute anxiety or panic results.[246]

The large majority of anxiety reactions occur in novices who have intense underlying anxiety concerning marihuana use, such as fears of arrest, of disruption of family and occupational relationships, and of possible physical or mental dangers. Individuals with relatively rigid personality structures appear to experience anxiety reactions more frequently than individuals who are members of the ''counterculture.''[278]

Simple episodes of neurotic depression may also be observed in this same type of individual during periods of unusual psychologic stress.[425] Both types of reactions are transient and abate as the drug wears off over a few hours. Treatment should consist of gentle but authoritative reassurance that nothing is seriously wrong and that the drug effects will wear off, leaving the individual to feel ''normal'' again.[278,425]

(5) *Effects of Marihuana Use on Concomitant Behavior*: Mendelson[408] analyzed the effects of acute marihuana intoxication on behavior on the basis of a variety of assessments, including simple operant tasks; mood states; individual and group observations before, during, and after smoking; and clinical psychologic evaluations.

Sleep-inducing properties were confirmed. Increased amounts were observed as to both number and length of shorter and longer blocks of consecutive hours of sleep.

The examination of mood assessments prior to, during, and after marihuana smoking indicates that the acute effects include a reduction of negative moods (anxiety, hostility, and guilt–shame) and an increase in positive moods (carefreeness and friendliness). Studies revealed that subjects tended to smoke marihuana when their moods were positive, in order to increase them. One paradoxic finding was that the subjects also reported feeling more depressed after smoking.

Acute effects of marihuana on cognitive and motor functions were studied with a battery of tests sensitive to brain function (Halstead Category Test, Tactile Performance Test, Seashore Rhythm Test, Finger Tapping Test, Trail Making Test, and the Weschler Adult Intelligence Scale). No alterations in performance as a result of acute intake of marihuana were noted in any of these.

The acute effect of marihuana smoking on social behavior was investigated by observing individuals and their interactions in small groups. The data strongly indicated that marihuana smoking, in addition to being a subjective drug experience, is also a social activity around which verbal interaction and other types of social behavior are centered.

But although marihuana smoking tended to be a group activity, subjects did not always engage in verbal communication while smoking. They were often observed withdrawing from social interactions and then participating in some type of noncommunicative passive activity, such as watching television, listening to music, reading, or staring at objects or people.

Heavy marihuana users tended to be more withdrawn than intermittent users, often listening to the stereo and focusing on the personal effects of the drug. The intermittent users tended to watch television, which provided group entertainment, and thus enhanced the social effects of the drug.

Verbal interaction in formal task-oriented discussion groups diminished when several group members were simultaneously intoxicated. However, groups engaged in problem-solving tasks performed more efficiently because fewer suggestions and less discussion ensued before a workable solution was proposed. Marihuana did not appear to increase hostility during these sessions but tended to change the nature of hostile communication from direct criticism to indirect sarcasm. Assessment of risk-taking behavior revealed that under the influence of marihuana, users tend to become more conservative in decision making.

In summary, it appears that marihuana does exert subtle effects on measurable components of social behavior and interaction.

(5) *Psychosis*: An alleged connection between mental illness and cannabis is based on studies from Africa, the Middle East, and India—although the findings or early studies are questionable because of lack of controls, biased sampling, poor data collection, and a failure to account for such variables as nutrition, living standard, cultural factors, and socioeconomic status. These areas are currently developing economically and scientifically, but for many years medical care, especially psychiatric care, has been given low priority. Well-trained psychiatrists and methodologists are very rare in mental hospitals in these countries.

India's mental institutions were widely quoted to support the connection between excessive cannabis consumption and insanity. The Indian Hemp Commission performed a thorough and objective investigation of this question, although methodologically it was not up to modern standards. The Commission was unconvinced of the reliability of hospital statistics, as the diagnoses were often made by policemen, not psychiatrists. In response to this, the Commission examined all admissions to Indian mental hospitals for one year. It found that cannabis use could not be considered a factor in more than 7 to 13 percent of all cases of both acute and chronic psychosis.

Chopra[426] carefully performed the same examination of admissions to Indian mental hospitals from 1928 through 1939 when cannabis use was extremely high. He found 600 cases of acute and chronic psychosis that could be traced to cannabis use. Other reports from India have produced varying estimates of the incidence of cannabis psychosis.[427–429] In Egypt 27 to 33 percent of mental hospital admissions were cannabis related.[430]

Kolansky and Moore,[431] in a widely publicized report of cases of individuals aged 13 to 24, claimed profound adverse psychologic effects from smoking marihuana two or more times a week. Of 38 individuals reported, all had decompensated personalities, eight had psychoses (four attempted suicide), and 13, according to the authors, became sexually promiscuous due to marihuana. These clinical impressions were all based on, at most, a few interviews with individuals who were referred to these psychiatrists for consultation for various problems (including one third by legal authorities after arrest for possession of marihuana).

Unfortunately the authors extended sweeping generalizations to all young adolescent marihuana users on the basis of this biased and nonrepresentative sample. No attempt was made to interview other young marihuana users who had not been referred for psychiatric help, and the high incidence of promiscuity and psychopathology in comparable adolescent populations was totally disregarded. In addition, case histories of previous mental health status were obtained retrospectively from the patients, their families, or the referral source. It is impossible to state unequivocally, as the authors do, that since marihuana use and psychiatric problems occurred at the same time, the former is causative of the latter.

Several authors have reported acute toxic psychosis following marihuana use by soldiers in Vietnam.[432-434] All cases represented transient reactions and cleared rapidly with treatment. In many cases, personality disorders or borderline personality states appeared to be predisposing factors in the development of the psychotic state. Often revealed were problems of identity diffusion, ego weakness, low self-esteem, and inability to form interpersonal relationships. The stressful conditions of the setting in which the drug was used should also be considered.

Halikas[435] performed intensive psychiatric interviews with a population of 100 regular marihuana users and a control group of 50 of their nonusing or casually using friends. Half of each group met the criteria for some psychiatric diagnosis. Psychiatric illness and antisocial behavior usually preceded marihuana use.

The Secretary of Health, Education and Welfare's 1972 report on *Marihuana and Health*, prepared by the National Institute of Mental Health, noted in summary that marihuana can clearly precipitate certain less serious adverse psychiatric reactions, such as simple depression and panic, particularly in inexperienced users. In these reactions, nondrug factors may be the most important determinants. Psychotic episodes also may be precipitated in persons with pre-existing borderline personalities or psychotic disorders or in persons under excessively stressful conditions. These acute psychoses appear to share considerable clinical similarities with the acute toxic psychoses noted in the Eastern literature. Both psychoses resemble an acute brain syndrome in that they occur primarily after heavier than usual usage and are self-limited and short lived after the drug is removed from the body.

Some reports describing a prolonged psychotic course after an initial acute episode cannot rule out the role of preexisting psychopathology. At the present time evidence that marihuana is a sufficient or contributory cause of chronic psychosis is weak.

(6) *Amotivational Syndrome*: Another type of possible mental deterioration of subtle personality and behavioral changes associated with heavy long-term cannabis use is the amotivational syndrome.

Many people throughout the world have described this syndrome in which the most potent preparations are used.[436-438] At this point the user shows a loss of interest in virtually all activities other than cannabis use. The resultant lethargy, social and personal deterioration, and drug preoccupation may be comparable to the skid row alcoholic's state.

Benabud[438] describes the occurrence of this syndrome in individuals chronically intoxicated with hashish. These individuals do not exhibit conventional levels of motivation, especially as the amount of time required to obtain and consume enough drug to maintain this state is not likely to leave much time for other pursuits. The passive user tends to lose interest in work and other long-term goals.

The question of whether there exists a significant causal, as opposed to an associative or correlational, relationship attracted attention only when the traditionally achievement-oriented Western youth adopted cannabis use. The traits of passivity or amotivation are commonly described among heavy cannabis users throughout the world.

In summary, if cannabis use produces personality and behavior changes, the extent of such changes is likely to be strongly related to the amount consumed and the age of the user. According to evidence found in Western literature, frequent use may be quite disruptive during the formative years of adolescence.

On the other hand, the Eastern literature indicates that, although the very heavy user (200 mg THC or more per day) is largely incapacitated, manual laborers often function adequately while consuming amounts containing 30 to 50 mg THC per day.[439] Similarly, many musicians and entertainers in the United States have lived productive lives while using marihuana.[440]

## G. CANNABIS AND PSYCHOPATHOLOGY

An acute panic anxiety reaction is the most common adverse psychologic reaction to use, especially when unexpectedly strong material is consumed. A number of clinicians have cautioned against use of marihuana by those with a history of serious psychologic problems or who have had drug-precipitated emotional disturbances (so-called "bad trips"). While more serious psychiatric problems such as a cannabis-related psychosis have been reported in countries with a long tradition of use, such reactions do not appear common here. Concern has been expressed that the recent availability of much stronger varieties of cannabis may result in more serious problems than in the past.

While there have been a number of overseas studies concerning the impact of chronic marihuana use on intellectual functioning, most of which have reported some impairment, the quality of such studies is highly variable and so the question remains in doubt. Studies of U.S. users have not generally reported such impairment, although the American experience has been limited to relatively highly motivated college populations using smaller amounts of cannabis for shorter periods of time.

More than five years ago, a report to Congress by the Secretary of Health, Education and Welfare[137] had the following to say about psychopathology:

> To date, well-controlled studies demonstrate few differences in psychopathology in carefully matched samples of users and non-users. However, a series of clinical and case reports associating marihuana use with a wide range of psychiatric symptomatology has appeared. The question of a causal role of cannabis still remains largely unresolved. Most such studies have reported on small self-selected samples many of whom were consuming other drugs in addition to marihuana. Previously reported (cf. earlier editions of *Marihuana and Health*), larger scale studies in countries where cannabis use is endemic which have described intellectual deficit or psychopathology associated with cannabis use have been poorly controlled, confounded by multiple drug use and used dubious diagnostic methods. Observations made in the last Report continue to appear sound. Serious psychiatric complications of use seem to be most common in those with a previous history of psychopathology who consume large doses of cannabis or inadvertently overdose. More recent findings tend to confirm the observation that American marihuana users who use heavily are somewhat more likely to come from populations with a higher preexisting risk for psychiatric problems than has the general population.

Other findings of cannabis-induced psychopathologic states include transient and paranoid feelings. It has been suggested that those who are characterized as having more paranoid defense mechanisms are less likely to experience other acute adverse reactions.

An acute brain syndrome associated with cannabis intoxication was reported and included such features as clouding of mental processes, disorientation, confusion, and marked memory impairment.[441] It is thought to be dose related and to be determined more by the size of the dose than by preexisting personality. This set of acute symptoms has not been frequently reported in the United States, possibly because until recently very strong cannabis materials were less readily available than in some overseas locations. Acute brain syndrome also diminishes as the toxic effects of the drug wear off.

Four cases of well-documented schizophrenia have been reported in which the use of marihuana is believed to have led to an exacerbation of psychotic symptoms in patients whose psychoses were in at least partial remission.[442] The author concludes that "while marihuana can perhaps be safely used by many persons, this is not so with the schizophrenic." He urges that schizophrenics be alerted to the special hazards he feels marihuana poses for them in the same way other patients would routinely be alerted to possible hazardous interactions between their illnesses and substances they might use.[442]

Abel,[443] in a detailed review of the relationship between cannabis and violence, concludes that while marihuana probably does not precipitate violent behavior in the majority of users, there may be some individuals who should be advised against its use because of a prior history of poor impulse control or special circumstances of stress which, combined with preexisting personality, can make it dangerous. He goes on to point out, however, that it is not clear that marihuana can be specifically blamed for precipitating violence any more than can a variety of other drugs.

Abruzzi,[444] based on his experience with some 5000 drug-related psychoses, summarized his clinical findings concerning adverse reactions to marihuana by pointing out that although marihuana-induced psychosis is rare, higher potency materials may induce a psychotic reaction. He concludes with some advice: ''Those with a history of emotional disturbances and especially 'bad trips' (i.e., previous drug precipitated emotional disturbances) should avoid intoxicants, including alcohol and marihuana.'' Finally, this author advises that emergency room and psychiatric hospital procedures be altered to create a less judgmental, less frightening and coercive, more compassionate and accepting atmosphere. He suggests more homelike and reassuring surroundings.[444]

Marihuana flashbacks—spontaneous recurrence of feelings and perceptions similar to those produced by the drug itself—have been reported. A survey of U.S. Army users found that flashbacks occurred in both frequent and infrequent users and were not necessarily related to a history of LSD use. Such occurrences may range from the quite vivid recreation of a drug-related experience to a mild evocation of a previous incident. The origin of such experiences is uncertain, but those who have had them typically appear to require little or no treatment.[445]

During a one-year period beginning in May 1976 and ending in April 1977, marihuana ranked 13th among the drugs mentioned in drug-related emergency room contacts—but by the year 1978 it had risen to sixth place. While such figures are not always easy to interpret, they do suggest that marihuana may be assuming a greater role in this respect, possibly because of an increase in the number of people using the drug or because of the increased availability of stronger materials more likely to precipitate adverse reactions.

## H. TOXICOLOGY

### 1. Acute Effects

#### *a. Central Nervous System*

A common toxic symptom secondary to marihuana overdose is nausea and vomiting. However, the hangover seen with alcohol is not present after a high on marihuana. The actual incidence of hallucination is difficult to determine, since many people will say they hallucinate when, in fact, they are experiencing perceptual alterations, illusions rather than true hallucinations. Some medical experts have attempted to classify marihuana as a mild hallucinogenic agent, and probably in certain susceptible individuals hallucinations can occur. As previously mentioned, Isbell[244] has definitely shown that one of the supposedly active ingredients of marihuana, $\Delta^9$-THC, is in fact a hallucinogenic agent in high doses. It seems reasonable to assume that marihuana in high doses in certain individuals can produce frank hallucination.

The literature has accumulated a large number of so-called psychotic reactions attributable to marihuana smoking. Again, these are difficult to substantiate scientifically, since many of the patients have been on multiple drugs and very little is written about the basic psychologic make-up of the marihuana user. The Haight-Ashbury experience has been that the primary marihuana psychosis is a very rare reaction, but that heavy marihuana smoking can precipitate a psychotic reaction in individuals with severe personality disturbances. In several of the Haight-Ashbury cases, psychotic reactions occurred in individuals who were members of the older establishment trying marihuana for the first time in unfamiliar environments. It was felt that psychotic reactions represented the user's negative attitude toward experimenting with an illegal drug in a peculiar environment rather than the pharmacologic properties of marihuana per se.[446,447] Acute toxic psychoses in 12 American soldiers in Vietnam after their first exposure to marihuana were reported.[432] Environmental factors appeared to be important.

### 2. Lethality

There is no conclusive evidence that short-term marihuana use alone directly results in any physical damage to humans. A few scattered fatalities associated with marihuana use are occasionally reported; most are from 19th century Indian experiences with large oral doses of charas.[448,449] Brill[450] and Smith[446] have noted that there have not been any reliable reports of human fatalities attributable purely to marihuana, even though very high doses have been administered.

Several case reports[451–455] noted severe physiologic disturbances and acute collapse (shock, chills, and fever) subsequent to intravenous injection of suspensions of marihuana. These symptoms may have been due to an allergic reaction to injected foreign plant material, to a bacteremia, and/or to the injection of insoluble particles that are filtered by the organs. The symptoms may be considered a complication of the mode of use rather than results of the drug.

Although a median lethal dose has not been established in humans,[450] one has been found in laboratory animals. Earlier reports[456,457] used materials of uncertain potency and composition. One group,[458] using THC extracted from marihuana, demonstrated the following $LD_{50}$ (the dose that causes death in 50 percent of the animals) in units of milligrams per kilogram of $\Delta^9$-THC for mice/rats: oral 481.9/666, intraperitoneal 454.9/372.9, intravenous 28.6/42.47.

Thompson et al.,[459] under contract to the National Institute of Mental Health, have carried out extensive studies in rats, dogs, and monkeys ιo define the range of toxicity of the drug. The group used synthetic $\Delta^9$- and $\Delta^8$-THC and a crude marihuana extract (CME) of carefully defined composition. Delta-9-THC was found to be more potent than $\Delta^8$-THC; CME was less potent that a similar quantity of $\Delta^9$-THC.

Acute toxicity was studied using intravenous, intraperitoneal, and oral routes of administration in rats. An $LD_{50}$ similar to that reported by Phillips[458] was found by the intravenous route (20 mg/kg of THC) and intraperitoneal route (400 mg/kg) but higher values were noted with oral administration (1140 mg/kg). Interestingly the $LD_{50}$ for males was 1400 mg/kg while for females it was 700 mg/kg by the oral route. The minimal lethal dose orally was between 225 and 450 mg/kg.

An $LD_{50}$ was not attainable in monkeys and dogs by the oral route. Enormous dose levels (over 3000 mg/kg of $\Delta^9$-THC) were administered without lethality to most animals. A dose of about 1000 mg/kg THC was the lowest dose that caused death in any animal. The completeness of intestinal absorption of THC at these high doses is unknown. Behavioral changes in the survivors included sedation, huddled posture, muscle tremors, hypersensitivity to sound, and hypermobility.

The cause of death in the rats and mice subsequent to oral THC was profound CNS depression dealing to dyspnea, prostration, weight loss, loss of righting reflex, ataxia, and severe fall in body temperature, which led to cessation of respiration from 10 to 40 hours after single-dose oral administration. No consistent pathologic changes were observed in any organs. The cause of death in the higher species (though it rarely occurred) did not appear to be related to the same mechanism as in the rats.

In summary, enormous doses of $\Delta^9$-THC, $\Delta^8$-THC, and concentrated marihuana extract ingested by mouth were unable to produce death or organ pathology in large mammals but did produce fatalities in smaller rodents as a result of profound CNS depression.

The nonfatal consumption of 3000 mg/kg $\Delta^9$-THC by the dog and monkey would be comparable to a 154-pound human eating approximately 46 pounds (21 kg) of 1 percent marihuana or 10 pounds of 5 percent hashish at one time. In addition, 92 mg/kg THC administered intravenously produced no fatalities in monkeys. These doses would be comparable to a 154-pound human smoking almost 3 pounds (1.28 kg) of 1 percent marihuana at one time or 250,000 times the usual smoked dose and over a million times the minimal effective dose, assuming 50 percent destruction of the THC by smoking.

Thus evidence from animal studies and human case reports appears to indicate that the ratio of lethal dose to effective dose is quite large. This ratio is much more favorable than that of many other common psychoactive agents, including alcohol and barbiturates.[450,458]

## 3. Birth Defects

There is recent evidence that exposure of adult mice to $\Delta^9$-THC, CBN, or CBD can influence fertility and induce chromosomal alterations in the testes. Moreover, there is an indication that these effects of Cannabinoids can be carried into the next generation as indicated by decreased fertility and cytogenetic defects in the male offspring or treated sires. Furthermore, the observation of severe congenital defects (e.g. exencephaly, spina bifida) in the third generation of these treated mice suggests that cannabinoids may have a mertagenic potential.[460] Although $\Delta^9$-THC does cross the placenta, there is no evidence that it produces birth defects in humans. There is also no evidence in humans that marihuana affects fetal development. However, it is unwise to use any drug during the childbearing age, especially during pregnancy.

There are at least three isolated case reports[461–463] of birth defects in the offspring of parents who had used marihuana and LSD. However, due to their complex gestational histories and the high level of birth defects seen in a "normal" population, a causal relationship cannot be attributed to cannabis. At present, there is no substantial evidence indicating that marihuana at the dose commonly used is a teratogen in humans.

Marihuana at high doses has been implicated as a teratogen in animals by several groups. One study[464] showed reduced fertility in rats impregnated after being fed a diet containing marihuana extract for several months. However, the offspring were normal. The reduced fertility may be related to the finding of a marked decrease rate of cellular division, but without chromosomal damage, when $\Delta^9$- or $\Delta^8$-THC is added to white blood cell cultures.[465,466]

Dorrance[467] and Gilmore[468] detected no significant difference in lymphocyte chromosomes in groups of users and nonusers. No significant differences were found in lymphocyte chromosomes between heavy, long-term Jamaican ganja users and matched nonusers.[469]

Does marihuana cause chromosomal structure malformation or birth defects? In 1980 Cohen[470] pointed out that "*in vitro* animal and human examinations of chromosome morphology indicate that chromosomal anomalies do not occur. Furthermore, when multiple drugs are abused, the number of abnormal cells tend to be increased. Scattered reports of birth defects of children born of marihuana-smoking mothers are available. Whether the number of congenital anomalies exceeds the 'normal' incidence (1 in 50 live births) is not known."

## 4. Organic Brain Damage

Deterioration of mental functioning allegedly due to long-term use of marihuana can be subdivided into four major categories: organic brain damage, mental illness-psychosis, amotivational syndrome, and recurrent phenomena. As with alcoholism, it is often impossible to distinguish whether the described effects result from drug use or represent personality traits or changes that would have been present without the drug.

When marihuana consumption was irregular, mental deterioration was not evidenced[471] in 310 users with an average history of seven years of use. Sixty-seven heavy users in New York showed no evidence of dementia attributable to drug use, although they did have underlying personality disorders. Another investigation[44] of individuals who used a daily average of seven marihuana cigarettes (two to 18 range) for an average of eight years (2½ to 16 range) showed no evidence of brain damage or mental deterioration.

Reports from India[472,473] relate minor impairment of judgment and memory, limited self-neglect, and insomnia when potent preparations are consumed regularly in large amounts for many years. No evidence of mental deterioration or brain damage has been noted.

Miras[464] has described a Greek population of heavy hashish smokers who appear to be outcasts from the community after 15 to 20 years of heavy hashish use. They seem mentally sluggish and depressed. They are reported to exhibit laziness, psychic instability, amorality, and an apparent lack of drive and ambition. Their speech and behavior have been described as peculiar. Some degree of responsibility is retained in that some work to cover their living and drug purchasing expenses. Some of them are still quite intelligent. Memory is not affected, except during the intoxication. They appear overly suspicious. Samples of their electroencephalograms were believed to demonstrate abnormalities.

However, Miras believes that this effect is related to the quantity and frequency of hashish use. He describes three categories of long-term hashish users. Type A uses low doses intermittently and is socially and mentally unaffected.

Type B[1] uses low doses daily and no interference is caused in function. Type B[2] uses high doses daily, causing dependence and performance decrements. Type C uses very high doses daily, allegedly causing mental deterioration and abnormal behavior.

A British research report, which originally appeared in 1971, attributed brain atrophy to cannabis use in a group of young male users. In the original study, ten patients, with histories of from three to 11 years of marihuana use, were examined by air encephalography, a neurologic technique used to detect gross brain changes. The authors concluded that their findings suggested that regular use of cannabis may produce brain atrophy.[474] This research was faulted on the grounds that all of the patients had used other drugs, making the causal connection with marihuana use questionable; and that the appropriateness of the comparison group and diagnostic technique was questionable. The potential significance of the original observations justifies a brief review of several subsequent studies bearing on the original British observations.

In a study of chronic Greek users, a different technique (echoencephalography) was employed to determine whether brain atrophy might be present in heavy users. The findings from the Greek study were negative; that is, users were not found to differ from nonusers in evidence of gross brain pathology.[475]

Two studies were subsequently conducted in Missouri and Massachusetts,[476,477] in which two samples of young men with histories of heavy cannabis smoking were examined by computerized transaxial tomography (CTT), a brain-scanning technique for visualizing the anatomy of the brain. In both studies the resulting brain scans were read by experienced neuroradiologists independently of the drug histories. Neither showed any evidence of cerebral atrophy. However, several additional points should be stressed. Neither study rules out the possibility that more subtle and lasting changes of brain function may occur as a result of heavy and continued marihuana smoking. It is entirely possible to have impairment of brain function from toxic or other causes that is not apparent on gross examination of the brain in the living organism. Nevertheless, virtually no studies completed as of late 1979 showed evidence of chronically impaired neuropsychologic test performance in humans at experimental dose levels.

A researcher who used electrodes implanted deep within the brains of monkeys instead of more conventional scalp recording techniques found persistent changes related to chronic use.[478] This same investigator reported that rhesus monkeys administered marihuana smoke from one joint daily for five days per week for six months showed persistent microscopic changes in brain cellular structure following this treatment.[386] While both these experiments demonstrate the possibility that more subtle changes in brain functioning or structure may occur as a result of marihuana smoking in animals, the implications of these changes for subsequent human or animal behavior are not certain. Other studies, using more conventional EEG techniques to measure brain electrical activity, have found changes temporarily associated with acute use, but no evidence of persistently abnormal EEG findings related to chronic cannabis use.[479,480]

## 5. Acute Psychoses

Rare cases of full-blown acute psychotic episodes precipitated by marihuana use are reported in individuals with histories of mental disorder, with marginal psychologic adjustments, or with poorly developed personality structures and ego defenses.[480–492]

Marihuana intoxication may hinder the ability of these individuals to maintain structural defenses to existing stresses, or alternatively produce a keener awareness of personality problems or existing stresses.[446] Psychotherapy and antipsychotic medications are useful in controlling and preventing this reaction.[425]

Exceptionally rare reports from North America of nonspecific toxic psychosis or acute brain syndrome have occurred after extremely high drug dose consumption, although such reports are more common in eastern countries. The conditions are self-limited and clear spontaneously as the drug effect abates.[248,254,493–495,519]

Finally, marihuana intoxication may trigger delayed anxiety reactions or psychotic episodes in a small percentage of persons who have had prior experience with the hallucinogenic drugs.[248,496–498]

The acute psychomotor-cognitive effects of marihuana intoxication are academically interesting to gain understanding of normal and abnormal mental function as well as for practically determining the risk factor for the individual—including determination of his/her functional level personally, vocationally, and socially in society. The effect on personal–social–vocational function is highly individualized and difficult to predict at present.

Although reports of anxiety attacks and psychotic episodes have become more frequent as marihuana use has spread, they are still exceedingly rare. For example, during the nine-year period of 1961–1969, out of 701,057 admissions to Los Angeles County Hospital, located in a city with very high marihuana use, only three patients required hospitalization for psychic sequelae of marihuana smoking.[454] During the academic year 1968–1969, eight students were seen in the mental hygiene division of a private eastern university student population (8500) with acute anxiety reactions.[419] The frequency of marihuana-associated acute adverse anxiety reactions requiring attention at Boston University Student Health Service (student population 20,000) is between five and seven annually.[403]

In a survey of newly admitted patients to a large mental hospital, marihuana was the direct cause of the hospitalization in only 0.9 per 1000 admissions.[375]

## 6. Persistent Effects After Acute Dose

Investigators have not noted persistent effects after smoking marihuana for periods of more than three to five hours.[403] Users report only minimal hangover effects[500,501] after very heavy use. Feelings of lassitude and heaviness of the head, lethargy, irritability, headaches, and loss of concentration are reported, especially when associated with lack of sleep.[437,439] This may be related to preliminary data[502] suggesting a subtle increase in REM sleep time primarily seen in the last one third of the night in individuals who smoked one to two cigarettes per day, usually at night, for at least a year.

## 7. Special Toxicologic Developments

The development of a better method for quantifying the amount of marihuana in the smoke administered to subjects has contributed to more accurate evaluation of the toxicity of marihuana. In a study comparing the $LD_{50}$ for $\Delta^9$-THC administered by three different routes (inhalation, parenteral, and oral), toxicity by smoking was equal to that obtained by the intravenous route (I.V.)—40 mg/kg when the inhalation $LD_{50}$ dose of 105.7 mg/kg was corrected for $\Delta^9$-THC losses in the rodent nasal passages. Toxicity by intragastric lavage was 20–30 times lower, depending on the type of preparation used to administer the $\Delta^9$-THC (i.e., emulsion or oil solution).[503]

That the toxicity or behavioral effects of $\Delta^9$-THC are significantly related to the solvent used was also reported by others using the intraperitoneal (I.P.) and/or subcutaneous route of administration on rodents.[504,505] In general, aqueous suspensions or emulsions in polysorbate or polyvinylpyrrolidone were found to be better absorbed than the oily solutions. A new formulation for I.V. administration using Emulphor, which can be sterilized and injected in a relatively small volume, has been found.[506]

An extensive study of the physiochemical properties, solubility, and protein binding of $\Delta^9$-THC provides some clarification of these findings and has specific implications for the planning of future clinical and preclinical studies.[181] The authors found that the bioavailability of $\Delta^9$-THC is influenced by a number of factors: The instability in acid solution implies that the compound may be significantly degraded in the stomach. Extremely low water solubility suggests that its solubility in plasma may be rapidly exceeded, thus producing precipitation and accumulation in a "deep compartment" (i.e., the body organs). Rapid diffusion into plastic containers and rubber stoppers and significant binding to glass stress the need for more careful techniques in the handling, storage, and assay, in aqueous and biologic fluids, of this compound. Finally, the high degree of binding to the plasma lipoprotein fraction may result in great individual variability in binding, depending on individual and species variations in lipoprotein and fat content.[181]

Chronic toxicity of $\Delta^9$-THC administered orally for 180 days to Fisher rats at lower dose levels of 2, 10, and 50 mg/kg showed no morphologic changes attributable to $\Delta^9$-THC. The same pattern of fighting aggression and neurotoxicity described previously after chronic administration at higher dose levels[507] occurred in this study. Tremors and clonic seizures, appearing in cyclic fashion and peaking in weeks 12, 18, and 21, were dose related: 50 percent showed seizures after 50 mg/kg, and 6 percent after 10 mg/kg. Except for a rise in liver function test indexes (SGOT and SGPT) suggestive of pathology in the higher dose males, clinical chemistry and hematologic and urinalysis parameters were within normal ranges. Anorexia and diminished water consumption in conjunction with a declining growth rate occurred in the second and third weeks at the high dose level, but were later reversed.[508]

Previously reported differences in toxicity between males and females were also found in the studies discussed above. However, the nature of these differences is inconsistent: At times females were more affected than males, and vice versa.[507,508] On the other hand, pharmacologic studies indicate that female rats may be more sensitive to $\Delta^9$-THC than male rats, but that testosterone or castration, respectively, can reverse this effect.[509] The mechanism by which $\Delta^9$-THC produces toxicity in animals is still uncertain but it seems to be related to the rate of absorption and the concentration of the parent compound, $\Delta^9$-THC, rather than the metabolites in the target tissues. Harbison[504] has shown that pretreatment with phenobarbital-antagonized THC induced lethality whereas pretreatment with SKF-525A, a metabolic inhibitor, produced liver damage and a marked increase in THC-induced lethality.

New data on the effects of marihuana and tobacco smoke on human lung explants[510,511] confirmed previous findings from studies with mice, conducted by the same laboratory, that both marihuana and tobacco "evoke not only abnormalities in DNA synthesis, mitosis and growth of fibroblastic cells of human lung explants, but also result in alterations of DNA."[511] The finding that these changes are observed very early and persist for prolonged periods after exposure indicates that they are not lethal to cells. Additional preclinical studies are being undertaken to determine whether inhaled marihuana smoke plays a role similar to that of tobacco smoke in pulmonary carcinogenesis, but Leuchtenberger and his colleagues[510] caution that no conclusions should be drawn until the results of epidemilogic studies and chronic preclinical inhalation experiments with marihuana cigarettes are completed. Confirmation of a previous report that marihuana tar painted on mice produces metaplasia of the sebaceous glands that often correlates with carcinogenicity indicates the need for additional studies in this area.[510] The improved techniques for administering marihuana smoke to animals from higher species should aid in the study of long-term toxic effects of marihuana smoking.

Studies regarding the effects of marihuana on reproduction and development have continued. Effects on the mother and the young are definitely related to dose, route of administration, and species used. The data are further confounded by differences between species, probably related to their differences in metabolism (i.e., the results in studies with rats usually were negative at behaviorally effective dose levels[512–514] while experiments with rabbits and mice indicate they may be more sensitive, especially at very high dose levels).[515,516]

For limited acute toxicity studies of cannabinoids, a simple new biologic method using as an indicator the process of regeneration in planarian worms has been developed.[517] This method allows determination of the activity of very small amounts of cannabinoids and could be used with advantage in structure-activity-type or neurochemical-type studies. For a recent review of the toxicologic aspects of marihuana, the work of Nahas and Patton is recommended.[518]

## 8. Chronic Effects[l]

There is little scientific evidence that long-term marihuana use produces chronic organ toxicity, that is, chronic brain damage, and the like. Reports from India indicate that chronic heavy use of potent preparations such as charas (equivalent to hashish) may result in increased susceptibility to respiratory (asthma, bronchitis, etc.) and digestive ailments, but use of bhang (equivalent to our marihuana) does not.

Two psychiatrists published reports on patients that suggest that moderate to heavy marihuana use may lead to ego decompensation ranging from mild ego disturbances to psychosis.[431,519] Patients consistently showed very poor social judgment, poor attention span, poor concentration, confusion, anxiety, depression, apathy, passiveness, indifference, and often slowed and slurred speech. There was usually a loss of interest in personal appearance and previous goals. However, these studies were uncontrolled and no definite conclusions can be made as to the role that marihuana played.

Another recent study reported evidence of cerebral atrophy (permanent brain damage) in ten patients who had used marihuana for extended periods of time.[474] The exact role played by marihuana, however, is unknown, since all patients were polydrug users.

An interesting report of gynecomastia (enlarged breasts) in three male, chronic marihuana users was presented.[520] The patients were between the ages of 23 and 26 years and had been intensive users of marihuana for several years. No other reason for the enlarged breasts could be discovered, and it was suggested that it was related to heavy marihuana use.

### *a. Dependence of the Marihuana Type*

The term "cannabis dependence" has often been used in an imprecise way, with meanings ranging from a vague desire to continue use, if available, to the manifestation of physical withdrawal symptoms following its discontinuance. If "dependence" is defined as experiencing definite physical symptoms following withdrawal of the drug, there is now experimental evidence that such symptoms can occur, at least under conditions of extremely heavy research ward administration that are atypical of social marihuana use in the United States. The changes noted after drug withdrawal under these experimental conditions include one or more of the following symptoms: irritability, restlessness, decreased appetite, sleep disturbance, sweating, tremor, nausea, vomiting, and diarrhea.[521,522] Some of these symptoms were experienced in a similar research study by users who selected their own smoked marihuana doses.[523] Such a "withdrawal syndrome" thus far has been reported clinically in only one formal research report.

### *b. Tolerance Development of the Marihuana Type*

Tolerance to cannabis, defined as either diminished response to a given repeated drug dose or an enhanced response (reverse tolerance), is complex. Tolerance development was originally suspected because experienced overseas users were able to use large quantities of the drug that would have been toxic to American users generally accustomed to smaller amounts of the drug. Carefully conducted studies with known doses of marihuana or THC leave little question that tolerance develops with prolonged use.

The novice has a moderate degree of tolerance. With increasing exposure, tolerance appears to decrease, so that the occasional user has a low degree of tolerance and can smoke less to get the desired results. With increasingly heavy use, it rises again so a high degree of tolerance is developed and the user can smoke ten or more joints daily and get only mildly high. Withdrawal of the drug, especially in the chronic user, may evoke a psychic response in that the individual feels the need for the drug and will seek it or some substitute. The anxiety, restlessness, insomnia, and other nonspecific symptoms of withdrawal are similar to those experienced by compulsive cigarette smokers. However, in social settings withdrawal does not produce a physical reaction as seen with the opiates or the sedative drugs. In most cases, the fear of withdrawal is not strong enough to provoke criminal acts to obtain the drug. The chronic user, or pothead, may exhibit a loss of interest in socially acceptable pursuits such as school work or office work. This is the so-called amotivational syndrome. It is not certain, however, to what degree the amotivational syndrome is the result of marihuana use *per se* or of a tendency for those who lack conventional motivations to find drugs attractive. Nonetheless, many express serious concern that the chronic use of marihuana may jeopardize the social and economic adjustments of adolescents. The heavy chronic use of any psychoactive drug would appear to constitute a high-risk behavior in this group.

Several detailed reviews of tolerance development to the behavioral and physiologic effects of marihuana in both animals and humans have been published.[524–526] Hofmann[401] has discussed physical dependence and tolerance to cannabis. He states that:

> Regardless of the pattern of usage, there are no involuntary physiological disturbances that typically follow sudden cessation of *THC* usage; therefore, it is said that physical dependence on the effects of THC does not develop. Heavy users of THC would probably be quite unhappy if abruptly denied access to it; this reflects their psychological dependence on THC. That unhappiness could psychogenically trigger a variety of somatic complaints (e.g., headaches, stomach cramps, feelings of lassitude, and so on) that would vary in type and intensity from one user to another.
>
> We still do not know if tolerance to the effects of THC can develop, and we have three possibilities to consider: tolerance, no tolerance, and "reverse" tolerance.

In America, there is no clear-cut evidence that 1) with chronic use there is a continuous increase in the amounts of THC to obtain effects, and 2) experienced users can better withstand higher doses of marihuana than novice users. Hofmann[40] suggests that therefore the typical American user of marihuana does not seem to develop significant tolerance to the effects of THC.

However, there is data to suggest rapid development of tolerance to the increased-heart-rate effect of marihuana when large quantities are used.[408] Likewise, with heavy use of marihuana many individuals report a diminution of the subjective level of intoxication with continued use of the drug. In support of this are the findings of Nahas[527] using synhexyl, a synthetic analog of THC related to its chemistry and pharmacologic actions. In humans, Nahas[527] reported that within four to six days of daily administration of synhexyl, many requested larger doses to compensate for the gradually weakening effects.

Other studies indicating tolerance to the effects of long-term use of marihuana, such as the work of Nowlan and Cohen,[291] point out tolerance to both tachycardia and eurphorgenic effects.

The work of Weil and associates[528] points toward the ideation of "reverse" tolerance. Reverse tolerance is a condition whereby repeated use might lead to an "inverse" tolerance. In Weil's studies experienced users seemed to be able to get high on lower quantities of marihuana than those needed by naive users. This area of tolerance is still questionable in terms of mechanism of action.

McMillan et al.[529] have suggested that tolerance to $\Delta^9$-THC is a pharmacodynamic tolerance based on cellular mechanisms. From more recent work by this group of researchers, it seems reasonable to conclude that $\Delta^9$-THC tolerance is not a metabolic or drug dispositional tolerance. When comparing the metabolic responses of tolerant and nontolerant pigeons to an injection of $\Delta^9$-THC, it was found that tolerant pigeons respond to $\Delta^9$-THC at the same rate and with the same pattern as nontolerant pigeons.[530] The levels of $\Delta^9$-THC and its metabolites were as high in the blood of tolerant animals as they were in nontolerant animals. Dewey et al.[531] found that radiolabeled $\Delta^9$-THC produces similar levels of radioactivity in the brains of tolerant and nontolerant pigeons. Thus tolerance to $\Delta^9$-THC does not seem to be due to distributional differences that produce a decreased concentration of total cannabinoids in the brain.

Several researchers[532–534] have suggested that learning or drug behavior interactions play a role in the development of tolerance to $\Delta^9$-THC as they have been shown to do in the development of tolerance to other psychotropic drugs. It is possible that learned and pharmacodynamic tolerance to $\Delta^9$-THC are simply manifestations of similar underlying mechanisms as suggested by Kalant et al.[535] However, on the basis of the literature, it seems evident that learning mechanisms can account for some—although by no means all—characteristics of tolerance to Δ$^9$-THC.

The role of behavioral adjustments to marihuana-produced effects on learned behavior has been emphasized by Ferraro.[512] Briefly stated, this position suggests that behavioral tolerance to marihuana should occur only when the drug produces impairment in performance or alters the environment to the detriment of the organism. Even in these instances, tolerance should only occur if the organism can learn to make behavioral adjustments that counteract the adverse behavioral effects produced by the drug.

Manning[536] found that if Δ$^9$-THC acted to increase the number of shocks received by rats under an avoidance schedule, then tolerance developed within six days. However, if the effects of the drug were to decrease shock rate, tolerance did not develop within up to 45 days. It was found that within-session tolerance to the effects of Δ$^9$-THC on monkeys' DRL responding were not the result of mere exposure to the drug, but rather were dependent upon the monkeys responding under the influence of the drug. These data are consistent with the hypothesis that organisms must learn the behavioral adjustments to the effects of cannabinoids for tolerance to be manifested. Additional evidence that the opportunity to respond under the influence of Δ$^9$-THC is an important factor in the development of tolerance was provided by Carder and Olson.[537] Rats were trained to lever press for food or water reinforcement and given I.P. injections of marihuana extract (4.0 mg/kg. Δ$^9$-THC) either prior to or after behavioral testing. Rats that responded under the influence of the drug developed tolerance while those who had received Δ$^9$-THC outside of the test situation did not. A related set of Δ$^9$-THC findings was obtained in chimpanzees by Ferraro and Grilly.[538]

The amount of prior training on a learning task has been shown to influence directly the magnitude of the behavioral effects produced by Δ$^9$-THC[538] and the rate of tolerance developed to the drug.[539] Olson and Carder[539] found that rats trained to run an alley under the influence of an oral dose of marihuana extract (6.0 mg/kg Δ$^9$-THC) showed a very slow improvement in performance during training. Those rats that received the marihuana extract, after asymptotic performance had been achieved, exhibited an initial disruption under the drug, and then rapidly developed tolerance.

In contrast to the rapid Δ$^9$-THC tolerance that typically develops in animals performing simple behavioral tasks, a lack of tolerance has been reported in animals working on more complex behavioral tasks. Failure to observe tolerance in a study wherein monkeys worked on a complex schedule of reinforcement after oral administration of 2.0 mg/kg Δ$^9$-THC was attributed to the complexity of the tasks.[540] Further, it was implied that the difficulty of learning responses, which compensate for drug-produced impairments in performance, is an increasing function of the complexity of the baseline task used. A similar conclusion was reached by Ferraro and Grilly,[541] who failed to observe tolerance to oral doses of Δ$^9$-THC (1.0 and 4.0 mg/kg) in chimpanzees working long-delay matching-to-sample problems.

In one of a series of experiments on delayed matching-to-sample performance in chimpanzees, Ferraro et al.[542] determined that tolerance to Δ$^9$-THC does occur under delayed matching-to-sample baselines, but only if the delay interval used is short. Similarly, Grilly et al.[543] found that chimpanzees administered oral doses (1.0 mg/kg) of Δ$^9$-THC developed tolerance at specific delay values of a matching-to-sample task. This tolerance did not transfer when the delay interval was increased. These researchers argued that if compensatory responses are learned under Δ$^9$-THC, then they should be specific to the particular stimulus situation used and should be relatively permanent. In other words, tolerance to Δ$^9$-THC, once established in a specific stimulus situation, should be at least partially retained in that situation even after prolonged abstinence from the drug is enforced. This implication was investigated with chimpanzees who had already developed tolerance to Δ$^9$-THC when involved with a short-delay matching-to-sample problem.[542] These chimpanzees were first exposed to a long-delay problem, where no tolerance was observed, and then given additional training in a drugfree state. Complete tolerance to Δ$^9$-THC was observed when the chimpanzees were returned to the original short-delay problem and administered the same oral dose of Δ$^{9}$-THC (0.75 or 1.0 mg/kg).

The literature pertaining to Δ$^{9}$-THC tolerance suggests that both pharmacodynamic and behavioral factors are important determinants in the development of marihuana tolerance.

Smith and Mehl's[275] clinical observations of many marihuana smokers suggest a J-shaped time curve of tolerance to marihuana. A novice marihuana smoker often reports feeling no high or requiring considerably more drug to get high on the first few trials with the drug than after more experience is gained. This phenomenon has been called "reverse tolerance." The clinicians believed this represented "learning to get high" or acquiring the ability to appreciate or become sensitive to the subtle aspects of the intoxication.

Goode[544] found that more frequent and longer term marihuana smokers tend to require fewer joints to get high, but differences were not statistically significant. Weil et al.[248] reported that experienced users of marihuana achieved a high after being given the same dose as naive persons who did not experience a high but did demonstrate objective physiologic and psychomotor drug effects.

Meyer et al.[249] found that heavy marihuana users (daily for three years) were most sensitive to the high and required less marihuana to achieve a social high than infrequent intermittent users (use one to four times per month for less than two years). An increase in severity of symptoms after repeated administration of THC to rats was reported by Phillips et al.[458] This "sensitization" may be a correlate of reverse tolerance.

Lemberger et al.[545] supplied additional evidence for reverse tolerance based on the intravenous administration of 0.5 mg of THC to experimental subjects. Naive subjects experienced no effect from this small dose. However, daily marihuana users, who were told they were receiving a nonpharmacologically active dose of THC, reported a marihuana high that lasted up to 90 minutes. Lemberger et al.[209] and Mechoulam[68] suggested the possibility that enzymes necessary to convert THC to a more active compound require prior use of marihuana.

Reverse tolerance is a complex phenomenon. Jones[277] presented evidence that stressed the importance of expectation, setting, and prior drug experience in learning to get high. As the user gains more experience with marihuana, the more the user's mind is able to respond to the expectation of the high by actually becoming high when given an inert material that smells and looks like marihuana.

Weil[546] believes that the capacity to get high is an inherent characteristic of one's mind. He says that marihuana facilitates the user's ability to achieve this altered state of consciousness.

Mendelson et al.[420] did not find evidence of reverse tolerance. In fact, the daily users were more likely than the intermittent users to smoke two cigarettes per occasion. Both groups had an average of five years of marihuana use. Several other investigators obtained no evidence of reverse tolerance after repetitive daily use in experienced subjects.[499,547]

In summary, since marihuana's metabolites (the transformation products that result as marihuana is metabolized) are persistent in body fat, it is also possible that repeated low-dosage use releases some of the previously stored material, enhancing the effects. Whatever the ultimate explanation of earlier impressions is, it seems that under conditions of heavier, more regular use, tolerance is well established.

### *c. Miscellaneous Chronic Effects of Marihuana*

One subject of debate is the amotivational syndrome described earlier as being the loss of drive, the increase in passivity, and the sluggish mentation of certain, but not all, chronic users. Cohen[547] succinctly points out "that large amounts of cannabis have a depressant effect upon the CNS, and equivalent amounts of alcohol or sedatives also would produce a decreased desire to work, poor performance, and a blunted emotional response. One difference is that THC is retained in the brain lipid phase for long periods because of its aqueous insolubility." In this regard, however, sufficient drive will overcome marihuana sedation whereas low drive levels will be overwhelmed by the drug.

With regard to cannabis-induced cerebral atrophy, Heath et al.[386] observed specific abnormal EEGs in monkeys. Postmortem examination of the limbic system in monkeys receiving marihuana indicated serious microscopic neuronal alterations.

A number of researchers have addressed themselves to earlier reports that $\Delta^9$-THC may produce physical dependence and abstinence in monkeys[548,549] and that monkeys will self-administer $\Delta^9$-THC. While the details of the experimental procedures vary in these studies, the fundamental approach is the same. Animals are first given forced exposure to $\Delta^9$-THC and then are tested to determine whether they will self-administer the drug or prefer the drug over a nondrug substance.

In one of these studies, monkeys prepared with indwelling jugular catheters were used to determine whether they would self-administer $\Delta^9$-THC.[550] A number of different procedures to induce self-administration were used. Among them were the substitution of $\Delta^9$-THC after the monkeys had been trained to respond for cocaine, gradually transferring the animals from a cocaine–THC mixture to THC alone, and infusing the monkeys for 30 days with 2.0 mg/kg $\Delta^9$-THC. In no instance did the animals self-administer $\Delta^9$-THC or show signs of withdrawal at the termination of a forced drug regimen.

Leite and Carlini performed four experiments with rats and concluded that rats do not self-administer a cannabis extract, nor do they show abstinence symptoms after prolonged ingestion of the drug.[551] In the longest experiment, rats were forced to drink a cannabis extract for 126 days. At various points in the drug regimen, the rats were withdrawn from the drug for up to 96 hours, and then were given a choice between the cannabis extract and a control solution. As in the other Leite and Carlini[551] experiments, the rats preferred the control solution and showed no behavioral symptoms of abstinence.

Two additional experiments demonstrated that rats and mice are reluctant to consume cannabinoid preparations. Rats forced to drink a hashish suspension for over 30 days rejected the drug when water was made available.[552] Maker et al.[553] found mice reluctant to consume food pellets containing $\Delta^9$-THC (5.0 mg/kg), even after subsisting on the pellets for over two months.

In addition, two long-term behavioral experiments failed to yield evidence of residual effects following termination of $\Delta^9$-THC administration. In one of these,[428] chimpanzees were administered oral doses of 1.0 mg/kg for five consecutive months on a delayed matching-to-sample baseline. In the second experiment,[554] the schedule-controlled operant responding in chimpanzees was drugged aperiodically with doses of marihuana extract over a seven-month period.

On the other hand, two reports suggest that dependence and abstinence symptoms may be produced by $\Delta^9$-THC. Two monkeys were treated orally for 50 days with 37.5 mg/kg $\Delta^9$-THC.[555] Upon termination of the drug treatment, both monkeys showed increased aggressiveness, and one exhibited "hallucinations." In another study, Hirschhorn and Rosencrans[556] treated rats for a five-week period with I.P. doses of $\Delta^9$-THC ranging from 8.0 mg/kg to 32.0 mg/kg. The rats exhibited narcotic-like withdrawal symptoms, including diarrhea, teeth chatter, "wet-dog" shakes, salivation, and ptosis. The existing literature clearly suggests that animals will voluntarily self-administer marihuana compounds only with reluctance, if at all. These findings conflict with the well-established widespread ingestion of marihuana by humans. It is hoped that further research on the reinforcing properties of marihuana in animals may serve to elucidate some of the factors that lead to the initiation and/or continued use of marihuana by humans.

One hypothesis in this regard is that marihuana is not reinforcing in and of itself, but instead produces secondary effects that indirectly reinforce humans. The experiments cited, which state that marihuana can produce state-dependent learning and can serve as the basis for discrimination learning, contribute to the likelihood of such a hypothesis. The research establishes that marihuana ingestion produces stimuli that are discriminable. Consequently these stimuli are available for conditioning to other events, including reinforcing ones.

It was concluded that the development of marihuana tolerance is influenced by both pharmacodynamic and learning factors. The cellular mechanisms underlying pharmacodynamic tolerance remain to be specified. And the compensatory responses to the deleterious effects of marihuana—which are presumed to be learned while responding under its influence—still need to be empirically identified. In this latter context, if it is to be assumed that organisms learn compensatory responses when suitable, then it should be possible to demonstrate that they do so (and develop tolerance) in situations designed explicitly to provide for compensatory behavior. Alternatively, no tolerance should be observed in situations designed specifically to block the acquisition of learned compensatory behavior. Given that such demonstrations are successful, a behavioral analysis of tolerance could help to account for some of the inconsistencies reported in the literature concerning the development of marihuana tolerance in humans. For example, learning mechanisms might, in part, account for the differences in performance obtained between ''marihuana-naive'' and ''marihuana-experienced'' human smokers when they are tested under the influence of marihuana during demanding real-life simulation tasks.

## I. PATTERNS OF MARIHUANA USE AND MISUSE[401,557]

### 1. Psychosocial Aspects

Within a relatively few years, marihuana usage has become widespread and, perhaps more important for the future, public attitudes toward marihuana have become more accepting. Even the legal institutions have demonstrated an increasing tolerance through statutory accommodation in ten states and a relaxation of the enforcement of existing statutes in other locales. By 1975 some observers were already interpreting these trends as irreversible: ''One thing is unmistakably clear: marihuana use is now a fact of American life''[558]; and ''Marijuana use will probably become a cultural norm within a few years for persons under 30.''[559] How quickly this transition has actually occurred is indicated by Akers'[560] recent description of the American scene, a description that would have elicited sharp disbelief even as recently as the late 1960s: ''Marijuana is smoked in an offhand, casual way . . . Before, during, or after sports events, dates, public gatherings, parties, music festivals, class or work will do; there is no special place, time, or occasion for marijuana smoking. The acceptable places and occasions are as varied as those for drinking alcohol.''

Such a description does not apply, of course, to all segments of the U.S. population or to all parts of the country. But it suggests that we are witnessing one aspect of cultural change that parallels others, including a relaxing of sexual attitudes and behavior. Whether the change will be an enduring one and whether the use of marihuana will, as with alcohol, become fully institutionalized in U.S. society is still a matter of considerable speculation and debate.

Ray[561] points out that, according to careful evaluation and epidemiologic surveys, marihuana has more or less become ''embedded in American culture.''

Research to date[557] suggests that social interaction and/or peer pressure of friends play a critical role in patterns of drug use, especially marihuana. However, others such as Huba et al.[562] suggest that the role that peers play in relation to marihuana use appears to be no different from the role they play in relation to various other domains—values, sexual behavior, styles of dress.

With regard to marihuana use and personality, users of marihuana differ from nonusers in a cluster of attributes reflecting their attitudes toward conventionality, tradition, and conformity. A second generalization about personality differences is that users tend to be more open to experience, more esthetically oriented, and more interested in creativity, play, novelty, and spontaneity.[563–570] These attributes are not unrelated to the preceding cluster, but what is emphasized more is a cognitive style of receptivity to uncertainty and change as against an emphasis on familiarity and inflexibility. Since marihuana is often sought specifically to initiate change in mood or outlook, this linkage with a general interest in sensation or experience seeking[6,65,571] is a logical one.

The connection between marihuana use and the use of other drugs, both licit and illicit, is well established in nearly all studies that assess a variety of drugs. Further, the greater the involvement with marihuana or the frequency of its use, the greater is the experience with other drugs.

In terms both of order of onset and prevalence of use, marihuana emerges as a "boundary" drug between the licit drugs, such as tobacco and alcohol, and the illicit drugs. This key position of marihuana in a developmental sequence has raised the question of whether it serves as a "stepping-stone" to other illicit drugs. What the stepping-stone notion implies is that experience with marihuana has inexorable implications for progressing to other illicit drugs. Although this issue cannot simply be dismissed,[572,573] and it is likely that engaging in the use of an illicit drug such as marihuana can stimulate the exploration of other illicit drugs, several considerations militate against assigning a "causal" role to marihuana use. First, the proportion of the population that has used marihuana is far greater than that with experience with any of the other illicit drugs; thus there is no inexorable progression. Second,[574] there has been an appreciable rise in marihuana use among youths in recent years without any concomitant increase in the proportion using other illicit substances. Third, it is logical to consider that the same factors that determined the use of marihuana may also influence the use of other illicit drugs, rather than that the influence on those other drugs necessarily stemmed from marihuana use itself. And finally, assigning cause to an antecedent permits an infinite regression in which it could be argued, for example, that since alcohol preceded marihuana, it is the more fundamental cause of other illicit drug use.[575]

According to social scientists, a salutary shift from an unsuccessful policy of prohibition to a policy of regulation might have greater relevance for the minimization of marihuana abuse.

## 2. Prevalence and Multiple Drug Usage

The overall use and/or abuse of marihuana continues to grow yearly, with the 12-to-25-year-old age group showing the highest prevalence. It has been seriously noted that approximately 10 percent of high school seniors surveyed smoked marihuana at least once a day. Preoccupation with this drug has in some cases resulted in poor grades as well as other psychological impairments.

Cannabinoid users are known to also abuse other psychoactive agents. However, sometimes unknowingly in the street they purchase contaminated "bags" of marihuana. PharmChem Laboratories, a San Francisco-based street detection organization, has found in these bags a variety of foreign substances—such as oregano, catnip, LSD, methamphetamine, PCP, strychnine, and atropine (or stramonium leaves containing atropine). These may induce unexpected, untoward effects in the user.[576,403] There are even allegations without evidence that marihuana "bags" have contained both heroin and cocaine.

The National Commission on Marihuana found that alcohol and tobacco were the two substances most commonly used with marihuana. Among those surveyed, 54 percent were concurrent cigarette smokers and 68 percent were concurrent alcohol users.

## 3. Special Marihuana Research

Cohen,[577] in discussing recent marihuana research, pointed out that, following alcohol, marihuana is the most widely used mind-altering substance. Furthermore, he states that in the United States 25 percent of the population have tried marihuana at least once, and between three and five million are daily users.

In this regard, penalties for simple possession are being reduced and vociferous proponents of ''pot'' advocate legalization. For a drug that has been around for millenia, reliable information is surprinsingly scanty. Aside from a few earlier studies, the scientific investigation of this plant is only about six years old. A report of the recent research findings seems worthwhile to develop an informed opinion about the social and medical issues involved.

### *a. The Plant*

When cannabis is kept at room temperature or exposed to light, the THC slowly changes to cannabinol, which is thought to be the end metabolite in the plant. In animals the first metabolite is 17-hydroxy-THC and it is biologically active.

Current typical THC values for various materials are as follow:

| | |
|---|---|
| Street THC | 0.0 percent THC |
| Fiber-type cannabis | 0.05 percent THC |
| Drug-type cannabis | 1.0–4.0 percent THC |
| Hashish (resin) | 10.0 percent THC |
| Red oil (cannabis distillate) | 20.0 percent THC |

The flowering tops and bracts contain the highest percentage of THC, leaves have a lesser amount, and seeds, stems, and roots contain negligible quantities. Contrary to the ancient lore, the male plant is as potent as the female. It is removed from cultivated areas to prevent fertilization and loss of THC.

### *b. Pharmacology*

The most recent research has indicated that no evidence exists of organ damage attributable to cannabis. However, chronic bronchitis has been noted in some regular users. The question of pulmonary carcinogenicity is still being researched.

Recent studies have indicated that marihuana in ordinary amounts induces feelings of relaxation, drowsiness, hunger, intensified sensory perceptions, emotional lability, and euphoria. Larger doses induce illusions, pseudo-hallucinations, paranoid delusions, depersonalization, driving decrements, and impairment of memory. With regard to ''flashbacks,'' this type of phenomenon is much less frequent with marihuana use than with the LSD-type hallucinogenic agents. However, another type of flashback may occur when a person takes marihuana some time after having had LSD.

In terms of chronic use, research findings reveal that long-term marihuana use may precipitate a prolonged psychotic schizophrenic reaction in predisposed individuals, but no real specific cannabis psychosis has been discovered in the United States.

The most current research findings on the cannabinoids can be found in the book entitled *Cannabinoids 82* edited by Agurell, Willette, and Dewey.[578] Areas covered in this volume include recent research of notable scientists from around the world in chemistry,[579–585] metabolism,[586–589] reproduction,[590–656] neuropharmacology,[140,597–600] pulmonary cytogenicity,[603] and kinetics.[604]

## J. THERAPEUTIC USES OF CANNABIS

A ''fringe benefit'' of the past decade's marihuana research has been a renewed interest in its potential as a therapeutic agent. Throughout history cannabis has been used in many parts of the world as a pharmaceutic preparation. As recently as 1937, tinctures of cannabis were still listed in the United States *Pharmacopoeia* and presumably were being used therapeutically. One limitation of the earlier preparations was the extreme variability of drug potency—ranging from inert, or nearly so, to unexpectedly potent.

Renewed interest in the potential usefulness of cannabis or of some synthetically related drugs has led to experimentation with them for a wide range of symptoms and disorders. Although several of these applications have shown promise, much remains to be learned about even those showing the greatest potential.

It is evident that cannabis itself will not be officially accepted by the U.S. Food and Drug Administration. It contains over 400 identified chemical entities, the great majority of which are unnecessary, or even undesirable, for any therapeutic activity. What is much more likely is that $\Delta^9$-THC, cannabidiol, or some synthetic variant will turn out to be the approved drug for specific therapeutic purposes.

## 1. Glaucoma

Since the original observation that marihuana is capable of reducing intraocular pressure (IOP), numerous subsequent research reports have substantiated it. At present, marihuana-related drugs have been shown to be capable of reducing IOP in people with glaucoma, alone and in combination with more conventional antiglaucoma medications. However, the long-term safety and efficacy of marihuana-related drugs administered chronically to glaucoma patients has not been established, nor are there any data from long-term controlled studies to demonstrate whether these preparations can actually preserve visual function in such individuals.

Oral $\Delta^9$-THC was used in 10- to 20-mg doses in 15 glaucoma patients.[614] When given alone, the drug was variably successful. When administered as a supplement to previously insufficiently effective medical treatment to eight patients, it was effective in five and partially effective in one. The psychic side effects were minor. Green et al.[606] have attempted to explain the mechanisms of action as a beta-adrenergic stimulation by $\Delta^9$-THC that dilates the efferent blood vessels of the anterior uvea. Alpha-adrenergic stimulation may also participate in the effect by reducing capillary pressure in the afferent vessels of the ciliary process. Those effects might be modulated through an inhibition of prostaglandin synthetase.[607]

Furthermore, $\Delta^8$-THC is at least as efficacious as the $\Delta^9$-analog, and it is less psychoactive; therefore, it may be preferable as an antiglaucoma preparation. Nabilone, a synthetic analog, also produces few psychic effects and reduces the average IOP by 35 percent in glaucoma patients in oral doses of 0.5 mg. Topical nabilone will induce an equivalent ocular hypotension in the rabbit, but the eye-drop preparation has been found irritating in humans. Except for its use as an ophthalmic topical preparation, nabilone is not being actively investigated because some dogs developed seizures and some humans manifested neurotoxicity.

Although formal studies have not yet been conducted on the issue, it appears from clinical notations that the effective cannabinoids show an additive effect when they are given with conventional antiglaucoma medications such as pilocarpine and acetazolamide (Diamox). This line of investigation might provide important clinical data in the future.

Continued work in both basic[608] and clinical[609] research is certainly warranted. As with other clinical applications, a synthesized drug with fewer of the side effects found with the natural material ultimately may prove more useful. Continued clinical trials to determine the most useful combinations with other drugs could be of value.

## 2. Asthma

Delta-9-THC is the major bronchodilator in cannabis, but it is a tracheobronchial irritant when smoked. Swallowed $\Delta^9$-THC has an antiasthmatic action, but it is delayed and unreliable due to variable absorption from the gastrointestinal tract. Tashkin and associates[610] developed a freon aerosol spray that was successful in producing bronchodilation in nonasthmatic subjects but caused irritation in asthmatic patients. Williams et al.[611] reported significant airway dilation in 100 percent asthmatic patients using 0.2 mg of an aerosolized $\Delta^9$-THC preparation.

A discouraging aspect of using cannabis for lung disorders is the finding that the smoke, like tobacco, contains carcinogens, cocarcinogens, and cilia-toxic components.[612] As with tobacco, skin tumors have been produced on mouse skin using coal tars from cannabis. Pulmonary macrophage inhibition after exposure of rats to marihuana smoke has been found.[613] Intrapulmonary bacterial inactivation to *Staphylococcus aureus* occurred in a dose-dependent manner. The cytotoxin in marihuana is not $\Delta^9$-THC but other constituents of the smoke. Impairment of the pulmonary defense system may be clinically significant by decreasing resistance to bacterial pulmonary infections.

Oral $\Delta^9$-THC offers no advantages over available antiasthmatic preparations, especially in the light of the cardiac-accelerating and sometimes unpleasant psychic effects of cannabis.

Finally, it is unknown whether an effective aerosol spray of THC can be developed. Natural or synthetic cannabinoids may prove to be more effective than THC with fewer side effects.

## 3. Control of Nausea in Cancer Chemotherapy

Use of marihuana, THC, or related drugs for the treatment of the extreme nausea and vomiting that often accompany cancer chemotherapy is probably the single most promising application of these drugs. While by no means invariably effective, they are sometimes valuable when other standard antinausea drugs are not. One of the earlier studies done in 1970 found that THC-treated cancer chemotherapy patients showed improved appetite and diminished weight loss.[614] A subsequent study done in Boston found that when compared with a placebo—that is, an inert substance—in a double-bind study in which neither patients nor physicians knew which drug was being administered, THC had an antiemetic effect in seven out of ten patients. The placebo-treated patients showed no improvement.[615] In one recent study of 15 patients receiving methotrexate for bone cancer, THC or placebo was randomly assigned. Fourteen of the 15 patients showed improvement following the use of THC. The amount of reduction in nausea and vomiting was closely related to the dose of THC given. At the highest THC dose employed, in 6 percent of the treatment sessions, patients experienced nausea and/or vomiting, compared with 44 percent when half the dosage was used. Such adverse symptoms were found in 72 percent of the sessions in which the pharmacologically inert placebo was employed. In a second phase of the same experiment, four patients who had shown excellent therapeutic response in the first phase were again treated with THC, but this time much less favorable results were achieved. The reasons for this are unclear, although the authors suggest the possibility that these patients developed a tolerance to the effect during the first phase of the experiment.[616] Other studies have attempted to compare marihuana-related drugs with other standard antinausea medication to determine their relative effectiveness. Nabilone, a drug chemically related to marihuana constituents, was compared with prochlorperazine, a standard antinausea drug, in a series of 113 patients receiving cancer chemotherapy. Eighty percent responded to nabilone, compared with 32 percent who responded to prochlorperazine.[617] Use of this experimental drug has been suspended, however, because of toxic effects observed in dogs.

A partial analysis of the responses of the first 66 patients in a series of 200 receiving prochlorperazine and THC in an experimental design in which each patient received trials of both found each was preferred by equal numbers (25), 12 had no preference, and four patients did not respond to the question. Sleepiness was the most common side effect of both drugs.[618]

Gross et al.[619] found that $\Delta^9$-THC did not significantly alter anorexia nervosa in a study on 11 patients comparing THC with diazepam.

The most recent work of McCarthy and colleagues[620] at Dartmouth Medical School revealed that the significantly altered chemically induced (cisplatin) vomiting in a cat bodes further support for its possible therapeutic value in the treatment of generalized emesis in humans.

## 4. Epilepsy

In general, antiseizure activity has been demonstrated to electrically induced, audiogenic, and pentylenetetrazol seizures.[621] The anticonvulsant profile resembles that of phenytoin (Dilantin) more than that of phenobarbital. Antiepileptic effects were obtained in amygdaloid-kindled rats with $\Delta^8$-THC and $\Delta^9$-THC.[622] Both isomers acutely suppressed kindled seizures, but consistent effects were obtained only with subtoxic doses. Repeated dosages of the cannabinoids resulted in tolerance development to the anticonvulsant action.

The hope that $\Delta^9$-THC might play a role in certain seizure disorders has been tempered by the reports of its convulsant properties in some animal species. Patterns of convulsive-like activity have been reported in EEGs of rodents, dogs, cats, rabbits, and monkeys.[623] In addition, behavioral convulsions have been reported at high doses in rats, dogs, and monkeys. Delta-

8-THC, SP-111A, cannabinol, and 11-hydroxy-$\Delta^9$-THC also produced convulsive episodes, but cannabidiol did not. Tolerance to the development of seizures occurred over a period of four to ten days. After a week without exposure to the cannabinoids, sensitivity to behavioral seizures was reinstated. Feeney[623] has obtained comparable results in two other species: in the naturally epileptic beagle dog and in cats with focal epilepsy induced by injections of alumina cream. He has also reported temporal lobe seizures and myoclonus in dogs given a single oral dose of 5 mg/kg. The fact that $\Delta^9$-THC has both convulsant and anticonvulsant effects is unique.

Cannabidiol (CBD), basically devoid of psychoactivity, is at least as effective as $\Delta^9$-THC as an antiseizure drug.[624] Insofar as synthetic analogs are concerned, Mechoulam and Carlini[625] prepared a series of oxygenated CBD derivatives and found that both the 6-oxo-CBD diacetate congener and CBD effectively protected mice from transcorneal electroshock convulsions. Finally, a survey of young epileptic patients who smoked marihuana revealed no particular effect of their cannabis use upon the seizure patterns.[626]

### 5. Antitumor Activity

In itself, $\Delta^9$-THC cannot be considered an effective antitumor agent despite an attractive differential in inhibition of tritiated thymidine into DNA between Lewis lung tumor cells and bone marrow cells.[627] The possibility remains that certain cannabinoids may prove to be useful as adjuncts to other chemotherapeutic agents. The impression that $\Delta^9$-THC and $\Delta^8$-THC are inferior to known antineoplastic drugs is reinforced by the equivocal findings of Friedman,[628] who did not find inhibition of thymidine-$^3$H incorporation into DNA, leucine-$^3$H uptake into protein, or cytidine-$^3$H into RNA in his *in vivo* Lewis lung carcinoma study.

### 6. Antibiotic Action

It has been found that $\Delta^9$-THC and cannabinol (CBN) are bacteriostatic or bacteriocidal against staphyllococci and streptococci *in vitro*.[629] When horse serum was introduced into a broth culture, it was noted that the antibacterial activity was essentially eliminated. Presumably binding of the CBN and $\Delta^9$-THC to plasma proteins could have accounted for the inactivation. They were ineffective against Gram-negative organisms. The possible clinical role of topical cannabis preparations as effective antibiotics requires additional investigation.

### 7. Antianxiety and Sleep-Inducing Effects

Like other sedatives, cannabis prolongs barbiturate sleeping time, reduces REM sleep periods, and may increase stage IV sleep[631]; REM rebound could occur after abrupt discontinuation of the drug. Neu et al.[632] found that, when used as a hypnotic, it decreased sleep latency with fewer awakenings. Doses of 10, 20, or 30 mg of $\Delta^9$-THC tended to produce hangover effects in some subjects. In a second study utilizing 5, 10, and 15 mg of $\Delta^9$-THC, 500 mg of chloral hydrate, or a placebo, no particular differences in sleep latency or duration were observed among the various drug schedules.

Work by Musty[633] reveals that cannabidiol similarly possesses possible anxiolytic properties.[633] Cannabis users occasionally relate that the prime reason that they use the drug is to relax, unwind, or decrease tensions. A few find it helpful in falling asleep. The sedative effect occurs most frequently; however, anxiety and dysphoria are also reported. This is especially true when intravenous $\Delta^9$-THC is taken, but it is also seen during oral ingestion and smoking. Somnolence is also listed as a side effect in many of the research studies in which sedation was not desired.

### 8. Muscle Relaxant

Only individual case reports are available to suggest a muscle relaxant effect of cannabis, and animal models for neuromuscular spasm have been rarely used.[634] A significant decrease of both twitch and tetanic contractions of the gastrocnemius muscle of adult mice following supermaximal stimulation of the sciatic nerve after chronic $\Delta^9$-THC treatment has been demonstrated.

When ten paraplegics were questioned[635] about the effects of their marihuana use upon symptoms, four reported a decrease in phantom pain sensations and five mentioned a decrease in muscle spasticity; three noted no improvement and two did not have significant spasticity. The results of smoking also had an inconsistent effect upon bladder spasms.

Fourteen patients with either lower motor neuron lesions due to spinal cord trauma or multiple sclerosis were said to have a reduced muscle spasticity in connection with their cannabis use.[636] Neurologic examinations before and after cannabis smoking showed evidence of decreased clonus and muscle spasticity.

## 9. Preanesthetic

The possibility that $\Delta^9$-THC could be employed as a preanesthetic agent has been explored by Smith and Kulp.[637] However, because of its cardiac-accelerating property, it is undesirable to use it prior to surgery.

## 10. Pain

The folk use of cannabis includes numerous references to its pain-allaying qualities. It was traditionally given for toothache, dysmenorrhea, difficult childbirth, neuralgia, and rheumatism in those lands where it grew wild.

Preclinical tests in general confirm an analgesic property by demonstrating an elevation of pain thresholds and an attenuation of the escape response to painful stimuli.[638] Delta-9-THC was found to be equipotent to morphine in some tests (hot plate, acetic acid writhing), but not in others (paw pressure).[639] Similarly, Cooler and Gregg[640] were unable to demonstrate an analgesic effect of $\Delta^9$-THC in human volunteers as measured by periosteal pressure stimulation or by cutaneous pair thresholds utilizing intravenous doses of 1.5 and 3 mg of $\Delta^9$-THC, 10 mg of diazepam, or a placebo.

Cancer patients requiring analgesics were treated with either a placebo or $\Delta^9$-THC, 10 or 20 mg orally, by Noyes et al.[641] It was concluded from the study that $\Delta^9$-THC is a mild analgesic. In a dose of 20 mg it was prohibitively sedating and intoxicating. The 10-mg dose only rarely presented such problems. Blurred vision and impaired thinking were also recorded. Appetite stimulation, mood elevation, and feelings of relaxation were occasionally noted.

Butler and Regelson,[642] in a broad study of $\Delta^9$-THC effects on advanced cancer patients, found no appreciable antipain response to 0.15 and 0.3 mg/kg of $\Delta^9$-THC as compared with a placebo. It was found that much of the analgesic effect of $\Delta^9$-THC was in its 11-hydroxy metabolite.[643] The 9-nor derivative that cannot form 11-hydroxy compounds *in vivo* does not possess analgetic action. Synthesis of 9-nor-9-β-hydroxyhexahydrocannabinol proved it to be a potent analgesic approximately equivalent to morphine. Harris[644] attempted to reverse the 9-nor-9-β-hydroxyhexahydrocannibinol antinociceptive effect with naloxone and was not able to reverse its activity completely; nor could cross-tolerance between this compound and morphine be demonstrated. However, in more recent work Kaymakcalaw[645] provided strong evidence that $\Delta^9$-THC has opiumlike effects.[645]

## 11. Antidepressant Action

Cannabis has been used for melancholia in many cultures in which it is a folk medicine. Pyrahexyl (Synhexyl) was used by physicians during the 1950s to treat depression; in fact, Parker and Wrigley's[646] study may have been the first in which a double-blind design was used with a cannabinoid. The results of this study were negative. Kotin et al.[647] did not find any difference from a placebo in their one-week study using 0.3 mg/kg of $\Delta^9$-THC in depressed patients. Many antidepressant drugs require longer periods of time before their therapeutic effect becomes discernible.

The studies performed on the amelioration of nausea and vomiting in cancer patients may be able to make a contribution to the question of an antidepressant action. Regelson et al.[614] found that $\Delta^9$-THC acted as a mood elevator and tranquilizer as measured by the Zung test. Decisive studies of unipolar and bipolar depressions utilizing $\Delta^9$-THC have not yet been done.

### 12. Alcoholism and Drug Dependence

Studies in animals reveal that THC can alter acute ethanol actions[648] as well as chronic alcohol abstinence.[649] The use of marihuana as a reward for certain alcoholics to stay on disulfiram (Antabuse) has been suggested by Rosenberg et al.[650] No drug interaction appears to occur between the two substances. However, cannabis alone or in combination with disulfiram was not particularly effective in inducing alcoholics to enter or remain in treatment. Some evidence exists that cannabis and alcohol produce cross-tolerance. Similarly, acute and chronic effects of cannabis on opiate actions have been reviewed by Siemans.[648]

Considering the past literature, the value of finding a new detoxification agent to ameliorate opiate withdrawal is not an important clinical need. A more important issue is whether the psychoactive cannabinoids interpose at the endorphin binding sites. This point is not yet settled.

## K. SUMMARY

According to Cohen,[654] 12 categories of symptoms or of disease states have been considered in relation to a potential ameliorative effect of cannabis or one of its derivatives. To summarize the state of the art insofar as the cannabinoids' role as therapeutic agents is concerned is difficult, but an overall impression will be attempted here.

Not only the effectiveness of the drug, but also the need for new treatment products, will be considered in the evaluation.

### 1. Indications

#### *a. Glaucoma*

An acceptable topical preparation will benefit certain patients not helped by the conventional medications. It will have to contain less than 0.5 percent of $\Delta^9$-THC. A superior synthetic analog may be found.

#### *b. Asthma*

Elucidating the mechanism of action of the cannabinoids may be more important than attempting to produce a nonirritating aerosol.

#### *c. Antiemetic*

It appears that cannabis has definite, but not invariable, antinauseant and antiemetic capabilities. It is at least comparable to standard antiemetics, and may offer relief to those who are currently not benefitted by them. Combinations of cannabis and the standard drugs used for vomiting should be tried in future studies.

#### *d. Epilepsy*

Cannabidiol deserves further clinical trials in humans as an anticonvulsant alone or with established antiseizure drugs.

#### *e. Tumor Growth Inhibition*

Although of interest, it does not appear that the cannabinoids will make a contribution in this area. What may be of concern is that tumor growth inhibitors are invariably cellular toxins to normal cells, depending on the dosage, since they interfere with cellular metabolism. Therefore $\Delta^9$-THC should be studied further for a possible cytotoxic effect in dosage levels used by humans.

#### *f. Topical Antibiotics*

The earlier Czechoslovakian work requires confirmation utilizing double-blind procedures and appropriate controls.

#### *g. Antianxiety and Insomnia*

While the cannabinoids seem to have sedative-hypnotic activity, they are inconstant and not comparable to existing medications for that purpose. Sometimes paradoxic anxiety and panic states intervene.

*h. Muscle Relaxant*

Although the work is quite preliminary, the effort to determine whether cannabis or its derivatives can make a contribution to the management of musculospastic disorders should continue.

*i. Preanesthetic*

It does not appear that the cannabinoids have any future for this indication.

*j. Pain*

Unless new synthetic compounds are found, it is difficult to believe that the available cannabinoids can compete with current analgesics.

*k. Depression*

This indication has not been convincingly investigated, and no conclusions can be drawn.

## 2. Cannabis as Treatment

It is not likely, judging from the work available, that the cannabis group will make a substantial impact on the treatment of the alcoholic or the drug-dependent person. According to Mikuriya,[652] former director of Marihuana Research at NIDA, "The development of nonirritating purified natural cannabinoid aerosol preparations should be a top priority effort."

Hollister[653] believes that the most promising therapeutic use of cannabis has been for control of nausea and vomiting associated with cancer chemotherapy. However, he points out that the new antiemetic metoclopramide may supersede the use of cannabis. Hollister also points out that the use of cannabis in the treatment of glaucoma looks promising but that the topical administration of cannabinoid has created difficulties. Furthermore, homologs of THC have been developed that separate the mental effects from analgesia and possibly THC may bind to opiate receptor sites, but it is too early to tell what these compounds will face in competition with the many new opioid analgesics. One homolog, nabolone, may soon be released.

Currently we cannot adequately appraise the therapeutic usefulness of cannabinoids because of the lack of clinical experience but continued research in this area is certainly warranted.

# L. GENERAL COMMENTS

There is no doubt that the use of marihuana in the United States has markedly increased in the past decade. Currently marihuana is used primarily for its psychoactive properties. The acute dangers of smoking marihuana are limited. Some people, probably only a small number, can experience severe anxiety and paranoia, but this does not usually last very long. Hashish, of course, which is ten times more potent than marihuana, can be hallucinogenic, and therefore can be more disruptive. Marihuana does not produce physical dependence in the sense that the opiates do, although it is evident that some marihuana users can become psychologically dependent on their drug. The long-term effects of marihuana are still in question. It would seem that the moderate social use of marihuana, similar to that with social drinking, is unlikely to result in harmful consequences. Chronic use of the drug, however, may pose a risk. Large numbers of new chemical derivatives of THC are being synthesized and will be evaluated in animals and humans. A great deal of time and effort is being, and will be, spent trying to determine whether these products have therapeutic usefulness. What chronic toxic effects of the drug will emerge also remains to be determined. Since marihuana has been in use for thousands of years, it would seem unlikely that gross physical abnormalities will occur. However, it should be remembered that although tobacco has been used for centuries, it is only within recent years that we have recognized that it is a major cause of cardiovascular disease, chronic lung disease, and lung cancer.

The *New York Times* published a letter written by six physicians at the College of Physicians and Surgeons, Columbia University, in its May 31, 1973, issue, which stated that marihuana contains toxic substances, soluble in fat that are stored in body tissues, including the brain, for weeks and months, as DDT is. The storage capacity of the tissues for these substances appears to be enormous, and explains the slow deleterious effects of marihuana in habitual smokers. The physicians stated that anyone using these substances more than once a week cannot be drugfree. They also pointed out that tolerance does develop, and therefore a significant number of habitual users of marihuana will require an increase in dosage or stronger preparations, such as hashish, or will escalate to more potent drugs. Marihuana smoke, they added, appears to induce cancer in tissue cultures of human lung, leads to cellular damage in humans, and decreases the ability of the user to respond to infection. They state that there is little evidence that this drug is innocuous.

It is obvious that there is a widespread difference of opinion as to the possible benefits and possible harm related to marihuana use. However, one thing appears clear: Marihuana is here to stay and we must be prepared to deal with its use in a rational and reasonable manner.

In the 1980s the tendency is to reduce penalties for possession of small amounts of marihuana while retaining controls over traffickers and dealers. At present federal, and many state, laws provide misdemeanor penalties for users or simple possessors. Some states already have enacted laws on decriminalization; among these are Oregon, Colorado, Maine, California, and Alaska. In fact, Alaska's Supreme Court has ruled that the constitutionally guaranteed right to privacy entails the right to possess marihuana for consumption in the citizen's own home. In the language of the court, "It appears that the use of marihuana, as it is presently used in the United States today, does not constitute a public health problem of any significant dimensions."

Legalization of marihuana, if and when it comes, would entail a legal manufacturing and distribution system with penalties only for selling to a juvenile, being intoxicated and disorderly, or driving under the influence, similar to the laws governing alcohol as a "social intoxicant." Certainly in view of the available data to date, the recommendation of the President's Commission on Marihuana to decriminalize private use and possession of small amounts of the drug is more rational than the severe penalty approved. However, caution concerning the legalization of this drug is recommended and should await further exploration into its potential harmful effects, especially in youths, and its long-term aspects.

As we are entering the "New Age of Pot," Albert Goldman[655] wonders, "What will happen when middle-class America gets the straight dope?" He has the following to say:

> The Age of Pot is upon us. The Day of the Reefer has dawned. After 40 years of trying to stamp out the dread weed with a steadily escalating law enforcement campaign that has become virtually a war, the various states of these United States are beginning to sue for peace. After spending millions of dollars, ruining thousands of young lives, and clogging our already overworked judicial and police apparatus with hundreds of thousands of petty crimes and misdemeanors, the men who make our laws are saying: "Let them smoke pot."

A real fallacy in the law is that marihuana has been classified with such dangerous and physically dependent drugs as the opiates (morphine and heroin). A hidden problem may lie with the phenomenon of being used to low-grade marihuana as in the past and the new age of very potent high-grade marihuana (high THC content). In this regard Goldman[655] further states:

> When marihuana is legalized, the days of people saying "I don't feel anything . . . do you feel anything?" will be over. Legalization will revolutionize the marihuana experience, making it another experience entirely. People will be able to buy unlimited quantities of marihuana in every conceivable form. There will be marihuana cigars, tins of marihuana tobacco, marihuana pastries and candies, marihuana drinks, and marihuana pills. Not only will the quantity and frequency of usage be altered drastically, but, most important, the quality of the dope will be different. High-grade marihuana, hashish, hash oil, and synthetic THC are different substances from the feeble grass known to most college students and Madison Avenue potheads. High-grade marihuana has powerful psychotropic effects. It can make you hallucinate, it can produce anxiety attacks, it can make you pass out. Even veteran potheads often panic when they encounter for the first time a grass like Colombian Wacky Weed, which turns your body to jelly, your mind to mush, as would, say a fistfull of Quaaludes. Hashish, which is simply the concen-

trated resin of marihuana, is often compared with marihuana by the analogy of whiskey to beer. Like so many cliches of the marihuana literature, this comparison is fallacious.

A signal of high-grade good-quality marihuana is the induction of "acute marihuana intoxication," under which even individuals familiar with its effects may become frightened. Most people tend to panic when they feel themselves losing control of their mind. And so the longer the loss of control persists and the more bizarre its manifestations in delusions, obsessions, and hallucinations, the greater is the panic.

It has been stated[655] that:

> Eventually, it is true, the approximately 250 million people who comprise this country may learn how to handle themselves when their heads fly off. But until that day comes—and considering the slowness of psychological and cultural change, it may take a long, long time—chances are great that widespread use of high-quality pot and hashish will produce some pretty crazy behavior. What whiskey did to the Indians, marihuana may do to white, middle-class America.

An important question to answer: Is marihuana another alcohol? Is it a social substance capable of providing us with "endless joy" and sexual zest or is it dependence producing and harmful physiologically as *alcohol* is? In terms of toxicity, at first glance marihuana does not seem as dangerous as alcohol. However, not until we have definitive evidence that a lifetime of inhaling deep into the lungs a hot, harsh, chemically irritating substance produces no harmful effects on the delicate membranes of the lips, mouth, esophagus, trachea, bronchial tubes, and lungs can we observe that smoking marihuana is only as harmful as smoking any other substance, such as tobacco.

Certain basic issues frequently arise in the course of a popular discussion about the pros and cons of marihuana use or abuse as:

1. Is it addictive?
2. Does it lead to crime?
3. Does it lead to sexual depravity?
4. Is it a stepping stone to heroin?
5. Does it enhance creativity?
6. Does it lead to psychosis?
7. Should it be legalized?
8. How much THC is needed to produce intoxication?
9. Does marihuana produce hangovers?
10. What marihuana preparations are used in the United States and elsewhere in the world?
11. Can marihuana be detected?
12. Does marihuana impair memory?
13. What effect does the smoking of marihuana have on driving skills?
14. What is a marihuana "contact high"?
15. Can marihuana cause brain damage?
16. Is there a cumulative effect from marihuana?
17. Does marihuana cause chromosomal structure malformation or [illegible] defects?
18. Does marihuana ex[illegible] cross-tolerance to other drugs?
19. Does tolerance or [illegible]verse tolerance to marihuana develop?
20. How much does [illegible] crave to continue the use of marihuana?
21. Is "pot" just a fad?
22. What would happen if pot were legalized?

The answers to most, if not all, of these questions should become obvious upon close scrutiny of this chapter; however, for a succinct review of the subject, the reader could refer to Cohen's book *The Substance Abuse Problems*.[470]

If marihuana were legalized, there are a number of future developments that we could predict.

Approximately 25 million more Americans would try marihuana, as it has been shown that 10 percent of students do not use it because of legal concerns. People over 25 years of age have desisted for similar reasons. In contrast, a few people who smoke pot as a symbolic gesture of defiance might stop using. Furthermore, there will be increased numbers of users who will become daily indulgers. The reason for this is that in every survey that showed an increased prevalence, the number of heavy users also increased. Thus in 2001 more than one million Americans will probably smoke pot daily, since approximately one million people in the United States smoke it daily now.

The potency of the cannabis used would also increase; already we are seeing evidence of this throughout the nation. In 2001 children would become involved in marihuana smoking at an early age; with greater availability they would mimic the behavior of their older siblings even sooner. Furthermore, although tobacco use will not be altered with the legalization of marihuana, the consumption of alcoholic beverages will not decrease. Among many cannabis smokers a preference for wine and beer rather than whiskeys is noted.

In 2001, with increased availability roughly a half billion dollars in taxes and licensing fees could be collected by regulating marihuana. Finally, an industry with sales of over $2 billion would be created. Thousands of acres would be sold for the cultivation of cannabis. This fact may have an impact on people's wellness as it related to drug abuse.[654]

In discussing the problems associated with decriminalization, Goldman[655] had this to say:

> Before decriminalization and legalization go any further, therefore, it might be a good idea if all the concerned parties—parents, children, cops, lawyers, legislators, and the president of the United States—took the testimony of those people who are already living in the Age of Free Dope. I refer to the potheads and dealers—they are one and the same people—who have for many years consumed unlimited quantities of grass of the highest quality, who have devoted their energies to tasting and comparing and trading various kinds of weed and who are therefore walking encyclopedias of the drug, as interesting for what they embody as for what they have to say about marihuana. By hearing their stories, examining their characters and personalities, observing their behavior, we can see today in miniature what someday we may see universally.

The notion of heaven and hell with regard to marihuana is best emphasized by the writings of Harry J. Anslinger and Ken Kesey.

> A person under the influence of marihuana can get so violent that it takes about five policemen to hold him down.
> *Harry J. Anslinger*
> *High Times, March 1976*

> To be just without being mad, to be peaceful without being stupid, to be interested without being compulsive to be happy without being hysterical—smoke grass.
> *Ken Kesey*
> *High Times, 1978*
> *Encyclopedia*

Whether we perceive marihuana to be heaven or hell, it is here to stay and we must learn more about its "magical" properties and be clever enough either to defoliate it completely or grow with it.

The real paradox concerning the use of marihuana is that most who rave about its aphrodisiac qualities (heaven) are at the same time faced with the inevitable pharmacologic effect to which abuse of the drug ultimately may lead—unwanted effects on male reproductive functions[656] (hell)—thereby providing impetus for some to continue in their search for the ultimate soma.

## REFERENCES


1. Briggs, A. H. Marihuana: Hades or god. In K. Blum and A. H. Briggs, eds. *Drugs: Use or Abuse*. Manual sponsored by U.S. Office of Education, Washington, D.C., 1970.
2. U.S. National Commission on Marihuana and Drug Abuse. *Marihuana: A Signal of Misunderstanding*. Vol. 1. Washington, D.C.: U.S. Government Printing Office, 1972.
3. Fishburne, P. M., Abelson, H. I., and Cisin, I. H. *National Survey on Drug Abuse: Main Findings: 1979*. Washington, D.C.: U.S. Government Printing Office, 1980, p. 43. DHHS publication no. (ADM)80-976.
4. Snyder, S. H. *Uses of Marihuana*. New York: Oxford University Press, 1971.
5. Sim, V. General discussion, summary and closing remarks. In D. H. Efron, ed. *Psychotomimetic Drugs*. Proceedings of a workshop, University of California, Irvine, January 25-26, 1969. New York: Raven Press, 1970, p. 332.
6. Li, H. L. The origin and use of cannabis in Eastern Asia: Linguistic-cultural implications. *Econ. Both*. 28(3):293, 1974.
7. Mikuriya, T. H. Marihuana in medicine: Past, present and future. *Calif. Med*. 110:34, 1969.
8. McMeens, R. R. Report of the Committee on

Cannabis Indica. In *Transactions of the 15th Annual Meeting of the Ohio State Medical Society*. Columbus, Ohio: Follett, Foster, 1860.
9. Hearings Before the Committee on Ways and Means, U.S. House of Representatives, Taxation of Marihuana, 75th Congress, First Session on H.R. 6385, 1937.
10. The cannabis problem: A note on the problem and the history of international action. *Bull Nar*. 14:4, 1962.
11. Chopra, I. S., and Chopra, R. N. The use of the cannabis drugs in India. *Bull Nar*. 9:1, 1957.
12. *Bull. Nar*. 1962:27.
13. Hollister, L. E. Marihuana in man: Three years later. *Science* 172:21, 1971.
14. Solomon, D. *The Marihuana Papers*. New York: New American Library, 1968.
15. *High Times Encyclopedia of Recreational Drugs*. New York: Stone Hill, 1978, p. 1.
16. Bloomquist, E. R. *Marihuana, The Second Trip*. Beverly Hills, Calif.: Glencoe Press, 1968.
17. Blum, R. H., et al. *Students and Drugs. Drugs II. College and High School Observations*. San Francisco: Jossey-Bass, 1969.
18. Curtis, B., and Simpson, O. D. Demographic characteristics of groups classified by patterns of multiple drug abuse. *Int. J. Addict*. 11:161, 1976.
19. Barber, T. X. *LSD, Marihuana, Yoga, and Hypnosis*. Chicago: Aldine, 1970.
20. Fort, J. *The Pleasure Seekers: The Drug Crisis, Youth and Society*. Indianapolis: Bobbs-Merrill, 1969.
21. Hepler, R. S., Frank, I. M., and Petrus, R. Ocular effects of marihuana smoking. In M. C. Braude and S. Szara, eds., *Pharmacology of Marihuana*. New York: Raven Press, 1976, p. 815.
22. Murphy, H. B. M. The cannabis habit: A review of recent psychiatric literature. *Bul. Nar*. 15:1, 1963.
23. Kabelikovi, J. Antibacterial action of cannabis indica. *Lekarske Listy* 15:7, 1952.
24. Krejci, J., Horak, M., and Santavy, F. Hemp (cannabis sativa)—Antibiotic drug, third report. *Pharmazie* 14, 1959.
25. Andrews, G., and Vinkenoog, S. (Editors) *The Book of Grass: An Anthology of Indian Hemp*. London: Peter Owen, 1967.
26. Kabelik, J., Drejci, Z., and Santavy, F. Cannabis as a medicant. *Bull. Nar*. 12:3, 1960.
27. Watt, J. M. Dagga in South Africa. *Bull Nar*. 13:3, 1961.
28. David, J. P., and Ramsey, H. H. Antiepileptic action of marihuana active substances. *Fed. Proc*. 8, 1949.
29. Lowe, S., and Goodman, L. S. Anticonvulsant action of marihuana active substances. *Fed. Proc*. 6, 1947.
30. Efron, D. H., (Editor) *Psychotomimetic drugs*: Proceedings of a workshop held at the University of California, Irvine, January 25–26, 1969. New York: Raven Press, 1969.
31. Walton, R. P. Marihuana: America's new drug problem. Philadelphia: Lippincott, 1938.
32. Adams, P. Marihuana. *Bull. N.Y. Acad. Med*. 1942.
33. Stockings, G. T. A new euphoriant for depressive mental states. *Br. Med. J*. 1:1947.
34. Parker, C. S., and Wrigley, F. Synthetic cannabis preparations in psychiatry: (I) Synhexyl. *J. Ment. Sci*. 6, 1950.
35. Report by the London Advisory Committee, 11, 1968.
36. Cardiac glycocides found cytotoxic. *Med. News* (London), Mar. 26, 1965.
37. Grinspoon, L. Marihuana. *Sci. Am*. 221:17, 1969.
38. *Marihuana and Health. a Report to the Congress from the Secretary, Department of Health, Education and Welfare*. Washington, D.C.: U.S. Government Printing Office, 1971.
39. Mikuriya, T. H. Cannabis substitution. An adjunctive therapeutic tool in the treatment of alcoholism. *Med. Times* 98:187, 1970.
40. Thompson, L. J., and Proctor, R. C. The use of pyrahexyl in the treatment of alcoholic and drug withdrawal conditions. *N.C. Med. J*. 14, 1953.
41. Blum, K., et al. Tetrahydrocannabinol: Inhibition of alcohol-induced withdrawal symptoms in mice. In J. M. Singh and L. Harbans, eds., *Drug Addiction: Neurobiology and Influences on Behavior*. New York: Stratton Intercontinental Medical Book Corp., 1974, p. 39.
42. Allentuck, S., and Bowman, K. M. The psychiatric aspects of marihuana intoxication. *Am. J. Psychiatry* 99:2, 1942.
43. Himmelsbach, C. J. Treatment of the morphine abstinence syndrome with a synthetic cannabis-like compound. *South. Med. J*. 37, 1944.
44. New York City. Mayor's Committee on Marihuana. *The Marihuana Problem in the City of New York: Sociological, Medical, Psychological and Pharmacological Studies*. Lancaster, Pa.: Jacques Cattell Press, 1944.
45. Watt, J. M., and Breyer-Brandwijk, M. G. *The Medicinal and Poisonous Plants of Southern*

*and Eastern Africa*, 2nd ed. Edinburgh, London: E. & S. Livingstone, 1962.
46. Chopra, R. N. Use of hemp drugs in India. *Indian Med. Gaz.* 1940.
47. Grinspoon, L. *Marihuana Reconsidered.* Cambridge, Mass.: Harvard University Press, 1971.
48. Geller, A., and Boas, M. *The Drug Beat.* New York: Cowles, 1969.
49. Reininger, W. Remnants from historic times. In G. Andrews and S. Vinkenoog, eds., *The Book of Grass: An Anthology on Indian Hemp.* London: Peter Owen, 1967, p. 14.
50. Reininger, W. Historical notes. In D. Solomon, ed., *The Marihuana Papers.* New York: New American Library, Signet Books, 1966.
51. Mikuriya, T. H. Marihuana in Morocco. In B. Aaronson and H. Osmond, eds., *Psychedelics, the Uses and Implications of Hallucinogenic Drugs.* Garden City, N.Y.: Doubleday, 1970.
52. Davies, A. Nigeria whispers. In G. Andrews and S. Vinkenoog, eds., *The Book of Grass: An Anthology on Indian Hemp.* London: Peter Owen, 1967, p. 229.
53. Dupont, R. L. Marihuana: An issue comes of age. In M. C. Braude and S. Szara, eds., *Pharmacology of Marihuana.* New York: Raven Press, 1976, p. 3.
54. Abelson, H. I., Fishburne, P. M., and Cisin, I. *National Survey on Drug Abuse: 1977.* Rockville, Md.: National Institute on Drug Abuse, 1977.
55. Johnston, L. D., Bachman, J. G., and O'Malley, P. M. *Drugs and the Class of '78: Behaviors, Attitudes, and Recent National Trends.* Rockville, Md.: National Institute on Drug Abuse, 1979.
56. Peterson, R. C. Marijuana and health: 1980. In R. C. Petersen, ed., *Marihuana Research Findings: 1980.* Rockville, Md.: National Institute on Drug Abuse, 1980, p. 7. (NIDA Research Monograph no. 31).
57. Doorenbos, N. J., et al. Cultivation, extraction and analysis of *Cannabis sativa L. Ann. N.Y. Acad. Sci.* 191:3, 1971.
58. Fetterman, P. S., et al. Mississippi-grown *Cannabis sativa L*: Preliminary observation on chemical definition of phenotype and variations in tetrahydrocannabinol content versus age, sex, and plant part. *J. Pharm. Sci.* 60:1246, 1971.
59. Ohlsson, A., et al. Cannabinoid constituents of male and female cannabis sativa. *Bull. Nar.* 23:29, 1971.
60. Phillips, R., et al. Seasonal variations in cannabinolic content of Indiana marihuana. *J. Forensic Sci.* 15:191, 1970.
61. Gaoni, Y., and Mechoulam, R. Isolation, structure, and partial synthesis of an active constituent of hashish. *J. Am. Chem. Soc.* 86:1646, 1964.
62. Mechoulam, R., and Gaoni, Y. The absolute configuration of delta-1-tetrahydrocannabinol, the major active constituent of hashish. *Tetrahedron Lett.* 12:1109, 1967.
63. Mechoulam, R., et al. Chemical basis of hashish activity. *Science* 169:611, 1970.
64. Hively, R. L., Mosher, W. A., and Hoffmann, F. W. Isolation of trans-delta-tetrahydrocannabinol from marihuana. *J. Am. Chem. Soc.* 88:1832, 1969.
65. Farenholtz, K. E., Lurie, M., and Kierstead, R. W. The total synthesis of dl-delta-9-tetrahydrocannabinol and four of its isomers. *J. Am. Chem. Soc.* 89:5934, 1967.
66. Petrzilka, T., and Sikemeier, C. Uber inhaltsstoffe des hashish II and III. *Helvetia Chim. Acta* 50:1410, 2111, 1967.
67. Mechoulam, R. Marihuana chemistry. *Science* 168:1159, 1970.
68. Mechoulam, R., et al. Chemical basis of hashish activity. *Science* 169:611, 1970.
69. Lemberger, L. The metabolism of the tetrahydrocannabinols. *Adv. Pharmacol. Chemother.* 10:221, 1972.
70. Paton, W. D. M., and Pertwee, R. G. The general pharmacology of cannabis. *Acta Pharma. Suec.* 8:691, 1971.
71. Waller, C. W. The chemistry of marihuana. *Proc. West. Pharmacol. Soc.* 14:1, 1971.
72. Gill, E. W. Propyl homologue of tetrahydrocannabinol: Its isolation from cannabis, properties and synthesis. *J. Chem. Soc. Organic* (3):579, 1971.
73. Merkus, F. W. Cannabivarin and tetrahydrocannabivarin, two new constituents of hashish. *Nature* 232:579, 1971.
74. Vree, T. B., et al. Identification of the methyl and propyl homologues of CBD, THC, CBN in hashish by a new method of combined gas chromatography-mass spectrometry. *Acta Pharm. Suec.* 8:683, 1971.
75. Gill, E. W., Paton, W. D., and Pertwee, R. G. Preliminary experiments on the chemistry and pharmacology of cannabis. *Nature* 228:134, 1970.
76. Bercht, C. A. L., et al. Constituents volatiles du cannabis satifa L. *U.N. ST/SOA/SER* 5/29:1, 1971.
77. Klein, F. K., Rapoport, H., and Elliott, H. W. Cannabis alkaloids. *Nature* 232:258, 1971.

78. Truitt, E., et al. Bioanalytical studies of cannabis smoking. Report to the National Institute of Mental Health, Contract no. PH-43-68-1338. Battelle Memorial Institute, Columbus, Ohio, 1970.
79. Magus, R. D., and Harris, L. S. Carcinogenic potential of marihuana smoke condensate. *Fed. Proc.* 30:277, 1971.
80. Domino, E. F., Hardman, H. F., and Seevers, M. H. Central nervous systems actions of some synthetic tetrahydrocannabinol derivatives. *Pharmacol. Rev.*
81. Sim, V. M., and Tucker, L. A. Summary Report on EA1476 and EA2233. Special Publication 1-44, U.S. Army Chemical Research and Development Laboratories, 1963.
82. Mechoulam, R. Marihuana chemistry. *Science* 168:1159, 1970.
83. Fentiman, A. F. Analytical techniques for determination of cannabinoids. Contract Report HSM-42-72-183, Oct. 8, 1973.
84. Turner, C. T. Shipment, analysis and storage of marihuana. Contract Report HSM-42-70-109, June 30, 1973.
85. Paris, M., et al. L'acide delta-1-tetrahydrocannabivarolique, nouveau constituant du cannabis sativa L. *Comptes Ronde Paris* 272:205, 1973.
86. Stromberg, L. Minor components of cannabis resin II. Separation by gas chromatography, mass spectra and molecular weights of some components with shorter retention times than cannabinol. *J. Chromatogr.* 68:248, 1972.
87. Shoyama, Y., et al. Cannabis IV: Cannabicyclolic acid. *Chem. Pharm. Bull.* 20:1927, 1972.
88. Bercht, C. A. L., et al. Cannabispirone and cannabispirerone, two naturally occurring spirocompounds. *Tetrahedron* 32:2938, 1976.
89. Fenselau, G., and Hermann, G. Identification of phytosterols in red oil extract of cannabis. *J. Forens. Sci.* 17:307, 1972.
90. Aldrich, M. R. The psychedelic underground. Hash oil and marihuana extracts. *L.A. Free Press* 10(1):24, 1974.
91. Erlich, D. Liquid hashish is uncovered. *J. Addict. Res. Found. (Toronto)* 31(1):11, 1974.
92. Massam, A. Increase in illicit hash oil has British police concerned. *J. Addict. Res. Found. (Toronto)* 3(4):10, 1974.
93. Mechoulam, R., Braun, P., and Gaoni, Y. Synthesis of delta-1-tetrahydrocannabinol and related cannabinoids. *J. Am. Chem. Soc.* 94:6159, 1972.
94. Abel, E. L., McMillan, D. E., and Harris, L. S. Tolerance to the behavioral and hypothermic effects of 1-9-tetrahydrocannabinol in neonatal chicks. *Experientia* 28:1188, 1972.
95. Mechoulam, R., et al. Synthesis and biological activity of five tetrahydrocannabinol metabolites. *J. Am. Chem. Soc.* 94:7930, 1972.
96. Pitt, C. G., et al. Synthesis of 11-hydroxy-6-tetrahydrocannabinol and other physiologically active metabolites of 8- and 9-tetrahydrocannabinol. *J. Am. Chem. Soc.* 94:8578, 1972.
97. Razdan, R. K., et al. Synthesis of 7-hydroxy-delta -tetrahydrocannabinol (THC): An important active metabolite of delta -THC in man. *J. Am. Chem. Soc.* 95:2361, 1973.
98. Turner, C. E., Elsohly, M. A., and Boeren, E. L. A review of the chemical constituents of *Cannabis sativa L. Lloydia* 43(2), 1980.
99. Wall, M. E. Synthesis of radiolabeled cannabinoids and metabolites. Contract Report HSM-42-71-108, Oct. 25, 1973.
100. Agurell, S., et al. Synthesis of tritium-labelled tetrahydrocannabinol and cannabidiol. *Acta Chem. Scand.* 27:1090, 1973.
101. Turner, C. E., et al. Constituents of *Cannabis sativa L.* XIV: Intrinsic problems in classifying cannabis based on a single cannabinoid analysis. *J. Nat. Prod.* 42(3):317, 1979.
102. Hollister, L. E. Structure–activity relationships in man of cannabis constituents, and homologs and metabolites of Delta-9-tetrahydrocannabinol. *Pharmacology* 11:3, 1974.
103. Perez-Reyes, M., et al. A comparison of the pharmacological activity in man of intravenously administered delta-9-tetrahydrocannabinol, cannabinol, and cannabidiol. *Experientia* 29:1368, 1973.
104. Karniol, I. G., and Carlini, E. A. The content of (−) 9-tetrahydrocannabinol (delta-9-THC) does not explain all biological activity of some Brazilian marihuana samples. *J. Pharm. Pharmacol.* 24:833, 1972.
105. Borgen, L. A., and Davis, W. M. Cannabidiol interaction with delta-9-tetrahydrocannabinol. *Res. Commun. Chem. Pathol. Pharmacol.* 7:663, 1974.
106. Siemens, A. J., Kalant, H., and deNie, J. C. Metabolic interactions between delta-9-tetrahydrocannabinol and other cannabinoids in rats. In M. C. Braude and S. Szara, eds., *The Pharmacology of Marihuana*. New York: Raven Press, 1976, p. 77.
107. Chan, W. R., Magnus, K. E., and Watson, H. A. The structure of cannabitriol. *Experientia* 32:283, 1976.
108. Elsohly, M. A., El-Feraly, F. S., and Turner, C. E. Isolation and characterization of (+)-

cannabitriol and (−)-10-ethoxy-9-hydroxy-delta 61 10a-tetrahydrocannabinol: Two new cannabinoids from *Cannabis sativa L.* extract. *Lloydia* 40:275, 1977.

109. Elsohly, M. A., et al. Anhydrocannabisativine, a new alkaloid from *Cannabis sativa L. J. Pharm. Sci.* 67:124, 1978.

110. Boeren, E. G., Elsohly, M. A., and Turner, C. E. Cannabiripsol: A novel cannabis constituent. *Experientia* 15:1278, 1979.

111. Coutts, R. T., and Jones, G. R. A comparative analysis of cannabis material. *J. Forensic Sci.* 24:291, 1979.

112. Turner, C. E., and Elsohly, M. A. Constituents of *Cannabis sativa L.* XVI. A possible decomposition pathway of delta-9-tetrahydrocannabinol to cannabinol. *J. Heterocyclic Chem.* 1979.

113. Preobraschensky, W. Cannabineae. *Jahresber Pharmacol. Toxicol.* 4:98, 1876.

114. Humphrey, J. The chemistry of cannabis indica. *Pharm. J.* 14:392, 1902.

115. Elsohly, M. A., and Turner, C. E. Screening of cannabis grown from seed of various geographical origins for the alkaloid hordenine, cannabisativine and anhydrocannabisativine. *U.N. Secretariat* ST/SOA/SER.S/54, 1977.

116. Ottersen, T., et al. X-ray structure of cannabispiran: A novel cannabis constituent. *J. Chem. Soc. Chem. Commun.* 580, 1976.

117. Turner, C. E. Chemistry and metabolism. In R. C. Petersen, ed., *Marihuana Research Findings: 1980*. Rockville, Md.: National Institute on Drug Abuse, 1980, p. 81. (NIDA Research Monograph no. 31).

118. Boeren, E. G., et al. Beta-Cannabispiranol: A new non-cannabinoid phenol from *Cannabis sativa L. Experientia* 33:848, 1977.

119. Kettenes-van den Bosch, J. J., and Salemink, C. A. Cannabis XI. Oxygenated 1, 2-diphenylethanes from marihuana. *J. Roy. Netherlands Chem. Soc.* 97:7, 1978.

120. Shoyama, Y., and Nishioka, I. Cannabis XIII. Two new spirocompounds, cannabispirol and acetyl cannabispirol. *Chem. Pharm. Bull.* 26:3641, 1978.

121. Crombie, L., Crombie, W. M. L., and Jamieson, S. V. Isolation of cannabispiradienone and cannabidihydrophenanthrene. Biosynthetic relationships between the spirans and dihydrostilbenes of Thailand cannabis. *Tetrahedron Lett.* 7:661, 1979.

122. Bailey, D. J., et al. Potentiation of the estrogenic activity of stilbestrol by spiro (cyclohexane-1, 2′-indan)-1′, 4-dione. *J. Med. Chem.* 19:438, 1976.

123. El-Feraly, F. S., et al. Crystal and molecular structure of cannabispiran and its correlation to dehydrocannabispiran. *Tetrahedron* 33:2373, 1977.

124. Burstein, S., et al. Identification of p-vinylphenol as a potent inhibitor of prostaglandin synthesis. *Biochem. Pharmacol.* 25:2003, 1976.

125. Ottersen, T., et al. The crystal and molecular structure of cannabinol. *Acta Chem. Scand. B.* 31:781, 1977.

126. Jones, P. G., et al. Cannabidiol. *Acta Cryst.* B33:3211, 1977.

127. Handrick, G. R., et al. Hashish. 1 Synthesis of (t/−)-delta 1 and delta 6-3, 4-cis-cannabidiols and their isomerization by acid catalysis. *J. Org. Chem.* 42:2563, 1977.

128. Uliss, D. B., et al. The conversion of 3,4-*cis*-to 3,4-*trans*-cannabinoids. *Tetrahedron* 34:1885, 1979.

129. Uliss, D. B., et al. A novel cannabinoid containing a 1,8-cineol moiety. *Experientia* 33:577, 1977.

130. Handrick, G. R., et al. Hashish. Synthesis of (−) delta 9-tetrahydrocannabinol (THC) and its biologically potent metabolite $3^1$-hydroxy-$\Delta^9$-THC. *Tetrahedron Lett.* 8:681, 1979.

131. Robertson, L. W., et al. Microbiological oxidation of the pentyl side chain of cannabinoids. *Experientia* 34:1020, 1978.

132. Pitt, C. G., et al. General synthesis of side chain derivative of cannabinoids. *J. Org. Chem.* 44(5):677, 1979.

133. Ohlsson, A., et al. Synthesis and psychotropic activity of side-chain hydroxylated Delta 6-tetrahydrocannabinol metabolites. *Acta Pharm. Succ.* 16:21, 1979.

134. Yagen, B., et al. Synthesis and enzymatic formation of a C-glucuronide of delta 6-tetrahydrocannabinol. (Letter) *J. Am. Chem. Soc.* 99:6444, 1977.

135. Harvey, D. J., Martin, B. R., and Paton, W. D. Identification of glucuronides as *in vivo* liver conjugates of seven cannabinoids and some of their hydroxy and acid metabolites. *Res. Commun. Chem. Pathol. Pharmacol.* 16:265, 1977.

136. Elsohly, M. A., Boeren, E. G., and Turner, C. E. Constituents of *Cannabis sativa L.* An improved method for the synthesis of *dl*-cannabichromene. *J. Heterocyclic Chem.* 15:699, 1978.

137. *Marihuana and Health.* Sixth Annual Report to Congress by the Secretary of Health, Education and Welfare, 1976. DHEW Publication no. (ADM) 77-443. Washington, D.C.: Su-

perintendent of Documents, U.S. Government Printing Office, 1977.

138. *Marihuana and Health*. Fifth Annual Report to Congress by the Secretary of Health, Education, and Welfare, 1975. DHEW Publication no (ADM) 76-314. Washington, D.C.: Superintendent of Documents, U.S. Government Printing Office, 1976.

139. Mikes, F., and Waser, P. G. Marihuana components: Effects of smoking on delta-9-tetrahydrocannabinol and cannabidiol. *Science* 172:1158, 1971.

140. Truitt, E. G., Jr. Biologic disposition of tetrahydrocannabinols. *Pharmacol. Rev.* 23:273, 1971.

141. Manno, J. E., et al. Comparative effects of smoking marihuana or placebo on human motor performance. *Clin. Pharmacol. Ther.* 11:808, 1970.

142. Fehr, O'Brien, K., and Kalant, H. Analysis of cannabis smoke obtained under different combustion conditions. *Can. J. Physiol. Pharmacol.* 50(8):761, 1972.

143. Lee, M. L., Novotny, M., and Bartle, K. D. Gas chromatography/mass spectrometric and nuclear magnetic resonance spectrometric studies on carcinogenic polynuclear aromatic hydrocarbons in tobacco and marijuana smoke condensate. *Anal. Chem.* 48(2):405, 1976.

144. Maskarinec, M. P., Alexander, G., and Novotny, M. Analysis of the acidic fraction of marijuana smoke condensate by capillary gas chromatography-mass spectrometry. *J. Chromatogr.* 126:559, 1976.

145. Novotny, M., Lee, M. L., and Bartle, K. D. A possible chemical basis for the higher mutagenicity of marihuana smoke as compared to tobacco smoke. *Experientia* 32:280, 1976.

146. Hofmann, D., et al. On the carcinogenicity of marihuana smoke. *Rec. Adv. Phytochem.* 9:63, 1976.

147. Kuppers, F. J., et al. Cannabis. XIV. Pyrolysis of cannabidiol-analysis of the volatile constituents. *J. Chromatogr.* 108:375, 1975.

148. Spronck, H. J. W., and Salemink, C. A. Cannabis XVII. Pyrolysis of cannabidiol. Structure elucidation of two pyrolytic conversion products. *J. Roy. Netherlands Chem. Soc.* 97:185, 1978.

149. Luteyn, J. M., Spronck, H. J. W., and Salemink, C. A. Cannabis XVIII. Isolation and synthesis of olivetol derivatives formed in the pyrolysis of cannabidiol. *J. Roy. Netherlands Chem. Soc.* 97:187, 1978.

150. Rosenkrantz, H., and Hayden, D. W. Acute and subacute inhalation toxicity of Turkish marihuana, cannabichromene, and cannabidiol in rats. *Toxicol. Appl. Pharmacol.* 48:375, 1979.

151. Fleischman, R. W., Baker, J. R., and Rosenkrantz, H. Pulmonary pathologic changes in rats exposed to marihuana smoke for 1 year. *Toxicol. Appl. Pharmacol.* 47:557, 1979.

152. Zwillich, G. W., et al. The effects of smoked marijuana on metabolism and respiratory control. *Am. Rev. Respic. Dis.* 118:885, 1978.

153. Zeeuw, R. D. de., Wijsbeck, J., and Malingre, T. M. Interference of alkanes in the gas chromatographic analysis of cannabis products. *J. Pharm. Pharmacol.* 25:21, 1973.

154. Fairbairn, J. W., and Liebmann, J. A. The extraction and estimation of the cannabinoids in cannabis sativa L. and its products. *J. Pharm. Pharmacol.* 25:150, 1973.

155. Waller, C. W., et al. *Marihuana: An Annotated Bibliography*. New York: Macmillan, 1976.

156. Hoffman, N. E., and Yang, R. K. Gas chromatography of delta-1-tetrahydrocannabinol. *Anal. Lett.* 5:7, 1972.

157. Masoud, A. N. and Doorenbos, N. J. Mississippi-grown *Cannabis sativa L.* 3 Cannabinoid and cannabinoid acid content. *J. Pharm. Sci.* 62:313, 1973.

158. Paris, M. R., and Paris, R. R. Importance de la chromatographie pour l'etude des constituants du cannabis sativa L. *Bull. Soc. Chem. France* 1:118, 1973.

159. Rasmussen, K. E., Rasmussen, S., and Svendsen, A. B. Gas-liquid chromatography of cannabinoids in micro quantities of cannabis by solid injection. *J. Chromatogr.* 69:381, 1972.

160. Vree, T. B., et al. Identification of cannabicyclol with a pentyl or propyl side-chain by means of combined gas chromatography-mass spectrometry. *J. Chromatogr.* 74:124, 1972.

161. Kuppers, F. J., et al. Cannabis-VIV: pyrolysis of cannabidiol, structure elucidation of the main pyrolytic product. *Tetrahedron* 29:2797, 1973.

162. Shani, A. and Mechoulam, R. New types of cannabinoid: Synthesis of cannabeilsoic acid A by a novel photo-chemical cyclization. *J. Chem. Soc.* 5:273, 1970.

163. Belgrave, B. E., et al. The effect of (−) trans-delta 9-tetrahydrocannabinol alone and in combination with ethanol, on human performance. *Psychopharmacology* (Berlin) 62:53, 1979.

164. Chao, F. C., et al. The passage of $^{14}$C-delta-9-tetrahydrocannabinol into the milk of lactating squirrel monkeys. *Res. Commun. Chem. Pa-*

*thol. Pharmacol.* 15(2)303, 1976.

165. Lewis, G. S., and Turner, C. E. Constituents of *Cannabis sativa L.* XIII. Stability of dosage form prepared by impregnating synthetic (−)-delta 9-trans-tetrahydrocannabinol on placebo cannabis plant material. *J. Pharm. Sci.* 67:876, 1978.
166. Ottersen, T., et al. The crystal and molecular structure of cannabidiol. *Acta Chem. Scand. B* 31:807, 1977.
167. Roth, S. H., and Williams, P. J. The non-specific membrane binding properties of delta 9-tetrahydrocannabinol and the effects of various solubilizers. *J. Pharm. Pharmacol.* 31:224, 1979.
168. Siemens, A. J., and Doyle, D. C. Cross-tolerance between delta-9-tetrahydrocannabinol and ethanol: The role of drug disposition. *Pharmacol. Biochem. Behav.* 10:49, 1979.
169. Siemens, A. J., and Khanna, J. M. Acute metabolic interactions between ethanol and cannabis. *Al. Clin. Exp. Res.* 1:343, 1977.
170. Stillman, R. C., et al. Low platelet monamine oxidase activity and chronic marijuana use. *Life Sci.* 23:1577, 1978.
171. Tamir, I., Lichtenberg, D., and Mechoulam, R. Interaction of cannabinoids with model membranes-NMR studies. In B. Pullman, ed., *Nuclear Magnetic Resonance Spectroscopy in Molecular Biology*. Dordrecht, Holland: P. Reidel, 1978, pp. 405–422.
172. Vardaris, R. M., et al. Chronic administration of delta-9-tetrahydrocannabinol to pregnant rats: Studies of pup behavior and placental transfer. *Pharmacol. Biochem. Behav.* 4:249, 1976.
173. Britofilho, D. Isolational cannabinol, cannabidiol and tetrahydrocannabinol from *Cannabis sativa L.* by thin layer chromatography. *Rev. Quim. Ind. (Rio de Janeiro)* 41:15, 1972.
174. Eskes, D., Verway, A. M., and Witte, A. H. Thin layer and gas chromatographic analysis of hashish samples containing opium. *Bull. Nar.* 25:41, 1973.
175. Friedrich-Fiechtl, J., et al. Zu Nachweis and identifizerung von tetrahydrocannabinol in biologischen flussigkeiten. [Demonstration and identification tetrahydrocannabinol in biological fluids]. *Naturwissenschaften* 60:207, 1973.
176. Just, W. W., Werner, G., and Wiechmann, M. Determination of delta-1- and delta-1 (16)-tetrahydrocannabinol in blood, urine, and saliva of hashish smokers. *Naturwissenschaft* 59:222, 1972.
177. Reiss, J. Thin-layer chromatographic separation of the constituents of hashish on pre-coated silica gel sheet. *Arch. Toxikol.* 29:265, 1972.
178. Segelman, A. B., *Cannabis sativa L.* (Marihuana). III. The RIM test: A reliable and useful procedure for the detection and identification of marihuana utilizing combined microscopy and thin-layer chromatography. *J. Chromatogr.* 82:151, 1973.
179. Gross, S. J., and Soares, J. R. Validated direct blood delta 9 THC radioimmune quantitation. *J. Anal. Toxicol.* 2:98, 1978.
180. Galanter, M., et al. Effects on humans of 9-tetrahydrocannabinol administered by smoking. *Science* 176:934, 1972.
181. Garrett, E. R., and Hunt, C. A. Picogram analysis of tetrahydrocannabinol and application to biological fluids. *J. Pharm. Sci.* 62:1211, 1973.
182. Chan, M. L., Whetsell, C., and McChesney, J. D. Use of high pressure liquid chromatography for the separation of drugs of abuse. *J. Chromatogr. Sci.* 12(9):512, 1974.
183. Karasch, F. W., Karasedk, D. E., and Kim, S. H. Detection of lysergic acid diethylamide, delta 9-tetrahydrocannabinol and related compounds by plasma chromatography. *J. Chromatogr.* 105(2):345, 197
184. Karler, R. Chemistry and metabolism. In R. C. Petersen, ed., *Marihuana Research Findings: 1976*. Rockville, Md.: National Institute on Drug Abuse, 1977, p. 55. (NIDA Research Monograph no. 14).
185. Agurell, S., Lindgren, J. E., and Ohlsson, A. Symposium on marihuana, Reims, France, July 22–23, 1978.
186. Fentiman, A. F., Foltz, R. B., and Foltz, R. L. Manual for quantitation of delta 9-tetrahydrocannabinol in biological media by gas chromatography/mass spectrometry. In *Report to NIDA*. Columbus, Ohio: Battelle Columbus Laboratories, 1978.
187. Rosenthal, P., et al. Comparison of gas chromatography mass spectrometry methods for the determination of delta 9-THC in plasma. *Biomed. Mass. Spect.* 5:312, 1978.
188. Foltz, R. L. Quantitative analysis of abused drugs in physiological fluids by gas chromatography/chemical ionization mass spectrometry. In A. P. de Leenheer, R. R. Roncucci, and C. van Peteghem, eds., *Quantitative Mass Spectrometry in Life Science. II*. Proceedings of the Second International Symposium, Ghent, June 13–16, 1978. Amsterdam: Elsevier Scientific, 1978, p. 39.
189. Pirl, J. N., Papa, V. M., and Spikes, J. J. The

detection of delta-9-tetrahydrocannabinol in postmortem blood samples. *J. Anal. Toxicol.* 3:129, 1979.

190. Kanter, S. L., Hollister, L. E., and Loeffler, K. O. Marihuana metabolites in the urine of man. VIII. Identification and quantitation of delta 9-tetrahydrocannabinol by thin layer chromatography and high pressure liquid chromatography. *J. Chromatogr.* 150:233, 1978.
191. Wall, M. E., et al. Analytical methods for the determination of cannabinoids in biological media. In R. E. Willette, ed., *Cannabinoid Assays in Humans*. Rockville, Md.: National Institute on Drug Abuse, 1976. (NIDA Research Monograph no. 7).
192. Rodgers, R., et al. Homogeneous enzyme immunoassay for cannabinoids in urine. *Clin. Chem.* 24:95, 1978.
193. Singer, A. J., Editor. Marihuana: Chemistry, pharmacology, and patterns of social use. *Ann. N.Y. Acad. Sci.* 191, 1971.
194. Lemberger, L., et al. Delta-tetrahydrocannabinol metabolism and disposition in long term marihuana smokers. *Science* 173:72, 1971.
195. Lemberger, L., Crabtree, R. E., and Rowe, H. M. 11-hydroxy-$^9$-tetrahydrocannabinol: Pharmacology disposition and metabolism of a major metabolite of marihuana in man. *Science* 177:62, 1972.
196. Razdan, R. An overview of chemistry of cannabinoids. In S. Agurell, R. Willette, and W. Dewey, eds., *Cannabinoids '82*. New York: Academic Press (in press).
197. Christensen, H. D., et al. Activity of delta 9- and delta 9-tetrahydrocannabinol and related compounds in the mouse. *Science* 172:165, 1971.
198. Burstein, S. H., et al. Metabolism of (6)-tetrahydrocannabinol. An active marihuana constituent. *Nature* 225:87, 1970.
199. Ben-Zui, Z., Mechoulam, R., and Burstein, S. Identification through synthesis of an active delta-1 (6)-tetrahydrocannabinol metabolite. *J. Am. Chem. Soc.* 92:3468, 1970.
200. Foltz, R. L., et al. Metabolite of (−)-trans-$^8$-tetrahydrocannabinol: identification and synthesis. *Science* 168:844, 1970.
201. Wall, M. E., et al. Isolation, structure, and biological activity of several metabolites of delta 9-tetrahydrocannabinol. *J. Am. Chem. Soc.* 92:3466, 1970.
202. Wall, M. E., et al. Studies on the *in vitro* and *in vivo* metabolism of $\Delta^9$-tetrahydrocannabinol. *Acta Pharm. Suec.* 8:702, 1971.
203. Nilsson, I. M., et al. Cannabidiol: Structure of three metabolites formed in rat liver. *Acta Pharm. Suec.* 8:701, 1971.
204. Miras, C. J., and Coutselinis, A. The distribution of tetrahydrocannabinol-$C^{14}$ in humans. Report no. 24. U.N. Secretariat *ST/SOA/SER.* S/25, Nov. 1970.
205. Klausner, H. A., and Dingell, J. V. The metabolism and excretion of delta-9-tetrahydrocannabinol in the rat. *Life Sci.* 10:49, 1971.
206. Agurell, S., and Leander, K. Stability, transfer and absorption of cannabinoid constituents of cannabis (hashish) during smoking. *Acta Pharm. Suec.* 8, 1971.
207. Burstein, S., and Rosenfeld, J. The isolation and characterization of a major metabolite of delta 9-THC. *Acta Pharma. Suec.* 8:699, 1971.
208. Nakazawa, K., and Costa, E. Induction by methylcholanthrene of delta 9-tetrahydrocannabinol (delta 9 THC) metabolism in rat lung. *Pharmacologist* 13:297, 1971.
209. Lemberger, L., et al. Delta-9-tetrahydrocannabinol temporal correlation of the physiological effects and blood levels after various routes of administration. *N. Engl. J. Med.* 226:685, 1972.
210. Galanter, M., et al. Delta-9-transtetrahydrocannabinol administered by smoking. *Science* 1972.
211. Perez-Reyes, M., and Lipton, M. A. The rate of absorption and excretion of orally administered delta-9-tetrahydrocannabinol to man. Prepared for the National Institute of Mental Health, Contract HSM 42-69-62, Department of Psychiatry, University of North Carolina, July 1971.
212. Lemberger, L., Axelrod, J., and Kopin, J. Metabolism and disposition of delta-$^9$-tetrahydrocannabinol in man. *Pharmacol. Rev.* 23:371, 1971.
213. Kiplinger, G. F., et al. Dose-response analysis of the effects of tetrahydrocannabinol in man. *Clin. Pharmacol. Ther.* 12:650, 1971.
214. Lemberger, L. Tetrahydrocannabinol metabolism in man. *Drug Metab. Dispos.* 1:461, 1973.
215. Wall, M. E., et al. Identification of delta-9-tetrahydrocannabinol and metabolites in man. *J. Am. Chem. Soc.* 94:8579, 1891, 1972.
216. Burstein, S., et al. The urinary metabolites of delta-1-THC. In W. D. M. Paton and J. Crown, eds., *Cannabis and Its Derivatives*. London: Oxford University Press, 1972.
217. Dingell, J. V., et al. The intracellular locationzation of 9-tetrahydrocannabinol in liver and its effects on drug metabolism in vitro.

*Biochem. Pharmacol.* 22:949, 1973.

218. Ho, B. T., et al. 9-Tetrahydrocannabinol and its metabolites in monkey brain. *J. Pharm. Pharmacol.* 24:414, 1972.

219. Lemberger, L., et al. Comparative pharmacology of delta 9-tetrahydrocannabinol and its metabolite, 11-hydroxy-delta 9-tetrahydrocannabinol. *J. Clin. Invest.* 52:2411, 1973.

220. Lemberger, L., et al. The *in vitro* and *in vivo* metabolism of delta-6a, 10a demethylheptyl tetrahydrocannabinol (DMHP). *J. Pharmacol. Exp. Ther.* 187:169, 1973.

221. Nilsson, I. M., et al. Metabolism of 7-hydroxy-delta-1(6)-tetrahydrocannabinol in the rabbit. *Acta Pharm. Suec.* 10:97, 1973.

222. Turk, R. F., Dewey, W. L., and Harris, L. S: Excretion of *trans*-delta-9-tetrahydrocannabinol and its metabolites in intact and bile duct-cannulated rats. *J. Pharm. Sci.* 62:737, 1973.

223. Dewey, W. L., et al. Distribution of radioactivity in brains of tolerant and intolerant pigeons treated with 3-H-delta-9-tetrahydrocannabinol. *Biochem. Pharmacol.* 22(3):399, 1973.

224. McMillan, D. E., et al. Blood levels of 3H-delta-9-tetrahydrocannabinol and its metabolites in tolerant and nontolerant pigeons. *Biochem. Pharmacol.* 22:383, 1973.

225. Meyers, F. H. Pharmacology effects of marihuana. *J. Psychedel. Drugs* 2:31, 1968.

226. Harvey, D. J., Martin, B. R., and Paton, W. D. M. Identification of metabolites of delta$^1$- and delta$^{1\ 6}$ -tetrahydrocannabinol containing a reduced double bond. *J. Pharm. Pharmacol.* 29:495, 1978.

227. Yisak, W., et al. *In vivo* metabolites of cannabinol identified as fatty acid conjugates. *J. Pharm. Pharmacol.* 30:462, 1978.

228. Harvey, D. J., and Paton, W. D. M. Identification of six substituted 4″-hydroxy-metabolites of $\Delta^1$-tetrahydrocannabinol in mouse liver. *Res. Commun. Chem. Pathol. Pharmacol.* 21:435, 1978.

229. Schou, J., et al. Penetration of delta-9-tetrahydrocannabinol and 11-OH-delta-9-tetrahydrocannabinol through the blood brain barrier. *Acta Pharmacol. Toxicol.* 41:33, 1977.

230. Johnson, K. M., and Dewey, W. L. The effect of delta$^9$-tetrahydrocannabinol on the conversion of [$^3$H] tryptophan to 5-[$^3$H] hydroxytryptamine in the mouse brain. *J. Pharmacol. Exp. Ther.* 207:140, 1978.

231. Myers, W. A., III, and Heath, R. A. *Cannabis sativa*: Ultrastructural changes in organelles or neurons in brain septal region of monkeys. *J. Neuro. Sci.* 4:9, 1979.

232. Uliss, D. B., et al. A terpenic synthon for $\Delta^1$-cannabinoids. *J. Am. Chem. Soc.* 100(9):2929, 1978.

233. Uliss, D. B., et al. Synthesis of racemic and optically active delta$^1$- and delta$^6$-3,4-*cis*-tetrahydrocannabinois. *Tetrahedron* 33:2055, 1977.

234. United Nations Division of Narcotic Drugs. The *Chemistry of Cannabis and Its Components.* MNAR/9/1974-GE, 74-11502, 1974.

235. United Nations Division of Narcotic Drugs. *The Chemistry of Cannabis Smoke.* MNAR/6/1975-GE, 75-5104, 1975.

236. Elsohly, M. A., Boeren, E. G., and Turner, C. E. 9,10-dihydroxy-$\Delta^{6a\ 10a}$ -tetrahydrocannabinol and (±)8,9-dihydroxy-delta$^{6a\ 10a}$ -tetrahydrocannabinol and (±)8,9-dihydroxy-delta(10a) 2 new cannabinoids from cannabinoids from *Cannabis sativa L. Experientia* 34:1127, 1978.

237. El-Feraly, F. S., and Turner, C. E. Alkaloids of *Cannabis sativa* leaves. *Psytochemistry* 14:2304, 1975.

238. Elsohly, M. A., and Turner, C. E. A review of nitrogen containing compounds from *Cannabis sativa L. Pharm. Weekblad* III, 1976.

239. Lotter, H. L., et al. Cannabisativine, a new alkaloid from *Cannabis sativa L.* root. *Tetrahedron Lett.* 33:2815, 1975.

240. Wall, M. E. Recent advances in the chemistry and metabolism of the cannabinoids. In *Recent Advancement in Phytochemistry* 1975.

241. Waller, C., Hadley, K., and Turner, C. Detection and identification of compounds in cannabis. In G. G. Nahas, ed., *Marihuana: Chemistry, Biochemistry and Cellular Effects.* New York: Springer-Verlag, 1976, p. 15.

242. Rosenfeld, J. A general approach to the analysis of ca-nabinoids from physiological sources. In J. A. Vinson, ed., *Cannabinoid Analysis in Physiologal Fluids.* American Chemical Symposium Series 58. Washington, D.C.: American Chemical Society, 1979, p. 81.

243. Rosenthal, D., and Brine, D. S. Quantitative determination of delta$^9$-tetrahydrocannabinol in cadaver blood. *J. Forens. Sci.* 24:282, 1979.

244. Isbell, H., et al. Effects of (−) delta-9-trans-tetrahydrocannabinol in man. *Psychopharmacologia* 11:184, 1967.

245. Rodin, E., and Domino, E. F. Effects of acute marihuana smoking in the electroencephalograms. *Electroenceph. Clin. Neurophysiol.* 29:321, 1970.

246. Melges, F. T., et al. Temporal disintegration

and depersonalization during marihuana intoxication. *Arch. Gen. Psychiatry* 23:204, 1970.

247. Tinklenberg, J. R., et al. Marihuana and immediate memory. *Nature* 226:1171, 1970.
248. Weil, A. T., Zinberg, N. E., and Nelsen, J. M. Clinical and psychological effects of marihuana in man. *Science* 162:1234, 1968.
249. Meyer, R. E., et al. Administration of marihuana to heavy and casual users. *Am. J. Psychiatry* 128:198, 1971.
250. Clark, L. D., and Nakashima, E. N. Experimental studies of marihuana. *Am. J. Psychiatry* 125:135, 1968.
251. Clark, L. D., Hugues, R., and Nakashima, E. N. Behavioral effects of marihuana. Experimental studies. *Arch. Gen. Psychiatry* 23:193, 1970.
252. Jones, R., and Stone, G. Psychological studies of marihuana and alcohol in man. *Psychopharmacologia (Berlin)* 18(1):108, 1970.
253. Manno, B. R., et al. Response of the isolated perfused rat heart to delta-9-tetrahydrocannabinol (THC). *Toxicol. Appl. Pharmacol.* 10:98, 1970.
254. Isbell, H., et al. Studies on tetrahydrocannabinol. *Bull. Prob. Drug Depend. Nat. Acad. Sci., Div. Med. Sci.* 4832, 1967.
255. Waskow, I. E., et al. Psychological effects of tetrahydrocannabinol. *Arch. Gen. Psychiatry* 22:97, 1970.
256. Hollister, L. E., Richards, R. K., and Gillespie, H. K. Comparison of tetrahydrocannabinol and synhexyl in man. *Clin. Pharmacol. Ther.* 9:783, 1968.
257. Lemberger, L., Axelrod, J., and Kopin, J. Metabolism and disposition of delta-9-tetrahydrocannabinol in naive subjects and chronic marihuana users. *Ann. N.Y. Acad. Sci.* 191:142, 1971.
258. Isbell, H., et al. Effects of (−) delta-9-*trans*-tetrahydrocannabinol in man. *Psychopharmacologia* 11:184, 1967.
259. Renault, P. F., et al. Marihuana: Standardized smoke administration and dose effect curves on heart rate in humans. *Science* 174(4009):589, 1971.
260. Hollister, L. E. Status report on clinical pharmacology of marihuana. *Ann. N.Y. Acad. Sci.* 191:132, 1971.
261. Hollister, L. E., and Gillespie, H. K. Marihuana, Ethanol and dextroamphetamine: Mood and mental function alterations. *Arch. Gen. Psychiatry* 23:199, 1970.
262. McIsaac, W., Harris, R. T., and Ho, B. T. Behavioral correlate of brain distribution of tetrahydrocannabinol. *Acta Pharm. Suec.* 8:703, 1971.
263. Ho, B. T., et al. Marihuana: Importance of the route of administration. *J. Pharm. Pharmacol.* 23:309, 1971.
264. Kennedy, J. S., and Waddell, W. J. Whole-body autoradiography of the pregnant mouse after administration of 14C-9-THC. *Toxicol. Appl. Pharmacol.* 22:252, 1971.
265. Idanpaan-Heikkila, J. E., McIsaac, W. M., and Ho, B. T. Delta 9-THC distribution in monkeys, mice and hamsters. Presented at the International Symposium on the Chemistry and Biological Activity of Cannabis, Stockholm, Oct. 1971.
266. *Marihuana and Health*, 1971, p. 171.
267. Ferraro, D. P., Grilly, D. M., and Lynch, W. C. Comparison of behavioral effects of synthetic -tetrahydrocannabinol and marihuana extract in chimpanzees. Prepared for the National Institute of Mental Health, Contract no. HSM 42-21-75, Department of Psychology, University of New Mexico, Albuquerque, Nov. 1971.
268. Harris, R. T., Watters, W. H., and McLendon, D. Behavioral effects in rhesus monkeys of repeated intravenous doses of marihuana extract distillate. Unpublished, 1972.
269. Lemberger, L., Axelrod, J., and Kopin, I. J. Clinical studies on the disposition and metabolism of delta 9 THC and their correlation with its pharmacological effects. *Acta Pharm. Suec.* 8:692, 1971.
270. Claussen, U., and Korte, F. Haschisch XV. *Liebigs Ann. Chem.* 713:162, 1968.
271. Ohlsson, A., et al. Quantification of tetrahydrocannabinol in human blood plasma by mass fragmentography. *Acta Pharm. Suec.* 14(suppl):60, 1977.
272. Miras, C. J., and Coutselinis, A. The distribution of tetrahydrocannabinol-$C^{14}$ in humans. Report no. 24. U.N. Secretariat publication ST/SOA/SER. S/24, Nov. 1970.
273. Wikler, A. Clinical and social aspects of marihuana intoxication. *Arch. Gen. Psychiatry* 23:320, 1970.
274. Jones, R. T. The marihuana induced "high": Influence of expectation, setting and previous drug experience. Presented at Annual Meeting of the Federations of American Societies for Experimental Biology, Chicago, Apr. 1971.
275. Smith, D. E., and Mehl, C. An analysis of marijuana toxicity. In D. E. Smith, ed., *The New Social Drug. Cultural, Medical, and Legal Perspectives on Marijuana.* Englewood Cliffs, N.J.: Prentice-Hall, 1970, p. 63.

276. U.S. Congress. National Commission on Marihuana and Drug Abuse. *Marihuana: A Signal of Misunderstanding*. Washington, D.C.: U.S. Government Printing Office, 1972.
277. Tinklenberg, J. R., et al. Marihuana and immediate memory. *Nature* 226:1171, 1970.
278. Petersen, R. C. Marihuana and health, 1980. In R. T. Peterson, ed., *Marihuana Research Findings: 1980*. Rockville, Md.: National Institute on Drug Abuse, 1980, p. 3 (NIDA Research Monograph no. 31).
279. Tinklenberg, J. R., and Darley, C. F. Psychological and cognitive effects of cannabis. In P. H. Connell and N. Dorn, eds., *Cannabis and Man*. Proceedings of the Third International Cannabis Conference, London, 1975. London: Churchill Livingstone, 1975.
280. Moskowitz, H., McGlothlin, W., and Hulbert, S. The effects of marihuana dosage on driver performance. Contract no. DOT-HS-150-2-236. University of California, Los Angeles, 1973.
281. Moskowitz, H. Marihuana and driving. *Accident Anal. Prev*. 8(1):21, 1976.
282. Klonoff, H. Effects of marijuana on driving in a restricted area and on city streets: Driving performance and physiological changes. In L. L. Miller, ed., *Marijuana: Effects on Human Behavior*. New York: Academic Press, 1974, pp. 359–397.
283. Klonoff, H. Marijuana and driving in real-life situations. *Science* 186:317, 1974.
284. Sterling-Smith, R. S. A special study of drivers most responsible in fatal accidents. Summary for Management Report, Contract no. DOT-HS-310-3-595, Apr. 1976.
285. Reeve, V. C. Incidence of marijuana in a California impaired driver population. State of California, Department of Justice, Division of Law Enforcement Investigative Services Branch, Sacramento, 1979.
286. Soueif, M. I. Chronic cannabis users: Further analysis of objective test results. *Bull. Narc*. 27(4):1, 1975.
287. Soueif, M. I. Some determinants of psychological deficits associated with chronic cannabis consumption. *Bull. Narc*. 28(1):25, 1976.
288. Fletcher, J. M., and Satz, P. A methodological commentary on the Egyptian study of chronic hashish use. *Bull. Narc*. 29:29, 1977.
289. Soueif, M. I. The Egyptian study of chronic cannabis use: A reply to Fletcher and Satz. *Bull. Narc*. 29:35, 1977.
290. Wig, N. N., and Varma, V. K. Patterns of long-term heavy cannabis use in North India and its effects on cognitive functions: A preliminary report. *Drug Alcohol Depend*. 2:211, 1977.
291. Nowlan, R., and Cohen, S. Tolerance to marihuana: Heart rate and subjective "high." *Clin. Pharmacol. Ther*. 22(5):550, 1976.
292. Prakash, R., and Aronow, W. S. Effects of marihuana in coronary disease. Reply. *Clin. Pharmacol. Ther*. 19(1):94, 1976.
293. Helper, R. S., and Frank, I. R. Marihuana smoking and intraocular pressure. *JAMA* 217:1392, 1971.
294. *Marijuana. Report of the Indian Hemp Drug Commission, 1893–1894*. Reprinted: Thomas Jefferson Publishing Co., Silver Spring, Md., 1969.
295. Tashkin, D. P., Calvarese, B., and Simmons, M. Respiratory status of 75 chronic marijuana smokers: Comparison with matched controls. UCLA School of Medicine, Los Angeles, California (abs.) *Am. Rev. Respir. Dis*. 117:(4, 2)261, 1978.
296. Cohen, S., et al. A 94-day cannabis study. In M. C. Braude and S. Szara, eds., *Pharmacology of Marihuana*. New York: Raven Press, 1976, pp. 621–626.
297. Hoffman, D., et al. On the carcinogenicity of marihuana smoke. *Res. Adv. Phytochem*. 9:63, 1975.
298. Novotny, M., Lee, M. C., and Bartle, K. D. A possible chemical basis for the higher mutagenicity of marihuana smoke as compared to tobacco smoke. *Experientia* 32(3):280, 1976.
299. Huber, G. L., et al. Depressant effect of marihuana smoke on antibactericidal activity of pulmonary alveolar macrophages. *Chest* 68:769, 1975.
300. Rosenkrantz, H., and Fleischman, R. W. Effects of cannabis on lungs. In G. G. Nahas and W. D. M. Paton, eds., *Marihuana: Biological Effects. Analysis, Metabolism, Cellular Responses, Reproduction and Brain*. Proceedings of the Satellite Symposium the 7th International Congress of Pharmacology, Paris, July 22–23, 1972. Oxford: Pergamon, 1979, p. 279 (Advances in the Biosciences, Vol. 22–23).
301. Chopra, G. S. Studies on psycho-clinical aspects of long-term marihuana use in 124 cases. *Int. J. Addict*. 8:1015, 1973.
302. Henderson, R. L., Tennant, F. S., and Guerry, R. Respiratory manifestations of hashish smoking. *Arch. Otolaryngol*. 95:248, 1972.
303. Tennat, F. S., et al. Medical manifestations associated with hashish. *JAMA* 216:1965, 1971.
304. Tennant, F. S., Jr. Histopathologic and clinical abnormalities of the respiratory system in

chronic hashish smokers. *Subst. Alcohol Action/Misuse* 1(1):93, 1980.
305. Harclerode, J. The effect of marihuana on reproduction and development. In R. C. Petersen, ed., *Marijuana Research Findings: 1980*. Rockville, Md.: National Institute on Drug Abuse, 1980, p. 137 (NIDA Research Monograph no. 31).
306. Hembree, W. C., III, et al. Changes in human spermatozoa associated with high dose marihuana smoking. In G. G. Nahas and W. D. M. Paton, eds., *Marihuana: Biological Effects. Analysis, Metabolism, Cellular Responses, Reproduction, and Brain*. Proceedings of the Satellite: Symposium of the 7th International Congress of Pharmacology, Paris, July 22–23, 1978. Oxford: Pergamon, 1979, p. 429 (Advances in the Biosciences, Vol. 22–23).
307. Issidorides, M. R. Observations in chronic hashish users: Nuclear aberrations in blood and sperm and abnormal acrosomes in spermatozoa. In G. G. Nahas and W. D. M. Paton, eds., *Marihuana: Biological Effects; Analysis Metabolism, Cellular Responses, Reproduction and Brain*. Proceedings of the Satellite Symposium of the 7th International Congress of Pharmacology, Paris, July 22–23, 1972. Oxford: Pergamon, 1979, p. 377 (Advances in the Biosciences, Vol. 22–23).
308. Sassenrath, E. N., Chapman, L. F., and Goo, G. P. Reproduction in rhesus monkeys chronically exposed to delta-9-tetrahydrocannabinol. In G. G. Nahas and W. D. M. Paton, eds., *Marihuana: Biological Effects; Analysis, Metabolism, Cellular Responses, Reproduction and Brain*. Proceedings of the Satellite Symposium of the 7th International Congress of Pharmacology, Paris, July 22–23, 1978. Oxford: Pergamon, 1979, p. 501 (Advances in the Biosciences, Vol. 22–23).
309. Dalterio, S., Steger, R., and Barthe, A. Effects of psychoactive or non-psychoactive cannabinoids on reproductive functions in male offspring. In S. Agurell, R. Willette, and W. Dewey, eds., *Cannabinoids '82*. New York: Academic Press (in press).
310. Strahilevitz, M., et al. Blocking of the effect of delta 1 tetrahydrocannabinol (delta 1 THC) on spontaneous motor activity in the rat by immunization with a protein conjugate of delta 1 THC. *Life Sci.* 14:1975, 1974.
311. Nahas, G. G., et al. Evidence for the possible immunogenicity of delta-9-tetrahydrocannabinol (THC) in rodents. *Nature* 243:407, 1973.
312. Nahas, G. G., et al. Inhibition of cellular mediated immunity in marihuana smokers. *Science* 183:419, 1974.
322. Herha, J., and Obe, G. Chromosomal damage in chronic users of cannabis. *Pharmakopsychiatric* 7:328, 1974.
323. Kumar, S., and Kunwar, K. B. Chromosome abnormalities in cannabis addicts. *J. Assoc. Physicians India* 19:193, 1972, 1971.
324. Stenchever, M. A., Kunysz, T. J., and Allen, M. A. Chromosome breakage in users of marihuana. *Am. J. Obstet. Gynecol.* 118:106, 1974.
325. Matsuyama, S. S., et al. Chromosome studies before and after supervised marijuana smoking. In M. C. Braude and S. Szara, eds., *Pharmacology of Marihuana*. New York: Raven Press, 1976, p. 723.
326. Matsuyama, S. S., et al. Marijuana exposure in vivo and human lyphocyte chromosomes. *Mutat. Res.* 48:255, 1977.
327. Nichols, W. W., et al. Cytogenetic studies on human subjects receiving marihuana and delta-9-tetrahydrocannabinol. *Mutation Res.* 26:413, 1974.
328. Leuchtenberger, C., and Leuchtenberger, R. Correlated cytological and cytochemical studies of the effects of fresh marihuana cigarette smoke on growth and DNA metabolism of animal and human lung cultures. In M. C. Braude and S. Szara, eds., *Pharmacology of Marihuana*. New York: Raven Press, 1976, p. 595.
329. Morishima, A., et al. Hypoploid metaphases in cultured lymphocytes of marihuana smokers. In G. G. Nahas and W. D. M. Paton, eds., *Marihuana: Biological Effects*. New York: Pergamon Press, 1979, pp. 371–376.
330. Boggan, W. O., Steele, R. A., and Freedman, D. 9-Tetrahydrocannabinol effect on audiogenic seizure susceptibility. *Psychopharmacologia* 29:101, 1973.
331. Carlini, E. A., et al. Letter. Cannabidiol and *Cannabis sativa* extract protect mice and rats against convulsive agents. *J. Pharm. Pharmacol.* 25:664, 1973.
332. Man, D. P., and Consroe, P. F. Anticonvulsant effect of delta-9-tetrahydrocannabinol sound-induced seizures in audiogenic rats. IRCS International Research System, Mar. 1973.
333. Corcoran, M. E., et al. Acute antiepileptic effects of delta-9-tetrahydrocannabinol in rats with kindled seizures. *Exp. Neurol.* 40(2):471, 1973.
334. Fried, P. A., and McIntyre, D. C. Electrical and behavioral attenuation of the anti-convulsant properties of delta-9-THC following chronic

administration. *Psychopharmacologia (Berlin)* 31(3):215, 1973.

335. Consroe, P. F., and Man, D. P. Effects of delta-8- and delta-9-tetrahydrocannabinol on experimentally induced seizures. *Life Sci.* 13:429, 1973.

336. Izquierdo, I., Orsingher, O. A., and Berardi, A. C. Effect of cannabidiol and of other *Cannabis sativa* compounds on hippocampal seizures. *Psychopharmacologia* 28:95, 1973.

338. Consroe, P. F. Effect of delta-9-tetrahydrocannabinol on a cholinergic-induced activation of the electroencephalogram in the rabbit. *Res. Commun. Chem. Pathol. Pharmacol.* 5:705, 1973.

339. Hattori, T., Jakubovic, A., and McGeer, P. L. The effect of cannabinoids on the number of nuclear membrane-attached ribosomes in infant rat brain. *Neuropharmacology* 12:995, 1973.

340. Wallach, M. B., and Gershon, S. The effects of delta-8-tetrahydrocannabinol on the electroencephalogram, reticular formation multiple unit activity and sleep in the rat. (In press.)

341. Fujimori, M., and Himwich, H. E. Delta-9-tetrahydrocannabinol and the sleep-wakefulness cycle in rabbits. *Physiol. Behav.* 11:291, 1973.

342. Barratt, E. S., and Adams, P. M. Chronic marihuana usage and sleep-wakefulness cycles in cats. *Biol. Psychiatry* 6(3):207, 1973.

343. Barratt, E., et al. The effects of the chronic use of marijuana on sleep and perceptual-motor performance in humans. In M. F. Lewis, ed., *Current Research in Marihuana*. New York: Academic, 1972, p. 163.

344. Boyd, E. S., Boyd, E. H., and Brown, L. E. The effects of some drugs on an evoked response sensitive to tetrahydrocannabinols. *J. Pharmacol. Exp. Ther.* 189:748, 1974.

345. Vasquex, A. J., and Sabelli, H. C. Electrophysiological studies with delta-9-tetrahydrocannabinol. In *Drug Addiction: Behavioral Aspects*. New York: Futura Press. (In press.)

346. Bieger, D., and Hockman, C. H. Differential effects produced by delta-1-tetrahydrocannabinol on lateral geniculate neurones. *Neuropharmacology* 12:269, 1973.

347. Pirch, J. H., et al. Studies on EEG tolerance to marihuana in the rat. *Arch. Int. Pharmacodyn.* 203:213, 1973.

348. Stadnicki, S. W., et al. Delta 9-tetrahydrocannabinol: Subcortical spike bursts and motor manifestations in a Fischer rat treated orally for 109 days. *Life Sci.* 74:463, 1974.

349. Brady, R. O., and Carbone, E. Comparison of the effects of 9-tetrahydrocannabinol, 11-hydroxy-delta 9-tetrahydrocannabinol and ethanol on the electrophysiological activity of the giant axon of the squid. *Neuropharmacology* 12:601, 1973.

350. Byck, R., and Ritchie, J. M. 9-tetrahydrocannabinol: Effects on mammalian nonmyelinated nerve fibers. *Science* 180:84, 1973.

351. Seeman, P., Chau-Wong, M., and Moyyen, S. The membrane binding of morphine, diphenylhydatoin, and tetrahydrocannabinol. *Can. J. Physiol. Pharmacol.* 50:1193, 1973.

352. Gascon, A., and Peres, A. L. Effect of delta-8- and delta-9-tetrahydrocannabinol on the peripheral autonomic nervous system in vitro. *Can. J. Physiol. Pharmacol.* 51:12, 1973.

353. Luthra, Y. K., Rosenkrantz, H., and Braude, M. C. Differential neurochemistry and temporal pattern in rats treated orally with delta-9-tetrahydrocannabinol for six months. (Submitted for publication.)

354. Ng, L. K., et al. Delta-9-tetrahydrocannabinol and ethanol: differential effects on sympathetic activity in differing environmental setting. *Science* 180:1368, 1973.

355. Lamprecht, F., et al. Effect of delta-9-tetrahydrocannabinol on immobilization-induced changes in rat adrenal medullary enzymes. *Eur. J. Pharmacol.* 21:249, 1973.

356. Neto, J. P., and Carvalho, F. V. The effects of chronic cannabis treatment on the aggressive behavior and the brain 5-hydroxy-tryptamine levels of rats with different temperaments. *Psychopharmacologia* 32:383, 1973.

357. Burstein, S., Levin, E., and Varanelli, C. Prostaglandins and cannabis. II. Inhibition of biosynthesis by the naturally occurring cannabinoids. *Biochem. Pharmacol.* 22:2905, 1973.

358. Smith, C. G., et al. Effects of tetrahydrocannabinol on prolactin levels in rhesus monkey. Presented at the NIDA Conference on Genetic, Perinatal, and Developmental Effects of Abused Substances, March 20–22, 1979, Airlie, Va.

359. Hembree, W. C., III, Zeidenberg, P., and Nahas, G. G. Marihuana's effects on human gonadal function. In G. G. Nahas, ed., *Marijuana—Chemistry, Biochemistry, and Cellular Effects*. New York: Springer-Verlag, 1976, p. 521.

360. Smith, C. G., et al. Effect of delta$^9$-tetrahydrocannabinol (THC) on female reproductive function. In G. G. Nahas and W. D. H. Paton, eds., *Marijuana—Biological Effects; Analysis, Metabolism, Cellular Responses, Reproduction*

*and Brain*. Proceedings of the Satellite Symposium of the 7th International Congress of Pharmacology, Paris, July 22–23, 1978. Oxford: Pergamon, 1979, p. 4. (Advances in the Biosciences, Vol. 22–23).

361. Tyrey, L. Delta-9-tetrahydrocannabinol suppression of episodic luteninizing hormone secretion in ovariectomized rat. *Endocrinology* 102:1808, 1978.

362. Smith, C. G., Ruppert, M. J., and Besch, N. F. Comparison of the effects of marijuana extract and delta 9-tetrahydrocannabinol on gonadotropin levels in the rhesus monkey. *Pharmacologist* 21:204, 1979.

363. Nir, I., et al. Suppression of the cyclic surge of luteninizing hormone secretion and of ovulation in the rat by $\Delta^1$-tetrahydrocannabinol. *Nature* (London) 243:470, 1973.

364. Asch, R. H., et al. Blockage of the ovulatory reflex in the rabbit with delta-9-tetrahydrocannabinol. *Fertil. Steril.* 31:331, 1979.

365. Lemberger, L., and Rubin, A. The physiologic disposition of marijuana in man. *Life Sci.* 17:1637, 1975.

366. Raine, J. M., Wing, D. R., and Paton, W. D. The effects of delta-1-tetrahydrocannabinol on mammary gland growth, enzyme activity and plasma prolactin levels in the mouse. *Eur. J. Pharmacol.* 51:11, 1978.

367. Daley, J. D., Branda, L. A., and Rosenfeld, J. Increase of serum prolactin in male rats by (minus)-trans-delta-9-tetrahydrocannabinol. *J. Endocrinol.* 63:415, 1974.

368. Lomax, P. The effect of marijuana on pituitary-thyroid activity in the rat. *Agents Actions* 1:5, 1970.

369. Dewey, W. L., Peng, T. C., and Harris, L. S. The effect of 1-*trans*-delta-9-tetrahydrocannabinol on the hypothalamic-hypophyseal-adrenal axis of cats. *Eur. J. Pharmacol.* 12:382, 1970.

370. Kubena, R. K., Perhach, J. L., Jr., and Berry, H. 3D. Corticosterone elevation mediated centrally by $delta^1$-tetrahydrocannabinol. *Eur. J. Pharmacol.* 14:89, 1971.

371. Hollister, L. E., et al. Delta $^1$-tetrahydrocannabinol, synhexyl, and marijuana extract administered orally in man: Catecholamine excretion, plasma cortisol levels and platelet serotonin content. *Psychopharmacologia* 17:354, 1970.

372. Knobil, E. On the control of gonadotropin secretion in the rhesus monkey. *Rec. Prog. Horm. Res.* 30:1, 1974.

373. Noel, G. L., Suh, H. K., and Frantz, A. G. L-dopa suppression of TRH-stimulated prolactin release in man. *J. Clin. Endocrinol. Metab.* 36:1255, 1973.

374. Labrie, F., et al. Control of prolactin secretion at the pituitary level: A model for postsynaptic dopaminergic systems. In R. Collu et al., eds., *Central Nervous System Effects of Hypothalamic Hormones and Other Peptides*. New York: Raven Press, 1979, p. 207.

375. Grimm, Y., and Reichlin, S. Thyrotropin-releasing hormone (TRH): neurotransmitter regulation of secretion by mouse hypothalamic tissue *in vitro*. *Endocrinology* 93:695, 1972.

377. Truitt, E. B., Jr., and Anderson, S. H. Biogenic amine alterations produced in the brain by tetrahydrocannabinol and their metabolites. *Ann. N.Y. Acad. Sci.* 191:68, 1972.

378. Welch, B. L., et al. Rapid depletion of adrenal epinephrine and elevation of telencephalic serotonin by (−)-*trans*-9-tetrahydrocannabinol in mice. *Res. Commun. Chem. Pathol. Pharmacol.* 4:382, 1971.

379. Howes, J., and Osgood, P. The effect of delta-9-tetrahydrocannabinol on the uptake and release of $^{14}$C-dopamine from crude striatal synaptosoma preparations. *Neuropharmacology* 13:1109, 1974.

380. Sofia, R. D., Dixit, B. W., and Barry, H. The effect of delta-1-tetrahydrocannabinol on serotonin metabolism in the rat brain. *Life Sci.* 10:425, 1971.

381. Revuelta, A. V., et al. GABAergic mediation in the inhibition of hippocampal acetylcholine turnover rate elicited by delta 9-tetrahydrocannabinol. *Neuropharmacology* 18:525, 1979.

382. Marks, B. H. Delta $^1$-THC and luteinizing hormone secretion. In E. Zimmerman, W. H. Gispen, B. H. Marks, and D. de Wied, eds., *Progress in Brain Research—Drug Effects on Neuroendocrine Regulation*, vol. 10. Amsterdam: Elsevier, 1973, p. 331.

383. Jakubovic, A., and McGeer, P. L. Inhibition of rat brain protein and nucleic acid synthesis by cannabinoids in vitro. *Can. J. Biochem.* 50:654, 1972.

384. Greenberg, J. H., Mellors, A., and McGowan, J. C. Molar volume relationships and the specific inhibition of a synaptosomal enzyme by psychoactive cannabinoids. *J. Med. Chem.* 21:1208, 1978.

385. Harper, J. W., Heath, R. G., and Myers, W. A. Effects of *Cannabis sativa* on ultrastructure of the synapse in monkey brain. *J. Neurosci. Res.* 3:87, 1977.

386. Heath, R. G., et al. Chronic marijuana smok-

ing: its effect on function and structure of the primate brain. In G. G. Nahas and W. D. M. Paton, eds., *Marijuana: Biological Effects; Analysis, Metabolism, Cellular Responses, Reproduction and Brain.* Proceedings of the Satellite Symposium of the 7th International Congress of Pharmacology, Paris, July 22–23, 1978. Oxford: Pergamon, 1979, p. 713. (Advances in the Biosciences, Vol. 22–23).

387. Birmingham, M. K. Reduction by delta-9-tetrahydrocannabinol in the blood pressure of hypertensive rats bearing regenerated adrenal glands. *Br. J. Pharmacol.* 48:169, 1973.

388. Babor, T. F., Mendelson, J. H., Greenberg, I., et al. Marihuana Consumption and Tolerance to Physiological and Subjective Effects. *Arch. Gen. Psychiatry* 32:1548, 1975.

389. Cavero, I., et al. Effects of (−)-delta-9-*trans*-tetrahydrocannabinol on regional blood flow in anesthetized dogs. *Eur. J. Pharmacol.* 20:373, 1972.

390. Graham, J. D., and Li, D. M. Cardiovascular and respiratory effects of cannabis in cat and rat. *Br. J. Pharmacol.* 49:1, 1973.

391. Cavero, I., et al. Studies of the hypotensive activity of (−)-delta-9-trans-tetrahydrocannabinol on anesthetized dogs. *Res. Commun. Chem. Pathol. Pharmacol.* 6(2):527, 1973.

392. Cavero, I., et al. Certain observations on the interrelations between respiratory and cardiovascular effects of (−)-delta-9-*trans*-tetrahydrocannabinol. *Res. Commun. Chem. Pathol. Pharmacol.* 3(2):483, 1972.

393. Sengstake, C. B. Interactive effects of marihuana and Na pentobarbital on heart rate in the rat. *Science* (submitted).

394. Sofia, R. D., and Knobloch, L. D. The interaction of delta-9-tetrahydrocannabinol pretreatment with various sedative-hypnotic drugs. *Psychopharmacologia* 30:185, 1973.

395. Sofia, R. D., Kubena, R. K., and Barry, H., 3D. Inactivity of delta-9-tetrahydrocannabinol in antidepressant screening tests. *Psychopharmacologia* 31:121, 1973.

396. Pirch, J. H., et al. Antagonism of amphetamine locomotor stimulation in rats by single doses of marijuana extract administered orally. *Neuropharmacology* 12:485, 1973.

397. Chesher, G. B., Jackson, D. M., and Starmer, G. A. Interaction of cannabis and general anesthetic agents in mice. Personal communication.

398. Adams, H. R., and Sofia, R. D. Interaction of chloramphenicol and delta-1-tetrahydrocannabinol in barbital-anesthetized mice. *Experientia* 29:181, 1973.

399. Rating, D., et al. Effect of subchronic treatment with (−) 8-trans-tetrahydrocannabinol (8-THC) on food intake, body temperature, hexobarbital sleeping time and hexobarbital elimination in rodents. *Psychopharmacologia* 27:349, 1972.

400. Poddar, M. K., and Ghosh, J. J. Effect of cannabis extract, Delta 9-tetrahydrocannabinol and lysergic acid diethylamide on rat liver enzymes. *Biochem. Pharmacol.* 21:3301, 1973.

401. Hofmann, F. G. *A Handbook on Drug and Alcohol Abuse: The Biomedical Aspects.* New York: Oxford University Press, 1975.

402. Klonoff, H. Strategy and tactics of marihuana research. *Can. Med. Assoc. J.* 108:145, 1973.

403. Pillard, R. C. Marihuana. *N. Engl. J. Med.* 283:294, 1970.

404. Dornbush, R. L., Fink, M., and Freedman, A. M. Marijuana, memory and perception. *Am. J. Psychiatry* 128:194, 1971.

405. McGlothlin, W. H., Arnold, D. O., and Rowan, P. K. Marihuana use among adults. *Psychiatry* 33:433, 1970.

406. Weil, A. T., and Zinberg, N. E. Acute effects of marihuana on speech. *Nature* 222:434, 1969.

407. Volavka, J., et al. Marihuana, EEG and behavior. *Ann. N.Y. Acad. Sci.* 191:205, 1971.

408. Mendelson, J. H., et al. Behavioral and biological concomitants of chronic marihuana smoking by heavy and casual users. Prepared for the National Commission on Marihuana and Drug Abuse, Department of Psychiatry, Boston City Hospital, Jan. 1972.

409. Crancer, A., Jr., et al. Comparison of the effects of marihuana and alcohol on simulated driving performance. Report 021, State of Washington, Department of Motor Vehicles, Apr. 1969. *Science* 164:851, 1969.

410. Abel, E. Marihuana and memory. *Nature* 227:1151, 1970.

411. Abel, E. L. Effects of marihuana on the solution of anagrams, memory and appetite. *Nature* 231:260, 1971.

412. Abel, E. L. Marihuana and memory: acquisition or retrieval. *Science* 173:1038, 1971.

413. Abel, E. L. Retrieval of information after use of marihuana. *Nature* 231(297):58, 1971.

414. Baker, A. A., and Lucas, E. G. Some hospital admissions associated with cannabis. *Lancet* 1:148, 1969.

415. Baker-Bates, E. T. A case of *Cannabis indica* intoxication. *Lancet* I:811, 1935.

416. Gaskill, H. S. Marihuana, an intoxicant. *Am. J. Psychiatry* 102:202, 1945.

417. Grossman, W. Adverse reactions associated with cannabis products in India. *Ann. Intern. Med.* 70:529, 1969.
418. Persyko, I. Marihuana psychosis. *JAMA* 212:1527, 1970.
419. Bialos, D. Adverse marihuana reactions: A critical examination of the literature with selected case material. *Am. J. Psychiatry* 127(6):119, 1970.
420. Sonnenreich, c., Goes, J. F. Marihuana and mental disturbances. *Neurobiologia* 25:69, 1962.
421. Sigg, B. W. *Le Cannabisme Chronique, Fruit de Sous-development et du Capitalisme: Etude Socio-economique et Psycho-pathologique.* Algiers, 1963.
422. Dally, P. Undesirable effects of marihuana. *Br. Med. J.* 367, 1967.
423. Hamaker, S. T. A. Case of overdose of *Cannabis indica. Ther. Gaz.* 7:808, 1891.
424. Marten, G. W. Case report. Adverse reaction to the use of marihuana. *J. Tenn. Med. Assoc.* 62:627, 1969.
425. Weil, A. T. Adverse reactions to marihuana. Classification and suggested treatment. *N. Engl. J. Med.* 282:997, 1970.
426. Chopra, R. N., Chopra, G. S., and Chopra, I. C. *Cannabis sativa* in relation to mental diseases and crime in India. *Indian J. Med. Res.* 30(1):155, 1942.
427. Peebles, A. S. M., and Mann, H. W. Ganja as a cause of insanity and crime in Bental. *Indian Med. Gaz.* 49:395, 1914.
428. Dhunjibhoy, J. E. The role of "Indian hemp" in causation of insanity in India. In *Transactions of 7th Session, Far Eastern Association of Tropical Medicine*, 1928, pp. 400–407.
429. Ewens, G. F. W. Insanity following the use of Indian hemp. *Indian Med. Gaz.* 39:401, 1904.
430. Warnock, J. Insanity from hasheesh. *J. Ment. Sci.* 49:96, 1902.
431. Kolansky, H., and Moore, W. T. Effects of marihuana on adolescents and young adults. *JAMA* 216:486, 1971.
432. Talbot, J. A., and Teague, J. W. Marihuana psychosis. Acute toxic psychosis associated with the use of cannabis derivatives. *JAMA* 210:299, 1969.
433. Colbach, E. M., and Crowe, R. R. Marihuana associated psychosis in Vietnam. *Mil. Med.* 135(7):571, 1970.
434. Bey, D. R., and Zecchinelli, V. A. Marijuana as a coping device in Vietnam. *Mil. Med.* 136:448, 1971.
435. Halikas, J. A., Goodman, D. W., and Guze, S. B. Marihuana effects: A survey of regular users. *JAMA* 217:692, 1971.
436. Christozov, C. Moroccan poisoning from the light of studies on chronic mental patients. *Maroc. Med.* 44:630, 1965.
437. *Indian Hemp Drug Commission Report 1893–1894.* Reprinted, Silver Spring, Md.: Thomas Jefferson Publishing, 1969, p. 3281.
438. Benabud, A. Psychopathological aspects of the cannabis situation in Morroco: Statistical data for 1956. *U.N. Bull Nar.* 9(4):1, 1957.
439. Chopra, R. N., and Chopra, G. S. The present position of hemp-drug addiction in India. *Indian Med. Res. Memoirs* (31):1, 1939.
440. Winick, C. Use of drugs by jazz musicians. *Soc. Probl.* 7:240, 1960.
441. Meyer, R. E. Psychiatric consequences of marihuana use: the state of the evidence. In J. R. Tinklenberg, ed., *Marihuana and Health Hazards: Methodological Issues in Current Research.* New York: Academic Press, 1975, p. 133.
442. Treffert, D. A. Marijuana use in schizophrenia: A clear hazard. *Am. J. Psychiatry* 135:10, 1978.
443. Abel, E. L. The relationship between cannabis and violence: A review. *Psychol. Bull.* 84:193, 1977.
444. Abruzzi, W. Drug-induced psychosis. *Int. J. Addict.* 121:183, 1977.
445. Stanton, M. D., Mintz, J., and Franklin, R. M. Drug flashbacks, II. Some additional findings. *Int. J. Addict.* 11(1):53, 1976.
446. Smith, D. E. Acute and chronic toxicity of marihuana. *J. Psychedel. Drugs* 2:37, 1968.
447. Ray, R., et al. Psychosocial correlates of chronic cannabis use. *Drug Alcohol Depend.* 3:235, 1978.
448. Deakin, S. Death from taking Indian hemp. *Indian Med. Gaz.* 71, 1880.
449. Bouquet, J. Cannabis. *U.N. Bull. Nar.* 2(4):14, 1950; 3(1):22, 1951.
450. Brill, N. O., et al. The marihuana problem. *Ann. Intern. Med.* 73(3):449, 1970.
451. Henderson, A. H., and Pugsley, D. J. Collapse after intravenous injection of hashish. *Br. Med. J.* 3:229, 1968.
452. King, A. B., and Cowen, D. L. Effect of intravenous injection of marihuana. *JAMA* 210:724, 1969.
453. King, A. B., Pechet, G. S., and Pechet, L. Intravenous injection of crude marihuana. *JAMA* 214:30, 1970.
454. Lundberg, G. D., Adelson, J., and Prosnitz, E. H. Marihuana-induced hospitalization. *JAMA* 215:121, 1971.

455. Gary, N. E., and Keylon, V. Intravenous administration of marihuana. *JAMA* 211:501, 1970.
456. Loewe, S. Studies on the pharmacology and acute toxicity of compounds with marihuana activity. *J. Pharmacol. Exp. Ther.* 88:154, 1946.
457. Joachimoglu, G. CIBA Foundation Study Group 21, 10, 1965.
458. Phillips, R. N., Turk, R. F., and Forney, R. B. Acute toxicity of delta-9-tetrahydrocannabinol in rats and mice. *Proc. Soc. Exp. Biol. Med.* 136:260, 1971.
459. Thompson, G. W., et al. Determine toxicity of delta-8- and delta-9-tetrahydrocannabinol and marihuana extract. Mason Research Institute, Worcester, Mass. Reports I–XIX to the National Institute of Mental Health. Contract no. HSM 42-70-95 (June 1970–June 1971), no. HSM 42-71-79 (June 1971–Jan. 1972).
460. Dalterio, S., et al. Cannabinoids in male mice: Effects on fertility and spermatogenesis. *Science* 216:315, 1982.
461. Carakushansky, G., Neu, R. L., and Gardner, L. I. Lysergide and cannabis as possible teratogens in man. *Lancet*, 1:150, 1969.
462. Hecht, F., et al. Lysergic-acid-diethylamide and cannabis as possible teratogens in man. *Lancet* 2:1087, 1968.
463. Gelehrter, I. D. Lysergic acid diethylamide (LSD) and estrophy of the bladder. *J. Pediatr.* 77:1065, 1970.
464. Miras, C. J. *Hashish, Its Chemistry and Pharmacology*. Boston: Little, Brown, 1965, pp. 37–52.
465. Neu, R. L., et al. Cannabis and chromosomes. *Lancet* 1:675, 1969.
466. Martin, P. A. Cannabis and chromosomes. *Lancet* 1:370, 1969.
467. Dorrance, D., Janiger, O., and Teplitz, R. L. *In vivo* effects of illicit hallucinogens in human lymphocyte chromosomes. *JAMA* 212:1488, 1970.
468. Gilmore, D. G., et al. Chromosomal aberrations in users of psychoactive drugs. *Arch. Gen. Psychiatry* 24:258, 1971.
469. Rubin, V., and Comitas, L. A study of the effects of chronic ganja smoking in Jamaica. Research Institute for the Study of Man, New York. In preparation for the National Institute of Mental Health, Contract no. HSM 42-70-77, 1972.
470. Cohen, S. *The Substance Abuse Problem*. New York: Haworth Press, 1980, p. 14.
471. Freedman, H. L., and Rockmore, M. J. Marihuana, a factor in personality evaluation and army maladjustment. *J. Clin. Psychopathol.* 7:765 (Part I); 8:221 (Part II), 1946.
472. Chopra, R. N. Drug addiction in India and its treatment. *Indian Med. Gaz.* 70(3):121, 1935.
473. Chopra, R. N. Use of hemp drugs in India. *Indian Med. Gaz.* 75(6):356, 1940.
474. Campbell, A. M., et al. Cerebral atrophy in young cannabis smokers. *Lancet* 1219, 1971.
475. Fink, M., et al. Quantitative EEG studies of marijuana, delta-9-tetrahydrocannabinol, and hashish in man. In M. C. Braude and S. Szara, eds., *Pharmacology of Marihuana*. New York: Raven Press, 1976, p. 383.
476. Co, B. T., et al. Absence of cerebral atrophy in chronic cannabis users. Evaluation by computerized transaxial tomography. *JAMA* 237:1229, 1977.
477. Kuehnle, J., et al. Computed tomographic examination of heavy marijuana smokers. *JAMA* 237:1231, 1977.
478. Heath, R. G. Marihuana and delta-9-tetrahydrocannabinol: acute and chronic effects on brain function of monkeys. In M. C. Braude and S. Szara, eds., *Pharmacology of Marihuana*. New York: Raven Press, 1976, p. 345.
479. Klonoff, H., and Low, M. D. Psychological and neurophysiological effects of marihuana in man: An interaction model. In L. L. Miller, ed., *Marihuana: Effects on Human Behavior*. New York: Academic Press, 1974, pp. 359–397.
480. Talbott, J. A. Pot reactions. *USARUV Med. Bull.* 40, 1968.
481. Heiman, E. M. Marihuana precipitated psychosis in patient evacuated to ConUS. *USARU Med. Bull.* 40(9):75, 1968.
482. Kaplan, H. S. Psychosis associated with marijuana. *N.Y. State J. Med.* 71(4):433, 1971.
483. Perna, D. Psychotogenic effect of marihuana. *JAMA* 209:1085, 1969.
484. Keeler, M. H. Marihuana induced hallucinations. *Dis. Nerv. Sys.* 29:314, 1968.
485. Defer, B., and Diehl, M. L. Acute psychoses due to cannabis Capropos of 560 cases. *Ann. Med. Psychol. (Paris)* 2:260, 1968.
486. Wurmser, L., Levin, L., and Lewis, A. Chronic paranoid symptoms and thought disorders in users of marihuana and LSD as observer in psychotherapy. *Bull. Prob. Drug. Depend.* 31:6154, 1969.
487. Bromberg, W. Marihuana, a psychiatric study. *JAMA* 113:4, 1939.
488. Bromberg, W. Marihuana intoxication, a clinical study of *Cannabis sativa* intoxication. *Am. J. Psychiatry* SCI(2):303, 1934.

489. Curtis, H.C., and Wolfe, J. R. Psychosis following the use of marihuana with report of cases. *J. Kans. Med. Soc.* 40:515, 526, 1939.
490. Hughes, J. E., Steachly, L. P., and Bier, M. M. Marihuana and the diabetic coma. *JAMA* 214(6):1113, 1970.
491. Keuip, W. Psychotic symptoms due to cannabis abuse. *Dis. Nerv. Sys.* 31(2):119, 1970.
492. Keeler, M. H., and Reifler, C. B. Grand mal convulsions subsequent to marihuana use: Case report. *Dis. Nerv. Sys.* 28:474, 1967.
493. Bartolucci, G., et al. Marihuana psychosis: A case report. *Can. Psychiatr. Assoc. J.* 14:77, 1969.
494. Ames, F. A clinical and metabolic study of acute intoxication with *Cannabis sativa* and its role in the model psychoses. *J. Ment. Sci.* 104(437):972, 1958.
495. Williams, E. G., et al. Studies on marihuana and pyrahexyl compound. *Pub. Health Rep.* 61(29):1059, 1946.
496. Ungerleider, J. T. Letter to the editor. *Am. J. Psychiatry* 125:1448, 1969.
497. Ungerleider, J. T., et al. A statistical survey of adverse reactions to LSD in Los Angeles County. *Am. J. Psychiatry* 125:108, 1968.
498. Favazza, A., and Domino, E. F. Recurrent LSD experience (flashbacks) triggered by marihuana. *Univ. Mich. Med. Center J.* 35:214, 1969.
499. Fink, M., et al. Interim Report: Study of Marihuana Users in Greece. Prepared for the National Institute of Mental Health, Contract no. HSM 42-70-98, Department of Psychiatry, New York Medical College, Oct. 1971.
500. Haines, L., and Green, W. Marihuana use patterns. *Br. J. Addict.* 65(4):347, 1970.
501. McGlothlin, W. H. Marihuana: An analysis of use, distribution and control. Prepared for the Department of Justice, Washington, D.C., June 1971.
502. Rickles, W. H., Kales, A., and Hanles, J. Psychophysiology of marihuana. Presented to Langley Porter Neuropsychiatric Institute, San Francisco, May 1970.
503. Rosenkrantz, H., Heyman, I. A., and Braude, M. C. Inhalation, parenteral and oral $LD_{50}$ doses of delta-9-tetrahydrocannabinol in Fischer rats. *Toxicol. Appl. Pharmacol.* (in press).
504. Mantilla-Plata, B., and Harbison, R. D. Alteration of delta$^9$-tetrahydrocannabinol-induced prenatal toxicity of phenobarbital and SKF-525A. In G. G. Nahas, ed., *Marihuana: Chemistry, Biochemistry and Cellular Effects*. New York: Springer-Verlag, 1976, p. 469.
505. Parker, J. M., and Dubas, T. C. Automatic determination of the pain threshold to electroshock and the effects of 9-THC. *Int. J. Clin. Pharmacol.* 7:75, 1973.
506. Olsen, J. L., et al. Preparation of 9-tetrahydrocannabinol for intravenous injection. *J. Pharm. Pharmacol.* 25:344, 1973.
507. Thompson, G. R., et al. Chronic oral toxicity of cannabinoids in rats. *Toxicol. Appl. Pharmacol.* 25:373, 1973.
508. Toxicological manifestations in Fischer rats treated orally with delta-9-tetrahydrocannabinol at doses equivalent to American marihuana and hashish for 180 consecutive days. Contract Report HSM-42-71-79, Mar. 9, 1973.
509. Cohn, R. A., Barratt, E. S., and Pirch, J. H. Marijuana responses in rats: Influence of castration or testosterone. *Proc. Soc. Exp. Biol. Med.* 146:109, 1974.
510. Leuchtenberger, C., Leuchtenberger, R., and Schneider, A. Effects of marihuana and tobacco smoke on human lung physiology. *Nature* 241:137, 1973.
511. Leuchtenberger, C., et al. Effects of marijuana and tobacco smoke on DNA and chromosomal complement in human lung explants. *Nature* 242:403, 1973.
512. Haley, L., et al. The effect of natural and synthetic delta-9-tetrahydrocannabinol on fetal development. *Toxicol. Appl. Pharmacol.* 21:450, 1973.
513. Pace, H. B., Davis, W. M., and Borgen, L. A. Teratogenesis and marihuana. *Ann. N.Y. Acad. Sci.* 191:123, 1971.
514. Uyeno, E. T. Delta-9-tetrahydrocannabinol administration during pregnancy in the rat. *Proc. West. Pharmacol. Soc.* 16:64, 1973.
515. Harbison, R. D., and Mantilla-Plata, B. Prenatal toxicity, maternal distribution and placental transfer of tetrahydrocannabinol. *J. Pharmacol. Exp. Ther.* 180(2):446, 1972.
516. Mantilla-Plata, B., Clewe, G. L., and Harbison, R. D. Teratogenic and mutagenetic studies of delta-9-tetrahydrocannabinol in mice. Abstract no. 2995. *Fed. Proc.* 32(3):746, 1973.
517. Lenicque, P. M., Paris, M. R., and Poulot, M. Effects of some components of *Cannabis sativa* on the regenerating planarian worm *dugesia tigrina*. *Experientia* 28:1399, 1972.
518. Nahas, G. G., and Paton, W. D. M., Editors. *Marihuana: Biological Effects; Analysis Metabolism, Cellular Responses, Reproduction and Brain*. Proceedings of the Satellite Symposium of the 7th International Congress of Pharmacology, Paris, July 22–23, 1978. Oxford: Pergamon, 1979 (Advances in the Bio-

sciences, Vol. 22–23).
519. Kolansky, H., and Moore, W. T. Toxic effects of chronic marihuana use. *JAMA* 222:35, 1972.
520. Harmon, J., and Aliapoulis, M. A. Gynecomastia in marihuana users. *N. Engl. J. Med.* 187:936, 1972.
521. Jones, R. Human effects. In R. C. Petersen, ed., *Marihuana Research Findings: 1976*. Rockville, Md.: National Institute on Drug Abuse, 1977, p. 128. (NIDA Research Monograph no. 14).
522. Jones, R. T., and Benowitz, N. The 30-day trip—Clinical studies of cannabis tolerance and dependence. In M. C. Braude and S. Szara, eds., *Pharmacology of Marihuana*. New York: Raven Press, 1976, p. 627.
523. Mendelson, J. H., Rossi, A. M., and Meyer, R. E., Editors. *The Use of Marihuana, a Psychological and Physiological Inquiry*. New York: Plenum, 1974.
524. Fried, P. A., Behavioral and electroencephalographic correlates of the use of marijuana—A review. *Behav. Biol.* 2:163, 1977.
525. Jones, R. T., and Benowitz, N. The 30-day trip—Clinical studies of cannabis tolerance and dependence. In M. C. Braude and S. Szara, eds., *Pharmacology of Marihuana*. New York: Raven Press, 1976, pp. 627–642.
526. Karler, R. Toxicological and pharmacological effects (of marihuana). In R. C. Petersen, ed., *Marihuana Research Findings: 1976*. Rockville, Md.: National Institute on Drug Abuse, 1977, p. 55. (NIDA Research Monograph no. 14).
527. Nahas, G. G. *Cannabis sativa*. the deceptive weed. *N.Y. State J. Med.* 72:856, 1972.
528. Weil, A. T., Zinberg, N. E., and Nelsen, J. M. Clinical and psychological effects of marihuana in man. *Science* 162:1234, 1968.
529. McMillan, D. E., Dewey, W. L., and Harris, L. S. Characteristics of tetrahydrocannabinol tolerance. *Ann. N.Y. Acad. Sci.* 191:89, 1971.
530. McMillan, D. E., et al. Blood levels of $^3$H- 9-tetrahydrocannabinol and its metabolites in tolerant and nontolerant pigeons. *Biochem. Pharmacol.* 22:383, 1973.
531. Dewey, W. L., et al. Distribution of radioactivity in brain of tolerant and nontolerant pigeons treated with 3H-9-tetrahydrocannabinol. *Biochem. Pharmacol.* 22:399, 1973.
532. Elsmore, T. F. Effects of delta-9-tetrahydrocannabinol on temporal and auditory discrimination performance of monkeys. *Psychopharmacologia* 26:62, 1972.
533. Ferraro, D. P., and Grisham, M. G. Tolerance to the behavioral effects of marihuana in chimpanzees. *Physiol. Behav.* 9:49, 1972.
534. Harris, R. T., Waters, W., and McLendon, D. Behavioral effects in rhesus monkeys of repeated intravenous doses of 9-tetrahydrocannabinol. *Psychopharmacologia* 26:297, 1972.
535. Kalant, H., LeBlanc, A. E., and Gibbons, R. J. Tolerance to, and dependence on, some nonopiate psychotropic drugs. *Pharmacol. Rev.* 23:135, 1971.
536. Manning, F. J. Tolerance to effects of delta-9-tetrahydrocannabinol (THC) on free-operant shock avoidance. *Fed. Proc.* 33:481, 1974.
537. Olson, J., and Carder, B. Behavioral tolerance to marihuana as a function of amount of prior training. *Pharmacol. Biochem. Behav.* 2:243, 1974.
538. Ferraro, D. P., and Grilly, D. M. Effects of chronic exposure to delta 9-tetrahydrocannabinol on delayed matching-to-sample in chimpanzees. *Psychopharmacologia* 37:127, 1974.
539. Carder, B., and Olson, J. Learned behavioral tolerance to marihuana in rats. *Pharmacol. Biochem. Behav.* 1:73, 1973.
540. Snyder, E. W., et al. Lack of behavioral tolerance to delta-9-tetrahydrocannabinol in stumptailed macaques. *Proc. Am. Psychol. Assoc.* 995, 1973.
541. Ferraro, D. P., and Grilly, D. M. Lack of tolerance to tetrahydrocannabinol in chimpanzees. *Science* 179:490, 1973.
542. Ferraro, D. P., Grilly, D. M., and Grisham, M. G. Delta-9-tetrahydrocannabinol and delayed matching-to-sample in chimpanzees. In J. M. Singh and H. Ca, eds., *Neurobiology and Influences on Behavior*. Second International Symposium on Drug Addiction, New Orleans, 1973. New York: Stratton Intercontinental Medical Book, 1975, p. 181. (Drug Addiction, Vol. 3).
543. Grilly, D. M. Ferraro, D. P., and Marriott, R. G. Long-term interactions of marijuana and behavior in chimpanzees. *Nature* 242:119, 1973.
544. Goode, E. Drug escalation. Marihuana use as related to the use of dangerous drugs. October 1971.
545. Lemberger, L., Axelrod, J., and Kopin, J. The metabolism and disposition of delta-9-tetrahydrocannabinol in man. *Fed. Proc.* 30, 1971.
546. Weil, A. T. Testimony before National Commission on Marihuana and Drug Abuse, Washington, D.C., May 1971.
547. Cohen, S. *The Substance Abuse Problems*. New York: Haworth, 1980, p. 37.

548. Deneau, G. A., and Kaymakcalan, S. Physiological and psychological dependence to synthetic delta-9-tetrahydrocannabinol (THC) in rhesus monkeys. *Pharmacologist* 13:246, 1971.
549. Kaymakcalan, S. Physiological and psychological dependence on THC in rhesus monkeys. In W. D. C. Paton and J. Crown, eds., *Cannabis and Its Derivatives*. London: Oxford University Press, 1972.
550. Harris, R. T., Waters, W., and McLendon, D. Evaluation of reinforcing capability of delta-9-tetrahydrocannabinol in rhesus monkeys. *Psychopharmacologia* 37:23, 1974.
551. Leite, J. R., and Carlini, E. A. Failure to obtain "cannabis-directed behavior" and abstinence syndrome in rats chronically treated with *Cannabis sativa* extracts. *Psychopharmacologia* 36:133, 1974.
552. Corcoran, M. E., and Amit, Z. Reluctance of rats to drink hashish suspensions: Free-choice and forced consumption, and the effects of hypothalamic stimulation. *Psychopharmacologia* 35:129, 1974.
553. Maker, H. S., Khan, M. A., and Lehrer, G. M. The effect of self-regulated delta-9-tetrahydrocannabinol consumption on pregnant mice and offspring. *Fed. Proc.* 33:540, 1974.
554. Ferraro, D. P., and Grilly, D. M. Marihuana extract in chimpanzees: Absence of long-term effects on operant behavior. *Psychol. Rep.* 32:473, 1973.
555. Stadnicki, S. W., et al. Crude marihuana extract: EEG and behavioral effects of chronic oral administration in rhesus monkeys. *Psychopharmacologia* 37:225, 1974.
556. Hirschhorn, I. D., and Rosencrans, J. A. Morphine and delta-9-tetrahydrocannabinol: Tolerance to the stimulus effects. *Psychopharmacologia* 36:243, 1974.
557. Jessor, R. Marihuana: A review of recent psychosocial research. In R. I. Dupont, A. Goldstein, and J. O'Donnell, eds., *Handbook on Drug Abuse*. Rockville, Md.: National Institute on Drug Abuse, 1979, p. 337.
558. Brotman, R., and Suffet, F. Marihuana use values, behavioral definitions and social control. In *National Commission on Marihuana and Drug Abuse, Drug Use in America: Problem in Perspective. Appendix, Volume 1, Patterns and Consequences of Drug Use*. Washington, D.C.: U.S. Government Printing Office, 1973, p. 1106.
559. Hochman, J. S., and Brill, N. Q. Chronic marihuana use and psychosocial adaptation. *Am. J. Psychiatry* 130(2):132, 1973.
560. Akers, R. L. *Deviant Behavior: A Social Learning Approach*, 2nd ed. Belmont, Calif.: Wadsworth, 1977.
561. Ray, O. S. *Drugs, Society and Human Behavior*, 2nd ed. St. Louis: C. V. Mosby, 1978.
562. Huba, G. J., Wingard, J. A., and Bentler, P.M. Adolescent drug use and peer and adult interaction patterns. Unpublished manuscript, University of California at Los Angeles, February 1978. Cited in R. I. Dupont, A. Goldstein, and J. O'Donnell, eds., *Handbook on Drug Abuse*. Washington, D.C.: U.S. Government Printing Office, 1979, p. 352.
563. Groves, W. E. Patterns of college student drug use and life-styles. In E. Josephson and E. E. Carroll, eds., *Drug Use: Epidemilogical and Sociological Approaches*. Washington, D.C.: Hemisphere (Halsted-Wiley), 1974, p. 241.
564. Stokes, J. P. Personality traits and attitudes and their relationship to student drug using behavior. *Int. J. Addict.* 9(2):267, 1979.
565. Segal, B. Personality factors related to drug and alcohol use. In D. J. Lettieri, ed., *Predicting Adolescent Drug Abuse: A Review of Issues, Methods and Correlates*. Rockville, Md.: National Institute on Drug Abuse, 1975, p. 165. (NIDA Research Issues no. 11).
566. Naditch, M. P. Ego mechanisms and marihuana usage. In D. J. Lettieri, ed., *Predicting Adolescent Drug Abuse: A Review of Issues, Methods and Correlates*. Rockville, Md.: National Institute on Drug Abuse, 1975, p. 207. (NIDA Research Issues, no. 11).
567. Weckowicz, T. E., and Janssen, D. V. Cognitive functions, personality traits, and social values in heavy marijuana smokers and nonsmoker controls. *J. Abnorm. Psychol.* 81(3):264, 1973.
568. Shibuya, R. R. Categorizing drug users and nonusers on selected social and personality variables. *J. Sch. Health* 44:442, 1974.
569. Mellinger, G. D., Somers, R. H., and Manheimer, D. I. Drug use research items pertaining to personality and interpersonal relations: a working paper for research investigators. In D. J. Lettieri, ed., *Predicting Adolescent Drug Abuse: A Review of Issues, Methods, and Correlates*. Rockville, Md.: National Institute on Drug Abuse, 1975, p. 299. (NIDA Research Issues no. 11).
570. Holroyd, K., and Kahn, M. Personality factors in student drug use. *J. Consult. Clin. Psychol.* 42:236, 1974.
571. Kohn, P. M., and Annis, H. M. Personality and social factors in adolescent marihuana use:

A path analytic study. *J. Consult. Clin. Psychol.* 40:366, 1978.

572. O'Donnell, J. A., et al. *Young Men and Drugs: A Nationwide Survey*. Rockville, Md.: National Institute on Drug Abuse, 1976. (NIDA Research Monograph no. 5).
573. Whitehead, P. C., and Cabral, R. M. Scaling the sequence of drug using behaviors: A test of the stepping-stone hypothesis. *Drug Forum* 5(1):45, 1975.
574. Johnston, L. D., Bachman, J. G., and O'Malley, P. M. *Drug Use Among American High School Abuse, 1975–1977*. National Institute on Drug Abuse. Washington, D.C.: U.S. Government Printing Office, 1977.
575. Goldstein, J. W., Gleason, T. C., and Korn, J. H. Whether the epidemic? Psychoactive drug-use career patterns of college students. *J. Appl. Soc. Psychol.* 5:16, 1975.
576. Keeler, M. H., Reifler, C. B., and Liptzin, M. B. Spontaneous recurrence of marihuana effect. *Am. J. Psychiatry* 125:384, 1968.
577. Cohen, S. *The Substance Abuse Problems*. New York: Haworth, 1980, p. 7.
578. Agurell, S., Willette, R., and Dewey, W. *Cannabinoids '82*. New York: Academic Press, 1982.
579. Turner, J. L., and Mahlberg, P. L. A simple HPLC method for separating acid neutral cannabinoids in *Cannabis sativa L.* In S. Agurell, R. Willette, and W. Dewey, eds., *Cannabinoids '82*. New York: Academic Press, (in press).
580. Mechoulam, R. Cannabidiol and THC as starting points in the search for new therapeutic agents. *Ibid.*
581. Elsohly, H. N., et al. Constituents of *Cannabis sativa L.* XXII. Isolation and characterization of channabiterol, a new cannabis constituent. *Ibid.*
582. Rosenfeld, J. Derivatization chemistry in the analysis of cannabinoids. *Ibid.*
583. Martin, B. R., Harris, L. S., and Dewey, W. L. Pharmacological activity of delta-0-THC metabolites and analogs of CBD, delta-8- and delta-9-THC. *Ibid.*
584. Weissman, A., Milne, G. M., and Melvin, L. S., Jr. Potent cannabiminetic activity from a derivative of 3-phenylcyclohexanol. *Ibid.*
585. Cook, C. E., et al. Radioimmunoassay for 11-hydroxy delta$^9$-tetrahydrocannabinol (HTHC), a major psychoactive metabolite of delta$^9$-tetrahydrocannabinol (THC). *Ibid.*
586. Agurell, S., et al. Recent studies on the pharmacokinetics and metabolism of cannabinoids in man—particularly $\Delta^1$-tetrahydrocannabinol (THC). *Ibid.*
587. Szeto, H. H., and Cook, C. E. Maternal-fetal pharmacokinetics and pharmacodynamics of tetrahydrocannabinol (THC). *Ibid.*
588. Haldin, M., and Widman, M. Urinary metabolites of $\Delta^1$-tetrahydrocannabinol in man. *Ibid.*
589. Wall, M. E., et al., Metabolism, disposition and pharmacokinetics of $\Delta^9$-tetrahydrocannabinol in male and female subjects. *Ibid.*
590. Heinrich, R. T., Schinohara, O., and Nogawa, T. Effects of chronic administration of THC on early embryonic development of mice. *Ibid.*
591. Albert, M., and Solomon, J. The effect of neonatal administration of $\Delta^9$-THC on reproductive development and function in the rodent. *Ibid.*
592. Fujimoto, G. I. Cannabinoid inhibition of androgenic and gonadotropic action. *Ibid.*
593. Dalterio, S., Steger, R., and Barthe, A. Effects of psychoactive or nonpsychoactive cannabinoids on reproductive functions in male offspring. *Ibid.*
594. Tilak, S., and Zimmerman, A. M. Effects of cannabinoids on spermatogenesis in mice: In vivo and in vitro studies. *Ibid.*
595. Husain, S., and Lowe, M. Possible mechanism of the cellular effects of marihuana on male reproduction. *Ibid.*
596. Smith, C. G., Almirez, R. G., and Ash, R. H. Tolerance develops to the disruptive effects of delta-9-tetrahydrocannabinol on the primate menstrual cycle. *Ibid.*
597. Ford, R. D., et al. Discriminate stimulus properties of the cannabinoids. *Ibid.*
598. Hosko, M. J., and Schmeling, W. T. $\Delta^9$-tetrahydrocannabinol: Site of action for autonomic effects. *Ibid.*
599. Turkanis, S. A., and Karlen, R. Electrophysiological mechanisms of CNS actions of $\Delta^9$-tetrahydrocannabinol. *Ibid.*
600. Consroe, P., and Fish, B. S. Behavioral pharmacogenetic studies of cannabinoids: Developmental effects in tetrahydrocannabinol-seizure susceptible rabbits. *Ibid.*
601. Young, G. A., et al. Acute effects of $\Delta^9$-THC, 11-OH-$\Delta^9$-THC and cannabinol on cortical EEL and EEG power spectron in the rat. *Ibid.*
602. Bloom, A. S. Effects of cannabinoids on neurotransmitter receptors in the brain. *Ibid.*
603. Huot, J., and Dufour, M. Biotransformation of $\Delta^1$-tetrahydrocannabinol by pulmonary cells isolated from lungs of normal hamsters and hamsters treated chronically with benzo-d-pyrne. *Ibid.*
604. Barnett, G. Interaction of THC and testoster-

one: Plasma data analysis and stimulation. *Ibid.*

605. Hepler, K. S., Frank, I. M., and Petrus, R. Ocular effects of marijuana smoking. In M. C. Braude and S. Szara, eds., *Pharmacology of Marijuana*. New York: Raven Press, 1976.
606. Green, K., Kim, K., and Bowman, K. Ocular effects of delta-9-tetrahydrocannabinol. In S. Cohen and R. C. Stillman, eds., *The Therapeutic Potential of Marijuana*. New York: Plenum, 1976, p. 4.
607. Burstein, S. Prostaglandins and cannabis: IV, a biochemical basis for therapeutic applications. In S. Cohen and R. C. Stillman, eds., *The Therapeutic Potential of Marijuana*. New York: Plenum, 1976, p. 19.
608. Waller, C. W., Benigni, D. A., and Harland, E. Cannabinoids in glaucoma III: The effects of different cannabinoids on intraocular pressure in the monkey. In S. Agurell, R. Willette, and W. Dewey, eds., *Cannabinoids '82*. New York: Academic Press, (in press).
609. Howes, J. F. Antiglaucoma effects of topically and orally administered cannabinoids. *Ibid.*
610. Tashkin, D. P., et al. Bronchial effects of aerosolized delta-9-tetrahydrocannabinol in healthy and asthmatic subjects. *Am. Rev. Respir. Dis.* 115:57, 1977.
611. Williams, S. J., Hartley, J. P., and Graham, J. D. Bronchodilator effect of tetrahydrocannabinol administered by aerosol of asthmatic patients. *Thorax* 31:720, 1977.
612. Cottrell, J. C., Sohn, S. S., and Vogel, W. H. Toxic effects of marihuana tar on mouse skin. *Arch. Environ. Health* 26:277, 1973.
613. Huber, G. L., et al. Marijuana, THC and pulmonary antibacterial defenses. Presented at the Seventh International Congress of Pharmacology, Reims, France, 1978.
614. Regelson, W., et al. Delta-9-tetrahydrocannabinol as an effective antidepressant and appetite stimulating agent in advanced cancer patients. In M. C. Braude and S. Szara, eds., *Pharmacology of Marijuana*. New York: Raven Press, 1976, p. 763.
615. Sallen, S. E., Zinberg, N. E., and Frei, E., 3D. Antiemetic effect of delta-9-tetrahydrocannabinol in patients receiving cancer chemotherapy. *N. Engl. J. Med.* 293:795, 1975.
616. Chang, A. E., et al. Evaluation of antiemetic effects of delta-9-THC during adjuvant chemotherapy in patients receiving high dose therapy. *Ann. Intern. Med.*, 1979.
617. Herman, T. S., et al. Superiority of nabilone over prochlorperazine as an antiemetic in patients receiving cancer chemotherapy. *N. Engl. J. Med.* 300:1295, 1979.
618. Ungerleider, J. T., and Andrysiak, T. Effect of inhaled delta-9-THC in reduction of nausea and vomiting associated with bone marrow transplant and chemotherapy. Personal communication, 1979. Cited in Cohen, S. Therapeutic agents. In R. C. Peterson, ed., *Marihuana Research Findings: 1980*. NIDA Monograph no. 31. Washington, D.C.: U.S. Government Printing Office, 1980, p. 199.
619. Gross, H. A., et al. A trial of delta-9-THC in primary anorexia nervosa. Presented at the Annual Meeting of the American Psychiatric Association, San Francisco, 1980.
620. McCarthy, L. E., and Borison, H. L. Antiemetic activity of nabilone, a cannabinol derivative. Reversed by naloxone in awake cats. *Pharmacologist* 19:230, 1977.
621. Consroe, P. F., Wood, G. C., and Buchsbaum, H. Anticonvulsant nature of marihuana smoking. *JAMA* 234:306, 1975.
622. Corcoran, M. E., McCaughran, J. A., Jr., and Wade, J. A. Antiepileptic and prophylactic effects of tetrahydrocannabinols in amygdaloid kindled rats. *Epilepsia* 19:47, 1978.
623. Feeney, D. M. Marihuana and epilepsy. *Science* 197:1301, 1977.
624. Karler, R., and Turkanis, S. The antiepileptic potential of the cannabinoids. In S. Cohen and R. C. Stillman, eds., *The Therapeutic Potential of Marijuana*. New York: Plenum, 1976, p. 383.
625. Mechoulam, R., and Carlini, E. A. Towards drugs derived from cannabis. *Naturwissenschaften* 65:174, 1978.
626. Feinberg, I., et al. Effects of marijuana extract and tetrahydrocannabinol on electroencephalographic sleep patterns. *Clin. Pharmacol. Ther.* 19:782, 1976.
627. Harris, L. S. Analgesic and antitumor potential of the cannabinoids. In S. Cohen and R. C. Stillman, eds., *The Therapeutic Potential of Marijuana*. New York: Plenum, 1976, p. 299.
628. Friedman, M. A. In vivo effects of cannabinoids on macromolecular biosynthesis in Lewis lung carcinomas. *Cancer Biochem. Biophys.* 2:51, 1977.
629. Van Klingerin, B., and ten Ham, M. Antibacterial activity of delta-9-tetrahydrocannabinol and cannabidiol. *Antonie van Leeuwenhoek* 42:9, 1976.
630. Krejci, Z. To the problem of substances with antibacterial action: Cannabis effect. *Casopis Lekaru Ceskych* 43:1351, 1961.
631. Freemon, F. R. The effect of delta-9-tetrahy-

drocannabinol on sleep. *Psychopharmacologia* 35:39, 1974.

632. Neu, C., Di Mascio, A., and Szilling, G. Hypnotic properties of THC: Experimental comparison of THC, chloral hydrate, and placebo. In S. Cohen and R. C. Stillman, eds., *The Therapeutic Potential of Marijuana*. New York: Plenum, 1976, p. 15.
633. Musty, R. E. Possible anxiolytic properties of cannabidiol. In S. Agurell, R. Willette, and W. Dewey, eds., *Cannabinoids '82*. New York: Academic Press (in press).
634. Passatore, M., et al. Effect of THC on the supramaximal stimulation of the mouse sciatic nerve. *Acta Med. Roma* 13:427, 1975.
635. Dunn, D., and Davis, R. The perceived effects of marihuana in spinal cord injuries. *Paraplegia* 12:175, 1974.
636. Petro, D. J., and Ellenberger, C. Marijuana (*Cannabis sativa*) as a therapeutic agent in patients with muscle spasms or spasticity: Case reports and literature review. Presented at the American Academy of Neurology meeting, Chicago, 1979.
637. Smith, T. C., and Kulp R. Respiratory and cardiovascular effects of delta-9-tetrahydrocannabinol alone and in combination with oxymorphone, pentobarbital and diazepam. In S. Cohen and R. C. Stillman, eds., *The Therapeutic Potential of Marijuana*. New York: Plenum, 1976, p. 123.
638. Parker, J. M., and Dubas, T. C. Automatic determination of the pain threshold to electroshock and the effects of 9-THC. *Int. J. Clin. Pharmacol. Ther. Toxicol.* 7:75, 1973.
639. Sofia, R. D., Vassar, H. B., and Knobloch, L. C. Comparative analgesic activity of various naturally occurring cannabinoids in mice and rats. *Psychopharmacologia* 40:285, 1975.
640. Cooler, P., and Gregg, J. The effect of delta-9-tetrahydrocannabinol on intraocular pressure in humans. In S. Cohen and R. C. Stillman, eds., *The Therapeutic Potential of Marihuana*. New York: Plenum, 1976, p. 77.
641. Noyes, R., Jr., et al. Analgesic effect of delta-9-tetrahydrocannabinol. *J. Clin. Pharmacol.* 15:139, 1975.
642. Butler, J. R., et al. Treatment effects of delta-9-THC in an advanced cancer population. In S. Cohen and R. C. Stillman, eds., *The Therapeutic Potential of Marijuana*. New York: Plenum, 1976, p. 313.
643. Wilson, R. S., and May, E. L. 9-*nor*-delta 8-tetrahydrocannabinol, a cannabinoid of metabolic interest. *J. Med. Chem.* 17:475, 1974.
644. Harris, L. S., Munson, A. E., and Carchman, R. A. Antitumor properties of cannabinoids. In M. C. Braude and S. Szara, eds., *The Pharmacology of Marijuana*. New York: Raven Press, 1976, p. 749.
645. Kaymakcalaw, S. Opioid-like effects of cannabinoids. In S. Agurell, R. Willette, and W. Dewey, eds., *Cannabinoids '82*. New York: Academic Press (in press).
646. Parker, C. S., and Wrigley, F. Synthetic cannabis preparations in psychiatry: Synhexyl. *J. Ment. Sci.* 96:275, 1950.
647. Kotin, J., Post, R. M., and Goodwin, F. K. 9-tetrahydrocannabinol in depressed patients. *Arch. Gen. Psychiatry* 28:345, 1973.
648. Siemens, A. J. Effects of cannabis in combination with ethanol and other drugs. In *Marijuana Research Findings: 1980*. Rockville, Md.: National Institute on Drug Abuse, 1980, p. 167. (NIDA Research Monograph no. 31).
649. Blum, K., et al. Tetrahydrocannabinol: Inhibition of alcohol-induced withdrawal symptoms in mice. In J. M. Singh and H. Lal, eds., *Neurobiologyand Influences on Behavior*. Second International Symposium on Drug Addiction, New Orleans, 1973. New York: Stratton Intercontinental Medical Book, 1975, p. 39 (Drug Addiction, vol. 3).
650. Rosenberg, C. M., Gerrein, J. R., and Schnell, C. Cannabis in the treatment of alcoholism. *J. Stud. Alcohol* 39:1955, 1978.
651. Cohen, S. Therapeutic aspects. In R. C. Petersen, ed., *Marijuana Research Findings: 1980*. Rockville, Md.: National Institute on Drug Abuse, 1980, p. 199. (NIDA Research Monograph, no. 31).
652. Mikuriya, J. Critique: Marihuana and health. *J. Psychoact. Drugs* 14(3):239, 1982.
653. Hollister, L. E. Present status of health aspects of cannabis use. In S. Agurell, R. Willette, and W. Dewey, eds., *Cannabinoids '82*. New York: Academic Press (in press).
654. Popenoe, C. *Wellness*. Washington, D.C.: Yes Inc., 1977, p. 366.
655. Goldman, A. *Entering the New Age of Pot: What Will Happen When Middle-Class America Gets the Straight Dope?* New York, 1975, p. 28.
656. Dalterio, S. L. Bartke, A., and Mayfield, D. Cannabinoids stimulate and inhibit testosterone production *in vitro* and *in vivo*. *Life Sci.* 32:605, 1983.

Chapter 18

# Psychedelics: Brave Old World

## A. INTRODUCTION

The term *psychotropic* has been used by academicians as a synonym for the more popular term *psychedelic*. A clear definition of psychotropic, as it relates to substances, has been adequately delineated in numerous publications.[1] Psychotropic substances are those that cause psychologic change or modify mental activity, either by use of a plant or by a chemical synthesis.[1] Delay[2] classified psychotropic drugs as: (1) psychic sedatives (narcotics, barbiturates, tranquilizers); (2) psychic stimulants (cocaine, caffeine, amphetamines); and (3) psychic derivatives or hallucinogens (LSD, mescaline, psilocybin, harmine).

This chapter focuses on the third type of psychotropic, the so-called psychedelics.

Anthropologic circles may testify to the fact that the use of chemical substances is not the only way in which humans attempt to alter states of consciousness. Highs are achieved through such activities as exercise, laughing, meditation, fasting, flaggelation, trance induction, and rhythmic dancing. However, as Ludwig[3] points out, hallucinogens are vehicles through which to achieve altered states of consciousness rapidly. In an era of space migration, rapid mass electronic communication, and computer technology, the desire to get there in a hurry is quite understandable.

In terms of a historic perspective on the search for and use and abuse of psychotropic drugs to achieve mental wellness (happiness, health, enjoyment), a brief review of the existing literature is presented in Table 18-1.

The lesson to be learned from this overview is that human beings seem to have two powerful needs that are at odds with each other: to keep things basically the same and to experience new challenge. As Barron and associates[4] stated in an article on hallucinogenic drugs, "We like to feel secure; yet, at times, we like to be surprised. Too much predictability leads to monotony, but too little may lead to anxiety." Thus our realization of the need to alter "ego" and change the state of our own minds better enables us to understand the search for psychoactive substances, both botanic and organically synthesized chemicals.

In spite of associated health hazards, in the United States alone, alcohol—which is consumed by approximately 100 million persons—has won the distinction of being the drug most sought after for these purposes. And this is true throughout the world, as alcohol

## TABLE 18-1

## Historic Perspectives on Addictive and Abused Substances

| | |
|---|---|
| **Alcohol** | Probable date of use by Indus Valley Egyptians and Indo-Aryan civilizations. Noah |
| 9400 B.C.–6400 B.C. | is said to have been drunk! |
| 1800 B.C. | Problems led to prohibition. Hammurabi's (Babylon) code of ethics prohibited it. |
| 1198 B.C. | Rameses III issued alcoholic drinks to his soldiers. |
| 600 B.C. | Used in chemical warfare by Cyaxares, who got the enemy (Scythians) drunk at a feast. Has been used in strategy many times! |
| **Ether** | High taxes and poverty of Irish peasants led to ether drinking. One small village, Omoah, consumed 225 gallons of ether in 1870. |
| 1800 A.D. | |
| **Chloroform** | Smaller and less well-documented consumption |
| **Nitrous oxide**<br>1777 A. D. | Synthesized by Humphrey Davy in England. Poets Coleridge and Southey, Roget (of *Roget's Thesaurus*), and Sir Josiah Wedgwood (of pottery fame) include those who inhaled it. In the United States, extensive use among the educated was also reported in the 18th and 19th centuries. |
| **Glue sniffing, acetone, petroleum products, etc.** | More recent peak around 1960–1965. In 1963, there were 2003 glue-sniffing offenses in New York City. |
| **Amphetamines**<br>1927–1932<br>(benzedrine, dexedrine, methedrine, etc.) | First synthetic work: 1877. Early pharmacologic tests and marketing as Benzedrine. Used in psychiatry, and as pep pills, and so on, but can itself cause a psychotic state that many believe is closer to schizophrenia than even the LSD psychosis. Sweden, as a psychiatrically advanced country, had severe problems with dependence and abuse of synthetic drugs, including phenacetin of APC (aspirin-phenacetin-caffeine) fame. |
| **Cocaine** | Isolated from coca leaves. |
| 1883 | First use by Bavarian soldiers. |
| 1884 | Sigmund Freud was certain about the great future for cocaine. |
| 1886 | Early observations of the harmful effects of cocaine. |
| 1914 | U.S. laws prohibiting cocaine. |
| **Barbiturates**<br>1903 | Barbituric acid synthesized in Germany by Von Mering and Fischer, led to a whole family of barbiturates that became extremely useful as sedatives, antiepileptic drugs, buffers, and the like. |
| 1942 | One and a half billion doses of barbiturates a year in 1942 and ten billion doses by 1969 were produced. |
| **Aspirin**<br>1853 | Synthesized by Gerhards, Medicinal value of plants and fruits containing salicylates was mentioned by Pliny in the first century B.C. Willow bark containing salicylates was used as a substitute for the Peruvian cinchona (quinine).<br>The first modern medicinal use of salicylates started in 1875. The name *aspirin* comes from acetyl and spirsaure.<br>While it is shown definitely not to be mind-altering, could its ever-increasing use in our civilization become "addictive"?<br>Realizing the billions of doses used, with reports of alleged ill effects in pregnancy, one cannot but think of its effects in prolonged course of its use on the evolution of the new humankind. |

## TABLE 18-1 (continued)
## Historic Perspectives on Addictive and Abused Substances

| | |
|---|---|
| **Marihuana** (*Cannabis sativa*, tetrahydro cannabinols) | Incense burning in Indus Valley civilizations. Possibly known to Chinese by 3000 B.C. |
| 3000 B.C. | Verdas of India. |
| 650 B.C. | Persia and Assyria. Nebuchadnezzar ate it. Herodotus mentions use by Scythians. |
| 400 B.C. | Rome. |
| 1545 A.D. | South America through Spanish traders. |
| 1804–1844 A.D. | Jacques-Joseph Moreau of France used it as a psychotropic drug. Club Haschischins of Paris. Baudelaire describes it in *Les Paradis Artificiels.* |
| **Opium** (*Papaver somniferum*) | Sumerians. 4000 B.C.<br>Egyptians. 3500 B.C.<br>Greek, Cretan, Mycenian. Religious rituals (Asclepia) 2000 B.C. |
| 850 B.C. | Persia and beginning of medicinal use. |
| 1511 A.D. | Cultivation in India. Use of a mixture of marihuana and opium by Babur, the Moghul emperor and great-great-grandfather of Shahjehan, who built the Taj Mahal (1631–1651). |
| 1843 | The hypodermic syringe was invented in 1843 and brought to the United States by 1856. The use of morphine was extensive among soldiers during the Civil War. By the end of the 19th century, one in 400 Americans (United States) was addicted to opium. |
| 1842–1858 | British defeated the Chinese into accepting imported opium. The Opium Wars and American Chinese Clippers. Millions of Chinese men were addicted, but by 1971, this seems to have disappeared. |
| 1851 | The "Yellow Peril" came to San Francisco. |
| 1850 *et seq.* | Widespread use of opium in England (laudanum, a mixture of wine and opium, was very popular, as illustrated in *Oliver Twist*) and in the United States. Hundreds of pounds were consumed by the working classes and "genteel" classes—men, women and children! |
| 1875 | First Narcotic Control Act posted in San Francisco. |
| **Mandragora plant** 700 B.C. *et seq.* | The mandrake root was referred to by the Assyrians. Was mentioned in *Genesis* as a fertility substance; in the "Song of Solomon," and by Hippocrates, Herodotus, and others. Mandrake roots, which look like the human figure, and have hair, were worn as talismans in 12th to 16th centuries in Europe and the Near East. |
| **Mimosa hastibis** | A hallucinogen used by Brazilian Indians, which contains dimethyltryptamine. |
| **Morning glory** | Used by the Indians of the New World. Contains chemicals related to LSD and chanoclavine. The U.S. variety of the morning glory is devoid of the hallucinogenic substance. |
| **Datura** (jimson weed, thorn apple, *Datura* spp.) | Used by early Incas and other Indians of South America in 38 A.D. Probably was the plant eaten by the Roman soldiers under Marc Antony on their retreat from Parthia. Caused stupor, insanity, and in large doses, death. Was used to stupefy victims. Some early settlers in the United States consumed it by accident, resulting in their "sitting naked in the corner like monkeys and making mews and wallowing in their own excreta." |

## TABLE 18-1 (continued)
## Historic Perspectives on Addictive and Abused Substances

| | |
|---|---|
| **Peyote** (*Lophophora williamsii, Anhalonium lewinii*) | Hallucinogenic cactus plant. Use must have been firmly entrenched for some centuries in some American Indian cultures as even some contemporary Indians use it as commonly as other people use aspirin. Rather unpleasant effects limit its attractiveness to the street user. The word *mescaline* is associated with its use by the Mescalero Apaches. |
| 1899 | Oklahoma outlawed peyote. |
| 1908 | Associated with ritualistic use and after testimony by Quanah Parker (a Commanche chief, who quit scalping whites after the Great Spirit revealed to him that He planted His flesh in the cactus pioniys), this law was repealed. |
| **Mushrooms** 1000 B.C. or earlier (*Amanita*) | Religious and tribal use of mushrooms. Also of phallic symbolism in the Americas. Warriors used to go beserk (wearing "ber sark" or bear skins) after consuming portions of this mushroom. |
| **Fly agaric** | Consumed in Siberia, especially by Koryaks. |
| Before 1100 A.D. | During carousing, men stayed intoxicated for several days at a time, even drinking their own urine to prolong the effects! Used in shamanistic rituals. |
| **Psilocybe** 1500 B.C. | Mushroom cultures of the "undiscovered" Americas. Teonanacatl (food or flesh of the gods) was used ceremonially. |
| **Tobacco** | |
| 1555 | First European observation in Brazil. |
| 1575 | Mexican edict prohibits it. Even priests smoked while performing mass! |
| 1590–1610 | Spread around the world to Europe, India, China, Japan, Africa. Took priority over price of slaves, women's bodies, and men's labor. A religious stricture prohibiting tobacco was of no avail. |
| 1614 | Some 7000 shops in London purveyed tobacco. |
| 1634 | Forbidden in Russia because of "stinking and infectious breath." |
| 1638 | Chinese prohibition, with the punishment decapitation. Apparently did not work. Prohibitions against tobacco by Pope Urban VIII (1642), Pope Innocent X (1650), Bavaria (1652), Zurich (1667), Czar Frodorovitch (1634). (In Russia, such penalties as slitting the nose did not prevent the people from selling their very shirts to buy tobacco.) Japan prohibited the growing of tobacco (1607–1609). Snuff used by Pope Benedict XIII (1725), Queen Anne (1702); 25 million pounds per year are used in the United States today. |
| 1914 | Thomas Alva Edison, addicted to cigars, did not wish to employ cigarette smokers! |
| 1921 | Fourteen states in the United States prohibited smoking. Repealed in 1927! |
| 1923–1939 | Freud underwent 33 operations in the mouth as a result of the unequivocal effects of smoking (oral satisfaction?). |
| 1973 | *The New York Times* reported women who smoke a pack or more of cigarettes a day die 19 years earlier than nonsmokers. |
| **Coffee** | Indigenous to Ethiopia and cultivated there. |
| 1300 A.D. | Initially used by dervishes for religious use. Prohibited by the Koran. |

## TABLE 18-1 (continued)

## Historic Perspectives on Addictive and Abused Substances

| | |
|---|---|
| 1500 A.D. | Introduction to Europe. |
| 1600–1700 | The world embraced coffee drinking. Coffee houses and parlors in cities. Frederick II of Prussia taxed coffee heavily to encourage beer drinking. Physical punishment was also decreed against coffee drinkers. |
| **Tea** | |
| 2700 B.C. | Known in China. |
| 1610 A.D. | Dutch brought tea to Europe. |
| 1658 | First English advertisement for tea. |
| 1660 | Queen Catherine of England was a confirmed tea drinker. The Dutchess of Bedford introduced the "afternoon tea" to decrease her "sinking feeling." |
| | What is being overlooked in the excessive use of coffee and tea is the not improbable carcinogenic activity of the coaltar-like substances produced in the roasting and curing of coffee. |
| **Colas**<br>1900 and later | Decocainized, but reportedly contains caffeine, acid, and pigments. Young people around the world are apparently as much addicted to colas as some others are to coffee and tea! |
| **Kava**<br>(Kawa-kawa, piper methysticum) | Widely drunk in Polynesia and Oceania as ritual. Alcohol and our modern civilization lessened the use. Active principle unknown. |
| **Betel** | |
| 340 B.C. | Theophrastus mentions it. |
| 600 A.D. | Some 30,000 betel shops in Persia alone. |
| 1940–1950 | The present author occasionally used to chew betel nuts, betel leaves, and lime after meals. It was not addictive and completely correct, but is still a major practice in India. |
| **Khat**<br>Before 1200 A.D. | Used in Ethiopia and East Africa. Causes several pathologic conditions. |
| **Coca** | Cultivated in Peru. Used by Incas. The Spanish paid for their lives in coca plants. |
| 1000 A.D. | Pope Leo XIII used coca to support his "ascetic retirement." |
| 1884 | Freud hailed coca as a cure for morphinism. "French Wine of Coca, the Ideal Tonic" was offered in the state of Georgia by a Dr. John Styth Pemberton in 1886, and introduced the forerunner of our present-day decocainized soft drink (colas). |
| **Miscellaneous** | Pitchery, an Australian drug containing nornicotine.<br>Acacia, from the Amazon basin.<br>Some types of mint.<br>Peganum harmala and Banisteri a cappi containing harmala alkaloids.<br>Piptadenic peregrina containing bufotenine and DMT. |

From C. Corti, *A History of Smoking.* New York: Harcourt, 1932.

retains its rank as first among the substances used to change mental experience. Opium and its derivatives, various cannabis preparations, such as hashish and marihuana, and cocaine are its closest rivals.

Although utilized on a more limited basis worldwide, evidence from recorded history indicates that the consciousness-altering substances, the hallucinogens or psychotomimetics, have stimulated the curiosity of even the deity.[5,6]

A psychotomimetic drug may be defined as one that will consistently produce changes in thought, perception, and mood, alone or in concert, without causing major disturbances of the autonomic nervous system or other serious disability. Dewsbery,[7] in remarking on the value of these substances, considers them important for three reasons:

1. They can give the investigator an approximate subjective experience of what mental disorder is like.
2. Model psychoses can be studied in the same way as mental disorders.
3. A study of their chemical nature can be expected to throw some light on the nature of the hypothetic substances believed to cause mental disorders.

It is important to realize that psychotomimetics, as the word implies, are substances which, in the animal body, cause symptoms similar to those of schizophrenia. They are not necessarily similar, and do not even act in a similar manner, to those substances that may be responsible for causing mental disorders.

Additionally the hallucinogens [the term primarily used here except for an occasional reference to "psychedelics" (mind-manifesting)[8]] cause visual, auditory, tactile, taste, and olfactory hallucinations and produce ecstatic states in some individuals. A variety of agents currently available (including LSD, mescaline, and psilocybin), which have been known in natural forms such as certain mushrooms, cactus buttons, and seeds, have the property of permitting experiences of expanding consciousness.

It has been noted that scientists will predictably conclude that the proper use of hallucinogens is for research and medical application, and the illicit abuse is for kicks and by cults.[9] Our puritanic nature prohibits us from exploring the use of hallucinogens to improve the healthy, or possibly transform Western society into a new Elysium.[10]

Whatever we may think, history does indeed record our urge to escape reality or anxiety with the aid of magic, drugs, festival rites, and dreams. The question is: What price must we pay for a chemically induced glimpse of paradise? In this regard, it has been stated that[11]: "It is remarkable that one characteristic which seems to separate man from the allegedly lower animals is a recurring desire to escape from reality."

There are more than 10,000 publications on hallucinogens in the literature and only selected papers are cited here to provide the reader with the quality of writing stimulated by these powerful chemicals. For example[12]:

> These substances have formed a bond of union between men of opposite hemispheres, the uncivilized and the civilized: they have forced passages which, once open, proved of use for other purposes: they produced, in ancient races, characteristics which have endured to the present day, evidencing the marvelous degree of intercourse that existed between different peoples just as certainly and exactly as a chemist can judge the relations of two substances by their reactions.

Also[13]:

> Man found it necessary to try to explain these extraordinary powers of some of the plants in his environment. In all primitive cultures, this explanation invariably ascribed to the plant some particular divinity or spirit which, in many instances, was thought to be efficacious as an intermediary between man's world of humdrum reality and the supernatural or spirit realm.

The use of psychedelics not only serves as a bridge between the supernatural and man's "world of humdrum reality," but also as a link between life and death. Primitive tribes buried their dead with such chemicals and related paraphernalia to accompany them on their voyage to the unknown. It is only sophisticated cultures which use drugs, the rest of the world, in touch with their primitive origins, use plants.
This is an important distinction. Drugs and

chemicals, although derived from plants, are not used in this way. Such groups use the plants themselves, which they believe to have a life, a resident divinity. Eating the plant means taking and acquiring the spiritual power.

One writer comments[14]: "The principle was true of even so mildly psychedelic a drug as tobacco. Originally, tobacco was always used in a sacred magico-religious context, and never for mere secular-indulgent enjoyment . . . And when . . . Indian chiefs . . . smoked the sacred calumet or peace pipe, the rite meant the invoking of the power of tobacco upon their sacred oath."

As we know, some of the psychoactive plants with long histories in western civilization have been adopted for "mere secular-indulgent enjoyment." Those who use drugs today in the search for religious experiences have voiced a similar concern[15]:

> To turn on means to find a sacrament which returns you to the temple of God, your own body, to go out of your mind. To tune in means to be reborn; to drop back in, to start a new sequence of behavior that reflects your vision; in other words, to manifest, in a behavioral way, the religious experience you have had . . . Today, the sacrament is LSD. However, sacraments wear out. They become part of the social game. Treasure LSD while it still works. In fifteen years, it will be a tame, socialized routine.

There is an impressive array of plants whose leaves, roots and flowers offer the psychedelic potential of a visionary reality to those who understand their folkloric mysteries. In the Western Hemisphere, nearly 100 plants have been used over the years by various cultural subgroups in search of psychoactive phenomena. It is not clear why the rest of the world has never experimented with more than seven species in its quest for psychedelic insight. Of the scores of plants that are classed as hallucinogens, they have as their outstanding similar characteristic the potential for altering perceptions in a bizarre manner and dramatically influencing states of consciousness. Most were included by Lewin[12] in his categorization of phantasticants. The few agents selected here will be described in terms of their interrelationship in society, as well as their impact on the individual.

Hallucinogenic drugs have been studied both as tools for the production of experimental psychosis and as possible therapeutic agents in mental disease. The striking effects of these drugs on the human mind have intrigued lay people and scientists alike. Some authorities believe that this class of drugs may prove to be valuable in the treatment of a variety of physical and mental diseases, and many of them have been used "medicinally" for centuries (mescaline, psilocybin, ololiuqui, and kava-kava).[16] The research undertaken to date, however, has not proved conclusive and, over the past ten years, publicity has created widespread interest in the psychedelics among the youth, and even among the so-called academicians or lay adults. According to Dr. Timothy Leary, "We have arranged transcendent experiences for over one thousand persons from all walks of life, including sixty-nine full-time religious professionals, two college deans, a divinity college president and several distinguished religious philosophers." Dr. D. Louria[17] believes that the consequence has been a drastic increase in the number of persons suffering temporary or long-term mental disorders as a direct result of strong, ego-destroying hallucinogenic experiences.

One of the most outspoken advocates of the LSD-type drugs was Aldous Huxley,[18] who once said: "Human beings will be able to achieve effortlessly what, in the past, could only be achieved with difficulty, by means of self-control and spiritual exercises." However, Huxley did question whether drug-induced changes in the human mind might be advantageous or harmful.

Many of those who have taken LSD trips are deeply affected by their experiences, and regard the use of psychedelics as a means not only of developing insights into their own "hang-ups," but into the nature and purpose of creation as well. Meher Baba,[19] who was born in Poona, India, and is hailed throughout the world as a God-realized being, is probably the best anti-drug authority available to compare the results of chemical-induced stimulation of deeper "spiritual" thoughts of being with those produced by special meditation techniques used by spiritual teachers. He has denounced the use of hallucinogens.

The hallucinogens are very powerful drugs

which, in carefully supervised settings, will induce, in some individuals, an experience reported as ecstatic. On the other hand, perhaps as many as half of those who indulge in these substances illicitly, alone or in the presence of unqualified "guides," will experience profound terror. Moreover, this terror can recur at any time, even without the drug, and the experience can have lasting and long-reaching effects. (In the street, these adverse reactions are referred to as "bummers" or "flashbacks.")

Although research in the past has focused on legitimate medicinal uses of hallucinogens, to date there is no evidence that drugs such as LSD can be employed safely in humans in a beneficial way. And, it is very unlikely that an understanding of the mechanisms of action of hallucinogenic drugs will be of much value in the study of the biochemical basis of mental function.

## B. HISTORY

The ingenuity of human beings in discovering natural drugs that alter consciousness seems inexhaustible. Mind-altering drugs have been found in virtually all parts of the world. Historically the predominant use of these drugs was for producing a mystical experience or a sense of communion with gods. They also were believed to have special healing powers and to enhance sociability. LaBarre[20] reported that throughout recorded history, the hallucinogenic plants were exalted to a highly sacred place and usually were reserved for a sacred role in magico-religious rites. Today we know that the so-called "resident divinities" of these sacred plants are chemical substances. The discovery of these new and potent psychotropic agents created the field of psychopharmacology. The basis for this discipline is defined from the early works of Ernst Freiherr von Bibra,[21] James F. Johnston,[22] Mordecai Cubit Cooke,[23] Emil Kraepelin,[24] Carl Hartwich,[25] William E. Safford,[26] Lewis Lewin,[12] Blas Pablo Reko,[27] and Kurt Beringer.[28]

In terms of a historic overview of psychopharmacology, Lewin grouped psychoactive plants in five categories: excitantia, inebriantia, hypnotica, euphorica, and phantastica. He defined the hallucinogenic drugs as *phantastica*. According to Lewin,[29] these drugs "bring about evident cerebral excitation in the form of hallucinations, illusions and visions. These phenomena may be accompanied or followed by disturbances of consciousness and other symptoms of altered cerebral functioning."

In more recent times, Diaz[30] has divided "psychodysleptics" (as he terms them) into six categories: (1) visionary psychodysleptics (the principal causative agents being phenylethylamines and indoles); (2) imagery-inducing psychodysleptics (mainly the cannabinoids, coumarins, and labiatae compounds); (3) trance-inducing psychodysleptics (ergot alkaloids, glucosides, Heimia alkaloids); (4) deliriant psychodysleptics (tropane alkaloids); (5) neurotoxic psychodysleptics (quinolizidone, pyrolizidine, Erythrina alkaloids); and (6) excitatory psychoanaleptics (ephedrine-like compounds, xanthines).

The following is a brief review of the history of these powerful hallucinogenic drugs, which produce "chemical psychosis" in those members of both primitive societies and sophisticated cultures who seek this means of escaping reality.

The most important of these drugs are mescaline, which comes from the peyote cactus *Lophophora williamsii*; psilocybin and psilocin, from such mushrooms as *Psilocybe mexicana* and *Stropharia cubensis*; and lysergic acid diethylamide (LSD), which is derived from ergot (*Claviceps purpurea*), a fungus that grows on rye and wheat.

In the western hemisphere, consumption of hallucinogenic plants in pre-Columbian times was limited to an area ranging from the southwestern part of the United States to the northwestern basin of the Amazon. The Aztecs achieved inspiration by eating peyote, called *teonanacatl* or "gods' flesh." Today "curanderos" of Mexico and southern parts of the United States still partake of *Psilocybe* and *Stropharia* in their rituals.

Shamans or Indian medicine men of the Rio Grande valley and central Mexico utilized "peyote buttons" in their tribal rituals, and "peyotism" spread rapidly through the Plains tribes, which eventually merged with Christianity. In 1918, recognizing the need for an effective organization to protect peyotism as a form of worship, several peyote churches joined to form the Native American Church, which, in 1964, had more than 225,000 members. Indian peyotists in the United States and Canada normally receive their supplies from Texas. The active principle of peyote, the alkaloid mescaline, was isolated in 1856, and by 1919, it was recognized that the molecular structure of mescaline was related to the structure of the adrenal hormone epinephrine.

In the 19th century, the works of such men as Francis Galton, J. M. Charcot, Sigmund Freud, William James, Havelock Ellis, and Silas Weir Mitchell stimulated scholarly interest. Pharmacologists began to explore these drugs as tools for investigating mental illnesses by evaluating hallucinogenic alkaloid–neurohormone interactions.

Professor Heinrich Klüver, in the foreword to the book *The Botany and Chemistry of Hallucinogens*,[31] summarized the historical perspective of mind-altering drugs in the following way:

> Psychoactive drugs, while spanning time and space psychically, cannot yet do so physically, by transporting us in a "flying carpet" from one region of the globe to another . . . It is a kind of "magic circle" that started with the synthesis of various lysergic acid amides and the discovery of the extraordinary psychotomimetic potency of LSD that led to an investigation of the search for Mexican mushrooms and the isolation of psilocyblin from teonanacatyl, ending finally with ololiuqui where, again, lysergic acid amides were encountered—thus closing the magic circle.

The brief review that follows should be read in the light of the French aphorism: "The more things change, the more they remain the same."[32]

## C. CHEMICAL CLASSIFICATION

Similar to other drug classification, the hallucinogens are grouped according to whether they are naturally occurring or synthetic, or of modern or ancient origin.

Hallucinogenic drugs for the most part can induce psychotic reactions characterized by visual or auditory hallucinations as well as other disturbances of perception. In terms of classification one can divide these drugs into two classes: 1) drugs such as atropine and diisopropylfluorophosphate (DFP) that induce delirium or organic psychosis, and 2) LSD- and mescaline-type drugs that mimic functional psychosis, such as mania and schizophrenia.

As can be predicted from the chemical structural similarity of mescaline to the neurotransmitter type of catecholamines, and the resemblance of LSD to the indoleamines such as serotonin, the psychedelic actions are probably attributable to their interaction with these neurotransmitter brain receptor sites. For example, it appears that LSD exerts its effects at presynaptic serotonin receptors in the mid-brain.

Figure 18–1 depicts the neurotransmitter serotonin which is based on the indole nucleus. LSD contains the indole moeity in its structure, and it is a synthetic compound related to the naturally occurring lysergic acid diethylamide found in morning glory seeds. Psilocybin is also based on the indole moeity and is an active ingredient in the magic Mexican mushroom.

Mescaline found in the peyote cactus religiously used by southwestern Indians in the United States is structurally related to the basic

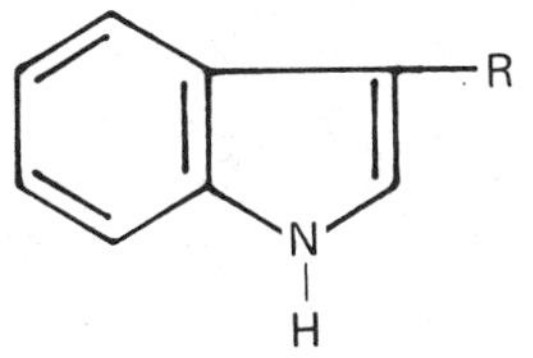

R
N
H

**Figure 18-1.**

catechol depicted in Figure 18–2. Noradrenaline and other adrenergic transmitters also contain this moeity. DOM (STP), another street hallucinogen, contains the catechol nucleus.

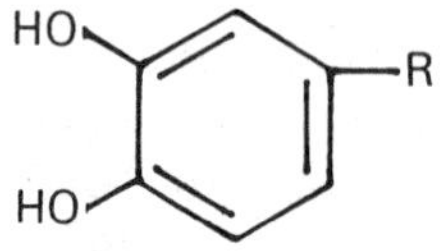

HO HO R

**Figure 18-2.**

The acetylcholine-like hallucinogens all contain the same moeity (as depicted in Figure 18–3), which consists of a positively charged atom a fixed distance from a carboxyl group. A synthetic hallucinogen in this group is ditran, whereas the naturally occurring plant cholinergic-type hallucinogens are represented by henbane, deadly nightshade, and datura.

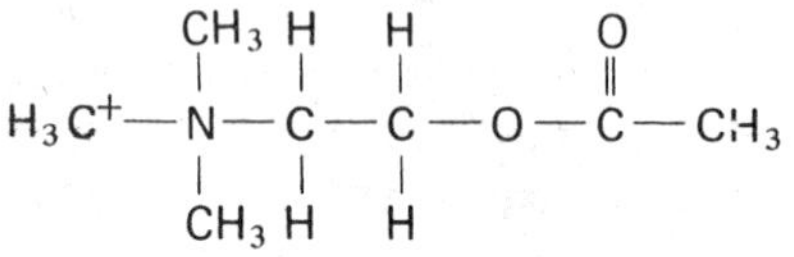

$$\begin{array}{ccccccccccc} & & CH_3 & & H & & H & & O & & \\ & & | & & | & & | & & \| & & \\ H_3C^{+} & — & N & — & C & — & C & — & O — C & — & CH_3 \\ & & | & & | & & | & & & & \\ & & CH_3 & & H & & H & & & & \end{array}$$

**Figure 18-3.**

## D. TYPES OF HALLUCINOGENIC DRUGS

There are, as previously stated, three major chemical classes of hallucinogens: those related to phenyethylamine, such as mescaline and 3,4,5-trimethoxyamphetamine (TMA); those resembling tryptamine, such as psilocin and LSD; and anticholinergic agents, such as atropine, scopolamine, and belladonna.

### 1. Plant B—Phenethylamines, Norepinephrine or Adrenergic Type

Two members of this class of chemicals, mescaline and adrenaline, typify the main properties of these compounds.

#### *a. Lophophora Williamsii (Peyote)*[35]

Peyote, or *Lophophora williamsii*, a small, grey-green napiform spineless cactus, was used by the pre-Columbian Mexican Indians to produce a ritual ecstatic state. The cactus grows in the deserts of central and northern Mexico and the adjacent United States and is concentrated in the area near the Rio Grande Valley.[36]

Peyote has been considered the "prototype" of New World hallucinogens, since it was one of the earliest discovered and was the most spectacular vision-inducing plant encountered by the Spanish conquerors of Mexico. The earliest European reports of peyote suggest that the Chichimecas and Toltecs were acquainted with it as early as 300 B.C.[37]

Sahagun[38] wrote that "petotl . . . is white, it is found in the north country; those who eat of it see visions either frightful or laughable; this intoxication lasts two or three days and then ceases."

Hernandez,[39] physician to the king of Spain, wrote that "both men and women are said to be harmed by it (peyote) . . . cut up and applied to painful joints, it is said to give relief . . . it causes those devouring it to be able to foresee and predict things."

Slotkin[40] described peyote worship by American Indians as a standardized religious ceremony consisting of an all-night ritual, often in a teepee, with singing, chanting, meditation, prayer, and usually a short "sermon" by the roadman or leader, ending in the morning with a communal meal.

Peyote is usually consumed in the form of the so-called mescal buttons, the dried tops of the dumpling cactus. According to Schultes and Hofmann,[41] "The name mescal, as applied to peyote, is a misnomer. Correctly the term refers to a strong distilled drink from a species of agave, the century plant. This error, unfortunately, is responsible also for the naming of the principal hallucinogenic alkaloid *mescaline*. Mescaline does not occur in agave, a member of the Amaryllidaceae.[11]

Peyote intoxication is characterized by brilliant colored visions in kaleidoscopic movement, often accompanied by auditory, taste, olfactory, and tactile hallucinations. The user also experiences sensations of weightlessness, macropsia, depersonalization, doubling of the ego, and alteration or loss of time perception. In 1940, Schultes[42] suggested that peyote's supernatural "medicinal" powers come from its ability, through visions, to put the user in contact with the spirit world.

There are differences in the nature and type of experience one obtains with peyote (which contains many alkaloids) and that induced by mescaline. The interested reader should refer to the writings of Kluver.[43]

Heffter[44] first suggested that mescaline was the chief constituent of peyote. Spath[45] determined the correct formula of mescaline. N-methyl and N-acetyl-mescaline have been isolated from other cactus species. N, N-dimethylmescaline has been similarly isolated and synthesized; however it has been found to have no sensory effect. The available analogs of mescaline that have been tested in general have less psychotomimetic activity than mescaline itself.

Variations of the possible synthesis of mescaline have been described by Banholzer et al.,[46] Dornow and Petsch,[47] and Tsao,[48] among others.

Fischer[49] reported that mescaline in humans causes a syndrome of central synaptic stimulation similar to that of LSD and psilocybin, characterized by increased pupillary size, increases in pulse rate and blood pressure, and elevated body temperature. In addition, it has been observed by Wollbach[50] that mescaline decreases the threshold for elicitation of the knee jerk. The early history of peyote and mescaline in modern pharmacology has been detailed by Bruhn and Holmstedt.[50]

Some users of psychedelics believe that the main difference between LSD and mescaline is that the latter is less potent and does not produce what they term a "head-stone"—or an intense mind experience—as LSD does.

A single dose may cost from $2.50 to $7.00 and the high lasts from four to 16 hours. Morselli[51] took 750 mg of mescaline while alone in his apartment. He suffered a severe psychotomimetic reaction that lasted about 16 hours. For the next two months, he had the delusion that a man in one of the pictures in his apartment was alive and was haunting him. Finally this delusion disappeared and he returned to normal.

A low dosage of mescaline would be 100 to 200 mg; a standard dose for an initial experience might be 500 to 800 mg. Mescaline is available on the illicit market as gelatin capsules or in a form to be mixed with water. It produces nausea, whereas this does not happen with other drugs such as LSD, except as a symptom of an undesirable trip. It is important to emphasize that synthetic mescaline is not readily available on the street market.

### *b. Mescaline Analogs*

In 1959, Alles[52] synthesized some methoxy derivatives of amphetamine that had effects similar to those of mescaline, but were more potent and had a longer duration of action. For example, TMA (3,4,5-trimethoxyamphetamine) and TMA-2 (2,4,5-trimethoxyamphetamine) are, respectively, about 2.0 times and 17 times more potent than mescaline as a hallucinogen, whereas TMA-3 (4,5,5-trimethoxyamphetamine) appears to be inactive.

1. DOM (2,5-dimethoxy-4-methylamphetamine) on the street is called STP, for serenity, tranquility, and peace. It is about 100 times as potent as mescaline, but only 1/13 as potent as LSD. A total dose of 1 to 3 mg most often yields euphoria and 3 to 5 mg results in a six- to eight-hour hallucinogenic period.

Pill forms of DOM obtained in the street contain rather high doses; as much as 10 mg has been reported. Because of this high dosage, users complain about its extraordinarily long duration of effect. Interestingly, unlike other hallucinogens, it has been suggested that DOM's effects are enhanced rather than blocked by chlorpromazine. The prime reason for this so-called paradox is that DOM is an amphetamine derivative and the neuropharmacologic actions indirectly are mediated by catecholamines. Chlorpromazine can enhance catecholamine effects; thus the paradoxic potentiation of DOM's actions. However, in controlled laboratory work with normal volunteers, chlorpromazine does attenuate the DOM experience.[53]

An excellent review[52] on the rise and fall of DOM use is derived from studies at the Haight-Ashbury Clinic. In 1969, Smith and Meyers[54] pointed out the following:

> It appears that DOM produces a higher incidence of acute and chronic toxic reactions than any of the other commonly used hallucinogens—it appears that the effects of DOM are like a combination of amphetamine and LSD with the hallucinogenic effects of the drug very often putting the peripheral amphetamine-like physiological effects out of perspective. . . .

DOM is often illicitly substituted for mescaline. In a study of 23 "mescaline" purchases, it was found that none contained mescaline but that several were DOM.

2. The chemical name of MDA is 3-methoxy-4,5-methylenedioxyamphetamine. According to Shulgin et al.,[55] MDA did not produce hallucinations in eight subjects, in up to 150-mg doses. However, MDA, like LSD, brought about an intensification of feelings, increased perceptions of self-insight, and heightened empathy with others during the experience. A toxicologic review of LSD has been provided but no similar review exists for MDA.[56] In the 1975 rock concert series in San Francisco and the surrounding Bay area, the rock medicine team had to handle numerous MDA "bummers" (bad experiences).[52]

MDA[52] was synthesized in the 1930s, when mescaline and related mescaline amphetamine compounds were becoming popular. The threshold for subjective psychologic effects is about 60 mg. At higher doses, near 120 mg, there occur such visual and related sensory changes as increased perceptions of self-insight and heightened empathy with others during the experience. Subjects also report an increased sense of ecstatic enjoyment.

As with other oral hallucinogenics, the onset of effects comes about 60 minutes after ingestion, with the effects peaking at the end of one and a half to two hours and having a duration of about eight hours. The experience is characterized as an "inward one," with many subjects focusing on their own lives and personalities. Contrary to many rumors, MDA is not a mixture of mescaline and amphetamine, but is actually a compound in its own right that is related structurally to both mescaline and amphetamine.

### *c. Epinephrine, Adrenochrome, and Amphetamine*

Some of the symptoms (fear, anxiety, tenseness) of epinephrine and norepinephrine poisoning following intravenous administration resemble those of the psychotomimetics. In large doses, ephedrine and amphetamine have similar effects, and it is believed that schizophrenic subjects are less able to control the destruction of injected adrenochrome than normal subjects.[57]

Along these lines, reports have appeared indicating that some individuals have attempted to reach a high with intravenous administration of epinephrine. That state was not reached, however, probably because the epinephrine did not penetrate the brain.

In summary, though the physiologic and psychic effects of these compounds are quantitatively similar, it is difficult to find components of chemical structure common to all of them (see Figure 18-4).

The most potent of the adrenergic hallucinogens, LSD, has at least a structural resemblance to other members of the group, and psilocybin is notable because it is a phosphorus-containing, quaternary ammonium compound.

All of these hallucinogens do contain nitrogen, and, in all but LSD, the grouping R′-C-C-N-R′ occurs. The structure of a central nervous system (CNS) stimulant, amphetamine, is provided to illustrate its general structural similarity to mescaline and DOM (2,5-dimethoxy-4-methylamphetamine.

In summing up the effects of mescaline, the prototype adrenergic hallucinogen, Aldous Huxley, in his book *The Doors of Perception*,[58] stated: "This is how one ought to see, how things really are. And yet, there were reservations. For, if one always saw like this, one would never want to do anything else."

## 2. Indole Types of Hallucinogens

According to Schultes and Hofmann,[59] when the structural types in Figure 18.4 are compared, indole structures appear and always in the form of tryptamine derivatives. In the indole class of hallucinogens, it includes tryptamines without any substitution in the indole nucleus or with hydroxymethoxy-o-phosphoryloxy groups in the phenyl ring of the indole, or else the tryptamine residue forms part of a polycyclic ring system, such as β-carboline, lysergic acid derivatives, and ibogaine. Hofmann[60] points out that the most specific and most potent hallucinogens, LSD and psilocybin, belong to the tryptamine type, which is related to serotonin, the neurotransmitter.

The compounds with isoxazole and with tropane structures are less typical and less specific hallucinogens than those of the tryptamine and phenylethylamine group (see Table 18-2) and do not resemble brain neurohormones.

The non-nitrogenous hallucinogens, unlike the indole type, induce marked euphoric states but, compared with mescaline and LSD, alterations of consciousness and hallucinations are much weaker.

### *a. Lysergic Acid Diethylamide (LSD-25)*

Much has been written on the so-called "psychedelic revolution" and the widespread use of psychedelics such as LSD. Many, however, are not aware that numerous seeds, trees, leaves,

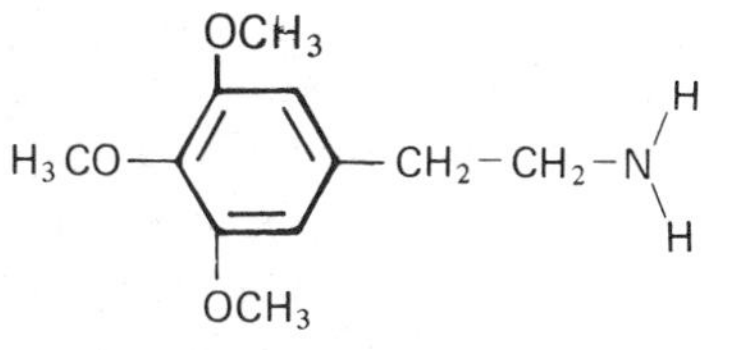

mescaline

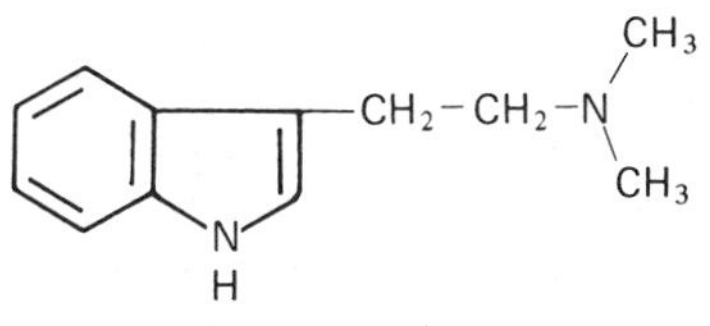

dimethyltryptamine (DMT)

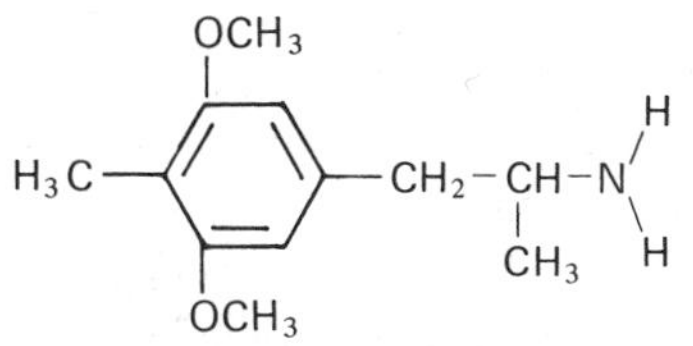

Dom ("STP")

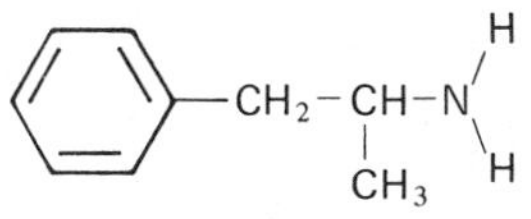

amphetamine

vines, cacti, and fungi are psychedelic resources. More than 100 species are known in the western hemisphere, about 20 in the eastern hemisphere, and more certainly will be discovered each year by ethnobotanists. These facts become even more significant when one considers the production of scores of synthetic psychedelics capable of dramatically altering the functioning of the 12 billion cells network of the human brain.

As previously mentioned, psychedelics have had, and most probably will continue to have, a great effect on the development of human perception and values. There is even archeologic evidence that people have been expanding their consciousness with psychedelic substances for as many as 35 centuries.

A brief example of some of the many writings concerning the use of psychedelic drugs is presented here.

From Lewis Carroll[61]:

> I know who I was when I got up this morning, but I must have been changed several times since then.

From John Paul Smith[62]:

> The wish for instant paradise is as old as man himself. For ages, people have searched for artificial means to improve their condition, and drugs have played an important role in this quest.

From Don McDonagh[63]:

> The LSD feeling would seem to have more fraternity with that tantalizing moment of total clarity, that complete understanding of what life is all about, that illuminates a man in the midst of an evenirg's alcoholic revels. He can't explain the way he feels, and doesn't even remember very clearly the next day, but he tries again and again to recapture that counterfeit moment of truth. Goaded like the gold-hungry conquistadores, whom El Dorado invisibly beckoned, he endures the ''bad'' trip or a ''morning after'' for a promise that is still there.

From David E. Smith[64]:

> The alchemists of the present day are the members of the drug cult. With LSD or something else exotic from the chemical retort, they believe this leaden old world can be turned into instant gold . . . What are the social consequences of several thousand young people regularly taking LSD, involving themselves with the psychedelic subculture . . . It is quite important for the adult community in the dominant culture to be aware of the ''psychedelic syndrome,'' primarily to shatter their stereotypes that ''hippiness'' is a fad, a passing phase similar to their adolescent rebellion of ''swallowing goldfish'' . . . The dominant attitudes of violence, competition, racism and exploitation in virtually every aspect of American life have produced intolerable conflicts in many intellectual, passive, noncompetitive youth and the only solution the individual can accept is to ''turn on, tune in and drop out'' into the antienvironment which may or may not resolve his own hate and disgust for ''straight'' society.

Writings such as these, together with the understanding that it was the accidental discovery of LSD only a generation ago that ''turned on'' western society to its roots, provide a plausible reason why humankind has chosen these agents as an artificial means to find the answers to cosmic questions.

### *b. History*[65]

LSD-25, commonly called LSD, is a derivative of ergot, a rye fungus that is the source of a number of compounds useful in contracting the uterus after childbirth and in the treatment of migraine headaches.[66] All of the ergot alkaloids contain lysergic acid as the basis of their chemical structure.

The use of ergot dates back to before Christ. Ergot, or *Secale cornutum*, refers to the brown protrusions from the ears of rye, which are the sclerotia of the fungus *Claviceps purpurea*. There are a few hundred host plants and 28 species of *Claviceps*.[67] The contaminating presence of ergot, particularly in rye bread, has been responsible for widespread outbreaks of the disease known as ''ergotism.'' In the Middle Ages, this disastrous disease was called ''St. Anthony's Fire.'' Symptoms of ergotism include vomiting, tremors, high temperature, convulsions and other associated problems. Countless people and animals were killed or maimed by the convulsive and gangrenous effects of the infected grain. For example, approximately 11,000 cases of ergotism were reported in Russia in 1926 to 1927.

As early as the 16th century, it was noted that ergot had the ability to induce pain in the uterus, and it became a valuable tool in European midwifery. In 1828, Dr. John Stearns introduced it as a therapeutic agent in America, as a remedy to cause contractions of the uterus and so hasten childbirth.

In 1875, the French chemist Charles Tannet was the first to isolate a crystalline substance from the extract of ergot. The nonpure extracted substance was named ergotine. It was Stoll,[68] in 1918, who isolated a pure crystalline substance, which he named ergotamine.

Several alkaloids are derived from ergot, which can be divided into two groups: lysergic acid and clavine. These are shown in Tables 18-2 and 18-3.

Lysergic acid, not the highly active diethylamide derivative referred to as LSD-25, was first synthesized in 1934 from ergotamine by Walter A. Jacobs and Lyman C. Craig of the Rockefeller Institute of New York.[69]

LSD was synthesized in 1938 by two Swiss chemists, Stoll and Hofmann, working for Sandoz Laboratories.[70] Its profound psychologic effects were not noted until 1943, by Dr. Hofmann, who accidentally took some of the compound and noted a kaleidoscopic play of vivid colors and some peculiar psychologic changes.

> I was seized by a peculiar sensation of vertigo and restlessness . . . Objects, as well as the shape of my associates in the laboratory, appeared to undergo optical changes. I was unable to concentrate on my

**TABLE 18-2**

**The Natural Alkaloids of Ergot (Lysergic Acid Group) and Their Isomers**

| *Name* | *Discoverer* |
|---|---|
| 1. *Ergotamine group* | |
| Ergotamine, ergotaminine | Stoll (1918) |
| Ergosine, ergosinine | Smith and Timmis (1936) |
| 2. *Ergotoxine group* | |
| Ergocristine, ergocristinine | Stoll and Burckhardt (1937) |
| Ergokryptine, ergokryptinine | Stoll and Burckhardt (1943) |
| Ergocornine, ergorcorninine | Stoll and Burckhardt (1943) |
| 3. *Ergometerine group* | |
| Ergometrine | Dudley and Moire |
| Ergometrinine | Kharasch and Legault |
| | Stoll and Burckhardt |
| | Thompson (1935) |

**TABLE 18-3**

**The Natural Ergot Alkaloids of the Clavine Group**

| *Name* | *Discoverer* |
|---|---|
| Ergoclavine | Abe (1951) |
| Elymoclavine | Abe, Yamamoto, Kozo, and Kusumoto (1952) |
| Festuclavine | Abe and Yamatodani (1954) |
| Pyroclavine | Abe, Yamatodani, Yamano, and |
| Costaclavine | Abe and Yamatodani (1954) |
| Secaclavine | Abe and Yamatodani (1955) |
| Molliclavine | Stoll, Brack, Kobel, |
| | Hoffman, and Brunner (1954) |
| Penniclavine | Hoffman, Brunner, |
| | Kobel, and Brack (1957) |
| Isopenniclavine | |
| Setoclavine | |
| Isosetoclavine | |
| Chanoclavine | |

From Sankar, D. V., *LSD—A Total Story*. Westbury, N.Y.: PJD Publications, 1975, pp. 52–53.

work. I left for home where an irresistible urge to lie down came over me. I immediately fell into a peculiar state similar to drunkenness; characterized by an exaggerated imagination . . . With my eyes closed, fantastic pictures of extraordinary plasticity and intensive color seemed to surge toward me. After two hours, this state gradually wore off.

Hofmann suspected that this peculiar state resulted from the ingestion of some of the compound with which he was working. Using other ergot alkaloids as a guide, he decided to be on the safe side and he took only 0.25 mg orally. This is now known to be five to ten times the dose of LSD required to cause disturbances in certain people.

His second experience with the drug confirmed his first impression—that this was indeed a substance with potentially profound psychologic effects.

LSD, and many of its consequences, have been extensively studied. LSD-25 is still the most potent and specific psychotogen of the indole class. It is noteworthy that most street preparations that are claimed to be mescaline are usually a mixture of STP and LSD or the aldehyde derivative of mescaline.

A lawyer working on a case involving a 26-year-old man accused of selling LSD to minors asked this writer to describe the difference between LSD and LSD-25. The answer was that lysergic acid diethylamide is the chemical name for LSD. There are two natural forms of LSD, a levo form and a dextro form. The levo form is inactive, but the dextro form is very active. The term LSD-25 refers to the dextro form of LSD.

Structurally LSD resembles serotonin (5-hydroxytryptamine), a substance found in the brain of animals and humans and suspected of involvement in the transmission of nervous impulses. Some investigators believe that LSD produces its effects by blocking the actions of serotonin in the brain.[71,72]

Following the first report by Dr. Hofmann of the psychologic effects of LSD, very little research on its profound CNS actions occurred until the 1950s. Aldous Huxley wrote of his mescaline experiences in *The Doors of Perception*[58] and *Heaven and Hell*.[73] The philosopher Alan Watts related his drug experiences in *This is It* and *The Joyous Cosmology*. His writings were more exuberant and less critical than Huxley's.[74] During this same time, the psychologists Leary and Alpert began experimenting with psilocybin, using Harvard students as subjects. Huxley, Leary, and others emphasized the personality-improving consciousness-expanding and mystic aspects of these agents. The publicity accompanying the Harvard experiments is considered to have triggered the current drug fad.[74]

Other hallucinogenic drugs, such as marihuana, peyote (mescaline), and mushrooms (psilocybin), have been used for centuries by primitive peoples. Havelock Ellis wrote more than 70 years ago about his experiences with peyote.[74] The Indians of the Native American Church have been using peyote in their religious ceremonies for many years, and have been subjected to a number of legal attacks, apparently motivated, at least partially, by a fear that the use of peyote might spread.[74]

LSD was made illegal by the Federal Drug Abuse Control Amendments of 1965, which went into effect February 1, 1966.[75] The use of psychedelic chemicals increased in 1967 by geometric proportions. In certain areas, such as the Haight-Ashbury district in its early days, usage approached 100 percent. LSD use spread across the country since then, but now has leveled off or decreased in incidence. College students are reducing their LSD intake because of anxieties about adverse reactions and chromosomal damage. Mescaline intake has increased, however; real increases in the 1980s seem to be in the use of psilocybin mushrooms.

## 3. Chemistry

The chemical structure of lysergic acid diethylamide is presented in Figure 18-5, together with the hallucinogens of the indole-type psilocybin.

In 1957, Freter and associates[76] reported that LSD had been oxidized chemically with $S_oCl_2$ in benzene to yield a dithio derivative.

The total synthesis of lysergic acid was carried out by Kornfeld and his associates at the Eli Lilly Laboratories, and first reported by Larbrecht[77]; it is shown in Figure 18-6.

In 1972, Stutz and Stadler[78] described methyl derivatives of LSD and Nakahara and Niwaguchi[79] synthesized N-6 dimethyl LSD.

Physical and chemical properties of LSD are adequately reviewed in the book by Sankar.[65] Briefly, in reported experiments, at least 50 percent of LSD-25 remained in the active form, even after baking it in a batter made from commercial Bisquick at 300°F for one hour and freezing it for several weeks.[80] In addition, boiling a solution of 1.0 mg/ml of LSD-25 in the dark for up to four hours did not lead to a significant destruction of LSD-25, although LSD-25 is very sensitive to light.

The numbering scheme for LSD, psilocin, and mescaline is presented in Figure 18-7.

In 1967, Arcamone et al.,[81] through acid catalyzed substitutions at the asymetric carbon atom in the side chains of lysergic acid, obtained epiners of lysergates such as lysergic acid α-hydroxyethylamide and dihydrolyseric acid α-dihydroxyethylanide. Blaha[82] and Inoue and coworkers[83] reported both optical properties and image spectra of LSD derivatives.

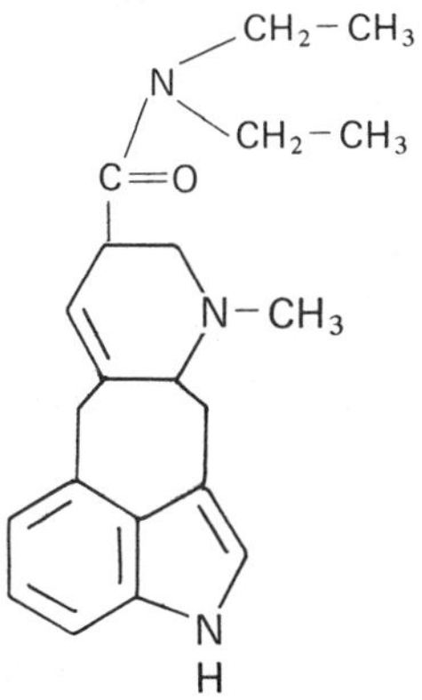

LSD

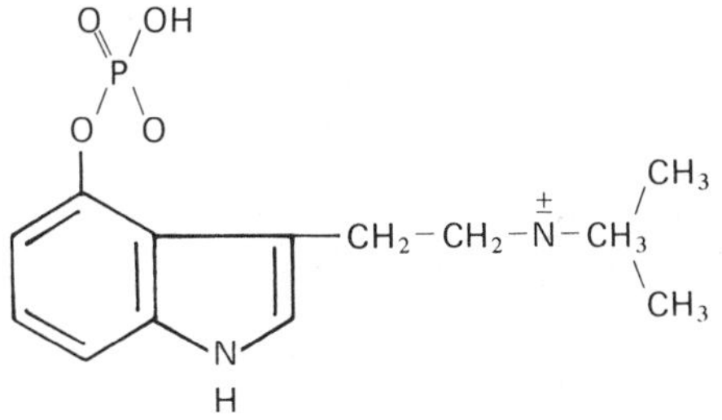

psilocybin

**Figure 18-5.**

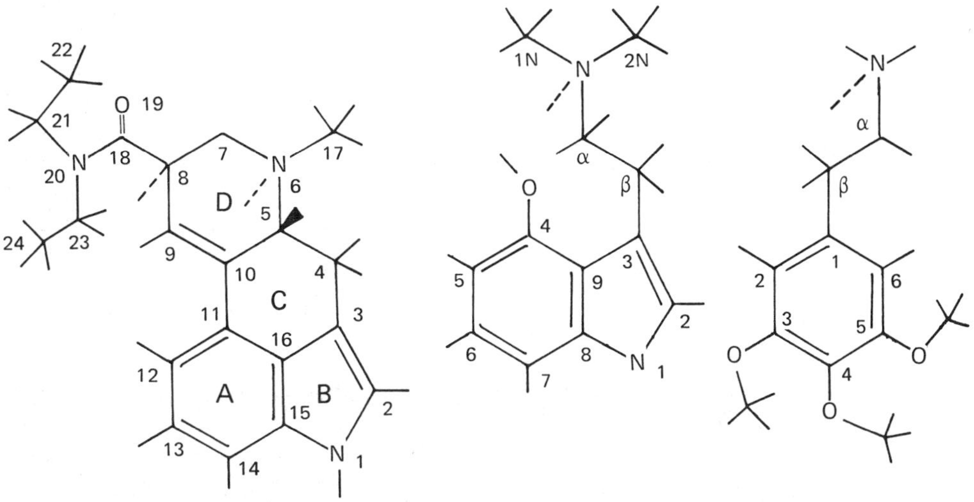

**Figure 18-7. Numbering scheme for LSD, psilocin, and mescaline.**

(From Sankar, D.V.S., *LSD: A Total Study*. Westbury, N.Y.: PJD Publications, 1975. With permission.)

$H_2/Ni$, $C_6H_5Cl$

$SOCl_2$, $AlCl_3$

$Br_2$

$HCl$, $EtO^-$

$(COCH_3)_2O$, $NaBH_4$

$SOCl_2$, $NaCN$

$CH_3OH/H$, $NaOH$, $-H_2$ (Ni)

*dl*-lysergic acid

**Figure 18-6. (From Sankar, D. V. S. *LSD—A Total Study*. Westbury, N.Y.: PJD Publications, 1975.)**

In 1972, Floss[84] proposed a hypothetic oxidative pathway for the formation of lysergates from simple precursors by oxidation, as illustrated in Figure 18-8.

A list of lysergate derivatives, including chemical names and toxicity ($LD_{50}$) in various animal species is illustrated in Table 18-4.

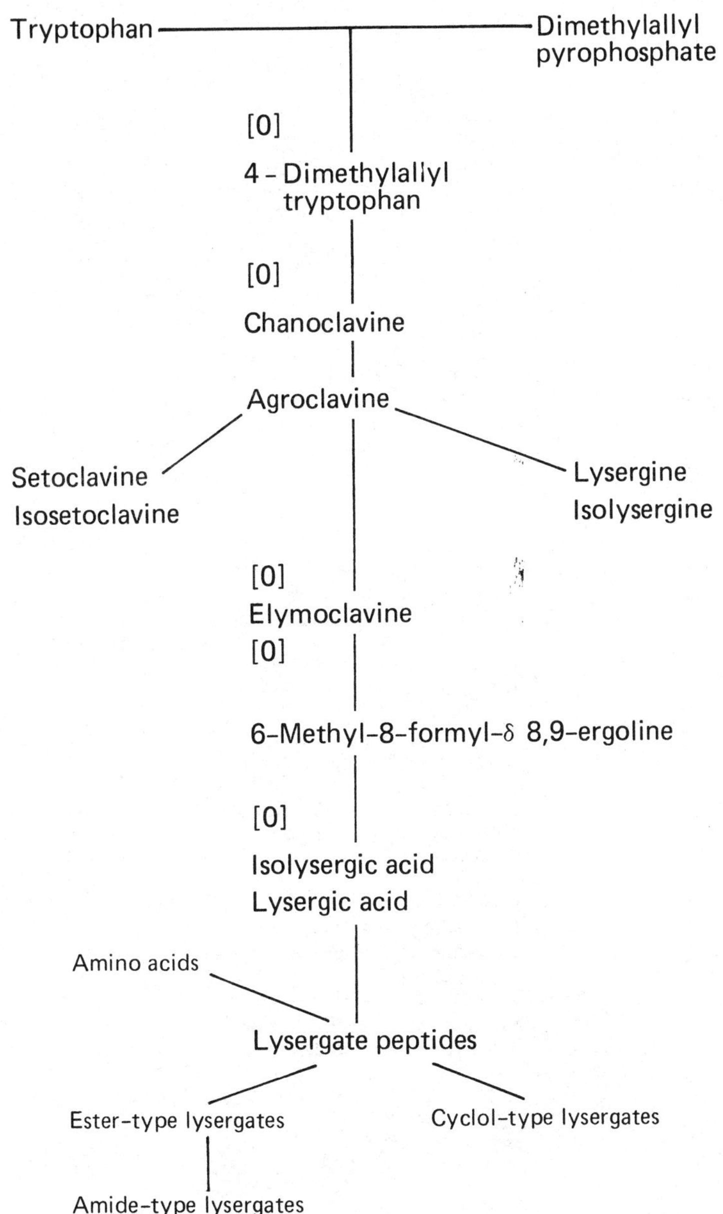


**Figure 18-8. (From Sankar, D. V. S. *LSD—A Total Study.* Westbury, N.Y.: PJD Publications, 1975.)**

## TABLE 18-4

| *COMPOUND* | *Chemical Name* | *$LD_{50}$* |
|---|---|---|
| 1-Acetyllysergic acid diethylamide | 1-Acetyl-9,10-didehydro-N,N-diethyl-6-methyl-ergoline—β-carboxamide bitartrate. | 1.6 mg/kg/I.V./R* |
| ALA-10 | 1-Acetyl-9,10-didehydro-N-ethyl-6-methyl-ergoline-8β-carboxamide. | 5.0 mg/kg/I.V./R |
| 2-Broolysergic acid diethylamide | 2-Bromo-9,10-didehydro-N,N-diethyl-6-methyl-ergoline-8β-carboxamide. | 20 mg/kg/I.V./m*<br>6 mg/kg/I.V./R |
| DAM-57 | 9,10-Didehydro-N,N,6-trimethylergoline-8 -carboxamide. | 0.4 mg/kg/I.V./R |
| Ergometrin(e) | 9,10-Didehydro-N-(α-(hydroxymethyl)ethyl)-6-methyl-ergoline-8β-carboxamide. | 7.5 mg/kg/I.V./R |
| 12-Hydroxylysergic acid diethylamide | 9,10-Didehydro-N,N-diethyl-6-methyl-12-hydroxy-ergoline-8β-carboxamide. | 0.3 mg/kg/I.V./R |
| IEC | N-Benzoxy Lysergamide | 0.05 mg/kg/I.V./R |
| LOL | 9,10-Didehydro-6-methyl-8-β hydroxymethyl-ergoline. | 0.32 mg/kg/I.V./R |
| LSM-775 | Lysergic acid morpholide. | 0.7 mg/kg/I.V./R |
| Lysergic acid amide | 9,10-Didehydro-6-methyl-ergoline-8β-carboxamide. | |
| Lysergic acid diethylamide | 9,10-Didehydro-N,N-diethyl-6-methyl-ergoline-8β-carboxamide. | 46 mg/kg/I.V./m<br>16.5 mg/kg/I.V./r*<br>0.3 mg/kg-I.V./R<br>65 mg/kg/I.V./m<br>*d*-isomer: 0.3 mg/kg/I.V./R<br>*l*-isomer: 17 mg/kg/I.V./R<br>*d*-iso isomer: 8.1 mg/kg/I.V./R |
| Lysergic acid ethylamide | 9,10-Didehydro-N-ethyl-6-methylergoline-8β-carboxamide. | 44 mg/kg/I.V./m<br>0.9 mg/kg/I.V./R |
| Lysergic acid pyrrolidate | D-Lysergic acid pyrrolidide. | 0.4 mg/kg/I.V./R<br>46 mg/kg/I.V./m |
| MBL-41 | 9,10-Didehydro-N,N-diethyl-2-bromo-6-methyl-ergoline-8β-carboxamide. | 15 mg/kg/I.V./R |
| 12-Methoxy lysergic acid diethylamide | 9,10-Didehydro-N,N-diethyl-6-methoxy-ergoline-8β-carboxamide. | 0.1 mg/kg/I.V./R |
| Methylergonovine | 9,10-Didehydro-N-(α-(hydroxymethyl)propyl)-6-methyl-ergoline-8 -carboxamide. | 85 mg/kg/I.V./m<br>187 mg/kg/P.O./m<br>23 mg/kg/I.V./r<br>93 mg/kg/P.O./r<br>2.6 mg/kg/I.V./R |
| 1-Methyl LSD | 9,10-Didehydro-N,N-diethyl-1,6-diemethyl-ergoline-8β-carboxamide dimaleate. | |
| Methysergid(e) | 9,10-Didehydro-N-(1-(hydroxymethyl)propyl)-1,6-dimethyl-ergoline-8β-carboxamide dimaleate. | 581 mg/kg/P.O./m<br>185 mg/kg/I.V./m<br>200 mg/kg/P.O./r<br>125 mg/kg/I.V./r<br>28 mg/kg/I.V./R |
| MLA-74 | 9,10-Didehydro-N-ethyl-1,6-dimethyl-ergoline-8β-carboxamide. | 9.4 mg/kg/I.V./R |
| MPD-75 | 1-Methyl-lysergic acid pyrrolidide. | 7.5 mg/kg/I.V./R |

*R = rabbit; m = mouse; r = rat.
From Sankar, D. V. S. *LSD—A Total Study*. Westbury, N.Y.: PJD Publications, 1975, pp. 80–82.

## 4. Pharmacokinetics and Metabolism

LSD is a polar compound (soluble in water) that is odorless, tasteless, and colorless. It is fairly rapidly absorbed from the gastrointestinal tract as evidenced by its effects being perceived within 30 to 40 minutes following oral ingestion. Aghanjanian and Bing[87] have calculated the half-life of LSD in human plasma to be approximately 175 minutes. Little is actually known about the distribution of LSD in human tissue except that the plasma concentrations of LSD following intravenous injections are higher than those that would be obtained if the drug were evenly distributed within the total pool of body water.[87]

Using the bromo analog of LSD known as BOL Kalbhen and Sargent[88] studied distribution patterns in humans. With radioactive bromine, they reported that the activity increased steadily in the blood for nine hours and then remained constant for 48 hours. The highest activity was found initially in the liver and later on in the lower abdomen. Formed blood elements contained 50 percent as much activity as plasma and over a six-day period 50 percent of the tracer bromine was excreted.

Various studies on the distribution of LSD in both animal and human tissues have been conducted. They include the work of Snyder and Reivich[89] in monkeys, Diab and associates[90] in rats, Wright[91] in choroid plexus of rodents, Freedman and Coquet[92] in rat brain, Faragella[93] in rat brain, and binding studies of LSD to subcellular fractions from rat brain were studied by Farrow and Van Vunakis.[94] In fact, Sankar[95] compared the LSD content of various regions of the brain.

### *a. Peripheral Effects*

Rothlin[97–99] reviewed the pharmacophysiologic effects of LSD *in vivo* and *in vitro*. He found that it contracted rabbit uterus; constricted perfused blood vessels of rat kidneys, rabbit ears, and cat spines, decreased blood pressure; selectively antagonized serotonin on rat uterus, smooth muscle of guinea pig gut, blood vessels, and bronchial muscles *in vivo*; increased the amplitude without changing sensitivity to acetylcholine and mimicked the serotonin effect on Venus mercenaria heart. LSD produced both sympathetic and parasympathetic activity. In normal volunteers, 1 or ½ μg/kg elevated the pulse rate. In animals, very high doses produced inhibition and paralysis.

Little is known about the metabolism and excretion of LSD in human beings, which is the case, by and large, for all ergot alkaloids and their semisynthetic cogeners. The fact that just 50 to 100 μg of LSD can exert effects that may last for 12 hours has led some to speculate that human metabolism and excretion of this compound occur very slowly; others suggest that LSD may act as a "trigger," setting in motion changes that persist for hours after the drug itself has been inactivated or excreted. This speculation stems largely from findings in laboratory animals in which the half-life of LSD in plasma is just 7.5 minutes.[87] Other animal studies have indicated that LSD is inactivated via hepatic oxidation and that little unchanged drug appears in the urine.[96]

In conclusion, immediately after the administration of LSD, it reaches a high concentration in the blood and subsequently in the brain. Sankar[95] points out that the eventual metabolism of LSD is carried through the hepatoenteric circulation of the bile. The major portion of LSD is excreted in approximately three days in the feces. There seems to be a higher concentration in the free supernatant fraction and strikingly smaller amounts in the mitochondrial synaptosomal fractions. The hypothalamic pituitary structures contain significantly larger concentrations of administered LSD than do the neocortical structures.

### *b. Central Effects*

The significant effects of LSD are almost entirely upon the CNS. In doses that affect the CNS in humans, little response is seen in other organ systems that can be attributed to a direct action of the drug. On the physiologic side, LSD produces marked effects on the nervous system. After it is taken, the pupils dilate, the blood pressure rises slightly, and the pulse quickens. At the doses actually employed by humans, the physiologic effects are quite minor, however, compared with the profound effects that are seen. Rothlin and others have reviewed the early work on the CNS pharmacology of LSD.[97–99]

The most sensitive and useful measure of LSD activity is mydriasis (pupillary dilation). According to Rinkel and co-workers,[100] the size of the subject's pupil is a very valuable measure of the intensity of the psychologic experience. In rabbits, the most sensitive test is its pyretogenic effect. Doses of 0.5 to 1 μg/kg elevate rabbit body temperature. This is the only animal measure sensitive to doses active in humans. The time sequence of the fever and the psychologic response in humans are similar.

In humans, LSD produces a prolonged period of analgesia. Kast and Collins[101] compared the analgesic property of 100 μg of LSD with 2 mg of dihydromorphinone HCl and 100 mg of peperidine CHl in patients suffering severe pain from terminal carcinoma. LSD produced the most painfree hours; however, the subjects refused to take it a second time.

### *c. Psychologic or Behavioral Effects*

Since the discovery of the powerful mind-altering effects of LSD some 40 years ago, its use has resulted in an extraordinary controversy. Many who have taken the substance report that they experienced an expansion of the mind and awareness of beauty, and that relative stability and security have been damaged beyond repair.

The effects of the drug are felt from 35 to 45 minutes after the injection of an average dose (150 to 200 μg). After the heart rate increases and the pupils dilate, a feeling of depersonalization and loss of body image is experienced. This earliest response in inexperienced users may cause great anxiety and is probably the most common cause of the bad trip or adverse experience. Subjects usually notice a change in their perceptions of their environment; they may notice that walls and other objects become a bit wavy or seem to move. Colors may appear to be much brighter and more intense. New colors, difficult to describe, are seen.[101] A rainbow effect is usually observed; white light may be much brighter and be surrounded by many colors.[102]

Hallucinations (false sensory perceptions without a basis in external reality) are surprisingly rare with LSD, but pseudo-hallucinations are common.[102] Fixed objects fuse and diffuse; there is often a perpetual flowing of geometric designs. Another outstanding perceptual change is synesthesia—one sensation merges into another, and one sense into another, so that the individual may report being able to taste color or touch sound. Sometimes an individual thinks he/she sees the actual notes of music moving or colors beating in rhythm with the music. The body image is distorted and ordinary sounds increase profoundly in intensity. Intense mood changes are experienced under the influence of LSD. An early stage in the LSD experience may often be euphoric. For example, the sight of blue sky can generate an ecstatic state, but if the sun goes behind a cloud, the subject's mood can change to one of sadness. Time stands still; also past, present, and future frequently become mixed up.[102,103]

It is well known that the type of experience one may achieve under the influence of LSD depends greatly on one's personality structure, one's "set" or attitude prior to the experience and the environment in which the drug experience takes place.

To some, the LSD trip is simply one of intense physical and erotic pleasure; to others, it has far greater meaning. Some claim an understanding of the universe and the meaning of God, of life beyond death, and of the whole concept of religion. The drug also has been hailed as a potent aphrodisiac.[104] A college youth referred to LSD as "God's gift to sex".[105] Vivid hallucinations with frightening environmental perceptions, such as seeing spiders, often occur.[103]

According to Dr. Smith,[103] "LSD users often seem to themselves to be conversing on a high, philosophical level, although they may be making no apparent sense to the listener. Paranoia may be generated, exhibiting itself in fear of friends, police officers and other real or imagined people who are 'following' or 'watching' the subject."

Despite the profound effects of the drug, the recognition of sensations remains intact, and the individual can perform coordinated acts. A chronic LSD user once described driving a car under the influence of LSD, something which, fortunately, is not done too often by most LSD users. Even though he was aware of the perceptual change in distance (100 feet converted to 10 feet), he noted that the reds were redder and the greens were greener, and so he was able to stop and go at appropriate times.

For many individuals, however, the LSD experience is so terrifying that the drug might be listed as one of the most dangerous known. Severe abnormal reactions have occurred when LSD was taken for kicks or indiscriminately under ill-controlled circumstances for "mind expansion."[106–109]

Consider the case of a man, aged 21, who had had a normal childhood and had done well at school until he was 17. He started taking amphetamines at 18, and this was succeeded by experimentation with other drugs such as heroin and cannabis. He tried LSD once and found the effects pleasant at the time:

> At first, it was a vague dream. I was semifloating. There is nothing you can't do. You throw your problems aside—think you are God. However, this pleasant experience was later superseded by severe panic attacks. The aftereffects were too terrifying. I would not want to repeat it. I was violently sick for a few days, my head was spinning, and I could hardly stand. I was in a deep depression, and thought someone was watching me all of the time. I would wake in a cold sweat, find myself lying paralyzed—it is frightening, you wake up and don't know if you are awake or not.

This individual had no desire to take LSD again. However, a bad experience (or trip) does not always turn off the user from further experimentation with LSD.

Taylor and associates[110] reviewed unfavorable reactions to LSD and concluded:

> By June 1967, 21 reports had been published in the literature relating to 225 adverse reactions to LSD. There were 142 cases of prolonged psychotic reactions, 63 non-psychotic reactions, 11 spontaneous recurrences, 19 attempted suicides, 11 successful suicides, 4 attempted homicides and 1 successful homicide. There were no clear cases of dependency, addiction or death due to toxic effects. About 80 percent of the prolonged psychotic reactions were outside therapeutic and experimental use, but two-thirds of the suicide attempts and the only successful homicide occurred in carefully protected settings. Previous personality disturbance may be as low as 23 percent. Spontaneous recurrence appears almost exclusively among heavy users. Users appear to be a population of predominantly male students and former students in their early twenties. Illicit use of LSD appears to be an urban phenomenon. Paid volunteers for a hallucinogenic study showed high rates of personality disturbance (41 percent needed psychiatric treatment and 20 percent had received such treatment in the past).

The psychotogenic effects of LSD in normals were considered comparable to clinical schizophrenia. However, Brengelmann[111] has shown that LSD psychosis is a drug-induced effect, whether short or long in its duration, even though it may precipitate a clinical psychosis in borderline schizophrenics.

Eisner[112] reported that LSD administered in a therapeutic setting showed a lessening of ego defensiveness, loosening of intellectual controls, better relations with the individuals present at the time of the experiment, and increased emergence of unconscious material. Similar to both meprobamate and several barbiturates, LSD significantly impairs performance in the digit symbol substitution test.[113]

Numerous studies have been reported on research dealing with the psychologic effects of LSD. In this regard, Kabes et al.[114] observed a biphasic action on spontaneous motor activity of small animals; and Cohen and Wakely[115] reported a dose-dependent decrease of mice maze performance with LSD. Other studies on the effects of LSD on open field and maze performance include the work of Dahdiya et al.,[116] Black et al.,[117] Uyeno and Mitoma,[118] Miller and Miller,[119] Songer and Rech,[120] Schechter and Rosecrans,[121] and Uyeno.[122] Studies on the effects of LSD on conditioned behavior include those of Olds,[123] Domino et al.,[124] Pawlowski,[125] Barry et al.,[126] Jarrard,[127] Caldwell and Domino,[128] Sparber and Tilson,[129] Appel and Freedman,[130] Miller et al.,[131] and Roberts and Bradley.[132]

LSD-induced disruption of discrimination was studied by Sharpe et al.[133] In other studies, LSD decreased the aggressiveness and the amplitude of the EEG waves of the optic lobes[134]; Horowitz et al.[135] found that LSD produced a biphasic effect on responding for internal hypothalamic self-stimulation; Siegel and Poole[136] observed a marked change in group aggregation and aggression in mice, leading to temporary disruption of social hierarchies.

The effect of LSD on psychosexual behavior includes the work of Bignami,[137] Herz,[138] Alpert,[139] Uyeno,[140] and Rosen and Iovino.[141] Deshon et al.[142] showed acceleration, retardation, or nonexistence of time as a result of LSD administration. Alexander et al.[143] found that LSD enhanced the incidence of seizures induced by high-frequency auditory stimuli. Paul[144] found that LSD caused an impairment in the ability to learn and retain connected verbal material; Jarvik and associates[145] showed that simple problem solving, attention and concentration, recognition, and recall were impaired by LSD. Other studies on the effects of LSD on anxiety, intellectual functions, learning, and memory include the research by McGlothin et al.,[146] Levine et al.,[147] Silverstein and Klee,[148] Lienert,[149] Goldberger,[150] Boyadzhieva and Mumdzhieva,[151] Wright and Hogan,[152] and Langs.[153]

To understand further the psychologic effects of LSD, one must first understand the effects LSD has on the psychedelic experience in humans. Five major kinds of potential psychedelic drug experiences have been described.

First is the psychotic psychedelic experience, characterized by the intense, negative experience of fear to the point of panic, paranoid delusions of suspicion or grandeur, toxic confusion, impairment of abstract reasoning, remorse, depression, and isolation or somatic discomfort, or both; all of these can be of very powerful magnitude.

Second is the cognitive psychedelic experience, characterized by astonishingly lucid thought. Problems can be seen from a novel perspective, and the inner relationships of many levels or dimensions can be seen all at once. The creative experience may have something in common with this kind of psychedelic experience, but such a possibility must await the results of future investigation.

Third is the esthetic psychedelic experience, characterized by a change and intensification of all sensory modalities. Fascinating changes in sensations and perception can occur—synthesia in which sounds can be "seen"; apparent pulsations or lifelike movements in objects, such as flowers or stones; the appearance of great beauty in ordinary things; release of powerful music; and eyes-closed visions of beautiful scenes, intricate geometric patterns, architectural forms, historic events, and almost anything imaginable.

Fourth is the psychodynamic psychedelic experience, characterized by a dramatic emergence into consciousness of material that was previously unconscious or preconscious. Abreaction and catharsis are elements of what may be experienced subjectively as an actual reliving of incidents from the past or a symbolic portrayal of important conflicts.

The fifth type of psychedelic experience has been called by various names: psychedelic peak, cosmic, transcendental, or mystical, and can be summarized under the following six major psychologic characteristics: (1) sense of unity or oneness (positive ego transcendence, loss of usual sense of self without loss of consciousness); (2) transcendence of time and space; (3) deeply felt positive mood (joy, peace, love); (4) sense of awesomeness, reverence, and wonder; (5) meaningfulness of psychologic or philosophic insight, or both; and (6) ineffability (sense of difficulty in communicating the experience by verbal description).

### *d. Effects of LSD on Electrical Activity of Brain*

Between 1943 and 1963, more than 2000 papers on LSD alone were published, involving the electrophysiologic, behavioral, biochemical, and sociologic fields of study. Extensive reviews on the subject have also appeared.[154,155]

Goldstein[154] discussed and reviewed the effects of LSD (and other hallucinogenic drugs) on single neuronal activity in populations of neurons subjected to artificial stimulation and spontaneous EEG. The major effects have been summarized by Sankar and are presented in Table 18-5. The more serious reader should refer to Goldstein's chapter in Sankar's book for complete references and discussion of this subject.

A review of the findings concerned with the effects of LSD on evoked potentials is presented in Table 18-6. Table 18-7 illustrates the effects of LSD on spontaneous brain electrical activity (cortex and subcortical structures) of animals.

The key contribution of neurophysiologic research on LSD is a fundamental knowledge of specific neurophysiologic systems and their mechanism of action.

### *e. Summary of LSD Effects*

A careful review of the literature reveals numerous studies on a multitude of biologic actions. Because of space limitations, and for brevity, the diverse (selective) properties of LSD-25 are summarized in Table 18-8.

### *f. Mode of Action*

The clinical resemblance of the syndromes produced by mescaline, psilocin, LSD, TMA, and other hallucinogens suggests that these drugs, despite differences in chemical structure, may share a common mechanism of action. The fact that the psychotropic effects of TMA, a methoxylated amphetamine, are unlike those of amphetamine but similar to those of LSD illustrates the complexity of structure–activity relationships of hallucinogens. The "hypothesis" that hallucinogens possess a common mechanism of action is supported by findings that cross-tolerance can develop between the hallu-

**TABLE 18-5**

**Summary of the Effects of LSD on Simple Neurons**

| *Site of Recording* | *Mode of Administration* | *Change in Firing Rates* | *Remarks* |
|---|---|---|---|
| Lateral geniculate body | Electrophoresis | Decrease | LSD less effective than 5-HT and bufotenine. More effective than psilocybin |
| Cerebral cortical cells | Iontophoresis | Long lasting decrease | Curarized rabbits |
| Septum (B-units) | I.V. 100 μg/kg* | No change | More marked effect with BOL and methysergide |
| Pyriform cortex | | Small decrease | |
| Renshaw cells, spinal cord | Electrophoresis | Decrease | Recovery after five minutes |
| Dorsal and median raphe nuclei | 25–50 μg/kg,* systemic | Inhibition | |

*μg/kg represents micrograms of substance per kilogram of body weight.
From Goldstein, L. The effect of LSD and other hallucinogens on the electrical activity of brain during wakefulness and sleep. In D. V. S. Sankar, ed., *LSD—A Total Study.* Westbury, N.Y.: PJD Publications, 1975, p. 399.

**TABLE 18-6**

**Effects of LSD on Evoked Potentials**

| *Site of Stimulation* | *Site of Recording* | *Dose* | *Route* | *Species* | *Effect Observed (Change in Relation to Drugfree Condition)* | *Remarks* |
|---|---|---|---|---|---|---|
| Cortex | Contralateral cortex | 10–50 μg/kg | Intracarotid | Cat | Decrease | "Transcallosal potential" |
| Optic nerve | Lateral gen. body | 10–30 μg/kg | Intracarotid | Cat | Marked decrease | Pentobarbital anesthetized |
| | | 0.5 mg/kg | I.V. | Cat | Marked decrease | Pentobarbital anesthetized |
| | | 1 mg/kg | I.V. | Cat | Marked decrease | Nonanesthetized |
| Visual | cortex | 35 μg/ animal | I.V. | Rabbit | Enhancement. Marked | Nonanesthetized |

## TABLE 18-7

## Effects of LSD on Spontaneous Brain Electrical Activity (Cortex and Subcortical Structures) in Animals

| *Dose (μg/kg)* | *Species* | *Effect Observed or Measured* | *Remarks* |
|---|---|---|---|
| 15–40 | Rabbit | Flattening of the waves | Unanesthetized |
| 15–25 oral | Cat | Arousal-type activity | Unanesthetized |
| 0.2 I.V. | Rabbit | 50% reversal of sedation | Mildly sedated with pentobarbital |
| 50–100 | Rabbit | Reversal of slow waves produced by barbiturates | |
| 100–200 g/animal intraventricular | | Cat | High-amplitude 4–7-Hz waves blocked by sensory stimulation |
| | 1–5 | Rabbit | Facilitation of arousal. Lowering of threshold for arousal by electrical stimulation of the RF |
| Curarized preparations | 10–15 | Rabbit | Spontaneous alerting patterns |
| | 20–60 | | Slow waves and spindles. Increase in threshold for RF arousal |
| No reversal of the effect with mescaline that remained stimulant at all doses | | | |
| 50–200 I.M. | Cat | Prolonged bursts of large sinusoidal waves, 3–4 Hz | Similar patterns in the hypothalamus including mammillary bodies and in the septum. No change in hippocampal activity |
| 100 | Cat | Activation pattern | Transient cerebral vasoconstriction. Same effect with smaller doses by intracarotid administration |
| 1–5 | Rabbit | Activation pattern. Marked decrease of variability of normal brain waves | |
| 850–1000 lateral ventricle | Cat | Slowing of cortical EEG with spindles. Reduction in amplitude in midbrain RF and dorsal hippocampus. Seizure-like pattern in medial geniculate body. Synchronized pattern in preoptic area, palladium, putamen, and amygdala. | Acute preparations immobilized with Flaxedil |
| 50 I.V. | Cat | Arousal patterns | Increase in amplitude of amygdala waves |
| 25 | Cat | Short episodes of seizure 4–5 Hz in hippocampal and entorhinal areas | Tolerance effect observed up to ten days post-administration |
| 50 chronic daily for 15 days | Rabbit | High-amplitude 5–6 Hz waves with superimposed fast rhythms | Effects persisting up to six days following cessation of treatment |

From Goldstein, L. The effect of LSD and other hallucinogens on the electrical activity of brain during wakefulness and sleep. In: D.V.S. Sankar, ed., *LSD—A Total Study*. Westbury, N.Y.: PJD Publications, 1975, p. 408.

cinogens, LSD, mescaline, and psilocybin but not between hallucinogens and amphetamine.[156]

A hypothesis for the structure mechanism of the hallucinogenic activity of drugs ideally should explain all the structure activity relationships described. Since norepinephrine and serotonin, the putative brain neurohumors, are structurally similar to phenylethylamine and tryptamine, it has been thought that hallucinogens might affect brain synaptic transmission. One theory, as previously mentioned, postulates that hallucinogens act in the brain as antimetabolites of serotonin. However, 2-brom-LSD, which has 50 percent more antiserotonin activity than LSD in the rat uterus, and which readily penetrates the brain, has no hallucinogenic activity.[157] For detailed reviews of the literature concerning the effects of LSD on CNS transmission, see Aghajanian[158] and others.[159,160]

Although LSD and other hallucinogens affect hormones, amines, and endocrine tissue, their effect on serotonin seems to be most profound.

## TABLE 18-8
## Effects of LSD-25

I. Effects on biogenic amines such as serotonin, histamine, and acetylcholine, on the one hand, and on the catecholamines, such as epinephrine, norepinephrine, and their metabolites, on the other.

II. Effects on hormones, especially the hypophyseal stimulating hormones, and TSH.

III. Effects on the autonomic nervous system
- Rise in body temperature
- Pilomotor reaction
- Mydriasis
- Tachycardia
- Other mesodiencephalic effects
- The following opposite type of effects are also known.
- Bradycardia
- Respiratory depression
- Lowering of blood pressure

IV. Somatomotor effects
- Ataxia
- Spastic paralysis (causes circular motions in animals)
- Pyramidal and extrapyramidal effects

V. Direct peripheral actions and effects on smooth muscles.
- Blood vessels
- Bronchi
- Uterus and vagina
- Adrenergic effects, and possibly effects on other systems such as the villi, intestines, rectum

VI. Psychic effects
- Excitation
- Changes in behavior and mood—euphoria, depression, megalomania, etc.
- Perceptual disturbances, disturbances in thought processes, cognition, objective and subjective structural organization, and size and body image
- Depersonalization, hallucinations
- Shizophrenia-like state

VII. Neurophysiologic effects
- Spindling and desynchronization of EEG
- No significant effect on sleep patterns

VIII. Genetic effects

In spite of a confusing mass of reports on the genetic effects of LSD, no significant mass of data seems to indicate genetic damage due to ingestion of pure LSD. However, as a *very potent* substance, LSD should be strictly avoided by the pregnant and the near-pregnant.

IX. Other effects include those on the binding and release of the several neurohormones, hyperglycemic action, effects of cholinesterase, etc. These may be found in greater detail later in this book.

From Sankar, D. V. S. *LSD—A Total Study.* Westbury, N.Y.: PJD Publications, 1975, p. 66.

Freedman[161] demonstrated an increase in whole-brain serotonin (5-hydroxytryptamine[5-HT]) following administration of LSD. The increase was later localized to a subsynaptosomal fraction consisting largely of synaptic vesicles.[162] Lovell and Freedman[163] showed that LSD binds directly to synaptic membranes. These authors also suggested that receptor sites for LSD appear to be present in both pre- and postsynaptic elements. Release of serotonin could be inhibited by LSD and thus lead to enhanced retention of serotonin by stimulating a presynaptic 5-HT receptor. Furthermore, displacement studies by Bennett and Snyder[164] show that serotonin and LSD can displace each other effectively from their respective binding sites. The work of Fillion et al.[165] postulated the existence of separate receptors for LSD and seronin.

Additionally, peripheral serotonin antagonists such as methiothepin, which are effective blockers of the LSD binding sites, do not prevent the raphe cell response to LSD.[166] Psilocybin, which inhibits both the firing and the increase of whole-brain 5-HT, binds only weakly to those receptors. However, the nonpsychoactive LSD congener 2-bromo-LSD (BOL) binds as strongly as LSD but it neither causes nor prevents the action of LSD in rapid firing.[167] Finally the work of Halavis et al.[160] clearly indicates that LSD has a direct effect on 5-HT receptors at the level of the presynaptic terminal.

### *g. Miscellaneous Facts*

1. *Dose and psychologic activity*

*Minimal recognizable dose.* The minimal effective dose seems to be about 25 μg per adult. Stoll[168] found that 20 to 30 μg were active. Hoffa[169] completed double-blind self-recognition trials in normal volunteers and found that the subjects could not detect 15-μg doses, but that most were able to detect 25 μg.

*Optimum psychotomimetic or psychedelic dose.* According to Hoffa and Osmond,[169] this dose varied from 100 to 1000 μg, depending upon a large number of variables. For example, the dose for nonalcoholics varied from 100 to 200 μg, but was higher for alcoholics, ranging from 200 to 500 μg.

2. *Maximum clinical dose.* The largest dose reported was 1.5 mg per adult. This seems to be close to the upper safe limit when given for the first time.[170]

3. *Variables that influence the LSD reaction.* The following is a list of factors which, in the opinion of Hoffa and Osmond, influence an individual's experience with LSD. For greater detail, see their book *The Hallucinogens*.[171]

a. *Education.* The level of education plays a decisive role in structuring the LSD experience. Subjects with minimal education have had psychedelic experience, as have scientists, but the quality of the subsequent account is very different.

b. *Reason for taking LSD.* Set and expectations are very important. If a psychedelic experience is desired, attention must be given to all the factors of space, color, sound, and other environmental matters that increase personal comfort.

c. *The subject's experience with hallucinogens.* It has been reported that the first LSD experience is the least typical, even though it may be the most vivid and most dramatic. Thereafter the reaction may be as rewarding or as fearful, but is seldom as memorable or as intense. Familiarity with other mind-altering drugs affect the LSD experience. Osmond and Hoffa have seen more anxiety, fear, tension, and panic in normal subjects than in alcoholics and drug addicts.

d. *Premedication.* Sedatives or tranquilizers may prevent the normal development of the experience and have been used as antidotes for so-called bad LSD "trips," but the talk-down method is recommended for unpleasant experiences.

e. *Circadian rhythm.* The time of day may be very important. Data suggest that fatigue plays a role and that evening sessions seem different from early morning sessions.

4. *Illegal forms of LSD (acid).* In the beginning, LSD—or the hawk, the chief, 25, the big D, the cube, or acid—was taken in the form of sugar cubes. Today, however, the black market LSD manufacturers use special brand names, shapes, and colors to single out their product from others. The following list includes the var-

ious street names and tablets available for the LSD seeker:

White lightning
Yellow dots
Purple wedges
Purple owsleys
Green caps
Yellow caps
Paisley caps
Blue dots
Pink dots
Purple flats
Orange wedges
Blue caps
Brown caps
Blue double domes

LSD is administered in doses ranging from 25 to 700 μg. The effects usually last from six to 18 hours, and up to 48 hours in certain cases.[172]

LSD usually is not injected intravenously but, in a few cases, this method has been employed; illicit users generally take it by mouth.

It is of interest to note the LSD may not be pure and may contain STP, strychnine, or other toxic stimulants, added to boost the effects of LSD. In fact, methamphetamine crystals, or speed, are often mixed with LSD and sold as pure acid. The tachycardia, muscle tremor, anxiety, and other sympathomimetic effects of amphetamine are magnified by the LSD and sometimes lead to a panic reaction.

The price of LSD varies from community to community, and so does the purity. The average price is between $2 and $10 nationwide.

### *h. Illicit Use and Street Cost*

As with the buying of narcotics, the purchase of LSD can be a risky business.[173] It is well established that street forms of LSD may contain little or no LSD up to perhaps as much as 80 percent of the declared amount.[174,175] One situation in which buyers received pharmacologically more than was bargained for occurred on November 11, 1967. In San Francisco, a preparation represented to be LSD and called "pink wedge" resulted in 18 cases of acute toxic psychoses clinically treated within a five-hour period following consumption of the tablets.[175] Advertised as 100 mg of LSD, the pink wedge was found to contain 270 mg and 900 mg DOM (STP). Another serious problem to consider is that when manufacturers are providing impure LSD, especially preparations containing LSD–methamphetamine mixtures, many more panic reactions occur compared with "standard doses" of pure LSD.[171]

Usually "street doses" of LSD range from 50 to 300 mg[174]; doses in excess of 35 mg are effectively hallucinogenic. The numerous forms of street doses of this compound include a powder, a solution, a capsule, and a pill with a distinctive shape or color, and drops of LSD solution have been placed in sugar cubes, animal crackers, and pieces of blotting paper.[176] Furthermore, LSD most commonly is taken by mouth, and only rarely injected subcutaneously or intravenously. LSD has also been mixed with tobacco and smoked, but the "high" obtained by this route is generally unsatisfactory.

It is known that a minority of drug users take LSD at short and regular intervals for sustained periods of time—once daily or once every two or three days. Ludwig and Levine,[176] in discussing patterns of LSD use, suggest that regular LSD users may be characterized as seeking "some personal, esoteric goal," which they disguise in mystical or religious terms. On the other hand, weekend users of the drug seem to seek feelings of greater insight, inspiration, sensory stimulation, and distortions, as well as to overcome apathy and social inhibitions and to facilitate meaningful conversations and interpersonal relationships.[176]

The synthesis of LSD is accomplished by clandestine chemists without much difficulty and the quantity for which a user may pay $10 probably costs no more than 10 cents to manufacture. Those same illicit chemists may also provide to the so-called "acid" salesperson other drugs, including amphetamines, barbiturates, and tetrahydrocannibinol (THC).

With the advent of polydrug abuse, the one true distinction between, for example, the heroin pusher and the seller of hallucinogens appears to be eroding. Although Dr. Timothy

Leary began to experiment with LSD at Harvard in the early 1960s, several large hospitals in Los Angeles have placed the date of the onset of the "LSD era" as September 1965. The reason for this was that their psychiatric emergency services, which previously had been observing patients with adverse reactions at the rate of about six per year in the early 1960s, began to see such patients at a rate of 60 to 100 per year.[178, 179]

In the 1980s, the use of LSD has significantly decreased; however, psychedelic mushrooms have apparently increased.

### *i. Toxicology of LSD*

1. *Acute toxicity*. Rothlin and Cerletti[180] have reviewed the toxicology of LSD. The $LD_{50}$ I.V. for mouse, rat, and rabbit was found to be 46, 16.5, and 0.3 mg/kg respectively. An elephant died after receiving 297 mg of LSD. For an elephant weighing 5000 kg, this would yield a $LD_{50}$ for elephants of about 0.15 mg/kg. It appears that the $LD_{50}$ decreases as the weight per animal species increases, which suggests that toxicity is related more closely to brain weight than it is to body weight. From this, it could be assumed that the $LD_{50}$ for humans is about 0.2 mg/kg, or 14,000 μg per average adult male.[171] According to Hoffa and Osmond,[171] LSD was given daily to young patients for over a year, without evidence of pathologic changes. There have been no reported deaths of humans from LSD, but death due to suicide has been documented.[181] Lucas and Jacques[182] found that LSD caused bleeding when given to anticoagulant-treated rats. The effect of LSD began 30 minutes after it was given, and lasted from four to six days. A dose of 0.1 mg per 200 grams of rat was administered. This is, of course, very much larger than human doses. This work suggests, however, that subjects taking anticoagulants should not be given LSD.

Other toxicologic effects (both acute and chronic) of LSD include emetic activity,[183] enhanced contractions of rat anterior tibial muscles,[184] increased cerebellum blood flow,[185] inhibition of adrenergic motor transmission in rat anococygeus muscles,[186] hypothermia[187] in rodents, decreased urinary excretion of dopamine and serotonin,[188] decreased DNA and RNA levels in cerebral tissues,[189] and in rat liver, kidney, and heart an initial increase followed by a decrease in the activity of glutamate dehydrogenase and glycophosphate dehydrogenase.[189] Other effects are an increase in acetylcholinesterase activity and a decrease in acetylcholine levels,[190] decreased conditioned avoidance response in rats,[191] and a decrease in the threshold of aggressive response in rodents.[192]

2. *Chronic toxicity*

a. *Tolerance*. Human beings and monkeys exhibit tolerance to the behavioral actions of LSD.[172] The pattern of use of LSD is determined, in part, by the dose-dependent tolerance induced. Three to four days are required for its full development or its full loss: Daily dosage leads to dramatically diminished effects unless the dose is increased. Cyclicity in tolerance is seen with higher dosages; for example, tolerance is lost and regained with every eighth or ninth consecutive daily dose. It is uncommon to find anyone who uses the drug more than twice a week, and most users prefer to wait at least four to six weeks before taking it again. The average price of an LSD tablet is between $3 and $5. This means that the individual can be a steady LSD user for a maximum of $10 a week. After a single dose, there is a "psychologic saturation," as McGlothlin[193] calls it. For some people, it may last for days, weeks, or even years.

b. *LSD and organic brain damages*. The fact that LSD ingestion has resulted in an acute brain syndrome characterized by paranoid thinking, panic, dysphoria, or confusion is well documented.[194] Similarly reports of prolonged schizophrenia-like psychosis following the LSD trip or a flashback are well known.[195] What is unknown is whether the prolonged use of LSD can lead to organic brain impairment.

In this regard, McGlothlin et al. examined the long-lasting effects of LSD on normal adults. They demonstrated subtle changes toward a passive and more introspective orientation with a greater appreciation for the esthetic in normal adults exposed to LSD, but found no evidence of enhanced artistic performance.

Recently it was reported that there was no evidence of a generalized psychoneurologic dysfunction attributable to chronic LSD use (at least 50 times). In the study, however, evidence exists that visual–spatial orientation is impaired. In addition, an inverse relationship between general intelligence and number of LSD exposures seems to be present.[196]

c. *Flashbacks*. There is no documented evidence of organic brain damage, but there does appear to be a serious long-term disruption in the personality structure in certain LSD users. The psychotic reaction is similar to an endogenous paranoid schizophrenic reaction.[197]

Another adverse side effect is the recurrence of the acute reaction, days, weeks, and years after the individual took LSD. The LSD acute reaction, commonly referred to as the flashback, has never been documented in the laboratory and was rarely observed in the early days of controlled LSD research.[198] The flashback, as defined by Shick and Smith, is a transient, spontaneous—usually multiple—recurrence of certain aspects of the psychedelic drug effect occurring after a period of relative normalcy following the original intoxication.''

Usually the flashback is transient and, during the intervening period, the individual returns to ''normal'' and is free of any toxic reactions of the drug. According to Shick and Smith, a true flashback reaction includes the patient visualizing geometric patterns (swimming or undulating fields of vision), depersonalization, derealization, and anesthesia or paresthesias (feelings of numbness) that creep or move over the body.[198]

Although a flashback may occur after a single experience with any psychedelic drug, it usually takes place after multiple exposures.[198] Interestingly enough, flashbacks may last from minutes to hours, may occur once a week or a few times a day, but most frequently happen during periods of psychologic stress. Many individuals have reported having flashbacks just before going to sleep, while driving, or while intoxicated with other psychoactive drugs (amphetamines, tranquilizers, marihuana, alcohol).

If the individual stops using psychedelic drugs, the intensity and frequency of the flashback will diminish. In one study, it was found that flashbacks may persist for up to six months, or as long as a year.[199]

Some people do not want the flashbacks to be interrupted, and may enjoy them as free LSD trips.[198] In most cases, therapy is mainly supportive and the patient is reassured that the flashbacks are not the result of brain damage.[198] Shick and Smith believe that the major tranquilizers do not control the recurrences of a flashback, and often may aggravate the anxiety state by producing a ''zombi-like'' depression characteristic of the major tranquilizers. It appears that the talk-down approach effectively decreases the incidence of subsequent debilitating flashback phenomena. The actual incidence of flashbacks in users is not really known. In one survey, approximately 60 percent of the patients reported a flashback occurrence.[199] One of the major problems in assessing the incidence of flashbacks is that the investigator is dependent upon a subjective rather than an objective response, since there is no way of accurately determining the validity of the patient's response.

Currently the mechanism of action of the flashback phenomenon is unknown. Flashbacks are not caused by the persistence of LSD in the CNS.

Flashbacks may be the result of long-lasting changes within the retina or optic pathway of the eyes. According to Shick and Smith,[198] LSD flashbacks represent a novel way of reacting to stress learned while in the LSD state. They also believe that the flashback is probably psychologic rather than chemically induced, and may be related to traumatic events within the LSD intoxication itself.

Shick and Smith, in their analysis of the LSD flashback, state that, in their opinion, the flashback does exist and it should be distinguished from prolonged nonpsychotic and psychotic reactions to LSD or psychedelic drugs in general.

The difference between the so-called bad trip and the flashback is that the bad trip is confined to the time period of the intoxication—for example, eight to 18 hours, and includes acute anxiety and panic states, along with paranoid reactions, whereas flashbacks are characterized by their high rate of recurrence and by a period of normality between the intoxication and the first flashback.

LSD is not the only drug known to induce the flashback. A variety of other psychedelic drugs, such as DOM (STP) and DMT, also have been reported to produce the flashback reaction.[198]

According to Shick and Smith,[198] they try to reassure all parties involved in treatment that the flashback phenomenon is not organic in nature but is psychologic. Drug treatment is limited to minor tranquilizers (Librium, Valium, phenobarbital) since the major tranquilizers (chlorpromazine) make flashbacks worse. Sometimes these clinicians will use a potent, short-acting hypnotic to induce sleep in cases where the flashbacks occur before sleep.

d. *Pregnancy, offspring, and chromosomal effects.* Throughout the years of research with LSD, many harmful physical effects have been suggested, but sound scientific evidence is lacking. The question of chromosomal damage and subsequent birth defects was raised following the positive *in vitro* findings in white blood cells by Cohen.[202] Since then, many papers have appeared in the literature. Chromosome breaks were noted in the peripheral white blood cells of individuals who had taken LSD.[203, 204] From those studies, it appeared that the chromosomal breaks in LSD users seemed to persist, in contrast to the transient chromosomal breaks in acute viral infections. Loughman,[205] however, found no significant difference in the number of chromosomal breaks between LSD users and appropriate controls. Pahnke et al.[206] reported no difference in the rate of chromosomal abberations before and after the administration of LSD to 37 individuals.

Currently there is no satisfactory answer to the question, "Does LSD cause permanent chromosomal damage?" Furthermore there are studies that do not support significant chromosomal effects with LSD usage. Animal studies by Amarose et al.[207] reveal a lack of any association between the acute and chronic administration of LSD to rabbits and pre- and postchromosome complements. The problem with research in this area, especially in humans, is the unsophistication of its approaches. Certainly experiments with humans who have taken LSD must include an investigation of their chromasomes before and after the usage of drugs to be a background parameter.

Human work in this area includes studies by Nielsen and associates,[208] who found more chromatid and isochromatid gaps and hyperdiploid cells in LSD users as compared with controls. Support for LSD-induced chromosonal damage is derived from the tissue culture works of Geiger et al.,[209] Quinn,[210] Gayer and Pribys,[211] and Kato and Jarvik.[212]

Furthermore the question of whether LSD induces birth defects is also waiting for a satisfactory answer. In this regard, Alexander et al.[213] report that LSD given to rats in the first trimester of pregnancy produced birth abnormalities in their offspring. This study was supported by Auerbach and Rugowski[214] in mice and by Geber in hamsters. Zellweger et al.[215] reported that LSD caused a birth abnormality in a woman who took the drug in the first trimester of pregnancy. The validity of such an uncontrolled study must be reconciled, since 2 percent of the population in this country gives birth to deformed offspring. It is interesting to note that aspirin produces birth abnormalities in rats, whereas thalidomide, although a powerful human teratogen, does nothing to the rat fetus.[216]

The radiomimetic properties of LSD were discussed in an article in the *New England Journal of Medicine*,[217] which pointed out that the average LSD user may experience somatic interactions and cell depletion at rates equivalent to a dose of 25 to 40 roentgens per day of chronic whole-body gamma radiation. The work further suggested the possibility that the chromosome breaks may be augmented synergistically without the ingestion of other drugs.

In an issue of *Look Magazine*,[57] David M. Rovik reviewed the recent work of Dr. Kurt Hirschhorn, chief of medical genetics at the Mount Sinai School of Medicine in New York. The article stated that, according to Dr. Hirschhorn, very few things will result in the kind of damage caused by LSD. LSD seems to differ in its effect on chromosomes from most of the drugs claimed by drug-culture folklore to cause chromosome changes, such as aspirin, amphetamine (speed), barbiturates, thorazine, and marihuana. These agents have been checked for chromosome breaks and chromosomal translocations. However, only LSD produced rearrangements of chromosome pieces and, in that sense, mimics radiation in producing long-term chromosomal translocations. The potential danger of these translocations is threefold: (1) for the person taking the drug, there is increased vulnerability to leukemia and other neoplasms;

(2) for an unborn child exposed *in utero*, there is the possibility of congenital malformations; and (3) if these rearrangements occur in the cells that produce the sperm and the eggs, there is danger of producing long-lasting genetic damage that persists into future generations.[218]

Along these lines, Jacobson and Magyar[219] found chromosomal breakage in more than 50 LSD users in the Washington, D.C., area. Other work includes reports by Eller and Morton,[220] Hsu et al.,[221] Sparkes et al.,[222] Lucas and Lehrnbeck and Corey and associates.[224] Negative findings with regard to LSD-induced chromosome breakage have been reported by Judd et al.[225] and Stenchever and Jarvis.[226]

Large populations must be surveyed to measure the actual effects of LSD on fetal deaths and congenital abnormalities and to see whether these effects might be genetically carried.

McGlothlin and coresearchers[227] reported that the frequencies of spontaneous abortions, premature births, and birth defects in 121 human pregnancies were within normal range with a low dose of medically administered LSD.

At the 32nd annual conference of the Committee on Problems of Drug Dependence, Dr. Uyeno[218] presented a paper concerned with the effects of LSD on viability and behavioral development of rat offspring. He reported that the percentages of nonproductive females who received LSD during pregnancy were significantly greater than that in the control group. The results of the behavioral tests, however, showed that the prenatal administration of 2 to 6 mg/kg of LSD-25 on the fourth day of gestation had no significant effect on the behavioral development of the offspring. The following germane conclusions were obtained from an article by Dishotsky et al.[228] concerning LSD and genetic damage.

> From our own work and from a review of the literature, we believe that pure LSD ingested in moderate doses does not damage, and is not a teratogen or a carcinogen in man. Within these bounds, therefore, we suggest that, other than during pregnancy, there is no present contraindication to the continued controlled experimental use of pure LSD.

Detailed reviews with regard to chromosomal and embryonic effects of the hallucinogens and marihuana can be found in a Stash publication,[229] an issue of the *Journal of Psychedelic Drugs*,[230] and in Sankar's book *LSD—A Total Study*.[231]

e. *LSD and violence*. Psychedelic drugs have been implicated as a major factor in such ritualistic killings as the murder of actress Sharon Tate and her guests in Los Angeles in 1969 and the California killings of a doctor and his family by a youth in 1970. Violent reactions have been reported by users of psychedelics such as LSD. A 24-year-old British student tried to "conquer time" by drilling a hole in his skull with a dental drill while under the influence of LSD. Nancy Moore, 24, after using LSD, set herself aflame. LSD ritual murders in Fort Bragg, North Carolina, alarmed and familiarized the general public with the rising trend toward "mystical murders."

On the other hand, Blocker[232] has described long-lasting LSD-induced personality changes with the emergence of an orientation to mysticism, but suggest that nonviolence is a dominant feature.

In discussing the question of whether drugs such as LSD or other psychedelic drugs (marihuana) lead to violence and crime, Dr. R. Blum, then director of the Psychopharmacology Project at Stanford University, had this to say, in a popular magazine[57]: "Let's get one thing straight immediately: drugs don't cause violence: people do. It makes me very angry how we tend to create a demonology around drugs, to say that it was the drug's fault, in the hope that this answer will let us off the hook." According to Dr. Blum, no drug can put murder into a person's heart, but if murder is already there, the drug might help unleash it. Other work by Blum supports this argument.[233]

Finally Smith, in a review of the subject,[234] concludes that: "In those cases where LSD has facilitated religious faith and blind obedience, the drug must be implicated in any subsequent violence. Although, by far, most individuals who become involved with psychedelic chemicals, tend toward non-violence." Caldwell,[235] however, points out that LSD can recall early experiences of sibling rivalry, possibly leading to a desire to murder. Since murder is not socially acceptable, the next best release of this emotion is a fantasized murder. The therapist could use this fantasy to rehabilitate the patient.

f. *Treatment of acute reactions—so-called "bummers."* Severe anxiety is probably the most frequent cause for panic reactions associated with acute LSD use.[194] However, other factors that contribute to an LSD panic reaction include environmental setting, the psychologic makeup of the individual, and unawareness that the drug is being taken. At a party in Austin, Texas, the potato chip dip was laced with LSD without the consumers' knowledge. Before the evening was over, a high percentage of these people "freaked out" because they did not expect any drug effects.

Terror, confusion, dissociation, and fear of going insane and of not coming back to reality are all common features of the acute panic reaction. During such reactions, some people actually feel that they have lost control of their experience and want to flee the situation and be taken out of the state immediately. Some patients believe that other people are staring at or plotting against them (a paranoid reaction). Bad trips can be divided into three categories:

1. Bad body trips (somatic distortions, that is, "my body is purple").
2. Bad environment trips (visual field distortion—pseudohallucinations). These seem real and so intense that the person thinks he or she is going crazy.
3. Bad mind trips (unexpected subconscious material bursts forth into consciousness, such as, "I'm responsible for my mother's death," or "I'm homosexual").

It is not possible to generalize as to the type of experience an individual obtains from LSD use. Sensations experienced by one individual may be perceived as frightening or threatening, whereas another person may perceive them as mystic or beautiful. Long-lasting complications may arise due to the great confusion, paranoid reaction, anxiety, and derealization experienced.

Treatment of the acute LSD reaction should be aimed at providing supportive care in the form of the talk-down method.

At the 1972 New Orleans Pop Festival, one of the medical students who was guarding the trip tent (a medical facility) reported that he spent four hours with a Tulane University football player, talking him down.

The therapist using talk-down methods reassures the patient that the distortions will terminate. But if the individual is in an advanced psychotic state and/or is extremely agitated, Dr. Smith recommends 50 mg I.M. or P.O. of chlorpromazine, which should be repeated every two hours depending on the patient's psychologic state. In the talk-down approach, the patient needs to be able to identify easily with the attendant, who must emphasize that the distorted and frightening feelings are induced by the drug and will disappear when the action of the drug terminates.[110]

The choice of treatment for acute reactions to LSD does not involve chemotherapy. If any drugs at all are used in an attempt to control anxiety, the minor tranquilizers Librium, Valium, or phenobarbital are recommended.[188]

According to Dr. David Smith[195]:

> The most common "bad trip" is the simple anxiety type of panic reaction. The inexperienced user is most susceptible to this reaction. The beginning of changes or perceptions are often frightening because they have little, if any, basis for comparison in everyday reality. A panic reaction, in the more experienced user, can often be credited to the high dosage he/she has taken. Some individuals under LSD show marked changes in cognition or very poor judgment. They may have the feeling that they can really fly, and go out of windows. Some have described a feeling of immortality.

### *j. Special Experimental Effects*

The experimental use of psychedelic drugs (LSD) has been going on since the early 1950s.[236] Busch and Johnson,[237] in their studies, found that patients were able to talk about their problems more easily during delirious states. They believed LSD is a deliriant and so studied its actions on various psychiatric conditions. They concluded that LSD may offer a method for gaining access to the chronically withdrawn, and that it may serve as a new tool for shortening psychotherapy. Since then, LSD has been used as a psychoadjuvant. Three major approaches have evolved: (1) psycholytic therapy, (2) psychedelic chemotherapy, and (3) psychedelic peak therapy. LSD has been used also to treat personality problems, addicts, and alcoholics.

It may induce a patient, under the care of a psychiatrist, to face certain depths in the subconscious mind. In essence, it seems to break down the resistance of the "ego" and to reactivate repressed memories.

Other work in this area has been conducted by numerous investigators, including Katzenelbogen and Fang,[238] Grof,[239] Unger,[240] Eisner and Cohen,[241] Chandler and Hartman,[242] Butterworth,[243] Baker,[244] and Whitaker.[245]

There are some data suggesting that LSD may be beneficial in the treatment of alcoholics. In several research centers, alcoholics given LSD one to three times abstained from alcohol for six to 12 months.[246] Pahnke et al.[206] reported that single high doses of LSD were similarly beneficial to 135 alcoholic patients.

The usefulness of LSD in the treatment of alcoholics has not gained much acceptance by the patients and thus has not become a part of the agenda for the treatment of alcoholism in the United States.

In humans, LSD produced a prolonged period of analgesia.[247] Kast and Collins[101] compared the analgesic property of 100 μg of LSD with 2 mg of dihydromorphinone and 100 mg of meperidine in patients suffering severe pain from terminal carcinoma. During the third hour postdrug, LSD was superior to both dihydromorphinone and meperidine, when their analgesia began to wear off. Meperidine produced 5.7 painfree 20-minute periods; dilaudid 8.4; and LSD 95.6 (32 hours). The authors pointed out, however, that even though many subjects were painfree for many hours, they refused to take LSD a second time.

A very important and still unanswered question is whether LSD or psychedelic drugs in general enhance creativity. Many users claim to obtain greater "insight" under the influence of such drugs, particularly LSD.[248]

In a popular magazine article it was cited that Dr. R. Hartmann,[233] a psychiatrist working at the Max Planck Institute for Psychiatry, enlisted the aid of 34 artists of varying styles. Each received 100 μg of LSD and then tried to create a painting based on an earlier work. Most of the artists found it difficult to concentrate on the task, some gave up completely, several found it difficult to hold their pencils and brushes in a proper way. Nearly all exhibited a decline in skill. In contrast, Dr. S. Krippner, then director of the Dean Laboratory, Maimonides Medical Center, New York, reviewed the effects of hallucinogenic drugs[233] (LSD, mescaline, psilocybin, and marihuana) on originality and artistic expression. The results of a survey of 180 professional artists and musicians were presented, with emphasis on the artists' subjective estimations of the effects of the drug on content, form, and production of the work. Krippner concludes that, though the use of psychoactive agents will have to be circumscribed and limited by society, the most rewarding utilization of these drugs will be by artists. Furthermore he believes that, under proper conditions, and in the hands of imaginative and responsible investigators, LSD may prove useful in enhancing creative functioning and may lead to a better understanding of our human potential.

Fisher and Scheib[249] and Krippner[250] reviewed some of the effects of hallucinogenic drugs on creative performance. Others[251] concluded that the administration of LSD to a relatively unselected group of people is not likely to increase their creative ability.

Sankar,[252] summing up the effects of LSD, points out that the concern over its abuse is completely justified on the basis of its effects on numerous biologic systems. Furthermore it is important to appreciate that basic research on LSD should not be hindered by government restraints because of the potent nature of a chemical that possibly could unravel the neurochemical mechanisms behind several psychophysiologic activities. The lesson to learn is that, if abuse of LSD were not so widespread, our knowledge about the drug would be much advanced.

## 5. Psilocybian Mushrooms (Agaricales)

The term "psilocybian" is used, since not all mushrooms containing psilocybin and/or psilocin belong to the Psilocybe genus.

The *Agaricales*, which contains the most familiar of the fungi—the mushrooms, is credited with 16 families and 197 to 200 genera by one systematist, and by another with seven families, about 275 genera, and 7000 species.

Intoxicating mushrooms—*Amanita, Cono-*

*cybe, Copelandin, Panaelous, Psilocybe*, and *Stropharia*—have classically been included in one broadly defined family, the Agaricaceae.

1. The genus Amanita comprises some 50 to 60 species. The hallucinogenic properties of the fly agaric (*A. muscaria*), a mushroom of the north temperate zone of Eurasia, is well known. Europeans discovered its narcotic use among primitive tribesmen of Siberia in the 18th century.

In the northern Siberian tundra regions, the mushrooms are usually expensive. Thus the tribesmen practice ritualistic drinking of the urine of intoxicated individuals, having learned that the inebriating constituents of the fungus are excreted unaltered or in the form of still active metabolites by the kidneys.[252]

In 1967, Wasson[253] described the intoxicating effects of this mushroom. These vary from person to person. Ingestion of from one to four mushrooms usually results in intoxication, which begins within 15 minutes to an hour. Intoxicating symptoms include twitching, trembling, slight convulsions of the limbs, numbness of the extremities, euphoria, lightness of the feet, a desire to dance, and colored visual hallucinations.

It is believed that *A. muscaria* played a vital magicoreligious role in India, suggesting that it contained the "soma[253]." Schmiedeberg and Koppe[254] discovered muscarine and believed that this compound was the main active principle in *A. muscaria*.

Subsequent investigations by Eugsten[255,256] and others led to the isolation of various amino acid derivatives with characteristic psychotropic activities corresponding to psychic effects induced by the ingestion of this mushroom. The chemicals, identified as ibotenic acid, muscimol, and muscazone, are illustrated in Figure 18-9.

Pharmacologic and experimental psychologic studies with ibotenic acid and muscimol have shown that there is no significant qualitative difference between these two substances. Quantitatively muscimol is at least five times more active than ibotenic acid.

In 1977, Eugsten (in a private communication to R. E. Schultes) reported that muscimol is a strong GABA mimeticum, which passes the blood–brain barrier.

Ibotenic acid and muscimol were detected in human urine within one hour after ingestion, and only 27 percent of the administered amounts were recovered in the urine excreted within the first 48 hours.[257]

According to Matsumoto et al.[258] and Schultes

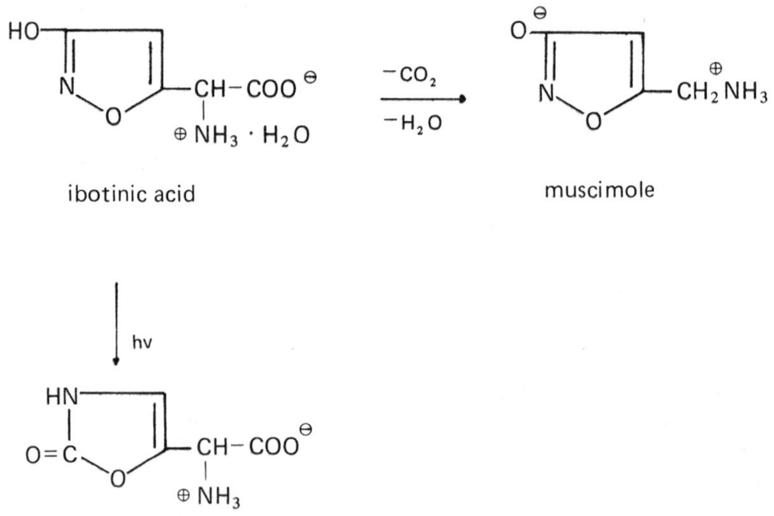

ibotinic acid $\xrightarrow[-H_2O]{-CO_2}$ muscimole

hv

**Figure 18-9. (From Schultes, R. E., and Hofmann. A. *The Botany and Chemistry of Hallucinogens.* Springfield, Ill.: Charles C. Thomas, 1980, p. 50.)**

and Hofmann,[259] two additional constituents of *A. muscaria* have been isolated: (−)-R-5-hydroxy-pyrolidone-(2) and an indolic compound, (−), 1,2,3,4-tetrahydro-1-methyl-β-carboline-carboxylic acid.

The hydropyrolidone possesses narcotic antagonizing activity, whereas the β-carboline compound was implicated as an endogenous human ligand for the benzodiazepine receptor and an inducer of human consumption of alcohol.

2. Among the numerous and diverse genera of fungi found in America, psilocybian mushrooms[260] are highly valued by some individuals for their psychoactive properties. The chemical substance known as psilocybin is one of the naturally occurring hallucinogens found in over 75 species of mushrooms belonging to the genera *Psilocybe, Panacelous*, and *Conocybe*.[261] These mushrooms grow throughout much of the world and at least 15 species can be found in the Pacific Northwest alone. A heightened awareness of psilocybian habitats, combined with indoor cultivation, has dramatically increased the availability of the mushrooms in recent years.[262]

### a. History

Psilocybian mushrooms have a long history of ritualistic use, particularly among the native populations of Mexico. The practice of incorporating a divine mushroom into religious ceremonies has been dated back to 1000 B.C., based on stone artifacts believed to represent mushrooms.[263] The mushroom was revered as a holy sacrament known as *teonanacatl* (''flesh of the gods'') and regarded as a divine key to religious communication.

As the Spanish conquered Mexico, they attempted to abolish the use of psilocybian mushrooms, believing them to be a pagan ritual. But their use continued in secret among the Native American populations. As late as 1915, it was conjectured that ''magic mushrooms'' were actually a myth, and that early Spanish priests had mistaken the peyote cactus for mushrooms.[264]

It was not until 1955 the westerners rediscovered the ancient ritual involved with psilocybian use among the Oaxacan Indians of Mexico. R. Gordon Wasson, a renowned ethnomycologist (one who studies the cultural aspects of mushroom use), experimented with the mushrooms, which were subsequently identified as belonging to the genus *Psilocybe*.[262] A short time later, Albert Hofmann (the discoverer of LSD-25) and his colleagues at Sandoz Laboratories successfully isolated two active principles in the mushrooms, psilocybin and psilocin.[265]

### b. Pharmacology and Physical Effects

Psilocybin (phosphorylated 4-hydroxydimethyltryptamine) is usually the major constituent found in the mushrooms. However, psilocin (4-hydroxydimethyltryptamine) is also often found in small amounts, and appears to possess about 1.4 times the strength of psilocybin. Research shows psilocybin to be relatively unstable and converted to psilocin upon ingestion by the enzyme, alkaline phosphatase. It thus appears that psilocin is actually responsible for the drug effects attributed to psilocybin.[266]

Two additional tryptamine derivatives, baeocystin and norbaeocystin, have been found in at least some of the psilocybian species, most notably *P. baeocystis*. Although they are very similar in chemical structure to psilocybin and psilocin, research is lacking concerning the pharmacology of these substances.[267]

Because of their chemical similarity to serotonin, psilocin and other indole hallucinogens are suspected of mimicking the feedback effect of serotonin on raphe cells. The net effect of their action is to decrease the modulation of sensory input and thereby increase the amount of information going to the higher brain centers, including those responsible for vision and emotion.[268]

One worker in this area has compared the raphe system to a sensory filter, which limits the amount of information entering higher brain centers. The inhibition of this sensory filter would help to explain the ''overwhelming'' sensory experience often reported by users of these drugs.[268]

Despite the similarities between psilocin and LSD, there are also some major differences. In contrast to LSD, which hardly penetrates the brain, psilocin is distributed uniformly throughout the body. Activity in the tissues reaches a peak about half an hour after ingestion, and then decreases gradually. Most of the metabolites are excreted within eight hours, although a small amount may still be present a week later.[270]

Pollock[271] noted that "hallucinogenic substances would reasonably be expected to have multiple sites and mechanisms of action." Though its effect on serotonin appears to be the primary action of psilocin, research has shown other mechanisms to be important as well. Activation of the sympathetic nervous system explains such effects as pupil enlargement, as well as slight increases in body temperatures, pulse rate, and blood pressure.[266]

As with LSD, there are surprisingly few significant physiologic effects from psilocybian use. In addition to the responses mentioned, dryness of mouth and a prominent tendency toward laughter have also been noted. During the initial stages of the experience, individuals often report stomach queasiness, muscular weakness, frequent yawning, and drowsiness.[270]

The toxicity of psilocybin is extremely low in comparison with the effective dose. Large doses have produced only slight increases in respiration and heart efficiency. The $LD_{50}$ (lethal dose for 50 percent of the subjects tested) for mice has been shown to be 280 mg/kg (milligrams of drug per kilogram of body weight).[266] This is more than 200 times the normally effective dose.

The only known human death associated with psilocybian use occurred in Oregon, where a small child died after consuming a large quantity of *P. baeocystis* in combination with other, unidentified mushrooms.[262] It is thought that children may be overly sensitive to the temperature increases induced by psilocybian mushrooms.[272]

Research has not demonstrated physical dependence with psilocybian use, although tolerance to the drug's effects develops rapidly when it is used continuously over a short period of time. In addition, psilocybin displays a cross-tolerance with LSD and mescaline.[266] This means that tolerance to any of these drugs will result in a lessened response to the others. Very limited research has demonstrated no apparent physiologic damage from the use of either psilocybin or psilocin.[268,273]

### *c. Psychologic Effects*

The most notable action of the psilocybian mushrooms is the altered state of consciousness they produce. In addition to complex cognitive changes, most individuals report changes in their auditory, visual, and touch senses. For example, colors appear brighter and there may be visual patterns, especially when the eyes are closed. Sounds are perceived more acutely, and synesthesia, a crossing of the senses ("seeing sounds," for example) may also be experienced.[268]

With the exception of very large doses, these perceptual changes are almost always recognized by the user as being a part of the drug experience. The sensory distortions, therefore, are not true hallucinations as experienced by schizophrenics, but are more accurately termed illusions.[274]

The subjective experience produced by psilocybian mushrooms is largely determined by the individual's mental *set* and the environmental *setting*. The set includes the personality of the user, and his/her expectations, mood, and preparation (such as background reading). The setting involves the user's comfort in the surroundings. Important considerations here include friends, music, type of lighting, and whether the drug is used outside or indoors.[274]

The dangers of psilocybin are primarily psychologic in nature. Anxiety, depression, disorientation, and an inability to distinguish between fantasy and reality may occur. These reactions are most often seen when very large doses are ingested or the drugs are taken in a potentially negative environment (such as at a rock concert). Prolonged psychotic reactions are quite rare, however, and are usually seen in individuals already psychologically disturbed.[267,273,274]

### *d. Treatment*

Treatment of adverse reactions should be symptomatic and supportive. The talk-down technique is most widely preferred, and involves giving personal support through a nonmoralizing, comforting approach. Limiting external stimulation, such as intense light or loud sounds, and having the individual lie down and relax, may also relieve some of the unpleasant effects.[274]

Although tranquilizers are sometimes used, they should be employed only as a last resort (if talking down has failed). In serious cases, minor tranquilizers (such as Valium and Librium) have been used with some success. Gastric lavage (stomach pump) is not required when it is certain that only psilocybian mushrooms have been ingested.[267]

### *e. Special Considerations*

Dosage is an extremely important consideration when dealing with powerful drugs such as LSD or psilocybin. Although the psychologic effects of psilocybin are similar to those of LSD, it is far less potent and has a shorter duration of action. Various researchers have estimated the effective dosage of psilocybin to be from 4 to 10 mg, making it apparently 200 times less potent than LSD.[266,270] At dosages in this range, the experience usually lasts between three and eight hours. The exact dosage is difficult to ascertain since mushrooms may vary greatly in the amount of psilocybin or psilocin they contain. Synthetic psilocybin is virtually nonexistent on the illicit market because of the high cost and complexity of manufacturing it.[270]

It is almost impossible to know exactly how much psilocybin or psilocin is contained in any particular mushroom. There is great variation in potency between the different species of psilocybian mushrooms, as well as significant differences between mushrooms of the same species. For example, the usual oral dose of *P. semilanceta* (liberty caps) may range from ten to 40 mushrooms, while the dose for *P. cyanescens* may be only two to seven mushrooms.[264] Thus the species must be accurately identified even to begin to determine an approximate dosage.

Because of the popularity of psilocybian mushrooms, the numbers of people collecting the fungi have increased dramatically over the past few years. Unfortunately this has led to problems with local property owners who do not appreciate "crazed hippies" trampling their fields and scaring livestock in search of the mind-altering mushrooms. A large number of "shroomers" have been prosecuted for trespassing, both in the Pacific Northwest and the southeastern United States. Users should also be aware that possession of psilocybin or psilocin (classified as a controlled substance under federal legal statutes) makes the individual liable to felony prosecution.[276] Up to this time, however, most individuals have been prosecuted for trespassing only.[277]

Another hazard of mushroom foraging is that of poisoning through mistaken identification. It is estimated that other toxic species outnumber psilocybian species by at least ten to one.[278] Many mushroom hunters do not realize that there are some extremely poisonous species which superficially resemble psilocybian mushrooms.

There has been an increase in the cultivation of certain psilocybian species. The most commonly grown species is *P. cubensis* (also known as *Stropharia cubensis*), which usually grows in the Gulf Coast states and southern Mexico. Spores of *P. cubensis*, complete with growing kits and instructions, are sold openly through magazines and are available in head shops in some states. This new dimension has significantly increased the availability of psilocybian mushrooms to almost anyone.[277,278]

In this regard, the late Dr. Steven Pollock probably possessed the largest collection of psychedelic mushrooms. Certainly the increasing popularity and availability of psilocybian mushrooms pose a difficult legal predicament.

## 6. DMT

N, N-dimethyltryptamine, commonly referred to as DMT, is present in the hallucinogenic drink prepared by some South American Indians from *Mimosa hostilis*, among others. This substance is very closely related chemically to psilocybin and is most often obtained soaked into parsley, which is then smoked in a pipe or as a cigarette. It can also be injected intramuscularly or intravenously, in which case the effects begin within minutes. Although the experience lasts for only half an hour, many who have tried DMT feel that it is the "granddaddy" of the hallucinogens in the power of experience it produces.[280] One needs a milligram of DMT, however, against the microgram needed with LSD. DMT is one of the easiest of hallucinogens for chemists to make in a home laboratory, and is as easy to obtain as LSD on the illicit market in the United States. Bufotenin (5-hydroxy-NN-dimethyltryptamine), another hallucinogen, was first isolated from many toad species.

## 7. Morning Glory

Morning glory seeds contain lysergic acid amide and are approximately one tenth as potent as LSD. Some of the toxic effects of the morning glory are attributable not only to the lysergic acid amide, but also to other ergot alkaloids in the seeds. Consumption of many hundred seeds, several days in a row, may lead to ergotism.[281] After the popularity of morning glory seeds was discovered by the seed companies, an additive was included in the seeds to make them unpalatable.

## 8. Anticholinergic Hallucinogens

Thus far not one of the hallucinogens discussed could trace its history to traditional Western culture. Briggs,[282] in reviewing the literature, indicated that anticholinergic drugs poisoned Hamlet's father as well as the Roman emperor Claudius, and these are the same agents that most likely made Cleopatra bright-eyed, gave witches lift-off power, and put the kick in Vietnam marihuana.

The anticholinergic hallucinogens are generally derived from the potato family and include four genera: (1) Atropa; (2) Hyoscyamus; (3) Mandragora; and (4) Datura.

The three pharmacologically active alkaloids that are responsible for the effects of the Solanaceae plant family are atropine (dl-hyoscyamine), scopolamine (l-hyoscine), and l-hyoscyamine. These agents are all potent central and peripheral cholinergic blocking agents. These substances are classified as parasympathetic system blockers by virtue of their occupancy of the acetylcholine receptor preventing the depolarization action of acetylcholine.

Scopolamine is as much as 100 times as potent as atropine in the central nervous system. In this regard, the l-form of hyoscyamine is up to 50 times as potent as atropine (dl-hyoscyamine) centrally. The structural formulas of atropine and scopolamine are depicted in Figure 18-10.

As cold remedy ingredients, the peripheral actions of these agents are also potent and include inhibition of mucus in the nose and throat, prevention of saliva, hyperthermia, and tachycardia (heart rate may show a 50-beat-per-minute increase with atropine). Infants have been known to reach fever levels of 109 degrees with atropine poisoning. In addition, moderate doses of these chemicals cause considerable dilation of the pupils of the eyes with a resulting inability to focus on nearby objects.

For the most part, these alkaloids are rapidly absorbed from the gastrointestinal tract and from the mucous membranes of the body and are excreted unchanged in the body. Overdoses induce death by paralysis of the respiratory muscles.

The CNS actions include depression of the reticular formation, slowing of the EEG, toxic

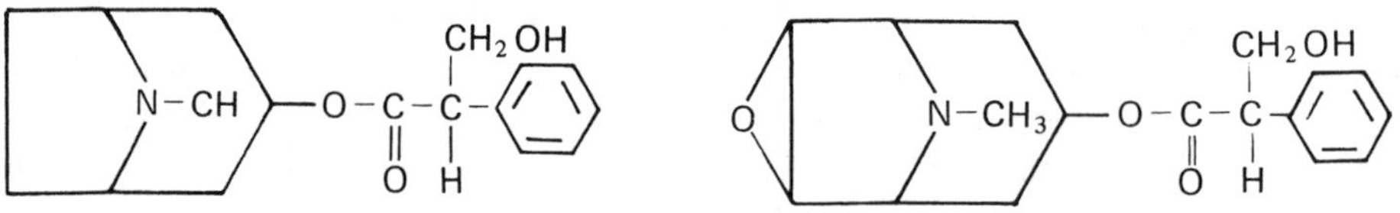

atropine (*dl*-hyoscyamine)
(1αH,5αH-tropan-3α-ol, [±] -tropate [ester])

scopolamine (*l*-hyoscine)
6β,7β-epoxy-1αH,5αH-tropan-3α-ol,
[−]-tropate [ester])

**Figure 18-10. Naturally occurring anticholinergic hallucinogens.**

(From Ray, O., *Drugs, Society and Human Behavior*. 3ed ed. St. Louis: The C.V. Mosby Co., 1983, p. 410. With Permission.)

psychosis, delirium, mental confusion, loss of attention, drowsiness, and loss of memory for recent events. These drugs differ from the indole and catechol hallucinogens and Lewin[12] classified them as hypnotics rather than phantasticants.

### *a. Atropa Belladonna*

In 1831, atropine was isolated from the deadly nightshade, *Atropa belladonna*. Certainly the name of the plant reflects its use as a poison. The word atropine was derived from Atropos, the eldest of the Three Fates in Greek mythology, whose duty it was to cut the thread of life at the appropriate time. There are many historical accounts referring to the use of the deadly nightshade. Roman and Egyptian women utilized belladonna to dilate their eyes and were referred to as "beautiful women." Interestingly, the plant used to kill Romeo—aconite, obtained from the buttercup family—contained atropine, which was an ingredient in a witches' brew reported to induce flying.[281]

It is believed that in some who use atropine, the feeling of levitation may come from the irregular heartbeat in conjunction with drowsiness. Briggs,[282] in his book *Pale Hecate's Team*, points out that some have indicated that changes in heart rate, coupled with falling asleep, sometimes result in a sensation of falling (or flying?).

Belladonna was also considered an aphrodisiac, probably because of its effect in increasing heart rate and causing sexual arousal.

### *b. Mandragora Officinarum*

The problem of drug abuse and the use of psychoactive materials date back to the beginnings of human history. A look at the Old Testament suggests that the tree in the Garden of Eden was actually a vine. Accordingly, the fruit given to Eve by the serpent was not an apple but a grape. This ancient Jewish legend states that, in fact, Eve became intoxicated by the vine of knowledge, and so Adam and Eve were cast out of the Garden of Eden, thus possibly providing future generations, by genetic legacy, with their first predilection for drug and alcohol abuse.

The mandrake plant (*Mandragora officinarum*) contains 0.4 percent of atropine-like alkaloids. It can be traced to the Bible and is associated therein with aphrodisiac properties.[284] Schultes[285] points out that mandrake is toxic but it has been used throughout time as a sedative and hypnotic agent in treating both pain and stress.

### *c. Hyoscyamus Niger*

*Hyoscyamus niger*, also known as henbane, contains the active substances, scopolamine and l-lyoscyamine. This plant material was not as popular as mandrake; however, it was used in the Middle Ages in association with sex orgies. Henbane's popularity in the Middle Ages was not sanctioned by the Church, and, in fact, people that participated in its use were considered witches. Approximately five leaves or more would prove fatal in most humans. Thus, the dose utilized to poison Hamlet's father was probably more than four.

### *d. Datura*

Datura species have a greater worldwide distribution than any of the indole or phenethylamine hallucinogens. These plants contain the alkaloids atropine, scopolamine, and hyoscyamine in differing amounts.

To aid in understanding the cultural exploration of Datura, an article[285] contains a quotation that suggests that the material has had a long use throughout history. "The Chinese valued this drug far back into the ancient times. A comparatively recent Chinese medical text, published in 1590, reported that 'when Buddha preaches a sermon, the heavens bedew the petals of this plant with rain drops.' "

Ray[33] points out that the text of this article suggests the importance of the plant *Datura metal* by associating it with Buddha, much as tea and Daruma were related in legend. Schmiedeberg and Koppe[254] relate tales of the use of Datura by virgins at Delphi, 2500 years before the Chinese text, to enhance their powers of divine possession.

Schultes described Datura as follows: "The real centre of the hallucinogenic use of Datura lies in the New World, where many more species play major roles in magic, medicine and religion in sundry cultures."[285] In this regard, Datura was even part of love potions in India, where the crushed seeds of *Datura metal* were mixed in tobacco and food—a practice that is still common in Asia today.

The common name of Datura is jimsonweed (Jamestown weed) and its properties and use have been recorded in the well-known account, *The History and Present State of Virginia*, first published in 1705 by Robert Beverly.[286]

It is noteworthy that in Southeast Asia it is believed[286] that marihuana is being spiked with Datura.

#### *e. Conclusion*

Belladonna, or deadly nightshade, means "beautiful lady," so named because of the drug's ability to dilate the pupils of the eyes. Belladonna alkaloids include the substances atropine, scopolamine, lyscyamine, and homatropine. Other plants that contain these belladonna alkaloids are jimsonweed and mandrake.

Dryness of mouth and mucous membranes, relaxation of muscles of the bronchial tract, dilated pupils, dryness and flushing of the skin, rapid heartbeat, blurred vision, and hallucinations are all possible side effects of belladonna alkaloids.

The main danger of using belladonna or similar drugs is that the psychologically effective dose is close to the toxic dose. Additionally, these alkaloidal-type compounds produce a general state of confusion and stupor that may lead to amnesia and also aphasia (an inability to speak coherently). Furthermore, belladonna alkaloids may induce a psychotic state in both normal individuals and preschizophrenic patients.

As a cautionary note, other hallucinogens are sometimes spiked with belladonna alkaloids and may make treatment of adverse reactions with chlorpromazine hazardous. It is well known that chlorpromazine potentiates the anticholinergic actions of the belladonna alkaloids. In fact this drug combination may lead to cardiorespiratory failure and coma.

Other known psychotomimetic substances include (1) harmine, (2) ibogaine (tryptaomaine nucleus), (3) piperidyl glycollates (Ditran), (4) kava-kava, and (5) anticholinesternase inhibitors—organo-phosphates (DFP; TEPP).

## 9. Miscellaneous

#### *a. Phencyclidine (PCP)*

Phencyclidine was first abused in oral form over a decade ago; today it is snorted or smoked and has become a serious problem that involves a significant number of users in America.

In the 1950s, PCP was investigated as an anesthetic agent. It was quite effective for both analgesia and anesthesia; however, certain side effects, especially postoperative agitation and delirium lasting for hours, precluded its final acceptance. Until the 1980s, the drug had been marketed as an animal anesthetic.

In the street, PCP is known as angel dust, and appears in many forms: as a crystalline powder, and as tablets and capsules in a variety of colors, shapes, and sizes. Kitchen chemists make this drug plentiful, since it is readily manufactured from available precursors.

1. *The material.* PCP, one of the group of arylcyclohexylamines, in pharmaceutically pure form, is a white powder that is soluble in water. On the street, PCP is commonly used as a substitute for less available psychedelics, such as mescaline. As a powder or liquid, it is often

placed on parsley or on other leaf mixtures to be smoked as cigarettes (joints). In fact, phencyclidine has been sold as psylocybin, LSD, mescaline, marihuana constituents such as cannabinol, amphetamine, and cocaine. A further complication in user identification of PCP is that it sometimes also is used in combination with such other drugs as barbiturates, heroin, cocaine, amphetamine, methaqualone, LSD, mescaline, and procaine.

In addition to the phencyclidine itself, there are over 30 chemically similar analogs, some of which are capable of producing similar psychedelic effects. These also can be synthesized with varying degrees of difficulty, and some have already appeared on the street. Those reportedly abused thus far include PCP, PCE, PHP, TCP, and the anesthetic ketamine. Details of their chemical formulas and structure are given in Figure 18-11. The addition of these compounds, and possibly others in the future, makes the problem of "tracking" PCP and related drug use more difficult.

Among the street names for PCP are angel dust, dust, crystal, cyclones, embalming fluid, elephant or horse tranquilizer, killer weed, superweed, mintweed, mist, monkey dust, peace pill, rocket fuel, goon, surfer, KW, and scuffle.

When PCP is sold as a granular powder (angel dust), it is usually relatively pure, consisting of perhaps 50 to 100 percent phencyclidine. Sold under a variety of other names or in other forms, the purity is from 5 to 30 percent, with leafy mixtures generally containing the smallest amounts of the drug.

Pharmacologic classification is difficult since PCP has stimulant, depressant, hallucinogenic, and pain-killing properties. One proposed classification is, like ketamine, as a "dissociative anesthetic."

Although originally ingested orally, PCP is now most commonly smoked or snorted. Intravenous use is much less frequent, but has been reported. By smoking, the experienced user is better able to limit the dose (self-titrate) to a level with which he/she is comfortable and is probably less likely to overdose. By contrast, when the drug is taken by mouth, there is a longer period before the drug takes effect; it continues to be absorbed after the user may have concluded he/she has had enough and the dose is frequently larger—all factors more likely to result in adverse reactions due to an overdose.

2. *Pharmacologic effects*. The major pharmacologic properties of PCP are summarized in Table 18-9.

Evidence of tolerance development or of a withdrawal syndrome is incomplete. Sympathomimetic effects such as tachycardia, hypertension, and increased deep reflexes are prominent. In addition, cholinergic activity, sweating, flushing, drooling, and pupillary constriction can be observed. Cerebellar signs include dizziness, ataxia, dysarthria, and mystagmus. In this regard, unlike with other hallucinogens, monkeys will self-administer phencyclidine. There is no evidence that PCP produces physical dependence comparable to that of the opiates or other CNS depressants.

Psychologic effects of PCP have been attributed to a defect in the integration of incoming stimuli. These effects have been compared to

## TABLE 18-9

*Central Nervous System effects**

1. Small doses lead to a "drunken" state with numbness of the extremities and, in some species, produce excitation.
2. In moderate doses, analgesia and anesthesia are produced.
3. A psychic state somewhat resembling sensory isolation is produced. Sensory impulses in grossly disoriented form do, however, reach the neocortex.
4. Cataleptiform motor responses occur.
5. Large doses, especially of PCP, may produce convulsions.
6. There are marked interspecies differences in effects. Primates and especially humans show predominantly depressant effects.

*Autonomic and cardiovascular system effects*

1. Sympathomimetic effects are produced, including increases in heart rate and blood pressure.
2. Catecolamines are potentiated through a cocaine-like action.

prolonged sensory deprivation. Acute responses to PCP because of an inability to process sensory information would give rise to secondary deficits, including a loss of reality and testing ability, dissolution of ego boundaries, and intellectual and emotional disorganization.

In humans, high doses can induce coma and major convulsions.[288] Cohen[289] pointed out that PCP-induced death may be from status epilepticus, cardiac or respiratory arrest, or a hypertensive hyperthermia crisis from rupture of a cerebral blood vessel. More than 19 phencycli-

phencyclidine (PCP)
1-(phenylcyclohexyl)
piperidine (CI--395)

cyclohexamine (PCE)
N-ethyl-phenylcyclo-
hexygamine (CI-400)

TCP
1-(1-2-thienylcyclohexyl)
piperidine

PHP
1-(1-phenylcyclohexyl)
pyrrolidine

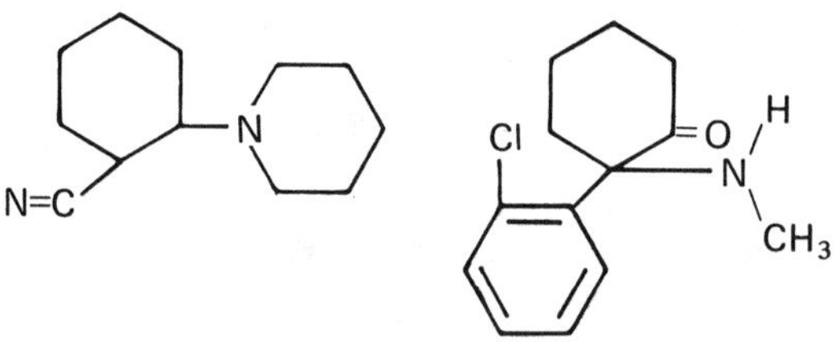


PCC
1-piperidinocyclohexane
carbonitrile

ketamine
2-(o-chlorophenyl)-2-
methylamine
cyclohexanone (CI-581)

**Figure 18-11. (From Domino, F. Neurobiology of phencyclidine. An update. In *PCP (Phencyclidine) Abuse: An Appraisal.* NIDA Research Monograph no. H21. Washington, D.C.: U.S. Department of Health, Education and Welfare.**

(From Domino, F., Neurobiology of Phencyclidine. An Update. In: PCP (Phencyclidine) Abuse: An Appraisal. NIDA Research Monograph No. H21. Washington, D.C. U.S. Department of Health, Education & Welfare.)

dine-related deaths have been reported.[290]

3. *Biotransformation.*[291] Figure 18-12 shows some of the proposed metabolites of phencyclidine. Lin et al.[292] have described some of the metabolites of phencyclidine they found in the urine of intoxicated human patients. Two conjugated hydroxylated compounds were found. These were 1-(1-phenyl-cyclohexyl)-piperidine (4-OH cyclo PCP) and 1-(1-phenyl-cyclohexyl)-4-hydroxylpiperidine (4-OH pip PCP). In addition, a dihydroxylated metabolite tentatively identified as 1-(1-phenyl-4-hydroxy-cyclohexyl)-4-hydroxy piperidine has been found in monkey urine. Wong and Biemann[293] have reported that 1-phenycyclohexylamine is also a metabolite of phencyclidine in humans and mice. These findings of Lin et al. are in partial agreement with those of Oer et al., who reported in 1963 that monkeys mainly excrete the dihydroxy metabolite. In their preliminary report,

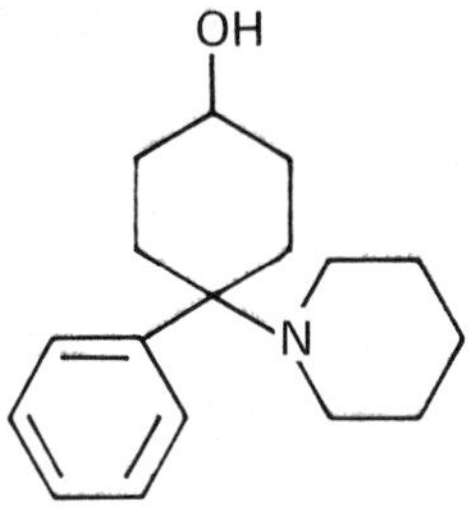

4-OH cyclo PCP

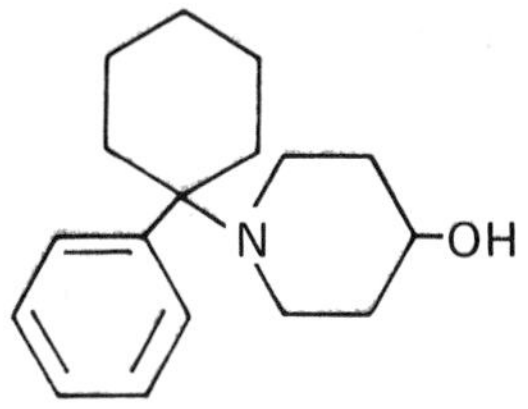

4-OH pip PCP

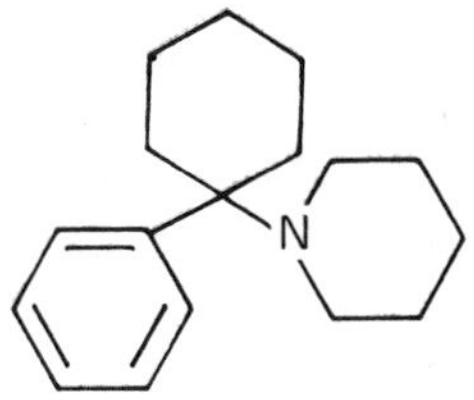

phenylcyclidine

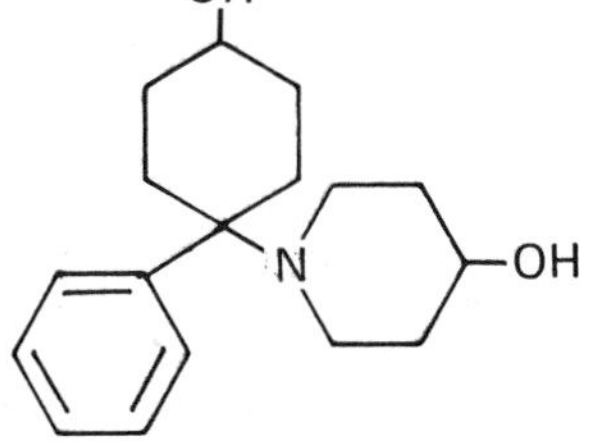

4-diOH cyclo, pip PCP

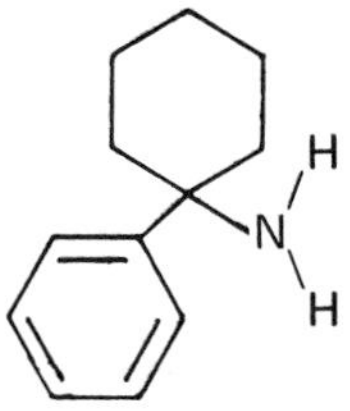

1-phenylcyclo-
hexylamine

**Figure 18-12. Some metabolites of phenecyclidine.**

(From Domino, F., Neurobiology of Phencyclidine. An Update. In: PCP (Phencyclidine) Abuse: An Appraisal. NIDA Research Monograph No. H21. Washington, D.C. U.S. Department of Health, Education & Welfare.)

they stated that the dihydroxy metabolite did not have any phencyclidine activity. Domino[294] reported that both 4-OH cyclo PCP and 4-OH pip PCP have biologic activity in the rat and the dog. One would expect the hydroxylated derivatives of phencyclidine to be more water soluble and to penetrate the blood–brain barrier less. Although these compounds are less potent than phencyclidine, they apparently cross the blood–brain barrier in sufficient amounts, as they have important convulsant components. Hence they may play a role in phencyclidine overdosage in humans. Much more work is obviously needed to determine not only the detailed biotransformation of phencyclidine, but also the pharmacologic properties of its metabolites

4. *Chemical analysis.* Phencyclidine has been analyzed chemically from biologic samples using both qualitative and quantitative techniques. Hawks and Willette[295] reviewed the methods utilized in this analysis. These techniques include thin-layer chromotography, gas chromatography, gas chromatography/mass spectroscopy, radioimmunoassays, and the dipstick.[296–300]

5. *Preclinical animal experimentation*

a. *Neurochemical actions.* The most complete review of the neurochemical effects of PCP has been written by Johnson.[301] Work in this area includes effects on brain serotonin,[302,303] catecholamines,[304–306] acetylcholine,[307–309] and γ-aminobutyric acid (GABA).[310]

Johnson has concluded that it is unlikely that the effects of PCP are caused by an alteration in the function of a single neurotransmitter.

In summary, these studies have only suggested that serotonin (5-HT), dopamine (DA), norepinephrine (NE), acetylcholine (ACH), and γ-aminobutyric acid (GABA) may be involved in the mediation of the behavioral effects produced by PCP.

b. *Behavioral studies.* A review of this subject can be found in the NIDA research monograph 21.[311] Specifically, chapters by Domino[291] and Balster and Chaiet[312] cover work in this area and include self-administration studies,[313] locomotor activities,[314] and drug discrimination experiments.[315]

Although some important research has been accomplished, the most important question, as to why animals and humans take PCP, has not been answered.

6. *Clinical problems*

a. *Acute effects.* Various clinical problems that arise in connection with PCP intake have been reported and can be classified, as illustrated in Table 18-10.

b. *Chronic effects.*

(1) *Symptoms*: After many exposures to PCP, some of the acute states may become chronic. For example, there is recurrent psychotic reactions in abusers; chronic depressive, anxiety, and confusional states also can be identified. In addition, chronic PCP abuse can lead to impairment of mental functioning, presumably of an organic nature (organic brain dysfunction). In fact, during sober intervals, the user demonstrates memory gaps, some disorientation, visual disturbances, and difficulty

**TABLE 18-10**

| *Type of Action* | *Dose (mg)* | *Effect* |
|---|---|---|
| Disinhibition | 1–5 | Euphoria and numbness |
| Toxic psychosis | 5–10 | Excited, confused, intoxicated, impaired communication and disoriented state |
| Schizophreniform psychosis | 10 and more | Symptoms reflecting schizophrenia |
| Stuporous catatonia | 10 and more | Mutism, grimacing, repetitive movements of the extremities, complete withdrawal (to "clam up") |
| Excited catatonia | 10 and more | Psychomotor agitation, incoherent profuse speech, destructiveness, bizarre actions, self-agression |
| Paranoid schizophrenia | 10 and more | Paranoid states, auditory hallucinations, depersonalization, impairment of ego functioning |
| Coma | 1000 | Comatose state and death; lower amounts lead to unresponsiveness to painful stimuli; amnesia, slowing of EEG |
| Other states | Unknown | Anxiety, panic, suicidal ideation, intense sensory blockade |

(From Domino, F., Neurobiology of Phencyclidine. An Update. In: PCP (Phencyclidine) Abuse: An Appraisal. NIDA Research Monograph No. H21. Washington, D.C. U.S. Department of Health, Education & Welfare.)

with speech. These effects may be reversible if PCP exposure does not recur. With chronic abuse of PCP, behavioral toxicity occurs, including outbursts at home and elsewhere, tantrums, aroused assaultiveness, unusual automobile accidents, criminal acts, uncontrolled belligerence, and antisocial behavior.

(2) *Diagnosis*: High dose intake is associated with leukocytosis at elevated CPK. In addition, the patient may present associated symptoms such as hypertension, tachycardia, and the aforementioned psychiatric disturbances. Certainly a direct urine measure of PCP presents a diagnosis, especially when other drugs such as amphetamines and cocaine are being used as well. Some cardinal signs of PCP overdose are ataxia, vertical and horizontal mystagmus, a catatonic staring, and generalized mysthesia. Severe convulsions may also occur with extremely heavy overdoses, leading to coma and death.

Aronow and Done[316] provide a useful summary as illustrated in Tables 18-11, 18-12, and 18-13 on the range of physical and psychologic symptoms likely to be encountered in the emergency room situation.

Psychologically the patient may have the following subjective responses: changes in body image, estrangement, disorganization of thought, feelings of inebriation, drowsiness, and apathy. The patient may show marked negativism and hostility, as well as bizarre behavior. Later the patient may be amnesic for the drug episode.

(3) *Extent of PCP abuse*: The major findings of the National Survey on Drug Abuse reveal that experience with PCP is reported by 3.9 percent of the youths, 14.5 percent of young adults, and 2.2 percent of older adults. Across-time comparisons indicate that lifetime prevalence among the 1979 youth is significantly less (3.9 percent) than the lifetime prevalence reported in the 12–17-year-olds in 1977 (5.8 percent). PCP experience for young adults has not changed significantly since 1977; however, for older adults, there has been a statistically significant increase (1.1 percent in 1977; 2.2 percent in 1979).

(4) *Treatment*: Since there is no specific antagonist for PCP, other treatments are symptomatic. Sometimes a nonstimulating environment may be all that is needed. Tranquilizers such as long intramuscular injections of diazepam will help control muscle spasms and restlessness. Vital signs require frequent recording in case cardiorespiratory intervention becomes necessary. An anticonvulsant such as phenytoin PCP actions. The phenothiazines can be employed for prolonged psychotic conditions. Control of hyperactivity with paraldehyde or parenteral barbiturates can be considered.

(5) *Summary*: The adverse effects of PCP seem to far outweigh its pleasure-inducing properties. Because of its unpredictable nature and uncontrolled belligerence, its use as a drug of

## TABLE 18-11

### Moderately Low Doses

At relatively low doses (of the order of 5 mg in the adult, leading to an estimated serum level of 20–30 ng/ml), the patient is described as likely to show the following symptoms:

**Agitation and excitement**
**Gross incoordination**
**Blank stare appearance**
**Catatonic rigidity**
**Catalepsy**
**Inability to speak**
**Horizontal or vertical nystagmus**
**Loss of response to pinprick**
**Flushing**
**Diaphoresis**
**Hyperacusis**

(From Domino, F., Neurobiology of Phencyclidine. An Update. In: PCP (Phencyclidine) Abuse: An Appraisal. NIDA Research Monograph No. H21. Washington, D.C. U.S. Department of Health, Education & Welfare.)

sodium (Dilantin) can be used as a prophylactic agent against convulsions. For most, antihypertensive therapy is rarely required. In addition, the induced aggressiveness, in some cases, can be controlled with major tranquilizers (phenothiazines); however, they might potentiate

**TABLE 18-12**

**Moderate Doses**

At moderate doses (approximately 5–10 mg, leading in the adult to serum levels of 30–100 ng/ml), the following symptoms are listed:

**Coma or stupor**
**Eyes remain open**
**Pupils in midposition and reactive**
**Nystagums**
**Vomiting**
**Hypersalivation**
**Repetitive motor movements**
**Myoclonus (shivering)**
**Muscle rigidity on stimulation**
**Flushing**
**Diaphoresis**
**Fever**
**Decreased peripheral sensations**
- **Pain**
- **Touch**
- **Position**

(From Domino, F., Neurobiology of Phencyclidine. An Update. In: PCP (Phencyclidine) Abuse: An Appraisal. NIDA Research Monograph No. H21. Washington, D.C. U.S. Department of Health, Education & Welfare.)

**TABLE 18-13**

**Higher Doses**

In still higher doses (over 10 mg, leading in the adult to serum levels of 100 ng/ml and higher), the following is noted:

**Prolonged coma (from 23 hours to many days)**
**Eyes closed**
**Variable pupil size, but reactive**
**Hypertension**
**Opisthotonic posturing**
**Decerebrate positioning**
**Repetitive motor movements**
**Muscular rigidity**
**Convulsions (at doses of 0.5–1 mg/kg)**
**Absent peripheral sensation**
**Decreased or absent gag and corneal reflexes**
**Diaphoresis**
**Hypersalivation**
**Flushing**
**Fever**

(The doses cited are rough guidelines; other investigators suggest that significantly higher doses of PCP are needed to produce each of these clinical pictures.)

(From Domino, F., Neurobiology of Phencyclidine. An Update. In: PCP (Phencyclidine) Abuse: An Appraisal. NIDA Research Monograph No. H21. Washington, D.C. U.S. Department of Health, Education & Welfare.)

abuse is of prime medical and criminal concern. Physicians who see only the undesirable side effects may question why anyone would deliberately consume such dangerous agents. One answer might reside in the knowledge that to some people, PCP use provides a new experience of a so-called "new reality." As Cohen[217] suggests, "The negative aspects of the PCP state could be relished by those seeking out-of-the-ordinary-states."

## E. GENERAL COMMENTS

A careful inspection of all of the available literature on drugs and our culture reveals, at least, that our culture takes drugs. For example, caffeine, nicotine, and alcohol are ubiquitous, but whereas the abuse of both nicotine and caffeine on a chronic basis is harmful, the abuse of alcohol on an acute or chronic basis is by far more common and more deleterious to society.

The desire to alter states of consciousness by either natural or artificial means, although initiated at the dawn of time, is still widespread. The artificial means include drugs such as cannabis, khat, morning glory seeds, mushrooms, weeds of the stramonium type, petroleum distillates, barbiturates, and amphetamines.

The basic rationale may include the use of a drug as a biogenetic substitute or simply for its effect on consciousness. Hollister[318] remarks that, "A number of takers do so as part of a special cult which uses drugs as a tool for religious and mystical exploration."

In light of the fact that psychotomimetic drugs induce many adverse reactions and involve a number of serious mental disorders, as well as physical problems leading to death, society is compelled to decree social controls. In considering such controls, it should always be emphasized that the reaction to these drugs depends not only on their chemical properties and biologic activity, but also on the context in which they are taken, the meaning of the act, and the personality and mood of the individual who takes them. The user of these drugs should be aware of their dangers and their potential to produce psychosis. However, even with mass knowledge of their potential dangers, widespread use of these drugs is creating many new legal problems.

In terms of their therapeutic usefulness, much research is warranted so that ways can be found to minimize or eliminate the hazards and to identify and develop further the constructive potentials of these powerful agents.

The acceptance of these mild-altering chemicals by Western society is a marked departure from our previous attitudes toward agents of this type.

Dr. Daniel X. Freedman, a world authority, had this to say about psychedelic use[319]:

> We should not forge to assess the cost of sustained euphoria or pleasure states; we have to wonder whether the mind of man is built to accommodate an excess, either of pleasure or of over-rationality. We do not know whether or not there are individuals with sufficient strength to take these drugs for growth or pleasure without enhanced and credulous alienation from it. Is a stable person really under sufficient control of his motives, let alone the dosage, to take these drugs as a civil right for whatever personal reasons he wishes? If so, who has to care for the consequences of his misjudgments?

The primary question to be answered is: Why do people, especially educated young people, "turn on" to psychedelic drugs to enter a new world filled with hope, optimism, and the feeling that people belong to each other and that love conquers all? The motives for the "phantasticants" are varied and include the following:

1. A "need to feel"—insight into oneself.
2. Clique activity—a "need to belong."
3. A need to be one up—to have "been there."
4. It is a challenge.
5. Others feel that they should confront themselves with an experience advertised to be so important.
6. Test of fitness.
7. Cult or religious reasons.
8. Fashionability—drug mystique.

Whatever the reasons for its use, LSD and other psychedelic drugs have found their place in the inevitable "greening of America" and their extensive use[286] has become part of that "future shock."[287]

A 1970 article in the *Minnesota Law Review*[320] discussed the research done with LSD. The author concluded that a solution to the problem of LSD use "is to be found, no doubt, where the answers to so many other social problems lie—in a general improvement of the quality of American society. If some such improvement came to pass, then either the need which LSD fills would disappear or its usage would become simply one very minor aspect of social life."

## REFERENCES


1. Dobkin, DeRios, M. The wilderness of minds: Sacred plants in cross-cultural perspective. *Sage Research Papers in the Social Sciences* 5. London: Sage Publications, 1976, p. 7.
2. Delay, J. Psychopharmacology and psychiatry: Towards a classification of psychotropic drugs. *Bul. Narcot.* 19:(1):1, 1967.
3. Ludwig, A. Altered states of consciousness. In C. T. Tart, ed., *Altered States of Consciousness.* New York: Wiley, 1969, p. 9.
4. Barron, F., Jarvik, M. E., and Bunnell, S., Jr. The hallucinogenic drugs. *Sci. Am.* 210:29, 1964.
5. LaBarre, W. Hallucinogens and the shamanic origins of religion. In P. T. Furst, ed., *Flesh of the Gods.* New York: Prager, 1972, pp. 261–278.
6. Wasson, R. G. The "divine" mushroom: Primitive religion and hallucinatory agents. *Proc. Am. Phil. Soc.* 102:221, 1958.
7. Dewsbery, J. P. Schizophrenia and the psychotomimetic drugs. *Endeavour* 19:20, 1960.
8. Osmond, H. A review of the clinical effects of psychotomimetic agents. *Ann. N.Y. Acad. Sci.* 66:418, 1957.
9. McGlothlin, W. H., and Arnold, D. O. LSD revisited: A 10-year followup of medical LSD use. *Arch. Gen. Psychiatry* 24:35, 1971.
10. Freedman, D. X. In D. H. Efron, B. Holmstedt, and N. S. Kline, eds., *Perspectives on the Use and Abuse of Psychedelic Drugs: Ethnopharmacologic Search for Psychoactive Drugs.* Washington, D.C.: U.S. Department Health, Education and Welfare, 1967, pp. 77–102.
11. Hornes, C. H. W., and McCluskie, J. A. W. *The Food of the Gods.* 1963.
12. Lewin, L. *Phantastica—Narcotic and Stimulating Drugs—Their Use and Abuse.* London: Paul, Trench, Trubner, 1964.
13. Schultes, R. E. Hallucinogenic plants of the New World. *Harvard Rev.* 1:18, 1963.
14. LaBarre, W. Old and new world narcotics: A statistical question and an ethnological reply. *Botany* 24:77, 1970.
15. Smith, D. E. Symposium: Psychedelic drugs and religion. *J. Psychedel. Drugs* 1:45, 1968.
16. Downing, D. F. The chemistry of the psychotomimetic substances. *Q. Rev.* 16:133, 1962.
17. Louria, D. *Nightmare Drugs.* New York: Pocket Books, 1966.
18. Huxley, A. Presentation to the New York Academy of Sciences, 1967.
19. Baba, M. L.S.D. and the highroads. *J. Psychedel. Drugs* 1:38, 1968.
20. LaBarre, W. The narcotic complex of the New World. *Diogenes* 48:125, 1964.
21. Von Bibra, E.F. Die narkotischen genussmittel und der mensch. Nürnberg: W. Schmid, 1855.
22. Johnston, J. F. *The Chemistry of Common Life.* New York: Appleton, 1855.
23. Cooke, M. C. *The Seven Sisters of Sleep.* London: Blackwood, 1860.
24. Kraepelin, E. Ueber die Beeinflussung einfacher psychischer Vorgänge durch einige Arzneimittel. Jena: Verlag von Gustav Fischer, 1892.
25. Hartwich, C. Die menschlichen Genussmittel. Leipzig: Chr. Herm. Tauchnitz, 1911.
26. Safford, W. E. An Aztec narcotic. *J. Heied.* 6:291, 1915.
27. Reko, B. P. Des los nombres botanicos aztecos. *El. Mex. Anat.* 1:136, 1919.
28. Beringer, K. *Der Meslcalinnausch.* Berlin: Springer-Verlag, 1927. Reprinted, New York: Springer-Verlag, 1969.
29. Lewin, L. Unterschunger über Banisteria caapi spr. (ein südanerikanisches Ranschmittel). *Arch. Exp. Path. Pharmakol* 129:133, 1928.
30. Diaz, J. L. Ethnopharmacology of sacred psychoactive plants used by the Indians of Mexico. *Ann. Rev. Pharmacol. Toxicol.* 17:647, 1977.
31. Klüver, H. Foreword. In R. E. Schultes and A. Hofmann, eds., *The Botany and Chemistry of Hallucinogens.* Springfield, Ill.: Charles C. Thomas, 1980, p. vii.
32. Hollister, L. E. *Chemical Psychoses: LSD and Related Drugs.* Springfield, Ill.: Charles C Thomas, 1968, p. 4.
33. Ray, O. S. The phantasticants. In *Drugs, Society and Human Behavior.* St. Louis: C. V. Mosby, 1972, p. 312.
34. Lipton, M. A. The relevance of chemically-

induced psychoses to schizophrenia. In D. H. Efron, ed., *Psychotomimetic Drugs*. New York: Raven Press, 1970, p. 236.
35. LaBarre, W. *The Peyote Cult*. Yale University publication no. 13. New Haven, Conn.: Yale University Press, 1938.
36. Bravo, H. H. Una revision del genero lophophora. *Cact. Succ. Mex*. 1967.
37. Rouhier, A. *La Plante Qui Faitles Yeux Emerveilles—le Peyoti*. Paris: Laton Doinet Cie, 1927.
38. Sahagun, B. *Historia General de las Cosas de la Nueva Espana*, vol. 3. Mexico: Editorial Pedro Robledo, 1938.
39. Hernandez, F. *Nova Plantrum, Animalium et Mineralium Mexicanorum Historia*. B. Deuersin and Z. Masohi, eds. Rowe, 1651.
40. Slotkin, J. S. *The Peyote Religion*. Glenroe, Ill: Free Press, 1963.
41. Schultes, R. E., and Hofmann, A. Plants of hallucinogenic use. In *The Botany and Chemistry of Hallucinogens*. Springfield, Ill.: Charles C. Thomas, 1980, p. 699.
42. Schultes, R. E. Teonanacatyl, the narcotic mushroom of the Aztecs. *Am. Anthropolog*. 42:429, 1940.
43. Kluver, H. *Mescal; the "Divine" Plant and Its Psychological Effects*. London: Paul, Trench, Trubner, 1928.
44. Heffter, A. *Ber Deut. Chem. Ges*. 38:3634, 1906.
45. Spath, E. *Monatsch. Chem*. 40:129, 1919.
46. Banholzer, K., Campbell, T. W., and Schmid, H. Synthesis of mescaline, N-methyl and N,N-dimethylmescaline. *Helv. Chim. Acta* 35:1577, 1952.
47. Dornow, A., and Petsch, G. Synthesis of 2-hydroxy-2(3,4,5-trimethoxyphenyl) ethylamine (hydroxymescaline), bis[2-(3,4,5-trimethoxyphenyl)-ethyl]amine (dimescaline) and 2-(3,4,5-trimethoxyphenyl)-ethylamine (Mescaline). *Arch. Pharm*. 284:160, 1951.
48. Tsao, M. T. A new synthesis of mescaline. *J. Am. Chem. Soc*. 73:5495, 1951.
49. Fischer, O. Ueber Hormin und Hormalin II. *Bevicht*. 22:637, 1889.
50. Bruhn, J. B., and Holmstedt, B. Early peyote research: An interdisciplinary study. *Elon. Bot*. 28:353, 1974.
51. Morselli, G. E. *J. Psychol*. 33:368, 1936.
52. Alles, C. A. In H. A. Abramson, ed., *Neuropharmacology*. New York: Josiah Macy, Jr., Foundation, 1952.
53. Snyder, S. H., Faillace, L., and Hollister, L. 2,5-dimethoxy-4-methyl-amphetamine (STP): A new hallucinogenic drug. *Science* 158:669, 1967.
54. Smith, D., and Meyers, F. The psychomimetic amphetamine with special reference to STP (DOM) toxicity. In D. Smith, ed., *Drug Abuse Papers*, section 4. Berkeley: University of California Press, 1969, p. 4.
55. Shulgin, A. T., Sargent, F., and Naranjo, C. The chemistry and psychopharmacology of nutmeg and of several related phenylisopropylamines. In D. H. Efron, B. Holmstedt, and N. S. Kline, eds., *Ethnopharmalogic Search for Psychoactive Drugs* (Public Health Service Publication #1645). Washington, D.C.: U.S. Government Printing Office, 1967, pp. 202–214.
56. Griffith, R. W., et al. Toxicological considerations. In B. Berde, and H. D. Schild, eds., *Ergot Alkaloids and Related Compounds*. New York: Springer-Verlag, 1978, p. 805.
57. Rorvik, D. M. Do drugs lead to violence? *Look Mag*. 58, Apr. 7, 1970.
58. Huxley, A. *The Doors of Perception*. London: Chotto & Windens, 1954. Reprinted: Redwood Press, 1972.
59. Schultes, R. E., and Hofmann, A. Hallucinogenic or psychotomimetic agents. In *The Botany and Chemistry of Hallucinogens*. Springfield, Ill.: Charles C Thomas, 1980, p. 25.
60. Hofmann, A. Psychotomimetic agents. In A. Burgen, ed., *Chemical Constitution and Pharmacodynamic Action*, 2nd ed. New York: Marcel Dekker, 1968, p. 169.
61. Carroll, L. *Alice in Wonderland*.
62. Smith, J. P., Personal Communication, 1967.
63. McDonagh, D., Personal Communication, 1968.
64. Smith, D. E., Personal Communication, 1967.
65. Sankar, D. V. S. Introduction—Early history of LSD. In *LSD—A Total Study*. Westbury, N.Y.: PJD Publications, 1975, p. 43.
66. Jarvik, M. E. Drugs used in the treatment of psychiatric disorders. In L. S. Goodman and A. Gilman, eds., *The Pharmacological Basis of Therapeutics*, 3rd ed. New York: Macmillan, 1965, pp. 205–207.
67. Brady, L. F. *Lloydien* 25(1), 1962.
68. Stoll, A. *Schwzic Apoth*. 60:341, 1922.
69. Jacobs, W. A., and Craig, L. C. The ergot alkaloids. II. The degraduation of ergotinine with alkali. Lysergic acid. *J. Biol. Chem*. 104:547, 1934.
70. Stoll, A., and Hofmann, A. Ergot alkaloids. III. Partial synthesis of ergobasine, a natural ergot alkaloid and its optical antipodes. *Z. Physiol. Chem*. 251:155, 1938.

71. Woolley, D. W. Manipulation of cerebral serotonin and its relationship to mental disorders. *Science* 125:752, 1957.
72. Boakes, R. J., et al. Effects of lysergic acid derivatives on 5-hydroxytryptamine excitation of brain stem neurones. *Br. J. Pharmacol.* 38:454, 1970.
73. Huxley, A. *Heaven and Hell*. London: Chatto & Winders, 1956. Reprinted: 1972.
74. Fact Sheets, Drug Enforcement Administration, U.S. Department of Justice, 1973, p. 45.
75. Dimijian, G. G. Contemporary drug abuse. In A. Goth, ed., *Medical Pharmacology*, 7th ed. St. Louis: C. V. Mosby, 1975, p. 314.
76. Freter, K., Axelrod, J., and Witkop, A. *J. Am. Chem. Soc.* 70:3191, 1957.
77. Larbrecht, W. L. Synthesis of amides of lysergic acid. *J. Organic Chem.* 24:368, 1959.
78. Stutz, P., and Stadler, P. A. Synthesis of 2-methyl-lysergic acid. Friedel-Craft method. 74. Ergot alkaloids. *Helv. Chim. Acta* 55:75, 1972.
79. Nakahara, Y., and Niwaguchi, T. *Chem. Pharmacol. Bull.* 11:2337, 1971.
80. Gettner, H. H., Rolo, A., and Abramson, H. A. Lysergic acid diethylamide (LSD25). 36. Comparison of effect of methysergide (UML 491) on gold fish and Siamese fighting fish. *J. Psychol.* 61:87, 1965.
81. Arcomone, F., et al. Studies concerning lysergic acid and dihydrolysergic acid alpha-hydroxyethylamides. *Tetrahedron* 23:11, 1967.
82. Blaha, K. Chloroptical properties of unsaturated derivatives of lysergic acid. *Col. Chezch. Chem. Commun.* 37:2473, 1972.
83. Inoue, T., Nakahara, Y., and Niwaguchi, T. Studies on lysergic acid diethylamine and related compounds. 2. Mass spectra of lysergic acid derivatives. *Chem. Pharmacol. Bull.* 20:409, 1972.
84. Aboutchoa, C. T., and Floss, H. G. Biosynthesis of ergot alkaloids—Incorporation of (5R) into chano clavines and tetracyclin ergolines. *Lloydia* 35:471, 1972.
85. Hofmann, F. G. *A Handbook on Drug and Alcohol Abuse: The Biomedical Aspects*. New York: Oxford University Press, 1975, p. 149.
86. Sankar, P. V. S. *LSD—A Total Study*. New York: PJD Publications, 1975, p. 255.
87. Aghanjanian, G. K., and Bing, D. H. L. Persistence of lysergic acid diethylamide in the plasma of human subjects. *Clin. Pharmacol. Ther.* 5:611, 1964.
88. Kalbhen, D. A., and Sargent, T. W. *Med. Eyptl.* 8:200, 1963.
89. Snyder, S. H., and Reivich, M. Regional localization of lysergic acid diethylamide in monkey brain. *Nature* 209:1093, 1966.
90. Diab, I. M., Freedman, D. X., and Roth, L. J. (3H) lysergic acid diethylamide: Cellular autoradiographic localization in rat brain. *Science* 173:1022, 1971.
91. Wright, E. M. Active transport of lysergic acid diethylamide. *Nature* 240:53, 1972.
92. Freedman, D. X., and Coquet, C. A. Regional and subcellular distribution of LSD and effects on 5-H-T levels. *Pharmacologist* 7:183, 1965.
93. Faragalla, F. F. The subcellular distribution of lysergic acid diethylamide in the rat brain. *Experientia* 28:1426, 1972.
94. Farrow, J. T., and Van Vunakis, H. Binding of D-lysergic acid diethylamide to subcellular fractions from rat brain. *Nature* 237:164, 1972.
95. Sankar, D. V. S. In *LSD—A Total Study*. Westbury, N.Y.: PJD Publications, 1975, p. 95.
96. Pfeiffer, C. C., and Murphee, H. B. Introduction to psychotropic drugs and hallucinogenic drugs. In J. D. DiPalma, ed., *Pharmacology in Medicine*, 3rd ed. New York: McGraw-Hill, 1965, p. 321.
97. Rothlin, E. Pharmacology of lysergic acid diethylamide and some of its related compounds. *J. Pharm. Pharmacol.* 9:569, 1957.
98. Rothlin, E.
99. Rothlin, E. In S. Garaltini and V. Ghetti, eds., *Psychotropic Drugs*. Amsterdam: Elsevier, 1957, p. 36.
100. Rinkel, M., Hyde, R. W., and Solomon, H. C. Experimental psychiatry IV: Hallucinogens: Tools in experimental psychiatry. *Dis. Nerv. Syst.* 16:229, 1955.
101. Kast, E. L., and Collins, V. S. A study of lysergic acid diethylamide as an analgesic agent. *Anaesth. Analg. Curr. Res.* 43:285, 1964.
102. Smith, D. E., and Rose, A. J. LSD: Its use, abuse and suggested treatment. (Observations by the Haight-Ashbury Medical Clinic). *J. Psychedel. Drugs* 1:117, 1968.
103. Fanchamps, A. Some compounds with hallucinogenic activity. In B. Berde, and H. D. Schild, eds., *Ergot Alkaloids and Related Compounds*. New York: Springer-Verlag, 1978, p. 567.
104. Louria, D. *Nightmare Drugs*. New York: Pocket Books in association with *This Week Magazine*, 1966, p. 46.
105. Henslin, J. M. Presented at 32nd Annual Conference of the Committee of Problems of Drug Dependence, Division of Medical Sciences,

National Academy of Science, Washington, D.C., 1970.

106. *High Times Encyclopedia of Recreational Drugs*. New York: Steve Lull, p. 179.
107. Cohen, S., and Ditman, K. S. Complications associated with lysergic acid diethylamide (LSD-25). *JAMA* 181:161, 1962.
108. Cohen, S., and Ditman, K. S. Prolonged adverse reactions to lysergic acid diethylamide. *Arch. Gen. Psychiatry* 8:475, 1963.
109. Frosch, W., Robbins, E. S., and Stern, M. Untoward reactions to lysergic acid diethylamide (LSD) resulting in hospitalization. *N. Engl. J. Med.* 273:1235, 1965.
110. Taylor, R. L., et al. Management of "bad trips" in an evolving drug scene. *JAMA* 213:422, 1970.
111. Brengelmann, J. C. Effects of LSD-25 on tests of personality. *J. Ment. Sci.* 104:1226, 1958.
112. Eisner, B. G. In P. Bradley, ed., *Neuropsychopharmacology*. Amsterdam: Elsevier, 1959, p. 438.
113. Mirsky, A. F., and Kornetsky, V. C. On the dissimilar effects of drugs on the digit symbol substitution and continuous performance. *Psychopharmacologia* 5:161, 1964.
114. Kabes, J., Fink, Z., and Roth, Z. A new device for measuring spontaneous motor activity—effects of lysergic acid diethylamide in rats. *Psychopharmacologia* 23:75, 1972.
115. Cohen, M., and Wakeley, H. A comparative behavioral study of ditran and LSD in mice, rats, and dogs. *Arch. Int. Pharmacodyn, Ther.* 173:316, 1968.
116. Dahdiya, P. C., et al. Effects of LSD on open field performance in rats. *Psychopharmacologia* 15:333, 1969.
117. Black, P., et al. In P. Black, ed., *Drugs and the Brain; Papers on the Action, Use, and Abuse of Psychotropic Agents*. Baltimore: Johns Hopkins Press, 1969, p. 291.
118. Uyeno, E. T., and Mitoma, C. The relative effectiveness of several hallucinogens in disrupting maze performance by rats. *Psychopharmacologia* 16:73, 1969.
119. Miller, R. C., and Miller, E. K. Lack of long-term effect of LSD on Y-maze learning in mice. *Nature (London)* 228:1107, 1970.
120. Swonger, A. K., and Rech, R. H. Serotonergic and cholinergic involvement in habituation of activity and spontaneous alternation of rats in a Y-maze. *J. Comp. Physiol. Psychol.* 81:509, 1972.
121. Schechter, M. D., and Rosecrans, J. A. Lysergic acid diethylamide (LSD) as a discriminative cue—Drugs with similar stimulus properties. *Psychopharmacologia* 26:313, 1972.
122. Uyeno, E. T. Lysergic acid diethylamide, chlorpromazine and maze performance. *Arch. Int. Pharmacodyn. Ther.* 184:389, 1970.
123. Olds, J. In P. Bradley, ed., *Neuropsychopharmacology*. Amsterdam: Elsevier-North Holland, 1959.
124. Domino, E. F., Caldwell, D. F., and Henke, R. Effects of psychoactive agents on acquisition of conditioned pole jumping in rats. *Psychopharmacologia* 8:285, 1965.
125. Pawlowski, A. A. Effects of lysergic acid diethylamide on the modification of a learned jumping response. *J. Neuropsychiatry* 4:81, 1963.
126. Barry, H., III, Wagner, S. A., and Miller, N. E. *Psychol. Rep.* 12:215, 1963.
127. Jarrard, L. E. Effects of D-lysergic acid diethylamide on operant behavior in the rat. *Psychopharmacologia (Berlin)* 5:39, 1963.
128. Caldwell, D. F., and Domino, E. F. Effect of LSD-25 in the rat on operant approach to a visual or auditory conditioned stimulus. *Psychol. Rep.* 20:199, 1967.
129. Sparber, S. B., and Tilson, H. A. Similarities and differences between mescaline, lysergic acid, diethylamide-25 (LSD) and D-amphetamine on various components of fixed interval responding in the rat. *J. Pharmacol. Exp. Ther.* 184:376, 1973.
130. Appel, J. B., and Freedman, D. X. The relative potencies of psychotomimetic drugs. *Life Sci.* 4:2181, 1965.
131. Miller, L. I., Drew, W. G., and Wikler, A. *Psychopharmacologia* 28:1, 1973.
132. Roberts, H. M. T., and Bradley, P. B. *Physiol. Behav.* 2:389, 1967.
133. Sharpe, L. G., Otis, L. S., and Schusterman, R. J. *Psychonomic. Sci.* 7:103, 1967.
134. Kostowski, W., and Tarchalska, B. The effects of some drugs affecting brain 5-HT on the aggressive behavior and spontaneous electrical activity of the central nervous system of the ant. *Rufa. Brain Res.* 38:143, 1972.
135. Horovitz, Z. P., et al. Behavioral and electroencephalographic effects of LSD. *J. Pharmacol. Sci.* 54:108, 1965.
136. Siegel, R. K., and Poole, J. *J. Psychol. Rep.* 25:704, 1969.
137. Bignani, C. *Psychopharmalogia* 10:44, 1966.
138. Herz, S. Behavioral patterns in sex and drug use on three campuses: Implications for education and society. *Psychiatr. Q. Suppl.* 42:258, 1968.

139. Alpert, R. *J. Sex Res.* 1:50, 1969.
140. Uyeno, E. T. Effects of lysergic acid diethylamide on the meternal behavior of the rat. *J. Psychol.* 75:271, 1970.
141. Rosen, E., and Iovino, A. Effect of lysergic acid diethylamide on the nesting behaviour of male pigeons. *Nature* 197:614, 1963.
142. DeShon, H. J., Rinkel, M., and Solomon, H. C. *Psychiat. Q.* 26:33, 1952.
143. Alexander, G. J., Gray, R., and Machizi, S. *Fed. Proc.* 31, 1972.
144. Paul, I. H. The effect of a drug-induced alteration in state of consciousness on retention of drive-related verbal material. *J. Nerv. Ment. Dis.* 138:367, 1964.
145. Jarvik, M. E., et al. *J. Physiol.* 39:465, 1955.
146. McGlothlin, W. H., Cohen, S., and McGlothlin, M. S. Short-term effects of LSD on anxiety, attitudes and performance. *J. Nerv. Ment. Dis.* 139:266, 1964.
147. Levine, A., et al. Lysergic acid diethylamide (LSD-25): XVI. The effect on intellectual functioning as measured by the Wechsler-Bellevue intelligence scale. *J. Psychol.* 40:385, 1955.
148. Silverstein, A. B., and Klee, G. D. Effects of lysergic acid diethylamide (LSD-25) on intellectual functions. *Arch. Neurol. Psychiatry* 80:477, 1958.
149. Liewert, G. A. In P. Bradley, ed., *Neuropsychopharmacology*. Amsterdam: Elsevier, 1959, p. 461.
150. Goldberger, L. Cognitive test performance under LSD-25, placebo and isolation. *J. Nerv. Ment. Dis.* 142:4, 1966.
151. Boyadzhieva, M., and Mumdzhieva, D. *Neurol. Psikhiatr. I Neurokhirurgiya (Sofia)* 8:63, 1969.
152. Wright, M., and Hogan, T. P. Repeated LSD ingestion and performance on neuropsychological tests. *J. Nerv. Ment. Dis.* 154:432, 1972.
153. Langs, R. J. Stability of earliest memories under LSD-25 and placebo. *J. Nerv. Ment. Dis.* 144:171, 1967.
154. Goldstein, L. The effect of LSD and other hallucinogens on the electrical activity of brain during wakefulness and sleep. In D. V. S. Sankar, ed., *LSD—A Total Study*. Westbury, N.Y.: PJD Publications, 1975, p. 395.
155. Brawley, P., and Duffield, J. C. The pharmacology of hallucinogens. *Pharmacol. Rev.* 24:31, 1972.
156. Isbell, H., et al. Cross-tolerance between LSD and psilocybin. *Psychopharmacologia* 2:147, 1961.
157. Foldes, V., et al. Histochemical demonstration of the inhibitory effect on d-lysergic acid diethylamide (LSD) and its congeners on brain cholinestermses. *Fed. Proc.* 18:381, 1959.
158. Aghanjanian, G. K. LSD and CNS transmission. *Ann. Rev. Pharmacol.* 12:157, 1972.
159. Sankar, D. V. Biochemical effects of LSD. In *LSD—A Total Study*. Westbury, N.Y.: PJD Publications, 1975, p. 802.
160. Halavis, A. E., et al. The raphe neuronal system and serotonergic effects of LSD. *Neuropharmacology* 21:811, 1982.
161. Freedman, D. X. Effects of LSD-25 on brain serotonin. *J. Pharmacol. Exp. Ther.* 134:160, 1961.
162. Halaris, A. E., and Freedman, D. X. Vesicular and juxtravesicular serotonin: Effects of lysergic acid diethylamide and reserpine. *J. Pharmacol. Exp. Ther.* 203:575, 1977.
163. Lovell, R. A., and Freedman, D. X. Stereospecific receptor sites for d-lysergic acid diethylamide in rat brain: Effect of neurotransmitters amine antagonist and other psychotropic drugs. *Molec. Pharmacol.* 12:620, 1976.
164. Bennett, J. P., Jr., and Snyder, S. H. Serotonin and lysergic acid diethylamide binding in rat brain membranes: Relationship to postsynaptic serotonin receptors. *Molec. Pharmacol.* 12:373, 1976.
165. Fillion, G. M. B., et al. High-affinity binding of 5-hydroxytryptamine to brain synaptosomal membranes: Comparison with (3H) lysergic acid diethylamide binding. *Molec. Pharmacol.* 14:50, 1978.
166. Freedman, D. X., and Halaris, A. E. Monoamines and the biochemical mode of action of LSD at synapses. In M. A. Lipton, A. DiMascio, and K. F. Killam, eds., *Psychopharmacology: A Generation of Progress*. New York: Raven Press, 1978, p. 347.
167. Aghajanian, G. K., Haigler, H. J., and Bloom, F. E. Lysergic acid diethylamide and serotonin direct actions on serotonin-containing neurons in rat brain. *Life Sci.* 11:615, 1972.
168. Stoll, W. Ein neues, in sehr kleinen Mengen wirksames Phantastikum. *Schweiz. Arch. f. Neuroll. Psychiatry* 64:483, 1947.
169. Hoffa, A. and Osmond, H. *The Hallucinogens*. New York: Academic Press, 1967, p. 103.
170. *Ibid.*, p. 104.
171. *Ibid.*, p. 95.
172. Jarvik, M. E. Drugs used in the treatment of psychiatric disorders. In L. S. Goodman and A. Gilman, eds., *The Pharmacological Basis of Therapeutics*, 3rd ed. New York: Macmil-

lan, 1965, p. 159.
173. Hofmann, F. G. *Handbook on Drugs of Abuse.*
174. Cheek, F. E., Newell, S., and Joffe, M. Deceptions in the illicit drug market. *Science* 167:1276, 1969.
175. Smith, D. E. Use of LSD in the Haight-Ashbury: Observations at a neighborhood clinic. *Calif. Med.* 110:472, 1969.
176. Ludwig, A. M., and Levine, J. Patterns of hallucinogenic drug abuse. *JAMA* 191:92, 1965.
177. Smith, D. E., and Rose, A. J. The use and abuse of LSD in Haight-Ashbury. (Observations by the Haight-Ashbury Medical Clinic.) *Clin. Pediatr.* 7:317, 1968.
178. Ungerleider, J. T., Fisher, D. D., and Fuller, M. The dangers of LSD. Analysis of seven months' experience in a university hospital's psychiatric service. *JAMA* 197:389, 1966.
179. Ungerleider, J. T., et al. The "bad trip"—the etiology of the adverse LSD reaction. *Am. J. Psychiatry* 124:1483, 1968.
180. Rothlin, E., and Cerletti, A. In L. Cholden, ed., *Lysergic Acid Diethylamide and Mescaline in Experimental Psychiatry*. New York: Grune & Stratton, 1956, p. 1.
181. Bewley, T. H. Adverse reactions from the illicit use of lysergide. *Br. Med. J.* 3:28, 1967.
182. Lucas, O. N., and Jaques, L. B. Effects of E-A.C.A. in spontaneous hemorrhage due to stress with anticoagulants in rats. *Can. J. Physiol. Pharmacol.* 42:803, 1964.
183. Johnson, F. N., et al. Emetic activity of reduced lysergamides. *J. Med. Chem.* 16:532, 1973.
184. Teuchmann, J. K., Kania, B. F., and Mulchar, T. Peripheral action of delyside tofranil and psychedrine. *Pol. Arch. Weter.* 15:527, 1972.
185. Goldman, H., et al. *Fed. Proc.* 33:256, 1974.
186. Scholes, N. W. Lysergic acid diethylamide (LSD-25) and gamma aminobutyric acid (GABA) interaction on spontaneous potentials and evoked response in the avian tectum. *Proc. Soc. Exp. Biol. Med.* 144:623, 1973.
187. Horita, A., and Hill, H. F. In E. Schoenbaum, ed., *Pharmacol. Thermoregul. Proc. Satel. Symp.* Basel, 1973, p. 417.
188. Messiha, F. S., and Grof, S. D-lysergic acid diethylamide (LSD)—effect on biogenic amines excretion in man. *Biochem. Pharmacol.* 22:2352, 1973.
189. Matveev, V. F., and Chudina, E. Kh. Gistoènzimologicheskoe issledouanie tkanei mozga vnutrennikk organico pri dlitel nom nvedenii diètlamida lizerginovoì kisloty—Zh nevropatol Psikhiatr. *Neuropathol. Pskikhiat. S.S. Korsakova* 73:1064, 1973.
190. Kabes, J., et al. Some biochemical aspects of LSD action on the central cholinergic system. *Activ. Nerv. Super.* 15:29, 1973.
191. Torre, M., and Fagiani, M. B. *Boll. Soc. Ital. Biol. Spec.* 48:590, 1972.
192. Krendal, F. P. Nekot probl. biofrematssi farmakokineti, tezisy dokl. nauch. font., 1973. *Chem. Abs.* 80:18, 1974.
193. McGlothlin, W. H., Cohen, S., and McGlothlin, M. S. Long-lasting effects of LSD on normals. *J. Psychedel. Drugs* 3:20, 1970.
194. Smart, R. G., and Bateman, K. Unfavorable reactions to LSD: A review and analysis of the available case reports. *Can. Med. Assoc. J.* 97:1214, 1967.
195. Smith, D. E. LSD, its use, abuse and suggested treatment. (Observations of the Haight-Ashbury Medical Clinic.) *J. Psychedel. Drugs* 1:117, 1968.
196. Cohen, S., and Edwards, A. E. *Drug Depend.* 2:1, 1969.
197. Smith, D. E., and Rose, A. J. LSD: Its use, abuse and suggested treatment. (Observations of the Haight-Ashbury Medical Clinic.) *J. Psychedel. Drugs* 1:117, 1968.
198. Shick, J. F. E., and Smith, D. E. Analysis of the LSD flashback. *J. Psychedel. Drugs* 3:13, 1970.
199. Louria, D. B. Lysergic acid diethylamide. *N. Engl. M. Med.* 278:435, 1968.
200. Ungerleider, J. T., et al. A statistical survey of adverse reactions to LSD in Los Angeles County.
201. Shick, J. F. E., and Smith, D. E. Analysis of the LSD flashback. *J. Psychedel. Drugs* 3:13, 1970.
202. Cohen, M. M., Marinello, M. J., and Back, N. Chromosomal damage in human leukocytes induced by lysergic acid diethylamide. *Science* 155:1417, 1967.
203. Cohen, M. M., Hirschhorn, K., and Frosch, W. A. *In vivo* and *in vitro* chromosomal damage induced by LSD-25. *N. Engl. J. Med.* 277:1043, 1967.
204. Egozcue, J., Irwin, S., and Maruffo, C. A. Chromosomal damage in LSD users. *JAMA* 204:214, 1968.
205. Loughman, W. D., Sargent, T. W., and Israelstam, D. M. Leucocytes of humans exposed to lysergic acid diethylamide: Lack of chromosomal damage. *Science* 158:508, 1967.
206. Pahnke, W. M., et al. The experimental use of psychedelic (LSD) psychotherapy. *JAMA* 212:1856, 1970.
207. Amarose, A. P., Schuster, C. R., and Muller,

T. P. Animal model for evaluation of drug-induced chromosome damage. *Oncology* 27:550, 1973.

208. Nielsen, J., et al. Lysergide and chromosome abnormalities. *Br. Med. J.* 68:801, 1968.
209. Geiger, R. S., et al. LSD effects on mature and immature brain cells in culture. *Fed. Proc.* 27:651, 1968.
210. Quinn, N. C. *Entomol. News* 81:241, 1970.
211. Gayer, J., and Pribys, R. *Experientia* 26:1332, 1970.
212. Kato, T., and Jarvik, L. F. LSD-25 and genetic damage. *Dis. Nerv. Sys.* 30:42, 1969.
213. Alexander, G. J., et al. LSD: Injection early in pregnancy produces abnormalities in offspring of rats. *Science* 157:459, 1967.
214. Auerbach, R., and Rugowski, J. A. Lysergic acid diethylamide: Effect on embryos. *Science* 157:1325, 1967.
215. Zellweger, H., McDonald, J. S., and Abbo, G. Is lysergic acid diethylamide a teratogen? *Lancet* 2:1066, 1967.
216. Smith, D. E. Editor's note. *J. Psychedel. Drugs* 1:1, 1968.
217. *N. Engl. J. Med.* 277:1090, 1967.
218. Uyeno, E. T. Presented at 32nd Annual Conference of the Committee on Problems of Drug Dependence. Division of Medical Sciences, National Academy of Sciences, National Research Council, Washington, D.C., February 16–17, 1970.
219. Jacobson, C. B., and Magyar, V. L. Genetic evaluation of LSD. *Clin. Proc. Child. Hosp. D.C.* 24:153, 1968.
220. Eller, J. L., and Morton, J. M. Bizarre deformities in offspring of user of lysergic acid diethylamide. *N. Engl. J. Med.* 283:395, 1970.
221. Hsu, L. Y., Strauss, L., and Hirschhorn, K. Chromosome abnormality in offspring of LSD user. D trisomy with D-D translocation. *JAMA* 211:987, 1970.
222. Sparkes, R. S., Melnyk, J., and Bozzetti, L. P. Chromosomal effect in vivo of exposure to lysergic acid diethylamide. *Science* 160:1343, 1968.
223. Lucas, G. J., and Lehrnbecker, W. Evaluation of chromosomal changes. *N. Engl. J. Med.* 281:1018, 1969.
224. Andrews, T. C., Meleod, M., Maclean, J. R., and Wilby, W. E. Chromosome studies on patients (in vivo) and cell (in vitro) treated with lysergic acid diethylamide. *N. Engl. J. Med.* 282:939, 1970.
225. Judd, L. L., Bradkamp, W. W., and McGlothlin, W. H. Comparison of the chromosomal patterns obtained from groups of continued users, former users, and nonusers of LSD-25. *Am. J. Psychiatry* 126:626, 1969.
226. Stenchever, M. A., and Jarvis, J. A. Lysergic acid diethylamide (LSD). Effect on human chromosomes in vivo. *Am. J. Obstet. Gynecol.* 106:485, 1970.
227. McGlothlin, W. H., Sparkes, R. S., and Arnold, D. O. Effect of LSD on human pregnancy. *JAMA* 212:1483, 1970.
228. Dishotsky, N. I., et al. LSD and genetic damage. *Science* 172:431, 1971.
229. Stash Capsules 4(6), Dec., 1972.
230. Egozcue, J., and Irwin, S. LSD-25 effects on chromosomes: A review. *J. Psychedel. Drugs* 3:10, 1970.
231. Sankar, D. V. S. Effects on pregnancy, chromosomes, offspring, etc. In *LSD—A Total Study*. Westbury, N.Y.: PJD Publications, 1975, p. 470.
232. Blocker, K. H. Aggression and the chronic use of LSD. *J. Psychedel. Drugs* 3:32, 1970.
233. Rorvik, D. M. Do drugs lead to violence? *Look Mag.* 58, April 7, 1970.
234. Smith, D. E. LSD, violence and radical religious beliefs. *J. Psychedel. Drugs* 3:38, 1970.
235. Caldwell, S. V. In W. Caldwell, ed., *LSD—Psychotherapy*. New York: Grove Press, 1969.
236. Abramson, H. A., and Evans, L. T. Lysergic acid diethylamide (LSD25): II. Psychobiological effects on the Siamese fighting fish. *Science* 120:990, 1954.
237. Busch, A. K., and Johnson, C. L.S.D.25 as an acid in psychotherapy. (Preliminary report of a new drug.) *Dis. Nerv. Sys.* 11:241, 1950.
238. Katzenelbogen, S., and Fang, A. D. Narocynthesis effects of sodium amytal, methadrine and L.S.D.-25. *Dis. Nerv. Sys.* 14:85, 1953.
239. Grof, S. The use of LSD in psychotherapy. *J. Psychedel. Drugs* 3:52, 1970.
240. Unger, S. M. In D. Solomon, ed., *LSD: The Consciousness Expanding Drug*. New York: Putnam, 1964, p. 257.
241. Eisner, B. G., and Cohen, S. Psychotherapy with lysergic acid diethylamide. *J. Nerv. Ment. Dis.* 127:528, 1958.
242. Chandler, A. L., and Hartman, M. A. Lysergic acid diethylamide (LSD-25) as a facilitating agent in psychotherapy. *Arch. Gen. Psychiatry* 2:286, 1960.
243. Butterworth, A. T. Some aspects of an office practice utilizing LSD 25. *Psychiat. Q.* 36:734, 1962.
244. Baker, E. F. W. The use of lysergic acid die-

thylamide (LSD) in psychotherapy. *Can. Med. Assoc. J.* 91:1200, 1964.
245. Whitaker, L. H. Lysergic acid diethylamide in psychotherapy. *Med. J. Aust.* 1:36, 1965.
246. Louria, D. *Nightmare Drugs*. New York: Pocket Books, 1966.
247. Kast, E. The analgesic action of lysergic acid compared with dihydromorphinone and meperidine. *Bull. Drug Addict. Narcot.* App. 27:3517, 1963.
248. Arana Gallegos, J. Anàlisis comparativo de la communicacion. Los process de interaccioǹ en las psicosis experimentales y en la esquizofreni. *Rev. Neuro-Psiqueat.* 31:26, 1969.
249. Fisher, R., and Scheib. *J. Calif. Psychiat.* 14:174, 1971.
250. Krippner, S. The influence of "psychedelic" experience of contemporary art and music. In J. A. Gamage and E. L. Zerkin, eds., *Hallucinogenic Drug Research: Impact on Science and Society*. Beloit, Wis.: Stash Press, 1970, pp. 83–114.
251. Zegans, L. S., Pollard, J. C., and Brown, D. The effects of LSD-25 on creativity and tolerance to regression. *Arch. Can. Psychiatry* 16:740, 1967.
252. Sankar, D. V. S. Epilogue. In D. V. S. Sankar, ed., *LSD—A Total Study*. Westbury, N.Y.: PJD Publications, 1975, p. 888.
253. Wasson, R. G. The fly agaric and man. In D. Efron, B. Holmstedt, and N. S. Kline, eds., *Ethnopharmacologic Search for Psychoactive Drugs*. (Public Health Service Publication #1645), Washington, D.C.: U.S. Government Printing Office, 1967, pp. 405–414.
254. Schmiedeberg, D., and Koppe, R. Das muscarin, das giftye alkaloid des Fliegenpilzes. *Leipzig Verlag Vogel R.C.* 1869.
255. Eugster, C. H. Active substances from the toadstool. *Naturwissenschaften* 55:305, 1968.
256. Eugsten, C. H., and Takemoto, T. Zur. nomenklatur der neven verbindungen aus amanita-arten. *Helv. Chim. Acta* 50:126, 1967.
257. Ott, J., et al. Neuvos datos sobre los supuestos licoperdaccos psicotropicos y dos cases de intoxicacion provacado por hongos del genero scleroderma en Mexic. *Biol. Soc. Mex. Mic.* 9:67, 1975.
258. Matsumoto, T., et al. Isolivung von (−)-R-4-ityhydroxy-pyrrolidon-(2) und einigen weiterew Verbinduage aus Amanita muscaria. *Helv. Chim. Acta.* 52:716, 1969.
259. Schultes, R. E., and Hofmann, A. Plants of hallucinogenic use. In *The Botany and Chemistry of Hallucinogens*. Springfield, Ill.: Charles C Thomas, 1980, p. 54.
260. Beck, J. E., and Gordon, D. V. Psilocybian mushrooms. *Pharmochem. Newsl.* 11:1, 1982.
261. Guzman, G. Presented at Pacific Northwest Hallucinogenic Mushroom Conference, Westlake, Oreg., Nov. 3, 1979.
262. Ott, J. A brief history of hallucinogenic mushrooms. In J. Ott and J. Bigwood, eds., *Teonanacatl: Hallucinogenic Mushrooms of North America*. Seattle: Madrona, 1978, pp. 5–22.
263. Wasson, R. G. The divine mushroom of immortality. In P. Furst, ed., *Flesh of the Gods*. New York: Praeger, pp. 185–200.
264. McLoud, D., et al. *Drug Information Primer*. Eugene, Oreg.: University of Oregon Press, 1977.
265. Hofmann, A. History of the basic chemical investigations on the sacred mushrooms of Mexico. In J. Ott and J. Bigwood, eds., *Teonanacatl: Hallucinogenic Mushrooms of North America*. Seattle: Madrona, 1978, pp. 45–61.
266. Schultes, R. E., and Hofmann, A. *The Botany and Chemistry of Hallucinogens*. Springfield, Ill.: Charles C Thomas, 1973.
267. Lincoff, G., and Mitchel, D. H. *Toxic and Hallucinogenic Mushroom Poisoning: A Handbook for Physicians and Mushroom Hunters*. New York: Van Nostrand Reinhold, 1977.
268. Grinspoon, L., and Bakalar, J. B. *Psychedelic Drugs Reconsidered*. New York: Basic Books, 1979.
269. Aghajanian, G. K., Foote, W. E., and Sheard, M. H. Lysergic acid diethylamide: Neuronal units in the midbrain. *Science* 161:706, 1968.
270. Stafford, P. *Psychedelics Encyclopedia*. Berkeley, Calif.: And/Or Press, 1977, p. 7.
271. Pollock, S. H. Psilocybian mycetismus with special reference to panaeolus. *J. Psychedel. Drugs* 8:43, 1976.
272. Menser, G. *Hallucinogenic and Poisonous Mushroom Field Guide*. Berkeley, Calif.: And/Or Press, 1977.
273. Pollock, S. H. Psilocybian mushroom pandemic. *J. Psychedel. Drugs* 7:73, 1975.
274. Stash Psilocybin. DHEW Reports Series 16, no. 1, May 1973.
275. Borhegyi, S. A. Miniature mushroom stones from Guatemala. *Am. Ant.* 26:498, 1961.
276. Triska, R. E. The legalities of mushroom experimentation. In T. Walters, ed., *Mushrooms and Man*. Albany, Oreg.: Linn-Benton Community College, 1977, p. 83–92.
277. Weil, A. The use of psychoactive mushrooms in the Pacific Northwest: An ethnopharmacologic report. *Botanical Museum Leaflets of Har-*

*vard University* 1977, pp. 131–149.
278. Stamets, P. *Psilocybe Mushrooms and Their Allies*. Seattle: Homestead, 1978.
279. Bigwood, J. Psilocybian mushroom cultivation. In J. Ott and J. Bigwood, eds., *Teonanacatl: Hallucinogenic Mushrooms of North America*. Seattle: Madrona, 1978, pp. 115–147.
280. Hofmann, H., et al. *F. Helv. Chim. Acta.* 42:1557, 1959.
281. Schoenfeld, E. *Dear Doctor Hippocrates; Advice Your Family Doctor Never Gave You*. New York: Grove Press, 1968.
282. Briggs, K. M. *Pale Hecate's Team*. New York: Humanities Press, 1962, p. 81.
283. Langdon-Brown, W. *From Witchcraft to Chemotherapy*. Cambridge, England: Cambridge University Press, 1941, p. 30.
284. Genesis 30:14-16. *The New English Bible*. New York: Oxford University Press, 1970, p. 33.
285. Schultes, R. E. The plant kingdom and hallucinogens (part III). *Bull. Narcot.* 22:43, 1970.
286. *Encyclopedia Brittanica*. 1929.
287. Evans, W. O., and Kline, N. S. Chairmen; Symposium and panel discussion on social patterns of drug use, historically and in nonwestern cultures, San Juan. American College of Neuropsychopharmacology, December 10, 1970.
288. Burns, R. S., and Lerner, S. E. Phencyclidine deaths. *JACEP*, 7:135, 1978.
289. Cohen, S. *The Substance Abuse Problems*. New York: Haworth Press, 1981, p. 62.
290. Kessler, G. E. Phencyclidine and fatal status epilepticus. *N. Engl. J. Med.* 291:979, 1974.
291. Domino, E. F. Neurobiology of phencyclidine—An update. In R. C. Peterson and R. C. Stillman, eds., *Phencyclidine (PCP) Abuse: An Appraisal* (NIDA Research Monograph 21). Washington, D.C.: NIDA, 1978, p. 28.
292. Lin, D. C. K., et al. Quantification of phencyclidine in body fluids by gas chromatography-chemical ionization mass spectrometry and identification of two metabolites. *Biomed. Mass Spectrom.* 2:206, 1975.
293. Wong, L. K., and Biemann, K. Metabolites of phencyclidine in humans. *Biomed. Mass Spectrom.* 2:204, 1975.
294. Domino, E. F. Some aspects of the pharmacology of phencyclidine. In R. C. Stillman and R. E. Willette, eds., *The Psychopharmacology of Hallucinogens*. New York: Pergamon, 1978, p. 105.
295. Hawks, R. L., and Willette, R. E. Phencyclidine: Analytical methodology. Research Technology Branch, Division of Research, National Institute on Drug Abuse, Rockville, Md., Dec. 1977.
296. Marshman, J. A., Ramsay, M. P., and Sellers, E. M. Quantitation of phencyclidine in biological fluids and application to human overdose. *Toxicol. Appl. Pharmacol.* 35:129, 1976.
297. Gupta, R. C., et al. Determination of phencyclidine (PCP) in urine and illicit street drug samples. *Clin. Toxicol.* 8:611, 1975.
298. Pearce, D. S. Detection and quantitation of phencyclidine in blood by use of [(2)H(5)] phencyclidine and select ion monitoring applied to non-fatal cases of phencyclidine intoxication. *Clin. Chem.* 22:1623, 1976.
299. Lau, S. S., and Domino, E. F. Gas chromotography mass spectrometry assay for ketamine and its metabolites in plasma. *Biomed. Mass. Spectrum.* 4:317, 1977.
300. Wallace, J., and Blum, K. An evaluation of the TRI DIPSTICK TEST for the detection of drugs of abuse in urine. *Subs. Alcohol Action/Misuse* 3:129, 1982.
301. Johnson, K. M. Neurochemical pharmacology of phencyclidine. In R. C. Petersen and R. C. Stillman, eds., *Phencyclidine (PCP) Abuse: An Appraisal.* (NIDA Research Monograph 21). Washington, D.C.: NIDA, 1978, p. 44.
302. 302. Tonge, S. R., and Leonard, B. E. Partial antagonism of the behavioral and neurochemical effects of phencyclidine by drugs affecting monoamine metabolism. *Psychopharmacologia* 24:516, 1972.
303. Johnson, K. M., and Balster, R. L. Acute and chronic phenaycliddine administration: Relationships between biodispositional factors and behavioral effects. *Subst. Alcohol Actions/Misuse* 2(3):131, 1982.
304. Smith, R. C., et al. Effects of phencyclidine on $^{3}$H-catecholamine and $^{3}$H-serotonin uptake in synaptosomal preparations from rat brain. *Biochem. Pharmacol.* 26:1435, 1977.
305. Finnegan, K. T., Kanner, M. I., and Meltzer, H. Y. Phencyclidine-induced rotational behavior in rats with nigrostrial lesions and its modulation by dopaminergic and cholinergic agents. *Pharmacol. Biochem. Behav.* 5:651, 1976.
306. Hitzemann, R. J., Loh, H. H., and Domino, E. F. Effect of phencyclidine on the accumulation of 14C-catecholamines formed from 14C-tyrosine. *Arch. Int. Pharmacodyn. Ther.* 202:252, 1973.
307. Weinstein, H., et al. Psychotomimetic drugs as anticholinergic agents (II). Quantum mechanical study of molecular interaction potentials of 1-cyclohexylpiperidine derivatives with

cholinergic receptor. *Molec. Pharmacol.* 73:820, 1973.

308. Maayani, S., et al. Psychotomimetics as anticholinergic agents (I). *Biochem. Pharmacol.* 23:1263, 1974.
309. Pinchasi, I., Maayani, S., and Sokolovsky, M. On the interactions of drugs with the cholinergic nervous system (III): Tolerance to phencyclidine derivatives: *in vivo* and *in vitro* studies. *Bhiochem. Pharmacol.* 26:1671, 1977.
310. Dye, D. J., and Taberner, P. V. The effects of some newer anesthetics on the *in vitro* activity of glutamate decarboxylase and GABA transaminase in crude brain extracts and on the levels of amino acids *in vivo*. *J. Neurochem.* 24:997, 1975.
311. Peterson, R. C., and Stillman, R. C., eds. *Phencyclidine (PCP) Abuse: An Appraisal* (NIDA Research Monograph 21). Washington, D.C.: NIDA, 1978.
312. Balster, R. L., and Chait, L. D. The behavioral effects of phencyclidine in animals. In R. C. Peterson and R. C. Stillman, eds., *Phencyclidine (PCP) Abuse: An Appraisal.* (NIDA Research Monograph 21) Washington, D.C.: NIDA, 1978, p. 53.
313. Moreton, E. J., et al. Ketamine self-administration by the Rhesus monkey. *J. Pharmacol. Exp. Ther.* 203:303, 1977.
314. Kanner, M., Finnegan, K., and Meltzer, H. Y. Dopaminergic effects of phencyclidine in rats with nigrostriatal lesions. *Psychopharmacol. Commun.* 1:393, 1975.
315. Balster, R. L., and Chait, L. D. The behavioral pharmacology of phencyclidine. *Clin. Toxicol.* 9:513, 1976.
316. Aronow, R., and Done, A. K. Phencyclidine overdose: An emergency concept of management. *JACEP* 7:56, 1978.
317. Cohen, S. *The Substance Abuse Problems*. New York: Haworth Press, 1981, p. 65.
318. Hollister, L. E. *Chemical Psychoses: LSD and Related Drugs*. Springfield, Ill.: Charles C Thomas, 1968, p. 157.
319. Freedman, D. X. Perspectives on the use and abuse of psychdedelic drugs. In D. H. Efrem, ed., *Ethnopharmacologic Search for Psychoactive Drugs*. (Public Health Service Pub. no. 1645). Washington, D.C.: National Institute of Mental Health, 1967, p. 77.
320. Ford, S. D. LSD and the law: A framework for policy making. *Minn. Law Rev.* 54:775, 1970.

Chapter 19

# Psychotropic Drug Interactions

## A. GENERAL INTRODUCTION

The development of many new therapeutic agents in recent years has represented considerable progress in the treatment of numerous disease entities. There is increasing recognition, however, of the drug-related problems that may accompany the therapeutic benefits of these agents. As drug therapy becomes more complex and more individuals are treated with several different drugs simultaneously, the ability to predict the probable magnitude of reaction to a specific therapeutic agent significantly diminishes.

Melmon[1] reports that 18 to 30 percent of all hospitalized patients experience a drug reaction. Three to 5 percent of all patient admissions to hospitals are primarily because of a drug reaction and 30 percent of these patients have a second drug reaction during their hospital stay.

One study[2] revealed that an adverse drug reaction either was responsible for or strongly influenced the hospitalization of 258 (3.7 percent) of 7017 medical inpatients. The drugs most commonly implicated in the report were acetylsalicylic acid, digoxin, guanethidine, prednisone, and warfarin. These agents are frequently reported to interact with other drugs.

The cost of these reactions is startling. Approximately one seventh of all hospital days is devoted to the care of drug toxicity at an estimated yearly cost of $3 billion.

There is no such thing as a safe drug. Drugs are like a double-edged sword, with a good side and a bad side. Successful treatment is a delicate balance between the beneficial and harmful effects, weighted in favor of the beneficial. In some cases, the original disease no longer is the problem. Instead the drug reaction becomes the major focus. The old dictum that "the cure is worse than the disease" frequently has been all too true.

Of the three million Americans who experience a severe drug reaction, it has been calculated that between 6000 and 140,000 die each year as a result.[3] In addition, there is evidence that about 4 percent of hospital admissions are for drug-induced illness.[4–6] Miller[7] reports that "in some U.S. hospitals, as many as 20 percent of their patients were admitted because of drug-provoked disease."

Americans spend about $11 billion on prescribed medications each year, and that does not include the $2.6 billion purchased as nonprescription, over-the-counter (OTC) pharmaceuticals.[8,9] In 1972, a Boston study[5] revealed that more than 75 million Americans consume a drug at least once a week, and usually every day.

According to the American Medical Association, the average doctor sees about 90 patients a week for roughly 17 minutes per patient.[8] Today the most prescribed drugs are tranquilizers (Valium and Librium are the top two on the list); the pain killer propoxyphene (Darvon) is third.

The lack of communication between doctor and patient has contributed to the drug-reaction dilemma. Dr. George Caranasos[10] observes that: ''Patients also cannot identify correctly 60 percent of their medicines. Forty percent of the patients receive drugs prescribed by two or more physicians, increasing the possibility of drug interactions. Twelve percent of patients take drugs prescribed for someone else and 60 percent of patients consider their drugs safe.''

Furthermore drug-taking errors are more common than most would imagine. As much as 58 percent of people studied at the University of North Carolina[11] made mistakes in the way they took their medication. It has been suggested that the problem may lie with the physician for not communicating clearly with the patient.

Graedon[12] points out that drug interactions are the Achilles' heel of the medical profession. A basic premise for understanding the phenomenon of drug–drug reactivity is that the law of nature no longer holds true and here one plus one equals three. Mixing medicines is very much like playing Russian roulette. For example, aspirin alone interacts with 24 other drugs to produce unexpected, and often unwanted, responses.

A major contribution to the problems associated with serious drug interactions is several physicians prescribing medicines for a single patient. Additional factors include diets, environment, and nonprescription or illicit agents that may influence the effects and interact directly with prescribed medications. The last include cold remedies, pain relievers, vitamins, antacids, and alcohol and other abusable drugs. Alcohol, by itself, as a special substance, cannot be ignored. It is known that alcohol can interact with 150 other drugs or chemicals in a potentially harmful way.

In simple terms, a chemical that modifies the actions of another drug can do so in numerous ways. It may potentiate the other drug and make the desired effect more powerful. Thus someone who takes a tranquilizer regularly could be destroyed by consuming excessive amounts of alcohol because the two together will sedate the individual more heavily than either drug alone. Another possibility is that one drug might decrease the beneficial effects of another medication and thereby diminish its therapeutic value.

An important site in the body where two or more drugs could influence each other is the liver. Hormones, antihistamines, tranquilizers, pain killers, and arthritis medications are but a few of the chemicals that can alter the liver's ability to metabolize or detoxify drugs. For example, in the presence of a tranquilizer, sedatives and anticoagulants are more rapidly eliminated via induction of metabolizing enzymes. In this case, it is necessary to elevate the dosage of anticonvulsants.

Many people, including doctors, are not aware of another unexpected interaction. Excessive consumption of licorice (of European origin) can induce headaches, high blood pressure, and even heart failure when amphetamines such as speed are taken concurrently.[13]

The only way one can improve the odds against an adverse drug interaction is to be knowledgeable about the potential drug–drug reactions of prescription drugs, nonprescription drugs, and illicit agents, as well as nutrition and other environmental factors.

For additional information, the reader should refer to other reviews.[11,14,15]

## B. TERMINOLOGY AND BIOPHARMACEUTICS OF DRUG INTERACTIONS

### 1. Terminology

Drug interaction is a phenomenon that occurs when the effects of one drug are modified by the prior or concurrent administration of another (or the same) drug(s). It takes place, more specifically, when the overall biologic response to the simultaneous (or nearly so) administration of two or more drugs is markedly different from the simple sum of the effect of each compound given singly. Drug interactions present a complex and proved problem, and may arise either from the alteration of the absorption, distribution, biotransformation, or excretion of one drug by another, or from a combination of their actions or effects.

Interestingly some individuals would extend the concept of drug interactions to include other conditions:

1. A dietary item influences the activity of a drug, for example, certain cheeses interact with monoamine oxidase (MAO) inhibitors.
2. A drug alters diagnostic laboratory test values.
3. A drug essentially interacts with itself, for example, by stimulating its own metabolism.

If, as one study has shown,[16] hospital patients receive an average of 14 different medications during their stay, what are the chances of one of these drugs affecting the organism's reactivity to another drug?

Although outpatients usually take fewer medications than hospital patients, the chances of drug interactions occurring are increased by several factors associated with the practice of medicine and the habits of patients.

1. The practice of polypharmacy is alive and well today. A patient who sees a physician expects more than one medication for the ailment. The tradition of prescribing a combination of drugs is still common. Indeed it is difficult adequately to treat many ailments with just one medication.
2. In this age of specialization, many patients see more than one physician, usually for different ailments.
3. Self-medication is prevalent and polypharmacy is practiced by individuals who take numerous OTC medications for various ailments.
4. Many modern drugs are polymechanistic and may affect several or many physiologic and biochemical systems of the body.

Although drug interactions do occur in the gastrointestinal tract, most of them take place after the drug has been absorbed and is being distributed, metabolized, and excreted by the body. The terms used to describe the effects of drug interactions are most ambiguous. Table 19-1 presents various terms used in describing the combined effects of drugs with regard to mechanism and locus of action. Although these terms may be the preferred and/or correct way of describing drug interactions, they are not necessarily the ones always used in the same context as shown here.

**TABLE 19-1**

**Terms Used to Describe the Combined Effects of Drugs**

I. Homoergic: Two drugs produce the same overt effect.
   - A. Summation. If the combined effects are equal to the sum of their individual effect.
   - B. Additive. If the combined effects are equal to those expected for drugs acting by the same mechanisms.
   - C. Synergism. Has various meanings and is best avoided for homoergic drugs.

II. Hetergic: Only one of a pair of drugs produces an effect.
   - A. Synergism. Combined effects of hetergic drugs that are greater than those of the active component alone.
   - B. Potentiation. Often a synonym for synergism; should be abandoned.
   - C. Antagonism. Combined effects of hetergic drugs that are less than that of the active component alone.
     - (1) Chemical antagonism. Interaction of an agonist and an antagonist to form an inactive complex (e.g. EDTA and lead; BAL and As and Hg; protamine sulfate and heparin sodium).
     - (2) Competitive antagonism. Antagonist acts reversibly at the same receptor site as the agonist (e.g., atropine and acetylcholine).
     - (3) Nonequilibrium antagonism. Receptor antagonist acts irreversibly.
     - (4) Noncompetitive antagonism. Agonist and antagonist act at different receptor sites.
     - (5) Physiologic or functional antagonism. Antagonism between drugs having overtly opposite effects (e.g., amphetamine and barbiturate).

(From Goodman, L. S., and Gilman, A. *The Pharmacological Basis of Therapeutics*. Macmillan, New York, 1970, p. 25.)

Several terms are employed to describe the properties of concurrently administered drugs. Two drugs are hetergic for a particular effect if such an effect is exhibited by one, but not the other, of the drugs. Two drugs are homoergic if they produce the same overt effect. These terms, however, are seldom employed.

Other terms, such as addition, summation, synergism, and potentiation, are used more frequently to describe an increased effect resulting from the concurrent use of two or more drugs. Antagonism and inhibition describe a decreased effect resulting from the concurrent use of two or more drugs.

As previously mentioned, drug interactions—alteration of the effects of one drug on another—will result in either (1) diminution of therapeutic efficacy or (2) an increase in drug activity and possible toxic drug reactions.

Several years ago, problems arising from drug interactions were classified as therapeutic incompatibilities. In retrospect, this was an unfortunate designation; although most drug interactions could be considered undesirable, some can be beneficial, as in the deliberate administration of one drug to modify the effects of another.

To understand the underlying principles of biopharmaceutics and the basic principles of drug interactions, it is necessary to understand the fundamentals of drug absorption, transport (distribution), metabolism (biotransformation), and excretion. This is the common ground for discussing and correlating biopharmaceutic phenomena and drug interactions.

## 2. Biopharmaceutics

The term *biopharmaceutics* and a definition of it first appeared in print in a review article by Dr. John Wagner, in the May 1961 issue of the *Journal of Pharmaceutical Sciences*.[17] In this article, Dr. Wagner included the following detailed definition.

> Biopharmaceutics encompasses the study of the relation between the nature and intensity of the biological effects observed in animals and man and the following factors:
>
> 1. The nature of the form of the drug (ester, salt, complex, etc.);
> 2. The physical state, particle size, and surface area;
> 3. Presence or absence of adjuvants with the drug;
> 4. The type of dosage form in which the drug is administered; and
> 5. The pharmaceutical process(es) used to make the dosage form.

Biopharmaceutics thus may be defined as the study of the influence of formulation on the therapeutic activity of a drug product. Or it may be defined as the study of the relationships between some of the physical and chemical properties of the drug and its dosage forms and the biologic effects observed following administration of the drug in its various dosage forms. Biopharmaceutics includes all possible effects of dosage forms on biologic response, and all possible physiologic factors that may affect the drug contained in the dosage form, and the dosage form of the drug itself.

The biologic availability of a drug may be greatly affected by its physical state and the form in which it is administered. A given drug may show different degrees of availability in different dosage forms even when given by the same route. For example, a drug might have different onsets of action or show different blood levels and concentrations depending on whether it is administered as a tablet, capsule, or suspension. Also a given drug might show different availability from the same dosage form made by two or more manufacturers, and there is the possibility of different availability from lot to lot of one drug product made by one manufacturer.

There are many and varied pharmaceutic factors that may alter drug availability. Some of the physiochemical ones are:

1. The particle size of the drug in solid dosage form can be an important factor. Some drugs such as griseofulvin are made available in a micronized form to increase their low dissolution rate. Inadequate particle size is one cause of the relatively poor availability of several generic-brand chloramphenicol capsules that were recalled several years ago.

2. The particle size of the dispersed phase in an emulsion is also important.

3. Tablet disintegration may depend not only on the type and quality of the disintegrating agent but also on the hardness of the tablet.

4. Tablet and capsule adjuncts such as diluents, binders, and lubricants may decrease water permeability and consequently reduce drug absorption.

5. Various tablet coatings may release drugs unevenly or not at all.

6. The crystalline or amorphous form of the drug may have a profound effect on the dissolution rate of the drug after ingestion. Cortisone acetate and novobiocin are examples of drugs whose availabilities are altered by changes in their crystalline forms.

The physiochemical properties of a compound are measurable characteristics by which the compound may interact with other systems. The physical and chemical properties of a molecule are determined by the number, the kind, and the arrangement of the atoms. Both properties are closely interrelated and, for this reason, the term *physiochemical* is a preferred expression of the properties that relate to biologic action, rather than physical properties or chemical properties. These properties are solubility, pH, surface activity, hydrogen binding, and partition coefficients.

In addition to physiochemical factors, of course, drug availability is also affected by various pharmacologic, physiologic, and biochemical factors.

## C. DRUG-INTERACTION MECHANISMS

In general, the following is a list of possible means by which drug interactions may occur.

1. Action—chemical or physical—of one compound directly upon another.

2. Modification of gastrointestinal absorption.

3. Competition for protein-binding sites during transport.

4. Modification of a drug's action at the receptor site.

5. Acceleration or retardation of the metabolism of a given drug-modify enzyme system.

6. Modification of the rate of urinary excretion–renal clearance.

Table 19-2 illustrates mechanisms that may contribute to diminution of therapeutic efficacy. In contrast, Table 19-3 illustrates mechanisms that may contribute to increases in drug activity.

## D. PSYCHOTROPIC DRUG INTERACTIONS

One area where drug interactions are liable to occur involves individuals who abuse or deliberately misuse drugs. It is conceiveable that some interactions may take place between drugs that are used for illicit purposes, but these are difficult to discern. Physicians who are called

**TABLE 19-2**

**Mechanism(s) That Contribute to Reduced Therapeutic Efficacy**

1. Chemical and physical antagonisms. Many drug interactions in the GI tract result from chemical reactions (complex formation) and physical antagonisms (adsorption of drugs on kaolin).
2. Protein-binding effects during transport. Displacement of a drug from protein-binding sites in plasma can result in the increased metabolism and excretion of the displaced drug.
3. Enzyme induction effects. The ability of some drugs to stimulate the production of drug-metabolizing enzymes in the liver can result in increased metabolism of the administered drug as well as other related or even unrelated drugs.
4. Antagonisms at receptor sites. Drug interactions can occur when an agent occupies the receptors normally used by an active drug, or acts on another site, either producing an opposite effect or blocking the effect of the drug.
5. Renal clearance effects. Changes in urinary pH can increase the excretion of weak acid and basic drugs.

upon in hospitals or treatment centers to treat deliberate abusers of drugs find it almost impossible to determine which drugs have been taken.

Certainly the drugs that act on mental processes are no different from other pharmaceutic agents in that they are capable of affecting the absorption, metabolism, and excretion of other drugs. Although such interactions are not always desirable, occasionally they are, and at other times may be of no clinical significance.

In this chapter, we explore certain types of drug interactions. The drugs discussed are alcohol, narcotics, narcotic antagonists, and psychotherapeutic agents. To systemize the available information on drug–drug interactions, a number of tables, mostly adapted from other sources, are presented.

## 1. Analgesics

The depressant effects of some opioids may be exaggerated and prolonged by phenothiazines, MAO inhibitors, and tricyclic antidepressants; the mechanisms of this supra-additive effect are not fully understood, but may involve alterations in the rate of metabolic transformation of the opioid or in the neurotransmitters involved in opioid actions. Some, but not all, phenothiazines reduce the amount of narcotic required to produce a given level of analgesia. However, the respiratory depressant effects seem also to be enhanced, the degree of sedation is increased, and the hypotensive effects of phenothiazines become an additional complication. Some phenothiazine derivatives enhance the sedative effects, but at the same time seem to be antianalgesic and to increase the amount of narcotic required to produce satisfactory relief from pain.[19]

There are documented experiences in both humans and animals that show profound and sometimes lethal interactions between MAOI's such as phenelzine, iproniazid, d- and l-amphetamines, SKF-525A, pargvline and tranylcypromine, and narcotic analgesics.[20-25] The above MAOI's inhibit meperidine N-demethylation or hydrolysis.[25] The combination of phenelzine, morphine, and meperidine causes semiconsciousness,[21-22] and in one case, death.[20] Other work showed a five-fold aug-

### TABLE 19-3
### Mechanism(s) That Contribute to Increases in Drug Activity

1. Addictive and synergistic effects—The concurrent or sequential administration of two or more agents possessing similar pharmacologic actions or side effects may give rise to drug interactions by the additive or synergistic effect of these properties. An additive effect would be produced by the concurrent administration of two barbiturates, phenobarbital and secobarbital. The concurrent administration of central nervous system (CNS) depressants, such as barbiturates and tranquilizers, or the administration of a sympathiomimetic (e.g. amphetamine) with an adrenergic sensitizer, e.g. imipramine (Tofranil) can produce additive or synergistic effects that may be dangerous. The effects of combining CNS depressants with alcohol have been called additive, synergistic and potentiated by various authors. It has been suggested that interactions involving drugs and alcohol be considered true drug interactions, with alcohol as one of the drugs.
2. Protein-binding during transport—Displacement of a drug from protein-binding sites in plasma can result in high and possible toxic blood levels of displaced drug.
3. Enzyme inhibition effects—The ability of some drugs to inhibit production of drug-metabolizing enzymes can result in high blood levels and prolonged activity of the more slowly detoxified drug. Also, two drugs may compete for the same metabolizing enzyme systems.
4. Biochemical effects—the administration of one drug with the potential to alter the basic mechanism of action of another drug can result in a drug interaction. The interaction is not a simple additive effect but is a result of drug-induced changes in the patient. For example, thiazide diuretics (Esidrix, Hydrodiuril), by producing potassium loss, can predispose patients to toxic reactions from cardiac glycosides, which affect ionic transfer in cardiac cells.
5. Renal clearance effects—Changes in urinary pH can decrease the renal clearance of weak acid and basic drugs.

mentation of not only analgesia but mortality with meperidine after the subject received an MAO inhibitor. The central stimulant amphetamine, and probably cocaine, are known poentiators of analgesics such as reported for peteridine[26] and codeine.[27] There is synergistic central depression between the antineoplastic, procarbazine and narcotic analgesics.[28] Antonita,[29] in an article concerned with important precautions when dispensing oral progestational durgs, cited oral proteins as inhibitors of meperidine metabolism.[29]

There are numerous studies,[30,31] which indicate that cholinergic drugs such as atropine, scopolamine, and neostigmine significantly alter both the duration and analgesic properties of meperidine and methadone.

Most recently, a highly publicized report appeared concerning 120 individuals in the San José, California, area who developed a parkinsonian-like syndrome as a result of utilizing an illicit synthetic analog of meperidine, known as 1-methyl-4-phenyl-1,2,5,6-tetrahydropryidine (MPTP). The chemist in a clandestine laboratory had overheated a batch of precursor chemicals to speed the slow chemical process, which resulted in the formation of the toxic by-product.[32]

Additionally, morphine analgesia is enhanced in rodents with synpathomimetics (dopamine, epinephrine, nethalide and methyldopa). In contrast, antiadrenergic drugs like guanethidine and reserpine reduced the pain-killing actions of morphine.[31]

Psychotropics, such as the major tranquilizers (chlorpomazine; aphenothiazine) potentiate both the sedative as well as the pain-killing properties of narcotic analgesics.[33,34] Generally, it appears that phenothiazines should be contraindicated in acute clinical utilization of morphine, since it is also recognized that the tranquilizers signficantly augment opioid-in-

**TABLE 19-4**

**Interactions of Narcotic Analgesics and Others**

| *Analgeisc* | *May Interact With* | *To Cause* | *Because* |
|---|---|---|---|
| Narcotic | Monoamine (oxidase inhibitors (including amphetamine and pyrocarbazine) | Restlessness, respiratory depression | Decreased metabolism of narcotics |
| Meperidine | Oral progestational drugs | Increased excretion of meperidine | |
| Narcotics | Autonomic drugs | Mixed reports (see text) | |
| Narcotics | Phenothiazines | Enhanced sedative effect, enhanced respiratory depression | Additive CNS depression |
| Meperidine | Tricyclic antidepressants | Increased respiratory depression | |
| Acetaminophen | Oral anticoagulants | Increased prothrombin time (high dose acetaminophen) | |
| Phenacetin | Halogenated hydrocarbon insecticides | No effect<br>Increased metabolism | Enzyme induction |
| Indomethacin | Probenecid | Increased plasma level of indomethacin | Inhibition of tubular secretion |
| Propoxyphene | Orphenadrine | Tremors, hallucinations | Additive side effects |
| Mefenamic Acid | Warfarin | Decreased binding of warfarin | Displacement from the binding site |
| Phenyramidol | Diphenylhydantoin, anticoagulants | Increased half-life decrease in protome | Microsomal enzyme inhibition |
| Colchicine | Vitamin $B_{12}$ | Decreased $B_{12}$ absorption | Alteration of ileal mucosa |
| Salicylamide | Salicylate | Decrease in glucuronate formation | Compatitive inhibition |

Taken from E. A. Hartshorn *Handbook on Drug Interactions.* Presented by CIBA, Hamilton Press, Hamilton, Illinois, 1973.

diced respiratory depression. This is also true with the tricyclic antidepressant imipramine.[36]

Another substance considered a synthetic analgesic of the narcotic type, propoxyphene, interacts with orphenadrine, and causes tremors and hallucinations.[36-39]

Table 19-4 represents typical drug interactions and the reader is reminded that this may serve as a useful source if any emergency should arise. Table 19-5 illustrates reported alterations in laboratory test results of analgesics.

## 2. Alcohol[40]

Since approximately 100 million Americans, about 60 to 70 percent of adults, consume alcohol in variable quantities for a number of reasons, it is inevitable that additional pharmacologic agents will be ingested concurrently with alcohol or while alcohol is still present in the body. It is important to note that, when considering a possible alcohol–drug interaction, many cough preparations contain both alcohol and other CNS depressants, and mouth washes, tonics, liquid vitamins, and OTC drugs may contain high concentrations of alcohol.

### *a. Direct Interactions*[40]

Becker et al.[40] have adequately reviewed this most important topic.

Ethyl alcohol and a variety of other drugs have been shown to include proliferation of the

**TABLE 19-5**

**Reported Alterations in Laboratory Test Results of Miscellaneous Analgesics**

| | |
|---|---|
| *NARCOTICS* | |
| Serum | |
| Meperidine: Amylase | Positive |
| Morphine, Codeine: BSP retention | Positive |
| Morphine: Blood Ammonia | Elevated |
| Urine Glucose | |
| Morphine: Benedict's | Positive |
| Morphine: UMA | Negative |
| *PARA-AMINOPHEN DERIVATIVES-PHENACETIN, ACETAMINOPHEN ACETANILID* | |
| Urine | |
| Phenacetin: 5HIAA | Positive |
| Acetaminophen: 5HIAA | Positive |
| Acetanilid: 5HIAA | Positive |
| Acetanilid: Benedict's | Brown Color |
| Phenacetin: Benedict's | Brown Color |
| Serum | |
| Phenacetin: NPN | Positive |
| Phenacetin: RBC or Hb | Negative |
| Phenacetin: Alters liver tests | |
| Phenacetin: WBC | Negative |
| Acetaminophen: WBC | Negative |
| Phenacetin: Serium bilirubin | Elevated |
| Acetaminophen: Serum Bilirubin | Elevated |
| Phenacetin: Blood Glucose | Decrease (toxic effect) |
| Acetaminophen: Blood Glucose | Decrease (toxic effect) |
| *INDOMETHACIN* | |
| Urine | |
| Glucose (Benedict's) | False Positive |
| RBC | Positive |

smooth endoplasmic reticulum in hepatic cells. Since many of these drugs are, in turn, metabolized in the endoplasmic reticulum, some investigators have suggested by analogy that alcohol may also be metabolized in the smooth endoplasmic reticulum, specifically in the hepatic microsomes. Such a metabolic pathway is considered to be present, in addition to an alcohol dehydrogenase pathway. Supportive evidence for the role of the microsomal enzyme system in alcohol metabolism has been drawn from such findings as the interference with alcohol metabolism by barbiturates. Furthermore, since alcohol seems to induce activity in the microsomal enzyme system, prolonged intake of alcohol may increase the effectiveness of this common drug-detoxifying pathway and therefore enhance the metabolic biotransformation of sedative-hypnotic drugs and tranquilizers. This would account for the observed decrease in clinical response to such drugs in the chronic alcoholic.

Enzyme induction in response to alcohol is apparently under genetic control, possibly polygenic in nature. As a consequence, enzyme induction is quite variable and may be clinically

**TABLE 19-5 (continued)**

**Reported Alterations in Laboratory Test Results of Miscellaneous Analgesics**

| | |
|---|---|
| Serum | |
| Alkaline Phosphatase | Positive |
| Amylase | Positive |
| Bilirubin | Positive |
| BUN | Positive |
| Cephalin flocculation | Positive |
| Glucose, fasting | Positive |
| SGOT | Positive |
| SGPT | Positive |
| Thymol turbidity | Positive |
| RBC or Hb | Negative |
| WBC | Negative |
| *MEFENAMIC ACID* | |
| Urine | |
| Porphyrins | Positive |
| RBC | Positive |
| Bilirubin | Interfere with test |
| Serum | |
| WBC | Negative |
| Thrombocyte | Negative |
| *PHENYRAMIDOL* | |
| Prothrombin Time | Positive |
| Decrease serum cholesterol | Positive |
| *COLCHICINE* | |
| Urine | |
| RBC | Positive |
| Steroids | Interfere with test |
| Serum | |
| Alkaline phosphatase | Positive |
| Thrombocytes | Negative |
| Decrease cholesterol | |
| SALICYLAMIDE | |
| PENTAZOCINE | |
| Serum amylase | Positive |

Taken from E. A. Hartshorn, *Handbook on Drug Interactions*, presented by Ciba, Hamilton Press, Hamilton, Illinois, 1973.

striking in some individuals. While evaluating the metabolic response to chronic alcohol administration, however, one must recognize that concomitant alcohol-induced hepatic damage may inhibit drug detoxification. When evaluating the metabolic response to acute alcohol administration where there has been insufficient time for enzyme induction, one should anticipate the effects of both the alcohol and the sedative-hypnotic drug or tranquilizer. Sedative-hypnotics and tranquilizers have potent additive effects with alcohol *in vivo* and the combinations are the two most common types of direct alcohol–drug interactions. They are most frequently implicated in vehicular accidents as well. Drugs other than sedative-hypnotics and tranquilizers that share the additive depressant effect include phenothiazines, antihistamines, tricyclic antidepressants, and narcotics.

Other direct alcohol–drug interactions of clinical interest include those of ethanol and MAO inhibitors, ethanol and drugs blocking acetaldehyde metabolism, ethanol and fructose, and ethanol and methyl alcohol. Monoamine oxidase inhibitors, such as pargyline (hydrochloride) and tranylcypromine, block the metabolism of catecholamines. Therefore, when an alcoholic beverage high in tyramine is ingested, such as Chianti, the catecholamines released in response to the tyramine cannot be metabolized and an acute hypertensive episode ensues. Some drugs block the metabolism of acetaldehyde, an intermediate in the metabolism of ethyl alcohol, causing its accumulation in the blood. This results in vasodilation, flushing, nausea, vomiting, and hypotension—"the acetaldehyde reaction." Drugs with this effect include disulfiram (used in the aversion therapy of binge-drinking abusers of alcohol) and several other agents, which, although used for other therapeutic indications, nevertheless have the same effect. Among these are metronidazole, furazolidone, procarbazine hydrochloride, quinacrine hydrochloride, tolazamide, and chloramphenicol.

Fructose has been found to enhance the rate of disappearance of alcohol from the blood by as much as 80 percent. This finding has been confirmed repeatedly, although it has not been duplicated by all investigators. Fructose appears to increase elimination of alcohol by rapid transformation of the fructose to D-glyceraldehyde. The glyceraldehyde is then reduced to glycerol by the hepatic alcohol dehydrogenase-reduced nicotinamide adenine dinucleotide (NADH) complex, and the complex, in turn, is converted into alcohol dehydrogenase-nicotinamide adenine dinucleotide (NAD). The final complex is that needed to oxidase more ethanol.

### *b. Indirect Interactions*[40]

The most common alcohol–drug interactions are those in which alcohol potentiates the anticipated pharmacologic effect of another drug. This type of interaction can occur in nonalcoholics, as well as alcoholics. Alcohol causes vasodilation, manifested by a decrease in blood pressure, an increase in pulse rate, and the cutaneous hallmark, the flushed face. As a consequence, alcohol may potentiate the effects of drugs that cause vasodilatation. For example, nitroglycerine, when taken in combination with alcohol, may exhibit enhanced effectiveness, leading, at times, to cardiovascular collapse. Antihypertensive drugs, whose mechanism of action is based either on alterations in the sympathetic nervous system or on direct vasodilation, are potentiated by the simultaneous administration of alcohol. In the clinical setting, this effect may be diagnosed inadvertently as labile hypertensive disease or ascribed to poor drug compliance when, in fact, simultaneous ingestion of alcohol is the underlying cause.

Alcohol affects carbohydrate metabolism in several ways. In brief, in the normal person, ingestion of alcohol causes mild hyperglycemia as a result of catecholamine release. Alcohol also directly inhibits gluconeogenesis, and in the starved alcoholic with depleted hepatic glycogen stores, its ingestion results in prolonged and profound hypoglycemia. The simultaneous use of oral hypoglycemic agents and alcohol may lead to an even more severe hypoglycemic episode. The frequency of glucose intolerance in alcoholics, whether caused by starvation, catechol release, pancreatic destruction, or heritable diabetes, makes the simultaneous ingestion of oral hypoglycemic agents and alcohol a fairly common event and increases the risk of severe or fatal hypoglycemia in the alcoholic population. Preliminary evidence also suggests that alcohol may alter the metabolism of some of the oral hypoglycemic agents and thus further potentiate this effect.

In the chronic alcoholic, alcohol consumption leads to the accumulation of lactate and mild-to-moderate hyperlactacidemia. The accumulation of lactic acid may be potentiated by the simultaneous use of phenformin, which leads to hyperlactacidemia by uncoupling oxidative phosphorylation and results in a severe, occasionally refractory, acidotic state. The lactacidemia also causes secondary hyperuricemia, as a result of direct competition for the renal tubular mechanisms responsible for the secretion of uric acid. The hyperuricemia frequently precipitates clinical gout, which, in turn, necessitates therapy with uricosuric agents or allopurinol. Sulfinpyrazone, a commonly used uricosuric agent, can have significant toxic effects on the bone marrow that are further potentiated by alcohol. Therefore, it should be remembered that the primary mode of therapy for the hyperuricemia of chronic alcohol abuse is abstinence from alcohol, not the use of other pharmacologic agents.

Other selected examples of indirect alcohol–drug interactions include those of alcohol with potent oral diuretics and alcohol with aspirin. Alcohol itself promotes diuresis, but the extent of the diuresis depends on the period of time during which the blood level of alcohol continues to increase. Once the blood alcohol concentration is maintained at a constant level, antidiuresis usually prevails. In the patient who also takes cardiotonic drugs, particularly digitalis preparations and oral diuretics, this initial loss of fluid and electrolytes may be significant and have morbid consequences. Hypokalemia may be an additional serious problem in patients whose only caloric source is an alcoholic beverage free of potassium (such as some cheap wines), who have diarrhea secondary to alcohol abuse or who continue to ingest alcohol and potent oral diuretics, or both.

The gastric irritant effects of both alcohol and aspirin are potentiated when the two agents are combined. Both affect the quality of the gastric mucous barrier and facilitate the back-diffusion of hydrogen into the mucosa. Since both aspirin and alcohol are among the most widely used drugs in modern society, their interactions are common. Other effects of alcohol–aspirin interaction icnlude several phenomena of metabolic significance. The effect of alcohol on the synthesis of vitamin K-dependent clotting factors, whether caused by hepatic damage or malabsorption of vitamin K, may be potentiated by aspirin's direct effect on the synthesis of the same factors, particularly factor VII, or proconvertin. The sequelae of alcohol-induced thrombocytopenia may be potentiated by aspirin's inhibition of platelet aggregation via inhibition of the second-phase release of adenosine diphosphate. The lactiacidemia produced by alcohol may be augmented by aspirin, which uncouples oxidative phosphorylation when ingested in therapeutic doses; the hyperuricemia produced is also potentiated by uric acid retention because of the direct effects of low-dose aspirin on the renal tubules. Several other alcohol–aspirin interactions are possible on a theoretic basis, but have not been shown to occur clinically. Additional interactions are summarized in Tables 19-6 and 19-7, taken from Martin[41] and Becker et al.[40] respectively.

### *c. Disulfiram and Disulfiram-like Reactions*[18,42]

There is a series of very serious toxic reactions between disulfiram and alcohol,[43] which have previously been discussed in Chapter 11.

To reiterate, the combination of this (antibuse) enzyme inhibitor of acetaldehyde dehydrogenase and alcohol results in the following adverse reactions: 1) changes in serum proteins[44] 2) hepatotoxicity[44] 3) hypotension 4) facial warmth 5) headache, and 6) breathlessness.

Other drugs may either increase or decrease the disulfiram/alcohol adverse interaction. For example, the antidepressant amitriptyline enhances, whereas diazepan (Valium) significantly lessens the reaction.[45] Of great interest is the report[28,46,47,48] that such a wide variety of substances (mushrooms, chlorpropamide, carbutamide, furaltadone and furazolidine, car-

## TABLE 19-6
## Alcohol Interactions

| *Primary Agent* | *Interactant* | *Possible Interaction* |
|---|---|---|
| Alcohol | See also CNS DEPRESSANTS | Alcohol induces some enzymes and inhibits others. |
| | Acetohexamide (Dymelor) | Alcohol, an enzyme inducer, inhibits acetohexamide. Patients receiving sulfonylureas (enzyme inhibitors) may experience the "disulfiram reaction" following ingestion of alcohol. See under ANTIDIABETICS, ORAL |
| | Adrenergics | Alcohol enhances adrenergic effects. |
| | Aminopyrine | Aminopyrine increases the toxic effects of alcohol |
| | Amitriptyline (Elavil) | Amitriptyline potentiates alcohol but the combination has no effect on driving skills other than that due to the alcohol itself after the first few days of therapy. Lethal. Contraindicated. See ANTIDEPRESSANTS, TRICYCLIC below. |
| | Amphetamines | See CNS STIMULANTS below |
| | Analgesic Agents | Alcohol potentiates analgesics such as codeine, morphine, propoxyphene, etc. See CNS DEPRESSANTS. Alcohol also potentiates acetaminophen, aspirin and related analgesics. |
| | Anesthetics, General | In patients with enhanced alcohol tolerance, larger amounts of anesthetic are required but alcohol and anesthetics have additive CNS depressant effects. See CNS DEPRESSANTS. |
| | Antabuse | See DISULFIRAM below. |
| | Anticoagulants, Oral (Coumadin, Dicumarol, Panwarfin, Sintrom) | Alcohol adversely affects the liver and patients with liver disease are sensitive to anticoagulants. Therefore, restrict intake of alcohol. Enzyme induction in alcoholics may decrease prothrombin time by inhibiting the anticoagulant but the response is unpredictable and variable. |
| | Antidepressants, tricyclic (Aventyl, Elavil, Norpramin, Pertofrane, Sinequan, Tofranil, etc.) | A lethal combination. Contraindicated. Tricyclic antidepressants potentiate sedation with alcohol: CNS depression and hypothermic coma. The combination adversely affects driving skills during the first few days of therapy. |
| | Antidiabetics, oral (Diabinese, Dymelor, Orinase, etc.) | Alcohol induces metabolism of oral antidiabetics, thus shortening half-life as much as 50% and inducing hyperglycemia. Antidiabetics (sulfonylureas) block alcohol metabolism and produce a disulfiram-like reaction. Angina pectoris from alcohol intolerance may be produced. See also INSULIN below. An antihistamine given an hour before a sulfonylurea alleviates the disulfiram-like symptoms. Excessive amounts of alcohol may produce hypoglycemic convulsions in children. |
| | Antihistamines | Antihistamines potentiate sedation with alcohol; alcohol potentiates the CNS depression caused by the antihistamines. See CNS DEPRESSANTS. |

## TABLE 19-6 (continued)
## Alcohol Interactions

| *Primary Agent* | *Interactant* | *Possible Interaction* |
|---|---|---|
| Alcohol | Antimalarials | Quinacrine, by inhibiting acetaldehyde oxidation, produces a disulfiram-like reaction. |
| | Aspirin | See SALICYLATES. |
| | Atabrine | See QUINACRINE below |
| | Ataractic agents | Alcohol potentiates CNS depressant effects in decreasing order: reserpine, chlorpromazine, propoxyphene, morphine, meprobamate, phenaglycodol, codeine, hydroxyzine. |
| | Atarax | See HYDROXYZINE below. |
| | Aventyl | See ANTIDEPRESSANTS, TRICYCLIC above |
| | Barbiturates | Barbiturates, especially rapidly acting ones, potentiate the sedative effects of alcohol; alcohol potentiates barbiturates. A potentially lethal combination. See CNS DEPRESSANTS. The synergistic CNS depressant action of a rapidly acting barbiturate like secobarbital (Seconal) and alcohol has resulted in many deaths. At least, reaction time is decreased and judgement is impaired while confidence in the judgements made is increased. |
| | Benzodiazepines (Librium, Serax, Valium) | Benzodiazepines potentiate the sedative effects of alcohol and decrease tolerance to alcohol and vice-versa. See CNS DEPRESSANTS. |
| | Caffeine | See CNS STIMULANTS below. |
| | Calcium barbimide citrated (Temposil) | Calcium carbimide (cyanamide) has an antialcoholic effect similar to disulfiram in alcoholics. See below. |
| | Carbamazepine (Tegretol) | Carbamazepine, chemically related to the tricyclic antidepressants, may potentiate the sedative effects of the alcohol. The combination with alcohol may be lethal. |
| | Carbon disulfide | Workers exposed to carbon disulfide, thiuram derivatives, etc. in the rubber industry and to n-butyraldoxime in the printing industry experience disulfiram-like reactions. |
| | Carbrital | Alcohol potentiates carbrital. May be a lethal combination. |
| | Carbutamide (Invenol, Nadisan) | A disulfiram-like reaction occurs. |
| | Carisoprodol (Rela, Soma) | This combination may cause decreased judgement, alertness, motor coordination and manual skills. See CNS DEPRESSANTS. |
| | Cartrax | Alcohol may enhance individual sensitivity to the hypotensive effects of PETN in Cartrax with severe responses (nausea, vomiting, collapse, etc.) |
| | Charcoal | Ingestion of animal charcoal produces a disulfiram-like reaction with alcohol. |

## TABLE 19-6 (continued)
## Alcohol Interactions

| *Primary Agent* | *Interactant* | *Possible Interaction* |
|---|---|---|
| Alcohol | Chloral hydrate | Chloral hydrate inhibits the metabolism of alcohol, thus producing a disulfiram-like reaction. Concomitant administration of chloral hydrate and alcohol, both of which are CNS depressants, may significantly potentiate the sedative effects. Respiratory arrest and death may occur with large doses. |
| | Chloramphenicol (Chloromycetin) | Chloramphenicol, by enzyme inhibition, produces a disulfiram-like reaction with alcohol. |
| | Chlordiazepoxide (Librium) | Alcohol potentiates the CNS depressant effects of chlordiazepoxide. See BENZODIAZEPINES above. |
| | Chlorpromazine | Alcohol potentiates the CNS depressant effects of chlorpromazine and vice-versa. The combination interferes with coordination and judgement. |
| | Chlorpropamide (Diabinese) | Intolerance to alcohol (disulfiram-like reaction) has been noted in many patients receiving chlorpropamide, a sulfonylurea (enzyme inhibitor). |
| | Chlorprothixene (Taractan) | Alcohol may potentiate the CNS depressant effects of chlorprothixene, an analog of chlorpromazine, and vice-versa. See CHLORPROMAZINE above and PHENOTHIAZINES, as well as CNS DEPRESSANTS. |
| | CNS Depressants | Alcohol combined with a psychotropic drug such as chlorpromazine, diazepam, phenobarbital, thioridazine, trifluoperazine or a tricyclic antidepressant increases the risk of death by impairing psychomotor skills. |
| | CNS Stimulants | CNS stimulants like the amphetamines and caffeine antagonize the CNS depressant effects of alcohol, except that they do not improve the decreased motor function induced by alcohol. |
| | Codeine | Alcohol potentiates codeine. See CNS DEPRESSANTS and NARCOTIC ANALGESICS. |
| | Compazine | See PHENOTHIAZINES below. |
| | Coumarin Antigoagulants | Alcohol has an unpredictable effect on coumarin anticoagulants. Alcohol, on the one hand, is a metabolizing enzyme inducer which may inhibit the anticoagulants. On the other hand, it may also adversely affect the liver and thereby make patients more sensitive to the drugs. Therefore, restrict intake of alcohol. |
| | Cyanocobalamin | See VITAMIN B below. |
| | Darvon | See PROPOXYPHENE below. |
| | Desipramine (Norpramin, Pertofrane) | The effects of alcohol may be exaggerated by desipramine. See ANTIDEPRESSANTS, TRICYCLIC above. |
| | Dextropropoxyphene | See PROPOXYPHENE below. |
| | Diabinese (Chlorpropamide) | See SULFONYLUREAS below. |

## TABLE 19-6 (continued)
## Alcohol Interactions

| *Primary Agent* | *Interactant* | *Possible Interaction* |
|---|---|---|
| Alcohol | Diazepam (Valium) | Diazepam may produce supra-additive hypotensive effects with alcohol. See BENZODIAZEPINES above. |
| | Diazepine derivatives | See BENZODIAZEPINES above. |
| | Dibenazpines (Elavin, Tofranil, etc.) | Dibenzazepines potentiate sedative effects of alcohol. See ANTIDEPRESSANTS, TRICYCLIC above. |
| | Dimethindene Maleate (Forhistal Maleate) | See ANTIHISTAMINES above. |
| | Diphenylhydantoin (Dilantin) | Alcohol may inhibit the anticonvulsant action of dipenylhydantoin in alcoholics, probably through enzyme induction. |
| | Diphenydramine (Benadryl) | See PHENOTHIAZINES below. |
| | Disulfiram (Antabuse) | Disulfiram, by inhibiting acetaldehyde dehydrogenase, increases acetaldehyde concentration in the blood. Severity of resulting unpleasant reaction varies with the individual and amount of alcohol. NEVER ADMINISTER TO A PATIENT WHEN HE IS IN A STATE OF ALCOHOL INTOXICATION OR WITHOUT HIS FULL KNOWLEDGE. The patient should carry an identification card and his physician should be prepared to institute supportive measures to restore blood pressure and to treat shock. Can be lethal. |
| | Diuretics (Thiazides, Chlorthalidone, Ethacrynic acid, Furosemide, Quinethazone, etc.). | Orthostatic hypotension may occur with these diuretics and it may be potentiated by alcohol. |
| | Doxepine (Sinequan) | See ANTIDEPRESSANTS, TRICYCLIC, above. |
| | Dymelor (Acetohexamide) | See ANTIDIABETICS, ORAL, above. |
| | Elavin (Amitriptylene) | See ANTIDEPRESSANTS, TRICYCLIC, above. |
| | Epinephrine | Alcohol causes increased urinary excretion of epinephrine, norepinephrine and their metabolites. |
| | Ethacrynic acid (Edecrin) | Ethacrynic acid may elevate blood levels of alcohol and potentiate its effects. |
| | Ethchlorvynol (Placidyl) | Potentiation of CNS depressant effects. See CNS DEPRESSANTS. |
| | Ethionamide (Trecator) | Ethionamide may potentiate the psychotoxic effects of alcohol. |
| | Eutonyl (pargyline) | See *MAO inhibitors.* |
| | Flagyl | See *Metronidazole.* |
| | Folic acid antagonists | See *Methotrexate.* |
| | Food | Foods (beer, milk, etc.) retard gastric but not intestinal absorption of alcohol. |

## TABLE 19-6 (continued)
## Alcohol Interactions

| *Primary Agent* | *Interactant* | *Possible Interaction* |
|---|---|---|
| Alcohol | Fructose | Fructose is a very effective compound for increasing the metabolism of ethyl alcohol and lowering blood concentrations. |
| | Furacin (Nitrofurazone) | See NITROFURANS, below. |
| | Furaltadone (Altafur) | Furaltadone, like furazolidone below, produces a disulfiram-like reaction (neurologic symptoms). |
| | Furazolidone (Furoxone) | Furazolidone, a MAO inhibitor, produces a disulfiram-like reaction (neurologic symptoms) and hypertension. Avoid alcohol during therapy and for 4 days after. |
| | Ganglionic blocking agents | Alcohol potentiates the antihypertensive effect. Hypotension. See CNS DEPRESSANTS. |
| | Glutethimide (Doriden) | This combination may enhance the central nervous system depressant effects. See CNS DEPRESSANTS. Proper supportive care (not dialysis) has prevented death in patients taking as much as 40 gm of glutethimide with f fifth of whiskey. |
| | Guanethidine (Ismelin) | Alcohol may aggrevate the orthostatic hypotension that is frequently seen with guanethidine therapy. See CNS DEPRESSANTS. |
| | Haloperidol (Halodol) | Haloperidol, a butyrophenone major tranquilizer, is potentiated by alcohol and is contraindicated in patients severely depressed by alcohol. |
| | Hexylresorcinol | Alcohol reduces the anthelmintic effects. |
| | Hydralazine (Apresoline) | Alcohol potentiates the postural hypotension produced by hydralazine. |
| | Hydrochlorothiazide (Hydrodiuril) | See DIURETICS above. |
| | Hydroxyzine (Atarax, Vistaril) | The CNS depression with hydroxyzine is potentiated by alcohol. See CNS DEPRESSANTS. |
| | Hypnotics | Toxic interaction; depressed cardiac activity, respiratory failure. See CNS DEPRESSANTS. |
| | Imipramine (Tofranil) | Imipramine prolongs alcohol narcosis. See ANTIDEPRESSANTS, TRYCYCLIC, above. |
| | Insulin | Alcohol, with its hypoglycemic effect, potentiates antidiabetics (insulin and oral agents). It may induce severe hypoglycemia in diabetics receiving these drugs and may induce irreversible neurological damage, coma and death. It inhibits glycogenesis and induces hypoglycemia when this mechanism is required to maintain normal glucose levels. It also inhibits the usual rebound of glucose after hypoglycemia.<br>Small amounts of alcohol have been used in the diet to decrease insulin requirements on the theory that alcohol provides energy without requiring insulin for its metabolism. |
| | Iproniazid (Marsilid) | Iproniazid potentiates effects of alcohol. See MAO INHIBITORS, below. |

## TABLE 19-6 (continued)
## Alcohol Interactions

| *Primary Agent* | *Interactant* | *Possible Interaction* |
|---|---|---|
| Alcohol | Isocarboxazid (Marplan) | Isocarboxazid potentiates sedative effects of alcohol. See MAO INHIBITORS, below. |
| | Isoniazid (Niconyl, Nydrazid, etc.) | Alcohol inhibits isoniazid; decreases its half-life by increasing its rate of metabolism. |
| | Levarterenol (Levophed, norepinephrine) | Alcohol increases the urinary excretion of levarterenol and its metabolites and thus inhibits the drug. |
| | MAO Inhibitors | MAO inhibitors potentiate the hypertensive effect of alcoholic beverages that contain pressor principles (beer, some wines, etc.). MAO inhibitors potentiate the CNS depressant effects of alcohol by inhibiting its metabolism and may cause a disulfiram-like reaction. See also TYRAMINE-RICH FOODS. |
| | Mebutamate (Capla) | Mebutamate may enhance the CNS depressant effects of alcohol. See CNS DEPRESSANTS. |
| | Meprobamate (Equanil, Miltown) | Mutual potentiation, when combined with alcohol; enhanced impairment of motor activity, coordination and judgement. Can cause drowsiness, lethargy, stupor, ataxia, coma, shock, vasomotor and respiratory collapse and, in some instances, death with excessive intake. |
| | Methaqualone (Quaalude) | Methaqualone potentiates the effects of alcohol, analgesics, sedatives and psychotherapeutic drugs. See CNS DEPRESSANTS. |
| | Methotrexate | Concomitant use of potentially hepatotoxic drugs like alcohol should be avoided. Respiratory failure and coma have occurred with one cocktail. |
| | Methyldopa (Aldomet) | Alcohol potentiates hypotensive effects. Hypotension may be severe. Also increased CNS depression. Better control of hypertension may be achieved in patients who do not drink tyramine-containing beverages like beer and Chianti wine. |
| | Metronidazole (Flagyl) | Metronidazole slows rate of metabolism of alcohol and produces a disulfiram-like intolerance to alcohol. |
| | Morphine analgesics | Morphine analgesics potentiate sedation with alcohol and they are potentiated by alcohol. Death may occur. |
| | Mushrooms | Mushrooms (COPRINUS ATRAMENTARIUS) cause a disulfiram-like reaction with alcohol. |
| | Muscle Relaxants | Additive effects occur with all centrally acting muscle relaxants; may cause increased CNS depression, respiratory arrest and death. |
| | Nalidixic acid (NegGram) | This combination may diminish alertness, judgement, motor coordination and manual skills. |
| | Nalorphine (Nalline) | Nalorphine may add to the depressant effects of alcohol. |
| | Naloxone (Naroan) | May antagonize depressant extracts or alcohol. |

## TABLE 19-6 (continued)
## Alcohol Interactions

| *Primary Agent* | *Interactant* | *Possible Interaction* |
|---|---|---|
| Alcohol | Narcotic analgesics | Narcotic analgesics prolong the CNS depressive effects of alcohol. |
| | Narcotics | Narcotics potentiate the CNS effects of alcohol; respiratory arrest may occur. |
| | Nifuroxime (Micofur) | Nifuroxime prevents the oxidation of acetaldehyde, a metabolite of alcohol, thereby producing a disulfiram-like reaction if sufficient of the topical agent is absorbed. See MAO INHIBITORS, above. |
| | Nitrates and nitrites | Vasodilating effect of nitrates and nitrites is potentiated by alcohol. May result in severe hypotension and cardiovascular collapse. |
| | Nitrazepam (Mogadon) | Nitrazepam potentiates the CNS depressant effects of alcohol. See CNS DEPRESSANTS. |
| | Nitrofurans (Furazolidone, Nitrofurantoin, Nitrofurazone) | Alcohol is potentiated by some nitrofurans (enzyme inhibitors). Contraindicated. See FURAZOLIDONE, a MAO inhibitor. It prevents the oxidation of acetaldehyde, a metabolite of alcohol, producing a disulfiram (Antabuse)-like reaction. |
| | Nitroglycerin | Severe hypotension when taken with alcohol, due to additive vasodilator effect; may cause cardiovascular collapse. May mistakenly be attributed to coronary insufficiency or occlusion. |
| | Norepinephrine | See LEVARTERENOL. |
| | Norpramin (Desipramine) | See ANTIDEPRESSANTS, TRICYCLIC. |
| | Opiates | See MORPHINE and NARCOTIC ANALGESICS, above. |
| | Orinase (Tolbutamine) | See ANTIDIABETICS, ORAL. |
| | Oxazepam (Serax) | Alcohol may potentiate the psychotropic oxazepam. See BENZODIAZEPINES, above and CNS DEPRESSANTS. |
| | Paraldehyde | This combination produces additive CNS depressant effects. See CNS DEPRESSANTS. |
| | Pargyline (Eutonyl) | Alcohol may induce hypotension (additive effects). Alcoholic beverages containing pressor agents are contraindicated. See TYRAMINE-RICH FOODS. |
| | Pentobarbital | Dual potentiation of CNS depressant effects occurs with alcohol and barbiturates. See BARBITURATES, above. |
| | Pentylenetetrazoe (Metrazol, etc.) | Alcohol suppresses convulsions induced by pentylenetetrazol, but only in amounts that cause general depression of the CNS. This combination is contraindicated. |
| | Phenaglycodol (Ultran) | The tranquilizer, phenaglycodol, is potentiated by alcohol. See CNS DEPRESSANTS. |

## TABLE 19-6 (continued)
## Alcohol Interactions

| *Primary Agent* | *Interactant* | *Possible Interaction* |
|---|---|---|
| Alcohol | Phenelzine (Nardil) | Some alcoholic beverages may precipitate a hypertensive crisis in patients on this drug. See MAO INHIBITORS, above. |
| | Phenformin (DBI) | Alcohol markedly increases the tendency of phenformin to produce lactic acidosis with nausea, vomiting, etc. |
| | Phenobarbital | Alcohol and phenobarbital mutually potentiate the CNS depressant effects. See BARBITURATES, above. |
| | Phenothiazines (Chlorpromazine, etc.) | Phenothiazines potentiate the CNS depressant effects of alcohol and vice-versa. Impaired psychomotor function. Alcohol blocks parkinsonism effects of phenothiazines. See CNS DEPRESSANTS. Some phenothiazines may inhibit the metabolism of alcohol. |
| | Procarbazine (Matulane) | Procarbazine may produce a disulfiram-like reaction with alcohol due to enzyme inhibition. |
| | Prochlorperazine (Compazine) | Prochlorperazine potentiates the CNS depressant effects of alcohol. See PHENOTHIAZINES, above. |
| | Promazine (Sparine) | Promazine potentiates the CNS depressant effects of alcohol. See PHENOTHIAZINES, above. |
| | Propoxyphene (Darvon) | Alcohol potentiates propoxyphene. See CNS DEPRESSANTS. |
| | Psychotropic drugs | Some psychotropic drugs may inhibit the metabolism of alcohol and thus potentiate its effects. See CNS DEPRESSANTS. |
| | Quinacrine (Atabrine, mepacrine) | Quinacrine, by inhibiting the oxidation of acetaldehyde, a metabolite of alcohol, produces a disulfiram-like reaction. |
| | Reserpine and derivatives | Reserpine and derivatives potentiate the sedative effects of alcohol. Reserpine is potentiated by alcohol. See CNS DEPRESSANTS. |
| | Salicylates (Aspirin, etc.) | Salicylates (aspirin, etc.) given with alcohol increases the probability of gastric hemorrhage. Salicylate buffering reduces the probability of the occurrence of this interaction. |
| | Sedatives and hypnotics (Barbiturates, bromides, chloral hydrate, paraldehyde, etc.) | Serious impairment of coordination may occur. Addiction, as well as tolerance, may develop. Cross-tolerance develops to sedative effects but not to the respiratory depressant effects. Thus, dangerous overdosage can easily occur. Possibly fatal. See CNS DEPRESSANTS. |
| | Sparine | See PHENOTHIAZINES. |
| | Stelazine | See PHENOTHIAZINES. |
| | Sulfonamides | Sulfonamides potentiate the psychotoxic effects of alcohol by inhibiting oxication of acetaldehyde (disulfiram-like reaction). |

## TABLE 19-6 (continued)
## Alcohol Interactions

| *Primary Agent* | *Interactant* | *Possible Interaction* |
|---|---|---|
| | Sulfonylurea hypoglycemics | See ANTIDIABETICS, ORAL, above in this Section. |
| | Temposil | See CALCIUM CARBIMIDE CITRATED, above. |
| | TETE (Tetraethylthiuram disulfide, Antabuse, disulfiram) | See DISULFIRAM, above. |
| | Tetrachloroethylene | Tetrachloroethylene can cause symptoms of inebriation; alcohol may enhance these effects and should not be ingested 24 hours before or after use of tetrachloroethylene. |
| | Tetracyclines | Tetracyclines Alcohol potentiates. |
| | Thiazide diuretics | Alcohol may potentiate the orthostatic hypotension caused by thiazide diuretics. |
| | Thioridazine (Mellaril) | Thioridazine potentiates the CNS depressant effects of alcohol. |
| | Thioxanthenes | Administration of thioxanthenes during alcohol withdrawal may lower the convulsive threshold. Caution is necessary. |
| | Thorazine (Chlorpromazine) | See PHENOTHIAZINES. |
| | Tofranil (Imipramine) | See ANTIDEPRESSANTS, TRICYCLIC. |
| | Tolazamide (Tolinase) | See ANTIDIABETICS, ORAL, above. |
| | Tolazoline (Priscoline) | Tolazoline, by preventing the oxidation of acetaldehyde, a metabolite of alcohol, produces a disulfiram-like effect. |
| | Tolbutamide (Orinase) | Tolbutamide, by enzyme inhibition, potentiates alcohol (disulfiram-like reaction). See ANTIDIABETICS, ORAL. The half-life of tolbutamide is reduced more than 2-fold in alcoholics through microsomal enzyme induction by alcohol. Effectiveness may be considerably reduced in diabetics who consume alcohol. |
| | Tranquilizers, minor | Tranquilizers may potentiate the CNS depressant effects (additive depression and secation). Severe hypotension may occur; also deep sedation. See CNS DEPRESSANTS. |
| | Tranylcypromine (Parnate) | Tranycypromine may potentiate the sedative effects of alcohol. See MAO INHIBITORS, above. |
| | Tricyclic Antidepressants | See ANTIDEPRESSANTS, TRICYCLIC, above. |
| | Urea derivatives | See BARBITURATES and CNS DEPRESSANTS (bromisovalum and carbromal). |
| | Vitamin $B_{12}$ | Alcohol causes malabsorption of Vitamin $B_{12}$. |

Taken from Martin, E. W. *Hazards of Medication*, J. B. Lippincott Company, Philadelphia, pg. 430-439, 1971.

## TABLE 19-7

## A Summary of Selected Alcohol–Drug Interactions

| Drug | Comment |
|---|---|
| *Alcohol-sensitizing agents* | |
| Disulfiram (Antabuse)<br>Calcium cyanamide citrated (Temposil) | Blockade of the metabolism of alcohol results in flushing of face, dyspnea, hypotention, tachycardia, nausea, and vomiting. Felt to be due to accumulation of acetaldehyde. |
| *Analgesics* | |
| Aspirin | See text. |
| D-Propoxyphene (Darvon) | Potentiation of CNS depressant effect of alcohol. |
| Opiates | Potentiation of CNS depressant effect of alcohol. |
| *Anticoagulants* | |
| Warfarin (Coumadin) | Half-life of warfarin decreased by chronic use of alcohol; however, anticoagulant effect may be enhanced in the presence of liver disease. Occasional moderate doses of ethanol unlikely to interfere with warfarin therapy in patients with normal liver function. |
| *Anticonvulsants* | |
| Diphenylhydantoin (Dilantin) | Half-life decreased with chronic ingestion of large doses of alcohol due to induction of microsomal enzymes. |
| *Phenobarbital* | See *Sedative-hypnotics* |
| *Antidepressants* | |
| Amitriptyline (Elavil)<br>Imipramine (Tofranil)<br>Nortriptylene (Aventyl)<br>Doxepin (Sinequan) | Potentiation of the CNS effects of alcohol. Deaths have been reported with tricyclics such as amitriptyline. |
| *Monoamine oxidase inhibitors* | Hypertensive crisis precipitated by alcoholic beverages containing tyramine. Potentiation of the CNS effect of alcohol. |
| *Antihistamines* | Potentiation of CNS depressant effect of alcohol. Sedation and decreased psychomotor performance. |
| *Antihypertensives* | |
| Guanethidine (Ismelin)<br>Hydralazine (Apresoline)<br>Methyldopa (Aldomet)<br>Rauwolfia alkaloids | Alcohol potentiates the postural hypotensive effects. |
| *Anti-infective agents* | |
| Chloramphenicol (Chloromycetin) | Disulfiram-like reaction. |
| Ethionamide (Trecator) | Psychologic abnormalities reported when use associated with heavy alcohol consumption. |
| Griseofulvin (Fulvicin, Grifulvin) | Possible disulfiram-like reaction. |
| Isoniazid (INH) | Chronic alcohol abuse may enhance metabolism. |
| Metronidazol (Flagyl) | Mild disulfiram-like effect. |
| Quinacrine (Atabrine) | Disulfiram-like effect. |

## TABLE 19-7 (continued)
## A Summary of Selected Alcohol–Drug Interactions

| *Drug* | *Comment* |
|---|---|
| Sulfonamides | May cause mild potentiation of CNS depressant effects of alcohol. |
| Tetrachloroethylene (perchlorethylene) | Potentiation of CNS depressant effects of alcohol. |
| *Antipsychotic agents* | |
| Chlorpromazine (Thorazine) | Potentiation of CNS depressant effects of alcohol. Significant impairment of psychomotor function. All phenothiazines have some potential. |
| Hydroxyzine (Atarax, Vistaril) | Possible potentiation of CNS depressant effects of alcohol. |
| *CNS stimulants* | |
| Amphetamine (Dexedrine)<br>Caffeine | No significant or constant antagonism of CNS depressant effect with alcohol. |
| *Hypoglycemic agents* | |
| Sulfonylurea drugs<br>Tolbutamide (Orinase)<br>Chlorpropamide (Diabinese)<br>Acetohexamide (Dymelor)<br>Tolazamide (Tolinase) | Alcohol causes potentiation of hypoglycemic effect. May also see disulfiram-like effect, particularly with chlorpropamide and tolbutamide. |
| Phenformin (DBI | Potentiation of the hyperlactiacidemia caused by chronic alcohol abuse. |
| *Sedative-hypnotics* | |
| Barbiturates | Additive effects with enhanced sedation, respiratory depression, and, occasionally, death. |
| Chloral hydrate (Noctec)<br>Ethchlorvynol (Placidyl)<br>Glutethimide (Doriden)<br>Meprobamate (Equanil, Miltown)<br>Methyprylon (Noludar)<br>Benzodiazepines (Valium, Librium, Dalmane) | All potentiate the CNS depressant effects of alcohol. Impair psychomotor function. Additive effect may be fatal. |
| *Sympatholytic drugs* | |
| Alpha-adrenergic blocker<br>Phenotolamine (Regitene) | Disulfiram-like effect. |
| *Vasodilators* | |
| Nitroglycerin | Alcohol potentiates hypotension; may cause cardiovascular collapse. |

(From Becker, C., Roe, R. L., and Scott, R. A. *Alcohol as a Drug: A Curriculum on Pharmacology, Neurology and Toxicology*, Medcom Press, New York, 1974, pp. 23–25.)

bazine and metronidazole) produce disulfiram-like reactions in combination with alcohol. Approximately, 10-20% of diabetic patients experience disulfiram-like reactions following treatment with sulfonylurea.[49] However, one of the hypoglycemic agents, tolbutamide, did not induce a reaction with alcohol.

*d. Miscellaneous Drugs*[18]

It is well documented that alcohol lowers glucose in diabetic patients and, furthermore, potentiates the hypoglycemic agents in their actions.[50-52] There are reports of phenformin-alcohol interactions resulting in severe abdominal pain, hyperkalemia, hypothermia, and acidosis, as well as increased lactate levels.[53,54]

there are a series of toxic reactions which have been noted when these miscellaneous drugs are taken in combination with alcohol. A partial list in included herein:

1) Nitroglycerin resulted in hypotension and cerebral vascular collapse[55] with alcohol.

2) Sulfonamides induce noxious effects[56] with alcohol.

3) With alcohol, isoniazid caused death due to pyridoxine deficiency and disturbances in tryptophan metabolism.[57]

4) Anticoagulants could enhance alcohol-induced changes in the clotting mechanism[58] and should be avoided with alcohol consumption.

5) Aspirin could intensify gastrointestinal irratation induced by alcohol.[59,60]

6) Ethionamide in combination with alcohol could produce psychotic reactions.[61]

7) Amphetamine and alcohol could result in unpredictable reactions.[62]

8) Alcohol alters folate metabolism.[64]

*e. Alcohol and Other CNS Depressants*

Alcohol and central nervous system depressants potentiate each other's depressive actions. Chronic abuse of alcohol induces a microsomal enzyme which reduces the half-life of a number of drugs such as diphenylhydantoin (anticonvulsant), warfarin (anticoagulant), and tolbutamide (oral hypoglycemic). Acute large amounts of alcohol even in alcoholics may result in enhanced absorption of sedatives and thereby augment acute potential depression.

## 3. Monoamine Oxidase Inhibitors[42]

Treatment practitioners in the substance abuse area are becoming more familiar with the use of psychotherapeutic agents, especially the antidepressants, since methadone, heroin, and amphetamine all produce postdrug depression.[65] Since drug-induced depression is treated with MAO inhibitors, attention is given to interactions of this drug class.

Monoamine oxidase is an endogenous enzyme that converts monoamine compounds into acids (—C—$NH_2$—COOH) by oxidative deamination. The enzyme is most commonly known for its ability to metabolize norepinephrine to its inactive metabolite, 3,4-dihydroxymandelic acid. The presence of MAO in the gut is important in preventing absorption of pharmacologically active substances found in foods.

Neurotransmitters, such as 5-hydroxytryptamine (serontonin, 5-HT), dopamine and norepinephrine are elevated in tissues following MAOI therapy for depression, among other clinical uses. MAOI's also inhibit liver microsomal enzymes. All enzyme deactivation effects by MAOI's terminate only after enzyme regeneration, which usually takes weeks. An example of a toxic effect of MAOI's is their blood-pressure-lowering action.

In terms of the pharmacodynamics of MAOI's, which has been detailed in Chapter 14, they are readily absorbed from the GI tract, and their urinary excretion is pH-dependent.[67]

The MAOI's include numerous agents with a variety of therapeutic actions as well as chemical structures. A partial list includes: antidepressants (tranylcypromine, phenelzine, isocarboxazid and nialamide); the antihypertensive, pargyline; the anti-infective, furazolidone; and the antineoplastic, procarbazine; sympathominetics, and amphetamines.[68,69] These MAOI's will increase sensitivty to the pressor effects of tyramine and will also augment tryptamine excretion.[70,71]

### a. Interactions of MAO Inhibitors and Foods

To understand the associated problems with MAOI's and certain foodstuff, a brief review of the neuroanatomy of the GI tract will be presented.

MAO, the enzyme, is found in the walls of the intestine as well as in the adrenergic nerve endings to destroy or inactivate norepinephrine. Normally when an individual ingests various foods, especially those containing the amino acid tyramine without the presence of MAOI's, no adverse effects are noticed. However, because tyramine causes a displacement or norepinephrine—a substance known to produce increases in blood pressure, which is, as mentioned above, inactivated by MAO—the lack of this enzyme by MAOI's results in a hypertensive reaction.

There are both animal as well as human experiments which confirm the associated adverse reactions of the cheese-MAOI interaction. In humans tyramine content was confirmed in cases suspected of this interaction. Its metabolite p-hydroxyphenyl-acetic acid was found in high quantities in the urine of these patients showing toxicity. Experiments in animals confirm this finding.[72-76]

Specifically involved in such reactions have been the MAO inhibitors tranylcypromine, phenelzine, and pargyline. Specific cheeses identified include New York State cheddar and Gruyere.[77,78] Provolone and Roquefort caused no reaction in one patient who reacted to New York sharp Cheddar.[77] A summary of the interactions of MAO inhibitors with food is presented in Table 19-8.

Goldberg[79] points out that although substantial quantities of tyramine are found in certain beers, no cases of adverse reactions involving beer have been reported.

It is noteworthy that as little as 20 grams of cheese produced a pressor response in an MAO-inhibitor-treated patient.[80] Horwitz and coworkers and Blackwell and Mabbitt assayed various foods for their tyramine content.[75,76,78] Their data are presented in Table 19-9.

### b. Mechanism of MAO Inhibition and Drug Interaction

Any drug which can significantly alter neurotransmitter functions would be a good candidate for adverse reactions with MAOI's. The drug types involved are as follows: 1) indirect-acting sympathomimetic amines act by causing norepinephrine release[81] 2) drugs which may have their inactivation altered by MAOI's, and 3) other drugs which are metabolized by microsomal enzymes which are inhibited by

MAOI's.[82] Interestingly, exogenously administered norepinephrine and epinephrine are metabolized by peripheral catechol-O-methyltransferase (COMT) and are not potentiated by MAOI's, but there are reports of hypersensitivity.[84] See Table 19-10 for a list of drug interactions on MAOI's.

(1) *MAOI's and Tricyclic Antidepressants*

There are serious toxic effects which result from the combination of MAOI's and various tricyclic antidepressants. A list of observed effects include: a) excitation b) delirium c) blurred vision d) hyperpyrexia e) paranoia f) delusions g) diarrhea h) sweating i) convulsions j) motor hyperactivity k) hyperthermia l) diorientation m) alternate hypertension and hypotension n) acute brain syndrome o) headache, and p) coma.

Drug combinations reported include: 1) amintriptyline-furazolidone-diphenoxylate[85] 2) tranylcypromine-imipramine[86,89,90,92] 3) imipramine-phenelzine[87,88] 4) imipramine-pargyline[91] 5) desimipramine-phenelzine[93] 6) phenelzine, isocarboxazid or iproniazid-amitriptyline, nortriptyline, or imipramine.[94]

(2) *Drepressants and MAOI's*

According to Hartshorn,[18] the combination of MAOI's and certain CNS-depressing drugs, such as meperidine, produce toxic reactions, including hyperpyrexia, restlessness and muscle twitching as reported by an anonymous source which appeared in 1969 in the pestigious *British Medical Journal*.[95] Certain durgs such as barbiturates, acetanilid, amphetamine (which is not a depressant), and aminopyrine, are more toxic when administered with an MAOI due to liver metabolism of the above drugs and respective inhibition by MAOI's. Liver disease would contribute significantly to potentiation of drug effects, especially when they are combined with MAOI's.[96]

Animal studies[98] found that MAOI's and d- and l-amphetamine and SKF-525A were competitive inhibitors of N-demethylation of narcotics, whereas pargyline and tranylcypromine were noncompetetive inhibitors.

## 4. Tricyclic Antidepressants

Replacement of the sulfur in the phenothiazine molecule with an ethylene linkage results in a compound that is ineffective in quieting agitated psychotic patients but apparently is of benefit in certain depressed patients. Such compounds are termed the *tricyclic antidepressants*.

The tricyclics are well-absorbed from the GI tract; excretion is rapid, in comparison with their long latency of onset of action. The tricyclics are excreted primarily in the urine as N-oxides or as unconjugated or conjugated hydroxyl derivatives. Approximately 70 percent of a dose is excreted in the first 72 hours. Desmethylimipramine metabolism has been studied. It is hydroxylated and extensively bound to plasma protein. It is claimed to be a powerful inhibitor of hydroxylating enzymes.[85]

Administration of the tricyclics causes feelings of fatigue accompanied by atropine-like symptoms (dryness of mouth, palpitation, blurred vision, urinary retention). On the cardiovascular system, the tricyclic antidepressants obtund various reflexes; orthostatic hypotension is commonly observed with therapeutic doses. The mechanisms whereby tricyclic antidepressants produce their effect is still not known; however, it has been shown that these agents block uptake of administered norepinephrine into the adrenergic neuron storage sites. Potentiation of the effect of norepinephrine has been demonstrated both *in vitro* and *in vivo* in animal studies.[99,100]

### *a. Interactions of the Tricyclics with Drugs*

A summary of interactions for tricyclics is presented in Table 19-10.

## TABLE 19-8

### Drug Interactions of Monoamine Oxidase Inhibitors

| *Antidepressant* | *Interacts with* | *To Cause* | *Reason* |
|---|---|---|---|
| *MAO Inhibitors* | *Sympathomimetic Amines* | | |
| Phenylezine, tranylcypromine | Ephedrine Phenylephrine | Increased blood pressure | Displacement of norepinephrine |
| Nialamide | Ephedrine | Subarachnoid hemorrhage | Same |
| Pargyline | Metaraminol | Increased blood pressure | Same |
| Tranylcypromine | d-Amphetamine—amobarbital | Agitation, convulsions | Same |
| Phenelzine | d-Amphetamine | Cerebral hemorrhage, death | Same |
| Iproniazid | Levarterenol | Myocardial injury | Unusual sensitivity to levarternol |
| Furazolidone | Tyramine | amphetamine | Sensitivity to drugs, increased urinary excretion of tryptamine |
| Phenelzine | Amphetamine, methamphetamine, meperidine | Potentiated drug effect (animal) | Displacement of norepinephrine |
| Debrisoquine | Phenylephrine | Hypertensive response | Same |
| Tranylcypromine | Phenylpropanolamine; cough syrup with phenylpropanolamine | Rapid rise in blood pressure | Same |
| Pargyline | Nasal decongestant containing phenylephrine | Hypertensive syndrome | Same |

**TABLE 19-8 (continued)**

**Drug Interactions of Monoamine Oxidase Inhibitors**

| *Antidepressant* | *Interacts with* | *To Cause* | *Reason* |
|---|---|---|---|
| Tranylcypromine | Phenylephrine | Increased blood pressure | Same |
| Phenelezine | "Mucron" (contains phenylpropanolamine) | Subarachnoid hemorrhage | Same |
| MAO inhibitor | "Procal" (contains phenylpropanolamine and isopropamide) | Severe reaction | Same |
| Phenelzine | "Romilar CF" (contains d-methorphan, phenylephrine) | Fatal adrenergic crisis | Same |
| *MAO Inhibitors* | *Tricyclics* | | |
| Furazolidone | Amitriptyline plus diphenoxylate | Blurred vision, sweating, delusions | Additive inhibition of metabolism of norepinephrine |
| Tranylcypromine | Imipramine | Rectal temperature of 107°F | Same |
| Phenelzine | Imipramine | Death | Same |
| Phenelzine | Amitriptyline (overdose) | Disorientation, hyper- and hypotension, hyperpyrexia | Same |
| Tranylcypromine | Imipramine | Comatose, seizures, death (two patients; one overdose) | Same |
| Pargyline | Imipramine (one 25-mg dose) | Acute brain syndrome | Same |
| Tranylcypromine | Imipramine (one tablet) | Headache, hyperpyrexia, coma, convulsions | Same |

**TABLE 19-8 (continued)**

**Drug Interactions of Monoamine Oxidase Inhibitors**

| *Antidepressant* | *Interacts with* | *To Cause* | *Reason* |
|---|---|---|---|
| *MAO Inhibitor* | *CNS Depressants* | | |
| Iproniazid | Barbiturates, amphetamine, aminopyrine, acetanilid | Increased effect of drugs | Microsomal enzyme inhibition by MAO inhibitor |
| Phenelzine, iproniazid, pargyline, tranylcypromine | Meperidine | Potentiated meperidine | Inhibits hydrolysis and N-demethylation of meperidine |
| MAO inhibitor | Meperidine | Respiratory depression, restlessness | Same |
| MAO inhibitor | Meperidine (mice) | Potentiated meperidine | |
| Phenelzine | Meperidine, morphine | Restlessness, hyperpyrexia, death | |
| Iproniazid | Meperidine | Cerebral excitement, restlessness, semiconsciousness (three patients) | |
| Pargyline | Meperidine | Comatose (one), hypotensive (one) | Microsomal inhibition |
| Nialamide | "Pethilorfan" (meperidine + levallorphan) | Deep sleep, coma, circulatory failure | Same |
| Phenelzine | Droperidol | Hypotension | Same |
| Phenelzine | Dextromethorphan | Toxic rigidity, hyperpyrexia, death | |
| Tranylcypromine | Amobarbital | Ataxia, headache, comatose (human) | Potentiates effect of barbiturates (animal) |

**TABLE 19-8 (continued)**

**Drug Interactions of Monoamine Oxidase Inhibitors**

| *Antidepressant* | *Interacts with* | *To Cause* | *Reason* |
|---|---|---|---|
| MAO inhibitor | Alcohol | Intensified CNS depression | |
| MAO inhibitor | Alcohol/disulfiram | Intensified disulfiram reaction | |
| MAO inhibitor | Other Drugs | | |
| Phenelzine | Levodopa | Increased blood pressure (two cases) | Increases in plasma catecholamines |
| Pargyline | Methyldopa | Hallucinations | Increase free cerebral catecholamines |
| Nialamide | Nitroman (reserpine-like) | Epileptiform attack, collapse | Rauwolfia releases bound serotonin; nialamide inhibits destruction |
| Nialamide | Guanethidine | Reverse hypotensive effect | MAO inhibitors displace guanethidine from binding site (human, animal) |
| Phenelzine, tranylcypromine | Guanethidine | Reverse hypotensive effect (animal data) | Same |
| Tranylcypromine | Ammonium chloride<br>Sodium bicarbonate | Excretion of tranylcypromine<br>Excretion | Effect of pH on ionization of weak base |
| Mebanazine, pheniprazine | Chlorpropamide<br>Tolbutamide | Hypoglycemia | |

**TABLE 19-8 (continued)**

**Drug Interactions of Monoamine Oxidase Inhibitors**

| *Antidepressant* | *Interacts with* | *To Cause* | *Reason* |
|---|---|---|---|
| Tranylcypromine, phenelzine | Cheese, especially N.Y. State Cheddar, Gũyere | Hypertensive reactions | Tyramine in food causes release of norepinephrine; inhibition of MAO permits supersensitivity reaction |
| Phenelzine | Beef liver | Hypertensive reaction | Same |
| Tranylcypromine | Chicken liver | Hypertensive reaction | Same |
| Tranylcypromine, phenelzine | Marmite (yeast) | Hypertensive reaction, intracranial hemorrhage | Same |
| MAO inhibitor | Stewed green bananas | Hypertensive reaction | Same |
| Tranylcypromine | Pickled herring | Increased blood pressure, palpitation, precordial pain | Same |
| Pargyline | Cheddar cheese | Hypertensive reaction (four patients) | Same |
| Debrisoquine | Gũyere cheese | Increased blood pressure | Same |
| Amphetamine | Tyramine | Increased blood pressure (animals) | Same |
| Procabazine | Seasoned cheese | Itchy papular skin eruption | |
| Pargyline | Broad beans | Hypertension, headache, palpitation (three patients) | Broad beans contain dopamine, precursor of norepinephrine |

(From Hartshorn, E. A. *Handbook of Drug Interactions* presented by CIBA. Hamilton Press, Hamilton, Ill., 1973.)

(1) *Alcohol*: Animal investigations reveal that tricyclic antidepressants, such as amitriptyline, potentiate the effects of alcohol, especially with regard to motor skills.[101-103] Studies on the effect of amitriptyline and alcohol/disulfiram combinations produced controversial results; one group argues for direct potentiation of the resultant adverse reactions,[104] whereas another group provides evidence for an indirect interaction.[105]

(2) *Psychotropic Drugs*: Drug-drug interactions of the anxiolytic-anti-depressant agents are well known.[106-107] The combination of chlordiazepofide (Librium) and amitriptyline induce a form of intoxication which makes the patient appear drunk.

Adverse reaction have occurred with tricyclic antidepressants and phenothiazines. Phenothiazines inhibit the metabolism of imipramine and nortriptyline. Haloperidol, as well as perphenazine and chlorpromazine (but not flupenthioxol) inhibit the metabolism of tricyclic compounds and especially enhance their anticholinergic action. In this regard, it was reported that even death resulted from the tricyclic-phenothiazine or butryophenone combination.[109]

The combination reported resulting in serious reactions primarily due to anticholinergic [110,111] actions are as follows: 1) imipramine-chlorpromazine 2) imipramine-thioridazine-trihexyphenidyl (an anticholinergic) 3) imipramine-diphenydramines-trihexyphendyl, and 4) imipramine-thioridazine.

(3) *Procaine*: Profound sedative properties of intravenously administered amitriptyline has a potentiating effect on procaine.[112]

## 4. Drug Interactions of Tricyclic Antidepressants

The basic pharmacology, biochemistry, pharmacodynamics and therapeutic uses of the

**TABLE 19-9**
**Tyramine Content of Foods**

| *Cheese* | *Tyramine Content* | *Other Food* | *Tyramine Content,* μg/ or ml* |
|---|---|---|---|
| English Cheddar | 0–953 | Yeast | ND |
| Canadian Cheddar | 231–535 | Yogurt | ND |
| New Zealand Cheddar | 471–500 | Beer A | 1.8 |
| Kraft, Cheshire | ND | Beer B | 2.3 |
| Camembert | 86 | Beer C | 4.4 |
| Stilton | 466 | Wines: | |
| Brie | 180 | Sherry | 3.6 |
| Ementaler | 225 | Sauterne | 0.4 |
| New York State Cheddar | 1416 | Reisling | 0.6 |
| Gruyere | 516 | Chianti | 25.4 |
| Processed American | ND | Port | ND |

*ND = Not demonstrable

(From Hartshorn, E. A. *Handbook of Drug Interactions.* CIBA. Hamilton Press, Hamilton, Ill., 1973.)

tricyclic antidepressants have been detailed in Chapter 14 of this book.

The fact that tricyclic antidepressants inhibit the biogenetic amine uptake pump into neurons provides the basis for its potentiation of neurotransmitters such as norepinephrine.[99,100]

A summary of interactions for tricyclics is presented in Table 19-10.

### 5. Stimulants

CNS stimulatns have been discussed in Chapter 12 in terms of their pharmacological as well as pharmacodynamic properties. Additional information on this topic is found in the drug interaction book by Hartshorn.[18]

A combination of amphetamine and ganglionic blockers of the guanethidine-type result in hypertension.[113-115] Bretylium, a guanethidine-like drug, is displaced by amphetamine.[116]

#### *a. Amphetamine*

Alcohol combination effects have already been discussed, especially the unpredicatble effects.[117]

#### *b. Caffeine*

Caffeine—Sodium benzoate is known to displace bilirubin and produces in premature infants a condition known as Kernicterus. Caffeine combinations with sodium benzoate may result in this bilirubin-albumin reaction. Sodium benzoate as well as benzoic acid as buffers with diazepam may cause this bilirubin-albumin effect, especially in heavy coffee drinkes.[121,123]

#### *c. Methyplhenidate*

Methylphenidate is a central stimulant with a similar drug-interaction profile of amphetamine. The drug inhibits microsomal enzyme activity, thereby prolonging the half-life of primidone, ethyl-bis-coumacetate and phenobarbital.[118] Clinical studies which support the positive effects of methylphenidate and tricyclic compounds have shown that the combination of imipramine-methylphenidate resulted in an enhanced therapeutic efficacy in refractive depressed patients.[119] Other studies show no change in metabolism of drugs with methylphenidate.[120]

#### *d. Anorexiants*

Rand and Day[123] indicate that certain amphetamine-like drugs, such as diethylpropion, an anorexiant, also interacts with guanethidien and produces hypotensive effects.

## E. DRUGS AND DRIVING[122]

In April 1982, President Ronald Reagan and the White House Office of Drug Abuse Policy decided to initiate a strong official policy concerning "drugs and driving." Certainly every person has a right to know when a drug can influence driving. Furthermore drivers have a right to drive safely without interactions with motorists with impaired judgment as a result of taking drugs. A group called MADD (Mothers Against Drunk Drivers) pushed certain states, such as California, to initiate harsh penalties (see Chapter II on alcohol-related problems) for these offenders.

**TABLE 19-10**

**Drug Interactions of Tricyclic Antidepressants**

| *Antidepressant* | *Interacts with* | *To Cause* | *Reason* |
|---|---|---|---|
| Imipramine desipramine, protriptyline | Norepinephrine | Supersensitization (increased blood pressure) | |
| Amitriptyline | Alcohol | Death (human) potentiation confirmed in animal data | Effect of alcohol potentiated |
| Amitriptyline | Alcohol | Impairment of motor skills | |
| Amitriptyline | Alcohol/disulfiram | Enhanced deterrent effect; does not enhance effect | |
| Imipramine | Guanethidine | Fatal cardiac standstill | Guanethidine depletes cardiac norepinephrine stores |
| Imipramine, desipramine, amitriptyline, protriptyline, nortriptyline | Guanethidine | Loss of blood pressure (confirmed in animal data, reference) | Tricyclic blocks pharmacologic effects of guanethidine |
| Imipramine, amitriptyline | Tri-iodothyronine | Faster response to antidepressant therapy | Increased receptor sensitivity |
| Amitriptyline | Chlordiazepoxide | Weakness, drowsiness, slurred speech, drunken appearance | Potentiates effect of chlordiazepoxide |
| Imipramine, nortriptyline | Perphenazine, haloperidol, chlorpromazine (but *not* flupenthioxol) | Excretion and plasma levels of metabolites; plasma level nortriptyline | Tranquilizers inhibit metabolism of tricyclics |

**TABLE 19-10 (continued)**

**Drug Interactions of Tricyclic Antidepressants**

| *Antidepressant* | *Interacts with* | *To Cause* | *Reason* |
|---|---|---|---|
| Imipramine | Chlorpromazine trihexyphenidyl, diphenhydramine | Excessive anticholinergic effect—dryness of mouth, dental caries, adynamic ileus (three deaths) | Additive anticholinergic effect |
| Imipramine | Thioridazine | Over sedation, rigidity, fast pulse | |
| Nortriptyline | Dicumarol | Prolonged half-life of dicumarol | Reduced rate of drug metabolism |
| Imipramine | Methylphenidate | Improvement of depression | Methylphenidate inhibits enzyme metabolism, increases blood level of tricyclic |
| Amitriptyline | Methyldopa | Agitation, fine tremors | |
| Amitriptyline | Procaine | Potentiation of procaine | "Depressant effect" |
| Imipramine | Ammonium chloride | Increased excretion of imipramine | pH effect on ionization of weak base |

(From Hartshorn, E. A. *Handbook of Drug Interactions.* CIBA. Hamilton Press, Hamilton, Ill., 1973.)

Traffic safety can be affected not only by alcohol, but also by preparations that can be obtained from a pharmacy without restrictions or even in a supermarket, and by some medicines prescribed by a physician.

It is unfortunate that the development of so many new drugs has made it difficult for the clinical practicioner to keep abreast of all of the research findings relevant to the use and abuse of drugs. In addition, the acceptance of large numbers of new drugs and mixtures by doctors and the public has led to the widespread use of more preparations than can be adequately tested. Sufficient information is available, however, to show that a doctor who has not issued the appropriate warnings to a patient later involved in an accident may face a civil action for negligence.

Milner[124] points out that drug effects represent a complex interaction between the chemical agent, the individual patient, and the environment in which the drug is taken. The environment for the majority of adults includes the frequent use of alcohol and the control of complex modern machinery, particularly the motor vehicle. When prescribing a drug, it is necessary to remember that this complex interaction is not constant, but involves an ever-changing psychologic, physiologic, and environmental pattern. Inherent drug variables often affect driving behavior less than variables related to the patient, such as the patient's personality traits, history of traffic code violations, criminal record, drinking and driving habits, and social circumstances.

Some traffic accidents may connote an adverse drug reaction. Because this reaction may be the result of the interplay of two drugs or environmental factors, inevitably associated with the patient's way of life, care in prescribing polydrugs is encouraged.

Polypharmacy is especially dangerous for motorists because of the difficulties in predicting the effects of drug combinations. Two drugs may be pharmacologically antagonistic, add to each other's activity, or unveil an unpredictable reaction. Their interaction will not be consistent, depending as it does on such factors as the relative times of taking the drugs, modifications of absorption rates by other drugs,[125] diet or disease, protein binding, and alteration of liver enzyme processes,[126,127] which will influence the rates of metabolism of each drug.

The effects of even one drug may differ greatly from one individual to another,[128] and even within the same individual. For instance, a certain dose of alcohol, taken under apparently similar circumstances, can result in a blood alcohol level that varies up to 2.5-fold.[129] Although tolerance to side effects often develops after a few days on alcohol, which affects attention,[130] the side effects of this drug cannot always be foreseen. Also many patients fail adequately to observe medical advice, often stopping and restarting therapy or altering their dose of tablets in a cavalier fashion.

A survey of 945 drivers performed by the Automobile Association in Great Britain showed that 14 percent had taken tablets or other medicine within the previous 24 hours.[131] Only four of those drivers had been told that their abilities might be affected in any way. Because of the widespread prescription of modern drugs, a substantial overlap of drug taking with driving seems inevitable. In the United States, half of the population of 200 million are licensed drivers.[132] In an affluent Australian state (Western Australia), 83 percent of adult men and 46 percent of the adult female population hold driving licenses.[133] Kibrick and Smart[134] of the Canadian Addiction Research Foundation in 1970 published a review and analysis of investigations into psychotropic drug use and driving risk. They concluded that as high a proportion as 35 to 50 percent of the general population run the risk of driving after drug use at least once per year. About 7 percent of these drivers are at risk because of drinking and driving while taking their prescribed drugs, and 11 to 15 percent of accidents involved drivers who had taken a psychotropic drug just prior to their crash.

Whereas information, even if still incomplete in some areas, does exist with regard to the role of alcohol in driver behavior and traffic safety, data have been relatively scanty concerning the possible role of drugs, or of combinations of alcohol and drugs, in traffic accidents. It is worth noting that the booklet *Accident Facts*, published by the American National Safety Council in 1945, claimed that alcohol accounted for 18 percent of traffic fatalities; in 1966, another edition of the same booklet declared that alcohol was the leading factor in 50 percent of traffic fatalities. The reader should refer to the section on drugs and driving in Chapter 11 of this text.

An editorial in *Traffic Laws Commentary* indicates that, in the United States, 10 to 20 percent of the population aged 16 years and over are using a prescribed drug, and that a further 15 to 30 percent are taking OTC medicines. Some 24 percent of the prescribed drugs are

**TABLE 19-11**
**Drug Interactions of CNS Stimulants and Anorexiants**

| *Drug* | *Interacts with* | *To Cause* | *Reason* |
|---|---|---|---|
| Amphetamine | Ammonium chloride<br>Sodium bicarbonate | Increased excretion<br>Decreased excretion | pH effect on ionization of weak base |
| Amphetamine, ephedrine, mephentermine, hydroxyamphetamine | Guanethidine, bretylium | Increase in blood pressure | Displacement of guanethidine from adrenergic binding site |
| Amphetamine | Alcohol | Unpredictable results | |
| Methylphenidate | Guanethidine | Increased blood pressure | Displacement |
| Methylphenidate | Primidone, phenobarbital, ethyl biscoumacetate | Prolonged blood level of drugs | Methylphenidate inhibits microsomal enzymes |
| | | No change in levels | No enzyme inhibition |
| Methylphenidate | Imipramine | Improvement in depression | Enzyme inhibition |
| Caffeine and sodium benzoate | Bilirubin | Kernicterus in premature infants (effect due to sodium benzoate, not caffeine) | Displaces bilirubin from albumin binding site |
| Caffeine | Serum glucose | Increase in serum glucose | |
| Diethylpropion | Guanethidine | Reverse hypotensive effect | Displacement |

(From Hartshorn, E. A. *Handbook of Drug Interactions.* Ciba. Hamilton Press, Hamilton, Ill., 1973)

probably psychotropic agents.[135] In addition, one must take into account the illegal use of drugs and the use of popular agents such as caffeine, nicotine, and alcohol, which properly may be regarded as "social" psychotropic drugs. Parry[136] has published a report of two surveys of the adult use of psychotropic drugs within the 12 months prior to the surveys, and a total of 48 percent had, at some time, used one of these agents.

It is unfortunate that some psychotropic drugs have not yet been adequately tested and that many physicians are not yet aware of their dangerous effects on sensory and motor functions. Thus the potential dangers of any new drugs are often not suspected until after they have been widely prescribed. The clinical investigation of some new drugs may be done by doctors who have little training in pharmacology or specialized laboratory techniques. Drugs that are valuable for bed patients may, even in small doses, be bad for ambulant patients. Extensive hospital trials will not, because of the rigid control of the subjects and their limited environment, reveal all of the possible adverse reactions to the drug, particularly in relation to fitness for driving.[137,138]

Many compound medicines are used, but with only a few of these is there evidence that they are more effective in treatment than a carefully chosen single drug.[139] As drinking moderate amounts of alcohol in conjunction with a sedative or tranquilizer may produce marked intoxication (while the same amount of alcohol alone might cause no apparent intoxication), due warning of the possible effects must be given.

Doctors have a responsibility to advise politicians and the public about public health problems in the areas of traffic, medicine, and drug and alcohol abuse. Unfortunately emotional conflicts and prejudiced attitudes about necessary legislative controls often make even the study of these problems difficult. Most doctors still subscribe to the myth of "social drinking," failing to recognize that the moderate drinker is heir to all the illnesses, accidents, and personal problems of the alcoholic,[140] in proportion to the amount the person drinks. Until alcohol is acknowledged to be a potent and dangerous drug (the ratio of the lethal to the therapeutic dose for alcohol is 10:1; for barbiturates, it is 20:1), doctors will continue to handle alcohol, and tend to regard other drugs, in a rather nonchalant manner. To inform a patient fully of a drug's effects on driving may "tend to vitiate essential rapport," but to neglect such advice may really indicate an indifference to safety.[141]

## F. CONCLUDING REMARKS

Psychotropic drugs are abundantly used legally by millions of Americans, and their illicit abuse is rampant and widespread throughout the world. Alcohol, because of its direct action on perception, thought, and mood, is a major factor in the complex etiology of traffic accidents. And enough barbiturates are produced each year for each American to take 30 capsules or tablets. The total distributed is in the millions, or 400 tons per year, on the average. Similarly tranquilizers, such as Valium and Librium, are pumped into the U.S. industrial complex each year, in amounts exceeding hundreds of tons.

## TABLE 19-12

## Examples of Psychotropic Drugs: Their Formulas, Chemical Grouping, Indications, Dosage, Principal Effects, and Principal Side Effects

| *GROUP* | *SYNONYMS* | *SUBGROUPS* | *PRINCIPAL INDICATIONS* |
|---|---|---|---|
| (1) Antipsychotic agent | Major tranquilizer<br>Neuroleptic<br>Neuroplegic<br>Psycholeptic<br>Psychoplegic | Phenothiazine derivative with aliphatic side chain<br>Chlorpromazine | Schizophrenia, mania, excitation |
| (2) Antipsychotic agent | Major tranquilizer<br>Neuroleptic<br>Neuroplegic<br>Psycholeptic<br>Psychoplegic | Phenothiazine derivative with piperidyl side chain<br>Thioridazine | Agitated depression, schizophrenia, mania |
| (3) Antipsychotic agent | Major tranquilizer<br>Neuroleptic<br>Neuroplegic<br>Psycholeptic<br>Psychoplegic | Phenothiazine derivative with piperazinyl–propyl side chain<br>Trifluoperazine | Schizophrenia |
| (4) Antianxiety agent | Minor tranquilizer<br>Ataractic<br>Anxiolytic<br>Tranquillo-sedative | Benzodiazepine derivative<br>Diazepam | Anxiety, tension, insomnia<br>Spasticity<br>Status epilepticus, tetanus |

## TABLE 19-12 (continued)

## Examples of Psychotropic Drugs: Their Formulas, Chemical Grouping, Indications, Dosage, Principal Effects, and Principal Side Effects

| *COMMON DAILY DOSAGE* | *PRINCIPAL EFFECTS* | *PRINCIPAL SIDE-EFFECTS* | *CHEMICAL FORMULA* |
|---|---|---|---|
| 75–600 mg | Antipsychotic, calming, sedative | Parkinsonism symptoms, jaundice, tachycardia, weight gain, agranulocytosis, photosensitivity | 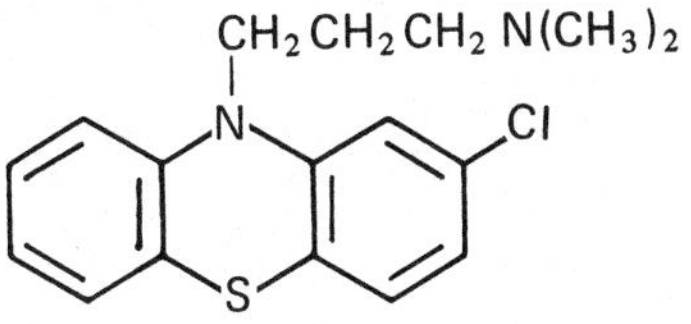 $CH_2CH_2CH_2N(CH_3)_2$; N; Cl; S |
| 75–600 mg | Antipsychotic, antidepressive, moderately sedative | Fatigue, weight gain, postural hypotension | 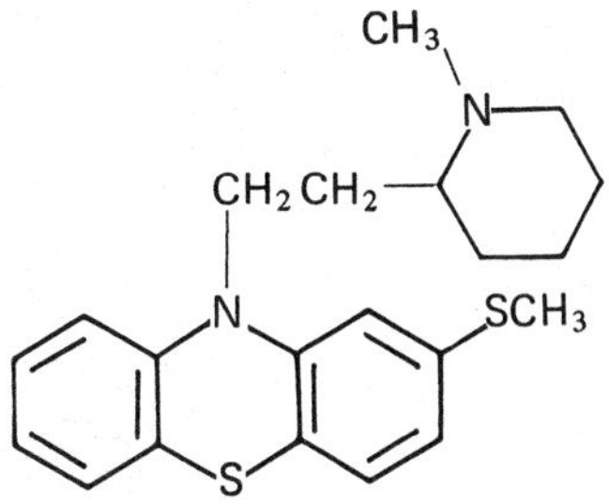 $CH_3$; N; $CH_2CH_2$; N; $SCH_3$; S |
| 5–30 mg | Antipsychotic | Extrapyramidal symptoms (drug-induced parkinsonism, dystonic reactions, akathisia) | 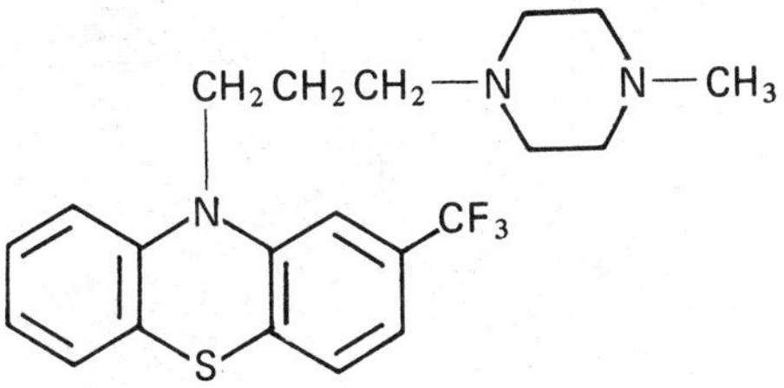 $CH_2CH_2CH_2$—N N—$CH_3$; N; $CF_3$; S |
| 6–40<br><br>4–30 mg<br>60–180 mg | Nonhypnotic sedative without antipsychotic effects, muscle relaxant | Drowsiness, disturbances of coordination, personality changes | 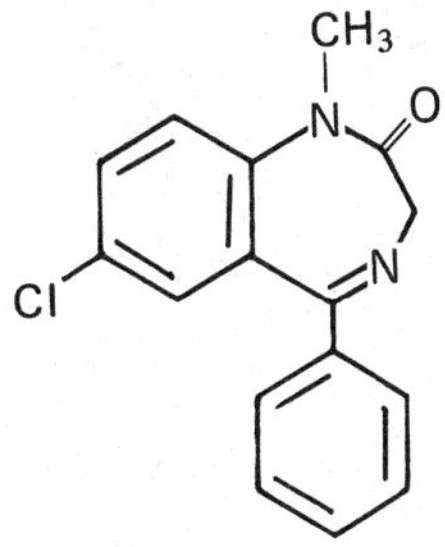 $CH_3$; N; O; N; Cl |

## TABLE 19-12 (continued)

## Examples of Psychotropic Drugs: Their Formulas, Chemical Grouping, Indications, Dosage, Principal Effects, and Principal Side Effects

| *GROUP* | *SYNONYMS* | *SUBGROUPS* | *PRINCIPAL INDICATIONS* |
|---|---|---|---|
| (5) Antianxiety agent | Minor tranquilizer<br>Ataractic<br>Anxiolytic<br>Tranquillo-sedative | Benzodiazepine derivative<br>Chlordiazepoxide | Anxiety, tension |
| (6) Tricyclic antidepressant | Thymoleptic<br>Thymoanaleptic<br>Psychoanaleptic<br>Antidepressant | Iminodibenzyl derivative<br>Imipramine | All types of psychotic depression, Melancholia with diurnal mood swings, retardation, enuresis |
| (7) Tricyclic antidepressant | Thymoleptic<br>Thymoanaleptic<br>Psychoanaleptic<br>Antidepressant | Iminodibenzyl derivative<br>Desipramine | All types of psychotic depression, melancholia with diurnal mood swings, retardation, enuresis |
| (8) Tricyclic antidepressant | Thymoleptic<br>Thymoanaleptic<br>Psychoanaleptic<br>Antidepressant | Iminodibenzyl derivative<br>Trimipramine | Psychotic depression with anxiety or agitation |

**TABLE 19-12 (continued)**

**Examples of Psychotropic Drugs: Their Formulas, Chemical Grouping, Indications, Dosage, Principal Effects, and Principal Side Effects**

| *COMMON DAILY DOSAGE* | *PRINCIPAL EFFECTS* | *PRINCIPAL SIDE-EFFECTS* | *CHEMICAL FORMULA* |
|---|---|---|---|
| 10–100 mg | Nonhypnotic without antipsychotic effects | Drowsiness, disturbances of coordination, personality changes | 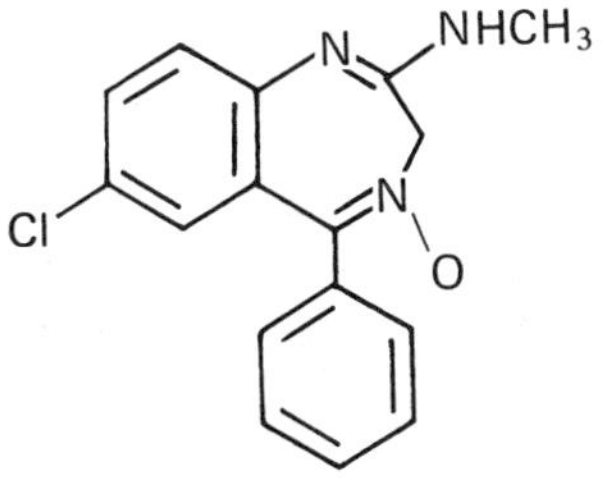 Cl; N; $NHCH_3$; N; O |
| 30–300 mg | Mood elevating | Dry mouth, sweating, tachycardia, tremor, constipation, blurred vision | 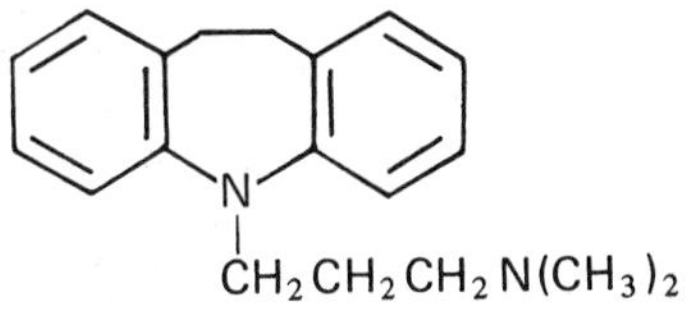 N; $CH_2CH_2CH_2N(CH_3)_2$ |
| 30–200 mg | Mood elevating | Dry mouth, sweating, tachycardia, tremor, constipation, blurred vision | 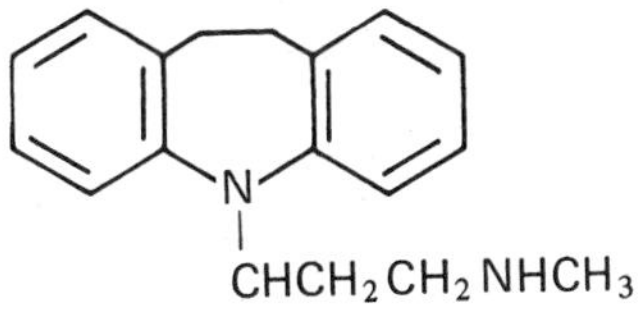 N; $CHCH_2CH_2NHCH_3$ |
| 30–300 mg | Mood elevating, sedative | Dry mouth, sweating, tachycardia, tremor, constipation, blurred vision, fatigue, drowsiness | 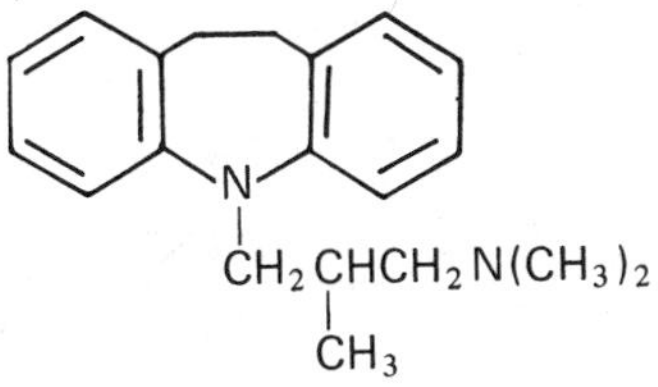 N; $CH_2CHCH_2N(CH_3)_2$; $CH_3$ |

## TABLE 19-12 (continued)

## Examples of Psychotropic Drugs: Their Formulas, Chemical Grouping, Indications, Dosage, Principal Effects, and Principal Side Effects

| GROUP | SYNONYMS | SUBGROUPS | PRINCIPAL INDICATIONS |
|---|---|---|---|
| (9) Tricyclic antidepressant | Thymoleptic<br>Thymoanaleptic<br>Psychoanaleptic<br>Antidepressant | Dibenzoxepin tricyclic derivative<br>Doxepin | Psychotic depression with anxiety or agitation |
| (10) Tricyclic antidepressant | Thymoleptic<br>Thymoanaleptic<br>Psychoanaleptic<br>Antidepressant | Dibenzo-cycloheptadiene derivative<br>Amitriptyline | Psychotic depression with anxiety or agitation |
| (11) Tricyclic antidepressant | Thymoleptic<br>Thymoanaleptic<br>Psychoanaleptic<br>Antidepressant | Dibenzo-cycloheptadiene derivative<br>Nortriptyline | Psychotic depression, enuresis |
| (12) Monamine oxidase inhibitor antidepressant | MAOI<br>Psychic energizer<br>Thymeretic | Hydrazine derivative<br>Phenelzine | Reactive depression |

## TABLE 19-12 (continued)

## Examples of Psychotropic Drugs: Their Formulas, Chemical Grouping, Indications, Dosage, Principal Effects, and Principal Side Effects

| *COMMON DAILY DOSAGE* | *PRINCIPAL EFFECTS* | *PRINCIPAL SIDE-EFFECTS* | *CHEMICAL FORMULA* |
|---|---|---|---|
| 30–300 mg | Mood elevating, sedative | Dry mouth, sweating, tachycardia, tremor, constipation, blurred vision, fatigue, drowsiness | 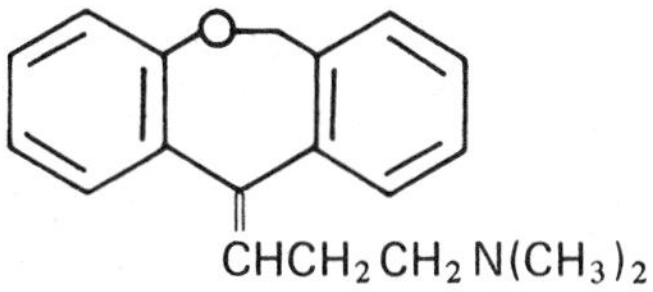 $CHCH_2CH_2N(CH_3)_2$ |
| 30–300 mg | Mood elevating, sedative | Dry mouth, sweating, tachycardia, tremor, constipation, blurred vision, fatigue, drowsiness | 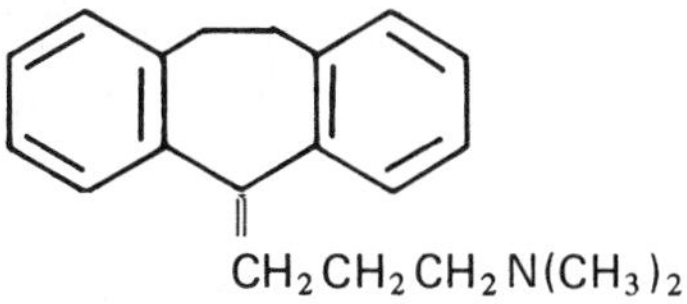 $CH_2CH_2CH_2N(CH_3)_2$ |
| 30–200 mg | Mood elevating | Dry mouth, sweating, tachycardia, tremor, constipation, blurred vision | 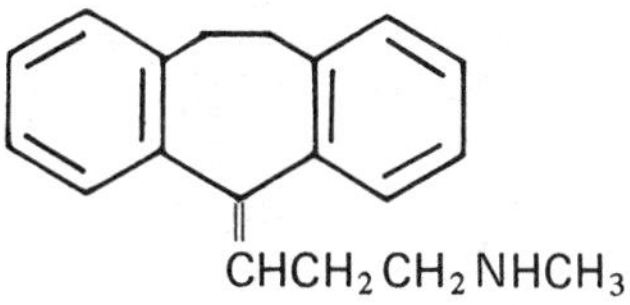 $CHCH_2CH_2NHCH_3$ |
| 45–150 mg | Antidepressant, disinhibition | Postural hypotension, dizziness, insomnia, agitation, jaundice, paroxysmal hypertension—parti cularly when certain foodstuffs or other drugs are taken concurrently | 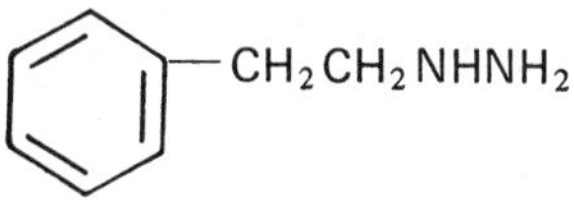 $CH_2CH_2NHNH_2$ |

**TABLE 19-12 (continued)**

**Examples of Psychotropic Drugs: Their Formulas, Chemical Grouping, Indications, Dosage, Principal Effects, and Principal Side Effects**

| *GROUP* | *SYNONYMS* | *SUBGROUPS* | *PRINCIPAL INDICATIONS* |
|---|---|---|---|
| (13) Stimulant | Psychotonic | Bicyclic compound<br>Methylphenidate | Physical exhaustion in convalescence, abreaction, hyperactive children |
| (14) Hypnosedative | Sedative<br>Hypnotic | Barbiturate<br>Phenobarbitone | Insomnia, anxiety, epilepsy |
| (15) Hypnosedative | Sedative<br>Hypnotic | Ethanol<br>Beers, wines, spirits, liquers | Used as a base in medicinal preparations, a tonic, a social euphoriant, oblivion |

## TABLE 19-12 (continued)

## Examples of Psychotropic Drugs: Their Formulas, Chemical Grouping, Indications, Dosage, Principal Effects, and Principal Side Effects

| *COMMON DAILY DOSAGE* | *PRINCIPAL EFFECTS* | *PRINCIPAL SIDE-EFFECTS* | *CHEMICAL FORMULA* |
|---|---|---|---|
| 5–30 mg | Excitant | Tachycardia, hypertension, insomnia, agitation | 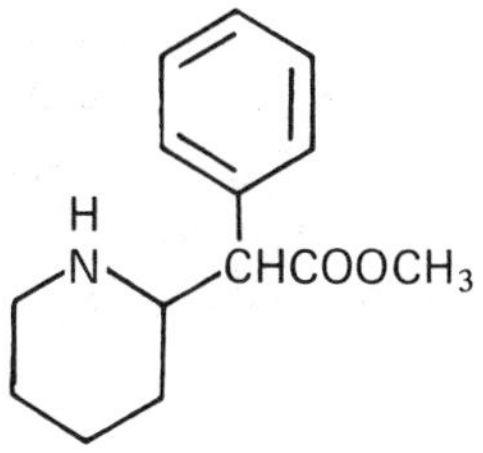 |
| 60–300 mg | Sedative, hypnotic, anticonvulsant | Dependency, suicide, toxic confusional states | 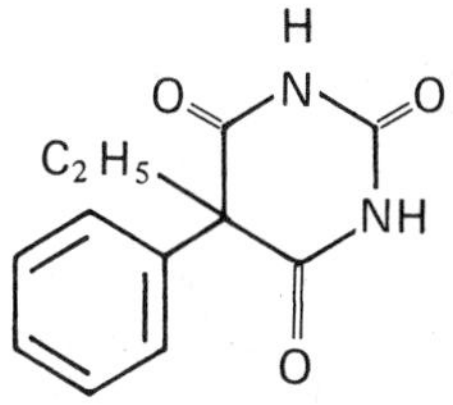 |
| 30 mg/100 ml blood is a social euphoriant level; 80 mg/100 ml causes marked intoxication; above 150 mg/100 ml indicates an "alcohol problem" | Sedative, hypnotic | Dependency, disturbances of equilibrium, judgment, sensation and perception, toxic confusional states | $C_2H_5OH$ |

Besides legal prescription drugs, other OTC agents, along with amphetamines (speed), psychedelics, marihuana, mushrooms, opiates, huge quantities of beer, wine, and whiskey, Quaaludes (other barbiturates), and even solvent inhalants, all significantly contribute to the drug–drug adverse reaction dilemma.

The polypharmacy approved by many physicians, sometimes unknowingly, also significantly contributes to drug adverse reactions. Furthermore there is still inadequate information concerning the exact mechanism of adverse drug reactions associated with polypharmacy, and drug interactions with various items of diet, despite increased interest in these problems. Over two decades ago, the World Health Organization affirmed that some psychotropic drugs had not yet been adequately tested, and that many physicians were not fully aware of some of their effects on sensory and motor functions. Finally, the potential dangers of any one drug often are not suspected until after it has been widely prescribed. Since there is no solution to eradicate the dangers of drug interactions, it is important at least to inform the public about the dangers.

More than any previous decade, the 1980s are being rapidly recognized as the decade most influential in changing laws that govern our safety on the road. Drugs and driving are a prime example. The dangers of this combination have been covered by numerous media presentations, including television, radio, newspapers, and popular magazines.

Another important aspect in the 1980s that relates to the problem of drug–drug interactions is the fashionable tampering with OTC products, such as the Chicago Tylenol incident (seven dead), the Denver Excedrin incident, the Sinutex contamination, and even the placing of needles in candy bars.

Does all of this add up to the fact that the only person one can trust is one's self? And what about those of us who inflict self-harm by abusing these drugs?

## REFERENCES


1. Melmon, K. L. Preventable drug reactions—causes and cures. L. Sherwood and E. Parris, eds. *N. Engl. J. Med.* 284:1361, 1971.
2. Miller, R. R. Hospital admission due to adverse drug reactions. *Arch. Intern. Med.* 134:219, 1974.
3. Koch-Wesser, J. Fatal reactions to drug therapy. *N. Engl. J. Med.* 291:302, 1974.
4. Hurwitz, N. Admissions to hospitals due to drugs. *Br. Med. J.* 1:539, 1969.
5. Jack, H. Drug—Remarkably nontoxic. *N. Engl. J. Med.* 291:824, 1974.
6. Gotti, E. W. Adverse drug reactions and the autopsy. *Arch. Pathol.* 97:201, 1974.
7. Miller, L. C. How good are our drugs? Distinguished Lecture delivered December 30, 1969, before the American Association for the Advancement of Science, Boston, Mass. *Am. J. Hosp. Pharm.* 27:367, 1970.
8. Muller, C. The overmedicated society: Forces on the marketplace for medical care. *Science* 176:488, 1972.
9. Rucker, P. T. Drug use data: Sources and limitations. *JAMA* 230:888, 1971.
10. Caranosos, G. J., Stewart, R. B., and Cluff, L. E. Drug-induced illness leading to hospitalization. *JAMA* 228:713, 1974.
11. Cohen, S. *The Substance Abuse Problem.* New York: Haworth Press, 1981, pp. 375–384.
12. Graedon, J. *The People's Pharmacy.* New York: Avon, 1976, pp. 1–6.
13. Lambert, M. L., Jr., Drug and diet interactions. *Am. J. Nursing* 75:402, 1975.
14. Cohen, S. N., and Armstrong, M. F. *Drug Interactions: A Handbook for Clinical Use.*

Baltimore: Williams & Wilkins, 1974.

15. Swidler, G. *Handbook of Drug Interactions*. New York: Wiley-Interscience, 1971.
16. Cluff, L. E., et al. Studies of the epidemiology of adverse drug reactions. *JAMA* 188:967, 1964.
17. Wagner, J. G. Biopharmaceutics: Absorption aspects. *J. Pharmaceut. Sci.* 50:359, 1961.
18. Hartshorn, E. A. *Handbook of Drug Interactions*. Hamilton, Ill.: Hamilton Press, 1973.
19. Moore, J., and Dundee, J. W. *Br. Anaesth.* 33:422, 1961.
20. Palmer, H. Potentiation of pethidine. *Br. Med. J.* 2:944, 1960.
21. Papp, C., and Benjamin, S. Toxic effects of ipromiazid in the patient with angina. *Br. Med. J.* 2:1070, 1958.
22. Slee, J. D. Dangerous potentiation of pethidine by iproniazid and its treatment. *Br. Med. J.* 2:507, 1960.
23. Brownlee, G., and Williams, G. W. Potentiation of amphetamine and pethidine by monoamine oxidase inhibitors. *Lancet* 1:669, 1963.
24. Churchill-Davidson, H. C. Anaesthesia and monoamine oxidase inhibitors. *Br. Med. J.* 1:520, 1965.
25. Eade, N. R., and Renton, K. W. Effect of monoamine oxidase inhibitors on the N-demethylation and hydrolysis of meperidine. *Biochem. Pharmacol.* 19:2245, 1970.
26. Goodman, L. L., and Gilman, A. *The Pharmacological Basis of Therapeutics*, 4th ed. New York: Macmillan, 1970, p. 258.
27. Ahmed, S. S., Joglekar, G. V., and Balwani, J. H. Potentiation of the analgesic effect of codeine in rats by d-amphetamine. *Arch. Inter. Pharmacodyn.* 159:185, 1969.
28. Roche Laboratories. Matulane (Procarbazine HCl), Aug. 1969.
29. Antonita, Sister M. Necessary precautions when dispensing oral progestational drugs to inpatients. *Hosp. Formulary Mgmt.* 3:34, 1968.
30. Christensen, E. M., and Gross, E. G. Analgesic effects in human subjects of morphine, meperidine and methadone. *JAMA* 137:594, 1948.
31. Contreras, E., and Tamaryo, L. Effects of drugs acting in relation to sympathetic functions of the analgesic action of morphine. *Arch. Inters. Pharmacodyn.* 160:312, 1966.
32. Langston, J. W., Ballard, P., Petrud, J. W., and Irwin, I., Chronic Parkinsonism in Humans Due to a Product of Meperidine Analog Synthesis. *Science* 219:979, 1983.
33. Wallis, R. Potentiation of hypnotics and analgesics: Clinical experience with chlorpromazine. *N.Y. State J. Med.* 55:247, 1955.
34. Keats, A. S., Telford, J., and Karosu, Y. Potentiation of meperidine by promethazine. *Anesthesiology* 22:34, 1961.
35. Goodman, L. S., and Gilman, A. *The Pharmacological Basis of Therapeutics*, 4th ed. New York: Macmillan, 1970, p. 245.
36. Wiederholt, I. D. Recurrent episodes of hyperglycemia induced by propoxyphene. *Neurology* 17:703, 1967.
37. Pearson, R. E., and Salter, F. J. Drug interactions, orphenadrine with propoxyphene. *N. Engl. J. Med.* 282:1215, 1970.
38. Puckett, W. H., and Visconti, J. A. Orphenadrine and propoxyphene. *N. Engl. J. Med.* 283:544, 1970.
39. Renforth, W. Orphenadrine and propoxyphene. *N. Engl. J. Med.* 283:998, 1970.
40. Becker, C., Roe, R. L., and Scott, R. A. *Alcohol as a Drug: A Curriculum on Pharmacology, Neurology and Toxicology*. New York: Medcom Press, 1974.
41. Martin, E. W. *Hazards of Medication: A Manual on Drug Interactions, Incompatibilities, Contraindications and Adverse Effects*. Philadelphia: Lippincott, 1971, pp. 430–439.
42. Lundwall, L., and Baekeland, F. Disulfiram treatment of alcoholism: A review. *J. Nerv. Ment. Dis.* 153:381, 1971.
43. Fox, R. Disulfiram-alcohol side effects. *JAMA* 204:271, 1968.
44. Burnett, G. B., and Reading, H. W. Drug interactions in alcoholism treatment. *Lancet* 1:415, 1969.
45. MacCallum, W. A. G. Drug interactions in alcoholism treatment. *Lancet* 1:313, 1969.
46. Perman, E. S. Intolerance to alcohol. *N. Engl. J. Med.* 273:114, 1965.

47. Parker, W. J. Clinically significant alcohol–drug interactions. *J. Am. Pharm. Assoc.* NS10:664, 1970.
48. Bhatia, S. K., Hadden, D. R., and Montgomery, D. A. D. Chlorpropamide in diabetes insipidus. *Lancet* 1:729, 1969.
49. Fitzgerald, M. C. Alcohol sensitivity in diabetics receiving chlorpropamide. *Diabetes* 11:40, 1962.
50. Arky, R. A. Irreversible hypoglycemia: A complication of alcohol and insulin. *JAMA* 206:575, 1968.
51. Arky, R. A., and Freinkel, N. Alcohol hypoglycemia. V. Alcohol infusion to test gluconeogenesis in starvation with special reference to obesity. *N. Engl. J. Med.* 274:426, 1966.
52. Kreisberg, R. A. Glucose-lactate inter-relations in man. *N. Engl. J. Med.* 287:132, 1972.
53. Isaacs, P. Alcohol and phenformin in diabetes. *Br. Med. J.* 3:773, 1970.
54. Johnson, H. K., and Waterhouse, C. Relationship of alcohol and hyperlactatemia in diabetic subjects treated with phenformin. *JAMA* 45:98, 1968.
55. Shafer, N. Hypotension due to nitroglycerin combined with alcohol. *N. Engl. J. Med.* 273:1169, 1965.
56. Shepherd, M. Psychotropic drugs (1) interaction between centrally acting drugs in man: Some general considerations. *Proc. Roy. Soc. Med.* 51:964, 1965.
57. Sfikakis, P. Isoniazid and alcohol. *Am. Rev. Respir. Dis.* 101:991, 1970.
58. Riedler, G. Einfluss des alkohols auf die antikoagulation—Therapeutic (Effect of alcohol on anticoagulant therapy). *Thromb. Diath. Haemorrhag.* 16:613, 1966.
59. Goulston, K., and Cooke, A. R. Alcohol, aspirin and gastrointestinal bleeding. *Br. Med. J.* 4:664, 1968.
60. Mould, G. Fecal blood-loss after sodium acetylsalicylate taken with alcohol. *Lancet* 1:1268, 1969.
61. Lansdown, F. S. Psychotropic reaction during ethionamide therapy. *Am. Rev. Respir. Dis.* 95:1053, 1967.
62. Wilson, L. The combined effects of ethanol and amphetamine sulfate on performance of human subjects. *Can. Med. Assoc. J.* 94:478, 1966.
63. Lindenbaum, J., and Lieber, C. S. Alcohol-induced malabsorption of vitamin B in man. *Nature* 224:806, 1969.
64. Gywn, R., Personal communication, 1982.
65. Blum, K. Depressive states induced by drugs of abuse: Clinical evidence, theoretical conclusions and proposed treatment. Part II. *J. Psychedel. Drugs* 235, 1976.
66. Reilly, M. J., editor. *American Hospital Formulary Service*. American Society of Hospital Pharmacists, Washington, D.C.
67. Turner, P. Influence of urinary pH on the excretion of tranylcypromine sulfate. *Nature* 215:881, 1967.
68. Eble, J. N., and Rudzik, A. D. Amphetamine: Augmentation of pressor effects of tyramine in rats. *Proc. Soc. Exp. Biol. Med.* 122:1059, 1966.
69. Aminu, J., D'Mello, A., and Vere, D. W. Interactions between debrisoquine and phenelephrine (letter). *Lancet* 2:935, 1970.
70. Pettinger, W. A., Soyangco, F. C., and Oates, J. A. Monoamine oxidase inhibition by furazolidone in man. *Clin. Res.* 14:258, 1966.
71. Pettinger, W. A., Soyangco, F. C., and Oates, J. A. Inhibition of monoamine oxidase in man by furazolidone. *Clin. Pharmacol. Ther.* 9:442, 1968.
72. Blackwell, B., and Marley, E. Interaction between cheese and monoamine oxidase inhibitors in rats and cats. *Lancet* 1:530, 1964.
73. Blackwell, B., and Mabbitt, L. A. Tyramine in cheese related to hypertensive crises after monoamine oxidase inhibition. *Lancet* 1:938, 1965.
74. Natoff, I. L. Cheese and monoamine oxidase inhibitors: Interaction in anaesthesized cats. *Lancet* 1:532, 1964.
75. Blackwell, B. Hypertensive interactions between monoamine oxidase inhibitors and foodstuffs. *Br. J. Psychiatry* 113:349, 1967.
76. Blackwell, B., Marley, E., and Mabbitt, L. A. Effects of yeast extract after monoamine oxidase inhibition. *Lancet* 1:940, 1965.
77. Leonard, J. W., Gifford, R. W., Jr., and Williams, G. H., Jr. Pargyline and cheese. *Lancet* 1:883, 1964.
78. Trevelyan, M. R. Monoamine oxidase inhibitors (letter). *Br. Dent. J.* 128:263, 1970.
79. Goldberg, L. J. Monoamine oxidase inhibitors: Adverse reactions and possible mechanisms. *JAMA* 190:456, 1964.
80. Horwitz, D. Monoamine oxidase inhibitors, tyramine and cheese. *JAMA* 188:1108, 1964.
81. Gelder, M. G., and Vane, J. R. Interaction of the effects of tyramine, amphetamine and reserpine in man. *Psychopharmacology* 3:231, 1962.
82. Sjoqvist, F. Psychotropic drugs (2) interaction between monoamine oxidase (MAO) inhibitors and other substances. *Proc. Roy. Soc. Med.* 58:967, 1965.
83. Elis, J. Modification by monoamine oxidase

inhibition of the effect of some sympathomimetics on blood pressure. *Br. Med. J.* 2:75, 1967.

84. Mond, E., and Mack, I. Cardiac toxicity of iproniazid (Marsilid): Report of myocardial injury in a patient receiving levarterenol. *Am. Heart J.* 59:134, 1960.
85. Aderhold, R. M., and Muniz, C. E. Acute psychosis with amitriptyline and furazolidone (letter). *JAMA* 213:2080, 1970.
86. Jenkins, L. C., and Graves, H. B. Potential hazards of psychoactive drugs in association with anesthesia. *Can. Anaesth. Soc. J.* 12:121, 1965.
87. Davies, G. Side effects of phenelzine. *Br. Med. J.* 2:1019, 1960.
88. Jarecki, H. G. Combined amitriptyline and phenelzine poisoning. *Am. J. Psychiatry* 120:189, 1963.
89. Luby, E. D., and Domino, E. F. Toxicity from large doses of imipramine and an MAO inhibitor in suicidal intent. *JAMA* 177:68, 1961.
90. Babick, W. Case fatality due to overdosage of a combination of tranylcypromine (Parnate) and imipramine (Tofranil). *Can. Med. Assoc. J.* 35:377, 1961.
91. McCurdy, R. L., and Kane, F. J. Transient brain syndrome as a non-fatal reaction to combined pargyline-imipramine treatment. *Am. J. Psychiatry* 121:397, 1963.
92. Brachfeld, J., Wirtshafter, A., and Wolfe, S. Imipramine-tranylcypromine incompatibility: Near-fatal toxic reaction. *JAMA* 186:1172, 1963.
93. Sargent, W. Combining the antidepressant drugs (letter). *Br. Med. J.* 1:251, 1965.
94. Gander, D. R. Treatment of depressive illnesses with combined antidepressants. *Lancet* 2:107, 1973.
95. Anonymous. Today's drugs: Monoamine oxidase inhibitors. *Br. Med. J.* 2:365, 1969.
96. Papp, C., and Beniam, S. Toxic effects of iproniazid in a patient with angina. *Br. Med. J.* 2:1070, 1958.
97. Eade, N. R., and Renton, K. W. Effects of monoamine oxidase inhibitors on the N-demethylation and hydrolysis of meperidine. *Biochem. Pharmacol.* 19:2243, 1970.
98. Brownlee, G., and Williams, G. W. Potentiation of amphetamine and pethidine by monoamine oxidase inhibitors (letter). *Lancet* 1:669, 1963.
99. Hrdina, P., and Garattini, S. Desipramine and potentiation of naradrenaline in the isolated perfused renal artery (letter). *J. Pharm. Pharmacol.* 18:259, 1966.
100. Jori, A., Carrara, M. C., and Garattini, S. Importance of noradrenaline synthesis for the interaction between desipramine and reserpine (letter). *J. Pharm. Pharmacol.* 18:619, 1966.
101. Lockett, M. F., and Milner, G. L. Combining the antidepressant drugs (letter). *Br. Med. J.* 1:921, 1965.
102. Milner, G. Cumulative lethal dose of alcohol in mice given amitriptyline. *J. Pharm. Sci.* 57:2005, 1968.
103. Landauer, A. A., Milner, G., and Patman, J. Alcohol and amitriptyline effects on skills related to driving behavior. *Science* 163:1467, 1969.
104. MacCallum, W. A. G. Drug interactions in alcoholism treatment (letter). *Lancet* 1:313, 1969.
105. Burnett, G. B., and Reading, H. W. Drug interactions in alcoholism treatment (letter). *Lancet* 1:415, 1969.
106. Kane, F. J., and Taylor, T. W. A toxic reaction to combined Elavil–Librium therapy. *Am. J. Psychiatry* 119:1179, 1963.
107. Abdou, F. A. Elavil–Librium combination. *Am. J. Psychiatry* 120:1204, 1966.
108. Gram, L. F., and Overo, K. F. Drug metabolism: Inhibitory effect of neuroleptics on metabolism of tricyclic antidepressants in man. *Br. Med. J.* 1:463, 1972.
109. Warnes, H., Lehman, H. E., and Ban, T. A. Adynamic ileus during psychoactive medication: A report of three fatal and five severe cases. *Can. Med. Assoc. J.* 96:1112, 1967.
110. Winer, J. A., and Bahn, S. Loss of teeth with antidepressant drug therapy. *Arch. Gen. Psychiatry* 16:239, 1967.
111. Witton, K. Severe toxic reaction to combined amitriptyline and thioridazine. *Am. J. Psychiatry* 121:812, 1965.
112. Lechat, P., Fontagne, J., and Giroud, J. Influence of a previous administration of tricyclic antidepressant compounds on the activity of local anesthetics. *Therapie* 24:393, 1969.
113. Chang, C. C., Costa, E., and Brodie, B. B. Interaction of guanethidine with adrenergic neurons. *J. Pharmacol. Exp. Ther.* 147:303, 1965.
114. Day, M. D., and Rand, M. J. Antagonism of guanethidine by dexamphetamine and other related sympathomimetic amines. *J. Pharm. Pharmacol.* 14:541, 1962.
115. Gulati, O. D., et al. Antagonism of adrenergic neuron blockade in hypertensive subjects. *Clin. Pharmacol. Ther.* 7:510, 1966.
116. Wilson, R., and Long, C. Action of bretylium antagonized by amphetamine (letter). *Lancet*

2:262, 1960.

117. Wilson, L., Taylor, J. D., and Nash, C. W. The combined effects of ethanol and amphetamine sulfate on performance of human subjects. *Can. Med. Assoc. J.* 94:478, 1966.

118. Milner, G. Interaction between barbiturates, alcohol and some psychotropic drugs. *Med. J. Aust.* 1:1204, 1970.

119. Wharton, R. N., Perel, J. M., and Dayton, P. Potential clinical use for methylphenidate with tricyclic antidepressants. *Am. J. Psychiatry* 127:1619, 1971.

120. Hague, D. E., Smith, M. E., and Ryan, J. Effect of methylphenidate and prolintane on the metabolism of ethyl biscoumacetate. *Clin. Pharmacol. Ther.* 12:259, 1971.

121. Done, A. K. Developmental pharmacology. *Clin. Pharmacol. Ther.* 5:432, 1974.

122. Cheraskin, E., and Ringsdorf, W. M., Jr. Caffeine versus placebo supplementation on blood-glucose concentration. *Lancet* 1:1299, 1967.

123. Day, M. D., and Rand, M. J. Antagonism of guanethidine and bretylium by various agents. *Lancet* 2:1282, 1962.

124. Milner, G. *Drugs and Driving*. Basel: S. Karger, 1972.

125. Forrest, F., Forrest, I., and Serra, M. Modification of chlorpromazine metabolism by some other drugs frequently administered to psychiatric patients. *Biolg. Psychiatry* 2:53, 1970.

126. Prescott, L. F. Pharmacokinetic drug interactions. *Lancet* 2:1239, 1969.

127. Rubin, E., et al. Induction and inhibition of hepatic microsomal and mitochondrial enzymes. *Lab. Inves.* 22:569, 1970.

128. Asberg, M., et al. Correlation of subjective side effects with plasma concentrations of nortriptyline. *Br. Med. J.* 4:18, 1970.

129. Enticknap, J. B. Driving and social drinking. *Br. Med. J.* 1:49, 1967.

130. Milner, G. Drugs and driving. *New Ethicals* 11:3:51, 4:59, 1970.

131. The drugged driver (could it be you?). *Drive, Motorist's Mag.* 30, Jan. 1969.

132. Rouse, K. A. *A Factual Summary for Responsible Drivers Who Drink and Drive and Who May Sometimes Do Both.* Chicago: Central Automobile Safety Committee Publications, Kemper Insurance Group, 1966.

133. Milner, G. Gastrointestinal side effects and psychotropic drugs. *Med. J. Aust.* 2:153, 1969.

134. Kibrick, E., and Smart, G. Psychotropic drug use and driving risk: A review and analysis. *J. Safety Res.* 2:73, 1970.

135. Cooperstock, R., and Sims, M. Hidden drug problems: Prescription drug use in urban population. Presented at North American Association of Alcoholism Program Annual Meeting, 1969.

136. Parry, J. H. Use of psychotropic drugs by U.S. adults. *Pub. Health Rep.* 33:799, 1968.

137. Barker, J. C. Drugs and driving. *Br. Med. J.* 2:109, 1967.

138. Smith, J. W., Seidl, L. G., and Cluff, L. E. Studies on the epidemiology of adverse drug reactions. V: Clinical factors influencing susceptibility. *Ann. Intern. Med.* 65:629, 1966.

139. Freeman, H. The therapeutic value of combinations of psychotropic drugs: A review. *Psychopharmacol. Bull.* 4:1, 1967.

140. Hayman, M. The myth of social drinking. *Am. J. Psychiatry* 124:585, 1967.

141. Allan, J. Drugs and driving. *Br. Med. J.* 2:739, 1967.

Chapter 20

# Influence of Psychopharmacologic Agents on Sexual Function: ''Psychopharmacosexology''

Ever since the dawn of history, man has been agonizing over and pursuing the answers to two questions: What is the meaning and purpose of life? and Where can I get a good aphrodisiac?

J. S. Margolis and R. Clorfene
*A Child's Garden of Grass, 1969*

## A. INTRODUCTION

Throughout time, the question of sexuality and the resultant ''battle of the sexes'' have baffled philosophers, enchanted wizards, and intrigued kings and peasants alike.

Along with the so-called ''sexual revolution'' of the 1960s came powerful substances which, when used licitly or illicitly, provoked the sexual appetite of even the puritanically reared individual. Drug use in the early 1960s gave us rock concerts and love-ins. Indiscriminate drug use and abuse was evident and drug devotees rallied around certain of these agents because of their so-called aphrodisiac qualities. Although most scientists would argue against the notion of a true aphrodisiac or sexual stimulant, results of college surveys in the 1960s and 1970s would support it. In this regard, certain substances such as marihuana, amphetamines, cocaine, LSD, opiates, alcohol, and methaqualone (Quaaludes) have been cited for their special effects on sexuality. For example, marihuana prolongs the sexual experience and releases inhibitions; amphetamines promote the coital urge; cocaine is considered the sexiest of the illicit drugs, and induces direct numbing of the sexual organs; LSD intensifies all sensual perceptions and induces, in some individuals, overwhelming sexual desire; opiates can stimulate the libido and erotic energy; alcohol liberates lust; methaqualone imparts a warm glow to one's sensibilities and releases inhibitions, especially in females.

The primary focus of this chapter is to provide the reader with a brief description of the current state of the art of the influence of various abusable drugs on sexual function and dysfunction. For an expanded review of the subject, the reader should refer to the *Journal of Psychoac-*

*tive Drugs*,[1] *the High Times Encyclopedia*,[2] and the work of Masters and Johnson[3] and others.[4–6]

## B. PHARMACOLOGY OF DRUG-INDUCED SEXUAL DYSFUNCTION

The subject of drug-induced effects on sexual dysfunction has not been very well researched, especially in humans. The area in the brain most associated with sexual behavior is the limbic system. Animal studies have revealed that an inverse relationship exists between brain serotonin and dopamine.[4] Weiss in 1972[7] reported that erection of the penis can occur as a result of psychogenic stimuli. Most researchers have accepted that erection and lubrication are mediated psychogenically by the sympathetic system and reflexogenically by the parasympathetic system.[7]

Consensus of the literature, however, seems to point toward an adrenergic rather than cholinergic control of erectile activity.[6,8–10] In terms of ejaculation, there are three separate components or reflexes involved in the process.[11] Both α- and β-adrenergic receptors and parasympathetic activity are involved.[12–16]

Peripheral sexual response mechanisms in females are believed to be similar to that in the male—namely, like penile erection, clitoral erection and swelling are governed by the parasympathetic and sympathetic systems[17] and orgasm is a combination of sympathetic and motor control.

Drug effects that produce sexual dysfunction in males include:

1. Decreased libido.
2. Decreased erection.
3. Decreased emission.
4. Retrograde ejaculation.
5. Delayed or inhibited orgasm.

Drug effects producing sexual dysfunction in females include:

1. Decreased libido.
2. Decreased lubrication.
3. Delayed or inhibited orgasm.

## C. ABUSABLE DRUGS PRODUCING EFFECTS ON SEXUAL FUNCTION

### 1. Opiates

In an article by the authors of the *High Times Encyclopedia*,[2] the following remarks concerning the aphrodisiac qualities of opium provide a general and concise, but liberal, overview.

> Opium, the dried exudate of the opium poppy (*Papaver somniferum*), can be smoked, eaten, taken in suppositories or introduced into any mucous corridor. Unfortunately, opium is becoming a rarity in many parts of the U.S.A., as scarce as primo hash or Jamaican weed, while its destructive derivatives continue to thrive.
>
> Although it has a generally relaxing effect, opium also stimulates erotic energy on both the mental and corporal levels. Voluptuous thoughts, visualizations, dreams and erotic imaginings from the bottom of the libido often accompany the opium high, and if opium is terrific for fantasy, it's even better for performance. According to the ancient Chinese ''Chin P'ing Mei'' (a pseudonym used collectively by a group of cognoscenti), even a little opium will give life to a tired lance, ''assuring the desideratum of at least 3,000 phallic thrusts.'' Step right up and count 'em. O also has a mild anesthetizing effect—strategically placed, it provides a pleasant numb feeling and delays orgasm to the benefit of both parties.

#### *a. Heroin*

In contrast, there are numerous reports on the synthetic morphine derivative, heroin, concerning its effect on human sexuality. Generally heroin has been reported to cause decreased libido, retarded ejaculation, and impotence.[18–24] Interestingly Bai et al.[25] report that 60 percent of heroin-using women noted decreased libido. Smith et al.[24] found that 45 percent of males had moderate or severe premature ejaculation before heroin use, as compared with only 12 percent after heroin use.

There are many investigators who have speculated on the mechanism of action and possible causes of heroin-induced changes in sexual function. These include studies on leutinizing hormone (LH),[23] testosterone,[19,26] α-adrenergic blocking action,[19] and histamine release.[27]

*b. Methadone*

Similar to other opiates, methadone has been reported to cause decreased libido as well as erection and ejaculation, and orgasm failure.[19,20,23,28–31] There is the question of whether heroin or methadone causes more sexual dysfunction. Studies that indicate that heroin is worse than methadone with regard to sexual dysfunction include the work of Cicero et al.,[19] Mintz et al.,[20] and Cushman,[23] whereas other studies show methadone to be more important in this respect.[19,29] Two studies show methadone as having a higher incidence of failure of orgasm than heroin.[19,29] Dosage seems to be a very important factor influencing the incidence of sexual side effects.

Methadone is more slowly detoxified in the body and this may be important in terms of its effect on the function of secondary sex organs. In this regard, the function of the secondary sex organs was found to be markedly impaired in the methadone patients as opposed to heroin users or controls, and in one study, ejaculate volume was reduced by over 50 percent in methadone clients.[19]

Soyka et al.,[32] based on their work in rats, suggest that the use of exogenous testosterone might be useful in humans on methadone, to prevent atrophy of accessory sex organs.

## 2. Depressants

*a. Alcohol*

Alcohol has been considered to be a drug that liberates lust in humans. Since it is socially acceptable, overindulgence in alcohol is involved in more sexual adventures than all the other substances combined. Curiously Masters and Johnson cite alcohol as one of the primary causes of secondary impotence and provide evidence for Shakespeare's observation in *Macbeth* (1623) that "alcohol provokes the desire but takes away the performance."

Alcohol has potent short-term and long-term effects on sexual function. Among its short-term effects are failure of erection and paradoxic enhanced libido, depending upon the blood alcohol level. Gordon and associates[33] found that alcohol impairs spinal reflexes, which can lead to both decreased sensation and decreased stimulus for erection.

Acute alcohol ingestion decreases plasma testosterone and increases LH.[34] It has been speculated that the increased libido associated with acute alcohol ingestion is the result of the increase in LH levels, whereas decreased serum testosterone levels may be the cause of the impotence.[34]

Mendelson and co-workers[34] believe that alcohol oxidation competes with testosterone biosynthesis in the testes. In addition, the decreased testosterone following alcohol ingestion could be attributable to alcohol-induced β-hydroxysteroid dehydrogenase/isomerase activity.[35] This enzyme is responsible for the rate-limiting step in testosterone production from pregnanalone.

Long-term effects in alcoholics include hyperestrogenization,[36,37] feminization, gynecomastia, sterility, impotence, and decreased libido.[38] Female alcoholics have been shown to have longer orgasmic latencies, decreased subjective intensity of orgasm, and vaginal vasoconstriction.[39,49] Paradoxically women reported significantly greater sexual arousal and orgasmic pleasurability under moderate or high alcohol intoxication.

*b. Barbiturates*

There are no specific or special sexual side effects with barbiturates that would not occur with other depressants. It has been noted that barbiturate-induced alteration of sexual function tends to be a biphasic response, with an initial beneficial effect on sexual desire followed by a decrease in the ability to maintain erection.[41,42]

*c. Benzodiazepines*

Usdin[43] in 1960 reported impotence in a series of 80 patients taking 15 to 75 mg/day of chlordiazepoxide (Librium). Hughes[44] has reported that chlordiazepoxide caused failure of ejaculation at a dose of 30 mg/day. Although this is not a very common finding, Hughes speculates that the explanation for this effect is depression of spinal reflexes induced by chlordiazepoxide.

### *d. Methaqualone*

In discussing the effects of methaqualone as a street aphrodisiac, numerous researchers report that this drug imparts a warm glow to one's sensibilities, loosens the tongue, frees the hands, and overrides the critical faculties of the mind.[2,45–49] Sold under the trade names of Quaalude, Mandrax, Sopor, and Parest, the drug produces a tingling numbness in the extremities and a rubberiness of the skin that pleasantly modify the physical sensations of sex.

Weissberg[48] reports that methaqualone seems to work better as an aphrodisiac in women and that high doses have deleterious effects on the male's desire and drive. Kochansky et al.[45] report that in a college survey, female students preferred methaqualone and men preferred marihuana as their aphrodisiac of choice. The increased libido is probably attributable to decreasing inhibitions. Ager[49] has observed that people on methaqualone tend to be ataxic, with weakness of the extremities. In this regard, in animals, the drug has been shown to have an inhibitory action on postsynaptic pathways and to produce hind limb weakness. According to Buffum,[17] this could be the cause of the impotence at higher doses.

## 3. Stimulants

Stimulants seem to promote the coital urge in both males and females—although more females than males report that stimulants make them feel sexier and have more orgasms. In fact, stimulants may promote sexual dysfunction in some men.

Injected methamphetamines give the strongest "sexual kick," but also the most dangerous and debilitating high. Extended overuse of any type of amphetamine can result in anxiety, paranoia, and physical deterioration.

### *a. Amphetamines*

Amphetamines cause increased libido, impotence, and delayed ejaculation in males.[50–52] Although consensus of the literature points toward enhanced sexuality in females and alteration of sexual function in males, findings are variable.[51,52] It is important to note that dosage, route of administration, habituation, and social setting play a large part in determining a user's sexual response to amphetamines.[50] Scrutiny of the literature reveals a dosage range from as low as 50 mg/day of amphetamine up to 1000 mg/day.

For example, in a study conducted by Smith and co-workers,[50] low oral doses tended to be associated with increased libido in both males and females. These low doses, however, sustained erections and produced some delay in ejaculation in males. High doses produced sexual dysfunction in both males and females. Males reported impotence and failure of orgasm while females reported failure of orgasm. But at higher intravenous doses, the pharmacogenic orgasm became a substitute for the sex act. Parr[18] has reported increased capacity for repeated orgasm in both sexes.

There is documented evidence that the incidence of sexual deviance increases under the influence of amphetamines.[50–52] As Dr. George Gay suggests, "Speed makes strange bedfellows."

There are numerous speculations concerning the mechanisms of the amphetamine-induced alteration of sexual function. Amphetamines act on dopaminergic systems[53] and peripheral $\alpha$- and $\beta$-adrenergic receptors,[54] inhibit monoamine oxidase (MAO), block neuronal uptake mechanism of catecholamines and serotonin, and cause a release of catecholamines from nerve endings.[53,55]

### *b. Cocaine*

According to the *High Times Encyclopedia*,[2]

> Cocaine is by far the sexiest of the illicit drugs, both in ambience and effect. "Power," according to Henry Kissinger, "is the ultimate aphrodisiac," and at current prices, cocaine is one of the most visible emblems of the wealthy and powerful hedonist. Though sometimes called "girl," the enchanting white powder is always thought of as a "lady"—seductive, sophisticated and exotically expensive.

Gawin[56] suggests that cocaine's effects on sexuality seem to be similar to those of amphetamine and may share similar mechanisms of action. Ellinwood and Rockwell[57] report that patients have claimed spontaneous erections following intravenous injection of both cocaine and amphetamine. Furthermore multiple orgasms have been reported to be facilitated by both cocaine and amphetamine.[56] Cocaine has the ability also to contract vaginal musculature.[57] Siegel,[58] in his study of 85 male social–recreational cocaine users, observed that 13 percent experienced sexual stimulation and 4 percent experienced situational sexual impotency.

Siegel[58] also found that 42 percent of males in his study used cocaine "to enhance performance at play (e.g., sports, hiking, sex)," whereas only 20 percent of females used cocaine knowingly to enhance sexual performance.

Finally, there are no controlled studies of the effects of cocaine on human sexuality.

## 4. Psychedelics

### *a. Lysergic Acid Diethylamide (LSD-25)*

The publication of Dr. Timothy Leary's famous 1966 *Playboy* interview calling LSD the most powerful aphrodisiac known to humanity probably sparked its widespread use in the 1960s. Leary said, "In a carefully prepared loving LSD session, a woman will inevitably have several hundred orgasms.'

Intense reaction to the interview came from many individuals, including Harry J. Anslinger, who pronounced that: "If we wanted to take Leary literally, we should call LSD 'Let's Start Degeneracy.' "

The sexual response to LSD and other hallucinogens of our culture varies widely among individuals. The uninhibiting nature of the psychedelics is probably the result of their profound effects on the five known senses so that people experience overwhelming sexual desire. It has been noted[2] that "many individuals born after World War II consider the most moving moments of their lives to be the ecstatic 'highs' of making love on good LSD."

In a similar vein, Richard Alpert (Baba Ram Dass) stated in *Playboy* in 1970: "Before taking LSD, I never stayed in a state of sexual ecstasy for hours on end, but I have done this under LSD. It heightens all of your senses and it means that you're living the sexual experience totally. Each caress or kiss is timeless."

A liberal, rather nonscientific overview of the effects of LSD on sexual function can be derived from the statement by Leary in the 1966 *Playboy* interview:

> The sexual impact is, of course, the open but private secret about LSD, which none of us has talked about in the last few years. . . . You can no more do research on LSD and leave out sexual ecstasy than you can do microscopic research on tissue and leave out cells. . . . The LSD session, you see, is an overwhelming awakening of experience; it releases potent, primal energies, and one of these is the sexual impulse, which is the strongest impulse at any level of organic life. . . ."

Scrutiny of the literature reveals that reports on the sexual side effects of LSD are conflicting. Although there are no adequate studies on the sexual effects of LSD, Gawin[56] and Gay et al.[42] report that some users have experienced no sexual feelings, whereas others have had deeply moving sexual–emotional experiences.

### *b. Phencyclidine (PCP)*

A dissociative anesthetic, PCP is discussed in detail in Chapter 18. Because of untoward reactions in initial tests with humans, the drug has been relegated to use in animals.[59] Most drug users do not use it for sexual purposes because it does not enhance sexual excitement. In one study, however, 50 percent of heavy chronic PCP abusers experienced more sexual desire after PCP use.[60]

In the same study, the authors observed that both recreational (light chronic users) and heavy abusers, after coming down from a PCP high, tended to have a decrease in sexual feelings following PCP use.

In homosexual males, PCP has been utilized to disinhibit and relieve pain associated with anal–manus intercourse (called "fisting").[59] Smith and associates[59] also found that high doses or chronic abuse has been linked with erectile and/or ejaculatory impairment, but less than that observed with heroin or amphetamine.

### c. *Ketamine Hydrochloride*

Ketamine, another dissociative anesthetic similar to PCP, is used mainly in surgery on children.[61] There are a few reports[62,63] indicating that its prime effect on sexual function is that it can prevent erections in patients. The mechanism of action of the erectile effects of ketamine is unknown.

### d. *3,4-Methylenedioxyamphetamine (MDA)*

An amphetamine derivative, MDA has been used as an adjunct in psychotherapy.[64,65]

According to Welti and Brodsky[66] and Gawin,[56] MDA facilitates sexual enhancement by increasing communication and emotional feelings. Although there have been no reports of sexual dysfunction because of its similarity to amphetamine, it is probably safe to assume that it may alter the erectile response in males, as with high doses of amphetamines, and may even interfere with libido.

Little is known about the sexual effects of other psychedelics (i.e., psilocybin, mescaline, and ibogaine).

## 5. Marihuana

Jaffe[67] and Hollister[68] suggest that the active ingredient of cannabis, D-9-tetrahydrocannabinol (THC), has properties of the sedatives, stimulants, and hallucinogens, and probably belongs in its own pharmacologic class.

Of the many social upheavals of the 1960s, only cannabis and sexual revolutions survived without major reversals.[2] The primary reason is that humans by nature are "pleasure seekers" and both marihuana and sex are positive reinforcers in this regard. Marihuana and hashish enhance *all* the perceptions, but specific sensual modifications depend upon the dose and the individual to a significant extent.

According to *High Times Encyclopedia*,[2] "a common sensation reported by cannabinol couples is that their sex organs feel larger." Generally, however, marihuana joints will slow both lovers down, but could make the experience more satisfying. The THC enhances the sexual experience in females by releasing inhibitions and allowing them to experience orgasm more freely while it overcomes premature orgasm in men.

An interesting quotation from Louisa M. Alcott's *Perilous Play* in 1869 seems to favor the use of hashish as a sexual aid: "He stretched his hand to her with his heart in his face, and she gave him hers with a look of tender submission, as he said ardently, 'Heaven bless hashish, if its dreams end like this.' "

After years of careful study, the Indian Hemp Drugs Commission Report[69] in 1894 concluded: "As a matter of fact, it is used by ascetics in this country [India] with the ostensible object of destroying sexual appetite."

These two opposing views present a noncomprehensible incongruity.

During the 1930s in the United States, such a mania about sex crazes arose that it was asserted that a reefer could drive its smoker to the depths of erotic depravity. Certainly even Harry Anslinger, the first Director of the Federal Bureau of Narcotics, would agree that marihuana intensifies sex.

Cohen[70] lists the various effects of marihuana on sexual function as follows:

*Sensory Enhancement*—The intensification of sensory awareness that is a component of many marihuana experiences can carry over into the sexual act. Tactile, visual, and auditory sensations may be amplified and sensualized.

*Prolongation of Time Sense*—Rather large amounts of cannabis are required to slow subjective time perception. This factor is part of the claims of increased coital satisfaction.

*Increased Dyadic Affectional Bonding*—At times, a loosening of emotional constraints develops during cannabis intoxication. This can lead to feelings of fusion and empathy as ego controls and superego surveillance are relaxed.

*Disinhibition*—Related to the above, a generalized disinhibition of behavior common to most consciousness-altering substances may permit certain activities to proceed that would evoke guilt feelings under sober conditions.

*Self-transcendence*—In high dose cannabis states, a diffusion of the ego boundaries can develop, and this might contribute to the experience of fusion with the partner.

*Sexualized Fantasy*—The cognitive shift during the

cannabis experience is toward increased reverie and fantasy-laden thinking. Sexualized imagery would tend to enhance enjoyment of the act.

In very high doses, such as those seen in chronic hashish abuse in India, it has been reported to cause both decreased libido and inability to perform.[68,71] In more moderate doses, however, it has been said to enhance sexual function, as discussed by Cohen,[70] Halikas et al.,[72] and Nowlis.[73]

Halikas and associates studied extensively the effects of regular marihuana use on sexual performance and concluded that, although 75 percent of males and 50 percent of females indicated that feelings of sexual pleasure and satisfaction were increased with marihuana, for only 35 percent of the males and 13 percent of the females was the duration of intercourse increased.

These authors[72] point out that, in terms of marihuana-induced effects on sexual performance, over half of the males and less frequent users reported an enhancement of quality of orgasm. The majority of subjects reported no effect of marihuana on duration of intercourse, number of orgasms, or ability to repeat, with only a very small percentage of males (not abusers or frequent users) indicating negative effects on their performance. (See Table 20-1.)

In the same study,[72] the modalities most affected by marihuana were the tactile-related senses of touching and physical closeness, which were reported to be enhancd, or variably enhanced, by 60 percent in the users. The next

**TABLE 20-1**

**Marihuana-Induced Effects on Sexual Performance**

| | **Gender** | | **Recent Usage** | | **Abuser Status** | |
|---|---|---|---|---|---|---|
| | *Males (N = 60), Percent* | *Females (N = 37), Percent* | *Less Frequent (N = 75) Percent* | *Frequent (N = 22) Percent* | *Male Nonabusers (N = 52) Percent)* | *Male Abusers (N = 8) Percent* |
| Duration of intercourse: | | | | | | |
| Increased | 27 | 8 | 22 | 14 | 28 | 25 |
| Decreased | 0 | 0 | 0 | 0 | 0 | 0 |
| Variable | 12 | 8 | 10 | 14 | 10,25 | No effect |
| 61 | 84 | 68 | 72 | 62 | 50 | |
| Group differences | $p = 0.05$ | | Not significant | | Not significant | |
| Quality of orgasm: | | | | | | |
| Enhanced | 58 | 32 | 51 | 36 | 57 | 63 |
| Decreased | 0 | 0 | 0 | 0 | 0 | 0 |
| Variable | 10 | 8 | 8 | 14 | 8 | 25 |
| No effect | 32 | 60 | 41 | 50,35,12 | | |
| Group differences | $p = 0.02$ | | Not significant | | Not significant | |
| Number of orgasms: | | | | | | |
| Increased | 12 | 16 | 16 | 5 | 12 | 13 |
| Decreased | 2 | 0 | 1 | 0 | 2 | 0 |
| Variable | 7 | 11 | 5 | 18 | 6 | 13 |
| No effect | 80 | 73 | 78 | 77 | 80 | 75 |
| Group differences | Not significant | | Not significant | | Not significant | |
| Ability to repeat: | | | | | | |
| Increased | 14 | 3 | 11 | 5 | 12 | 25 |
| Decreased | 3 | 0 | 3 | 0 | 4 | 0 |
| Variable | 3 | 5 | 4 | 5 | 4 | 0 |
| No effect | 80 | 92 | 82 | 90 | 80 | 75 |
| Group differences | Not significant | | Not significant | | Not significant | |

*Source G. & L. (with permission)

From Halikas, J., Wellen, R., and Morse, C. Effects of regular marijuana use on sexual performance, *J. Psychoact. Drugs* 14(1–2):65, 1982. (With permission.)

most affected was snuggling (50 percent), followed by taste (29 percent), smell (19 percent), hearing (17 percent), and sight (10 percent). Two male subjects said that marihuana decreased their sense of smell. Males and females did not differ significantly in their reports of any of these sensory effects. (See Table 20-2.)

Furthermore, in the Halikas study,[72] more than 70 percent of the users felt that marihuana acts as an aphrodisiac, but only about 9 percent

## TABLE 20-2

### Marihuana-Induced Effects on Specific Senses During Sexual Activity*

| | **Gender** | | **Recent Usage** | | **Abuser Status** | |
|---|---|---|---|---|---|---|
| | *Males (N = 60) Percent* | *Females (N = 37) Percent* | *Less Frequent (N = 75) Percent* | *Frequent (N = 22), Percent* | *Male Nonabusers (N = 52), Percent* | *Male Abusers (N = 8), Percent* |
| Touching: | | | | | | |
| Enhanced | 59 | 57 | 62 | 47 | 60 | 50 |
| Decreased | 0 | 0 | 0 | 0 | 0 | 0 |
| Variable | 3 | 3 | 4 | 0 | 3 | 0 |
| No effect | 39 | 40 | 35 | 53 | 37 | 50 |
| Physical closeness: | | | | | | |
| Enhanced | 51 | 56 | 50 | 67 | 55 | 25 |
| Decreased | 0 | 0 | 0 | 0 | 0 | 0 |
| Variable | 9 | 4 | 8 | 0 | 10 | 0 |
| No effect | 40 | 41 | 42 | 33 | 36 | 75 |
| Snuggling: | | | | | | |
| Enhanced | 34 | 56 | 42 | 50 | 36 | 25 |
| Decreased | 0 | 0 | 0 | 0 | 0 | 0 |
| Variable | 9 | 4 | 8 | 0 | 7 | 25 |
| No effect | 57 | 41 | 50 | 50 | 58 | 50 |
| Taste: | | | | | | |
| Enhanced | 23 | 33 | 24 | 42 | 23 | 25 |
| Decreased | 0 | 0 | 0 | 0 | 0 | 0 |
| Variable | 0 | 4 | 2 | 0 | 0 | 0 |
| No effect | 77 | 63 | 74 | 58 | 77 | 75 |
| Smell: | | | | | | |
| Enhanced | 23 | 7 | 16 | 17 | 23 | 25 |
| Decreased | 3 | 0 | 0 | 8 | 3 | 0 |
| Variable | 0 | 4 | 2 | 0 | 0 | 0 |
| No effect | 74 | 89 | 82 | 75 | 74 | 75 |
| Hearing: | | | | | | |
| Enhanced | 17 | 11 | 16 | 8 | 19 | 0 |
| Decreased | 0 | 0 | 0 | 0 | 0 | 0 |
| Variable | 3 | 0 | 2 | 0 | 0 | 25 |
| No effect | 80 | 89 | 82 | 92 | 81 | 75 |
| Sight: | | | | | | |
| Enhanced | 11 | 7 | 10 | 8 | 13 | 0 |
| Decreased | 0 | 0 | 0 | 0 | 0 | 0 |
| Variable | 0 | 4 | 0 | 0 | 0 | 0 |
| No effect | 89 | 93 | 90 | 92 | 87 | 100 |

*No group differences significant at or above 0.05 level.

From Halikas, J., Weller, R., and Morse, C. Effects of regular marijuana use in sexual performance. *J. Psychoact. Drugs* 14(1–2):65, 1982. (With permission.)

rated the effect as strong. (See Tables 20-3 and 20-4.)

With regard to an explanation for the sexual enhancement effects of marihuana, Dalterio and associates[74] found that low-dose oral administration of THC results in a rapid sustained elevation of serum testosterone, whereas high doses result in an initial rise followed by a decrease below baseline serum levels. This mechanism could explain why low doses are associated with sexual enhancement, but high doses with sexual dysfunction.

Recent research has provided evidence that would caution against the indiscriminate use of

**TABLE 20-3**

**Is Marihuana an Aphrodisiac?**

| | **Gender** | | **Recent Usage** | | **Abuser Status** | |
|---|---|---|---|---|---|---|
| | *Males (N = 60), Percent* | *Females (N = 37), Percent* | *Less Frequent (N = 75), Percent* | *Frequent (N = 22), Percent* | *Male Nonabusers (N = 52), Percent* | *Male Abusers (N = 8), Percent* |
| Yes, mild | 36 | 34 | 33 | 54 | 38 | 25 |
| Yes, strong | 8 | 11 | 10 | 8 | 9 | 0 |
| Variable effect | 28 | 21 | 26 | 23 | 25 | 50 |
| No effect | 28 | 29 | 31 | 15 | 28 | 25 |
| Group differences | Not significant | | Not significant | | Not significant | |

From Halikas, J., Weller, R., and Morse, C. Effects of regular marijuana use on sexual performance. *J. Psychoact. Drugs* 14(1–2):68, 1982. (With permission.)

**TABLE 20-4**

**Marihuana-Induced Effects on Sexual Enjoyment***

| | **Gender** | | **Recent Usage** | | **Abuser Status** | |
|---|---|---|---|---|---|---|
| | *Males (N = 60), Percent* | *Females (N = 37), Percent* | *Less Frequent (N = 75), Percent* | *Frequent (N = 22), Percent* | *Male Nonabusers (N = 52), Percent* | *Male Abusers (N = 8), Percent* |
| Feelings of sexual pleasure and satisfaction: | | | | | | |
| Increased | 70 | 76 | 75 | 65 | 72 | 50 |
| Decreased | 3 | 0 | 2 | 0 | 3 | 0 |
| Variable | 5 | 14 | 8 | 12 | 6 | 0 |
| No effect | 23 | 10 | 15 | 24 | 19 | 50 |
| Feelings of emotional closeness and intimacy: | | | | | | |
| Increased | 46 | 63 | 52 | 58 | 48 | 25 |
| Decreased | 3 | 0 | 2 | 0 | 3 | 0 |
| Variable | 14 | 7 | 10 | 17 | 13 | 25 |
| No effect | 37 | 30 | 36 | 25 | 36 | 50 |

*No group differences reached 0.05 level of significance.

From Halikas, J., Weller, R., and Morse, C. Effects of regular marijuana use on sexual performance. *J. Psychoact. Drugs* 14(1–2):68, 1982. (With permission.)

cannabis as an aphrodisiac.[70] The following is a list of research results on the effects of THC on gonadal hormones.

- Large doses of THC (equivalent to seven NIDA joints a day for nine days in humans) produced decreased testosterone production in male rats along with a reduction in testicular weight.[75]
- After four weeks of heavy marihuana use (eight to 20 cigarettes a day), healthy human male smokers produced a decrease in sperm count and a reduction of sperm with normal structure. These changes seem to be reversible.[76] A rat study revealed similar findings.[77]
- There are conflicting reports of testosterone reduction in male humans. A number of studies have been positive, and an equal number negative. Even if it turns out that chronic heavy smoking does reduce testosterone levels over time, the decrement is from normal to low-normal levels. This should not interfere with normal sexual functioning.
- Single large doses (50 to 350 mg of THC equivalent in women) can decrease LH and follicle-stimulating hormone in female monkeys.[78]
- Female monkeys receiving 2.4 mg/kg of THC orally for up to five years lost 42 percent of pregnancies as compared with a control group that had an 8 to 11 percent loss.[79] No effects were cited on male monkeys. No difference in sexual function was observed.

Although there are cautions against the indiscriminate use of marihuana, which may be backed by scientific fact, and even known negative effects on sexual function with high doses, young adults are not ready to stop abusing this sexual stimulant.

Cohen[70] points out that:

> The indiscriminate use or abuse of marihuana for sex-related activities may well have been termed ''promiscuous'' by a preceding generation or two. However, because of the general loosening of morality, the erosion of family, church and other authoritarian controls, the Pill, antibiotics, anti-Herpes pills and other developments have contributed to the acceptance of its current use. In short, marihuana is not the ultimate aphrodisiac, but for over two decades now has become as commonplace as the use of alcohol as a social intoxicant in people under the age of 35, searching for a sexual stimulant.

## 6. Volatile Nitrites

Lowry[80] suggests that the inhalable nitrites may be the nearest thing to a true aphrodisiac. If Lowry's suggestion is not scientifically accurate, approximately 250 million recreational doses have been consumed yearly in the United States for erroneous reasons.

The volatile nitrites are yellowish flammable liquids with an odor described as fruity or unpleasant. The nitrites are unstable and decompose to heat, oxygen, and light. There are two marketable forms of volatile nitrites: (1) amyl nitrite, a prescription drug used in cardiology, in conditions such as angina pectoris; and (2) butyl nitrite, which is marketed as a ''room odorizer'' under such trade names as Quicksilver and Hardware; its street use as a sexual stimulant includes such names as Rush, Bolt, Locker Room, Bullet, Aroma of Men, and Dr. Bananas.

In 1969, amyl nitrite was removed as an over-the-counter product and became a prescription drug once again. Users in the Southwest now travel to Mexico where no prescription is required. In contrast, butyl nitrite can be purchased at head shops and adult bookstores, by mail, and at a few liquor stores. It is available in 12-ml screw-top bottles; amyl nitrite is sold in 0.3-ml crushable ampules (''poppers,'' ''snappers'').

Nitrites relax vascular smooth muscles, and produce beneficial effects on the heart by relaxing systemic arterioles, thus resulting in a fall in blood pressure, reflex tachycardia, and a decrease in left ventricular work. In terms of peripheral effects that may impinge upon sexual response, the nitrites produce in the user a sense of warmth, giddiness, and a pounding heart. The major central nervous system (CNS) effect is dilation of the retinal and pial arteries and veins, an increase in brain volume, and an increased cerebral blood flow.

Lowry[80] reports that social uses of the nitrites involve dancing and sexuality. It is well known that in discos (especially gay discos), individuals sniff nitrites on the dance floor, thus enjoying a combined high of lights, rhythm, drugs, and social–sexual excitement.

Nitrites induce a release of inhibitions during foreplay, which enables the user to experience total skin-surface sensuality. In females, it has been noted that nitrites reduce the primary female sexual dysfunction—distraction—in which peripheral thoughts of unfinished business, child care, body self-consciousness, and domestic duties interfere with sexual sensations. In short, nitrites may facilitate the process of "letting go." Additional effects include a sensation of timelessness and the enhancement of penetration, especially anal. Nitrites reduce the pain of penetration because muscles are relaxed and there is decreased pain perception. When nitrites are inhaled shortly before orgasm, the user may experience a sense of exhiliration and acceleration, a freeing of inhibition of movement and vocalization, and a perception of orgasm as being greatly prolonged, intense, and exalted. Headaches seem to be the prime toxicologic problem associated with their use.

According to Lowry,[81] the Drug Abuse Warning Network (DAWN) found that of 1,350,000 drug-related emergency visits, only 67 were related to volatile nitrites. There were no deaths reported when the substance was inhaled, but deaths have occurred when it was ingested.[82]

In summary, the volatile nitrites have positive effects on sexual function, with limited toxicity, when inhaled, but are quite dangerous when swallowed.

## 7. Nitrous Oxide

Impotence in approximately 50 percent (seven of 15) dental personnel using available nitrous oxide for recreational purposes has been seen. The impotence was one of many symptoms found when myeloneuropathy developed as a result of exposure to nitrous oxide.

## 8. Tobacco

The advertising industry has attempted to link cigarette smoking and human sexuality. In reality, there is only one negative report, by Forsberg and co-workers,[83] associated with erectile dysfunction in two young men. It appears that tobacco, when smoked, may reduce penile blood flow, resulting in a reversible inhibition of erectile capacity.

## 9. Disulfiram (Antabuse)

As discussed in Chapter 11 on alcohol, disulfiram is described as an aldehyde dehydrogenase inhibitor that is used clinically in the treatment of alcoholism. Van Thiel and associates[84] report that disulfiram alters the hypothalamic–pituitary–gonadal function. Ewing et al.[85] point out that, if disulfiram is used clinically at doses of 2 grams per day, one might expect a 10 to 12 percent incidence of impotence. Today much lower doses are usually employed, with little or no reports of sexual dysfunction.

## 10. Naloxone (Narcaon)

Naloxone, the narcotic antagonist used clinically to block the central effects of illicit opiates, was seen to increase copulatory behavior in sexually inactive rats by blocking the endogenous endorphins, which could otherwise block sexual behavior.[86] Goldstein and Hamsteen[87] observed no alteration in the sexual arousal, penile erection, ejaculation, or orgasm in a 35-year-old male receiving 10 mg of naloxone intravenously administered. They concluded that endorphins are not involved in sexual behavior.

## 11. Antipsychotics

Antipsychotics block dopamine in the CNS, which could adversely affect libido through hypothalamic–pituitary–gonadal axis suppression.[88,89] As $\alpha$-adrenergic blocking agents, they could block neural innervation of the internal genital organs. Finally, the vasodilating properties of some antipsychotics could block erectile response by shunting blood away from the genitals. The following antipsychotic agents are reported to affect human sexuality.

- Thioridazine (Mellaril)
- Mesoridazine (Serentil)
- Chlorpromazine (Thorazine)
- Chlorprothixene (Taractan)
- Fluphenazine (Prolixin)
- Perphenazine (Trilafon)
- Trifluoperazine (Stelazine)
- Butaperazine (Repoise)
- Haloperidol (Haldol)

### 12. Antidepressants

Both the tricyclic and MAO inhibitors block the reuptake of catecholamines and serotonin.[90,91] Tricyclics also possess peripheral anticholinergic effects.[92] Although decreased libido, inhibition of erection, and inhibition of ejaculation have been reported with tricyclics[93] and MAO inhibitors,[94] the exact mechanisms are not clear. Since decreased libido is associated with depression, it becomes very difficult to differentiate disease-induced suppression of sexual activity from drug-induced effects. The following is a list of antidepressants cited for effects on induction of sexual dysfunction.

- Imipramine (Tofranil)
- Amitriptyline (Elavil)
- Protriptyline (Vivactyl)
- Desipramine (Norpramin)
- Clomipramine (Anatranil)
- Amoxapine (Asendin)
- Tranylcypromine (Parnate)
- Phenelzine (Nardil)
- Isocarboxazid (Marplan)
- Pargyline (Eutonyl)

### 13. Antimania Drugs (Lithium—Eskalith)

Vinarova et al.[95] observed that lithium in patients caused "impaired sexual function and decreased sexual appetite." In this study, sexual function did return to normal when the lithium was terminated. Interestingly Buffum[17] points out that because hypersexuality is a symptom of mania, a decrease in sexual function might be attributable either to a resolution of the manic state or to a toxic effect of the drug.

### 14. Other Drugs

There are other psychoactive substances that enhance sexuality in animals, but may or may not affect human sexual function. For completion only, the reader should refer to the review by Buffum[17] and inspect Table 20-5 for additional details on drug effects on sexual function in males.

## D. SUMMARY

This chapter briefly reviews the effects of psychoactive agents on sexual function and dysfunction. Certainly clinically useful drugs have sexual side effects. Additionally, illicit use of central acting agents also produces both sexual enhancement and sexual dysfunction, depending on many critical factors (i.e., dose, frequency, setting, etc.).

Throughout history, there has been a search for the so-called "true" aphrodisiac. No drug known today can fulfill all the critical requirements, yet young and old alike continue to explore, experiment, indulge in, and abuse certain of these substances for sexual recreational stimulation as a substitute for or enhancer of sexuality. For the most part, it appears that chronic abuse of popular drugs such as opiates, alcohol, and cocaine results in impotence and has profound negative effects on sexual functions in both males and females.

The explosion of drug use and the sexual revolution of the 1960s paved the way for the development of a new discipline known as "pharmacosexology." There are numerous unanswered questions concerning both effects and mechanisms of drug-induced alterations of sexual function. The era of the 1980s inevitably will result in furthering the phenomena of psychopharmacosexology, and will provide, through laborious research, those answers so urgently needed by street drug *aficionados*.

## TABLE 20-5

## Drug Effects on Sexual Function in Males

| | *Decreases Desire* | *Erectile Dysfunction* | *Ejaculatory Dysfunction* |
|---|---|---|---|
| *Antihypertensives* | | | |
| Diuretics | | | |
| Thiazides (bendroflumethiazide) | None | 9–20% | None |
| Spironolactone (Aldactone) | Common | 4–30% (high dose) | None |
| Chlorthalidone (Hygroton) | None | Occurs | None |
| Nondiuretics | | | |
| Methyldopa (Aldomet) | 7–14% | 2–80% | 7–19% |
| Propranolol (Inderal) | 1–4% | Up to 28% | None |
| Clonidine (Catapres) | Occurs | 4–70% | None |
| Guanethidine (Ismelin) | 29% | 4–100% | 2–100% |
| Hydralazine (Apresoline) | None | None | None |
| Prazosin (Minipres) | None | 0.6–4% | None |
| Reserpine (Serpasil) | 7% (small study) | 11–33% | 14% |
| Metoprolol (Lopressor) | None | None | None |
| Minoxidil (Loniten) | None | None | None |
| Phenoxybenzamine (Dibenzylene) | None | None | 4.5–100% (retrograde ejaculation rarely occurs) |
| Atenolol (Tenormin) | None | 0.2% | None |
| Timolol (Blocadren) | 0.6% | Occurs | None |
| Nadolol (Corgard) | "Sexual dysfunction" occurs | "Sexual dysfunction" occurs | "Sexual dysfunction" occurs |
| *Antipsychotics* | | | |
| Thioridazine (Mellaril) | Occurs | 54% | 30–57% |
| Other antipsychotics | Isolated cases | Isolated cases | Isolated cases |
| Mesoridazine (Serentil) | | | |
| Chlorpromazine (Thorazine) | | | |
| Fluphenazine (Prolixin) | | | |
| Perphenazine (Trilafon) | | | |
| Trifluoperazine (Stelazine) | | | |
| Butaperazine (Repoise) | | | |
| Haloperidol (Haldol) | | | |
| Chlorprothixene (Taractan) | | | |
| *Antidepressants* | | | |
| Tricyclics | | | |
| Increased/decreased desire | | | |
| Isolated cases | | | |
| Isolated cases | | | |
| Amitriptyline (Elavil) | | | |
| Protriptyline (Vivactil) | | | |
| Imipramine (Tofranil) | | | |
| Desipramine (Norpramin) | | | |
| Amoxapine (Asendin) | | | |
| MAO Inhibitors | Increased desire | Occurs | Occurs |
| Tranylcypromine (Parnate) | | | |
| Phenelzine (Nardil) | | | |
| Lithium carbonate | Two cases | Two cases | None |
| *Hormones* | | | |
| Progestins | Common | 24–70% | Occurs |
| Estrogens | Common | Common | Occurs |
| Corticosteroids | None | None | None |
| Antiandrogens | Common | Common | Occurs |
| Androgens | Increased/decreased desire | Increased/decreased erections | None |
| *Sedative-hypnotics* | | | |
| Benzodiazepines | | | |
| Diazepam (Valium) | None | None | None |
| Chlordiazepoxide (Librium) | None | None | None |

## TABLE 20-5 (continued)
## Drug Effects on Sexual Function in Males

| | *Decreases Desire* | *Erectile Dysfunction* | *Ejaculatory Dysfunction* |
|---|---|---|---|
| Barbiturates | Increase†/ Decrease | Common | None |
| Methaqualone (Quaalude) | Increase†/ Decrease | Common | None |
| Ethyl alcohol | Increase†/ decrease | Common | Occurs |
| *Stimulants* | | | |
| Amphetamine | Increase | Occurs | Occurs |
| Cocaine | Increase | Occurs | Occurs |
| *Opiates* | | | |
| Heroin | 60% | 39% | 70% |
| Methadone (Dolophine) | 6–38% | 6–50% | 5–88% |
| *Other drugs and chemicals* | | | |
| Marihjuana | Increase/ decrease | Increase/ decrease | None |
| LSD (lysergic acid diethylamide) | Increase/ decrease | Occurs | Occurs |
| MDA (3,4-methylenedioxyamphetamine) | Increase/ decrease | Occurs | Occurs |
| Cimetidine (Tagamet) | 31 cases | 31 cases | None |
| Aminocaproic acid (Amicar) | None | None | 24% |
| Disopyramide (Norpace) | None | 2 cases | None |
| Thiabendazole (Minitezol) | None | 9% | None |
| Clofibrate (Atromid-S) | None | 3% | None |
| Methantheline (Banthine) | None | Occurs | None |
| Ketamine (Ketoject) | None | Occurs | None |
| Insecticides and herbicides (type not known) | None | Four cases | One case |
| Nitrous oxide | None | Seven cases | None |
| Disulfiram (Antabuse) | None | 10–12%† | None |
| Digoxin (Lanoxin) | 36% | 36% | None |
| Tobacco | None | Two cases | None |
| Cancer chemotherapy agents | Occurs | Occurs | None |
| Phencyclidine (PCP) | Increase/ decrease | Occurs | Occurs |
| Naproxen (Naprosyn) | None | None | One case |
| Carbonic anhydrase inhibitors | 32 cases | Three cases | None |
| Carbon disulfide | None | Occurs (60%) | None |
| *Drugs used to enhance sexual function* | | | |
| Levodopa (L-Dopa) | Increase (occurs) | None | Two cases |
| Volatile nitrites (amyl nitrite) | Increase (occurs) | Occurs | None |
| Bromocriptine (Parlodel) | Increase (occurs) | None | None |
| Zinc salts | Increase (occurs) | None | None |
| Parachlorophenylalanine (PCPA) | Increase (occurs) | None | None |
| L-Tryptophan | None | None | None |
| Yohimbine | None | None | None |
| Pheromones | Increase thought to occur | None | None |
| Clomiphene (Clomid) | Increase (one case) | Increase (one case) | None |
| Luteinizing hormone (LH) | Increase (occurs) | Increase (occurs) | None |
| Naloxone (Narcan) | Insufficient data | Insufficient data | Insufficient data |

*"None" indicates that there are currently no reports in the literature.
†Any increase in sexual desire secondary to sedative-hypnotics is probably due to disinhibition.
‡Erectile failure is seen only with high doses (2 grams/day); none is seen at low doses (500 mg/day).
From Buffum, J. Pharmacosexology: The effects of drugs on sexual function: A review, *J. Psychoact. Drugs*, 14(1–2):42, 1982. (With permission.)

## REFERENCES


1. Smith, D. E., et al. A clinical guide to the diagnosis and treatment of heroin-related sexual dysfunction. *J. Psychoactive Drugs* 14:91, 1982.
2. *High Times Encyclopedia of Recreational Drugs*. New York: Stonehill, 1978.
3. Masters, W. H., and Johnson, V. E. *Human Sexual Response*. Boston: Little Brown, 1966.
4. Hyyppä, M. T., et al. Neuroendocrine regulation of gonadotropin secretion and sexual motivation after l-tryptophan administration in man. In M. Sandler and D. L. Gessa, eds., *Sexual Behavior: Pharmacology and Biochemistry*. New York: Raven Press, 1975.
5. Newman, H. F., and Northrup, J. D. Mechanism of human penile erection: An overview. *Urology* 17:399, 1981.
6. Wagner, G., and Levin, R. J. Effect of atropine and methylatropine on human vaginal blood flow, sexual arousal and climax. *Acta Pharmacol. Toxicol.* 46:321, 1980.
7. Weiss, H. B. Physiology of human penile erections. *Ann. Intern. Med.* 76:793, 1972.
8. Domer, F., et al. Involvement of the sympathetic nervous system in the urinary bladder internal sphincter and in penile erection in the anesthetized cat. *Invest. Urol.* 15:404, 1978.
9. Dorr, L. D., and Brody, M. J. Hemodynamic mechanisms of erection in the canine penis. *Am. J. Physiol.* 213:1526, 1967.
10. Melman, A., et al. Alteration of the penile corpora in patients with erectile impotence. *Invest. Urol.* 17:474, 1980.
11. Marberger, H. The mechanisms of ejaculation. *Basic Life Sci.* 4(pt. B):99, 1974.
12. McLeod, D. G., Reynolds, D. G., and Demaree, G. E. Some pharmacologic characteristics of the human vas deferens. *Invest. Urol.* 10:338, 1973.
13. Kimura, Y., et al. The role of alpha-adrenergic receptor mechanism in ejaculation. *Tohoku J. Exp. Med.* 108:337, 1972.
14. Baumgarten, H. G., et al. Adrenergic innervation of the human testis, epididymus, ductus deferens and prostate: A fluorescence microscopic and fluorimetric study. *Z. Zellforsch. Mikrosk. Anat.* 90:81, 1968.
15. Kimura, Y., et al. The role of alpha-andrenergic receptor mechanism in closure of the internal urethral orifice during ejaculation. *Urol. Int.* 30:341, 1975.
16. Kolle, G. B. Neurohumoral transmission and the autonomic nervous system. In L. Goodman and A. Gilman, eds., *The Pharmacological Basis of Therapeutics*. New York: Macmillan, 1975.
17. Buffum, J. Pharmacosexology: The effects of drugs on sexual function. *J. Psychoactive Drugs* 14:5, 1982.
18. Parr, D. Sexual aspects of drug abuse in narcotic addicts. *Br. J. Addict.* 71:261, 1976.
19. Cicero, T. J., et al. Function of the male sex organs in heroin and methadone users. *N. Engl. J. Med.* 292:882, 1975.
20. Mintz, J., et al. Sexual problems of heroin addicts. *Arch. Gen. Psychiatry* 31:700, 1974.
22. DeLeon, G., and Wexler, H. K. Heroin addiction: Its relation to sexual behavior and sexual experience. *J. Abnorm. Psychol.* 31:36, 1973.
23. Cushman, P. Sexual behavior in heroin addiction and methadone maintenance. *N.Y. State J. Med.* 72:1261, 1972.
24. Smith, D. E., et al. A clinical guide to the diagnosis and treatment of heroin-related sexual dysfunction. *J. Psychoactive Drugs* 14:91, 1982.
25. Bai, J., et al. Drug-related menstrual aberrations. *Obstet. Gynec.* 44:713, 1974.
26. Mirin, S. M., et al. Opiate use and sexual function. *Am. J. Psychiatry* 137:909, 1980.
27. Jaffe, J. H., and Martin, W. R. Narcotic analgesics and antagonists. In L. Goodman and A. Gilman, eds., *The Pharamcological Basis of Therapeutics*. New York: Macmillan, 1975.
28. Espejo, R., Hogben, G., and Stimmel, B. Sexual performance of men on methadone maintenance. In *Proceedings of the National Conference of Methadone Treatment, New York City*, vol. 1, 1973, pp. 490–493.
29. Handbury, R., Cohen, M., and Stimmel, B. Adequacy of sexual performance in men maintained on methadone. *Am. J. Drug Alcohol Abuse* 4:13, 1977.
30. Kreek, M. J. Medical safety and side effects of methadone in tolerant individuals. *JAMA* 223:665, 1973.
31. Cassidy, W. J. Maintenance methadone treatment of drug dependency. *Can. Psychiatr. Assoc. J.*. 17:107, 1972.
32. Soyka, L., Joffe, J., and Smith, S. Adverse effects of methadone (meth) on progeny acting through sires: Block by testosterone. *Fed. Proc.* 38:437, 1979.
33. Gordon, G. G., et al. The effect of alcohol (ethanol) administration on sex-hormone metabolism in normal men. *N. Engl. J. Med.* 295:793, 1976.
34. Mendelson, J. H., Mello, N. K., and Ellingboe, J. Effects of acute alcohol intake on pituitary-gonadal hormones in normal human males. *J. Pharmacol. Exp. Ther.* 202:676, 1977.
35. Chiao, Y. B., et al. Effect of chronic ethanol feeding on testicular content of enzymes required

for testosteronogenesis. *Alcoholism*. 5:230, 1981.
36. Gordon, G. G., Southren, A. L., and Lieber, C. S. Hypogonadism and feminization in the male: A triple effect of alcohol. *Alcohol. Clin. Exp. Res.* 3:210–211, 1979.
37. Van Thiel, D. H., and Lester, R. Sex and alcohol: A second peek. *N. Engl. J. Med.* 295:835, 1976.
38. Lemere, F., and Smith, J. W. Alcohol-induced sexual impotence. *Am. J. Psychiatry* 130:212, 1973.
39. Wilson, G. T., and Lawson, D. Effects of alcohol on sexual arousal in women. *J. Abnorm. Psychol.* 85:489, 1976.
40. Malatesta, V., et al. Acute alcohol intoxication and female orgasmic response. *J. Sex. Res.* 18:1, 1982.
41. Harvey, S. C. Hypnotics and sedatives (the barbiturates). In L. Goodman and A. Gilman, eds., *The Pharmacological Basis of Therapeutics*. New York: Macmillan, 1975.
42. Gay, G. R., et al. Drug-sex practices in the Haight-Ashbury, or the "sensuous hippie," In M. Sandler and D. L. Gessa, eds., *Sexual Behavior: Pharmacology and Biochemistry*. New York: Raven Press, 1975.
43. Usdin, G. L. Preliminary report on librium: A new psychopharmacologic agent. *J. La. State Med. Soc.* 112:142, 1960.
44. Hughes, J. M. Failure to ejaculate with chlordiazepoxide. *Am. J. Psychiatry* 121:610, 1964.
45. Kochansky, G. E., et. al. Methaqualone abusers: A preliminary survey of college students. *Dis. Nerv. Sys.* 36:348, 1975.
46. Gerald, M. C., and Schwirian, P. M. Nonmedical use of methaqualone. *Arch. Gen. Psychiatry* 28:627, 1973.
47. Inaba, D. S., et al. Methaqualone abuse—"Luding out." *JAMA* 224:1505, 1973.
48. Weissberg, K. Sopors are a bummer. *Berkeley Barb* Sept. 1-7:13, 1972.
49. Ager, S. A. Luding out. *N. Engl. J. Med.* 287:51, 1972.
50. Smith, D. E., Buxton, M. E., and Dammann, G. Amphetamine abuse and sexual dysfunction: Clinical and research considerations. In D. E. Smith, ed., *Amphetamine Use, Misuse and Abuse*. Cambridge, Mass.: G. K. Hall, 1979.
51. Angrist, B., and Gershon, S. Clinical effects of amphetamine and L-dopa on sexuality and aggression. Comp. Psychiatry 17:715, 1976.
52. Bell, D. S., and Trethowan, W. H. Amphetamine addiction and disturbed sexuality. *Arch. Gen. Psychiatry* 4:76, 1961.
53. Patrick, R. L. Amphetamine and cocaine: Biological mechanisms. In J. D. Barkas et al., eds., *Psychopharmacology: From Theory to Practice*. New York: Oxford University Press, 1977.
54. Innes, I. R., and Nickerson, M. Atropine, scopolamine and related antimuscarinic drugs. In L. S. Goodman and A. Gilman, eds. *The Pharmacological Basis of Therapeutics*. New York: Macmillan, 1975.
55. Weiner, N. Norepinephrine, epinephrine and the sympathomenetic amines. In L. S. Goodman and A. Gilman, eds., *The Pharmacological Basis of Therapeutics*, 6th ed. New York: Macmillan, 1980.
56. Gawin, F. H. Drugs and eros: Reflection on aphrodisiacs. *J. Psychedel. Drugs* 10(3):227, 1978.
57. Ellinwood, E. H., and Rockwell, K. The effect of drug use on sexual behavior. *Med. Aspects Hum. Sex.* 9:10, 1975.
58. Siegel, R. K. Cocaine: Recreational use and intoxication. In R. C. Petersen and R. C. Stillman, eds., *Cocaine: 1977*. NIDA Research Monograph no. 13. Rockville, Md.: NIDA, 1977.
59. Smith, D. E., et al. PCP and sexual dysfunction. *J. Psychedel. Drugs* 12:269, 1980.
60. Graeven, D., Sharp, J., and Glatt, A. Acute effects of phencyclidine (PCP) on chronic and recreational users. *Am. J. Drug Alcohol Abuse* 8:39, 1981.
61. Price, H. L. General anesthetics (intravenous anesthetics). In L. Goodman and A. Gilman, eds., *The Pharmacological Basis of Therapeutics*. New York: Macmillan, 1975.
62. Pietras, J., Cromie, W., and Duckett, J. Ketamine as a detumescence agent during hypospadias repair. *J. Urol.* 121:654, 1979.
63. Gale, A. S. Ketamine prevention of penile turgescence. *JAMA* 219:1629, 1972.
64. Di Leo, F. B. Psychotherapy with psychedelic drugs: A case report. *J. Psychoactive Drugs* 13:319, 1982.
65. Naranjo, C. *The Healing Journal*. New York: Pantheon, 1974.
66. Welti, R., and Brodsky, J. Treatment of intraoperative penile tumescence. *J. Urol.* 124:925, 1980.
67. Jaffe, J. H. Drug addiction and drug abuse. In L. Goodman and A. Gilman, eds., *The Pharmacological Basis of Therapeutics*. New York: Macmillan, 1975.
68. Hollister, L. E. The mystique of social drugs and sex. In M. Sandler and D. L. Gessa, eds., *Sexual Behavior: Pharmacology and Biochemistry*. New York: Raven Press, 1975.

69. *Indian Hemp Drugs Commission Report*. Government Central Printing Office, Simla, India, 1894.
70. Cohen, S. Cannabis and sex: Multifaceted paradoxes. *J. Psychoactive Drugs* 14:55, 1982.
71. Chopra, G. S. Man and marijuana. *Int. J. Addict.* 4:215, 1969.
72. Halikas, J., Weller, R., and Morse, C. Effects of regular marijuana use on sexual performance. *J. Psychoactive Drugs* 14:59, 1982.
73. Nowlis, V. Categories of interest in the scientific search for relationships (i.e., interactions, associations, comparisons) in human sexual behavior and drug use. In M. Sandler and D. L. Gessa, eds., *Sexual Behavior: Pharmacology and Biochemistry*. New York: Raven Press, 1975.
74. Dalterio, S., Bartke, A., and Mayfield, D. Delta 9-tetrahydrocannabinol increase plasma testosterone concentrations in mice. *Science* 213:581, 1981.
75. deHarcler, J., et al. Effect of cannabis on sex hormones and testicular enzymes of the rodent. In G. G. Nahas and W. D. M. Paton, eds., *Marijuana: Biological Effects*. New York: Pergamon Press, 1979.
76. Hembree, W. C., et al. Changes in human spermatazoa associated with high dose marijuana smoking. *Ibid.*
77. Huang, H. F. S., Nahas, G. G., and Hembree, W. C. Effects of marijuana inhalation on spermatogenesis of the rat. *Ibid.*
78. Smith, C. G., et al. Effects of delta-9-tetrahydrocannabinol on female reproductive function. *Ibid.*
79. Sassenrath, E. N., Chapman, L. F., and Goo, G. P. Reproduction of rhesus monkeys chronically exposed to delta-9-THC. *Ibid.*
80. Lowry, T. P. Psychosexual aspects of the volatile nitrites. *J. Psychoactive Drugs* 14:77, 1982.
81. Lowry, T. P. Amyl nitrite: A toxicological survey. In M. Nickerson, ed., *Isobutyl Nitrite and Related Compounds*. San Francisco: Pharmex.
82. Shesser, R., et al. Fatal methemoglobinemia from butyl nitrite ingestion. *Ann. Intern. Med.* 92:131, 1980.
83. Forsberg, L., et al. Impotence, smoking and beta-blocking drugs. *Fertil. Steril.* 31:589, 1979.
84. Van Thiel, D. H., et al. Disulfiram-induced disturbances in hypothalamic-pituitary function. *Alcoholism (NY)*, 3:230, 1979.
85. Ewing, J. A., et al., Roundtable: Alcohol, drugs and sex. *Med. Aspects Hum. Sex.* 4:18, 1970.
86. Gessa, G., and Paglietti, E. Induction of copulatory behavior in sexually inactive rats by naloxone. *Science* 204:203, 1979.
88. Arató, M., Erdös, A., and Polgár, M. Endocrinological changes in patients with sexual dysfunction under long-term neuroleptic treatment. *Pharmakopsychiatr. Neuropsychopharmacol.* 12:426, 1979.
89. Laughren, T., Brown, W., and Petrucci, J. Effects of thioridazine on serum testosterone. *Am. J. Psychiatry* 135:982, 1978.
90. Snyder, S. H., and Yamamura, H. I. Antidepressant and the muscarinic acetylcholine receptor. *Arch. Gen. Psychiatry* 34:236, 1977.
91. Hollister, L. E. Treatment of depression with drugs. *Ann. Intern. Med.* 89:78, 1978.
92. Byck, R. Drugs and the treatment of psychiatric disorders. In L. Goodman and A. Gilman, eds., *The Pharmacological Basis of Therapeutics*. New York: Macmillan, 1975.
93. Petrie, W. M. Sexual effects of antidepressants and psychomotor stimulant drugs. *Mod. Probl. Pharmacopsychiatry* 15:77, 1980.
94. Glass, R. Ejaculatory impairment from both phenelzine and imipramine, with tinnitus from phenelzine. *J. Clin. Psychopharmacol.* 1:152, 1981.
95. Vinarova, E., et al. Side effects of lithium administration. *Act. Nerv. Sup.* 14:105, 1972.

# CHAPTER 21

# Epilogue: ''Drug Odyssey 2001''

The area of psychopharmacology provides the fundamental principles that enable drugologists and/or alcohologists to understand the basic mechanisms of cellular actions of psychoactive compounds. But even if we eventually unravel all of the mysteries of how these drugs act in the body we will be left with the most illusive question: what in the everyday lives of human beings makes them take refuge in the drug world?

While a careful look at the work of neuroscientists reveals that strides are being made toward the understanding of the ''mind,'' we are still far from an exact definition or consensus on what it means. The studies are fraught with incomplete data. However, they have begun to comprehend the chemical messengers hurled—by nerve cells, across synapses—sending signals that process information, sustain emotions, and breathe life into our very existence. Our knowledge of the brain and its parallel science of psychology is in its infancy. Little more than a century ago, researchers were unable to interpret cellular forms lying under their microscopes. Today investigators chemically identify genetic inborn errors of metabolism, regenerate tissues, grow nerve cells, transplant organs, split molecules and atoms, clone, and produce color pictures of the living brain at work. Afficionados of brain science continue to encourage researchers in their tireless efforts to provide answers to the most basic questions: Who are we? Why do we respond in a particular fashion? Where do love, anger, joy, aggression lie in our ''minds'' and how do the feelings emerge? What do enzymes, hormones, and genes really do? Even with all our sophisticated scientific know-how, these remain ''mystical'' questions for most.

How far have scientists progressed since the ''father of psychoanalytic theory,'' Sigmund Freud, laid the groundwork? Freud created a symbionic relationship between psychoanalysts and biologists. Today a tribute to this concept is the documented evidence for a biochemic linkage of various brain ''molecules'' and ''addictive'' behavior and mental disorders.

Progress is dramatic; yet most of us are unaware of the wonders in the cranium. Joseph Conrad in *Heart of Darkness* said: ''The mind of man is capable of anything—because everything is in it, all the past as well as all the future.''

A fundamental premise about the brain is that its workings—sometimes referred to as the ''mind''—are the result of its anatomy, physiology, and neurochemistry, and that is all. The mind, therefore, is a consequence of the brain and of the action of its constituents. The entire scope of recent history and biology points to the conclusion that we are, to a remarkable degree, chemically identified as nucleic acids, DNA and RNA, and other operational agents referred to as the proteins. If we accept that we are made up basically of genetic material, then what makes us so different from other organisms of the universe?

In his book on the evolution of human intelligence, *The Dragons of Eden*, Carl Sagan[1] speculated that most complex organisms on earth today contain substantially more stored information, both genetic and extragenetic, than the most complex organisms of 200 million years ago. According to Sagan, the basic means for capturing this information lies within something termed "genetic memory."

In this regard, consider the possibility that all organisms on planet earth have chromosomes that contain genetic material passed on from generation to generation, whether those organisms are fruit flies or human beings. Factual material presented in this book suggests that although certain brain mechanisms seem to explain the biologic effects of specific psychotropic agents, certain actions are unexplained as yet. For example, what are the mechanisms of drug-induced hallucinations? If we apply concepts of genetic memory, these unexplained actions become more comprehensible.

Theoretically a cave dweller imbibing some *Mandragova officionarum* (mandrake root)—a psychoactive substance with extreme aphrodisiac powers—may have experienced an effect that passed through genetic memory to any offspring. The experience, being pleasant and stored, may or may not be experienced in the recipient offspring. However, appropriate extragenetic stimuli may trigger awareness of that stored pleasure state, in one degree or another, in future generations. Given that extragenetic triggering action, the recipient offspring may believe it to be a "fantasy" or "hallucination" but its origin might actually be traced as far back as the beginnings of recorded history.

Where is this genetic information stored? It is scientifically apparent that the brain is not equipotent in its capacity to store bits of information for memory purposes. Studies on the limbic system reveal that electrical activity of that part of the brain—termed "theta activity"—appears to be related to short-term memory. Drugs such as nicotine, that increase memory, are a good example.

A review of the pertinent literature tells us that—at least in humans—memories are stored somewhere in the cerebral cortex (activated somehow within the limbic system), waiting to be retrieved by electric impulses generated through the ingestion of psychoactive plant materials such as cocoa root (*Colocasin ontiguorum*), poppy (*Papaver somniferum*), nutmeg (*Nigella sativa*), nightshade (*Solanum coagulans*), hemp (*Cannabis sativa*), and jasmine (*Sasminum officianale*)—or, of course, generated within the brain itself by endogenous substances (internal opiates) or processes.

It is well known that the human brain consists of a right and left hemisphere and that the synaptic densities of these two brain spheres differ significantly between the sexes. Humans exhibit an interesting separation of musical and verbal skills and this may be linked with how drugs act in the brain. A further extension could be that people explore various psychoactive substances for either musical (creative) or verbal (cognitive) reasons.

It is noteworthy that patients with lesions of the right hemisphere are significantly impaired in musical, but not in verbal, ability. Sagan[1] suggests that on the basis of scientifically sound experiments, those functions we ordinarily describe as "rational" live mainly in the left hemisphere, while those we consider "intuitive" dwell mainly in the right. In this regard, it has been claimed[1] that as normal people change from analytic to creative intellectual activities, the electroencephalographic activity of the corresponding cerebral hemispheres varies in the predicted way: When a subject is performing mental arithmetic, the right hemisphere exhibits the alpha rhythm characteristic of an "idling" cerebral hemisphere. It has been suggested[1] that our awareness of right-hemisphere function is a little like our ability to see stars in the daytime. Sagan further describes this hypothesis: "The sun is so bright that the stars are invisible, despite the fact that they are just as present in our sky in the daytime as at night. When the sun sets, we are able to perceive the stars."

In essence inhibition of the left hemisphere releases our potent "intuitive" side of the brain, reflecting our most primitive desires, feelings, and appetites. Keeping this view in mind, it is not surprising that moments of real anxiety could drive modern people to experimentation with consciousness-altering substances in the hope that they might reach back to the roots of *homo sapiens*' intuitive powers. For example, a close look at the plant psychotropic marihuana reveals that it is often described as improving our appreciation for music, art, dance, sex, and sign and symbol recognition, and our sensitivity for nonverbal communications.

On the other hand, marihuana is seldom reported to improve abilities for cognitive calculation. It is more commonly observed that rather than enhancing human powers, the cannabinols simply suppress the left hemisphere. This also may be true for other psychoactive substances, such as opiates derived from poppy, cocaine from cocoa root, or even alcohol. This inhibition/release mechanism may not only be the objective of meditation in many oriental religions, but also the basis for the seeking of pleasure states via natural or unnatural means. In other words, the "high" would simply be the suppression of the left hemisphere. Barrett[2] has suggested that people's preoccupation with left-hemisphere concerns in contemporary society creates alienation and loneliness. To alleviate these feelings, many fall into psychoactive chemical abuse.

How can we communicate with the right hemisphere of our brain without the use of drugs? Dreams may be one key method. We must consider the possibility that psychotropic substances induce in the subject dreamlike states of a creative nature—sometimes referred to as hallucinations. It may follow that if dreams are the result of right-hemisphere dominance, and if there is an alteration of the level of consciousness in a positive way (feeling good), then the high one obtains from drugs or herbs may be due to their effect of inhibiting the left hemisphere. Sagan[1] points out that in dreams "we are sometimes aware that a small portion of us is placidly watching; often, off in a corner of the dream, there is a kind of observer." In psychedelic drug experiences—for example, with *Cannabis sativa* or lysergic acid (LSD)—the presence of such a "watcher" is frequently reported. LSD experiences may be quite terrifying, and it is the "watcher" who acts to buffer the terror with the reassurance that the experience is just a dream.

The desire to feel good is basic in all humankind. It is no surprise that getting high, according to Weil,[3] is a time-honored tradition. Weil[4] points out that human beings are born with an innate need to get high, to experience periodically other states of consciousness, and the capacity for this experience is a capacity of the human nervous system. Often external things, such as drugs, seem to cause highs, but this is an illusion. External factors may elicit highs, but the experiences are latent in our nervous systems, and their true causes are internal.

It is possible to be high spontaneously and to learn to get high with less and less external stimulation. But we must accept that many people are going to rely on external things, including drugs and plant psychotropics. From the beginning, humankind has devoted considerable energy and ingenuity to "turning on" under such labels as "altering levels of consciousness" or "opening psychedelic doors to perception." Through smoking, sniffing, eating, drinking, or mainlining, people of all cultures and times have sought a little something more than the standard view of reality.

Adam tried it with a bite from the forbidden apple. Bacchus glorified it with the deification of the grape. Some are behind bars for their explorations with hallucinogens while others who engage in "socially acceptable" drugs such as alcohol, are free to, if not encouraged to, continue their use.

Certainly the problem of psychoactive use, misuse, or abuse throughout the world is symptomatic of more general societal problems. The drug scene is nothing new; it is the American way—a billion dollar complex that pushes and pumps its products into all facets of our life. The neon "come-ons" of the fast-food chains cannot compare to the blazing Rx flicker sign in the sky. The only real difference is that corporate drug dealers shy away from the figures of how many "pill-burgers" they have actually sold us.

It is clear now, as Cohen[5] puts it, "that a

drug-free Eden, if it ever existed, will never return.'' He further points out: ''We can expect ebbs and surges of psychochemical usage for what is called 'recreation,' but a return to an era when adolescent drug abuse did not exist is difficult to visualize.'' There are two possible reasons for this: (1) the fact that, in spite of governmental intervention, it seems impossible to interdict more than a ''fraction'' of the traffic; and (2) social acceptance of relaxed social taboos against the nonmedical use of psychoactive chemicals for recreational purposes.

The question of whether we should give drugs to people is really being decided by juveniles themselves. Now the issues at hand are: ''What quantity of drugs can we afford, and what is the system of barter?''

A review of the literature reveals that the number of 18- to 25-year-olds who at some time tried marihuana rose from 7 percent in 1962 to 68 percent in 1980. In the same age group the statistics for illicit drugs other than marihuana went from 3 percent to 33 percent during the same time interval. How many of these first-time experimenters go on to use drugs dysfunctionally? According to Cohen[3] this number is more difficult to obtain, because it includes not only the heavy user of any drug that is intoxicating, but also the one-time user who happens to drive a car ineptly while under the influence.

Recognizing that psychoactive chemical abuse will almost definitely continue, we must consider what can be done to keep the morbidity and mortality down. Some major forces that can influence drug-seeking behavior can be listed:

1. Family
2. Peers
3. Teachers
4. The electronic media
5. Entertainment and sports figures
6. Religion

For the most part these forces have not been too successful in providing positive, life-enhancing, drug-deterring guidance. In fact, as Cohen[3] points out, some of these forces have had negative consequences as far as drug usage is concerned.

On the other hand, certainly groups such as AA (Alcoholics Anonymous), NA (Narcotics Anonymous), and Synanon, as well as therapeutic communities and transcendental meditation modalities, have been quite influential both in preventing the involvement of young people in drugs and in rehabilitating the substance abuser. This would seem to reinforce the idea that drug or plant psychotropic abuse is not the real issue—people are. Lack of human interaction and of faith in one's self and in existence may be basic to many of what we call ''causes'' of substance abuse. These would include depression, anxiety, hopelessness, poor self-esteem, directionlessness, and inability to trust.

People provide the real highs. However, in today's psychedelic world, loneliness and alienation are commonplace. Where love, compassion, and friendship are lacking, there is always synthetic chemistry to turn you on to a synthetic high. In whatever way happiness is sought, whether through other people, drugs, or sugar-coated placebos, the end result is that an individual strives in his/her own way to achieve happiness. While Marx said that ''religion is the opium of the people,'' it may actually be that ''opium is the religion of the unbelieving people.''[5] It is interesting that certain drugs such as hallucinogens and alcohol have sometimes been used to induce what could be called transcendental states. William James in his *Principles of Psychology* in 1907 wrote: ''It is the power of alcohol to stimulate the mystical consciousness that has made it such an important substance in man's history.''

Although the use of certain deliriants by youth in many cultures has been in the context of a rite of passage there are no such rituals in the United States. It has been noted[5] that affluent juveniles in the Western world can afford marihuana at \$100 an ounce, methaqualone at \$5 a tablet, and even high-priced cocaine at \$100 a snort or two; this is a new but remarkable phenomenon and significantly contributes to the partaking of the psychotropic ''smorgasbord.''

Pharmacologically there is evidence that some of the drug-metabolizing enzyme systems in young people are not as developed as in older people and this may be the cause of their inability to handle psychochemicals in the same way. This fact, along with the clinical observation that the earlier a drug habit starts, the more unfavorable is the long-term outlook, warrants strong support for intelligent governmental strategies. The 1980s will see harsher laws governing the use, misuse, and abuse of drugs. Already many states have returned the drinking age to 21 years old and have made penalties tougher for those driving while intoxicated. But it will take more than more rigid law enforcement to dissuade us from being a chemically oriented society; it will take a revolution of values and a new morality to pass down to our children.[5] The ultimate answer actually lies in our cranium, since the essential ingredient is *pleasure* and most of us always want just a little bit more.

There is a basic need in humans to achieve pleasure states, and some think that drugs provide a means of getting there. One person drinks a couple of martinis, while another chews coca leaves. We have not yet learned to curtail or control the abuse of various kinds of pleasure—whether drinking or smoking pot or gambling or watching TV—but sooner or later society is going to have to learn to deal with drugs and pleasure and altered states in ways other than by sheer emotional reaction.[6]

A review of work presented in this book reveals that there are naturally occurring chemicals, hormones, peptides, and other unidentifiable material in our brain that can induce "mind" alterations. For example, the discovery of an opiate-like polypeptide (endorphins, enkephalins) raises interesting questions about the addictive process. What happens chemically when a person has a natural deficiency of these potentially euphoric-producing endorphins? Can this sort of deficiency drive some people into seeking another kind of euphorogenic-producing substance to make up for that deficiency? Are imbalances in the production of natural opiatelike substances responsible for certain "abnormal" behavior that we label psychoses (schizophrenia, etc.)? It has been suggested[7] that some people who are prone to addiction may have certain deficiencies in their natural abilities to produce these substances and that the chemical deficiencies may be inheritable.[8] Additional research should provide insight into the notion of "reward versus punishment" states as natural entities, potentially being mediated via naturally occurring substances.

This creates a most frustrating paradox. On the one hand we seek fulfillment and satisfaction through the attainment of pleasure states—naturally or synthetically induced. On the other hand, we can easily overload our pleasure circuits through abuse, misuse, or simple miscalculation. Society does not condone pleasure if it does not fall within current social mores. Thus the unresolved issue is: If drugs induce pleasure states, and if pleasure states are natural, then how responsible or guilty are people who turn to artificial forms of euphorogenic-producing substances? Are our laws really adequate for dealing with this human reality? Are we making laws against drugs or against nature?

In 1970, when the Controlled Substances Act became federal law, the psychotropic drugs came under a new system of legal controls. No longer are drugs controlled according to pharmacologic class,[9] but are categorized according to five schedules, into which many, but not all, of the mood-altering drugs are placed. Cohen[7] suggests that the purpose is to permit proper medical usage while attempting to deter nonmedical abuse of these drugs.

Other factors considered prior to scheduling include the actual or potential abuse of a drug as determined by its pharmacologic properties, the pattern of abuse, and the drug's dependence-producing liability.

## SCHEDULE I

Schedule I includes those drugs that have a high potential for abuse and have no current medical use in the United States; all of the other schedules contain drugs that do have such medical usefulness. This schedule also contains drugs that can be used to make Schedule I substances, and others that have an action so similar to Schedule I drugs that it is reasonable to believe they will also be abused if they become available.

These drugs can be used for research purposes under a special license. A prescription cannot be written for them and they are not available in pharmacies, except in certain research hospital pharmacies. Almost 100 chemicals are named in I, and this number increases markedly when their salts and isomers are included.

These agents are either narcotics or hallucinogens. They have variable abuse potential, but because they have no established medical utility, they must all be placed here (Table 21-1).

## SCHEDULE II

Schedule II drugs have a high abuse potential that may lead to severe psychologic or psychic dependence. They have a current, accepted therapeutic use. Schedule II substances require a special prescription that must be written and signed by a doctor. It cannot be telephoned in, except in an emergency. In that instance, the written prescription must be supplied within 72 hours. Refills are not permitted and the patient must see the doctor to obtain a new prescription. Like Schedule I items, these drugs must be kept in a secure, locked place.

The opiates, some stimulants, and certain hypnotics are placed in Schedule II (Table 21-2).

## SCHEDULE III

Assignment of a drug to Schedule III requires that it have an abuse potential less than for those drugs in I and II. Abuse of these drugs may lead to moderate or low physical dependence or high levels of psychic dependence. Schedule III drugs require a prescription in writing or telephoned to the pharmacy. If so authorized, the prescription can be refilled up to five times within six months after the original date of the prescription.

The less abusable sedative-hypnotics and so-called class B narcotics are found here (Table 21-3).

**TABLE 21-1**

**Examples of Schedule I Drugs***

| | |
|---|---|
| Heroin (diacetylmorphine) | LSD (lysergic acid diethylamide) |
| Alpha-acetylmethadol (LAAM) | Marihuana *(cannabis sativa)* |
| Ibogaine | THC (delta-9-tetrahydrocannabinol) |
| Psilocybin | DMT (dimethyltryptamine) |
| Peyote *(Lophophora williamsii)* | Mescaline |

*From Cohen, S., *The Substance Abuse Problems.* New York: Haworth Press, 1981, p. 370.

**TABLE 21-2**

**Examples of Schedule II Drugs***

| | |
|---|---|
| Opium *(Papaver somniferum)* | Eskatrol (dextroamphetamine + prochlorperazine) |
| | Biphetamine (amphetamine + dextroamphetamine) |
| Morphine | Desbutal (methamphetamine + pentobarbital) |
| Codeine | Methedrine (methamphetamine) |
| Percodan (oxycodone) | Obedrin (methamphetamine + pentobarbital + vitamins) |
| Pantopon (opium alkaloids) | |
| Dilaudid (dihydromorphinone) | Amytal (amobarbital) |
| Dolophine (methadone) | Nembutal (pentobarbital) |
| Demerol (meperidine) | Quaalude (methaqualone) |
| Seconal (secobarbital) | Tuinal (secobarbital + amobarbital) |
| Cocaine | Preludin (phenmetrazine) |
| Benzedrine (amphetamine) | Ritalin (methylphenidate) |
| Dexamyl (dextroamphetamine + amobarbital) | |
| Dexedrine (dextroamphetamine) | |

*From Cohen, S., *The Substance Abuse Problems.* New York: Haworth Press, 1981, p. 371.

## SCHEDULE IV

Drugs with a low abuse potential relative to those in III, and whose abuse leads to limited physical or psychologic dependence, are placed in Schedule IV. Prescription requirements are the same as for III.

Certain of the hypnosedatives, weight-reducing substances, and minor tranquilizers are included here (Table 21-4).

## SCHEDULE V

To be placed in Schedule V the drug must have a lower abuse potential than those in IV. Only a limited psychologic or physical dependence might result from its abuse. A prescription is not needed for many compounds in V, but the purchaser must be at least 18 years of age. Identification must be shown and the buyer's name entered into a special log book kept by the pharmacist.

The exempt narcotics make up Schedule V and consist of those with small amounts of opium, codeine, or other narcotics in a large quantity of some vehicle (Table 21-5).

Some unscheduled drugs are listed in Table 21-6.

Although the control of abusable drugs is costly in terms of time and money, the general community benefits because a reduced supply of abusable drugs is available on the black marketplace. For example, it was the rescheduling of the amphetamines and methaqualone, bringing them under tighter controls, that markedly reduced their street availability. (See Table 21-7.) On the other hand, the softening of laws against the use of marihuana reduces the number of so-called paper criminals.

In discussing the coming of age in America and associated contemporary adolescent problems, Cohen[5] had the following to say:

**TABLE 21-3**

**Examples of Schedule III Drugs***

| | |
|---|---|
| Empirin with codeine | Nodular (methyprylon) |
| A.S.A. with codeine | Doriden (glutethimide) |
| Tylenol with codeine | Butisol (butabarbital) |
| Hycodon (hycodan + homatropine) | Florinal |
| Paragoric (tincture of camphorated opium) | Carbrital |

*From Cohen, S., *The Substance Abuse Problems.* New York: Haworth Press, 1981, p. 372.

**TABLE 21-4**

**Examples of Schedule IV Drugs***

| | |
|---|---|
| Luminal (phenobarbital) | Placidyl (ethchlorvynol) |
| Veronal (barbital) | Valmid (ethinamate) |
| Noctec (chloral hydrate) | Pondimin (fenfluramine) |
| Paraldehyde | Dalmane (flurazepam) |
| Talwin (pentazocine) | Tranxene (chlorazepate) |
| Darvon (propoxyphene) | Miltown (meprobamate) |
| Valium (diazepam) | Tenuate (diethylpropion) |
| Librium (chlordiazepoxide) | Serax (oxazepam) |

*From Cohen, S., *The Substance Abuse Problems.* New York: Haworth Press, 1981, p. 372.

**TABLE 21-5**

**Examples of Schedule V Drugs***

| | |
|---|---|
| Cheracol with codeine | Cosadein |
| Robitussin A-C | Terpinhydrate with codeine |

*From Cohen, S., *The Substance Abuse Problems.* New York, Haworth Press, New York, 1981, p. 372.

The adolescent hazards of the past, starvation, pestilence and poverty have given way to the modern plagues of youth, accidents, suicides and homicides. The interaction of drugs and alcohol with these three current disasters is obvious. The common denominator is the degree of freedom, the lack of responsibility and the failure of faith that adolescents cannot handle or endure.

Coming of age in America before the present era was far from ideal. Although we do not want to go back to the child labor practices of those "good old days," we must be aware that something has gone wrong. In the effort to make things better for our children, according to Cohen,[5] we have succeeded only in making things easier, and that may not be better for now or for their future.

If it is true that we do not expect exudication of the human search for rapid relief of central "pain" via artificial or natural means in the near future, then it might be prudent to look into the future insofar as our use of mind-altering chemicals is concerned. In this regard, the well-known sociologists Newett, Singer, and Kahn[10] discussed the uses of mind-affecting drugs in America in the year 2001. According to them, alcohol will retain a secure position as the most favored intoxicant because of its many and strong traditional associations and uses, its infinite variety of forms and potencies, and other factors (not the least, beer's thirst-quenching properties). Possibly there will be available synthetic spirits matching in quality the finest French vintages, and Newett and associates believe that this development will somewhat blur the distinction between alcohol and other pleasure-giving drugs.

Although there is growing concern about the harmful effects of cannabis, there is probably a less than even chance that marihuana and hashish will be legally available to adults. Patterns of use—solitary and social, light, medium, and heavy—will closely resemble those for alcohol. Underage use and minimum-legal-age use will have similar coming-of-age connotations as drinking beer and whiskey have today. It is predicted that these drugs will have become acculturated.[10] If this is true, there may well be a new drug or something else (see Figure 21-1)

**TABLE 21-6**

**Some Examples of Unscheduled Drugs***

| | |
|---|---|
| Tylenol (acetaminophen) | Mellaril (thioridazine) |
| Atarax (hydroxyzine) | Stelazine (trifluoperazine) |
| Vistaril (hydroxyzine pamoate) | Haldol (haloperidol) |
| Solacen (tybamate) | Navane (thiotixene) |
| Thorazine (chlorpromazine) | Tofranil (imipramine) |
| | Elavil (amitriptyline) |

*From Cohen, S., *The Substance Abuse Problems.* New York: Haworth Press, 1981, p. 372.

**TABLE 21-7**

**Some Examples of Rescheduled Drugs***

| *Drug* | *From* | *To* | *Year* |
|---|---|---|---|
| Benzedrine (amphetamine) and related drugs | III | II | 1971 |
| Preludin (phenmetrazine) | III | II | 1971 |
| Ritalin (methylphenidate) | III | II | 1971 |
| Tenuate (diethylproprion) and certain other anorectics | Unscheduled | IV | 1975 |
| Cylert (pemoline) | Unscheduled | IV | 1975 |
| Seconal (secobarbital) and other barbiturate hypnotics | III | II | 1973 |
| Quaalude (methaqualone) | III | II | 1973 |
| Valium (diazepam) and other benzodiazepines | Unscheduled | IV | 1975 |
| Propoxyphene (Darvon) | Unscheduled | IV | 1977 |
| Pentazocine (Talwin) | Unscheduled | IV | 1977 |
| Naloxone (Narcan) | I | Unscheduled | 1971 |
| Phencyclidine (PCP) | Unscheduled | II | 1978 |

*From Cohen, S., *The Substance Abuse Problems.* New York: Haworth Press, 1981, p. 374.

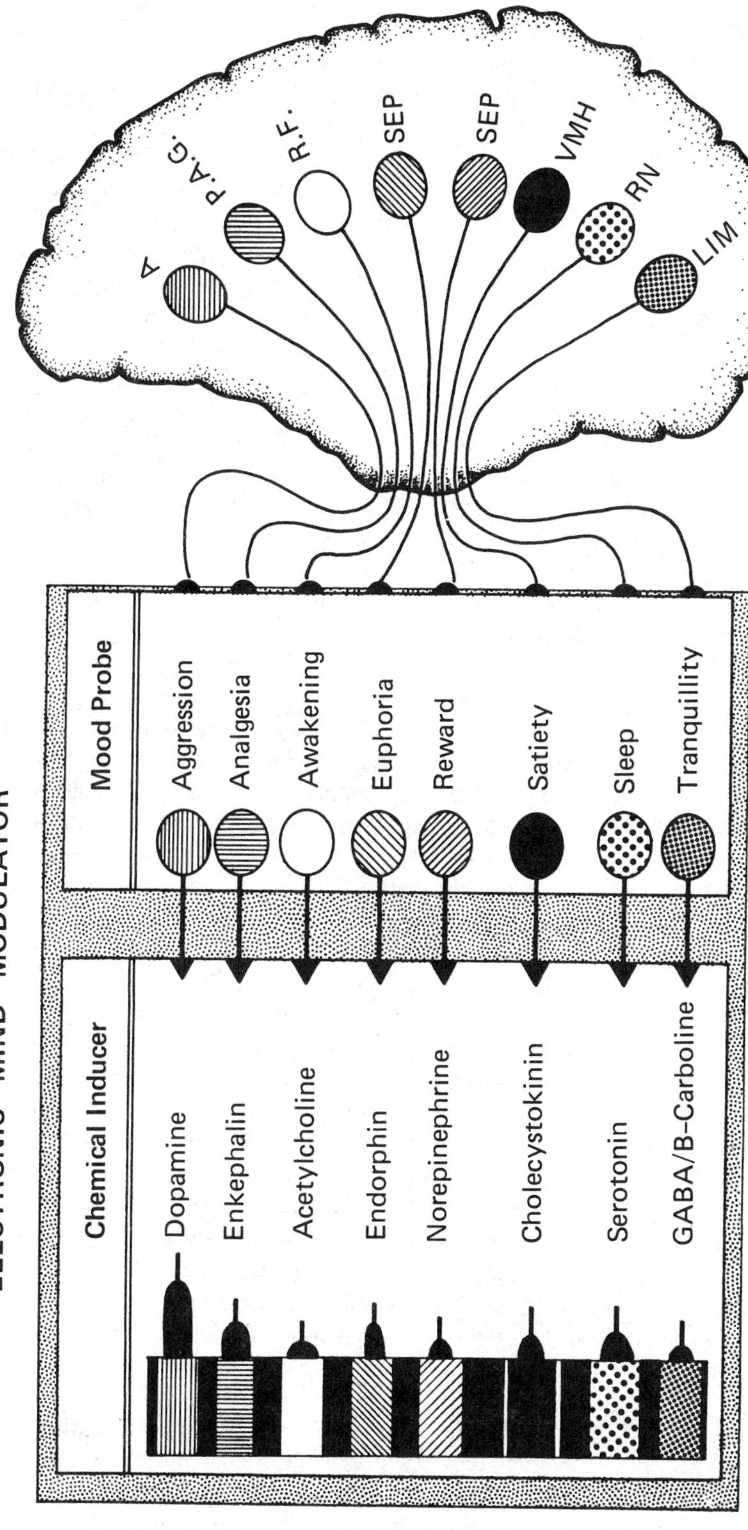


Key:
A = Amygdala
P.A.G. = Peri Aqueductal Gray
R.F. = Reticular Formation
SEP = Septal
VMH = Ventral Medial Hypothalamus
RN = Raphe Nucleus
LIM = Limbic

**Figure 21-1**

that performs some of the symbolic functions now performed by cannabis.

It is suspected that the casualty rates and other social costs of legalizing marihuana might be comparable to those with alcohol, although not identical in all particulars. For example, cannabis will not be implicated in crimes of passion and violence, as liquor is, but the availability of potent forms will mean more stoned drivers, industrial accidents, and psychologic if not physiologic dependence.

In an alternative version,[10] the marihuana fad will have waned. Again, use, possibly legal, will be largely restricted to "old fashioned" experimental youth and to a few well-defined cultural subgroups, including fastidious ritualists and counterparts of the wine connoisseur and the gourmet, as well as artists, mystics, the underclass, and indiscriminately drug-prone individuals.

In discussing the hallucinogens, Newett and associates[10] predict that we may expect a new generation of synthetics to have replaced those in use today. These will be biochemically less hazardous, but their appeal and acceptance will continue to be limited by the intensity and variability of effects. While it may prove possible to develop a hallucinogen that will carry a guarantee of "no bad trips," this may not be considered a genuine advantage by most of the people who are drawn to the hallucinogenic type of drug experience. What is sought here is an adventure, not an overwhelming, reliable euphoria such as heroin can provide.

Although illicit spree use of hallucinogens by adolescents will continue, according to Newett and associates,[10] the characteristic form of "tripping" will be by licensed groups of adults, generally of a religious or quasi-religious nature. Membership in such groups will be open to almost anyone and there will be comparable periodic efforts to tighten regulations. In terms of future hallucinogenic drug use, a much larger percentage of the adult population than today will have had the hallucinogenic type of drug experience—perhaps 30 percent, as compared with the 5–10 percent of youth today (probably only a small minority will use these drugs regularly). Furthermore, Newett et al.[10] speculate that the introspective person who finds the chemical manipulation of moods attractive will exhaust interest in the hallucinogens at a relatively early age and later will rely on marihuana or alcohol or some analog of the endogenous opiate peptides or natural manipulation of brain chemicals.

In the year 2001, alternatives in the use of drugs for pleasure will probably increase and there will be wide diversification of available means for getting high. The drug mystique and countless drug issues will probably defuse, and this will greatly reduce the current pressures on young people.

By the year 2001, it is conjectured that societal problems will have greatly escalated and intensified. The despair that so many feel now will worsen as economic strife increases; world war becomes more imminent; famine increases; pollution permeates our streams and air; crime becomes rampant in our streets; assassination haunts our leaders; prejudice worsens; education deteriorates, especially for the poor; unemployment throughout the world reaches endemic proportions; street rioting and looting become commonplace; police brutality inevitably substitutes for law and order; natural disasters such as weather, floods, and earthquakes shock the earth repeatedly because of radiation-induced shifts; stress-induced psychosomatic diseases inflict millions as daily life struggles become more difficult; government spending in social areas is drastically reduced; OPEC prices surge to unprecedented highs; the Federal Reserve Bank through the Trilateral Commission controls international currency flow and interest rates become fixed at 20 percent or above; and as the world in 2001 seems entirely without hope. As our existence becomes more fragile, it is only logical that even more people will reach for rapid ways to ease tensions, escape from reality, and relieve "central pain" under the guise of quasi-medical motives, resulting in the spread of drug use.

Furthermore, we can expect an increase in knowledge and discrimination, a sorting out of drugs and drug uses, and a development of grass-roots mechanisms for limiting and coping with the entire phenomenon of drug abuse.

A closer look into the future is rather shocking if we consider the biologic implications of recent findings of neuroscientists concerning the mechanisms of neurochemical-induced mood alterations.

If we are not successful in dealing with stronger governmental controls, the age of "mood" regulation by governmental order may come to fruition 20 years from now. In this regard, knowledge of mind mechanisms and understanding of its chemistry may provide the armamentarium (newly developed centrally acting drugs) to control so-called deviant behavior. It is easy to visualize that, for example, in certain "hot" spot areas in New York, Los Angeles, and Miami, among others, the government could order tranquilizer-laced water supplies in an attempt to ease anguished inhabitants as one would tame animals. Certainly one could predict the enhanced usage of "mind" drugs for criminals in our jails, for mentally imbalanced individuals in our hospitals, for drug- and alcohol-dependent individuals, and for calming rebellious youth. In fact, governmental abuse of these "mind drugs" has already been considered (people's protest against police utilization of "tranquilizer guns") and could eventually result in their use as "war weapons" sprayed on entire populations for takeover or control by aggressive powers.

The implications are frightening but there is also a more optimistic view to consider. Neuroscientific advances may yield the discovery and mass implementation of a biomechanical device to tap into our brain chemistry for the specific purpose of "mind control" in relation to positive behavior modification.

*The electronic "mind" modulator* (EEM) is proposed in Figure 21-1 as a plausible example of how we could "turn on" or "turn off" these potent brain chemical modulators at will. In fact, with the flick of a switch, one could affect an entire spectrum of behavior—including aggression (antishyness), analgesia (antipain), awakeness (antifatigue), euphoria (antidysphoria), reward (antidepression or punishment), sleep (anti-insomnia), and tranquility (antianxiety). The concomitant chemicals identified with each behavior have already been investigated and strong evidence exists for each chemical depicted in Figure 21-1. In this regard, it has been shown that the amygdala is the area of the brain identified with aggressive behavior and dopamine seems to mediate this response[11]; the periacqueductal grey matter has been identified with pain mechanisms and the opiate peptide enkephalin has been found to mediate this response[12,13]; the reticular activating center is associated with the behavior of wakefulness and acetylcholine (ACH) has been firmly established as the mediator of this response[14]; the septal area of the brain has been identified with both euphoria and reward where the hormone beta-endorphin[15] and the neurotransmitter norepinephrine (NE)[16,17] have been proposed as mediators of these behaviors respectively; the Raphe nuclei, well known as the brain area most responsible for sleep induction, are mediated by the chemical serotonin (5-HT)[18]; the hypothalamus identified as the brain part responsible for the function of satiety contains high amounts of the cholecystokinin peptide (CCK), which has been proposed to mediate the feeding response[19]; and finally, the limbic system is dense with benzodiazepine receptors and is most identified with "calming" behavior and, although not fully accepted, the neurotransmitter gamma-amino-butyric acid (GABA)[20] and a proposed ligand for the so-called tranquilizer receptor beta carboline,[21] have been implicated as tranquilizer mediators.

One way to influence substance- and alcohol-seeking behavior is to encourage the blending of biomechanical engineers and research psychiatrists to develop the electronic "mind" modulator (a possible analogy being the extender telephone, a cordless modulator of frequency waves) and subsequent governmental recommendation of its use. Already we have seen progress in this area with the development of the transentaneous electrical stimulator (TENS) for the release of enkephalins to control pain in humans, which provides impetus for research along these lines. It must be similarly conjectured that with the advent of the EEM people eventually could learn to abuse these "mind chemicals" in the same way they have learned to abuse drugs, but it would be less costly than buying drugs illicitly from black market sources and would significantly reduce crime. In essence, introduction of EEM in society may result in the abuse of "mind masturbation," our new-age dilemma.

It is always interesting to imagine our future, but first and foremost we must deal with contemporary problems. Chemical abuse is a subject of great contemporary concern and must include accidental poisoning, volutionary indulgence, and maniac contamination of our products with poisons. In 1982, over a half million children accidentally swallowed, inhaled, or came in contact with various kinds of poisons or other harmful substances. Adults hardly fared better, falling victim to the dangers of poisoning, both at home and on the job, accidentally or intentionally. Medications, cleaners, petroleum products, insecticides, and automotive products are among the potential killers found in every household. Fluids, gases, and many solid wastes threaten workers every day, whether in factories, in offices, or on their way to and from their jobs.[22]

The recent increase in contaminated drug and consumer products has spread the fear of poisoning throughout the country. Over-the-counter drugs are now associated with a degree of risk. Shoppers are looking closely at the packaging of food products before making a purchase. Kids are warned to avoid eating Halloween candy. But although people are becoming more aware of poisoning and contamination, very few know how to avoid the danger or what to do if someone falls victim to a toxic substance.

Health officials and the media have agonized over the problem of informing the public about the dangers of poisoning without causing undue alarm. In the case of contaminated products, there is a fear of triggering mass paranoia or even ''copycat'' contaminations. Nevertheless, the medical community and the press both realize that the problem of poisoning, contamination, and drug abuse must be faced. ''We are approaching an epidemic in the contamination of products and reports of poisonings, both at home and on the job,'' says Dr. Richard Weisman, director of the New York City Department of Health's Poison Control Center. ''If it's not quite an epidemic, it is being perceived by the public as an epidemic and that's almost as bad. It is causing people to be extremely cautious, almost bordering on paranoia.''

Reports of poisonings and contaminated products carry with them an unusually high potential for disturbing the lives of people of all ages. Unfortunately we cannot count on a decrease of these incidents to ease the public's fear of poisoning and contamination. What we can hope for, however, is to provide the public with peace of mind by informing it about poisoning—how to reduce the risk, where to look for help, and how to provide first aid. Governmental regulation and ''tamper''-proof containers are certainly a step in the right direction. One way toward a healthier society is to educate its people about the potential dangers and uses of all drugs—illicit and approved, black market and prescribed, popular and obscure. *Public awareness can save lives.*

Blum and Tilton,[23] in their article entitled ''Understanding the High Mind,'' provide an interesting summary of the problem of abusable drugs.

> What is needed at this juncture is a holistic approach to the process of life that approaches the intuitive forces unleashed in more primitive societies, before civilization took upon itself the role of arbitrator and rule-maker over the seeking of pleasure states. The complexity of modern society brings down technological barriers between our inner strivings and those elusive pleasure states which seem always to dance just beyond our reach. We need to get in touch with our own identities, grasp the meanings of symbols which lie beyond our current language and mathematics, and once again confront ourselves in the unconscious and nearly forgotten well-springs of our origin. Rather than allow ourselves to become castaways of a genetic legacy which passes us by on the way to some ultimate and unknown fulfillment, it is time for us to pause, to listen to the voices of our past while going to the pleasure states which comprise our ultimate destiny. Perhaps the answer lies in a leaf, alkaloids found in herbs and plants. Perhaps the answer has been there all along.

Finally, some experts view ''addiction'' prevention as not simply a matter of saying no. In this regard, probably we cannot overcome the natural desire to reach ''higher states of consciousness'' or even curtail the indiscriminate use or abuse of psychoactive agents. If we accept the view that for many ''addiction'' proneness viz genetic determinants serves as an explanation of the biological disease concept and ultimately leads to drug seeking behavior in some, then we must also assume that very little could be achieved to totally eliminate addictive behavior in these people. Should we then support the idea that something positive could be ascribed to compulsive behavior? In search for a solution it is tempting to suggest that we begin to explore the nature of a new term—Euaddiction—not as a definitive answer, but rather a point of departure. Let us begin. . . .

## REFERENCES


1. Sagan, C. *The Dragons of Eden: Speculations on the Evolution of Human Intelligence*. New York: Random House, 1977.
2. Barrett, W. *Irrational Man*. Garden City, N.Y.: Doubleday, 1962.
3. Weil, A. T. Botanical vs chemical drugs: Pros and cons. In C. G. Meyer, K. Blum, and J. C. Cull, eds., *Folk Medicine and Herbal Healing*. Springfield, Ill.: Charles C. Thomas, 1981, p. 287.
4. Weil, A. *The Natural Mind*. Boston: Houghton, Mifflin, 1972.
5. Cohen, S. Coming of age in America—with drugs: Contemporary adolescence. *Drug Abuse Alcoholism Newsl.* 11(9):November 1982.
6. Fort, J. *The Pleasure Seekers: The Drug Crisis, Youth and Society*. Indianapolis: Bobbs-Merrill, 1969.
7. Goldstein, A. Future research on opiate peptides (endorphins): A preview. In K. Blum, ed., *Alcohol and Opiates: Neurochemical and Behavioral Mechanisms*. New York: Academic Press, 1977.
8. Blum, K., et al. Psychogenetics of drug seeking behavior. *Subs. Alcohol Act. Use/Misuse* 1:255, 1980.
9. Cohen, S. *The Substance Abuse Problems*. New York: Haworth Press, 1981, p. 369.
10. Newitt, J., Singer, M., and Kahn, H. Some speculations on U.S. drug use. *J. Social Issues* 27(3), 1971.
11. Cooper J. R., Bloom, F. E., and Roth, R. H. *The Biochemical Basis of Neuropharmacology*, 3rd ed. New York: Oxford University Press, 1978.
12. Graf, L., et al. Comparative study of analgesic effect of met$^5$-enkephalin and related lipotropin fragments. *Nature* 263:240, 1976.
13. Guillemin, R. Peptides in the brain: The new endocrinology of the neuron. *Science* 202:390, 1978.
14. Iversen, S. D., and Iversen, L. L. *Behavioral Pharmacology*. New York: Oxford University Press, 1975.
15. Catlin, D. H., et al. Pharmacologic activity of beta-endorphin in man. *Commun. Psychopharmacol.* 1:452, 1977.
16. Baldessarini, R. J. The basis for amine hypothesis in affective disorders: A critical evaluation. *Arch. Gen. Psychiatry* 32:1087, 1975.
17. U'Pritchard, D. C., et al. Tricyclic antidepressants: Therapeutic properties and affinity for alpha-noradrenergic receptor binding sites in the brain. *Science* 197:199, 1978.
18. Kay, D. C., et al. Human pharmacology of sleep. In R. L. Williams and I. Karacan, eds., *Pharmacology of Sleep*. New York: Wiley, 1976, pp. 83–210.
19. Myers, R. D., and McCaleb, M. Peripheral and intrahypothalmic cholecystokin act on the noradrenergic feeding circuit in that diencephalon. *Neuroscience* 6:645, 1981.
20. Iversen, L. L. Biochemical psychopharmacology of GABA. In M. A. Lipton, A. Dimascio, and K. F. Kivam, eds., *Psychopharmacology: A Generation of Progress*. New York: Raven Press, 1978, p. 25.
21. Bloom, F., et al. *Beta-Carbolines and Tetrahydroisoquirolines*. New York: Alan Liss, 1982.
22. The Apogee Communications Group. "Poison Prevention and Control," a proposal for video production. Copyright 1982.
23. Blum, K., and Tilton, J. E. Understanding the high mind. In G. G. Meyer, K. Blum, and J. L. Cull, eds., *Folk Medicine and Herbal Healing*. Springfield, Ill.: Charles C. Thomas, 1981, p. 261.

# Appendix I

# Glossary of Street and Scientific Terms

''A rose is a rose is a rose.''
*Gertrude Stein, ''Sacred Everly,'' 1913*

## A. INTRODUCTION

The identity of a drug may be denoted by several different types of names. For example, ''legal'' drugs are denoted by scientific chemical names which are difficult to remember; quasi-official names used by scientists are termed ''generic''; and finally ''trade names'' are the patented property of drug manufacturers. Some drugs have more than one trade name; in fact, some drugs have been known to have as many as five or more.

Within the medical profession sometimes drug names are purposely chosen to hide their real pharmacologic properties so that the ''mystique'' of the profession is maintained. On the other hand, in terms of the illicit street market drug names become code words. In attempting to understand the phenomenology of street names, it has been suggested that for some street drug afficionados the code becomes an important part of membership in a special drug fraternity. Names of drugs are also a method by which drug users baffle or identify ''squares''. Additionally, teenagers feel different, rebellious and somewhat more knowledgeable about something that adults are not privy to in their use of street names. These feelings are most bluntly exemplified by a drug preparation that was given the name FUK. Also, drug names are devised by basement chemists for sale purposes to describe the type of response expected to their concocted mixtures.

In some cases, certain street names are used to baffle the nonuser and may even mislead the user. The name of a drug may differ from one locale to another and may not gain general acceptance worldwide. For example, there are numerous names for marihuana; in general (pot, tea, grass), names that denote high potency (Acapulco gold, gold-leaf special), names that refer to the quantity of the drug offered for sale (dime bag, ki, or kilo), and names that refer to cigaretttes containing marihuana (reefer, joint).

Sometimes, street names are short-lived and tend to serve no purpose when the code has been broken.

Basement chemists are aware of the competitive market and to stimulate sales of a particular illicit drug like LSD, for example, may prepare the drug in special shapes and colors and give it names like "purple dot, wedges, owsleys, flats, orange carborators among others."[2] Most clandestine manufacturers are too small to produce large batches so that the original preparation becomes quickly exhausted.

Sometimes, one name may be used for a pharmacologic class such as "speed" or "crank" used for amphetamine and methamphetamine or other stimulants.

Sometimes, street names are not short-lived, such as the name "acid" for LSD, first used in the 1960s.

Certainly, the terminology of drugs represents a minor aspect of the drug dilemma. Furthermore, their use by well-meaning inexperienced adults or health professionals may tend to turn off adolescents and provide them with additional reasons to proclaim hypocrisy and dishonesty on the part of the older generation.[3]

With tighter drug controls came the advent of the so-called look-alikes for such drugs as amphetamines and barbiturates. A major problem with these drugs is that at the dosages needed to obtain euphoria, they have as many dangers as the amphetamines and barbiturates. Fortunately, these look-alike drugs have received poor publicity and their production and use have declined.[4–6]

According to Cohen[7]:

> The point to be learned from the look-alike caper is that control of supplies, important as it is, is not enough. In a modern society there are always substitutes or analogues to be found or chemists who will make them, and citizens who will deal in them.

Since people will continue to explore the world of psychomeric drugs, other chemical substitutions discovered by chemists will be sold to anxious fans under new exciting names. Possibly in the future governments will allow patented recreational euphoriants.

## B. STREET TERMS

The following section is primarily of cultural interest and not intended to be comprehensive or precise, but is a glossary of some commonly used street slang referring to drugs, drug use, and subcultural concomitants of the drug scene. If someone uses a term that escapes your understanding, do not be afraid to ask questions; they will always evoke a meaningful explanation.

**A-bomb**—Joint dusted with opium or heroin.

**Acapulco gold**—Marihuana of gold color, high potency, and said to be grown around Acapulco, Mexico.

**Acid**—LSD-25.

**Acid freak**—User of LSD whose behavior is bizarrely affected.

**Acid head**—Habitual user (possibly exclusively) of LSD.

**Acid rock**—Kind of music, noted to be loud, frenetic, electronic, fast-moving rock and roll.

**"A head"**—Habitual user (possibly exclusively) of amphetamines.

**A la canona**—Abrupt withdrawal from heroin without medication or treatment (Puerto Rican slang).

**Ames**—Small glass vials of amyl nitrite (also *pearls* or *snappers*).

**Angel off**—To arrest the buyers from a dealer (in drugs) who is being watched.

**Anywhere**—Possessing illegal drugs (also *holding*).

**Baby**—Marihuana.

**Backwards**—Tranquilizers (to bring one back from acid or speed).

**Bador**—Hallucinogenic seed from the morning glory plant (Aztec slang).

**Bad seed**—Peyote.

**Bad trip**—Unpleasant experience with a drug (usually hallucinogens).

**Bag**—"Measured" amount of a street drug (usually heroin) indicated by the price; or can be one's life-style.

**Bagman**—Drug dealer.

**Bale**—Pound of marihuana.

**Bam**—Amphetamine to be injected or taken orally.

**Banana smoking**—Previously a fad. One smoked the inner fibrous peelings of the banana to get high, although psychotropic activity not proven (mellow yellow).

**Bang**—To inject drugs intravenously (usually speed or heroin).

**Bank bandit pills**—Barbiturates or other sedative pills.

**Bar**—Solid block of marihuana stuck together with honey or sugar water (brick).

**B-bombs**—Benzedrine inhalers (removed from the market in 1949).

**B.C. (or BCP)**—Birth control pills.

**Beast, The**—LSD-25 (Harlem slang since 1965).

**Beat**—Cheat or rob someone of money or goods (*beat* the system).

**Bee**—Box or bag of marihuana.

**Belly habit**—Heroin withdrawal pains subjectively centered in the stomach.

**Bennies**—Benzedrine pills.

**Bent**—High, stoned, plastered, ripped, or intoxicated from drugs.

**Bernies**—Cocaine.

**Bhang**—From India; the marihuana plant, and the drink made with the plant used to produce psychotropic effects.

**Big bags**—$5 to $10 bags of heroin. (Price varies.)

**Big bloke**—Cocaine.

**Big chief, The**—Mescaline.

**Big "D," The**—LSD-25.

**Big man, The**—Distributor of wholesale illegal drugs to other dealers.

**Big supplier**—Same as *big man*.

**Bindle**—Small folded paper containing heroin.

**Bingle**—Dope dealer.

**Black beauties**—Biamphetamine capsules.

**Black gunion**—Extra thick, potent, dark, gummy marihuana.

**Black pills**—Pellets of opium heated over a flame and smoked.

**Black Russian**—Dark-colored, very potent hashish.

**Blank**—Container of white powder that was sold as heroin but was not (also called *dummy* and *lemonade*).

**Blast**—To smoke a drug.

**Blast party**—Party gathered to smoke dope (marihuana).

**Blockbusters**—White and yellow striped pills of barbiturates.

**Blotter acid**—LSD on porous paper.

**Blow**—To smoke marihuana; to inhale cocaine or heroin into the nose; to miss a vein while trying to inject drugs intravenously.

**Blow snow**—To inhale cocaine into one's nose.

**Blow your mind**—To alter one's consciousness drastically (possibly with drugs).

**Blow your mind roulette**—Game played with barbiturate and amphetamine pills.

**Blue acid**—LSD.

**Bluebirds**—Amytal sodium capsules.

**Blue heavens**—Amytal sodium capsules.

**Blue velvets**—Combination of terpin hydrate elixir, codeine, and tripelennamine.

**Body drugs**—Drugs that produce physical dependence.

**Body trip**—Drug experience that seems physical rather than mental (that is, one is speeded up or slowed down physically, or possibly sexually aroused).

**Bogue**—Withdrawal from physical-dependence-producing drugs.

**Bolsa**—Bag of heroin.

**Bombed out**—High, ripped, stoned, blasted, intoxicated on drugs.

**Boo**—Marihuana.

**Booting**—Technique of injecting heroin a little at a time in order to prolong the initial pleasurable sensation.

**Bouncing powder**—Cocaine.

**Boxed**—Same as being high.

**Brain ticklers**—Amphetamine or barbiturate pills.

**Bread**—Money.

**Brick**—Pressed block of marihuana, heroin, or opium, usually in pounds or kilograms.

**Brownies**—Amphetamines, especially dexedrine capsules.

**Bum bend**—Bad trip, unpleasant experience with a drug.

**Bum kicks**—Troubled, worried, or depressed.

**Bummer**—Bad trip, unpleasant experience with a drug.

**Bundle**—Package of twenty-five $5 bags of heroin stacked together.

**Burese**—Cocaine.

**Burn, To**—To cheat or steal.

**Burning**—Smoking marihuana.

**Burn out**—To overexploit or overuse a drug, person, or place so that it is no longer desirable to continue with it.

**Bush**—Marihuana.

**Businessman's trip**—DMT, due to its short duration of action.

**Bust**—To arrest, or to be arrested by the police.

**Button**—Surface growth of the peyote cactus; peyote.

**Buy**—To purchase drugs.

**Buzz**—Moderate high from any drug without hallucinations.

**Buzz, rolling**—A moderate high from a drug that continues after the intake of the drug has stopped.

**C.**—Cocaine.

**Caapi**—Hallucenogenic tea made from the vine, banisteriopsis.

**Ca-ca**—Shit; counterfeit or very-poor-quality drugs (Puerto Rican slang).

**Canadian black**—Variety of marihuana grown in Canada.

**Candy man**—Drug dealer.

**Cannabis**—Family of plants called marihuana.

**Cap**—Capsule of a drug.

**Carry, To**—To have drugs on one's person (also *to hold*).

**Cartwheels**—Amphetamine tablets (also *crossroads*).

**Catnip**—Strong-smelling herb sometimes sold as marihuana to unsuspecting buyers.

**Chalk**—Amphetamine tablets.

**Charas**—Resin exuded by the flowering tops of female hemp plants (cannabis plants) in India; it is very potent (also called *hashish*).

**Charles**—Cocaine.

**Charlie**—A dollar.

**Chasing the bag**—Hustling for heroin, or physically dependent on heroin.

**Chasing the dragon**—Inhaling the fumes of heroin and barbiturate mixture that has been placed in tinfoil and heated over a flame.

**Chief, The**—LSD-25.

**Chill, To**—To ignore or refuse to deal with someone in terms of drugs.

**Chipping**—Using heroin irregularly to avoid physical dependence.

**Chota**—An informer, a rat (Puerto Rican slang).

**Cibas**—Glutethimide.

**Clean**—Free from suspicion; not having narcotics in one's possession; marihuana with seeds and stems removed.

**Coasting**—Somnolent, nodding state of heroin user after recent injection of the drug.

**Cocktail**—Ordinary cigarette used to smoke the end of a joint; made by removing a bit of tobacco from the plain cigarette (see *Roach*).

**Coke**—Cocaine.

**Coke head**—Habitual user of cocaine, possibly exclusively.

**Cold turkey**—Abrupt withdrawal from drugs that have produced physical dependence, with no medication or treatment.

**Collar**—To arrest (by the police).

**Come down** (or **Coming down**)—The gradual loss of effect of a drug on one's consciousness.

**Connect, To**—To find a source of drugs, or to buy drugs (to score).

**Contact**—A drug supplier or dealer.

**Contact habit**—Experiencing the effects of physical dependence on a drug by constantly associating with those who use it and are dependent.

**Cook**—To heat a mixture of heroin and water until the heroin is dissolved.

**Cooker**—A small metal container in which heroin and water are heated (a spoon).

**Cop**—To connect, or score; to buy narcotics.

**Co-pilot**—One who stays with a person who has taken a powerful drug (usually LSD) to help and/or comfort that person if necessary.

**Corrine**—Cocaine.

**Courage pills**—Barbiturates or other sedative pills.

**Crap**—Low-quality drugs of any type, but usually heroin or marihuana.

**Crash**—To go to sleep or to bed; to come down after using a stimulating drug.

**Creep**—Person using heroin who does not engage in risky activities to pay for the drugs.

**Crossroads**—Amphetamine tablets (cartwheels).

**Crutch**—Anything used to hold the last bit of a joint so it can be smoked (also a *roach clip*).

**Crystal**—Methedrine or desoxyn (also *speed* or *amphetamines*).

**Cut, To**—To dilute a drug with another substance to make more quantity (also *cutting*).

**D.**—Doriden (glutethimide).

**Dabbling**—Using drugs that produce physical dependence irregularly so that one does not become dependent.

**Dagga**—Marihuana (South Africa).

**Datura**—Jimson weed; found in Mexico, the United States, India, South America. Has psychotropic properties (also *Devil's weed*).

**Deadly nightshade**—Belladonna.

**Deal, To**—To buy or sell drugs (also *dealer, dealing*).

**Dealer's band**—Rubberband around the wrist that secures packets of drugs (usually heroin) so that if the wrist is flipped violently, the drugs will fall from the wrist.

**Deck**—Folded paper or glassine envelope containing drugs (usually heroin or cocaine).

**Deeda**—LSD-25.

**Dexies**—Dexedrine tablets.

**Dime**—Ten dollars.

**Dirty**—Person or place that contains illegal drugs.

**Djamba**—Marihuana (Brazil).

**Djomba**—Marihuana (also *diamba, liamba, lianda,* and *maconha*) (Central Africa).

**DMT**—Short for N,N-dimethyltrypyamine, a fast-acting, hallucenogenic drug with a short duration of action or effect.

**Dogie**—Heroin (also *doojee, duji*).

**Dollies**—Dolophine pills.

**Dolls**—Barbiturate or amphetamine pills.

**Dolophine**—Methadone; synthetic opiate slightly more potent than morphine, and with much longer duration of action.

**Dom**—STP.

**Dope**—Any drug that will produce a change in mental state (including alcohol).

**Dope fiend**—Term ironically and defiantly applied to themselves by those physically dependent on drugs.

**Do**, or **Doing**—Refers to the state in which someone is using a drug ("doing" acid).

**Do up**—To inject a drug intravenously (usually heroin).

**Downer**—Barbiturate or tranquilizer, or sedative drug (also *down, downie*).

**Down trip**—Depression or boring experience.

**Dragged**—To be frightened or hysterical after using a drug (usually marihuana).

**Dreamer**—Morphine.

**Dried out**—Detoxified, no longer physically dependent on a drug or drugs.

**Drop**—To swallow a pill, capsule, or tablet of a drug (also to *eat*).

**Dropper**—Medicine dropper used as a syringe for injecting drugs.

**Druggies**—People who experiment widely with many different drugs; regular drug users; heads.

**Duby**—Marihuana.

**Dummy** or **Dummies**—Counterfeit heroin or cocaine (also *shit, blank, lemonade, crap, garbage*).

**Dusting**—Putting a drug on another substance to be smoked (opium-dusted marihuana).

**Dynamite**—Very potent version of any drug (dynamite dope); or cocaine and heroin taken in combination.

**Eighth**—One-eighth ounce of a drug, usually heroin or cocaine.

**Electric**—Containing either marihuana or a hallucenogenic drug (also *magic*).

**Electric Kool-Aid**—A liquid beverage made with

regular Kool-Aid to which a hallucinogenic drug has been added.

**Embalao**—Strongly addicted, strung out (Puerto Rican slang).

**Enchaioui**—Man who has centered his life around marihuana (Arabic slang).

**Epena**—Hallucenogenic stuff made from the bark of trees and used by Indians in Brazil.

**Esrar**—Marihuana (Turkish).

**Explorer's club**—A circle of illicit LSD users.

**F-40's**—Secobarbital.

**Factory**—Place in which drugs are made, diluted, or cleaned for sale.

**Falling out**—Dozing off or going to sleep under the influence of a drug.

**Fatty**—Thickly rolled joint (also a *bomber*).

**Feds**—Federal Bureau of Narcotics agents.

**Five cent paper**—A $5 bag of heroin.

**Five dollar bag**—Bag of heroin sold for $5, and containing five grains of from 0 to 80 percent pure heroin.

**Fives**—Tablets containing 5 milligrams of a drug.

**Fix, To**—To inject a drug intravenously (usually heroin, amphetamines, or cocaine); also to *fix up*.

**Flake**—Cocaine.

**Flash**—Sudden onset of the effects of a drug (usually injected), but in the case of hallucinogens, can be produced by some intense external stimulus.

**Flashing**—Same as *flash*; also glue sniffing.

**Flea powder**—Very poor drug (also *shit, crap, blank, dummy, garbage*, etc.).

**Flip out**—State of fear and loss of control produced by a drug or some external stimulus.

**Floating**—High, stoned, ripped, fucked, fucked up, etc.

**Flower power**—Power of love rather than force.

**Flush**—Sudden onset of euphoria from a drug (usually injected).

**Flying**—High, stoned, etc.

**Flying saucers**—Variety of morning glory plant, the seeds of which are hallucinogenic.

**Footballs**—Diamphetamine pills; or dilaudid, a synthetic opiate.

**Forwards**—Amphetamine pills.

**Freak**—Person whose life-style, behavior, appearance, or ideas determine that the person is different, usually in an unacceptable way, from the rest of society; or a person who prefers a particular drug or behavior (speed freak, acid freak, television freak).

**Freaking freely**—Spontaneous, random behavior, usually hallucinogenic produced.

**Freak-out**—Panic reaction from the effects of a drug or experience.

**Frisco speedball**—Heroin, cocaine, and LSD, mixed and taken.

**Fruit salad**—Game in which each participant takes one pill from every bottle in the medicine cabinet.

**Full moon**—Large peyote chunk greater than four inches in diameter.

**Fuzz**—Pigs, cops, the man, turds, narcs, the police, especially narcotics officers.

**Gage**—Marihuana (also *gauge*).

**Gammon**—One microgram (one millionth of one gram) of LSD.

**Ganga**—Marihuana of high potency, also *gunga, gunja* (Jamaica).

**Gangster**—Marihuana.

**Gangster pills**—Barbiturates or other sedative pills.

**Gaping**—Experiencing withdrawal symptoms.

**Garbage**—Shit, crap, blank, lemonade, etc.; very poor drugs of any type.

**G.B.**—Goofball, barbiturates.

**Gee head**—Person physically dependent on paregoric.

**Get down**—Use heroin.

**Get off**—To experience a change in consciousness or mental state as a result of the intake of a drug.

**Get on**—To use drugs for the first time.

**Ghanja**—Active principle of marihuana in highly concentrated form.

**Ghost, The**—LSD.

**Giggle weed**—Marihuana.

**Girl**—Cocaine.

**Globetrotter**—Person who goes to various drug dealers looking for the best drugs (heroin).

**Glow**—High, stoned, etc.

**Going down**—Going well.

**Going high**—Continuing state of intoxication from drugs, not necessitating more drugs.

**Gold, Acapulco**—Marihuana.

**Gold dust**—Cocaine (also *gold duster*).

**Golden leaf**—Acapulco gold marihuana.

**Goods**—Any kind of drugs.

**Good stuff**—Best drugs of any kind.

**Goofball**—Barbiturate pill.

**Gorilla pills**—Barbiturate, or other sedative pills.

**Grass**—Marihuana.

**Gravy**—Mixture of blood from vein and heroin that is reheated because it has coagulated.

**Greasy junkie**—Passive, indolent person who is physically dependent on heroin, but who will make no great effort to obtain money for drugs.

**Green**—Cheapest form of marihuana.

**Grefa**—Marihuana; also *Greta, grifa* and *griffe*.

**Ground control**—One who helps or talks to a person under the influence of a hallucinogenic drug, in order for that person to have a good experience.

**Guide**—One who helps or guides another person who is under the influence of a hallucinogenic drug through the experience.

**Guru**—Same as *guide*.

**H.**—Heroin.

**Half load**—Fifteen packages of heroin, wrapped together for resale.

**Hand to hand, Go**—Transfer of drugs at the point of sale.

**Haraz**—Policeman or cop (Puerto Rican slang).

**Hard stuff** (or **hard drugs** or **hard narcotics)**—Derivatives of opium, especially heroin, cocaine, sometimes hallucinogens, depending on person using the term.

**Harry**—Heroin.

**Hash** (or **hashish**)—Pure resinous extract from the marihuana plant, *Cannabis sativa*.

**Hawk, The**—LSD-25.

**Hay**—Marihuana.

**H-caps**—Gelatin capsules of heroin.

**Head**—One who uses drugs.

**Head drugs**—Those that appear to affect one's mind, and not the body (hallucinogens, mostly, but sometimes amphetamines and marihuana).

**Hearts**—Amphetamines.

**Heat**—Fuzz, pigs, cops, policemen.

**Heaven dust**—Cocaine.

**Heavenly blue**—Variety of morning glory seeds that have hallucinogenic properties.

**Hemp**—Marihuana.

**Henry**—Heroin.

**Hep**—Hepatitis.

**Her**—Cocaine.

**Herb**—Marihuana.

**Him**—Heroin.

**Hit**—To inject intravenously (any drugs).

**Hold** (or **holding**)—Possessing drugs.

**Hookah**—Pipe for smoking marihuana.

**Hooked**—Physically dependent on drugs.

**Hop**—Opium.

**Hophead**—Person physically dependent on heroin or opium.

**Horse**—Heroin.

**Hot shot**—Injection that is supposed to be heroin, but is actually poison.

**Hungry croaker**—Doctor who will prescribe drugs to a person who is physically dependent on them, for money.

**Hustling**—Prostitution, stealing, or otherwise getting money for drugs.

**Ice cream habit**—Infrequent or moderate use of drugs producing physical dependence.

**Idiot pills**—Barbiturate or other sedative pills.

**Indian hay**—Marihuana.

**Indian hemp**—Marihuana.

**Into**—Using or paying special attention to something, usually drugs.

**In transit**—On an LSD trip.

**Jag**—Prolonged state of consciousness caused by a drug (usually marihuana, amphetamines, or barbiturates).

**Jammed up**—Having taken an overdose of drugs.

**J.** or **"Jay"**—Short for joint or a marihuana cigarette.

**Jerk off**—Injecting a little heroin at a time in order to prolong the initial euphoria.

**Joint**—Marihuana cigarette.

**Jones**—Physical dependence on drugs.

**Joy juice**—Chloral hydrate, appetizers, or tonics.

**Joypop**—Irregular use of heroin so that one is not physically dependent, but will experience the euphoria.

**Juanita**—Marihuana.

**Juice**—Any alcoholic beverage.

**Juice-head**—One who prefers alcoholic beverages, an alcoholic (also *juice freak*).

**Junk**—Heroin.

**Junkie**—One who is physically dependent on heroin.

**Kava**—Mild, psychotropic beverage drunk by the people of New Guinea.

**Key**—Or (ki) kilogram, an amount of a drug (usually marihuana, cocaine, or heroin); also *kilo*.

**Kick**—To withdraw from physical dependence on drugs (kicking).

**Kicks**—Pleasure or pleasureable experience.

**Kick the habit on the elevator**—Refers to one who is so very slightly physically dependent on drugs that withdrawal would be very easy.

**Kilo**—Same as *key*, a kilogram of drugs.

**Kilter**—Marihuana.

**King-Kong pills**—Barbiturates or other sedative pills.

**L.**—LSD-25.

**Lady Snow**—Cocaine.

**Leapers**—Amphetamines.

**Lemonade**—Shit, blank, crap, garbage, etc.—poor-quality drugs.

**Lid**—One ounce of marihuana.

**Lid poppers**—Amphetamines.

**Life**—Characteristic pattern of the life of one whose existence revolves around the use of drugs.

**Light stuff**—Marihuana or other non-dependence-producing hallucinogenic drugs.

**Light up**—To smoke marihuana.

**Line**—Vein used to inject drugs (usually heroin or amphetamine).

**Load**—Some 25 to 30 packets of heroin stacked and held together with a rubberband for delivery.

**Loco**—Marihuana.

**LSD-25**—D-lysergic acid diethylamide tartrate 25.

**Lush**—Heavy drinker or an alcoholic.

**M.**—Morphine.

**Magic mushrooms**—Mushrooms containing psilocybin or psilocin.

**Mainline**—Large vein (used to inject drugs, usually heroin or amphetamines). Also called *mainlining*.

**Majoon**—Hashish produced in the Middle East (also *majoun*).

**Making a croaker for a reader**—Bribing a doctor to write an illegal prescription for drugs.

**Man, The**—Police, fuzz, pigs, the heat, etc.

**Mary**—Morphine.

**Mary Ann**—Marihuana (also *Mary Jane, Mary Warner, Mary Weaver*).

**Matchbox**—A small one-penny matchbox full of marihuana for sale.

**Mellow yellow**—Inner fibrous layer of banana peels that are scraped and smoked, and thought to have psychotropic effects.

**Mesc**—Hallucinogenic drug made from peyote cactus (also *mescal, mescaline*).

**Methamphetamine**—A very powerful amphetamine (also *methedrine* and *desoxyn*).

**Meth freak**—(*speed freak*) one who uses methamphetamines habitually, and possibly exclusively.

**Mexican brown**—A grade of marihuana, also called *Mexican green*.

**Mexican locoweed**—Marihuana.

**Mexican mushroom**—Hallucinogenic mushroom containing psilocybin.

**Microdot**—Tiny tablet of LSD.

**Mike**—One microgram (one millionth of a gram) of drugs, usually LSD.

**Milk sugar**—Also *mannite*, used to cut drugs that come in powdered form, such as heroin.

**Milligram**—One thousandth of one gram.

**Mind detergent, The**—LSD-25.

**Mind trippers**—People who use drugs to explore their minds.

**Miss Emma**—Morphine.

**M.J.**—Marihuana.

**MDA**—A powerful amphetamine that also has powerful hallucinogenic properties (3-methoxy-4,5 methylenedioxyamphetamine).

**Mojo**—Heroin, cocaine, or morphine.

**Monkey**—Physical addiction to a drug, usually heroin.

**Moon**—Peyote cactus top, or cake or bulk hashish.

**Morning shot**—Wake-up injection, usually of heroin.

**Morph**—Morphine.

**Mota**—Marihuana.

**Mother**—Drug dealer.

**Mu**—Marihuana.

**Muggles**—Marihuana joints or cigarettes.

**Nab**—Same as *bust*, or arrest by the police.

**Nail**—Hypodermic needle used for injection of drugs (also *spike*).

**Narc(s)**—Narcotics police officer (also *narco* and *narco fuzz*).

**Natch, On the**—Not using drugs, being natural.

**Needle park**—Place used for shooting up drugs, usually heroin.

**Nemish** (or **nemmies**)—Nembutal capsules (also *numby*).

**Nickel**—Five dollars.

**Nodding** (also **nod**, or **on the nod**)—Drowsy, dreamy, dozing state following injection of heroin characterized by the head lolling forward, and slowly jerking up and down.

**O.**—Opium.

**O.D.**—Overdose.

**Ololiuqui**—Aztec name for morning glory seeds.

**On**—Using drugs.

**On the needle**—Injecting drugs.

**Opiate** (also **opioid**)—Opium and its derivatives (morphine, heroin, codeine, and methadone).

**Outfit**—Equipment used for injecting drugs (also rigs, gimmicks, works).

**Overjolt**—Overdose.

**O.Z.**—An ounce.

**P.**—Peyote.

**Panama**—Short for Panama Red, a kind of marihuana.

**Panama Red**—See *Panama*.

**Paper**—Folded piece of paper containing drugs, usually heroin.

**Peaches**—Benzedrine tablets.

**Pearls**—Amyl nitrite.

**Pellets**—LSD capsules.

**People, The**—Sometimes used as synonym for fuzz, police, etc.

**Pep pills**—Amphetamines.

**Peyote**—Small grey-green cactus, *Lophophora williamsii*, from which the hallucinogenic drug mescaline is derived, also called peyote.

**Phenos**—Barbiturates, especially phenobarbital and seconal.

**Picked up**—Smoked marihuana.

**Piece**—Measure or part of a quantity of drugs.

**Pill (Pill head)**—Barbiturate or amphetamine pill; one who uses them.

**Pin**—Very thin marihuana cigarette.

**Pinks**—Seconal, a barbiturate.

**Pinned**—Constricted, as "The pupils of his eyes are *pinned* after he injects the heroin."

**Plant**—Stash or cache of drugs, hiding place for drugs.

**Poison**—Heroin.

**Poison people**—Those physically dependent on heroin.

**Poke**—A puff of a marihuana cigarette.

**Pop**—To swallow a pill, or to inject heroin subcutaneously.

**Popped**—Busted or arrested by the police.

**Poppers**—Small vials of amyl nitrite that are broken and inhaled.

**Popping**—See *Pop*.

**Pot**—Marihuana.

**Potlikker**—Tea brewed with marihuana seeds and stems.

**Potsville**—Using marihuana.

**Primo**—Very good drug, usually marihuana.

**Psychedelic art**—Art that tries to mimic hallucinations experienced from the use of psychedelic drugs.

**Psychotropic**—Mind-changing, altering the consciousness.

**Purple hearts**—Luminal tablets; or a combination of barbiturates and amphetamines.

**Pusher**—Drug dealer, one who sells drugs; also *push, deal, pushing, dealing*.

**Quarter bag**—A bag of drugs that sells for $25.

**Quill**—Folded matchbook cover used to sniff a drug into the nose.

**Rainbow**—Tuinal capsule.

**Rainy day woman**—Marihuana cigarette.

**Rap**—To talk (also *rapping*).

**Rat**—An informer, or one who gives information to the police.

**Reader**—Prescription for drugs.

**Red and blues**—Tuinal capsules.

**Red birds**—Seconal capsules.

**Red devils**—Seconal capsules.

**Red dirt marihuana**—Marihuana that grows wild.

**Reds**—Seconal capsules.

**Reefer**—Marihuana cigarette, joint, number, J., etc.

**Rig**—Hypodermic equipment.

**Righteous bush**—Marihuana.

**Ripped**—Stoned, high, floating, intoxicated, etc.

**Roach**—The last bit of a joint or marihuana cigarette that is too small and hot to be held in the fingers.

**Roach clip**—Instrument used to hold the roach so that it can be smoked down entirely (also *roach holder, roach pick*).

**Root**—Marihuana cigarette.

**Roses**—Benzedrine tablets.

**Run, A**—A period of time in which one uses a particular drug successively, without stopping. Especially a speed run.

**Rush**—Initial onset or feelings of euphoria after taking a drug.

**Sacred mushrooms**—Mushrooms containing psilocybin, a hallucinogen.

**Salt shot**—Injection, intravenously, of salt and water into the vein of someone who has overdosed on heroin, believed to revive the person, but actually, it does not.

**Scag**—Heroin.

**Scars**—Needle marks that cause scars on the body.

**Schmack (smack)**—Heroin, but can be cocaine or any drug.

**Schmeck**—Heroin.

**Scissors**—Marihuana.

**Scoff**—To eat, food.

**Scoop**—Folded matchbook cover used to sniff drugs (cocaine or heroin) into the nose.

**Score, To**—To connect, to buy drugs successfully.

**Scratch(ing)**—Being physically dependent on drugs.

**Scrip (script)**—Drug prescription.

**Seccy** (or **seggy**)—Seconal capsules.

**Shit**—Garbage, crap, lemonade, etc.—very-poor-quality drugs.

**Shlook (poke, toke, toak)**—A puff of a marihuana cigarette or joint.

**Shooting gallery**—Place where people gather to inject heroin in a group, most of them being physically dependent on the drug.

**Shoot up**—To inject drugs, usually heroin.

**Sick**—Heroin withdrawal symptoms.

**Sizzle**—Drugs carried on one's person.

**Skid bag**—Bag containing highly diluted heroin.

**Skin**—Cigarette paper used to make marihuana cigarette (rolling joints).

**Skinning (skin popping)**—To inject heroin subcutaneously, not intravenously.

**Sleep walker**—Person who is physically dependent on heroin.

**Smack**—Heroin, or one who uses heroin (smacker).

**Snappers**—Glass vials of amyl nitrite.

**Sniffing**—Inhaling heroin or cocaine into the nose.

**Snop**—Marihuana.

**Snort**—To inhale heroin or cocaine into the nose.

**Snow**—Cocaine crystals.

**Source, The**—Supplier of drugs.

**Spaced**—High, stoned, ripped, intoxicated, *spaced out* on drugs.

**Sparkle plenties**—Amphetamines.

**Speed**—Amphetamines, methamphetamine, or methedrine.

**Speedball**—Injected mixture of heroin and cocaine.

**Spike**—Hypodermic needle.

**Splash**—Amphetamines.

**Split**—To go, run away, to leave.

**Splits**—Tranquilizers.

**Spoon**—Usually 1/16 ounce of heroin.

**Star dust**—Cocaine.

**Stash**—A hiding place for drugs.

**Steamboat**—To inhale marihuana through any special instrument to give more and cooler smoke.

**Stick**—Marihuana cigarette.

**Stone (stoned)**—High, ripped, flying, etc.

**Stone addict**—One who is physically dependent on drugs of a very potent nature, very rapidly acquired.

**Stool or Stoolie**—Informer or rat.

**STP**—DOM, very-long-acting, 36 to 72 hours, hallucinogenic drug (4 methyl-2,5-dimethoxy-α-methylphenethylamine).

**Straight**—Not using drugs; not intoxicated with them or under their influence.

**Strung, Strung out**—Physically dependent on a drug.

**Stuff**—Heroin.

**Super pot**—Very potent marihuana.

**Sunshine**—LSD as an orange tablet.

**Sweet Lucy**—Marihuana.

**Swingman**—Drug dealer or pusher.

**Tabs**—Short for tablets.

**Tall**—High or euphoric.

**Tapita**—Bottle cap used for cooking heroin.

**Taste**—Small amount of a drug, usually heroin, given as a gift.

**Tea**—Marihuana.

**Tea bag**—State of smoking marihuana.

**Tea head**—One who regularly uses marihuana.

**Tecata**—Heroin.

**Ten-cent pistol**—A heroin bag that actually contains poison.

**Tetrahydrocannabinol**—Active psychotropic ingredient in marihuana and hashish.

**Texas tea**—Marihuana.

**THC**—Tetrahydrocannabinol.

**Thrusters**—Amphetamine pills.

**Thumb**—A fat marihuana cigarette.

**Ticket, The**—LSD-25.

**Tin**—Small amount of opium.

**Tingle**—Rush, or first onset of effects of a drug.

**TMA**—A synthetic hallucinogen of greater potency than mescaline (3,4,5-trimethoxyphenyl-β-aminopropane).

**Toak (toke)**—Puff of a joint.

**Toke**—Same as *toak.*

**Toke pipes**—Short-stemmed pipes in which marihuana is smoked.

**Tooies**—Tuinal capsules.

**Tools**—Rig, works, equipment for shooting drugs.

**Topi**—Peyote cactus that contains mescaline as the hallucinogen.

**Torn up**—Ripped, stoned, floating, intoxicated with drugs.

**Toss out**—To feign withdrawal symptoms to a doctor in order to obtain a prescription for the drug.

**Tracked up**—Having needle marks or scars on the body from previous injections of drugs.

**Tracks**—Needle marks or scars from injecting drugs.

**Travel agent**—Drug dealer who supplies LSD (for a *trip*).

**Trip**—To take hallucinogenic drugs; the experience one has using hallucinogenic drugs.

**Trips**—Drugs that give one a hallucinogenic experience.

**Turn on to**—To introduce someone to a drug or experience for the first time.

**Twenty-five**—LSD-25.

**Twist**—Marihuana.

**Twisted**—Suffering withdrawal symptoms.

**Tying up**—Putting something around the upper arm so the veins will stand out more clearly in the lower arm, thus facilitating injection.

**Up**—High, stoned, ripped, intoxicated with drugs.

**Upper**—Amphetamine pill (also *uppie, ups*).

**Up-tight**—Tense, worried, anxious.

**Using**—To take drugs of any type.

**Vipe**—Marihuana.

**Viper**—Marihuana smoker.

**Voyager**—Person under the influence of LSD.

**Wake-up**—Person who is physically dependent on a heroin injection first thing in the morning.

**Waste**—Destroy, pulverize, or kill someone.

**Wasted**—Very intoxicated from a drug.

**Weed**—Marihuana.

**Weeding out**—Smoking marihuana.

**White cross**—X-scored tablet, 15 to 20 mg of methamphetamine.

**White Lady, The**—Heroin.

**White light**—Very beautiful enlightening experience gained by using hallucinogenic drugs under special circumstances.

**Whites**—Benzedrine pills.

**White stuff**—Heroin.

**Wired**—Highly stimulated, usually under the influence of a stimulant.

**Wingoing**—Physical withdrawal symptoms from drug dependence.

**Wings**—First intravenous injection.

**Window pane**—LSD in small squares of coated plastic or stiffened gel.

**Works**—Equipment for dilution and injection of drugs (*rig, gimmicks*).

**Wrap**—Innocent looking covering for drugs.

**Yellow jackets**—Nembutal capsules (also *yellows*).

**Yen (ing)**—Withdrawal symptoms from physical dependence on drugs.

**Zonked**—High, stoned, ripped, intoxicated with drugs.

## C. SCIENTIFIC TERMS

This is a sample of the commonly used terms in the substance abuse field that need definition. It in no way represents a complete list of scientific terminology, but is presented so that a person working in this field can have a handy reference source.

**Acidosis**—A condition of reduced alkalai reserve (bicarbonate) of the blood and other body fluids, with or without an actual decrease in the pH. If untreated and allowed to worsen, this condition can be lethal.

**Addiction**—A behavioral pattern of compulsive drug use, characterized by overwhelming involvement with the use of a drug, the securing of its supply, and a high tendency to relapse after withdrawal. This does not necessarily imply physical dependence; as it is a very nebulous word, its general use and clinical applications are being discontinued.

**Addition (drug)**—A state produced by the simultaneous administration of two or more drugs, and their independent effects on the same organism under the same conditions.

**Adrenal medulla**—Innermost portion of the adrenal glands that produces sympathetic hormones (i.e., adrenalin or epinephrine and noradrenalin or norepinephrine).

**Adrenergic**—Of or pertaining to the sympathetic nervous system and the synthesis, storage, and release of sympathomimetic substances.

**Adrenergic receptors**—Those components of a cell that are responsive to adrenergic substances and are directly involved with the initial action of the adrenergic.

a. **Alpha adrenergic receptors**—That part of the dual adrenergic receptive mechanism that is specifically blocked by either phenoxybenzamine or phentolamine, which are specific alpha adrenergic blockers.

b. **Beta adrenergic receptors**—That part of the dual adrenergic receptive mechanism specifically blocked by dichloroisoproterenol or propanolol effects. The "alpha effects" are blocked by an alpha adrenergic blocker, and the "beta effects" are blocked by a beta adrenergic blocker, so that if both alpha and beta adrenergic blockers are administered, and then an adrenergic substance is administered, there will be no effect of the adrenergic substance on the organism.

**Adverse reaction**—A reaction of an organism to a drug that is different from the desired reaction, and is determined to be detrimental to the organism.

**Albuminuria**—The presence of protein in the urine, chiefly albumin; usually indicative of disease, but sometimes resulting from a temporary dysfunction of the kidneys (as opposed to a truly pathologic condition).

**Alcohol dehydrodgenase**—An enzyme manufactured in the body that plays an important role in the metabolism of alcohol by the body.

**Alkaline phosphatase test**—A test that measures the blood level of the enzyme alkaline phosphatase, and thereby determines the potential presence or absence of certain disease states.

**Allergic reaction**—Any abnormal or altered reaction to a substance upon contact with that substance. The quality and quantity of the reaction can range from simple sneezing or a slight skin rash, to anaphylactic shock and death within minutes.

**Allergy (drug)**—A state in which a particular organism will react with an "allergic reaction" (see above) when exposed to a particular drug (that is, a person can be allergic to penicillin).

**Alpha adrenergic receptor**—See *Adrenergic receptor, alpha.*

**Amino acid**—An organic acid in which one of the hydrogen atoms has been replaced by an $NH_2$ group, the smaller molecules of which proteins are built.

**Analgesic agent**—A drug which, when administered to an organism, causes relief from pain, or a sensation of decreased pain intensity.

**Anesthesia**—Total loss of sensation in a part or all of the body, especially the sense of touch in the skin and mucous membranes as the result of the administration of a drug to an organism or in certain disease states of an organism.

**Anorexia**—Loss or lack of appetite.

**Anticholinergic**—Of or pertaining to any of a number of drugs that block or suppress the action of acetylcholine, which is a substance that transmits nervous impulses.

**Anticoagulant**—Any of a group of drugs that inhibit or suppress the clotting of blood.

**Aplastic anemia**—A condition in which there is a reduction of circulating red blood cells in the bloodstream because of a lack of regeneration or destruction of the bone marrow by certain chemical agents (benzene or arsenic) or physical factors (radiation, etc.).

**Arrythmias**—As referred to the heart; loss of normal rhythm or heart beat or irregularities that can be lethal.

**Behavioral pharmacology**—See *Pharmacology, Behavioral.*

**Beta adrenergic receptor**—See *Adrenergic receptors, Beta.*

**Biochemical pharmacology**—See *Pharmacology, Biochemical.*

**Blood alcohol concentration**—The percentage of alcohol per unit volume of blood (that is, if the blood were 0.15% alcohol, that person would be legally drunk in most states).

**Carcinogen**—Any cancer-producing substance or force.

**Carcinogenesis**—Originating or producing a cancer.

**Cardiac palpitations**—An abnormally rapid or violent fluttering or throbbing pulsation of the heart.

**Catecholamines**—Biologically active substances (specifically epinephrine and norepinephrine) that have marked effects on the nervous system, cardiovascular system, muscles, temperature, and metabolism.

**Cerebellar dysfunction**—An abnormality manifested by lack of control of some or all voluntary muscular actions (walking, moving the arms, etc.).

**Cerebral dysfunction**—An abnormality of that part of the brain concerned with processing and interpreting outside impulses and forming modes of action concerning them (hence thought); therefore some abnormality of the thought processes that can have thousands of manifestations.

**Central nervous system**—Brain and spinal cord, including their nerves and end organs.

**Centrilobular necrosis**—Disease of the liver in which one or more cells near the center of a liver lobule are irreversibly destroyed; especially as in the case of exposure to substances such as chloroform, carbon tetrachloride, and naphthalenes.

**Cholinergic**—Of or pertaining to the nerve endings and their end organs, which are involved in the synthesis, production, storage, release, or response to the substance acetylcholine (acetylcholine is a neurotransmitter substance and has different effects depending on the nerves involved and what organs they are innervating).

**Circadian rhythm**—Of or pertaining to events that occur at approximately 24-hour intervals.

**Classical pharmacology**—See *Pharmacology, Classical.*

**Complex drug action**—Drug action manifested by more than one mechanism, effect, dose, or biochemical metabolism.

**Conjunctival blood vessels**—Blood vessels of the inner portions of the upper and lower parts of the eyelids.

**Coronary arteries**—Those arteries that directly supply the heart with blood, oxygen, and nutrients.

**Cross-tolerance**—A state in which an organism, after developing simple tolerance to one drug through its repeated administration, then develops a "tolerance" also to another drug, though it was not administered at all. This cross-tolerance is attributable to similarities that the two or more drugs share in some facet.

**Cumulative effects**—A strong, often intense, effect of the last of a series of doses of a drug, the preceding doses of which had a moderate, mild, or even negligible effect.

**Delirium tremens**—A psychic disorder involving hallucinations, both visual and auditory, found in habitual and excessive users of alcohol and sometimes manifested by shaking tremors of the hands or total body.

**Delusion**—False belief or perception involving one or more of the senses (a person believes him/herself to be an elephant, or a person sees an object and perceives it to be other than what it is).

**Dependence (drug)**—That state of being during which an organism needs a particular drug in order to function without profound alternations of behavior in the absence of the drug. This does not necessarily cause physical withdrawal symptoms.

**Dependence, Physical**—A state characterized by the appearance of a physiologically disruptive withdrawal illness when administration of the drug is stopped completely. This state usually involves tolerance as a requisite.

**Dependence, Psychologic**—A state characterized by a drive or craving that requires periodic or chronic administration of a drug for pleasure or for relief of psychologic discomfort.

**Depersonalization**—A state in which one loses the feeling of one's reality or feels one's own body to be unreal.

**Derealization**—A state of being characterized by a person losing awareness of tangible and measurable reality on which our physical laws are based. The person may feel that he or she is dead or in another universe.

**Detoxification**—Literally, to remove the poison or toxin. When applied to a drug, it is those biochemical or internal metabolic reactions that convert pharmacologically active drugs into pharmacologically less active or inactive drugs. When applied to a human subject, it is that process of recovery from the acute and immediate toxic effects of a drug.

**Diuresis**—Urine excretion in excess of the usual amount, as induced by water drinking, drugs, or disease states.

**Disinhibition**—The removal of an inhibitory effect by a stimulus or a drug. The inhibition of an inhibition.

**Dosage**—The determination of the proper amount of a given remedy (a drug, or other treatment modality).

**Dose**—The quantity of a drug or other remedy to be taken or applied all at one time, or in fractional amounts within a given period.

**Dose–effect relationship**—The relationship between the quantity of a drug being administered and the amount of the observed effect. This relationship is such that there are usually one or more points at which, for a given quantity of drug, there is a maximum observed effect such that, if one administered more or less of the same drug, the effect would be less per unit of the drug administered.

**Dose–response relationship**—See *Dose–effect relationship*.

**Drug antagonist**—Any means (usually another drug) of neutralizing, preventing the action of, or destroying the effects of a certain other drug.

**Drug hunger**—A common manifestation of psychologic drug dependence in which the subject has a drive or craving for a particular drug, or for the past, subjectively pleasurable effects of a particular drug.

**Drug interaction**—A state characterized by modification of the effects of one drug by prior or concurrent administration of another drug. (This interaction can be either advantageous or adverse, depending on the drugs used and the effect desired.)

**Drug metabolism**—That process which is the sum total of all bodily processing of a drug; including uptake, biotransformation, distribution throughout the body, storage, and excretion of the drug or its byproducts.

**Drug receptor complex**—Those components of a cell which are directly involved with the initial action of a drug.

**Dysphoria**—Restlessness; a feeling of being ill at ease.

**Effective dose ($ED_{50}$)**—That amount of drug which produces the desired or looked-for effect in 50 percent of the test animals or subjects.

**Electrocardiograph**—An instrument for measuring the potential of the electric currents that traverse the heart and initiate its beat. It is used to measure the quality and quantity of the heart beat, and in many cases to ascertain whether the heart is functioning properly.

**Electroencephalograph**—An instrument that records the alternating currents of the brain, and in some cases can be used to determine whether the brain is functioning properly.

**Embolization**—The obstruction of a blood vessel by a transported piece of matter, be it blood clot, vegetation, bacteria, or other foreign material.

**Endogenous paranoid schizophrenic reaction**—A state of mind such that the person experiencing it, through no overt external stimuli, will manifest the symptoms of paranoid schizophrenia (that is, ambivalence, autism, loose associations, and flat or labile affect, with an overriding fear that he or she is in grave danger from an external force that may or may not be identifiable).

**Enzyme**—A protein secreted by the body cells that acts as a catalyst for certain chemical changes in other substances, while apparently remaining unchanged itself.

**Enzyme induction**—A state or process by which certain enzymes are more active after the administration of certain drugs or disease states.

**Enzyme inhibition**—A process by which certain enzymes are rendered less active by the administration of certain drugs or disease states.

**Ergotism**—Poisoning by toxic substances containing the fungus *Claviceps purpurea* (from which the drug LSD is purified). The symptoms are lameness and necrosis of the extremities resulting from contraction of the peripheral vascular bed.

**Euphoria**—A feeling of well being, commonly exaggerated and not necessarily well founded.

**Glaucoma**—A disease of the eye characterized by increased intraocular pressure that results in defects in the field of vision, and eventually potential total blindness.

**Granulomatous reaction**—Any one of a rather large group of distinctive focal reactions characterized by formation, as a result of inflammation due to biologic, chemical, or physical agents, of gross granule-like appearance (appearance at some time of large mononuclear phagocytes) which persists in the tissue as slow smoldering reactions or inflammations.

**Habituation (drug)**—That process of learning to use a drug by habit such that physical or psychologic dependence is much more likely to occur.

**Hallucination**—A subjective perception that has no basis in tangible and measurable reality such as is subject to present physical laws (as opposed to a delusion).

**Hematuria**—Any condition in which the urine contains blood or red blood cells.

**Hepatic cirrhosis**—A disease of the liver of many causes characterized by degeneration, fatty infiltration, atrophy, and inflammation that gives rise to a deformity that interferes with liver function and circulation of the blood and bile.

**Hyperglycemia**—An abnormally high level of glucose in the blood.

**Hypoglycemia**—An abnormally low level of glucose in the blood.

**Hypotension**—An abnormally low arterial blood pressure.

**Inhibitory center**—The part of the brain that controls the quality and quantity of inhibitions to particular actions or thought patterns of an organism.

**Initial response**—The first response, subjective or objective, to the administration of a particular drug.

**$K_i$**—Is numerically equal to the concentration of an inhibitor required to displace 50 percent of a bound ligand (or drug) to its receptor site. $[K_i = l + F/k_D]$

**Microsomal ethanol oxidizing system**—An additional system concerned with the breakdown of alcohol in the body.

**Minimal effective dose**—The particular amount of a particular drug, less than which will *not* produce the desired quantity of the desired effect.

**Mucous membrane**—The lining of passages and cavities in communication with the air (mouth and lungs, vagina, penis, rectum, nasal passages).

**Mucarinic**—Having a mucarine-like action, that is, producing effects that resemble postganglionic parasympathetic stimulation.

**Mutagenesis**—The origin or production of a mutation in an organism.

**Narcolepsy**—Uncontrollable and suddenly oncoming sleep.

**Narcotics**—Drugs which, when used in moderate doses, produce stupor, insensibility, or sound sleep.

**Neurohumors**—A chemical substance liberated in the tissues by a nerve impulse.

**Nicotinic effects**—Of or pertaining to cholinergic receptor theory.

**Nucleic acids**—A family of substances of large molecular weight found in chromosomes, mitochondria, and viruses that is thought to be the ultimate carrier of genetic inheritance or physical characteristics, and to control enzyme pattern characteristics of cells of which nucleis acids form a part.

**Pain threshold**—The level of painful stimulation, particular to each individual organism, at which the organism subjectively experiences the sensation of pain.

**Paranoid delusions of grandeur**—Thoughts or perceptions of oneself or one's plans that are greatly exaggerated and have as their stimulating basis a fear of some external force.

**Paranoid psychosis**—State of mind such that a person is so frightened of being harmed by some external force that the person experiences an inability to continue with some previous normal functions.

**Pharmacodynamics**—The study of the actions of drugs on the living organism.

**Pharmacogenetics**—The study of genetically determined variations in responses to drugs in humans or laboratory animals.

**Pharmacology, Behavioral**—The study of the alteration of behavior by certain drugs.

**Pharmacology, Biochemical**—The study of the mechanism and metabolism by which certain drugs manifest their effects.

**Pharmacology, Classical**—The study of the effect of certain drugs on test subjects or laboratory animals, under controlled conditions.

**Physical dependence**—See *Dependence, Physical.*

**Postganglionic nerve ending**—Those nerve endings denoting autonomic fibers of the second order arising from the cells in the peripheral autonomic ganglia.

**Potentiation**—A state of drug action in which two drugs are administered simultaneously, and have greater than their additive effect, See *Addiction.*

**Protein binding**—That state of an administered drug in which it becomes bound to the protein found in the blood or other body fluids.

**Proteins**—One of a group of substances constituting the greater part of the nitrogen-containing components of animal and vegetable matter.

**Pseudo-hallucinations**—Similar to delusions; the perception of an object that already exists as something other than what it is (a person perceives a brown desk to be a multicolored miniature rocket).

**Psychoadjuvant**—A remedy or drug added to the main type or mode of psychotherapy to assist or aid or increase the efficacy of the main mode or type of psychotherapy.

**Psychologic dependence**—See *Dependence, Psychologic.*

**Psychosis**—A severe emotional or psychologic illness of such proportions that the afflicted individual cannot function or care for himself or herself in a fashion that was previously normal for that individual.

**Psychotic**—Of or pertaining to psychosis and/or behavior associated with psychosis.

**Psychotogen**—Drug that produces psychotic manifestations.

**Psychotomimetic**—Of or pertaining to drugs that produce psychosis-like symptoms.

**Psychotropic**—Of or pertaining to drugs that have an observable effect on the psychologic state of the individual ingesting the drug.

**Pulmonary edema**—A perceptible accumulation of excessive clear watery fluid in the tissues of the lungs, pulmonary arteries, and bronchii.

**Pulmonary hypertension**—High arterial blood pressure in the pulmonary circuit (the circuit of the pulmonary arteries, pulmonary veins, both sides of the heart). It can cause pulmonary edema and can be lethal.

**Pulmonary talc granulomatosis**—A granulomatous inflammation of the lungs caused by the inhalation of talc granules. It can interfere with respiration and lead to respiratory failure and death if left untreated with continuing insult.

**Quantitative analysis**—The determination of amount as well as the nature of each of the elements that composes a compound being investigated.

**Receptor complex**—See *Drug receptor complex.*

**Receptor concept**—See *Adrenergic receptor.*

**Reticular activating system**—The core of the brain stem, which contains neurons and is involved in the maintenance of consciousness of the subject. It contains both activating and inhibitory capabilities, and thus can affect the conscious thinking processes of the individual in either manner. It also can be blocked by certain drugs as in anesthesia.

**Reversed tolerance**—A state produced by a particular drug, process, or individual, such that lower doses of the same drug produce the same amount and quality of the desired or observed effect that previously was observed only with higher doses of the same drug (see *Tolerance*).

**Schizophrenia-like psychosis**—A psychosis-like state resembling the named disease schizophrenia (the subject is ambivalent, autistic, has loose association, a labile or flat affect, and has nebulous ego boundaries). (The reader is now probably more confused about this definition than ever.)

**Seminiferous tubules**—Those tubules from the testicles that carry the semen and sperm.

**Sensitizing contact**—Contact with a drug or substance that triggers the "immune system" such that any further contact with the same substance will result in an allergic or hypersensitive reaction to that substance. (See *Allergic reaction.*)

**Serial sevens**—A mental dexterity test during which the subject is given a two-digit number and then told by the person administering the test either to add or subtract 7 from that number many times in succession as rapidly as possible, stating each new number aloud (a subject given the number 64 plus 7 is 71 plus 7 is 78 plus 7 is 85 plus 7 is 92, and so on). The speed and accuracy with which the subject produces the answers gives the tester a good estimation of the intactness of the subject's thinking processes.

**Somatotype**—Literally, body type of an individual (tall and thin, short and fat, etc.). Each body type has a scientific name and certain general correlations that go with it.

**Supersensitivity**—That state of being such that the organism in question has an increased susceptibility to a drug (usually a protein-type drug) after being administered the drug initially. This continues until the organism develops anaphylactic shock whenever the drug is administered; anaphylactic shock, when untreated, is fatal.

**Sympathomimetic agent**—An agent which, when administered, will stimulate the autonomic nervous system; specifically the adrenergic aspect (see *Adrenergic receptor*).

**Synergy**—Literally, working together. With regard to drugs, it is that state which, when two drugs are administered to a subject simultaneously, the combined effect is greater than the additive effect of the drugs if they had been administered alone (a case of the whole being greater than the individual parts algebraically added).

**Tachycardia**—State characterized by an increased pulse rate or heart beat, defined as being greater than 100 beats per minute in human subjects.

**Teratogen**—A drug or process that produces a monster (refers to those drugs acting on the fetus while it is still in the uterus).

**Teratogenesis**—The process of producing a monster from a normal human fetus; the disturbed growth processes involved in production of a monster.

**Therapeutic index**—The relationship between the desired and undesired effects of any given drug; also called *margin of safety* or *selectivity*. In laboratory animal studies, this is the ratio of the lethal dose$_{50}$ to the effective dose$_{50}$ ($LD_{50}/ED_{50}$). A drug does not have one therapeutic index, but many, depending on how many different effects it has and how the therapist wishes to define the index in a particular given case. There are so many different definitions for humans that it would be foolish to try to enumerate them all here.

**Therapeutics**—The practical branch of medicine dealing with the treatment of disease, and in this case the use of drugs to treat certain diseases.

**Tolerance**—A state developed in an individual such that after repeated administration of a given constant dose of a given drug, that drug produces a decreasing effect, or conversely, a state such that increasingly larger doses of the same drug must be administered in order to obtain the same effects observed with the original dose (related to *Physical dependence*).

**Toxic agent**—An agent that is poisonous when given in certain dose amounts, or to certain individuals, or under certain conditions. (Therefore any agent can be toxic, only some are more toxic than others, such as arsenic and cyanide).

**Toxicity**—A state of being poisonous; or those measurable conditions, doses, and circumstances during which a particular drug or agent is toxic.

**Toxicology**—The study of the noxious or poisonous effects of certain drugs, agents, or processes.

**Toxic reaction**—A reaction to a drug, agent, or process that indicates that the subject in question is under the influence of the noxious undesirable effects of that particular drug, agent, or process (certain poisons cause convulsions; a toxic effect of heroin in high enough doses would be respiratory depression and death).

**Toxin**—Literally, poison. Any noxious or poisonous substance that is an integral part of a cell or tissue, is an extracellular product, represents a combination of the two situations, formed or elaborated during metabolism and growth of certain microorganisms, as well as some of the higher plant and animal species; or can be a drug or metabolic product of a drug.

**Vascular sclerosis**—A hardening of the arteries and potentially narrowing of the bore of the arteries. (Also called *arteriosclerosis*.)

**Vasodilitation**—Dilation of the blood vessels.

**Vasomotor system**—That system of nerves and chemicals which cause either dilation or constriction of the blood vessels.

**Ventricular fibrillation**—Fine, very rapid twitching movements of the muscles of the largest chambers of the heart. This replaces normal heart contractions; if it persists, it is 100 percent fatal, because the heart is not contracting as a unit, and there is very little, if any, movement of the blood in the vessels.

## REFERENCES

1. Hofmann, F. G. Introduction. In *Handbook on Drug and Alcohol Abuse: The Biomedical Aspects*. New York: Oxford University Press, 1975, p. 3.
2. Smith, D. E. Use of LSD in the Haight-Ashbury. *Calif. Med.* 110:472, 1969.
3. Solursh, L. P., and Clement, W. R. Hallucinogenic drug abuse: Manifestations and management. *Can. Med. Assoc. J.* 98:407, 1968.
4. *California Society for Treatment and Other Drug Dependencies News*. Stimulant look-alikes 9:(3-4) Oct. 1982.
5. Siegel, R. K. Cocaine smoking. *J. Psychoactive drugs* 14:271 1982.
6. *Pharm. Chem. Newsletter*. The look-alikes explosion. 2:(3) May, June 1982.
7. Cohen, S. The rise and fall of the look-alikes. *Drug Abuse and Alcoholism Newsletter* 12:(4) June 1983.

Appendix II

# Psychopharmacologic Classification of Drugs

I. Narcotics
II. CNS depressants:
 Barbiturates
 Alcohol
 Solvent inhalants
III. Psychostimulants:
 Amphetamines (speed)
IV. Psychotomimetics:
 Marihuana
 LSD
V. Other:
 Tobacco

## I. NARCOTICS

*Representatives*

Opium—derived from the poppy plant (*Papaver somniferum*)
Opium derivatives—codeine and morphine
Synthetic narcotics:
 Meperidine (Demerol)
 Oxycodone (Percodan)
 Methadone (Dolophine)
Semisynthetics:
 Heroin
 Nalorphine

*CNS Inhibitory Actions*

CNS depressions
Narcosis (sleep)
Depression
Depression of respiratory center (raises threshold to carbon dioxide)
Sedation
Depression of cough reflex
Depression of vomiting center (late depression)

*CNS Stimulatory Actions*

Spinal cord (strychnine-like tonic convulsions)
Vomiting center (early stimulation)
Slowing of heart (bradycardia; stimulates tenth cranial nerve)
Pinpoint pupils (stimulates third cranial nerve)

*Behavioral Actions*

Mental clouding
Reduced hunger
Euphoria
Reduced ability to concentrate
Reduced sex drive
Drowsiness
Apathy

Reduced activity
Reduced aggressive drives

### *Peripheral Nervous System Actions*

Body warmth
Heaviness of limbs
Itchiness of nose
Constipation
Vomiting
Lowered blood pressure
Nausea
Pupillary constriction

### *Acute Narcotic Toxicity*

Increasing depression
Pinpoint pupils
Respiratory failure
Slowed respiration
Flushing and cyanosis
Death

### *Chronic Narcotic Toxicity*

Psychologic dependence
Physical dependence
Tolerance (not to constipation and pupilary constriction)

### *Withdrawal (Bad Case of the Flu)*

Frequent yawning
Gooseflesh skin
Watery eyes
Nausea and vomiting
Abdominal muscle cramps
Limb tremors (jerks)
Weight loss
Anxiety
Irritability
Loss of appetite
Dilated pupils
Muscle spasms
Convulsions (occasional)
Coma and death (rare)

### *Symptoms of Use*

Initial signs:
- Nausea and vomiting
- Slight stimulation

Later signs:
- Being "on the nod"
- Slowness of breath
- Unresponsiveness to pain
- Constricted pupils
- Lethargy

### *Overuse*

Social and personal deterioration

### *Main Dangers*

Accidental death from overdose
High potential for psychologic and physical dependence (less with codeine or methadone)
Social deterioration
Reduced motivation
Infection from nonsterile injections (VD or hepatitis)
Rapid development of tolerance and high physical dependence
High cost of procurement leading to criminal activities

### *Antidote*

Narcotic antagonists: nalorphine (Nalline), naloxone
- Reverses depressant effects of the opiates
- Naloxone test—unmasks withdrawal symptoms in physically dependent persons

### *Treatment*

Development of self-help programs
Use of methadone maintenance
Specific opiate antagonists

### *Route of Administration*

Oral form
Injectable form

*Medical Uses*

To relieve pain
To relieve cough
To relieve diarrhea
Preanesthetic medication (to reduce anxiety and depression and to promote sleep)

*Physical Signs of Use*

Needle marks with scarring
Glassine envelopes
Burned bottle caps or spoons
Blood stains on sleeves
Hypodermic syringe
Empty bottles of cough medicine containing narcotics

## II. CNS DEPRESSANTS

### Barbiturates

*Representatives*

Pentobarbital (Nembutal)
Secobarbital (Seconal)
Amobarbital (Amytal)
Glutethimide (Doriden and Tuinal), combined amobarbital and secobarbital

*CNS Actions*

General depression
Respiratory depression
Sedation
Antianxiety (antiepileptic)
Hypnotic
Spinal cord depression

*Behavioral Actions*

Drowsiness
Difficulty in thinking
Incoordinate gait
Loss of inhibitions
Faulty judgment
Emotional lability
Euphoria
Talkativeness
Slurred speech
Poor memory
Quarrelsomeness

*Acute Toxicity*

Severe depression
Unconsciousness
Respiratory cessation
Serious drop in blood pressure
Coma
Death

*Chronic Toxicity*

Psychologic dependence
Physical dependence (potentially more lethal than heroin)
Tolerance (does not occur to the lethal dose)
Number abusing hypnotic drugs exceeds number abusing opiates

### Alcohol

*Representatives*

Whiskey, about 50 percent ETOH (volume)
Wine, about 14 to 20 percent ETOH (volume)
Beer, about 4.5 percent ETOH (volume)

*CNS Actions and Behavioral Actions (Graded Dose Response)*

Three ounces of 90 proof whiskey produce:
- Relaxation
- Slight reduction in reflexes
- Increased talkativeness
- No impairment in driving skills

Six ounces of 90 proof whiskey produce:
- Slightly slurred speech
- Impaired judgment
- Sixfold increase in driving fatalities and accidents

Incoordination of movement
Reduced inhibitions
Less emotional control

Nine ounces of 90 proof whiskey produce:
Gross intoxication
Distorted judgment
Impaired gait
Quarrelsomeness
Gross effects on thinking and memory

Eighteen to 30 ounces of 90 proof whiskey produce:
Coma
Respiratory cessation
Death

### *Peripheral Nervous System Actions*

Increased feeling of warmth
Vasodilation
Diuretic to kidneys
Minor effects on circulation
Stimulation of gastric secretions

### *Acute Toxicity*

Acute death due to respiratory paralysis from high doses

### *Chronic Toxicity*

Dependence—psychologic and physical
Tolerance develops partly to its depressant effects, but not as greatly to its lethal dose.
Withdrawal from alcohol dependence is more dangerous and more potentially fatal than the withdrawal from heroin.

### *Withdrawal*

Increasing tremors
Anxiety
Cramps
Increased reflex actions
Major convulsions
Exhaustion
Nausea
Perspiration
Vomiting
Terrifying hallucinations
Delirium
Circulatory and heart failure
Death

### *Symptoms of Use*

Nausea
Incoordination
Emotional lability
Aggressiveness
Vomiting
Slurring of speech
Loss of inhibitions

### *Main Dangers*

Faulty judgment
Emotional lability
Incoordination
Increased aggressiveness
Death from overdosage (alone or in combination with other depressants)
Social and personal deterioration
Antisocial and homicidal behavior
Irreversible damage to body tissues (brain, liver, pancreas, kidney)
Possible vitamin deficiency from use

### *Antidote*

Empty stomach contents (gastric lavage)
Administer hot black coffee
Maintain body heat
Artificial respiration
Other symptomatic support as needed

### *Medical Uses*

To sedate
To promote sleep
As a food source for energy (in limited cases)
By lay people to arrest head colds and anxiety

### *Physical Signs of Use*

Odor of alcohol on breath
Alcohol blood level test

## Solvent Inhalants

*Representatives*

Toluene
Xylene
Benzene
Gasoline
Paint thinner
Lighter fluid

*CNS Actions*

CNS depression
Dizziness
Floating sensations
Breakdown of inhibitions
Exhiliration and intense feelings of well-being
Inebriation
Loss of appetite
Grandiose feelings

*Behavioral Actions*

Aggressiveness
Visual hallucinations
Insomnia
Display of bizarre behavior
Similar to alcohol
Depression
Mental confusion

*Peripheral Nervous System Actions*

Nausea and vomiting
Increased salivation
Local irritation (eyes and mucous membranes)
Lack of coordination
Anorexia (loss of appetite)

*Acute Toxicity*

Like alcohol and other CNS depressants
Disinhibition excitement, followed by depression
Euphoria
Excitement
Delusions and visual hallucinations
Slurred speech
Ringing in the ears
Blackout (spotty-type amnesia)

*Chronic Toxicity*

Dependence—moderate psychologic
Little physical dependence
Tolerance after three months of continued weekly usage

*Withdrawal Symptoms (Temporary)*

Delirium tremens
Tremors
Hallucinations
Increased irritability
Difficulty in sleeping

*Antidote*

Artificial respiration

*Symptoms of Use*

Strong odor of glue or of other chemicals
Symptoms of intoxication:
  Euphoria
  Incoordinate gait
  Slurred speech
All similar to alcohol

*Physical Signs of Use*

Tubes of glue
Large paper or plastic bags
Glue smears on handkerchiefs
Various volatile products

*Main Dangers*

Impaired judgment
Increased possibility of dangerous accidents
Certain solvent chlorinated hydrocarbons such as triethylene may lead to damage to bone marrow, liver, kidneys, and possibly to brain.

Propellants or aerosol sprays lead to sudden death.

*Route of Administration*

Sniffing
Inhalation

## III. PSYCHOSTIMULANTS (SPEED)

*Representatives*

Methamphetamine (Methedrine)
*d*- and *d,l*-amphetamine (Dexedrine, Benzedrine)
Cocaine, methylphenidate (Ritalin); caffeine (in coffee, tea, and cola)

*CNS Actions*

Stimulation
Stimulation of respiration
Reduction in appetite
Antagonizes barbiturate depression
Mood elevation
Convulsions
Increased motor activity

*Behavioral Actions*

Increased talkativeness
Anxiety
Excitement
Delusions
Confusion
Irritability
Suspiciousness (paranoid)
Increase in initiative
Confidence
Prolonged use followed by mental depression
Restlessness
Aggressiveness
Mania
Delirium
Dizziness
Increase in pleasurable sensations
Auditory hallucinations
Precipitation of paranoid schizophrenia
Euphoria

*Peripheral Nervous System Actions*

Dilated pupils
Headaches
Tremors (shaking hands)
Increased sweating
Palpitations
Quickened breathing
Decreased fatigue
Reflex slowing of heart rate
Rise in blood pressure
Cardiac arrhythmias
A peripheral flash (likened to a sexual orgasm)

*Chronic Toxicity*

High potential for psychologic dependence, but not physical dependence
Tolerance develops to its use (sometimes to a great degree)
Psychotic-like behavior (paranoia and schizophrenia)
Suicidal tendency
Substitute for heroin (tendency to switch from speed to heroin)

*Withdrawal Symptoms*

Severe depression
Severe cramping of abdominal muscles
Symptoms resembling asthmatic attack
Changes in brain-wave patterns
Collapse from exhaustion

*Medical Uses*

To reduce appetite
To improve mood
As motivation for work and learning
To overcome fatigue and sleepiness
To increase attentiveness
To reduce the overactivity and distractability of hyperactive children

*Antidote*

Chlorpromazine (Thorazine) or thioridazine (Mellaril)

*Symptoms of Use*

Dilated pupils
Loss of appetite
Overactivity
Belligerence
Confusion
Mania
Hallucinations
Rapid speech
Suspiciousness
Bizarre behavior
Fatigue from lack of sleep (insomnia)

*Physical Signs of Use*

Pills of varying colors
Chain-smoking because of restlessness

*Main Dangers*

High levels of pleasurable feelings
Feelings of greatly increased power
Sexually orgiastic experiences (I.V. route)
Marked impairment of judgment
Paranoia
Aggressive behavior
Interruption of eating and sleeping habits

*Route of Administration*

Oral
Injectable

# IV. PSYCHOTOMIMETICS

## Cannabis Sativa—Marihuana

*Representatives*

Marihuana
Hashish
Mary Jane
Texas tea
Charas
Sweet Lucy
Bhang
THC

*CNS Actions*

Small doses of the drug (one-half joint of good quality) produce:
Mild alcohol-like intoxication
Increased talkativeness
Feeling of calm
Disinhibition or excitement
Pleasurable feelings of well-being
Gaiety
Relaxation
Anesthesia
Respiratory and vasomotor (medullary) depression

*Behavioral Actions*

Effect of marihuana on sensory perception (one and one-half joints of good quality):
Tendency to heightened sensory perception
Increased awareness and involvement
Increased visual imagery (with eyes open or closed)
Intensified sense of taste and touch
Intensified colors and sounds taking on new dimensions (users may think they hear colors and see sounds)
Possible impaired depth perception
Impaired tactile—distorted distance
Impaired immediate memory
Distortion of time (minutes to hours)
Psychologic effects of high marihuana dosage

(three joints of good quality):
Hallucinations (pseudo)
Panic states (rare)
Failures in judgment and coordination
Strong bodily perception

### *Peripheral Nervous System Actions*

No prominent cardiovascular effects
Reddening of the eyes
No change in pupil size
Diuresis (dryness of mouth)
Nausea, vomiting, diarrhea

### *Chronic Toxicity*

Moderate potential for psychologic dependence
No physical dependence
Possible reverse tolerance in humans
Liability for abuse
Chronic use may lead to reduced motivation, neglect of personal hygiene, social deterioration

### *Withdrawal Symptoms*

No noticeable physical signs

### *Medical Uses*

Before 1930, the drug was used for relief of depression, headache, loss of appetite, insomnia, withdrawal from opiates, epilepsy, and the common cold.

### *Drug Identification*

Liquid pot
Synthetic grass
THC
Liquid pot sold on the illicit market is probably not THC; instead, what is commonly sold are other psychoactive compounds, such as Sernyl and belladonna alkaloids.
Percent of THC in varieties of marihuana:
Indian hemp, 6 percent
South Vientam pot, 10 percent
Hashish, greater than 20 percent
Pharmacognosy of marihuana:
Mixture of leaves, stems, and flowers from the plant
Potency determinants:
Climate, manner of cultivation, method of manufacture
Male and female leaves are equal in potency.
Female flowering tops are more potent than male.

### *Antidote*

Limit the stimulation coming into the individual from the environment:
Darken the lights.
Turn down the music.
Have the patient lie down.
Tell patient to close eyes and relax.
Use the talk-down method.

### *Symptoms of Use*

Intoxication and euphoria without drastic impairment of judgment or gait, depending on the dose
Reddening of the eyes
Unusual hilarity
Increased appetite for food (usually sweets)
Slightly increased pulse rate
Dreamy state

### *Physical Signs of Use*

Odor of burned rope
Cigarette paper and roller
Specialized pipes
Small seeds in pocket linings
Roach clamp
Discolored fingers

### *Treatment*

Unpleasant reactions requiring hospitalization and treatment are very infrequent. Since the lethal dose of marihuana is almost unattainable, few, if any, deaths due to overdose have been reported.

*Main Dangers*

High doses used by inexperienced person may lead to:
- Impulsive behavior
- Panic
- Anxiety
- Psychotic reactions (rare)

*Route of Administration*

Smoke
Ingestion
Snuff

## LSD

*Representatives*

LSD-25
Dimethyltryptamine (DMT)
Mescaline (peyote)
THC
DOM (STP)
Psilocybin
Diethyltryptamine (DET)
PCP (Sernyl)
MDA

*CNS Actions*

Altered perception (hear colors, see sounds)
Intensified emotional activity
Relative sense of timelessness
Dreamy states
Extraordinary sensitivity to stimuli
Visual, auditory, tactile hallucinations

*Behavioral Actions*

Paradoxic and ambivalent symptoms. (Person feels relaxed and peaceful, but at the same time, feels anxious and tense; one is happy and sad all in the same moment.)
Schizophrenia
Multipotential behavior (panic or tranquility)
Psychologic makeup dictates behavioral effects. (Individuals who are rigid, anxious, or fearful may have intense panic reactions; other people may achieve deep personal insights, religious or mystical, union or intensified creativity.)

*Peripheral Nervous System Actions*

Sympathetic predominance:
- Pupilary dilation
- Piloerection
- Tachycardia
- Hyperthermia
- Hyperglycemia

*Acute Toxicity*

Mice tolerate highest dose
Rabbits most sensitive (excluding humans)
Respiratory failure (death in animals)
In humans, no reported deaths (suicide attempts)
Convulsions (high dose)
Panic (fear reactions)
Flashbacks (18 months later)

*Chronic Toxicity*

Dependence
Slight dependence for psychologic dependence, and no potential for physiologic dependence.
Tolerance rapidly builds up in a cyclic manner (four- to five-day continued use leads to tolerance, cycle broken after eight days).

*Withdrawal Symptoms*

None observed

*Medical Uses (Proposed)*

Reactivate repressed memories
"Death" therapy
Alcoholism
Model psychosis
Analgesic

*Drug Identification*

Names of street forms:
- White lightning
- Purple wedges
- Purple owsleys
- Paisley tops
- Window panes
- Blue dots
- Orange sunshine
- Orange wedges
- Blue double domes

*Antidote*

Talk-down method
Tranquilizers—chlordiazepoxide (Librium), diazepam (Valium), chlorpromazine
Nicotinic acid and vitamin treatment (poor treatment)
Tranquilizers are not recommended as these drugs may be psychologically disruptive and may increase the chances of the person later experiencing flashbacks.

*Symptoms of Use*

Markedly dilated pupils
Emotional swings
Bizarre behavior
Unusual hilarity
Suspiciousness
Nausea and vomiting (primarily with peyote)
Increased pulse and blood pressure (primarily with DMT)

*Physical Signs of Use*

Pills of varying colors, sizes, and shapes

*Treatment*

No known treatment, except proper rest and psychotherapy

*Main Dangers*

Intense anxiety
Depressive and paranoid reaction
Confusion
Panic
Mood changes
Flashbacks
Inability to discriminate between "reality" and "fantasy"
Impairment of normal motivation (to study, work, and otherwise contribute to society)
Some prolonged psychotic reactions
Reoccurrences of drug effects after drugfree period
Chromosomal effects probably negligible
Possible greater occurrence of miscarriage
Social changes seen in chronic users
"Dropping out and doing one's own thing"

## V. OTHER

### Tobacco

*Representatives*

Cigarettes
Pipe tobacco
Cigars

*CNS Actions*

Initial stimulation followed by depression
Increasing doses produce tremor, increase breathing
High doses produce paralysis of breathing, convulsions, death

*Behavioral Actions*

Facilitates learning
Calms down, relaxes

*Peripheral Nervous System Actions*

Constriction of blood vessels
Increased heart rate
Increased blood pressure
Enlarged pupils

*Chronic toxicity*

Physical dependence in some genetically prone individuals
High psychologic dependence
Tolerance—moderate development

*Withdrawal Symtpoms*

Irritability
Impatience
Anxiety
Headaches
Loss of concentration
Drowsiness or insomnia
Cramps
Hunger
Tremors
Energy Loss
Fatigue

*Antidote*

Gastric lavage (empty stomach contents) with 1:10,000 solution of potassium permanganate; artificial respiration and symptomatic support as needed.

*Drug Identification*

Nicotine is an active chemical.
Cigarette tobacco contains 1.5 percent nicotine.
The smoke of an average cigarette yields 6 to 8 mg of the drug.
A cigar contains 120 mg of nicotine, twice the dose necessary to kill a person.

*Physical Signs of Use*

Tobacco lines in pockets
Tobacco odor
Burned matches

*Treatment*

Symptoms reversed by smoking tobacco or administering nicotine.

*Main Dangers*

Cancer of lungs, larynx, mouth
Irritation of respiratory system
Chronic bronchitis
Pulmonary emphysema
Impaired vision
Air pollution
Fire
Damage to heart and blood vessels
If nicotine is taken orally, death occurs within a few minutes.

*Route of Administration*

Chewed
Snuffed
Smoked

# Author Index

# Subject Index

# Drug Index

## About The Author

KENNETH BLUM is Chairman of the Board and Director of Scientific Affairs of the Pharmogen Corporation of San Antonio, Texas and Adjunct Professor of Pharmacology at the University of Texas Health Science Center, San Antonio. Dr. Blum received his B.S. from Columbia University, his M.S. from New Jersey School of Medicine and his doctorate from the New York Medical College.

Dr. Blum is President of the National Foundation on Addictive Diseases, Editor-in-Chief of the international journal, *Substance and Alcohol Actions/Misuse*, and is a Council Member of the Gordon Research Conferences.

Dr. Blum has published over 150 scientific articles in journals and dozens of chapters in contributed books. He is also the editor of several research books.